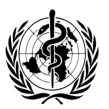

World Health Organization Classification of Tumours

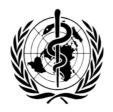

WHO   OMS

International Agency for Research on Cancer (IARC)

Revised 4th Edition

WHO Classification of Tumours of Haematopoietic and Lymphoid Tissues

Edited by

Steven H. Swerdlow

Elias Campo

Nancy Lee Harris

Elaine S. Jaffe

Stefano A. Pileri

Harald Stein

Jürgen Thiele

International Agency for Research on Cancer

Lyon, 2017

World Health Organization Classification of Tumours

Series Editors   Fred T. Bosman, MD, PhD
Elaine S. Jaffe, MD
Sunil R. Lakhani, MD, FRCPath
Hiroko Ohgaki, PhD

WHO Classification of Tumours of Haematopoietic and Lymphoid Tissues

Editors   Steven H. Swerdlow, MD
Elias Campo, MD, PhD
Nancy Lee Harris, MD
Elaine S. Jaffe, MD
Stefano A. Pileri, MD, PhD
Harald Stein, MD
Jürgen Thiele, MD, PhD

Senior Advisors   Daniel A. Arber, MD
Robert P. Hasserjian, MD
Michelle M. Le Beau, PhD
Attilio Orazi, MD
Reiner Siebert, MD

Project Coordinator   Paul Kleihues, MD

Project Assistants   Asiedua Asante
Anne-Sophie Hameau

Technical Editor   Jessica Cox

Database   Kees Kleihues-van Tol

Layout   Markus Fessler

Printed by   Maestro
38330 Saint-Ismier, France

Publisher   International Agency for
Research on Cancer (IARC)
69372 Lyon Cedex 08, France

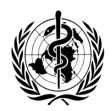

This volume was produced with support from the following organizations:
American Society of Hematology
Fondazione Italiana Linfomi ONLUS
Fondation José Carreras pour la lutte contre la leucémie, Genève
University of Chicago Medicine Comprehensive Cancer Center
Leukemia Clinical Research Foundation

Published by the International Agency for Research on Cancer (IARC),
150 Cours Albert Thomas, 69372 Lyon Cedex 08, France

© International Agency for Research on Cancer, 2017

Distributed by
WHO Press, World Health Organization, 20 Avenue Appia, 1211 Geneva 27, Switzerland
Tel.: +41 22 791 3264; Fax: +41 22 791 4857; email: bookorders@who.int

Second print run (15000 copies), with minor corrections:
http://publications.iarc.fr/Book-And-Report-Series/Who-Iarc-Classification-Of-Tumours/

Format for bibliographic citations:
Swerdlow SH, Campo E, Harris NL, Jaffe ES, Pileri SA, Stein H, Thiele J (Eds):
WHO Classification of Tumours of Haematopoietic and Lymphoid Tissues (Revised 4th edition).
IARC: Lyon 2017

IARC Library Cataloguing in Publication Data

WHO classification of tumours of haematopoietic and lymphoid tissues / edited by Steven H. Swerdlow, Elias Campo,
Nancy Lee Harris, Elaine S. Jaffe, Stefano A. Pileri, Harald Stein, Jürgen Thiele. – Revised 4th edition.

(World Health Organization classification of tumours)

1. Hematologic Neoplasms – classification   2. Hematologic Neoplasms – genetics
3. Hematologic Neoplasms – pathology

I. Swerdlow, Steven H. II. Series

ISBN 978-92-832-4494-3   (NLM Classification: WH 525)

Contents

WHO classification of tumours of haematopoietic and lymphoid tissues

Myeloproliferative neoplasms

Chronic myeloid leukaemia, BCR-ABL1–positive	9875/3
Chronic neutrophilic leukaemia	9963/3
Polycythaemia vera	9950/3
Primary myelofibrosis	9961/3
Essential thrombocythaemia	9962/3
Chronic eosinophilic leukaemia, NOS	9964/3
Myeloproliferative neoplasm, unclassifiable	9975/3

Mastocytosis

Cutaneous mastocytosis	9740/1
Indolent systemic mastocytosis	9741/1
Systemic mastocytosis with an associated haematological neoplasm	9741/3
Aggressive systemic mastocytosis	9741/3
Mast cell leukaemia	9742/3
Mast cell sarcoma	9740/3

Myeloid/lymphoid neoplasms with eosinophilia and gene rearrangement

Myeloid/lymphoid neoplasms with PDGFRA rearrangement	9965/3
Myeloid/lymphoid neoplasms with PDGFRB rearrangement	9966/3
Myeloid/lymphoid neoplasms with FGFR1 rearrangement	9967/3
Myeloid/lymphoid neoplasms with PCM1-JAK2	9968/3*

Myelodysplastic/myeloproliferative neoplasms

Chronic myelomonocytic leukaemia	9945/3
Atypical chronic myeloid leukaemia, BCR-ABL1–negative	9876/3
Juvenile myelomonocytic leukaemia	9946/3
Myelodysplastic/myeloproliferative neoplasm with ring sideroblasts and thrombocytosis	9982/3
Myelodysplastic/myeloproliferative neoplasm, unclassifiable	9975/3

Myelodysplastic syndromes

Myelodysplastic syndrome with single lineage dysplasia	9980/3
Myelodysplastic syndrome with ring sideroblasts and single lineage dysplasia	9982/3
Myelodysplastic syndrome with ring sideroblasts and multilineage dysplasia	9993/3*
Myelodysplastic syndrome with multilineage dysplasia	9985/3
Myelodysplastic syndrome with excess blasts	9983/3
Myelodysplastic syndrome with isolated del(5q)	9986/3
Myelodysplastic syndrome, unclassifiable	9989/3
Refractory cytopenia of childhood	9985/3

Myeloid neoplasms with germline predisposition

Acute myeloid leukaemia with germline CEBPA mutation	
Myeloid neoplasms with germline DDX41 mutation	
Myeloid neoplasms with germline RUNX1 mutation	
Myeloid neoplasms with germline ANKRD26 mutation	
Myeloid neoplasms with germline ETV6 mutation	
Myeloid neoplasms with germline GATA2 mutation	

Acute myeloid leukaemia (AML) and related precursor neoplasms

AML with recurrent genetic abnormalities

AML with t(8;21)(q22;q22.1); RUNX1-RUNX1T1	9896/3
AML with inv(16)(p13.1q22) or t(16;16)(p13.1;q22); CBFB-MYH11	9871/3
Acute promyelocytic leukaemia with PML-RARA	9866/3
AML with t(9;11)(p21.3;q23.3); KMT2A-MLLT3	9897/3
AML with t(6;9)(p23;q34.1); DEK-NUP214	9865/3
AML with inv(3)(q21.3q26.2) or t(3;3)(q21.3;q26.2); GATA2, MECOM	9869/3
AML (megakaryoblastic) with t(1;22)(p13.3;q13.1); RBM15-MKL1	9911/3
AML with BCR-ABL1	9912/3*
AML with mutated NPM1	9877/3*
AML with biallelic mutation of CEBPA	9878/3*
AML with mutated RUNX1	9879/3*

AML with myelodysplasia-related changes	9895/3

Therapy-related myeloid neoplasms	9920/3

Acute myeloid leukaemia, NOS

Acute myeloid leukaemia, NOS	9861/3
AML with minimal differentiation	9872/3
AML without maturation	9873/3
AML with maturation	9874/3
Acute myelomonocytic leukaemia	9867/3
Acute monoblastic and monocytic leukaemia	9891/3
Pure erythroid leukaemia	9840/3
Acute megakaryoblastic leukaemia	9910/3
Acute basophilic leukaemia	9870/3
Acute panmyelosis with myelofibrosis	9931/3

Myeloid sarcoma	9930/3

Myeloid proliferations associated with Down syndrome

Transient abnormal myelopoiesis associated with Down syndrome	9898/1
Myeloid leukaemia associated with Down syndrome	9898/3

Blastic plasmacytoid dendritic cell neoplasm	9727/3

Acute leukaemias of ambiguous lineage

Acute undifferentiated leukaemia	9801/3
Mixed-phenotype acute leukaemia with t(9;22)(q34.1;q11.2); *BCR-ABL1*	9806/3
Mixed-phenotype acute leukaemia with t(v;11q23.3); *KMT2A*-rearranged	9807/3
Mixed-phenotype acute leukaemia, B/myeloid, NOS	9808/3
Mixed-phenotype acute leukaemia, T/myeloid, NOS	9809/3
Mixed-phenotype acute leukaemia, NOS, rare types	
Acute leukaemias of ambiguous lineage, NOS	

Precursor lymphoid neoplasms

B-lymphoblastic leukaemia/lymphoma, NOS	9811/3
B-lymphoblastic leukaemia/lymphoma with t(9;22)(q34.1;q11.2); *BCR-ABL1*	9812/3
B-lymphoblastic leukaemia/lymphoma with t(v;11q23.3); *KMT2A*-rearranged	9813/3
B-lymphoblastic leukaemia/lymphoma with t(12;21)(p13.2;q22.1); *ETV6-RUNX1*	9814/3
B-lymphoblastic leukaemia/lymphoma with hyperdiploidy	9815/3
B-lymphoblastic leukaemia/lymphoma with hypodiploidy (hypodiploid ALL)	9816/3
B-lymphoblastic leukaemia/lymphoma with t(5;14)(q31.1;q32.1); IGH/*IL3*	9817/3
B-lymphoblastic leukaemia/lymphoma with t(1;19)(q23;p13.3); *TCF3-PBX1*	9818/3
B-lymphoblastic leukaemia/lymphoma, BCR-ABL1–like	9819/3*
B-lymphoblastic leukaemia/lymphoma with iAMP21	9811/3
T-lymphoblastic leukaemia/lymphoma	9837/3
Early T-cell precursor lymphoblastic leukaemia	9837/3
NK-lymphoblastic leukaemia/lymphoma	

Mature B-cell neoplasms

Chronic lymphocytic leukaemia (CLL)/ small lymphocytic lymphoma	9823/3
Monoclonal B-cell lymphocytosis, CLL-type	9823/1*
Monoclonal B-cell lymphocytosis, non-CLL-type	9591/1*
B-cell prolymphocytic leukaemia	9833/3
Splenic marginal zone lymphoma	9689/3
Hairy cell leukaemia	9940/3
Splenic B-cell lymphoma/leukaemia, unclassifiable	9591/3
Splenic diffuse red pulp small B-cell lymphoma	9591/3
Hairy cell leukaemia variant	9591/3
Lymphoplasmacytic lymphoma	9671/3
Waldentröm macroglobulinemia	9761/3
IgM monoclonal gammopathy of undetermined significance	9761/1*
Heavy chain diseases	
Mu heavy chain disease	9762/3
Gamma heavy chain disease	9762/3

Alpha heavy chain disease	9762/3
Plasma cell neoplasms	
Non-IgM monoclonal gammopathy of undetermined significance	9765/1
Plasma cell myeloma	9732/3
Solitary plasmacytoma of bone	9731/3
Extraosseous plasmacytoma	9734/3
Monoclonal immunoglobulin deposition diseases	
Primary amyloidosis	9769/1
Light chain and heavy chain deposition diseases	9769/1
Extranodal marginal zone lymphoma of mucosa-associated lymphoid tissue (MALT lymphoma)	9699/3
Nodal marginal zone lymphoma	9699/3
Paediatric nodal marginal zone lymphoma	9699/3
Follicular lymphoma	9690/3
In situ follicular neoplasia	9695/1*
Duodenal-type follicular lymphoma	9695/3
Testicular follicular lymphoma	9690/3
Paediatric-type follicular lymphoma	9690/3
Large B-cell lymphoma with IRF4 rearrangement	9698/3
Primary cutaneous follicle centre lymphoma	9597/3
Mantle cell lymphoma	9673/3
In situ mantle cell neoplasia	9673/1*
Diffuse large B-cell lymphoma (DLBCL), NOS	9680/3
Germinal centre B-cell subtype	9680/3
Activated B-cell subtype	9680/3
T-cell/histiocyte-rich large B-cell lymphoma	9688/3
Primary DLBCL of the CNS	9680/3
Primary cutaneous DLBCL, leg type	9680/3
EBV-positive DLBCL, NOS	9680/3
EBV-positive mucocutaneous ulcer	9680/1*
DLBCL associated with chronic inflammation	9680/3
Fibrin-associated diffuse large B-cell lymphoma	
Lymphomatoid granulomatosis, grade 1, 2	9766/1
Lymphomatoid granulomatosis, grade 3	9766/3*
Primary mediastinal (thymic) large B-cell lymphoma	9679/3
Intravascular large B-cell lymphoma	9712/3
ALK-positive large B-cell lymphoma	9737/3
Plasmablastic lymphoma	9735/3
Primary effusion lymphoma	9678/3
Multicentric Castleman disease	
HHV8-positive DLBCL, NOS	9738/3
HHV8-positive germinotropic lymphoproliferative disorder	9738/1*
Burkitt lymphoma	9687/3
Burkitt-like lymphoma with 11q aberration	9687/3*
High-grade B-cell lymphoma	
High-grade B-cell lymphoma with *MYC* and *BCL2* and/or *BCL6* rearrangements	9680/3
High-grade B-cell lymphoma, NOS	9680/3
B-cell lymphoma, unclassifiable, with features intermediate between DLBCL and classic Hodgkin lymphoma	9596/3

Mature T- and NK-cell neoplasms

T-cell prolymphocytic leukaemia	9834/3
T-cell large granular lymphocytic leukaemia	9831/3
Chronic lymphoproliferative disorder of NK cells	9831/3
Aggressive NK-cell leukaemia	9948/3
Systemic EBV-positive T-cell lymphoma of childhood	9724/3
Chronic active EBV infection of T- and NK-cell type, systemic form	
Hydroa vacciniforme–like lymphoproliferative disorder	9725/1*
Severe mosquito bite allergy	
Adult T-cell leukaemia/lymphoma	9827/3
Extranodal NK/T-cell lymphoma, nasal type	9719/3
Enteropathy-associated T-cell lymphoma	9717/3
Monomorphic epitheliotropic intestinal T-cell lymphoma	9717/3
Intestinal T-cell lymphoma, NOS	9717/3
Indolent T-cell lymphoproliferative disorder of the gastrointestinal tract	9702/1*
Hepatosplenic T-cell lymphoma	9716/3
Subcutaneous panniculitis-like T-cell lymphoma	9708/3
Mycosis fungoides	9700/3
Sézary syndrome	9701/3
Primary cutaneous CD30-positive T-cell lymphoproliferative disorders	
Lymphomatoid papulosis	9718/1*
Primary cutaneous anaplastic large cell lymphoma	9718/3
Primary cutaneous gamma delta T-cell lymphoma	9726/3
Primary cutaneous CD8-positive aggressive epidermotropic cytotoxic T-cell lymphoma	9709/3
Primary cutaneous acral CD8-positive T-cell lymphoma	9709/3*
Primary cutaneous CD4-positive small/medium T-cell lymphoproliferative disorder	9709/1
Peripheral T-cell lymphoma, NOS	9702/3
Angioimmunoblastic T-cell lymphoma	9705/3
Follicular T-cell lymphoma	9702/3
Nodal peripheral T-cell lymphoma with T follicular helper phenotype	9702/3
Anaplastic large cell lymphoma, ALK-positive	9714/3
Anaplastic large cell lymphoma, ALK-negative	9715/3*
Breast implant–associated anaplastic large cell lymphoma	9715/3*

Hodgkin lymphomas

Nodular lymphocyte predominant Hodgkin lymphoma	9659/3
Classic Hodgkin lymphoma	9650/3
Nodular sclerosis classic Hodgkin lymphoma	9663/3
Lymphocyte-rich classic Hodgkin lymphoma	9651/3
Mixed cellularity classic Hodgkin lymphoma	9652/3
Lymphocyte-depleted classic Hodgkin lymphoma	9653/3

Immunodeficiency-associated lymphoproliferative disorders

Post-transplant lymphoproliferative disorders (PTLD)	
Non-destructive PTLD	
Plasmacytic hyperplasia PTLD	
Infectious mononucleosis PTLD	
Florid follicular hyperplasia	
Polymorphic PTLD	9971/1
Monomorphic PTLD	**
Classic Hodgkin Lymphoma PTLD	9650/3
Other iatrogenic immunodeficiency-associated lymphoproliferative disorders	

Histiocytic and dendritic cell neoplasms

Histiocytic sarcoma	9755/3
Langerhans cell histiocytosis, NOS	9751/1
Langerhans cell histiocytosis, monostotic	9751/1
Langerhans cell histiocytosis, polystotic	9751/1
Langerhans cell histiocytosis, disseminated	9751/3
Langerhans cell sarcoma	9756/3
Indeterminate dendritic cell tumour	9757/3
Interdigitating dendritic cell sarcoma	9757/3
Follicular dendritic cell sarcoma	9758/3
Fibroblastic reticular cell tumour	9759/3
Disseminated juvenile xanthogranuloma	
Erdheim–Chester disease	9749/3

The morphology codes are from the International Classification of Diseases for Oncology (ICD-O) {1257A}. Behaviour is coded /0 for benign tumours; /1 for unspecified, borderline, or uncertain behaviour; /2 for carcinoma in situ and grade III intraepithelial neoplasia; and /3 for malignant tumours. The classification is modified from the previous WHO classification, taking into account changes in our understanding of these lesions.

* These new codes were approved by the IARC/WHO Committee for ICD-O.
** These lesions are classified according to the lymphoma to which they correspond, and are assigned the respective ICD-O code.

Italics: Provisional tumour entities.

Introduction to the WHO classification of tumours of haematopoietic and lymphoid tissues

Harris N.L.
Arber D.A.
Campo E.
Hasserjian R.P.
Jaffe E.S.
Orazi A.

Pileri S.A.
Stein H.
Swerdlow S.H.
Thiele J.
Vardiman J.W.

Why classify? Classification is the language of medicine; diseases must be described, defined, and named before they can be diagnosed, treated, and studied. A consensus on definitions and terminology is essential for both clinical practice and investigation. A classification should contain diseases that are clearly defined, clinically distinctive, and non-overlapping (i.e. mutually exclusive), and that together constitute all known entities (i.e. are collectively exhaustive). A classification should provide a basis for future investigation and should be able to incorporate new information as it becomes available. Disease classification involves two distinct processes: class discovery (the process of identifying categories of diseases) and class prediction (the process of determining to which category individual cases belong). The work of pathologists is essential for both processes.

The 2008 *WHO classification of tumours of the haematopoietic and lymphoid tissues* (4th edition) {3848} was a collaborative project of the European Association for Haematopathology and the Society for Hematopathology. It was a revision and update of the 3rd edition {1820}, which was the first true worldwide consensus classification of haematological malignancies. The 4th edition had an eight-member steering committee composed of members of both societies. Through a series of meetings and discussions, with input from both societies, the steering committee agreed on a proposed list of diseases and chapters and chose authors. As was done for the 3rd edition, the advice of clinical haematologists and oncologists was obtained to ensure that the classification would be clinically useful {1556}. Two clinical advisory committees were convened: one for myeloid neoplasms and other acute leukaemias and one for lymphoid neoplasms. The meetings were organized around a series of questions, which addressed topics such as disease definitions, nomenclature, grading, and clinical relevance. The committees were able to reach consensus on most of the questions posed, and much of the input from the committees was incorporated into the classification. More than

130 pathologists and haematologists from around the world were involved in writing the chapters.

It has now been more than 8 years since the publication of the 4th edition, and numerous basic and clinical investigations have since led to many advances in the field that warrant an update to the classification. Important contributions have been made through the application of high-throughput genetic technologies such as gene expression profiling and next-generation sequencing. These technologies have led to new diagnostic tools and have revealed new mechanisms of tumorigenesis and new potential therapeutic targets. Because the 4th edition of the *WHO classification of tumours* series is not yet complete (with several volumes yet to be released), the 5th edition cannot yet be started, so the editors and authors have instead undertaken a major update to the existing 4th edition of the *WHO classification of tumours of the haematopoietic and lymphoid tissues*. This process has involved many of the original editors as well as an additional three senior advisors specializing in myeloid neoplasms and two senior advisors with expertise in molecular and cytogenetic issues. Clinical advisory committee meetings were held regarding both myeloid and lymphoid neoplasms, as was done for prior editions. The key features of this revision have been summarized in recent review articles {129A,3848A}.

The *WHO classification of tumours of haematopoietic and lymphoid tissues* is based on the principles initially defined in the *Revised European-American classification of lymphoid neoplasms* (REAL), proposed by the International Lymphoma Study Group (ILSG) {1557}. In the WHO classification, these principles have also been applied to the classification of myeloid and histiocytic neoplasms. The guiding principle of both the REAL and the WHO classification is the importance of defining 'real' diseases that can be recognized by pathologists using the available techniques, and that appear to be distinct clinical entities. There are three important components of this process.

The first component is the recognition that the underlying causes of these neoplasms are often unknown and may vary. Therefore, the WHO approach to classification incorporates all available information – morphology, immunophenotype, genetic features, and clinical features – to define the diseases. The relative importance of each of these features varies by disease, depending on the current state of knowledge; there is no single gold standard by which all diseases are defined.

The second important component of this classification process is the recognition that the complexity of the field makes it impossible for any single expert or small group of experts to be completely authoritative; for a classification to be widely accepted, broad agreement is necessary. Therefore, the WHO approach to classification relies on building a consensus on the definitions and nomenclature of the diseases among as many experts as possible. We recognize that compromise is essential for establishing a consensus, but we believe that even an imperfect single classification is better than multiple competing classifications.

The final important component of this classification process is the understanding that although pathologists must take primary responsibility for developing a classification, the involvement of clinicians is also essential, to ensure the classification's usefulness and acceptance in daily practice {1556}. When the 3rd edition of the WHO classification was published, previous proponents of other classifications of haematological neoplasms agreed to accept and use the new classification, ending decades of controversy over the classification of these tumours {338A,339,340, 1165,1330A,1643A,2412A,2836,3310A}.

As stated above, there is no single gold standard by which all diseases are defined in the WHO classification. Morphology is always important; many diseases have characteristic or even diagnostic morphological features. Immunophenotype and genetic features are also important aspects of the definition of tumours of haematopoietic and lymphoid tissues, and the availability of this information means that it is now easier to establish consensus definitions than it was when only subjective morphological criteria were available. Immunophenotyping is used in the routine diagnosis of the vast majority of haematological malignancies, both to determine lineage in malignant processes and to distinguish between benign and malignant processes. Many diseases have an immunophenotype so characteristic that it is essential (or nearly essential) for the diagnosis; for other diseases, the immunophenotype plays a smaller diagnostic role. For some lymphoid and many myeloid neoplasms, a specific genetic abnormality is the key defining criterion, whereas other neoplasms lack known specific genetic abnormalities. Some genetic abnormalities are characteristic of a given disease or disease group but are not specific, such as MYC, CCND1, and BCL2 rearrangements and JAK2 mutations; others are prognostic factors for several diseases, such as TP53 mutations and FLT3 internal tandem duplication (FLT3-ITD). The use of immunophenotypic features and genetic abnormalities to define entities not only provides objective criteria for diagnosis, but has also enabled the identification of antigens, genes, and pathways that can be targeted for therapy. The success of the anti-CD20 monoclonal antibody rituximab for the treatment of B-cell neoplasms and the success of the tyrosine kinase inhibitor imatinib for the treatment of leukaemias associated with rearrangements in ABL1 and other tyrosine kinase genes are testament to this approach. Finally, the diagnosis of some diseases requires knowledge of clinical features such as patient age, nodal versus extranodal presentation, specific anatomical site, and history of cytotoxic and other therapies. Most of the diseases described in the WHO classification are considered to be distinct entities; however, some are not as clearly defined, and these are listed as provisional entities. In addition, borderline categories have been created for cases that do not clearly fit into a single category, so that well-defined categories can be kept homogeneous and borderline cases can be studied further.

The WHO classification classifies neoplasms primarily according to lineage – myeloid, lymphoid, or histiocytic/dendritic – and a normal counterpart is postulated for each neoplasm. Although the goal is to define the lineage of each neoplasm, lineage plasticity can occur in precursor or immature neoplasms, and has also been identified in some mature haematolymphoid neoplasms. In addition, genetic abnormalities such as rearrangements in FGFR1, PDGFRA, and PDGFRB, or PCM1-JAK2 fusion, can give rise to neoplasms of either myeloid or lymphoid lineage associated with eosinophilia; these disorders are recognized as a separate group. Precursor neoplasms (i.e. acute myeloid leukaemias, lymphoblastic leukaemias/lymphomas, acute leukaemias of ambiguous lineage, and blastic plasmacytoid dendritic cell neoplasm) are discussed separately from more-mature neoplasms (i.e. myeloproliferative neoplasms, mastocytosis, myelodysplastic/myeloproliferative neoplasms, myelodysplastic syndromes, mature [peripheral] B-cell and T/NK-cell neoplasms, Hodgkin lymphomas, and histiocytic and dendritic cell neoplasms). The mature myeloid neoplasms are classified according to their biological features (i.e. myeloproliferative neoplasms with effective haematopoiesis vs myelodysplastic neoplasms with ineffective haematopoiesis), as well as by their genetic features. Within the category of mature lymphoid neoplasms, the diseases are generally listed according to their clinical presentation (i.e. disseminated often leukaemic, extranodal, indolent, or aggressive), and to some extent according to the stage of differentiation when this can be postulated. However, the order in which the diseases are listed is in part arbitrary, and is not an integral aspect of the classification.

This revised 4th edition of the WHO classification incorporates new information that has emerged since the publication of the original 4th edition. It includes some changes in terminology related to our improved understanding of certain disease entities and presents revised defining criteria for some neoplasms. In addition, a number of previously provisional entities have now been accepted as definite entities, and new provisional entities have been added – some defined by genetic criteria (particularly among the myeloid neoplasms) and others by a combination of morphology, immunophenotype, and clinical features. The frequent application of immunophenotyping and genetic studies using peripheral blood, bone marrow, and lymph node samples has led to the detection of small clonal populations in asymptomatic individuals. These clonal populations include small clones of cells with the BCR-ABL1 translocation seen in chronic myeloid leukaemia, small clones of cells with IGH/BCL2 rearrangement, and small populations of cells that have the immunophenotype of chronic lymphocytic leukaemia or follicular lymphoma (i.e. monoclonal B-cell lymphocytosis, in situ follicular and mantle cell neoplasia, paediatric follicular hyperplasia with monoclonal B cells, and more recently, mutations in haematopoietic cells in older individuals, without evidence of a haematological malignancy – so-called clonal haematopoiesis of indeterminate potential {3772}). It is not always clear whether these clonal proliferations constitute early involvement by a neoplasm, a precursor lesion, or an inconsequential finding. These situations are somewhat analogous to the identification of small monoclonal immunoglobulin components in serum (i.e. monoclonal gammopathy of undetermined significance). The chapters on these neoplasms include updated recommendations for dealing with these situations. The recommendations of international consensus groups have also been updated, with regard to criteria for the diagnosis of chronic lymphocytic leukaemia and plasma cell myeloma.

Any classification of diseases must be periodically reviewed and updated to incorporate new information. The Society for Hematopathology and the European Association for Haematopathology now have a record of nearly two decades of collaboration and cooperation in this effort. The societies are committed to updating and revising the classification as needed, with input from clinicians and in collaboration with the International Agency for Research on Cancer (IARC) and WHO. The process of developing and updating the WHO classification has generated a new and exciting degree of cooperation and communication among pathologists and oncologists from around the world, which will facilitate our continued progress in the understanding and treatment of haematological malignancies. The multiparameter classification approach that has been adopted by the WHO classification, with its emphasis on defining real disease entities, has been shown in international studies to be reproducible; the diseases defined are clinically distinctive, and the uniform definitions and terminology used facilitate the interpretation of clinical and translational studies {1, 148}. In addition, the accurate and precise classification of disease entities has facilitated the discovery of the genetic basis of myeloid and lymphoid neoplasms in the basic science laboratory.

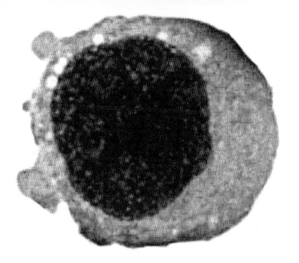
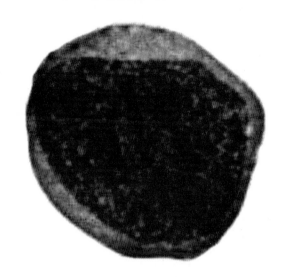

CHAPTER 1

Introduction and overview of the classification of myeloid neoplasms

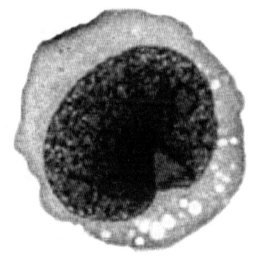
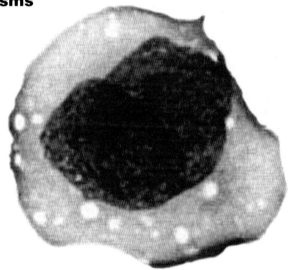

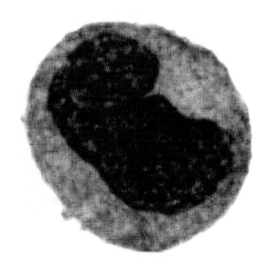
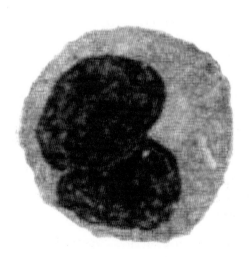

Introduction and overview of the classification of myeloid neoplasms

Arber D.A.
Orazi A.
Hasserjian R.P.
Brunning R.D.
Le Beau M.M.
Porwit A.

Tefferi A.
Levine R.
Bloomfield C.D.
Cazzola M.
Thiele J.

The 2001 *WHO Classification of Tumours: Pathology and Genetics of Tumours of Haematopoietic and Lymphoid Tissues* (3rd edition) reflected a paradigm shift in the approach to the classification of myeloid neoplasms {1820}. For the first time, genetic information was incorporated into diagnostic algorithms provided for the various entities. The publication was prefaced with a comment predicting future revisions necessitated by rapidly emerging genetic information relevant to the diagnosis and classification of myeloid malignancies. The 4th edition (published in 2008) and the current 4th edition revision reflect the significant new molecular insights that have become available since the publication of the 2001 edition.

The first entity described in this volume, chronic myeloid leukaemia, remains the prototype for the identification and classification of myeloid neoplasms. This leukaemia is recognized by its clinical and morphological features, and its natural progression is characterized by an increase in blasts of myeloid, lymphoid, or mixed myeloid–lymphoid immunophenotype. It is always associated with the *BCR-ABL1* fusion gene, which results in the production of an abnormal protein tyrosine kinase with enhanced enzymatic activity. This oncoprotein is sufficient to cause the disease and is also a target for protein tyrosine kinase inhibitor therapy, which has prolonged the lives of thousands of patients with this previously fatal illness {1040}. This successful integration of clinical, morphological, and genetic information embodies the goal of the WHO classification scheme.

In this revision, the combination of clinical, morphological, immunophenotypic, and genetic features continues to be used in an attempt to define disease entities, such as chronic myeloid leukaemia, that are biologically homogeneous and clinically relevant – the same approach used in the 3rd and 4th editions of the classification. The previous classification schemes opened the door to including genetic abnormalities as criteria for classifying myeloid neoplasms, and the

current revision explicitly acknowledges that recurrent genetic abnormalities not only provide objective criteria for recognition of specific entities but are also vital for the identification of abnormal gene products and pathways that are potential therapeutic targets. Several disease subgroups and sets of defining criteria have been expanded to include not only neoplasms associated with chromosomal abnormalities recognizable by conventional karyotyping, but also those with gene mutations with or without a cytogenetic correlate. However, the importance of careful clinical, morphological, and immunophenotypic characterization of every myeloid neoplasm, and correlation with the genetic findings, cannot be overemphasized. The discoveries of activating *JAK2* mutations and mutations in *CALR* and *MPL* have revolutionized the diagnostic approach to myeloproliferative neoplasms (MPNs) {299,1831,2014, 2037,2099,2290,2823}. However, these mutations are not specific for any single clinical or morphological MPN phenotype, and some are also reported in certain cases of myelodysplastic syndromes (MDSs), myelodysplastic/myeloproliferative neoplasms (MDS/MPNs), and acute myeloid leukaemia (AML). Therefore, an integrated, multimodality approach is necessary for the classification of all myeloid neoplasms. It is also critical to elucidate how molecular testing can be used to inform the diagnosis and treatment of myeloid malignancies, and to articulate how these tests should be incorporated into clinical practice, on the basis of current and evolving scientific evidence.

With so much yet to be learned, there may be some missteps as traditional approaches to categorization are fused with more molecularly oriented classification schemes. But the authors, senior advisors and editors of this revision of the WHO classification, as well as the clinicians who served as members of its clinical advisory committees, have worked diligently to develop an updated, evidence-based classification that can be used in daily practice for therapeutic

decision-making and that also provides a flexible framework for integration of new data.

Prerequisites for the classification of myeloid neoplasms by WHO criteria

The WHO classification of myeloid neoplasms relies on the morphological, cytochemical, and immunophenotypic features of the neoplastic cells to establish their lineage and degree of maturation, and to determine whether the cellular appearance is cytologically normal, dysplastic, or otherwise morphologically abnormal. The classification is based on criteria applied strictly to initial specimens obtained prior to any therapy. Blast percentages in the peripheral blood, bone marrow, and other involved tissues remain of practical importance for categorizing myeloid neoplasms and determining their progression. Cytogenetic and molecular genetic studies are required at the time of diagnosis not only for recognition of specific genetically defined entities, but also for establishing a baseline against which follow-up studies can be interpreted to assess disease progression. Given the integrated, multimodality approach required for diagnosing and classifying these neoplasms, it is recommended that the various diagnostic studies be correlated with the clinical findings and communicated in a single integrated report. If a definitive classification cannot be determined, the report should indicate why and provide guidance for additional studies that may clarify the diagnosis.

For the purpose of achieving consistency, the following guidelines are recommended for the evaluation of specimens when a myeloid neoplasm is suspected. In this context, a standardized approach to the processing, documentation, and reporting of bone marrow findings is emphasized {2253}. It is assumed that the evaluation will be performed with full knowledge of the clinical history and pertinent laboratory data.

Morphology

Peripheral blood

A peripheral blood smear should be examined and correlated with the results of a complete blood count. Freshly made smears should be stained with May-Grün-wald-Giemsa or Wright-Giemsa stain and examined for white blood cell, red blood cell, and platelet abnormalities. It is important to ensure that smears are well stained. Evaluation of neutrophil granularity is important when a myeloid disorder is suspected; the designation of neutrophils as abnormal on the basis of hypogranular cytoplasm alone should not be considered unless the stain is well controlled. Manual 200-cell leukocyte differential counts are recommended as part of the peripheral blood smear evaluation in patients with a myeloid neoplasm when the white blood cell count permits. The presence of abnormal erythrocytes (e.g. tear-drop cells) as well as platelet size and granularity should also be taken into account.

Bone marrow aspiration

Aspirate smears should be stained with May-Grünwald-Giemsa or Wright-Giemsa stain for optimal visualization of cytoplasmic granules and nuclear chromatin. Because the WHO classification relies on percentages of blasts and other specific cells to categorize some entities, it is rec-ommended that 500 nucleated bone marrow cells be counted on cellular aspirate smears in an area as close to the particle and as undiluted with blood as possible. Counting from multiple smears may reduce sampling error due to irregular distribution of cells. The cells to be counted include blasts and promonocytes (as defined below), promyelocytes, myelocytes, meta-myelocytes, band neutrophils, segmented neutrophils, eosinophils, basophils, monocytes, lymphocytes, plasma cells, erythroid precursors, and mast cells. Megakaryocytes (including dysplastic forms) should not be counted. If a concomitant non-myeloid neoplasm (e.g. plasma cell myeloma) is present, it is reasonable to exclude those neoplastic cells from the count for the purpose of classifying the myeloid neoplasm. If an aspirate cannot be obtained due to fibrosis or cellular packing, touch preparations of the biopsy may yield valuable cytological information, but differential counts from touch preparations may not be representative. When performing touch preparations, care must be taken to avoid crush artefact or damage to the core biopsy. The differential counts obtained from marrow aspirates should be compared with an estimate of the proportions of cells observed in available corresponding biopsy sections.

Bone marrow trephine biopsy

The importance of adequate bone mar-row biopsy sections for the diagnosis of myeloid neoplasms cannot be overstated. The bone marrow biopsy provides information regarding overall (age-matched) cellularity, histotopography, and the proportion and maturation of haematopoietic cells and also enables evaluation of bone marrow stroma and cancellous bone structure. The biopsy also provides material for immunohistochemical studies that may be of diagnostic and prognostic importance. A biopsy is essential whenever there is myelofibrosis, and the classification of some entities, in particular MPNs, relies heavily on histology sections. The specimen must be adequate, be taken at a right angle from the cortical bone, and be ≥1.5 cm in length (to enable evaluation of ≥10 partially preserved intertrabecular areas {2253}. It should be well fixed, thinly sectioned (at 3–4 μm), and stained with H&E and/or a stain such as Giemsa that allows for detailed morphological evaluation. A silver impregnation method (including reticulin and collagen assessment) is recommended for evaluation for marrow fibrosis, which should be graded according to the European consensus scoring system {2148,3975}. Periodic acid–Schiff (PAS) staining may facilitate the detection of megakaryocytes. Immunohistochemical study of the biopsy (discussed below) can be very useful in the evaluation of myeloid neoplasms.

Blasts

The percentage of myeloid blasts is very important for the diagnosis and classification of myeloid neoplasms. In the peripheral blood, the blast percentage should be determined from a 200-cell leukocyte differential count and in the bone marrow, from a 500-cell count using cellular bone marrow aspirate smears as described above. The blast percentage determined from the bone marrow aspirate should correlate with an estimate of

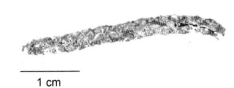

1 cm

Fig. 1.02 Bone marrow trephine biopsies of suspected myeloid neoplasms should be ≥1.5 cm in length and obtained at right angles to the cortical bone.

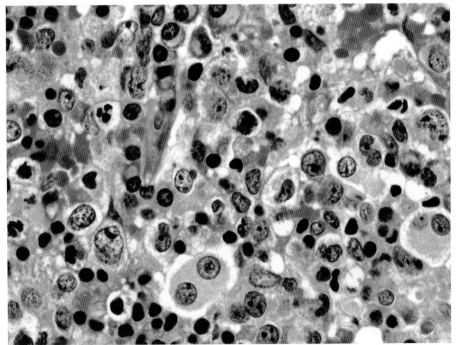

Fig. 1.01 Myelodysplastic syndrome. Bone marrow biopsies should be well fixed, and thin (3–4 μm) sections should be stained with H&E and/or Giemsa stain to enable optimal evaluation of histological details.

the blast percentage in the trephine biopsy. Immunohistochemical staining of the bone marrow biopsy for CD34+ blasts is often helpful in correlating aspirate and trephine biopsy findings (particularly focal clusters or sheets of blasts), although in some myeloid neoplasms the blasts do not express CD34. Flow cytometry determination of blast percentage should not be used as a substitute for visual counting of blasts: flow cytometry samples are often haemodilute, and they can be affected by a number of preanalytic variables; in addition, as noted above, not all blasts express CD34.

Myeloblasts, monoblasts, and megakaryoblasts are included in the blast count. Myeloblasts range from slightly larger than mature lymphocytes to the size of monocytes or larger, with scant to abundant dark-blue to bluish-grey cytoplasm. The nuclei are round to oval, with finely granular chromatin and usually several nucleoli; in some, nuclear irregularities are prominent. The cytoplasm may contain a few azurophilic granules.

Monoblasts are large cells with abundant cytoplasm that can be light grey to deep blue and may show pseudopod formation. Their nuclei are usually round, with delicate, lacy chromatin and one or more large, prominent nucleoli. They are usually strongly positive for non-specific esterase (NSE), but have no or only weak myeloperoxidase (MPO) activity. Promonocytes have a delicately convoluted, folded, or grooved nucleus with finely dispersed chromatin; a small, indistinct, or absent nucleolus; and finely granulated cytoplasm. Most promonocytes express NSE and have MPO activity. Promonocytes are considered to be monoblast equivalents when the requisite percentage of blasts is tallied for the diagnosis of acute monoblastic, acute monocytic, or acute myelomonocytic leukaemia and in subclassifying chronic

myelomonocytic leukaemia. Distinguishing between monoblasts and promonocytes is often difficult, but because both cell types are regarded as monoblasts for the purpose of rendering a diagnosis of AML, the distinction between a monoblast and a promonocyte is not always critical. Distinguishing promonocytes from more mature but abnormal leukaemic monocytes can also be difficult, but is critical, because the designation of a case as acute monocytic or acute myelomonocytic leukaemia versus chronic myelomonocytic leukaemia often hinges on this distinction. Abnormal monocytes have more clumped chromatin than promonocytes, variably indented folded nuclei, and grey cytoplasm with more abundant lilac-coloured granules. Nucleoli are usually absent or indistinct. Abnormal monocytes are not considered to be monoblast equivalents.

Megakaryoblasts are usually small to medium-sized, with a round, indented, or irregular nucleus with fine reticular chromatin and 1–3 nucleoli. The cytoplasm is basophilic, is usually agranular, and may show cytoplasmic blebs (see *Acute megakaryoblastic leukaemia*, p. 162). Small dysplastic megakaryocytes and micromegakaryocytes are not blasts.

In acute promyelocytic leukaemia, the blast equivalent is the abnormal promyelocyte. Early erythroid precursors (proerythroblasts) are not included in the blast count, except in the rare setting of pure erythroid leukaemia.

Cytochemistry and other special stains
Cytochemical studies are useful in determining the lineage of blasts, although in some laboratories they have been supplanted by immunological studies using flow cytometry and/or immunohistochemistry. Cytochemical studies are usually performed on peripheral blood and bone marrow aspirate smears, but some can

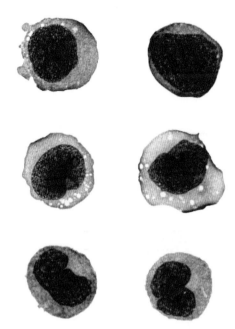

Fig. 1.04 Monoblasts, promonocytes, and abnormal monocytes from a case of acute monocytic leukaemia. *Top:* The monoblasts are large, with abundant cytoplasm that may contain a few vacuoles or fine granules and have round nuclei with lacy chromatin and one or more variably prominent nucleoli. *Middle:* Promonocytes have more irregular and delicately folded nuclei, with fine chromatin, small indistinct nucleoli, and finely granulated cytoplasm. *Bottom:* Abnormal monocytes appear immature, but have more condensed nuclear chromatin, convoluted or folded nuclei, and more cytoplasmic granulation.

be performed on histological sections of bone marrow or other tissues. Detection of MPO indicates myeloid differentiation, but its absence does not exclude a myeloid lineage, because early myeloblasts as well as monoblasts can lack MPO. The MPO activity in myeloblasts is usually granular and is often concentrated in the Golgi region, whereas monoblasts (although usually MPO-negative) may show fine, scattered MPO-positive granules, a pattern that becomes more pronounced in promonocytes. Erythroid blasts, megakaryoblasts, and lymphoblasts are also MPO-negative. Sudan Black B staining parallels MPO staining but is less specific. In the occasional cases of lymphoblastic leukaemia that exhibit Sudan Black B positivity, light-grey granules are seen rather than the black granules that characterize myeloblasts. The NSEs (alpha-naphthyl butyrate esterase and alpha-naphthyl acetate esterase) show diffuse cytoplasmic activity in monoblasts and monocytes. Lympho-

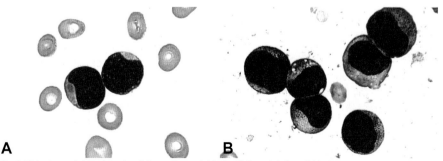

Fig. 1.03 Acute myeloid leukaemia. **A** Agranular myeloblasts. **B** Granulated myeloblasts.

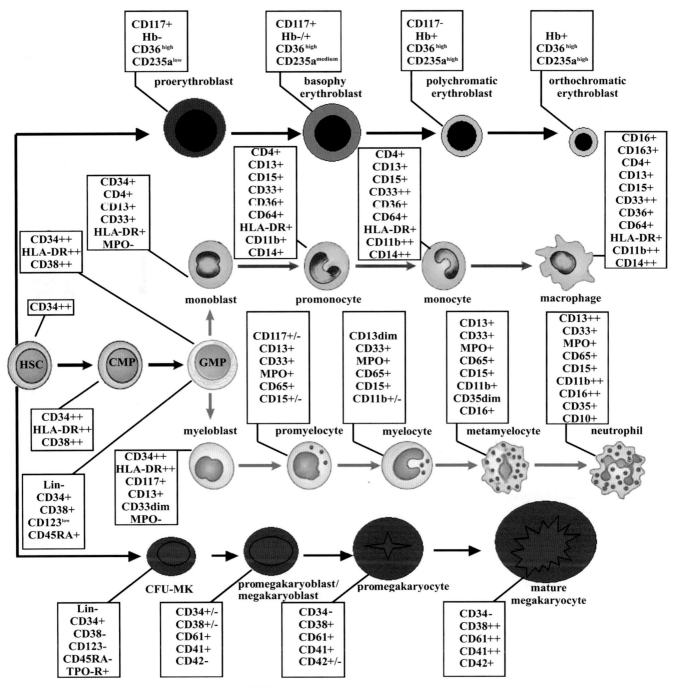

Fig. 1.05 Antigen expression at various stages of normal myeloid differentiation.

blasts may have focal punctate activity with NSEs, but neutrophils are usually negative. Megakaryoblasts and erythroid blasts may have some multifocal, punctate alpha-naphthyl acetate positivity, but the reactivity is partially resistant to sodium fluoride inhibition, whereas monocyte reactivity is totally inhibited by sodium fluoride. The combined use of an NSE and the specific esterase naphthol AS-D chloroacetate esterase (CAE), which pri-

marily stains cells of the neutrophil line-age and mast cells, enables identification of monocytes and immature and mature neutrophils simultaneously. Some cells, particularly in myelomonocytic leukae-mias, may exhibit simultaneous activity with NSEs and CAE. Although normal eo-sinophils lack CAE, it may be expressed by neoplastic eosinophils. CAE staining can be performed on tissue sections (providing the sections are not acid de-

calcified) as well as on peripheral blood or bone marrow aspirate smears. In pure erythroid leukaemia, periodic acid–Schiff (PAS) staining may be helpful because the cytoplasm of the leukaemic pro-erythroblasts may show large globules of PAS positivity. Well-controlled iron stains should always be performed on the bone marrow aspirate to detect iron stores, nor-mal sideroblasts, and ring sideroblasts; ring sideroblasts are defined as erythroid precursors with ≥5 granules of iron, encircling one third or more of the nucleus.

Immunophenotype

Immunophenotypic analysis by either multiparameter flow cytometry or immunohistochemistry is an essential tool in the characterization of myeloid neoplasms. Differentiation antigens that appear at various stages of haematopoietic development and in corresponding myeloid neoplasms are illustrated in Fig. 1.05, and a thorough description of the lineage assignment criteria is provided in the sections on mixed-phenotype acute leukaemia (See *Acute leukaemias of ambiguous lineage*, p. 179). The techniques used and the antigens analysed vary according to the myeloid neoplasm suspected and the information required to best characterize it, as well as by the tissue available. Immunophenotyping is often important in the diagnosis of any haematological neoplasm; in myeloid neoplasms, it is most commonly required to identify mixed-phenotype acute leukaemia, to distinguish between AML with minimal differentiation and lymphoblastic leukaemia, to detect monocytic differentiation in AML, and in determining the phenotype of blasts at the time of transformation of chronic myeloid leukaemia, MDS, MDS/MPN, and MPN.

Multiparameter flow cytometry is the preferred method of immunophenotypic analysis in AML due to the ability to analyse large numbers of cells in a relatively short period of time with simultaneous recording of information about several antigens for each individual cell. Extensive panels of monoclonal antibodies directed against leukocyte differentiation antigens are usually applied, due to the limited utility of individual markers in identifying the commitment of leukaemic cells to the various haematopoietic lineages. Evaluation of the expression patterns of several antigens, both membrane and cytoplasmic, is necessary for determining lineage, identifying mixed-phenotype acute leukaemia, and detecting aberrant phenotypes that will facilitate the evaluation of follow-up specimens for minimal residual disease.

Immunophenotypic analysis has a central role in distinguishing between AML with minimal differentiation and lymphoblastic leukaemia, and in chronic myeloid leukaemia in distinguishing the myeloid blast phase from the lymphoid blast phase. Among the AMLs with recurrent genetic abnormalities, several have characteristic phenotypes. These patterns, described in the respective sections, can facilitate the planning of molecular cytogenetic (FISH) and molecular genetic investigations for individual patients. The immunophenotypic features of the other AML categories are extremely heterogeneous, probably due to high genetic diversity. It has been suggested that the expression of certain antigens (e.g. CD7, CD9, CD11b, CD14, CD56, and CD34) could be associated with an adverse prognosis in AML, but their independent prognostic value is still controversial, and cytogenetic and molecular genetic abnormalities are generally more reliable prognostic markers than is immunophenotype. With 8- or 10-colour flow cytometry, aberrant or unusual immunophenotypes have been found in as many as 90% of cases of AML; these aberrancies include cross-lineage antigen expression, maturational asynchronous expression of antigens, antigen overexpression, and the reduction or absence of antigen expression. Similar aberrancies have been reported in MDS, and their presence can be used to support the diagnosis in early or morphologically difficult cases; however, aberrant flow cytometry immunophenotypes should not be used to diagnose MDS in the absence of standard diagnostic criteria.

Immunophenotyping by immunohistochemistry on bone marrow biopsy sections can be performed, provided that appropriate methods for fixation and decalcification have been applied. Antibodies reactive with paraffin-embedded bone marrow biopsy tissue are available for many lineage-associated markers (e.g. MPO, KIT [CD117], CD33, CD68R, CD14, lysozyme, glycophorin A and C, CD71, CD61, CD42b, CD19, CD3, PAX5, CD79a, and tryptase). As noted previously, CD34 staining of the biopsy can facilitate the detection of blasts and enable assessment of their distribution (provided the blasts express CD34) {2989}. For cases rich in megaloblastoid erythroblasts, immunohistochemistry for glycophorin, CD71, E-cadherin, or haemoglobin may be helpful in distinguishing those cells from myeloblasts in MDS with excess blasts or pure erythroid leukaemia, and CD61 or CD42b staining often facilitates the identification of abnormal megakaryocytes and megakaryoblasts.

Genetics

The WHO classification includes a number of entities defined in part by specific genetic abnormalities, including gene rearrangements due to chromosomal translocations, deletions, and specific gene mutations; therefore, the determination of genetic features of the neoplastic cells is of critical importance for a comprehensive clinicopathological evaluation. A complete cytogenetic analysis of bone marrow by conventional karyotyping should be performed at the time of initial evaluation to establish the cytogenetic profile and at regular intervals thereafter to detect evidence of genetic evolution. Additional diagnostic genetic studies should be guided by the diagnosis suspected on the basis of clinical, morphological, and immunophenotypic studies. In cases with variants of typical cytogenetic abnormalities and cases in which the abnormality is cryptic (e.g. the *FIP1L1-PDGFRA* fusion in myeloid neoplasms associated with eosinophilia), RT-PCR and/or FISH may detect gene rearrangements that are not apparent in the initial chromosomal analysis. Depending on the abnormality, quantitative PCR and/or RT-PCR performed at the time of diagnosis may also provide a baseline against which the response to therapy can be monitored. In addition, the use of array-based and next-generation sequencing technologies enables the sensitive and accurate detection of many common gene rearrangements and has emerged as an alternative to RT-PCR and FISH for the detection of pathogenic fusion genes in haematological malignancies.

A rapidly increasing number of somatic gene mutations detected by gene sequencing, allele-specific PCR, and other techniques have emerged as important diagnostic and prognostic markers for all categories of myeloid neoplasms. Mutations in *JAK2*, *MPL*, *CALR*, *NRAS*, *NF1*, *PTPN11*, *ASXL1*, and *KIT* in MPN and MDS/MPN; *TP53*, *SF3B1*, *ASXL1*, *RUNX1*, *EZH2*, and *ETV6* (among others) in MDS; and *NPM1*, *CEBPA*, *FLT3*, *RUNX1*, *IDH1*, *IDH2*, *ASXL1*, and *KIT* (among others) in AML are important for diagnosis and prognosis. In particular, *JAK2*, *MPL*, *CALR*, *CSF3R*, *SF3B1*, *FLT3*, *NPM1*, *RUNX1*, and *CEBPA* figure prominently in this revised classification. In addition, many recently characterized somatic disease alleles (e.g. recurrent mutations in *TET2*, *ASXL1*, and *DNMT3A*) can serve as definitive markers of clonal haematopoiesis, which can be used as an adjunct to the diagnosis of myeloid malignancies, despite the fact that these alleles are neither specific for a particular disease nor sufficient to diagnose a myeloid neoplasm. These mutations and others seen in myeloid malignancies can also be observed in healthy individuals with clonal haematopoiesis, which appears to constitute a premalignant, clonal state with a variable risk of progression to overt, clinical disease, and has important implications for interpreting genetic profiling in the context of clinical, laboratory, and pathological evaluation to make a specific diagnosis.

Next-generation sequencing continues to emerge as a standard technology for mutational profiling; it is therefore critical to establish methods for identifying alleles with diagnostic, prognostic, and therapeutic relevance, and to use best practices (including informational annotation and paired sequencing of tumour and normal material when possible) to ascertain which alleles are present as acquired mutations and which are present in the germline. In particular, given the likelihood of tumour-derived contamination of paired normal material collected at diagnosis and the frequent presence of antecedent, premalignant clonal haematopoiesis at the time of clinical remission, the choice and timing of collection of non-haematopoietic reference DNA are of critical importance for best-practice genomic profiling. The current approaches to genomic profiling include focused, gene-specific tests for a small set of genes tailored to a specific disease and/or clinical scenario, as well as panel-based assays that query all genes implicated in the pathogenesis of myeloid malignancies, or even more broadly, of all haematological malignancies. Both approaches have clinical value in the current context, but we expect the use of panel-based assays and whole-genome/exome sequencing to increase as the cost and throughput of clinical genomic profiling continue to improve.

Gene over- and underexpression, as well as loss of heterozygosity (LOH) and copy number variants detected by array-based approaches, are only now being recognized as important abnormalities, and may influence diagnostic and prognostic models in the near future {2770}. It will be critical to develop gene-specific and panel-based assays to query for differential expression of specific biomarkers and to assess for copy number and zygosity alterations at specific loci with diagnostic, prognostic, and therapeutic relevance.

Revised WHO classification of myeloid neoplasms

Myeloproliferative neoplasms

The major subgroups of MPNs are listed in the WHO classification table at the beginning of this volume (p. 10). Note that the name of the entity previously called 'chronic myelogenous leukaemia, BCR-ABL1 positive' has been changed to 'chronic myeloid leukaemia, BCR-ABL1–positive'.

The MPNs are clonal haematopoietic stem cell disorders characterized by the proliferation of cells of one or more of the myeloid lineages (i.e. granulocytic, erythroid, and megakaryocytic). They primarily occur in adults, with incidence peaking in the fifth to seventh decades of life, but some subtypes are also reported in children. The annual incidence of all subtypes combined is 6 cases per 100 000 population {1375,1864,2764,4010}.

Most MPNs are initially characterized by varying degrees of age-matched hypercellularity of the bone marrow, with effective haematopoietic maturation and increased numbers of granulocytes, red blood cells, and/or platelets in the peripheral blood. Splenomegaly and hepatomegaly, caused by sequestration of excess blood cells and/or proliferation

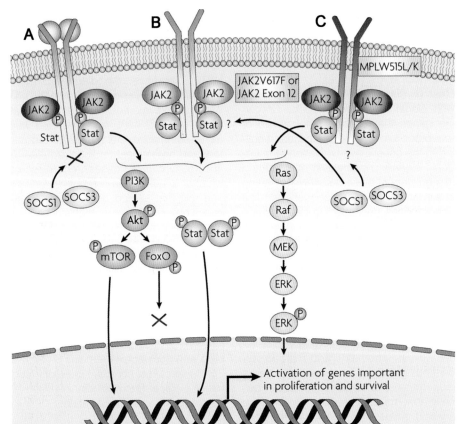

Fig. 1.06 Mechanism of activation of JAK2 kinase activity by mutations in the JAK2 signalling pathway. **A** Cytokine ligands normally bind cytokine receptors, which results in JAK2 phosphorylation, recruitment of STAT signalling proteins, and phosphorylation and activation of downstream signalling pathway components such as STAT transcription factors, MAPK (ERK) signalling proteins, and the PI3K-AKT pathway. **B** The V617F-mutant and exon 12–mutant JAK2 kinases bind cytokine receptors and are phosphorylated in the absence of ligand, leading to ligand-independent activation of downstream signalling pathways. **C** In contrast, MPL W515L/K–mutant thrombopoietin receptors can phosphorylate wildtype JAK2 in the absence of thrombopoietin, resulting in the activation of signalling pathways downstream of JAK2; negative regulation of JAK2 signalling is normally mediated by suppressor of cytokine signalling proteins, most notably SOCS1 and SOCS3; recent data indicate that the JAK2 V617F allele might escape negative feedback by SOCS3. Reproduced from Levine RL et al. {2289}.

of abnormal haematopoietic progenitor cells, are common. Despite an insidious onset, each MPN has the potential to undergo a stepwise progression that terminates in marrow failure due to myelofibrosis, ineffective haematopoiesis, or transformation to an acute blast phase. Evidence of genetic evolution usually heralds disease progression, as may increasing organomegaly, increasing or decreasing blood counts, myelofibrosis, and the onset of myelodysplasia. The finding of 10–19% blasts in the peripheral blood or bone marrow generally signifies accelerated disease, and a proportion of ≥20% is sufficient for the diagnosis of blast phase.

Rationale for and problems with diagnosis and classification of myeloproliferative neoplasms

The revisions to the 2008 criteria for the classification of MPNs have been influenced by three main factors {258}:

1. The recent discovery of genetic abnormalities has provided diagnostic and prognostic markers and novel insights into the pathobiology of *BCR-ABL1*–negative MPNs {3920,3932}.

2. Improved characterization and standardization of morphological features aiding in histological pattern recognition and differentiation of disease groups has increased the reliability and reproducibility of diagnosis {257,1361,1379, 2433,3977}.

3. A number of clinicopathological studies have now validated the WHO postulate of an integrated approach that includes haematological, morphological, and molecular genetic findings {251,266, 1363,1379,1380,2433,3977}.

Reports of controversial aspects have mainly focused on subjectivity and lack of interobserver reproducibility regarding the morphological criteria, especially their validity in distinguishing essential thrombocythaemia (ET) from prefibrotic/early phases of primary myelofibrosis (pre-PMF) and polycythaemia vera (PV). A critical evaluation of these studies suggests that the failure to use a standardized approach to recognizing the distinctive bone marrow features of these disorders resulted in incorrect histological pattern recognition {255,257,3977}. However, several studies on large cohorts of patients have reported consensus rates for the correct diagnosis of MPNs of 76–88%, which are significantly dependent on study design; for example, inclusion of all subtypes of MPN as opposed to restriction to ET vs pre-PMF, inclusion of control cases with reactive changes, and blinded morphological evaluation vs evaluation together with clinical data as recommended by the WHO diagnostic guidelines {257,1361,1379,2433}. In this context, the learning effects of a workshop exercise including interobserver consensus among six haematopathologists included an increase in consensus from 49% to 72% and an agreement rate of 83% between blinded histological and clinical diagnoses {2434}. A number of problems and pitfalls associated with assessing the fibrous matrix of the bone marrow, including the differentiation between reticulin and collagen fibres and the grading of osteosclerosis, must be taken into account {2148}. A multicentre study that compared the results of fibre grading between local pathologists and a panel of experts showed an overall agreement rate of only 56%, supporting the concept of central pathology review for clinical studies {3228}.

Most (if not all) MPNs are associated with clonal abnormalities either involving genes that encode cytoplasmic or receptor protein tyrosine kinases (resulting in the constitutive activation of oncogenic signalling pathways) or occurring in regulators of these pathways (resulting in similar biological consequences). The abnormalities described to date include translocations, insertions, deletions, and point mutations of genes resulting in abnormal, constitutively activated protein tyrosine kinases that activate signal transduction pathways, leading to abnormal proliferation. In some cases, these genetic abnormalities (e.g. the *BCR-ABL1* fusion gene in chronic myeloid leukaemia) are associated with consistent clinical, laboratory, and morphological findings, which enables their use as major criteria for classification; other genetic abnormalities provide proof that the myeloid proliferation is neoplastic rather than reactive.

Acquired somatic mutations in *JAK2*, at chromosome band 9p24, have been shown to play a pivotal role in the pathogenesis of many cases of *BCR-ABL1*–negative MPNs {1831,2045,2099,2289, 2290}. The most common mutation, *JAK2* V617F, results in a constitutively active cytoplasmic JAK2, which activates STAT, MAPK, and PI3K signalling pathways to promote transformation and proliferation of haematopoietic progenitors. The *JAK2* V617F mutation is found in almost all patients with PV and in nearly half of those with PMF and ET. In the few patients with PV who lack the *JAK2* V617F mutation, activating *JAK2* exon 12 mutations may be found; these can be missense or insertion/deletion mutations that are not always detectable by standard *JAK2* mutation assays. In a small proportion of cases of PMF and ET, an activating *MPL* W515L or W515K mutation is seen, and somatic mutations in *CALR* are found in most ET and PMF cases with wildtype *JAK2* and *MPL*. *CALR* and *MPL* mutations are therefore important diagnostic criteria for *JAK2*-wildtype ET and PMF. It is important to note that *JAK2* V617F is not specific for any MPN, nor does its absence exclude MPN. The mutation can also be found in some cases of MDS/MPN and in rare cases of de novo AML and MDS, and can occur in combination with other well-defined genetic abnormalities, such as *BCR-ABL1* {1872}. Therefore, the diagnostic algorithms for PV, ET, and PMF have been updated to take into account the mutational status of *JAK2*, *MPL*, and *CALR*, as well as to summarize the additional laboratory and histological findings required to accurately classify cases, regardless of whether a mutation is present.

The role that altered protein tyrosine kinases play in the pathogenesis of chronic myeloid leukaemia, PV, ET, and PMF supports the inclusion of similar chronic myeloid proliferations related to protein tyrosine kinase abnormalities under the MPN umbrella; however, the molecular pathogenesis of some cases of ET and PMF, a subset of chronic neutrophilic leukaemia cases that lack *CSF3R* mutation, and a number of myeloid neoplasms associated with eosinophilia remains unknown. For these cases, clinical, laboratory, and morphological features remain essential for diagnosis and classification.

Mastocytosis

Due to its unique clinical and pathological features, mastocytosis (which ranges from indolent cutaneous disease to aggressive systemic disease) is no longer considered a subgroup of the MPNs. It is now a separate disease category in the WHO classification.

Myeloid/lymphoid neoplasms with eosinophilia and gene rearrangement

This category of the classification remains largely unchanged, except for the addition of the provisional entity of myeloid/lymphoid neoplasms with t(8;9)(p22;p24.1) resulting in PCM1-JAK2 {230,3108}. The finding of a rearrangement of PDGFRA, PDGFRB, or FGFR1, or of PCM1-JAK2 places a case in this category regardless of the morphological classification; eosinophilia is absent in a subset of cases. Myeloid neoplasms with eosinophilia that lack all of these abnormalities and that meet the criteria for chronic eosinophilic leukaemia, not otherwise specified (NOS), should be placed in that MPN subgroup. Other JAK2-rearranged neoplasms, such as those with t(9;12)(p24.1;p13.2), resulting in ETV6-JAK2, and t(9;22)(p24.1;q11.2), resulting in BCR-JAK2, may have similar features, but are uncommon and are not included as formal entities in this classification. Many cases with BCR-JAK2 present primarily as B-lymphoblastic leukaemia, and these are best classified as B-lymphoblastic leukaemia/lymphoma, BCR-ABL1-like (a new provisional category of B-lymphoblastic leukaemia/lymphoma) {230}.

Myelodysplastic/myeloproliferative neoplasms

The MDS/MPNs include clonal myeloid neoplasms that at the time of initial presentation are associated with some findings that support the diagnosis of an MDS and other findings more consistent with an MPN {2987}. These neoplasms are usually characterized by hypercellularity of the bone marrow due to proliferation in one or more of the myeloid lineages. Often, the proliferation is effective in some lineages, with increased numbers of circulating cells that may be morphologically and/or functionally dysplastic. Simultaneously, one or more of the other lineages may exhibit ineffective proliferation, so that cytopenia may be present as well. The blast percentage in the bone marrow and blood is always < 20%. Although hepatosplenomegaly is common, the clinical and laboratory findings vary along a continuum between those usually associated with MDSs and those usually associated with MPNs. Cases of well-defined MPNs in which dysplasia and ineffective haematopoiesis develop as part of the natural history of the disease or af-

ter chemotherapy should not be placed in this category. Rarely, MPNs may present as accelerated phase in which the chronic phase was not recognized, and may have findings that suggest they belong to the MDS/MPN group. In such cases, if clinical and laboratory studies fail to reveal the nature of the underlying process, the designation 'MDS/MPN unclassifiable' may be appropriate. Cases with BCR-ABL1; with rearrangement of PDGFRA, PDGFRB, or FGFR1; or with PCM1-JAK2 should not be categorized as MDS/MPNs. Mutations in non-kinase genes, including in epigenetic regulators such as TET2 and ASXL1, are very common in MDS/MPNs; they can be used to establish clonality, but are neither diagnostic nor specific for this disease subset {1795,2779}.

Rationale for diagnosis and classification of myelodysplastic/myeloproliferative neoplasms

A diagnosis of chronic myelomonocytic leukaemia (CMML) requires both the presence of persistent peripheral blood monocytosis (monocyte count $\geq 1 \times 10^9$/L) and monocytes accounting for $\geq 10\%$ of white blood cells on the differential count. As a result of the discovery of molecular and clinical differences between the so-called proliferative type (white blood cell count $\geq 13 \times 10^9$/L) and the dysplastic type (white blood cell count $< 13 \times 10^9$/L) {620,3349,3827}, these cases have been separated into two subtypes, myelodysplastic and myeloproliferative, in this classification update. Cases of CMML with eosinophilia associated with PDGFRB rearrangement are excluded, but rare cases of CMML with eosinophilia that do not exhibit such rearrangement are included in this category. The category 'CMML-0' has also been added, for cases with low peripheral blood and bone marrow blast cell counts {2978,3587,3805}.

In juvenile myelomonocytic leukaemia, nearly 80% of cases demonstrate mutually exclusive mutations of PTPN11, NRAS or KRAS, or NF1 {2382,3796,3906}, all of which encode components of RAS-dependent pathways; approximately 30–40% of cases of CMML and atypical chronic myeloid leukaemia, BCR-ABL1-negative, exhibit NRAS mutations {3053,4152,4329}. Given the lack of any specific genetic abnormality to suggest that these entities should be relocated to

another myeloid subgroup, they remain in this mixed category, which acknowledges the overlap that may occur between MDS and MPN.

In the original version of the 4th edition of the WHO classification, refractory anaemia with ring sideroblasts associated with marked thrombocytosis was proposed as a provisional entity to encompass cases with the clinical and morphological features of MDS with ring sideroblasts but also with thrombocytosis associated with abnormal megakaryocytes similar to those observed in BCR-ABL1-negative MPNs. More recently, and in particular after the discovery of a strong association with SF3B1 and concurrent JAK2 V617F, MPL, or CALR mutations, MDS/MPN with ring sideroblasts and thrombocytosis, the new term for the former refractory anaemia with ring sideroblasts associated with marked thrombocytosis category, has become a distinct, well-characterized MDS/MPN overlap entity {2460,2461,3102}.

The classification of myeloid neoplasms that carry an isolated isochromosome of 17q and that have < 20% blasts in the peripheral blood and bone marrow has proven difficult {1913}. Some authors suggest that this cytogenetic defect defines a unique disorder characterized by mixed MDS and MPN features associated with prominent pseudo–Pelger–Huët anomaly of the neutrophils, a low bone marrow blast count, and a rapidly progressive clinical course. A proportion of cases are reported to have prominent monocytosis that meets the criteria for CMML, but in some, the peripheral blood monocyte count does not reach the threshold for that diagnosis {1220,2594}. For cases that do not fulfil the criteria for CMML or another well-defined myeloid neoplasm category, designation as MDS/MPN, unclassifiable, with isolated isochromosome 17q abnormality is most appropriate {1912}.

Myelodysplastic syndromes

These neoplasms are characterized by the simultaneous proliferation and apoptosis of haematopoietic cells that result in a normocellular or hypercellular bone marrow and peripheral blood cytopenia. MDSs are among the most diagnostically challenging of the myeloid neoplasms, both in terms of their distinction from the numerous other (often non-neoplastic) causes of cytopenia and in terms of the

Table 1.01 Diagnostic approach to myeloid neoplasms in which erythroid precursors constitute ≥50% of the nucleated bone marrow (BM) cells

Percentage of BM cells that are erythroid precursors	Percentage of BM (or PB) cells that are myeloblasts	Prior therapy	Defining WHO genetic abnormality present	Meets criteria for AML with myelo-dysplasia-related changes	4th Edition diagnosis (2008)	Revised 4th edition diagnosis (2017)
≥ 50%	n/a	yes	n/a	n/a	Therapy-related myeloid neoplasm	Therapy-related myeloid neoplasm
≥ 50%	≥ 20%	no	yes	n/a	AML with recurrent genetic abnormality	AML with recurrent genetic abnormality
≥ 50%	≥ 20%	no	no	yes	AML with myelodysplasia-related changes	AML with myelodysplasia-related changes
≥ 50%	≥ 20%	no	no	no	AML, NOS; acute erythroid leukaemia (erythroid/myeloid subtype)	AML, NOS (a non-erythroid subtype)
≥ 50%	< 20%, but ≥ 20% of non-erythroid cells	no	no[a]	n/a	AML, NOS; acute erythroid leukaemia (erythroid/myeloid subtype)	MDS[b]
≥ 50%	< 20%, and < 20% of non-erythroid cells	no	no[a]	n/a	MDS[b]	MDS[b]
> 80% immature erythroid precursors with > 30% proerythroblasts	< 20%	no	no[a]	n/a	AML, NOS; acute erythroid leukaemia (pure erythroid subtype)	AML, NOS; pure erythroid leukaemia

AML, acute myeloid leukaemia; BM, bone marrow; MDS, myelodysplastic syndrome; n/a, not applicable; NOS, not otherwise specified; PB, peripheral blood.

[a] Cases of AML with t(8;21)(q22;q22.1) resulting in the *RUNX1-RUNX1T1* fusion protein, AML with inv(16)(p13.1q22) or t(16;16)(p13.1;q22) resulting in the *CBFB-MYH11* fusion protein, or acute promyelocytic leukaemia with the *PML-RARA* fusion protein may rarely occur in this setting with < 20% blasts, and those diagnoses take precedence over the diagnosis of either AML, NOS or MDS.
[b] Classify according to the myeloblast percentage of all BM cells and PB leukocytes, along with other MDS criteria.

proper classification to guide the clinical approach. The general features of MDS, as well as specific guidelines for their diagnosis and classification, are outlined in Chapter 6, *Myelodysplastic syndromes: Overview* (p. 98).

In this revised WHO classification, new terminology has been introduced. In the original 4th edition, MDS disease names included references to cytopenia or specific types of cytopenia (e.g. refractory anaemia). Although cytopenia is a sine qua non of any MDS diagnosis, the WHO classification relies mainly on the degree of dysplasia and blast percentages for MDS classification; specific cytopenias have only a minor impact on classification. Moreover, the lineage(s) manifesting significant morphological dysplasia often do not correlate with the specific cytopenias seen in individual MDS cases. For these reasons, the updated MDS names do not refer to cytopenia. All diagnostic entity names start with 'myelodysplastic syndrome', with further qualifiers specified: single lineage versus multilineage dysplasia, ring sideroblasts, excess blasts, or the defining del(5q) cytogenetic abnormality. No new disease entities have been introduced, but the diagnostic criteria for some entities have been refined, as detailed in Table 6.01 (p. 101) in the *Myelodysplastic syndromes* chapter and in the sections on each MDS entity. MDS cases with multilineage dysplasia, ring sideroblasts, and no excess of blasts or isolated del(5q) cytogenetic abnormality are now categorized as a subgroup of MDS with ring sideroblasts rather than being grouped with MDS with multilineage dysplasia lacking ring sideroblasts as in the original 4th edition. MDS in children has features that differ from those of most MDS in adults, and the provisional entity refractory cytopenia of childhood remains in this updated classification. Although this entity is still provisional, its morphological features and distinction from severe aplastic anaemia are now better defined. An important change in this revision that affects MDS diagnosis is in the diagnostic criteria for myeloid neoplasms in which ≥50% of the bone marrow cells are erythroid precursors. In the original 4th edition WHO classification, erythroid/myeloid-type acute erythroid leukaemia (erythroleukaemia) was diagnosed if blasts accounted for ≥20% of the non-erythroid cells in the bone marrow; if blasts accounted for <20% of the non-erythroid cells, the case was considered to be MDS and subclassified on the basis of the blast count among all nucleated bone marrow cells. Due to the apparent close biological relationship of erythroleukaemia to MDS and the poor reproducibility and potential lability of non-erythroid blast counts, and in an attempt to achieve consistency in expressing blast percentages across all myeloid neoplasms, non-erythroid blast counting has been eliminated from the diagnostic criteria for all myeloid neoplasms. For all cases (even those with ≥50% bone marrow erythroid cells), the bone marrow blast percentage is now expressed as a percentage of all nucleated marrow cells. This will result in most cases that previously would have been classified as erythroleukaemia (i.e. those in which blasts constitute < 20% of all nucleated marrow cells) now being classified as MDS with excess blasts, rather than as a subtype of AML. The diagnostic approach to dealing with myeloid proliferations with increased numbers of erythroid cells is summarized in Table 1.01.

The prognostic relevance of many somatic mutations in MDS has led to the increasing use of genomic profiling in this clinical context; the optimal integration of mutational information into existing MDS risk-stratification schemes and its impact on clinical management are evolving issues. Specifically, mutations in *SF3B1* are now considered in the diagnosis of MDS with ring sideroblasts.

The revised classification of MDS is shown in the WHO classification table at the beginning of this volume (p. 10); the rationale for the changes is provided in the sections on each MDS entity.

Acute myeloid leukaemia

AML results from the clonal expansion of myeloid blasts in the peripheral blood, bone marrow, or other tissue. It is a heterogeneous disease clinically, morphologically, and genetically and can involve a single or all myeloid lineages. Worldwide, the annual incidence is approximately 2.5–3 cases per 100 000 population per year, and is reportedly highest in Australia, western Europe, and the USA. The median patient age at diagnosis is 65 years, and there is a slight male predominance in most countries. In children aged < 15 years, AML constitutes 15–20% of all cases of acute leukaemia, with peak incidence in the first 3–4 years of life {960,4409}.

The requisite blast percentage for a diagnosis of AML is ≥ 20% myeloblasts, monoblasts/promonocytes, and/or megakaryoblasts in the peripheral blood or bone marrow. The diagnosis of myeloid sarcoma is synonymous with AML regardless of the number of blasts in the peripheral blood or bone marrow. If there is a prior history of MPN or MDS/MPN, myeloid sarcoma is evidence of acute transformation (blast phase). A diagnosis of AML can also be made when the blast percentage in the peripheral blood and/or bone marrow is < 20% if

there is an associated t(8;21)(q22;q22.1), inv(16)(p13.1q22), or t(16;16)(p13.1;q22) chromosomal abnormality or *PML-RARA* fusion. Although the line between AML and MDS when other recurrent cytogenetic abnormalities are present is increasingly blurred, such cases continue to be classified on the basis of peripheral blood and bone marrow blast cell counts. The revised classification also continues to place a high proportion of cases into the AML, NOS category, for which the prognosis is variable. This is particularly true in paediatric AML {3503}, but studies seeking additional prognostic markers in all age groups are probably warranted.

Although the diagnosis of AML according to the above guidelines is operationally useful by indicating an underlying defect in myeloid maturation, the diagnosis does not necessarily confer a mandate to treat the patient for AML; clinical factors, including the pace of progression of the disease, must always be taken into consideration when choosing therapy.

Rationale for the diagnosis and classification of acute myeloid leukaemia
The 3rd edition of the WHO classification ushered in the era of formal incorporation of genetic abnormalities in the diagnostic algorithms for AML. The abnormalities included were mainly chromosomal translocations involving transcription factors and associated with characteristic clinical, morphological, and immunophenotypic features that defined a clinicopathological and genetic entity. As our knowledge about leukaemogenesis has increased, so has the acceptance that the genetic abnormalities leading to leukaemia are not only heterogeneous, but also complex; multiple aberrations often contribute in a multistep process to initiate the complete leukaemia phenotype. Experimental evidence suggests that in cases with rearrangements or mutations in genes (e.g. *RUNX1*, *CBFB*, and *RARA*) that encode transcription factors implicated in myeloid differentiation, an additional genetic abnormality is necessary to promote proliferation or survival of the neoplastic clone {1984}. Often, this additional abnormality is a mutation of a gene (e.g. *FLT3* or *KIT*) that encodes proteins that activate signal transduction pathways to promote proliferation/survival. A similar multistep process is also evident in AML that evolves from MDS or that has myelodysplasia-related features,

often characterized by loss of genetic material and haploinsufficiency of genes. Within the past few years, novel genetic mutations have also been identified in essentially all types of AML {545,2774}, and our approach to and understanding of gene mutations in AML has evolved (see Table 1.02, p. 26). Some of the mutations, such as those of *CEBPA* and perhaps *NPM1*, involve transcription factors; others, including those of *FLT3*, *NRAS*, and *KRAS*, affect signal transduction. An emerging class of mutations in epigenetic regulators, including *TET2*, *IDH1*, *IDH2*, *ASXL1*, *DNMT3A*, and cohesin complex family members, are seen in nearly half of all AML cases. These discoveries have improved our understanding of the pathogenesis of AML and suggest that many cases are driven by mutations in ≥ 3 distinct biological pathways, which act in concert to induce progression from normal haematopoietic stem/progenitor cells to clonal, preleukaemic stem/progenitor cells, to overtly transformed leukaemic cells. Not only have these mutations informed our understanding of leukaemogenesis in cytogenetically normal AML, they have also proved to be powerful prognostic factors {2774}. Genetic abnormalities in AML elucidate the pathogenesis of the neoplasm, provide the most reliable prognostic information, and will likely lead to the development of more-successful targeted therapies. Therefore, the use of genomic profiling is a critical aspect of the evaluation and risk stratification of AML in the clinical context.

One of the challenges in this revision and in the original 4th edition has been how to incorporate important and/or recently acquired genetic information into a classification scheme for AML and yet adhere to the WHO principle of defining homogeneous, biologically relevant entities based not only on genetic studies or their prognostic value, but also on clinical, morphological, and/or immunophenotypic studies. This was particularly problematic with the most frequent and prognostically important mutations in cytogenetically normal AML: mutations in *FLT3*, *NPM1*, *RUNX1* and *CEBPA*. Cases with these mutations have few or variably consistent morphological, immunophenotypic, and clinical features reported to date, and the mutations are not mutually exclusive. For the most part, the framework established in the 3rd edition and

Table 1.02 Functional complementation groups of genetic alterations in acute myeloid leukaemia

Period	Before 2008	2008–2012	From 2013
Analysis	**Cytogenetic and molecular genetic analysis**	**Next-generation sequencing approaches**	**The Cancer Genome Atlas (TCGA) project {545}**
Functional groups	**Class I** Activated signalling e.g. *FLT3*, *KIT*, RAS mutations	**Class I** Activated signalling e.g. *FLT3*, *KIT*, and RAS mutations	**Class 1** – Transcription factor fusions e.g. t(8;21), inv(16), and t(15;17)
			Class 2 – Nucleophosmin 1 *NPM1* mutations
			Class 3 – Tumour suppressor genes e.g. *TP53* and *PHF6* mutations
		Class II Transcription and differentiation e.g. t(8;21), inv(16), t(15;17), *CEBPA* and *RUNX1* mutations	**Class 4** – DNA methylation–related genes DNA hydroxymethylation e.g. *TET2*, *IDH1*, and *IDH2* DNA methyltransferases e.g. *DNMT3A*
			Class 5 – Activated signalling genes e.g. *FLT3*, *KIT*, RAS mutations
			Class 6 – Chromatin-modifying genes e.g. *ASXL1* and *EZH2* mutations, *KMT2A* fusions, *KMT2A*-PTD
	Class II Transcription and differentiation e.g. t(8;21), inv(16), t(15;17), and *CEBPA* mutations	**Epigenetic modifiers** (so-called 'Class III') e.g. *TET2*, *DNMT3A*, and *ASXL1* mutations	**Class 7** – Myeloid transcription factor genes e.g. *CEBPA*, *RUNX1* mutations
			Class 8 – Cohesin complex genes e.g. *STAG2*, *RAD21*, *SMC1*, *SMC2* mutations
			Class 9 – Spliceosome-complex genes e.g. *SRSF2*, *U2AF1*, *ZRSR2* mutations

used in the 4th edition proved flexible enough to incorporate the new entities proposed by members of the WHO and clinical advisory committees. The original entities described in the subgroup 'acute myeloid leukaemia with recurrent genetic abnormalities' remain (with only minor modifications), and two provisional entities have been added. A new provisional category, AML with *BCR-ABL1*, has been added to recognize these rare de novo cases {2082,2801,3740}, which may benefit from tyrosine kinase inhibitor therapy and must be distinguished from blast transformation of chronic myeloid leukaemia. AMLs with mutated *NPM1* and *CEBPA* are now full entities, but a biallelic mutation is required for the revised category now known as AML with biallelic mutation of *CEBPA*. Additionally, multilineage dysplasia alone no longer supersedes a diagnosis of AML with mutated *NPM1* or AML with biallelic mutation of *CEBPA*, because recent

studies have shown no difference in de novo cases with and without this finding {211,975,1145}. Lastly, the provisional category of AML with mutated *RUNX1* has been added for de novo cases with this mutation that are not associated with MDS-related cytogenetic abnormalities. This provisional category appears to represent a biologically distinct form of AML {1274,2627,3576,3897}. AML with mutated *FLT3* is not included as a separate entity, because *FLT3* mutation occurs across multiple AML subtypes; however, the significance of this mutation should not be underestimated, and it should be tested for in essentially all cases, including those with *NPM1* or *CEBPA* mutation or other recurrent genetic abnormalities. Broader gene panels are becoming increasingly available and are probably indicated in most, if not all, types of AML. Modifications have been made to the AML with myelodysplasia-related changes subgroup. Cases should still be

assigned to this category if they evolve from previously documented MDS, have specific myelodysplasia-related cytogenetic abnormalities, or exhibit morphological multilineage dysplasia. However, these features do not supersede therapy-related disease or the defined cytogenetic categories of AML. As mentioned above, de novo cases with *NPM1* or biallelic *CEBPA* mutation with no MDS-related cytogenetic abnormalities, but with multilineage dysplasia, are now classified as either AML with mutated *NPM1* or AML with biallelic mutation of *CEBPA*. The cytogenetic abnormalities that define MDS-associated disease have also been modified: del(9q), which does not appear to have prognostic significance in the setting of *NPM1* or biallelic *CEBPA* mutation, has been removed from the list {1511,3562}, as has monosomy 5; del(5q) and unbalanced translocation involving 5q remain {1559,4209}.

Therapy-related myeloid neoplasms (i.e. therapy-related AML, MDS, and MDS/MPN) remain in the revised classification as a distinct subgroup. Most patients who develop therapy-related neoplasms have received therapy with both alkylating agents and topoisomerase II inhibitors, so division according to type of therapy remains impractical. It has been argued that ≥90% of cases of therapy-related AML have cytogenetic abnormalities similar to those seen in AML with recurrent genetic abnormalities or AML with myelodysplasia-related changes, and could be assigned to those categories. However, in most reported series, therapy-related myeloid neoplasms – except therapy-related AML with inv(16)(p13.1q22), t(16;16)(p13.1;q22), or *PML-RARA* – have a significantly worse clinical outcome than do their de novo counterparts with the same genetic abnormalities {94,392,3435,3699,3709}, suggesting some biological differences between the two groups. The study of therapy-related neoplasms may provide valuable insight into the pathogenesis of de novo disease by providing clues as to why certain patients develop leukaemia whereas most patients treated with the same therapies do not. Therefore, cases of therapy-related neoplasms should always be designated as such, and any specific genetic abnormality should also be listed as part of the diagnosis; for example, therapy-related AML with t(9;11)(p21.3;q23.3).

The category 'acute myeloid leukaemia, NOS' encompasses the cases that do not fulfil the specific criteria for any of the other entities. This group currently accounts for 25–30% of all AML cases. If cases of AML with mutated *NPM1* or biallelic mutation of *CEBPA* are removed from this group as is advocated in this revised classification, the subtypes of AML, NOS, no longer have prognostic significance {4233}. The number of cases that fall into the AML, NOS, category will continue to diminish as more genetic subgroups are identified. As mentioned above, the category 'acute erythroid leukaemia (erythroid/myeloid)' has been removed from the classification, and most of these cases are now classified as MDS.

Myeloid sarcoma, an extramedullary tumour mass consisting of myeloid blasts, is included in the classification as a distinct pathological entity. However, when myeloid sarcoma occurs de novo, the diagnosis is equivalent to a diagnosis of AML, and further evaluation (including genetic analysis) is necessary to determine the appropriate classification of the leukaemia {3177}. When the peripheral blood and/or bone marrow are concurrently involved by AML, these specimens can be used for analysis and further classification. However, when the myeloid sarcoma precedes evidence of peripheral blood or bone marrow involvement, the immunophenotype should be ascertained by flow cytometry and/or immunohistochemistry, and the genotype determined by cytogenetic analysis or (in the absence of fresh tissue) by FISH or molecular analysis for recurrent genetic abnormalities. Myeloid sarcoma may also be the initial indication of relapse in a patient previously diagnosed with AML, or may indicate disease progression to AML or to the blast phase in patients with a prior diagnosis of MDS, MDS/MPN, or MPN

As in the original 4th edition, the unique features of myeloid proliferations associated with Down syndrome are addressed in a separate category, which encompasses transient abnormal myelopoiesis associated with Down syndrome and myeloid leukaemia associated with Down syndrome.

A section on myeloid neoplasms with germline predisposition {1390,4301} has been added to the classification to address cases of AML, MDS, and MDS/MPN that have germline genetic abnormalities. The recognition of such cases should lead to screening of family members, which may enable earlier disease detection in affected individuals.

CHAPTER 2

Myeloproliferative neoplasms

Chronic myeloid leukaemia, *BCR-ABL1*–positive

Chronic neutrophilic leukaemia

Polycythaemia vera

Primary myelofibrosis

Essential thrombocythaemia

Chronic eosinophilic leukaemia, NOS

Myeloproliferative neoplasm, unclassifiable

Chronic myeloid leukaemia, *BCR-ABL1*–positive

Vardiman J.W.
Melo J.V.
Baccarani M.
Radich J.P.
Kvasnicka H.M.

Definition

Chronic myeloid leukaemia (CML), *BCR-ABL1*–positive, is a myeloproliferative neoplasm (MPN) in which granulocytes are the major proliferative component. It arises in a haematopoietic stem cell and is characterized by the chromosomal translocation t(9;22)(q34.1;q11.2), which results in the formation of the Philadelphia (Ph) chromosome, containing the *BCR-ABL1* fusion gene {282,2620,2905,3433}. In CML, *BCR-ABL1* is found in all myeloid lineages and in some lymphoid and endothelial cells {1210,1496}. The natural history of untreated CML is biphasic or triphasic: an initial indolent chronic phase (CP) is followed by an accelerated phase (AP), a blast phase (BP), or both. The diagnosis requires detection of the Ph chromosome and/or *BCR-ABL1* in the appropriate clinical and laboratory settings.

ICD-O code   9875/3

Synonyms

Chronic myelogenous leukaemia, *BCR-ABL1*–positive; chronic granulocytic leukaemia, *BCR-ABL1*–positive (9863/3); chronic myelogenous leukaemia, Philadelphia chromosome–positive (Ph+); chronic myelogenous leukaemia, t(9;22)(q34;q11); chronic granulocytic leukaemia, Philadelphia chromosome–positive (Ph+); chronic granulocytic leukaemia, t(9;22)(q34;q11); chronic granulocytic leukaemia, *BCR/ABL1*; chronic myeloid leukaemia (9863/3)

Epidemiology

Worldwide, CML has an annual incidence of 1–2 cases per 100 000 population, with a slight male predominance. The annual incidence increases with age, from < 0.1 cases per 100 000 children to ≥ 2.5 cases per 100 000 elderly individuals {1662,1749}. Significant ethnic or geographical variations in incidence have not been reported, but an earlier patient age at onset has been reported in areas where socioeconomic status is lower {2626}. Due to the success of tyrosine kinase inhibitor (TKI) therapy in reducing mortality rates (down to only 2–3% per year), the prevalence of CML is expected to increase considerably {1725}.

Etiology

The predisposing factors for CML are largely unknown. Acute radiation exposure has been implicated, largely due to the reported increased incidence of CML among atomic bomb survivors {387,815}. Unlike other MPNs, there is slight, if any, inherited predisposition {2209,3306}.

Localization

In CP, the leukaemia cells are minimally invasive and mostly confined to the blood, bone marrow, spleen, and liver. In BP, the blasts can infiltrate any extramedullary site, with a predilection for spleen, liver, lymph nodes, skin, and soft tissue {822,1810,2776}.

Clinical features

Most patients with CML are diagnosed in CP, which usually has an insidious onset. Nearly 50% of newly diagnosed cases are asymptomatic and discovered when a white blood cell (WBC) count performed as part of a routine medical examination is found to be abnormal {822, 1809}. Common findings at presentation include fatigue, malaise, weight loss, night sweats, and anaemia, and about 50% of patients have palpable splenomegaly {822,1662,1809,3534}. Atypical presentations include marked thrombocytosis without leukocytosis that mimics essential thrombocythaemia or other types of MPN {512,618,3732}. About 5% of cases are diagnosed in AP or BP without a recognized CP {1662,3534}.

Without effective therapy, most cases of CML progress from CP to BP (directly or via AP) within 3–5 years after diagnosis {822,1602}. These transformed stages are characterized clinically by declining performance status, constitutional signs such as fever and weight loss, and symptoms related to severe anaemia, thrombocytopenia, increased WBC count, splenic enlargement, and in BP, a dismal outcome {1601,1809}. With targeted TKI therapy and careful disease monitoring, the incidence of AP and BP has decreased, and the 10-year overall survival rate for CML is 80–90% {207, 573,1602,1904}.

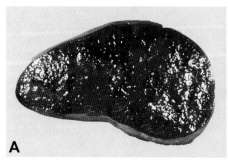
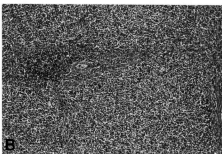
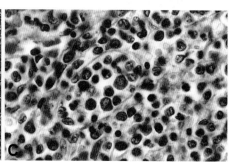

Fig. 2.01 Splenomegaly in chronic myeloid leukaemia, *BCR-ABL1*–positive. **A** The gross appearance of the spleen is solid and uniformly deep red, although areas of infarction may appear as lighter-coloured regions. **B** The red pulp distribution of the infiltrate usually compresses and obliterates the white pulp. **C** The leukaemic cells are present in the splenic cords and sinuses. In this case the cells are shifted towards immature forms; care must be taken to assess the maturity of the cells in splenectomy specimen, because enlarging spleens, particularly in the face of TKI therapy, may be associated with disease progression.

Microscopy

Chronic phase

In CP, the peripheral blood shows leukocytosis (12–1000 × 10⁹/L, median: ~80 × 10⁹/L) due to neutrophils in various stages of maturation, with peaks in the proportions of myelocytes and segmented neutrophils {1662,3534,3753}; children often have higher WBC counts than adults (median: ~250 × 10⁹/L) {1374,2665,3836}. Significant granulocytic dysplasia is absent. Blasts typically account for <2% of the WBCs. Absolute basophilia and eosinophilia are common {1662,3753}. Absolute monocytosis may be present, but the proportion of monocytes is usually <3% {339}, except in rare cases with the p190 BCR-ABL1 isoform, which often mimic chronic myelomonocytic leukaemia {2623}. Platelet counts are normal or increased to ≥1000 × 10⁹/L; marked thrombocytopenia is uncommon in CP {1662}.

Most cases of CML can be diagnosed on the basis of peripheral blood findings combined with detection of the Ph chromosome and/or *BCR-ABL1* by cytogenetic and molecular genetic techniques. However, bone marrow aspiration is essential to ensure sufficient material for a complete karyotype and for morphological evaluation to confirm the phase of disease. Bone marrow biopsy is not required to diagnose CML in most cases, but should be done if the findings in the peripheral blood are atypical or if a cellular aspirate cannot be obtained {1662, 2911}.

In CP, bone marrow specimens are hypercellular, with marked granulocytic proliferation and a maturation pattern similar to that in the blood, including expansion at the myelocyte stage {822}. There is no significant dysplasia. Blasts usually account for <5% of the marrow cells; ≥10% suggests advanced disease {817}. The proportion of erythroid precursors is usually significantly decreased. Megakaryocytes may be normal or slightly decreased in number, but 40–50% of cases exhibit moderate to marked megakaryocytic proliferation {495,3976,3982}. In CP, the megakaryocytes are smaller than normal and have hyposegmented nuclei; they are referred to as 'dwarf' megakaryocytes, but are not true micromegakaryocytes such as those seen in myelodysplastic syndromes {853,3982}. Eosinophils and basophils are usually increased in number, and pseudo-Gau-

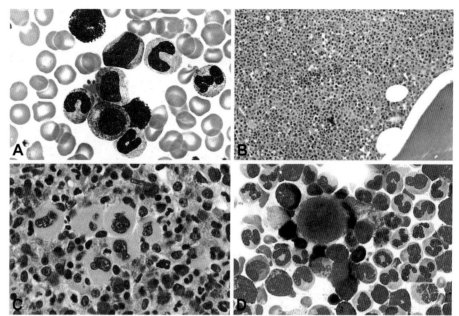

Fig. 2.02 Chronic myeloid leukaemia (CML), *BCR-ABL1*–positive (chronic phase). **A** Peripheral blood smear showing leukocytosis and neutrophilic cells at various stages of maturation; basophilia is prominent; no dysplasia is present. **B** Bone marrow biopsy showing marked hypercellularity due to granulocytic proliferation. **C** The megakaryocytes in CML are characteristically smaller than normal megakaryocytes. **D** Bone marrow aspirate smear shows expansion and maturation of the neutrophil lineage, increased basophils and a small 'dwarf' megakaryocyte, which is smaller than a normal megakaryocyte but larger than the micromegakaryocytes seen in myelodysplastic syndromes, although micromegakaryocytes are sometimes seen in CML in the accelerated or myeloid blast phase.

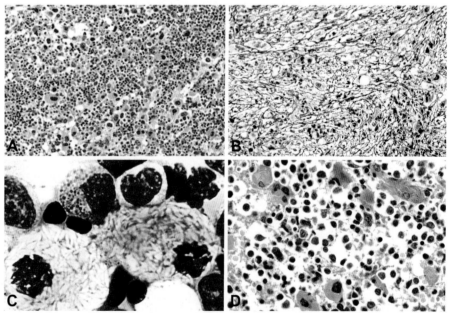

Fig. 2.03 Chronic myeloid leukaemia (CML), *BCR-ABL1*–positive (chronic phase). **A** There may be morphological variability in the initial bone marrow biopsy specimens of patients with CML. In this case there is a prominent increase in the number of 'dwarf' megakaryocytes that are dispersed throughout the marrow. Such cases are sometimes referred to as 'megakaryocyte-rich' CML. **B** Up to 30% of cases of CML may have reticulin fibrosis of variable degree at presentation. **C** Pseudo-Gaucher cells in CML. Pseudo-Gaucher cells are commonly observed in the marrow aspirates of patients with CML. **D** They may also be appreciated as foamy or striated cells in marrow biopsy sections. These histiocytes are secondary to increased cell turnover, are derived from the neoplastic clone and are easily distinguished from the 'dwarf' megakaryocytes seen in the lower middle margin of the photograph.

cher cells are common. These features are mirrored in marrow biopsy sections, in which a layer of immature granulo-

cytes (5–10 cells in thickness) is common around the bone trabeculae, in contrast to the normal thickness of 2–3 cells {853}.

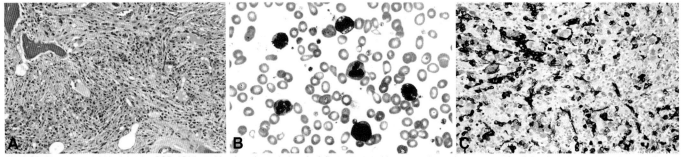

Fig. 2.04 Chronic myeloid leukaemia, *BCR-ABL1*–positive (accelerated phase). **A** Bone marrow biopsy specimen shows areas of cellular depletion and prominence of small megakaryocytes. The swirling appearance of the cells is caused by an increase in underlying reticulin fibres. **B** Basophils accounted for more than 20% of the WBCs in this case, with occasional blasts. **C** An increase in blasts is appreciated in the biopsy with CD34; an aspirate could not be obtained due to increased reticulin fibres.

Moderate to marked reticulin fibrosis, which correlates with increased numbers of megakaryocytes and may be associated with an enlarged spleen, has been reported in 30–40% of biopsies at diagnosis {490,495,1329,3982}. Although the presence of fibrosis at the time of diagnosis was reported to be associated with a worse outcome in the pre-TKI era, it reportedly has no substantial impact on prognosis in patients treated with TKIs {926,1932}.

Splenic enlargement in CP is due to infiltration of the red pulp cords by mature and immature granulocytes. A similar infiltrate can be seen in hepatic sinuses and portal areas.

Disease phases

Disease progression: accelerated phase and blast phase

Recognition of disease progression is important for treatment and prognostic purposes, but the clinical and morphological boundaries between CP, AP, and BP are not always sharp, and the parameters used to define them differ between investigators. These categories were of substantial prognostic importance in the pre-TKI era, when effective treatment without allogeneic transplant was not available, but the effectiveness of TKIs has further blurred the lines between these phases of CML. For example, some studies show that newly diagnosed patients who initially present in AP may have similar outcomes, when treated with TKIs, as those of patients with newly diagnosed CP {2939,3324}. In contrast, AP

disease that develops during TKI therapy has a poor outcome. Furthermore, gene expression studies of CP, AP, and BP suggest that progression of CP to AP and/or BP is more consistent with a two-step process, with new gene expression profiles occurring early in AP (or late in CP), before the accumulation of blasts and other features often used to define AP {3277}. BP continues to have a very poor outcome, even with TKI therapy {1601}. Death occurs due to bleeding or infectious complications, as normal haematopoiesis is increasingly disrupted by the malignant cells. In BP, the increase in blasts not only indicates a loss of response to therapy, but also signifies that the disease has acquired characteristics of acute leukaemia.

Accelerated phase

In the original 4th edition of the classification, it was recommended that the diagnosis of AP be made if any of the following parameters were present: (1) a persistent or increasing high WBC count ($> 10 \times 10^9$/L) and/or persistent or increasing splenomegaly, unresponsive to therapy; (2) persistent thrombocytosis ($> 1000 \times 10^9$/L), unresponsive to therapy; (3) persistent thrombocytopenia ($< 100 \times 10^9$/L), unrelated to therapy; (4) evidence of clonal cytogenetic evolution, defined by cells harbouring the Ph chromosome and additional cytogenetic changes; (5) ≥ 20% basophils in the peripheral blood; and (6) 10–19% blasts in the peripheral blood and/or bone marrow. In addition, large clusters or sheets of small, abnormal megakaryocytes associated with marked reticulin or collagen fibrosis were considered to be presumptive evidence of AP, particularly if accompanied by any of the haematological parameters listed above. Although other defining criteria for AP have been

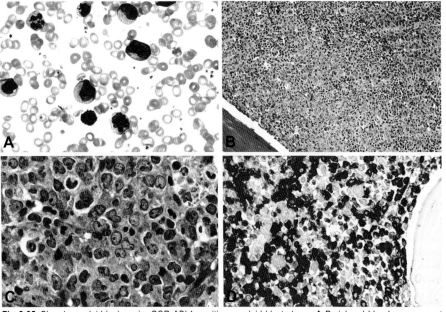

Fig. 2.05 Chronic myeloid leukaemia, *BCR-ABL1*–positive, myeloid blast phase. **A** Peripheral blood smear; most of the white blood cells are blasts. **B** and **C** Sheets of blasts in the bone marrow biopsy. **D** Myeloperoxidase (MPO) immunohistochemistry proving the myeloid origin of the blasts.

suggested {817}, these clinical, haematological, morphological, and genetic parameters are evidence of disease progression (Table 2.01).

When defined as above, however, AP includes a very heterogeneous group of cases, so these parameters alone are insufficient for prognostic purposes. However, their utility may be increased by the consideration of additional response-defined parameters {1535}. Response to therapy (e.g. TKIs or allogeneic transplant) is linked to the phase of disease. For example, the rare cases defined at diagnosis as AP solely on the basis of additional cytogenetic changes {1124} but who do not have an increase in blasts respond to therapy similarly to patients with CP disease, whereas patients with newly diagnosed AP disease with additional cytogenetic abnormalities and increased blasts do appreciably worse {3324}. Moreover, cases in clinical and morphological CP that develop resistant *BCR-ABL1* mutations have gene expression patterns similar to those seen in advanced disease {2605,3277}. Therefore, response-to-therapy parameters are now included as provisional criteria for AP, pending verification of their validity. According to these provisional criteria, CP cases can be considered to be functionally in AP (with poor rates of long-term, progression-free survival) if there is (1) haematological resistance to the first TKI, (2) any grade of resistance to two sequential TKIs, or (3) occurrence of two or more *BCR-ABL1* mutations (Table 2.01).

In AP, bone marrow specimens are often hypercellular, and dysplastic changes may be seen in any of the myeloid lineages {2776,4395}. Clusters of small megakaryocytes (including true micromegakaryocytes similar to those seen in myelodysplastic syndromes) may be

Table 2.01 Defining criteria for the accelerated phase (AP) of chronic myeloid leukaemia (CML)

CML-AP is defined by the presence of ≥ 1 of the following haematological/cytogenetic criteria or provisional criteria concerning response to tyrosine kinase inhibitor (TKI) therapy

Haematological/cytogenetic criteria[a]

- Persistent or increasing high white blood cell count (> 10 × 10^9/L), unresponsive to therapy
- Persistent or increasing splenomegaly, unresponsive to therapy
- Persistent thrombocytosis (> 1000 × 10^9/L), unresponsive to therapy
- Persistent thrombocytopenia (< 100 × 10^9/L), unrelated to therapy
- ≥ 20% basophils in the peripheral blood
- 10–19% blasts in the peripheral blood and/or bone marrow[b,c]
- Additional clonal chromosomal abnormalities in Philadelphia (Ph) chromosome–positive (Ph+) cells at diagnosis, including so-called major route abnormalities (a second Ph chromosome, trisomy 8, isochromosome 17q, trisomy 19), complex karyotype, and abnormalities of 3q26.2
- Any new clonal chromosomal abnormality in Ph+ cells that occurs during therapy

Provisional response-to-TKI criteria

- Haematological resistance (or failure to achieve a complete haematological response[d]) to the first TKI
- Any haematological, cytogenetic, or molecular indications of resistance to two sequential TKIs
- Occurrence of two or more mutations in the *BCR-ABL1* fusion gene during TKI therapy

---

[a] Large clusters or sheets of small, abnormal megakaryocytes associated with marked reticulin or collagen fibrosis in biopsy specimens may be considered presumptive evidence of AP, although these findings are usually associated with one or more of the criteria listed above.
[b] The finding of bona fide lymphoblasts in the peripheral blood or bone marrow (even if < 10%) should prompt concern that lymphoblastic transformation may be imminent, and warrants further clinical and genetic investigation.
[c] ≥ 20% blasts in the peripheral blood or bone marrow, or an infiltrative proliferation of blasts in an extramedullary site, is diagnostic of the blast phase of CML.
[d] Complete haematological response is defined as white blood cell count < 10 × 10^9/L, platelet count < 450 × 10^9/L, no immature granulocytes in the differential, and spleen not palpable.

present and may be associated with significant reticulin and/or collagen fibrosis, which is best assessed in biopsy sections. The increased proportion of blasts in AP (10–19%) may be highlighted with immunohistochemical staining for CD34 {2989,3960}. In most cases, the blasts have a myeloid phenotype {1131}. Lymphoid blasts may be seen, but some data suggest that the finding of any bona fide lymphoblasts in the blood and/or bone marrow in CP or AP should raise concern that a lymphoblastic crisis may be imminent, because lymphoblastic BP is reported to sometimes have an abrupt onset, without a preceding AP {66,619, 1087,1931}.

Blast phase

The criteria for BP include (1) ≥ 20% blasts in the blood or bone marrow or (2) the presence of an extramedullary proliferation of blasts. Some investigators and clinical trials have instead used a threshold of ≥ 30% blasts in the blood and/or bone marrow to define BP, but most patients in BP have a very poor prognosis regardless of which cut-off point is used {817,1601}.

In most BP cases, the blast lineage is myeloid, and may include neutrophilic, monocytic, megakaryocytic, basophilic, eosinophilic, or erythroid blasts, or any combination thereof {1131,1601,1997, 2806}. In approximately 20–30% of BP

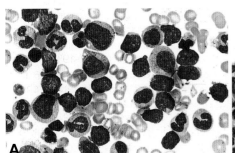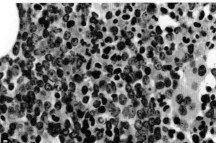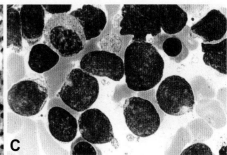

Fig. 2.06 Chronic myeloid leukaemia, *BCR-ABL1*–positive (lymphoid blast phase). **A** Peripheral blood smear with numerous lymphoid-morphology blasts among leukaemic myelocytes. **B** Bone marrow biopsy of the same case. **C** Marrow aspirate smear. By flow cytometry, the blasts coexpressed CD19, CD10, CD22, terminal deoxynucleotidyl transferase (TdT), and CD13, but there was no expression of MPO.

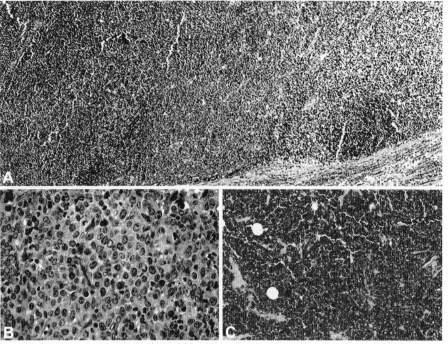

Fig. 2.07 Chronic myeloid leukaemia (CML), *BCR-ABL1*–positive (myeloid blast phase), in an extramedullary site. **A** and **B** On lymph node biopsy obtained from a patient with a 3-year history of CML, the lymph node architecture is effaced by a proliferation of medium-sized to large cells. **C** Lysozyme immunohistochemistry confirms the myeloid lineage of the blasts.

cases, the blasts are lymphoblasts (usually of B-cell origin, although cases of T-lymphoblastic and NK-cell transformation have been reported) {682,2015, 4261}. Sequential lymphoblastic and myeloblastic crises have also been reported. In BP, the blast lineage may be morphologically obvious, but the blasts are often primitive and/or heterogeneous, and expression of antigens of more than one lineage is common {1997, 3335}; therefore, cytochemical and immunophenotypic analysis of the blasts is recommended.

Extramedullary blast proliferations are most common in the skin, lymph nodes, bone, and CNS, but can occur anywhere; they may be of myeloid, lymphoid, or mixed-lineage phenotype {682,1810}. In bone marrow biopsy specimens, sheets of blasts that occupy focal but substantial areas of the bone marrow (e.g. an entire intertrabecular space or more) can be considered presumptive evidence of BP even if the rest of the marrow shows CP.

Immunophenotype

Immunophenotypic data on CML-CP suggest that the expression of CD7 on CD34+ cells has adverse prognostic significance, whereas a normal CD34+ stem-cell population, lacking expression of abnormal markers (e.g. CD7, CD56, or CD11b), predicts a better response to TKI therapy {2089,3393,4427}. However, the main role of immunophenotyping in CML is analysis of the blasts in BP. In myeloid BP, the blasts have strong, weak, or no MPO activity but express one or more antigens associated with granulocytic, monocytic, megakaryocytic, and/or erythroid differentiation, such as CD33, CD13, CD14, CD11b, CD11c, KIT (CD117), CD15, CD41, CD61, and glycophorin A and C. However, in many myeloid BP cases, the blasts also express one or more lymphoid-related antigens {1997,3335,3480}. Most lymphoblastic BP blasts are of precursor–B-cell origin and express terminal deoxynucleotidyl transferase (TdT) in addition to B-cell–related antigens (e.g. CD19, CD10, CD79a, PAX5, and CD20), but a minority of lymphoblastic BP blasts are of T-cell origin and express T-cell–related antigens (e.g. CD3, CD2, CD5, CD4, CD8, and CD7). Expression of one or more myeloid-related antigens by the blasts is common in both B- and T-cell–derived blast transformations {2015,4261}. Bilineage cases (i.e. with distinct populations of myeloid and lymphoid blasts) also occur {682, 3480}, and sequential lymphoblastic BP and myeloblastic BP have been reported {525}. A recent study showed a higher frequency of unusual blast types and immunophenotypes (e.g. basophil blasts or megakaryoblasts) after the introduction of TKI therapy {3647}. Flow cytometry is the preferred technique for phenotypic analysis in order to detect mixed phenotypes, but immunohistochemical stains can also be applied if a marrow aspirate cannot be obtained and there are insufficient numbers of blasts in the blood.

Cell of origin

CML originates from an abnormal pluripotent bone marrow stem cell. However, disease progression may originate in more committed precursors than previously supposed, given that myeloid BP has been reported to involve the granulocyte–macrophage progenitor pool rather than the haematopoietic stem cell pool {2655}. It is unknown whether this is also the case with lymphoid BP. Recent data have shown that the quiescent leukaemic stem cells do not rely on BCR-ABL1 for survival, and are refractory to TKI therapy {808,1529}.

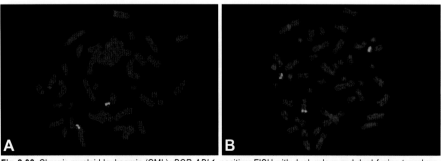

Fig. 2.08 Chronic myeloid leukaemia (CML), *BCR-ABL1*–positive: FISH with dual-colour and dual-fusion translocation probes for *ABL1* (red) and *BCR* (green). **A** In a normal metaphase cell, there are two red signals labelling *ABL1* at 9q34.1 and two green signals labelling *BCR* at 22q11.2. **B** On a metaphase preparation from a patient with CML and t(9;22)(q34.1;q11.2), there are one red signal (normal 9q34.1), one green signal (normal 22q11.2), and two orange/green (yellow) signals labelling derivative 9q34.1 and 22q11.2, respectively.

Genetic profile

At diagnosis, 90–95% of cases of CML have the characteristic t(9;22) (q34.1;q11.2) reciprocal translocation that results in the Ph chromosome, der(22) t(9;22) {3433}. This translocation fuses sequences of the *BCR* gene on chromosome 22 with regions of *ABL1* on chromosome 9 {282}. The remaining cases have either variant translocations that involve a third or even a fourth chromosome in addition to chromosomes 9 and 22, or a cryptic translocation of 9q34.1 and 22q11.2 that cannot be identified by routine cytogenetic analysis. In such cases, the *BCR-ABL1* fusion gene is present and can be detected by FISH analysis and/or RT-PCR {2619}.

The site of the breakpoint in chromosome 22 may influence the phenotype of the disease {2619}. In CML, the breakpoint cluster region (BCR) is almost always in the major BCR (M-BCR), spanning exons 12–16 (previously known as b1–b5) and an abnormal fusion protein, p210, is formed, which has increased tyrosine kinase activity. Rarely, the breakpoint in the *BCR* gene occurs in the μ-BCR region, spanning exons 17–20 (previously known as c1–c4), and a larger fusion protein, p230, is encoded. Patients with this fusion may demonstrate prominent neutrophilic maturation and/or conspicuous thrombocytosis {2619,3048}. Although breaks in the minor breakpoint region, m-BCR (exons 1–2) lead to a short fusion proteins (p190) and is most frequently associated with Ph chromosome–positive ALL, small amounts of the p190 transcript can be detected in more than 90% of patients with CML as well, due to alternative splicing of the BCR gene (4140). However, this breakpoint may also be seen in rare cases of CML associated with increased numbers of monocytes, which can resemble chronic myelomonocytic leukaemia {2623}.

It is generally accepted that the increased tyrosine kinase activity of BCR-ABL1 is necessary and sufficient to cause CML-CP through the constitutive activation of proteins in several signal transduction pathways. Among the many pathways affected are the JAK/STAT

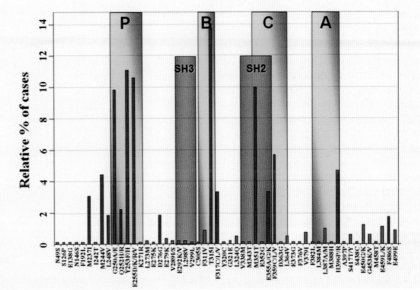

Fig. 2.09 Chronic myeloid leukaemia, *BCR-ABL1*–positive (chronic phase): incidence of reported mutations within the kinase domain by percentage of the total. The seven most frequent mutations are depicted in red and the next eight in blue. The mutations shown in green have been reported in < 2% of clinical resistance cases. Specific regions of the kinase domain are indicated as a P-loop or ATP-binding site (P), an imatinib-binding site (B), a catalytic domain (C), and an activation loop (A). The contact regions with SH2 and SH3 domain–containing proteins are also shown. Based on data from Apperley JF {122} and Soverini S et al. {3743A}.

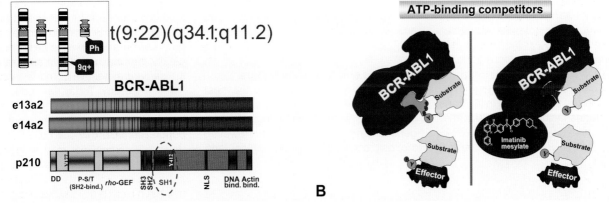

Fig. 2.10 Chronic myeloid leukaemia, *BCR-ABL1*–positive. **A** Schematic representation of the t(9;22) chromosomal translocation, the fusion mRNA transcripts encoded by the *BCR-ABL1* fusion gene generated in the changed chromosome 22 and the Philadelphia (Ph) chromosome, and the translated BCR-ABL1 fusion protein (p210) – whose oncogenic properties are due primarily to its constitutively activated tyrosine kinase, encoded by the SH1 domain (indicated in red). Some of the other important functional domains contributed by the BCR and ABL1 portions of the oncoprotein are also shown: the dimerization domain (DD); Y177, which is the autophosphorylation site crucial for binding to GRB2; the phospho-serine/threonine (P-S/T) SH2-binding domain; a region homologous to Rho guanine nucleotide exchange factors (rho-GEF); the ABL1 regulatory SH3 and SH2 domains; Y412, which is the major site of autophosphorylation within the SH1 kinase domain; nuclear localization signals (NLS); and the DNA-binding and actin-binding domains. **B** Mechanism of action of BCR-ABL1 tyrosine kinase inhibitors. The physiological binding of ATP to its pocket allows BCR-ABL1 to phosphorylate selected tyrosine residues on its substrates (left panel); a synthetic ATP mimic such as imatinib fits the pocket (right panel), but does not provide the essential phosphate group to be transferred to the substrate. The downstream chain of reactions is then halted because, with its tyrosines in the unphosphorylated form, the substrate does not assume the necessary conformation to ensure association with its effector.

(cell growth and survival), PI3K/AKT (cell growth, cell survival, and inhibition of apoptosis), and RAS/MEK (activation of transcription factors, including NF-κB) pathways {689,3771}. The understanding of the abnormal signalling in CML cells led to the design and synthesis of small molecules that target the tyrosine kinase activity of BCR-ABL1, of which imatinib was the first to be successfully used to treat CML {1041,1042}. Imatinib competes with ATP for binding to the BCR-ABL1 kinase domain, thus preventing phosphorylation of tyrosine residues on its substrates. Interruption of the oncogenic signal in this way is effective for control of the disease, particularly when used early in CP. However, the emergence of subclones of leukaemic progenitor cells that have *BCR-ABL1* point mutations that alter amino acids and prevent the binding of the inhibitor to the BCR-ABL1 kinase domain can lead to drug resistance, particularly in AP and BP {122}. The second and third generations of TKIs (i.e. nilotinib, dasatinib, bosutinib, and ponatinib) can circumvent this form of drug failure in the presence of most kinase domain mutations {4281}.

The molecular basis of transformation is still largely unknown {2620}. Progression is usually associated with clonal evolution; at the time of transformation to AP or BP, 80% of cases demonstrate cytogenetic changes in addition to the Ph chromosome, including an extra Ph chromosome, isochromosome 17q, and gain of chromosome 8 or 19, the so-called major route karyotypic abnormalities. The presence of any of these abnormalities in the karyotype at the time of initial diagnosis of CML has been reported to be an adverse prognostic finding, and places a case in the AP category {1161}. Genes reported to be altered in the transformed stages include *TP53*, *RB1*, *MYC*, *CDKN2A* (also called *p16INK4a*), *NRAS*, *KRAS*, *RUNX1* (also called *AML1*),

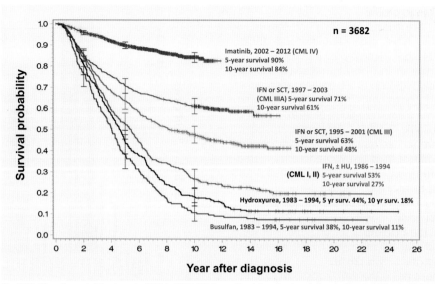

Fig. 2.11 Chronic myeloid leukaemia (CML), *BCR-ABL1*–positive (chronic phase). Survival probabilities in CML over time as observed in five consecutive randomized treatment-optimization studies (1983–2014) of the German CML Study Group using different treatment modalities, showing marked improvement in survival with tyrosine kinase inhibitor therapy. Similar results have been published by other cooperative groups. From: Hehlmann R {1602}.

MECOM (also called *EVI1*), *TET2*, *CBL*, *ASXL1*, *IDH1*, and *IDH2*, but their exact role (if any) in the transformation is unknown {2453,3743}. The introduction of genome-wide expression profiling by microarray technology has revealed other candidate genes associated with the advanced stages, and has also revealed similar gene expression patterns in AP and BP, suggesting that the genetic events leading to transformation in AP and BP occur in late CP or early AP {4426}. These studies have also shown that progression to advanced-phase disease often shares biological features associated with resistance to TKI therapy {3277}.

Prognosis and predictive factors
In the current era of TKI therapy, the most important prognostic indicator is response to treatment at the haematological, cytogenetic, and molecular level. However, the risk scores based on clinical and haematological findings (the Sokal score {3716} and EUTOS score {1582}) are also valid, with low-risk patients responding to TKIs significantly better than high-risk patients {207}. Overall, the complete cytogenetic response rate to first-line TKI is 70–90%, with 5-year progression-free and overall survival rates of 80–95%. A major molecular response (*BCR-ABL1* < 0.1% on the international scale) and a deeper molecular response (*BCR-ABL1* ≤ 0.01%) are achieved faster and more frequently with second-generation TKIs, predicting that a condition of treatment-free remission will be achieved in more patients than with imatinib. However, the progression-free survival rate is only marginally improved, and overall survival is the same irrespective of the TKI used as first-line therapy. Today, few patients die from leukaemia, and the overall survival is similar to that of the non-leukaemic population {207,1602}.

Chronic neutrophilic leukaemia

Bain B.J.
Brunning R.D.
Orazi A.
Thiele J.

Definition

Chronic neutrophilic leukaemia is a rare myeloproliferative neoplasm characterized by sustained peripheral blood neutrophilia, bone marrow hypercellularity due to neutrophilic granulocyte proliferation, and hepatosplenomegaly. There is no Philadelphia (Ph) chromosome or *BCR-ABL1* fusion gene. The diagnosis requires exclusion of reactive neutrophilia and other myeloproliferative and myelodysplastic/myeloproliferative neoplasms (Table 2.02, p.38).

ICD-O code 9963/3

Epidemiology

The true incidence of chronic neutrophilic leukaemia is unknown; >200 cases have been reported, but only about 150 of these meet the current diagnostic criteria {231}. In one study of 660 cases of chronic leukaemias of myeloid origin, not a single case of chronic neutrophilic leukaemia was observed {3642}. Chronic neutrophilic leukaemia generally affects older adults, but has also been reported rarely in adolescents and young adults {1588,4441,4501}. In 116 patients whose age and sex were reported, the median age at presentation was 66 years and the male-to-female ratio was 1.6:1 {231}.

Etiology

The cause of chronic neutrophilic leukaemia is unknown. Some cases have followed cytotoxic chemotherapy {1095}. Its occurrence in a father and son has been reported {2072}. In about a quarter of reported cases of chronic neutrophilic leukaemia or an apparently similar condition, the neutrophilia was associated with an underlying neoplasm, most often multiple myeloma or monoclonal gammopathy of undetermined significance. The majority of such cases constitute a neutrophilic leukaemoid reaction resulting from synthesis of granulocyte colony-stimulating factor by neoplastic plasma cells. A very small number of patients appear to have had both a plasma cell neoplasm and true chronic neutrophilic leukaemia {391,2845}, but there is no reason to postulate a relationship between the two conditions. Acute myeloid leukaemia has supervened in 3 cases of a chronic neutrophilic leukaemia–like condition associated with a plasma cell neoplasm, but all 3 patients had been exposed to leukaemogenic drugs before the emergence of acute myeloid leukaemia {995, 2294,4079}. The association of a condition resembling chronic neutrophilic leukaemia with other neoplasms is also likely to reflect a leukaemoid reaction.

Localization

The peripheral blood and bone marrow are always involved, and the spleen and liver usually show leukaemic infiltrates. However, any tissue can be infiltrated {4035,4441,4501}.

Clinical features

The most constant clinical feature reported is splenomegaly, which may be symptomatic. Hepatomegaly is usually present as well {4441,4501}. There may be bruising and purpura. A history of bleeding from mucocutaneous surfaces or from the gastrointestinal tract is reported in 25–30% of cases {1588,4501}. Gout and pruritus are other possible features {4501}. Serum vitamin B12 and uric acid are often elevated.

Imaging

Imaging may show enlargement of the liver or spleen.

Microscopy

The peripheral blood shows neutrophilia, with a white blood cell count ≥25 × 10⁹/L. The neutrophils are usually segmented, but there may also be a substantial increase in band forms. In almost all cases, neutrophil precursors (promyelocytes, myelocytes, and metamyelocytes) account for <5% of the white blood cells, but occasionally they may account for as much as 10% {515,1094,1096A,1588, 4441,4501}. Myeloblasts are almost

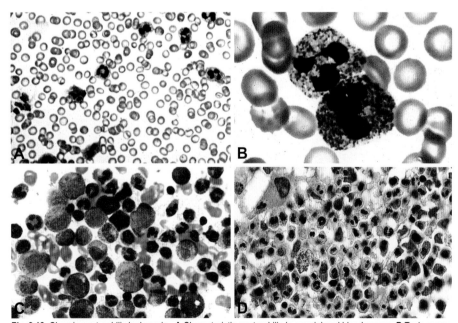

Fig. 2.12 Chronic neutrophilic leukaemia. **A** Characteristic neutrophilia in a peripheral blood smear. **B** Toxic granulation is commonly observed. **C** Bone marrow aspirate smear demonstrates neutrophil proliferation from myelocytes to segmented forms with toxic granulation, but no other significant abnormalities. **D** The bone marrow biopsy specimen is hypercellular, showing a markedly elevated myeloid-to-erythroid ratio, with increased numbers of neutrophils, in particular mature segmented forms.

never observed in the blood. The neutrophils often show toxic granulation and Döhle bodies, but they may also appear normal. However, it should be noted that toxic granulation and Döhle bodies appear to be more consistently present in plasma cell–associated leukaemoid reactions than in chronic neutrophilic leukaemia {231}. Neutrophil dysplasia is not present. Red blood cell and platelet morphology is usually normal.

Bone marrow biopsy shows hypercellularity, with neutrophilic proliferation. The myeloid-to-erythroid ratio may reach ≥20:1. Myeloblasts and promyelocytes are not increased in percentage at the time of diagnosis, but the proportion of myelocytes and mature neutrophils is increased. Erythroid and megakaryocytic proliferation may also occur {515, 4441}. Megakaryocytes may be cytologically normal or there may be increased smaller forms. Significant dysplasia is not present in any of the cell lineages; therefore, if it is found, another diagnosis, such as atypical chronic myeloid leukaemia, BCR-ABL1–negative (aCML), should be considered. Reticulin fibrosis is uncommon {515,1094,4441,4501}.

Given the frequency of neutrophilic leukaemoid reaction in association with multiple myeloma and monoclonal gammopathy of undetermined significance, the bone marrow should be examined for evidence of a plasma cell neoplasm {231,595,995,3764,3765}. If plasma cell abnormalities are present, clonality of the neutrophil lineage should be demonstrated by cytogenetic or molecular techniques before a diagnosis of chronic neutrophilic leukaemia is made.

Splenomegaly and hepatomegaly result from tissue infiltration by neutrophils. In the spleen, the infiltrate is mainly confined to the red pulp; in the liver, infiltration may affect the sinusoids, portal areas or both {4441,4501}.

Cytochemistry

The neutrophil alkaline phosphatase score is usually elevated, but is occasionally normal or even low {231}. However, because the score is also usually elevated in neutrophilic leukaemoid reactions, this is not a diagnostically useful test.

Table 2.02 Diagnostic criteria for chronic neutrophilic leukaemia

1. - Peripheral blood white blood cell count ≥ 25 × 10^9/L
   - Segmented neutrophils plus banded neutrophils constitute ≥ 80% of the white blood cells
   - Neutrophil precursors (promyelocytes, myelocytes, and metamyelocytes) constitute < 10% of the white blood cells
   - Myeloblasts rarely observed
   - Monocyte count < 1 × 10^9/L
   - No dysgranulopoiesis

2. - Hypercellular bone marrow
   - Neutrophil granulocytes increased in percentage and number
   - Neutrophil maturation appears normal
   - Myeloblasts constitute < 5% of the nucleated cells

3. Not meeting WHO criteria for BCR-ABL1–positive chronic myeloid leukaemia, polycythaemia vera, essential thrombocythaemia, or primary myelofibrosis

4. No rearrangement of PDGFRA, PDGFRB, or FGFR1, and no PCM1-JAK2 fusion

5. CSF3R T618I or another activating CSF3R mutation
   or
   Persistent neutrophilia (≥ 3 months), splenomegaly, and no identifiable cause of reactive neutrophilia including absence of a plasma cell neoplasm or, if a plasma cell neoplasm is present, demonstration of clonality of myeloid cells by cytogenetic or molecular studies

The distinction of chronic neutrophilic leukaemia from the neutrophilic variant of BCR-ABL1–positive CML should rely on molecular analysis. No other cytochemical abnormality has been reported {1588, 4501}.

Cell of origin

A haematopoietic stem cell, which may have limited lineage potential {1259,4417}

Genetic profile

Cytogenetic studies are normal in nearly 90% of cases. In the remaining cases, reported clonal karyotypic abnormalities include gains of chromosomes 8, 9, and 21; del(7q); del(20q) (the most frequently observed abnormality); del(11q); del(12p); nullisomy 17; a complex karyotype; and several non-recurrent translocations {735,846,970,1094,1259,2553, 3475,4417}. Clonal cytogenetic abnormalities may appear during the course of the disease. There is no Ph chromosome or BCR-ABL1 fusion. Cases with the neutrophilic variant of CML have a variant fusion gene and a variant BCR-ABL1 fusion protein (p230), and are classified as CML rather than chronic neutrophilic leukaemia. Chronic neutrophilic leukaemia is now known to be strongly associated with CSF3R mutation {2588,3057}, often together with mutation of SETBP1

or ASXL1 {846,1096A,2226,2588,2630}. Coexisting ASXL1 mutation is associated with a worse prognosis {1095}. CSF3R mutation was reported in 8 of 20 patients with a diagnosis of aCML in an initial study {2588}, but this high prevalence was not confirmed in subsequent investigations {3057,4248}. JAK2 V617F has been reported in at least a dozen patients {231,2591} and is sometimes homozygous {1902}; this appears to be an alternative mechanism of leukaemogenesis. Complete cytogenetic remission with imatinib was reported in a patient with chronic neutrophilic leukaemia and t(15;19)(q13;p13.3), suggesting the possibility of an unidentified fusion gene in some cases {735}.

Prognosis and predictive factors

Although generally considered a slowly progressive disorder, chronic neutrophilic leukaemia is associated with variable survival, ranging from 6 months to > 20 years. The neutrophilia is usually progressive, and anaemia and thrombocytopenia may follow. The development of myelodysplastic features may signal a transformation of the disease to acute myeloid leukaemia {1588,4501}. Transformation has been reported following cytotoxic therapy, but also in its absence.

Polycythaemia vera

Thiele J.
Kvasnicka H.M.
Orazi A.
Tefferi A.
Birgegård G.
Barbui T.

Definition

Polycythaemia vera (PV) is a chronic myeloproliferative neoplasm (MPN) characterized by increased red blood cell (RBC) production independent of the mechanisms that normally regulate erythropoiesis.

Virtually all patients carry the somatic *JAK2* V617F gain-of-function mutation or another functionally similar *JAK2* mutation that results in proliferation not only of the erythroid lineage but also of granulocytes and megakaryocytes (i.e. panmyelosis). Generally, two phases of PV are recognized: a polycythaemic phase, associated with elevated haemoglobin level, elevated haematocrit, and increased RBC mass, and a spent phase or post-polycythaemic myelofibrosis phase (post-PV myelofibrosis), in which cytopenias, including anaemia, are associated with ineffective haematopoiesis, bone marrow fibrosis, extramedullary haematopoiesis, and hypersplenism.

The natural progression of PV also includes a low incidence of evolution to a myelodysplastic/pre-leukaemic phase and/or blast phase (i.e. acute leukaemia). All causes of secondary erythrocytosis, heritable polycythaemia, and other MPNs must be excluded. The diagnosis requires integration of clinical, laboratory, and bone marrow histological features, as outlined in Table 2.03.

ICD-O code   9950/3

Synonyms

Polycythaemia rubra vera; proliferative polycythaemia (no longer recommended); chronic erythraemia (obsolete)

Epidemiology

The reported annual incidence of PV increases with advanced age and ranges from 0.01 to 2.8 cases per 100 000 population in Europe and North America; the lowest incidence rates are reported in Japan and Israel {1864,2764,4010}. Most reports indicate a slight male predominance, with a male-to-female ratio of 1–2:1 {2500,3209}. The median patient age at

Table 2.03 Diagnostic criteria for polycythaemia vera

The diagnosis of polycythaemia vera requires either all 3 major criteria or the first 2 major criteria plus the minor criterion[a].

Major criteria

1. Elevated haemoglobin concentration (> 16.5 g/dL in men; > 16.0 g/dL in women) or
   Elevated haematocrit (> 49% in men; > 48% in women) or
   Increased red blood cell mass (> 25% above mean normal predicted value)
2. Bone marrow biopsy showing age-adjusted hypercellularity with trilineage growth (panmyelosis), including prominent erythroid, granulocytic, and megakaryocytic proliferation with pleomorphic, mature megakaryocytes (differences in size)
3. Presence of *JAK2* V617F or *JAK2* exon 12 mutation

Minor criterion

Subnormal serum erythropoietin level

[a] Major criterion 2 (bone marrow biopsy) may not be required in patients with sustained absolute erythrocytosis (haemoglobin concentrations of > 18.5 g/dL in men or > 16.5 g/dL in women and haematocrit values of > 55.5% in men or > 49.5% in women), if major criterion 3 and the minor criterion are present. However, initial myelofibrosis (present in as many as 20% of patients) can only be detected by bone marrow biopsy, and this finding may predict a more rapid progression to overt myelofibrosis (post-PV myelofibrosis) {253}.

diagnosis is 60 years {2500,3209,3929}; cases in patients aged < 20 years are rarely reported {1375,3087}. The reported worldwide annual incidence of MPNs is 0.44–5.87 cases per 100 000 population, with annual rates of 0.84, 1.03, and 0.47 cases per 100 000 population for PV, essential thrombocythaemia, and primary myelofibrosis, respectively {1864}.

Etiology

The underlying cause is unknown in most cases. A genetic predisposition has been reported in some families {1411,1677,3457}. Ionizing radiation and occupational exposure to toxins have been suggested as possible causes in some cases {526,3606}.

Localization

The blood and bone marrow are the major sites of involvement, but the spleen and liver are also affected and are the major sites of extramedullary haematopoiesis in later stages. However, any organ can be damaged as a result of the vascular consequences of the increased RBC mass.

Clinical features

The major symptoms of PV are related to hypertension or vascular abnormalities caused by the increased RBC mass (i.e.

increased viscosity of blood). In nearly 20% of cases, an episode of venous or arterial thrombosis (such as deep vein thrombosis, myocardial ischaemia, or stroke) is documented in the medical history, and may be the first manifestation of PV {1103,2500,3209,3929}. Mesenteric, portal, or splenic vein thrombosis or Budd–Chiari syndrome should always lead to consideration of PV as an underlying cause, and may precede the onset of overt polycythaemic disease manifestations {1022,1362,2012,3240, 3702}. Headache, dizziness, visual disturbances, and paraesthesias are major symptoms; pruritus, erythromelalgia, and gout are also common. In PV, physical findings usually include plethora and palpable splenomegaly {2603}, and may also include hepatomegaly depending on the diagnostic criteria used {2602, 3758,3917,3929}. There is debate as to which of the three RBC variables (haemoglobin, haematocrit, or RBC mass) should be used to define the diagnostic hallmark of PV {256}. In the original 4th edition of the WHO classification, the first major diagnostic criterion for PV was haemoglobin concentration > 18.5 g/dL in men or > 16.5 g/dL in women, haemoglobin concentration > 17 g/dL in men or

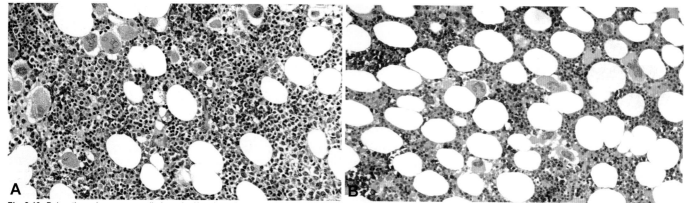

Fig. 2.13 Polycythaemia vera, so-called masked/prodromal presentation. **A** Mildly hypercellular bone marrow showing a predominance of large megakaryocytes in the bone marrow biopsy section. **B** Many large and giant hypersegmented (essential thrombocythaemia–like) megakaryocytes in a case clinically mimicking ET, because of a platelet count > 1000 × 10⁹/L). Note the only mildly increased granulo- and erythropoiesis (panmyelosis), better demonstrated by naphthol-AS-D-chloroacetate esterase (CAE) reaction.

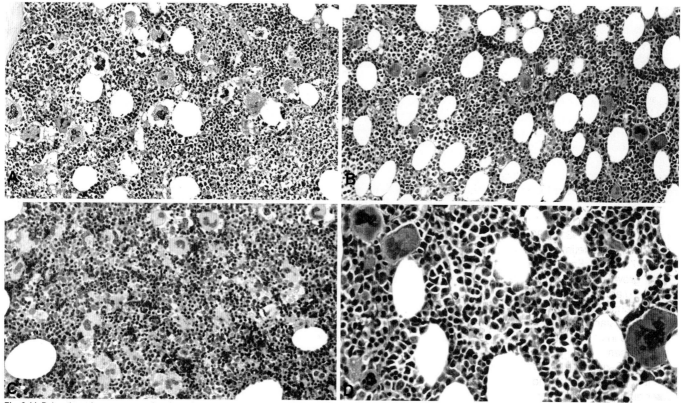

Fig. 2.14 Polycythaemia vera, overt polycythaemic presentation. **A** Bone marrow biopsy shows a characteristically hypercellular marrow characterizing the overt polycythaemic presentation (panmyelosis). **B** Megakaryocytes revealing different sizes are always a prominent feature. The cells are more easily evaluated by using the periodic acid–Schiff (PAS) staining reaction. **C** Panmyelosis (trilineage proliferation) as demonstrated by the naphthol-ASD-chloroacetate (CAE) stain which, by accurately identifying the granulocytic cells (red reaction product), helps in the assessment of the relative proportion of the two major marrow lineages (erythropoietic and granulopoietic). **D** At this disease stage, the megakaryocytes show increased pleomorphism, with significant differences in size but no relevant maturation defects such as nuclear or cytoplasmic differentiation, as shown with PAS staining.

> 15 g/dL in women associated with a sustained increase of ≥2 g/dL from baseline that cannot be attributed to correction of iron deficiency, or RBC mass > 25% above the mean normal predicted value {3931}. However, it has been argued that the application of these criteria may result in the underdiagnosis of PV due to exclusion of patients with an actual RBC mass > 25% above the mean

normal predicted value, but with haemoglobin levels and haematocrit below the cut-off points {2602,3677,3758}. For this reason, the term 'masked PV' was introduced {82,251} for *JAK2*-mutated cases in patients with latent (initial, occult prepolycythaemic) disease manifestations who have persistently elevated haemoglobin concentrations (> 16.5 g/dL in men; > 16.0 g/dL in women) or that fulfil

the diagnostic criteria for PV proposed in the 2007 British Committee for Standards in Haematology (BCSH) guidelines {248,2603}. Cut-off points were determined to be the optimal thresholds for distinguishing *JAK2*-mutated essential thrombocythaemia from PV {249,252}. Consequently, these values have been included in the revised WHO criteria {3932} (see Table 2.03, p. 39).

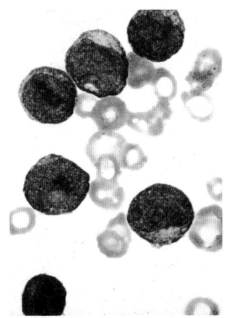

Fig. 2.15 Acute leukaemia in polycythaemia vera. Blood smear from a patient with a long-standing history of PV. The patient had been treated with alkylating agents during the polycythaemic stage. The blasts expressed CD13, CD33, CD117 and CD34, and had a complex karyotype.

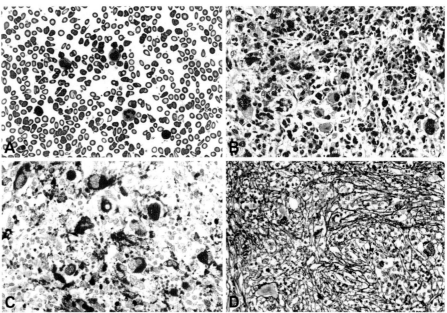

Fig. 2.16 Polycythaemia vera, post-polycythaemic myelofibrosis (post-PV MF) and myeloid metaplasia stage. **A** Peripheral blood smear demonstrates leukoerythroblastosis with numerous teardrop-shaped red blood cells (dacryocytes). **B** Bone marrow biopsy shows conspicuously abnormal megakaryocytic proliferation and depletion of the erythroid and granulocytic cells. **C** Immunostaining for CD61 illustrates the atypia in the megakaryocytic population, including a population of small immature megakaryocytes. **D** Overt reticulin fibrosis that is invariably present in post-PV MF with myeloid metaplasia.

Clinical laboratory studies that facilitate the diagnosis of PV include detection of *JAK2* V617F or functionally similar mutations (e.g. *JAK2* exon 12 mutations) {2603,3056,3929,3931,3932} and subnormal erythropoietin levels {251,2602, 2760,3677,3929}. Endogenous erythroid colony growth is no longer included as a minor diagnostic criterion, due to its limited practicality {3932}; it is time-consuming, unstandardized, restricted to specialized institutions, and costly.

Some cases (in particular cases in *JAK2* V617F–mutated patients with prominent thrombocytosis and initially low haemoglobin levels and/or haematocrit) can clinically mimic essential thrombocythaemia at onset {249}, despite showing bone marrow histopathology characteristic of PV and later increases in the RBC parameters {1364,2152,3972}. Therefore, determination of *JAK2* and *CALR* mutation status alone (without morphological examination) is not sufficient to differentiate PV from *JAK2*-mutated essential thrombocythaemia {3920}.

Microscopy

In PV, the major features in the peripheral blood and bone marrow are attributable to effective proliferation in the erythroid, granulocytic, and megakaryocytic

lineages; i.e. there is a panmyelosis.

The peripheral blood shows a mild to overt excess of normochromic, normocytic RBCs. If there is iron deficiency due to bleeding, the RBCs may be hypochromic and microcytic. Neutrophilia and rarely basophilia may be present. Occasional immature granulocytes may be detectable, but circulating blasts are generally not observed.

Bone marrow cellularity is usually increased {3975}. Hypercellularity is espe-

cially noteworthy in the subcortical marrow space, which is normally hypocellular {1329,3964}. Panmyelosis accounts for the increased haematopoietic cellularity, but increased numbers of erythroid precursors and megakaryocytes are often most prominent {1098,1329,3964,3978}. Using standardized prominent bone marrow features {3969,3973}, several groups have succeeded in identifying histological patterns that are characteristic of WHO-defined PV, including so-called

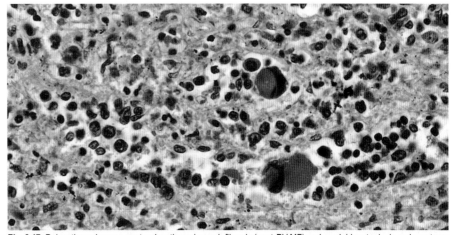

Fig. 2.17 Polycythaemia vera, post-polycythaemic myelofibrosis (post-PV MF) and myeloid metaplasia, splenectomy specimen. The splenic enlargement in the post-polycythaemic phase is due mainly to extramedullary haematopoiesis that occurs in the splenic sinuses, as well as fibrosis and entrapment of platelets and haematopoietic cells in the splenic cords.

Table 2.04 Relative incidence of discriminating features according to standardized WHO morphological criteria generating histological patterns in initially performed bone marrow biopsy specimens. Modified and adapted from Thiele J. and Kvasnicka H.M. {3969}

Bone marrow morphology features		Relative frequency of features			
		PV	ET	Pre-PMF	Overt PMF
Cellularity	Age-related increase	>80%	10–19%	>80%	10–19%
Granulopoiesis	Increased in quantity	>80%	<10%	50–80%	0%
	Left-shifted	<10%	<10%	20–49%	10–19%
Erythropoiesis	Increased in quantity	>80%	<10%	<10%	0%
	Left-shifted	>80%	<10%	10–19%	<10%
Megakaryopoiesis	Increased in quantity	50–80%	>80%	50–80%	20–49%
Size of cells	Small	20–49%	<5%	20–49%	20–49%
	Medium	20–49%	10–19%	10–19%	10–19%
	Large	20–49%	20–49%	20–49%	10–19%
	Giant	10–19%	20–49%	10–19%	<10%
Histotopography Cluster formation	Endosteal translocation	10–19%	10–19%	20–49%	20–49%
	Small clusters (>3 cells)	10–19%	10–19%	50–80%	50–80%
	Large clusters (>7 cells)	<10%	0%	20–49%	20–49%
	Dense clusters	<10%	<5%	20–49%	50–80%
	Loose clusters	20–49%	20–49%	50–80%	10–19%
Nuclear features	Hypolobulation (bulbous)	10–19%	<10%	50–80%	50–80%
	Hyperlobulation (staghorn-like)	50–80%	50–80%	<10%	0%
	Maturation defects	0%	0%	50–80%	>80%
	Naked nuclei	20–49%	20–49%	50–80%	>80%
Fibrosis	Increased reticulin	10–19%	<5%	20–49%	>80%
	Increased collagen	0%	0%	0%	50–80%
	Osteosclerosis	0%	0%	0%	20–49%
Stroma	Iron deposits	0%	20–49%	10–19%	<10%
	Lymphoid nodules	10–19%	<5%	10–19%	<10%

PV, polycythaemia vera; ET, essential thrombocythaemia; pre-PMF, prefibrotic / early primary myelofibrosis; Overt PMF, overt primary myelofibrosis

masked PV {251,1361,1364,3677,3964, 3972,3978,3983}. Erythropoiesis is usually normoblastic, erythroid precursors form large islets or sheets, and granulopoiesis is morphologically normal. The proportion of myeloblasts is not increased. Megakaryocytes are increased in number (particularly in cases with an excess of platelets) and frequently display hypersegmented nuclei. Cases with high platelet counts and low haemoglobin or haematocrit values may mimic essential thrombocythaemia at onset {1364, 2152,3972}. Megakaryocytes tend to form loose clusters or lie close to the bone trabeculae, and often show a significant degree of pleomorphism, resulting in a mixture of sizes. Most of the megakaryocytes exhibit normally folded or deeply lobed nuclei, and they usually lack significant atypia, although a minority may show bulbous nuclei and other nuclear abnormalities, particularly when associated

with a minor increase in reticulin {3964}. Marrow sinuses are dilated and often densely filled by erythrocytes. It is usually possible to distinguish PV from essential thrombocythaemia, primary myelofibrosis, and reactive erythrocytosis and thrombocytosis {1361,1380,2147,2433, 3964,3983} on the basis of the characteristic histological pattern of PV (Table 2.04) {3969}. Therefore, WHO has adopted bone marrow morphology as one of the major diagnostic criteria for PV {257,3932}. Reticulin staining reveals a normal reticulin fibre network in about 80% of cases, but the remainder may display increased reticulin and even mild to moderate collagen fibrosis {11,253, 496,1329,2105,3964,3983}, depending on the stage of disease at initial diagnosis. Even a minor increase in reticulin fibres (reticulin grade 1) {3975} at initial presentation of PV has been associated with a more rapid progression to post-PV

myelofibrosis, underscoring the value of bone marrow biopsy {11,253}. Reactive nodular lymphoid aggregates are found in as many as 20% of cases {3964,3969}. In >95% of cases, stainable iron is absent in bone marrow aspirate and biopsy specimens {1098,3978,3983}.

Spent phase and post-polycythaemic myelofibrosis (post-PV MF)
During the later phases of PV, erythropoiesis progressively decreases. As a result, the RBC mass normalizes and then decreases, and the spleen further enlarges. Persistent leukocytosis occurring at or around the time of progression to post-PV MF has been reported to be associated with an overall more aggressive course of disease {405}. These changes are usually accompanied by corresponding bone marrow alterations {407,1098, 3511,3758}. The most common pattern of disease progression is post-PV MF

Table 2.05 Diagnostic criteria for post–polycythaemia vera (PV) myelofibrosis {265}

Required criteria

1. Documentation of a previous diagnosis of WHO-defined PV

2. Bone marrow fibrosis of:
   grade 2–3 on a 0–3 scale {3975} or
   grade 3–4 on a 0–4 scale {2146}

Additional criteria (2 are required)

1. Anaemia (i.e. below the reference range given age, sex, and altitude considerations) or sustained loss of requirement of either phlebotomy (in the absence of cytoreductive therapy) or cytoreductive treatment for erythrocytosis

2. Leukoerythroblastosis

3. Increasing splenomegaly, defined as either an increase in palpable splenomegaly of > 5 cm from baseline (distance from the left costal margin) or the development of a newly palpable splenomegaly

4. Development of any 2 (or all 3) of the following constitutional symptoms: > 10% weight loss in 6 months, night sweats, unexplained fever (> 37.5 °C)

Reprinted by permission from Macmillan Publishers Ltd: Leukemia. Barosi G, Mesa RA, Thiele J, Cervantes F, Campbell PJ, Verstovsek S, et al. Proposed criteria for the diagnosis of post-polycythemia vera and post-essential thrombocythemia myelofibrosis: a consensus statement from the International Working Group for Myelofibrosis Research and Treatment. Leukemia. 2008;22:437-8. Copyright 2008.

accompanied by myeloid metaplasia, which is characterized by a leukoerythroblastic peripheral blood smear, poikilocytosis with teardrop-shaped RBCs, and splenomegaly due to extramedullary haematopoiesis, as defined in Table 2.05, p. 38 {265}. In two large series of patients with WHO-defined myelofibrosis, post-PV MF was found to account for about 20% of the cases {3920}. The morphological hallmark of this disease stage is overt reticulin {3983} and collagen fibrosis {407,1098,3511,3964} of the bone marrow. Cellularity varies in this terminal stage, but hypocellular specimens are common. Clusters of megakaryocytes, often with hyperchromatic and very dysmorphic nuclei, are prominent; however, cases retaining PV-like features have also been described {407}. Erythropoiesis and granulopoiesis are decreased in quantity; RBCs, granulocytes, and megakaryocytes are sometimes found lying within dilated marrow sinusoids {3511, 3964}. Bone marrow fibrosis is usually of grade 2–3 on a 0–3 scale {2148,3975} or grade 3–4 on a 0–4 scale {2146}. Osteosclerosis may occur {1098,3511}. There is disagreement about the degree to which advanced post-PV MF resembles overt primary myelofibrosis in terms of clinical and morphological features {407,3511}. The splenic enlargement is a consequence of extramedullary haematopoiesis, which is characterized by the presence of erythroid, granulocytic, and megakaryocytic elements in the splenic sinuses and cords of Billroth. An increase

in the number of immature cells may be observed in these stages, but the finding of ≥ 10% blasts in the peripheral blood or bone marrow or the presence of substantial myelodysplasia is unusual, and most likely indicates transformation to an accelerated phase. Cases with ≥ 20% blasts are considered to be blast-phase post-PV MF, formerly called acute leukaemia {3089,3758,3964}.

Cell of origin
The postulated cell of origin is a haematopoietic stem cell.

Genetic profile
The most common genetic abnormality in PV is the somatic gain-of-function mutation JAK2 V617F {2099}. Although this mutation occurs in > 95% of patients with PV {3915,3929}, it is not specific for this entity; it is found in other MPNs {3915, 3920} and is also seen in a small subset (< 5%) of cases of acute myeloid leukaemia, myelodysplastic syndromes, chronic myelomonocytic leukaemia, and other myeloid malignancies {3775}. Rare cases of JAK2-mutant PV acquire a BCR-ABL1 rearrangement; however, the clinical significance of this is uncertain. Due to this additional phenotypic mutation, a morphological and haematological shift capable of producing a chronic myeloid leukaemia–like evolution may occur {1740, 3190}. Functionally similar mutations in exon 12 of JAK2 are found in about 3% of cases, which generally show a predominant erythroid haematopoiesis {2194,

3056,3604}. Mutations similar to those described in MPNs {3915} have also been found at very low frequencies in elderly patients with no haematological malignancy {1326,1830,4386}. At diagnosis, cytogenetic abnormalities are detectable in as many as 20% of cases {3920}. The most common recurrent abnormalities are gain of chromosome 8 or 9, del(20q), del(13q), and del(9p); gains of chromosomes 8 and 9 are sometimes found together {102,4307}. There is no Philadelphia (Ph) chromosome or BCR-ABL1 fusion. The frequency of chromosomal abnormalities increases with disease progression; they are seen in nearly 80–90% of cases of post-PV myelofibrosis {102}. Cases that progress to the accelerated phase or blast phase often have cytogenetic abnormalities, including those commonly observed in therapy-related myelodysplastic syndrome and acute myeloid leukaemia (see *Acute myeloid leukaemia and related precursor neoplasms*, p. 129).

Genetic susceptibility
A genetic predisposition has been reported in some families {1411,1677,3457}.

Prognosis and predictive factors
With currently available treatment, median survival times > 10 years are commonly reported {2150,3090,3209,3758}. Recent studies using WHO criteria have found median survivals of > 13 years overall and about 24 years in patients aged < 60 years {3920,3929}. Prognostic factors other than older age remain controversial {2150,2500,3090}. It has been shown that survival is adversely affected by leukocytosis and abnormal karyotype {405,3929}. Most patients die from thrombotic complications or second malignancies, but as many as 20% succumb to myelodysplastic syndrome or blast phase / acute myeloid leukaemia {2500,3209, 3758}. In large series of cases defined per the WHO criteria, 3–7% of cases were found to be in the blast phase {3920}. The factors that predict the risk of thrombosis or haemorrhage are not well defined, but age and previous thrombosis have been shown to indicate a higher thrombotic risk {247,2500,2501,3087,3758}. The incidence of myelodysplastic syndrome and the blast phase is only 2–3% in patients who have not been treated with cytotoxic agents, but increases to ≥ 10% following certain types of chemotherapy {1216,2500,3087,3089,3758,3929}.

Primary myelofibrosis

Thiele J.
Kvasnicka H.M.
Orazi A.
Gianelli U.

Barbui T.
Barosi G.
Tefferi A.

Definition

Primary myelofibrosis (PMF) is a clonal myeloproliferative neoplasm (MPN) characterized by a proliferation of predominantly abnormal megakaryocytes and granulocytes in the bone marrow, which in fully developed disease is associated with reactive deposition of fibrous connective tissue and with extramedullary haematopoiesis.

There is a stepwise evolution from an initial prefibrotic/early stage, characterized by hypercellular bone marrow with absent or minimal reticulin fibrosis, to an overt fibrotic stage with marked reticulin or collagen fibrosis in the bone marrow, and often osteosclerosis. The fibrotic stage of PMF is clinically characterized by leukoerythroblastosis in the blood (with teardrop-shaped red blood cells), hepatomegaly, and splenomegaly. The diagnostic criteria for prefibrotic/early PMF (pre-PMF) are summarized in Table 2.06 and those of overt (classic) PMF in Table 2.07.

ICD-O codes

Primary myelofibrosis	9961/3
Primary myelofibrosis, prefibrotic/early stage	9961/3
Primary myelofibrosis, overt fibrotic stage	9961/3

Synonyms

Chronic idiopathic myelofibrosis; myelofibrosis/sclerosis with myeloid metaplasia; agnogenic myeloid metaplasia; megakaryocytic myelosclerosis; idiopathic myelofibrosis; myelofibrosis with myeloid metaplasia; myelofibrosis as a result of myeloproliferative disease

Epidemiology

The estimated annual incidence of overt PMF is 0.5–1.5 cases per 100 000 population {2613,2764,3916,4010}. Valid data on the incidence of pre-PMF are not available, but data from reference centres suggest that the prefibrotic/early stage accounts for 30–50% of all PMF cases. There are few reliable estimates of prevalence {2764,4010}. The preva-

lence of PMF is probably increasing, due to earlier diagnosis (i.e. of pre-PMF) and prolonged survival {615}. PMF affects men and women nearly equally {3916}. It occurs most commonly in the sixth to seventh decades of life, and only about 10% of overt PMF cases are diagnosed in patients aged < 40 years {614}. Children are rarely affected {81,614}.

Etiology

Exposure to benzene or ionizing radiation has been documented in some cases {998}. Rare familial cases of bone marrow fibrosis in young children have been reported; how many of these constitute MPNs is unknown, but at least some cases appear to constitute an autosomal recessive inherited condition {3457}. In other families, with a somewhat older patient age at onset, the features have been consistent with an MPN, suggesting a

familial predisposition to PMF {617,3418}.

Localization

The blood and bone marrow are always involved. In the later stages of the disease, extramedullary haematopoiesis (also known as myeloid metaplasia) becomes prominent, particularly in the spleen {267}, which harbours neoplastic stem cells {4255}. In the initial stages, the number of randomly distributed CD34+ progenitors is slightly increased in the bone marrow, but not in the peripheral blood. The frequency of bone marrow CD34+ cells is inversely related to the number of circulating CD34+ cells {2864, 3971}; only in the later stages do they appear in large numbers in the peripheral blood. This increase in the number of circulating CD34+ cells is a phenomenon largely restricted to overt PMF; it is not seen in non-fibrotic polycythaemia vera

Table 2.06 Diagnostic criteria for primary myelofibrosis, prefibrotic/early stage

The diagnosis of prefibrotic/early primary myelofibrosis requires that all 3 major criteria and at least 1 minor criterion are met.

Major criteria

1. Megakaryocytic proliferation and atypia, without reticulin fibrosis grade > 1[a], accompanied by increased age-adjusted bone marrow cellularity, granulocytic proliferation, and (often) decreased erythropoiesis
2. WHO criteria for BCR-ABL1–positive chronic myeloid leukaemia, polycythaemia vera, essential thrombocythaemia, myelodysplastic syndromes, or other myeloid neoplasms are not met
3. JAK2, CALR, or MPL mutation

   or

   Presence of another clonal marker[b]

   or

   Absence of minor reactive bone marrow reticulin fibrosis[c]

Minor criteria

Presence of at least one of the following, confirmed in 2 consecutive determinations:
- Anaemia not attributed to a comorbid condition
- Leukocytosis $\geq 11 \times 10^9$/L
- Palpable splenomegaly
- Lactate dehydrogenase level above the upper limit of the institutional reference range

[a] See Table 2.09 (p. 47).
[b] In the absence of any of the 3 major clonal mutations, a search for other mutations associated with myeloid neoplasms (e.g. ASXL1, EZH2, TET2, IDH1, IDH2, SRSF2, and SF3B1 mutations) may be of help in determining the clonal nature of the disease.
[c] Minor (grade 1) reticulin fibrosis secondary to infection, autoimmune disorder or other chronic inflammatory conditions, hairy cell leukaemia or another lymphoid neoplasm, metastatic malignancy, or toxic (chronic) myelopathies.

or essential thrombocythaemia {101,268, 3091}. It has been postulated that extramedullary haematopoiesis is a consequence of the unique ability of the spleen to sequester the numerous circulating CD34+ cells {3970,4255}. Other possible sites of extramedullary haematopoiesis are the liver, lymph nodes, kidneys, adrenal glands, dura mater, gastrointestinal tract, lungs and pleura, breasts, skin, and soft tissue {3916}.

Clinical features

As many as 30% of cases are asymptomatic at the time of diagnosis and are discovered by detection of splenomegaly during a routine physical examination or when a routine blood count reveals anaemia, leukocytosis, and/or thrombocytosis. Less commonly, the diagnosis results from discovery of unexplained leukoerythroblastosis or an increased lactate dehydrogenase level {613,3916,3931}. In the initial prefibrotic stage of PMF, the only finding may be marked thrombocytosis mimicking essential thrombocythaemia, because the other clinical features may be either within the normal range or only borderline abnormal {254,266,3931, 3962,3966,3977}. Therefore, neither sustained thrombocytosis nor positive mutation status alone can distinguish prefibrotic PMF from essential thrombocythaemia; careful analysis of bone marrow morphology is necessary (see Table 2.04, p. 42, and Table 2.08, p. 47) {254,257,263,1366, 1380,3933,3965}.

More than 50% of patients with PMF experience constitutional symptoms, including fatigue, dyspnoea, weight loss, night sweats, low-grade fever, and cachexia {2643}. These symptoms, which reflect the biological activity of the disease, compromise quality of life and are associated with prognosis {616}. Gouty arthritis and renal stones due to hyperuricaemia can also occur. Splenomegaly of various degrees is detected in as many as 90% of patients, and can be massive. Nearly 50% of patients have hepatomegaly, depending on the stage of disease {264,613,614,3916}.

In WHO-defined PMF, *JAK2* V617F mutation is found in 50–60% of early-stage cases {254} (as well as in advanced stages); *CALR* mutations are found in about 24% of PMF cases and *MPL* mutations in 8%. About 12% of cases are triple-negative for mutations in *JAK2*, *CALR*, and MPL {3920,3932,3933}.

Although these mutations are helpful in distinguishing PMF from reactive conditions that can result in bone marrow fibrosis, they are not specific for PMF; mutations in these genes can also be found in essential thrombocythaemia, and *JAK2* V617F can be found in polycythaemia vera {3920}.

Microscopy

The classic picture of overt (advanced) PMF includes a peripheral blood smear that shows leukoerythroblastosis and anisopoikilocytosis (typically with teardrop-shaped red blood cells) associated with a hypocellular bone marrow with marked reticulin and/or collagen fibrosis and organomegaly caused by extramedullary

Table 2.07 Diagnostic criteria for primary myelofibrosis, overt fibrotic stage

The diagnosis of overt primary myelofibrosis requires that all 3 major criteria and at least 1 minor criterion are met.

Major criteria

1. Megakaryocytic proliferation and atypia, accompanied by reticulin and/or collagen fibrosis grades 2 or 3[a]
2. WHO criteria for essential thrombocythaemia, polycythaemia vera, *BCR-ABL1*–positive chronic myeloid leukaemia, myelodysplastic syndrome, or other myeloid neoplasms[b] are not met
3. *JAK2, CALR, or MPL* mutation

   or

   Presence of another clonal marker[c]

   or

   Absence of reactive myelofibrosis[d]

Minor criteria

Presence of at least one of the following, confirmed in 2 consecutive determinations:
- Anaemia not attributed to a comorbid condition
- Leukocytosis ≥ 11 × 10⁹/L
- Palpable splenomegaly
- Lactate dehydrogenase level above the upper limit of the institutional reference range
- Leukoerythroblastosis

[a] See Table 2.09 (p. 47).
[b] Myeloproliferative neoplasms can be associated with monocytosis or they can develop it during the course of the disease; these cases may mimic chronic myelomonocytic leukaemia (CMML); in these rare instances, a history of MPN excludes CMML, whereas the presence of MPN features in the bone marrow and/or MPN-associated mutations (in *JAK2, CALR,* or *MPL*) tend to support the diagnosis of MPN with monocytosis rather than CMML.
[c] In the absence of any of the 3 major clonal mutations, a search for other mutations associated with myeloid neoplasms (e.g. *ASXL1, EZH2, TET2, IDH1, IDH2, SRSF2,* and *SF3B1* mutations) may be of help in determining the clonal nature of the disease.
[d] Bone marrow fibrosis secondary to infection, autoimmune disorder or another chronic inflammatory condition, hairy cell leukaemia or another lymphoid neoplasm, metastatic malignancy, or toxic (chronic) myelopathy.

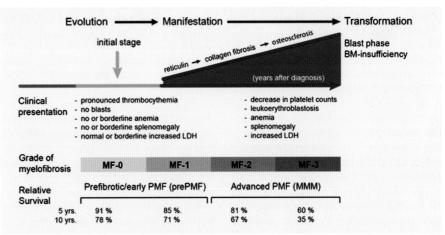

Fig. 2.18 Primary myelofibrosis (PMF). Dynamics of the disease process, with haematological presentation and associated bone marrow fibrosis (MF) grading and relative survival rates.
BM, bone marrow; LDH, lactate dehydrogenase; MMM, myelofibrosis with myeloid metaplasia.

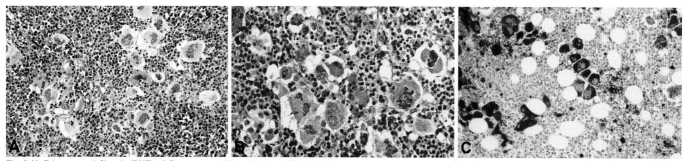

Fig. 2.19 Primary myelofibrosis (PMF). **A** Bone marrow biopsy in this prefibrotic/early-stage case shows megakaryocytic and granulocytic proliferation. Naphthol AS-D chloro-acetate esterase (CAE) staining identifies the granulocytic component (red reaction product); megakaryocytes show extensive clustering and condensed nuclei with conspicu-ously clumped chromatin and abnormal nuclear:cytoplasmic ratios (N:C). **B** Megakaryocytic abnormalities are the key finding in diagnosing PMF and in its distinction from other myeloproliferative and reactive disorders; in this prefibrotic/early-stage case, note the abnormalities of megakaryopoiesis, including anisocytosis, abnormal N:C ratios, abnormal chromatin clumping with hyperchromatic nuclei, plump lobation of some nuclei (cloud-like nuclei), and clustering. **C** Immunohistochemistry for CD61 highlights abnormal mega-karyocytes, including small forms.

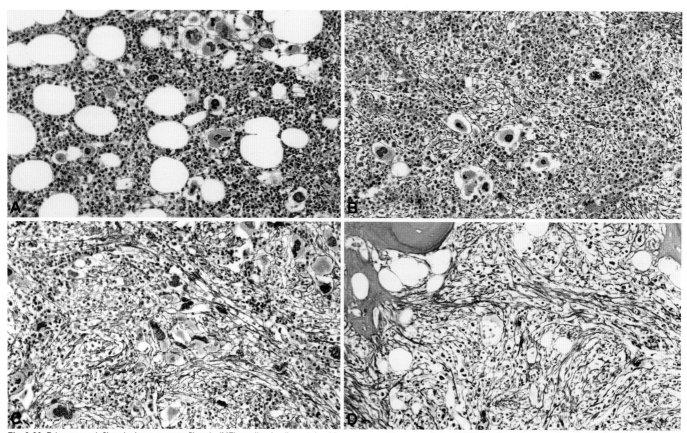

Fig. 2.20 Primary myelofibrosis: bone marrow fibrosis (MF) grading in silver-stained bone marrow biopsy sections. **A** MF-0, with no increase in reticulin. **B** MF-1, with a very loose network of reticulin fibres. **C** MF-2, showing a more diffuse and dense increase in reticulin fibres and some coarse collagen fibres. **D** MF-3, with coarse bundles of collagen fibres intermingled with dense reticulin, accompanied by initial osteosclerosis.

haematopoiesis. However, the morpholog-ical and clinical findings can vary signifi-cantly at diagnosis, depending on whether the case is first encountered during the prefibrotic/early stage or the overt fibrotic stage {254,264,266,613,3931,3977}. Be-cause the progressive accumulation of fibrous tissue (including reticulin and col-lagen) and the development of osteoscle-rosis parallel disease progression {3967}, reproducible, sequential grading of bone

marrow fibrosis is important. A simplified, semiquantitative grading system (recently slightly modified), is presented in Ta-ble 2.09 {2148,3975}. For cases present-ing with higher fibre grades (2 and 3), and particularly for clinical studies, an addition-al trichrome stain is recommended, to es-tablish the grade of collagen (Table 2.10) {2148}. In this context, a corresponding grading system for osteosclerosis may also be useful (Table 2.11) {2148}.

Prefibrotic/early primary myelofibrosis

No registry-based prevalence or inci-dence data are available for this prodro-mal stage of PMF, but series from refer-ence centres show that 30–50% of PMF cases are first detected in the prefibrotic/early stage {263,496,3963,3965}, with no significant increase in reticulin and/or col-lagen fibres (i.e. fibrosis grades 0 and 1) {2148,3975}. In these cases, the bone marrow biopsy usually shows hypercellularity, with an increase in the number of neutrophils and atypical megakaryocytes. There may be a minor left shift in granulopoiesis, but metamyelocytes, bands, and segmented neutrophils usually predominate. Myeloblasts are not increased in percentage, and conspicuous clusters of blasts are not observed; however, the number of randomly distributed CD34+ progenitors is slightly increased {3965,3971}. In most cases, erythropoiesis is reduced but the erythrocytes show no dysplastic features {3963,3965}. The megakaryocytes are markedly abnormal, and their morphological atypia and topographical distribution within the bone marrow are critical for the recognition of pre-PMF. The megakaryocytes often form dense clusters, which are frequently adjacent to the bone marrow vascular sinuses and bone trabeculae {496,2147,2152, 3965,3969,3978}. Most megakaryocytes are enlarged, but small megakaryocytes may also be seen; their detection is facilitated by immunohistochemistry with antibodies reactive with megakaryocytic antigens {3962,3965}. Deviations from the normal N:C ratio (an indication of defective maturation), abnormal patterns of chromatin clumping (including hyperchromatic forms and bulbous, cloud-like, or balloon-shaped nuclei), and the frequent occurrence of bare (naked) megakaryocytic nuclei are typical findings. Overall, in pre-PMF, the megakaryocytes are more atypical than in any other type of MPN (Table 2.04, p. 42, and Table 2.08). Vascular proliferation is only mildly increased in the bone marrow, with no gross abnormalities of vessel shape {2149}. Lymphoid nodules are found in as many as 20% of cases {3962,3965}.

Careful morphological examination of the bone marrow is particularly crucial for distinguishing pre-PMF with accompanying thrombocytosis from essential thrombocythaemia, as has been demonstrated by a number of groups {254,1227,1361, 1366,1379,1380,2105,2147,2433,3962, 3966,3977}. No single morphological feature is pathognomonic of a specific subtype, but the identification of characteristic morphological patterns is key for the differential diagnosis between pre-PMF and essential thrombocythaemia (Table 2.04, p. 42, and Table 2.08). Most cases of pre-PMF eventually transform into overt fibrotic/sclerotic myelofibrosis associated with extramedullary haematopoiesis {494,2105,2152,3965,3980}.

Table 2.08 Morphological features helpful in distinguishing essential thrombocythaemia (ET) from prefibrotic/early primary myelofibrosis (pre-PMF)[a]

Morphological feature	ET	Pre-PMF
Cellularity (age-adjusted)	Normal	Increased
Myeloid-to-erythroid ratio	Normal	Increased
Dense megakaryocyte clusters	Rare	Frequent
Megakaryocyte size	Large/giant	Variable
Megakaryocyte nuclear lobulation	Hyperlobulated	Bulbous/hypolobulated
Reticulin fibrosis, grade 1[b]	Very rare	More frequent

[a] On the basis of a representative, artifact-free bone marrow biopsy (> 1.5 cm) taken at a right angle (90°) from the cortical bone.
[b] According to WHO grading {3975}: see Table 2.09.

Table 2.09 Semiquantitative bone marrow fibrosis (MF) grading system proposed by Thiele J et al. {3975}, with minor modifications concerning collagen and osteosclerosis[a]

Grade	Definition
MF-0	Scattered linear reticulin with no intersections (cross-overs), corresponding to normal bone marrow
MF-1	Loose network of reticulin with many intersections, especially in perivascular areas
MF-2	Diffuse and dense increase in reticulin with extensive intersections, occasionally with focal bundles of thick fibres mostly consistent with collagen and/or associated with focal osteosclerosis[b]
MF-3	Diffuse and dense increase in reticulin with extensive intersections and coarse bundles of thick fibres consistent with collagen, usually associated with osteosclerosis[b]

[a] Fibre density should be assessed only in haematopoietic areas; if the pattern is heterogeneous, the final grade is determined by the highest grade present in ≥ 30% of the marrow area.
[b] In grades MF-2 and MF-3, an additional trichrome stain is recommended (Table 2.10).

Table 2.10 Semiquantitative grading of collagen[a]

Grade	Definition
0	Perivascular collagen only (normal)
1	Focal paratrabecular or central collagen deposition with no connecting meshwork
2	Paratrabecular or central deposition of collagen with focally connecting meshwork or generalized paratrabecular apposition of collagen
3	Diffuse (complete) connecting meshwork of collagen in > 30% of marrow spaces

[a] If the pattern is heterogeneous, the final grade is determined by the highest grade present in ≥ 30% of the marrow area.

Table 2.11 Semiquantitative grading of osteosclerosis[a,b]

Grade	Definition
0	Regular bone trabeculae (distinct paratrabecular borders)
1	Focal budding, hooks, spikes, or paratrabecular apposition of new bone
2	Diffuse paratrabecular formation of new bone with thickening of trabeculae, occasionally with focal interconnections
3	Extensive interconnecting meshwork of new bone with overall effacement of marrow spaces

[a] If the pattern is heterogeneous, the final grade is determined by the highest grade present in ≥ 30% of the marrow area.
[b] Bone marrow core biopsy of sufficient length, taken at a right angle (90°) from the cortical bone, without fragmentation, is mandatory for the grading of osteosclerosis.

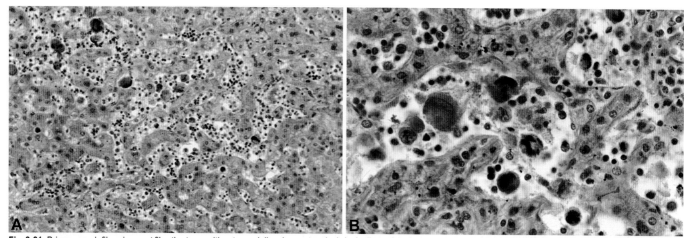

Fig. 2.21 Primary myelofibrosis, overt fibrotic stage, with extramedullary haematopoiesis in the liver. **A** In the liver, the sinusoids are prominently involved by trilineage proliferation. **B** Abnormal megakaryocytes are the hallmark of abnormal intrasinusoidal haematopoiesis.

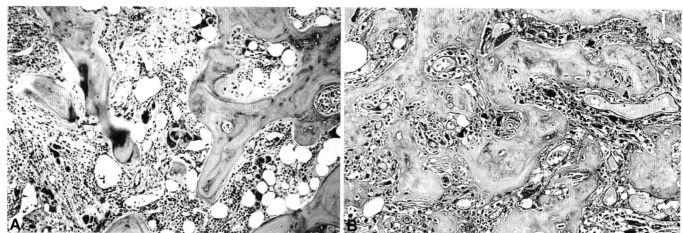

Fig. 2.22 Primary myelofibrosis (PMF), overt fibrotic stage. **A** Bone marrow biopsy specimen showing hypocellularity, markedly dilated sinuses, and severe marrow fibrosis with osteosclerosis, findings typical of advanced-stage PMF. **B** PMF with osteomyelosclerosis characterized by broad, irregular bone trabeculae, which can occupy as much as 50% of the marrow space; fibrosis, cellular depletion, sinusoidal dilatation, and megakaryocytic proliferation are prominent in the intertrabecular areas.

Overt primary myelofibrosis

Most cases of PMF are initially diagnosed in the overt fibrotic stage {264,613,3916}. In this stage, the bone marrow biopsy shows clear-cut reticulin or collagen fibrosis (i.e. fibrosis grades 2 and 3) {2148, 3975}, often associated with various degrees of collagen fibrosis and osteosclerosis (see Table 2.10 and Table 2.11, p. 47). The bone marrow may still be focally hypercellular, but is more often normocellular or hypocellular, with patches of active haematopoiesis alternating with hypocellular regions of loose connective tissue and/or fat. Foci of immature cells may be more prominent, although myeloblasts account for < 10% of the bone marrow cells {3965}. Atypical megakaryocytes are often the most conspicuous finding; they occur in large clusters or sheets, often within dilated vascular sinuses {494,3965}. In some cases, the bone marrow is almost devoid of hae-

matopoietic cells, showing mainly dense reticulin or collagen fibrosis, with small islands of haematopoietic precursors situated mostly within the vascular sinuses. Associated with the development of myelofibrosis is a significant proliferation of vessels showing marked tortuosity and luminal distension, often also associated with conspicuous intrasinusoidal haematopoiesis {438,2149,2642,2863}. Osteoid seams or appositional new bone formation in bud-like endophytic plaques may be observed {3965}. In this osteosclerotic phase, the bone may form broad, irregular trabeculae that can occupy > 50% of the bone marrow space.

The development of overt fibrosis in PMF is related to disease progression {494, 3979,3980}, and is not significantly influenced by standard cytoreductive treatment modalities (with the exception of allogeneic stem cell transplantation {2125,2864,3974}). However, it has been

reported that interferon {744,3204} and *JAK1/JAK2* inhibitor {1563A,1798,1800, 1833,2543A,4316} therapy may delay or even reverse bone marrow fibrosis progression across all aspects of the fibrotic process (i.e. reticulin fibrosis, collagen deposition, and osteosclerosis).

The development of monocytosis in PMF may indicate disease progression {404}. In patients with a previously established diagnosis of PMF, the finding of 10–19% blasts in the peripheral blood and/or bone marrow and the detection by immunohistochemistry of an increased number of CD34+ cells with cluster formation and/or an abnormal endosteal location in the bone marrow {3965,3971} indicate an accelerated phase of the disease, whereas the finding of ≥20% blasts is diagnostic of blast transformation. Patients with PMF may rarely present initially in the accelerated phase or blast phase.

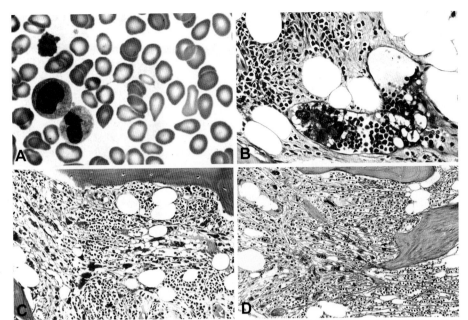

Fig. 2.23 Primary myelofibrosis (PMF), overt fibrotic stage. **A** Peripheral blood smear showing dacryocytes, occasional nucleated red blood cells, and immature granulocytes (leukoerythroblastosis). **B** Dilated sinus containing immature haematopoietic elements, most notably megakaryocytes, as demonstrated by periodic acid–Schiff (PAS) staining. This intrasinusoidal haematopoiesis together with vascular proliferation is characteristic (but not diagnostic) of PMF with myeloid metaplasia. **C** Megakaryocytes are often the most conspicuous haematopoietic element in the marrow; the cells often appear to stream through the marrow, due to the underlying fibrosis. **D** Silver staining highlights the marked reticulin and collagen fibrosis associated with a stream-like arrangement of megakaryocytes and initial osteosclerosis.

Extramedullary haematopoiesis
The most common site of extramedullary haematopoiesis is the spleen, followed by the liver. The spleen shows an expansion of the red pulp by erythroid, granulocytic, and megakaryocytic cells {3232}. The identification of these cells can be facilitated by immunohistochemistry {2918,3959}, which also facilitates the identification of neoangiogenesis {267}. Megakaryocytes are often the most conspicuous component of the extramedullary haematopoiesis. Occasionally, large aggregates of megakaryocytes growing cohesively can produce macroscopically evident tumoural lesions. In the presence of nodular lesions and in any advanced-stage disease with large amounts of extramedullary haematopoiesis in general, the possibility of a myeloid sarcoma should be considered and carefully excluded through immunohistochemical studies with CD34 and KIT (CD117) {3970,4255}. The red pulp cords may exhibit fibrosis and pooling of platelets. Hepatic sinuses also show prominent extramedullary haematopoiesis, and cirrhosis of the liver may occur {3916}.

Cell of origin
The postulated cell of origin is a haematopoietic stem cell.

Genetic profile
No genetic defect specific for PMF has been identified. Approximately 50–60% of WHO-defined PMF cases carry JAK2 V617F or a functionally similar mutation, about 30% of cases have a mutation in CALR and 8% in MPL, and about 12% of cases are triple-negative for these mutations {3915,3920,3933}. A subset of triple-negative cases have been found to have gain-of-function mutations (e.g. MPL S204P and MPL Y591N) through whole-exome sequencing or other sensitive molecular techniques {2666}. This finding is consistent with the assumption that JAK2/CALR/MPL-wild-type PMF is not a homogeneous entity and that cases with polyclonal haematopoiesis probably constitute a hereditary disorder {2666}. Although the presence of the JAK2 mutation confirms the clonality of the proliferation, the mutation is also found in polycythaemia vera and essential thrombocythaemia, and therefore does not distinguish PMF from these MPNs {3920,3933}. CALR mutation has been reported to have a favourable im-

pact on survival {3920,3924,3934}, in contrast to the negative prognostic value of the triple-negative mutation status (i.e. JAK2, CALR, and MPL wild-type) {3920, 3924} and other, less frequent mutations {1486,3921,4149}. Mutations similar to those described in MPNs {3915} have also been found at very low frequencies in elderly patients with no haematological malignancy {1326,1830,4386}. Very rarely, cases of PMF acquire a BCR-ABL1 rearrangement; however, the clinical significance of this is uncertain. Due to this additional phenotypic mutation, a morphological and haematological shift capable of producing a chronic myeloid leukaemia–like evolution may occur {1740}. Cytogenetic abnormalities occur in as many as 30% of cases {3920}. There is no Philadelphia (Ph) chromosome or BCR-ABL1 fusion gene. The presence of either del(13)(q12-22) or der(6)t(1;6)(q21-23;p21.3) is strongly suggestive (but not diagnostic) of PMF {996}. The most common recurrent abnormalities are del(20q) and partial trisomy 1q; gains of chromosomes 9 and/or 8 have also been reported {3336,3926}. Deletions affecting the long arms of chromosomes 7 and 5 occur as well, but may be associated with prior cytotoxic therapy used to treat the myeloproliferative process.

Prognosis and predictive factors
The time of survival with PMF ranges from months to decades. Overall prognosis depends on the stage at which the neoplasm is initially diagnosed {2150, 3965} and the corresponding risk status, which can be determined using several prognostic scoring systems {616,1290, 3086,3923}. The median overall survival time for patients diagnosed in the overt fibrotic stage (myelofibrosis with myeloid metaplasia) is approximately 3–7 years {264,613,3914}, whereas diagnosis in the prefibrotic/early stage is associated with 10-year and 15-year relative survival rates of 72% and 59%, respectively {254, 2150,3965,3967,4173}. The widely used refined Dynamic International Prognostic Scoring System (DIPSS Plus) includes eight predictors of inferior survival: patient age >65 years, haemoglobin concentration <10 g/dL, leukocytes >25 × 10⁹/L, circulating blasts ≥1%, constitutional symptoms, red blood cell transfusion dependency, platelet count <100 × 10⁹/L, and unfavourable karyotype (i.e. a complex karyotype or 1–2 of the following

abnormalities: gain of chromosome 8, loss of chromosome 7/7q, isochromosome 17q, inv(3q), loss of 5q or 12p, or 11q23.3 rearrangement). Risk status is defined by the number of adverse prognostic factors present: 0 (low risk), 1 (intermediate-1 risk), 2 or 3 (intermediate-2 risk), or ≥4 (high risk), with respective median survival times of approximately 15.4, 6.5, 2.9, and 1.3 years {1290, 3916}. High-risk disease is also defined by a *CALR*-negative and *ASXL1*-positive mutation status {1486,3920,3921,3924}.

In the context of these risk models, the prognostic value of bone marrow fibrosis reflecting the stage of disease (pre-PMF vs overt PMF) is emphasized {2150, 3923,3967,4173}. The findings of a study investigating the relationship between DIPSS score {3086} and marrow fibrosis grading {3975} in patients with PMF suggested that better prognostication could be achieved by considering morphological parameters in addition to clinical and mutation data {1365}. Major causes of morbidity and mortality are bone marrow

failure (infection, haemorrhage), thromboembolic events, portal hypertension, cardiac failure, and blast-phase disease (i.e. secondary acute myeloid leukaemia). The reported frequency of the blast phase is 5–30% {264,613,3914,3916, 3920}. Although some blast-phase cases are related to prior cytotoxic therapy, many have been reported in patients who have never been treated, confirming that blast transformation is part of the natural history of PMF.

Essential thrombocythaemia

Thiele J.
Kvasnicka H.M.
Orazi A.
Gianelli U.

Tefferi A.
Gisslinger H.
Barbui T.

Definition

Essential thrombocythaemia (ET) is a chronic myeloproliferative neoplasm (MPN) that primarily involves the megakaryocytic lineage. It is characterized by sustained thrombocytosis (platelet count ≥450 × 10⁹/L) in the peripheral blood and increased numbers of large, mature megakaryocytes in the bone marrow and clinically by the occurrence of thrombosis and/or haemorrhage. Because there is no known genetic or biological marker specific for ET, other causes of thrombocytosis must be excluded, including other MPNs, inflammatory and infectious disorders, haemorrhage, and other types of haematopoietic and non-haematopoietic neoplasms. The presence of *BCR-ABL1* gene fusion excludes the diagnosis of ET. The diagnostic criteria for ET are listed in Table 2.12.

ICD-O code   9962/3

Synonyms

Idiopathic thrombocythaemia/ thrombocytosis; essential haemorrhagic thrombocythaemia; idiopathic haemorrhagic thrombocythaemia; idiopathic thrombocythaemia

Table 2.12 Diagnostic criteria for essential thrombocythaemia

The diagnosis of essential thrombocythaemia requires that either all major criteria or the first 3 major criteria plus the minor criterion are met.

Major criteria

1. Platelet count ≥450 × 10⁹/L

2. Bone marrow biopsy showing proliferation mainly of the megakaryocytic lineage, with increased numbers of enlarged, mature megakaryocytes with hyperlobulated nuclei; no significant increase or left shift in neutrophil granulopoiesis or erythropoiesis; very rarely a minor (grade 1ᵃ) increase in reticulin fibres

3. WHO criteria for *BCR-ABL1*–positive chronic myeloid leukaemia, polycythaemia vera, primary myelofibrosis, or other myeloid neoplasms are not met

4. *JAK2*, *CALR*, or *MPL* mutation

Minor criterion

Presence of a clonal marker or
Absence of evidence of reactive thrombocytosis

ᵃ See Table 2.09 (p. 47).

Epidemiology

The true overall incidence of ET is unknown, but the annual incidence in Europe and the USA of cases diagnosed per the guidelines of the Polycythemia Vera Study Group (PVSG) {2791} is estimated to be 0.2–2.3 cases per 100 000 population {2613,2764,4010}. Most cases occur in patients aged 50–60 years, and a slight female predilection was found in a series of strictly WHO-defined cas-

es {254,3933,3977}. There is a second peak in incidence among patients (in particular women) aged about 30 years {1217,1563}. ET also occurs (infrequently) in children, in whom it must be distinguished from rare cases of hereditary thrombocytosis {1375,3302}.

Etiology

In most patients, the etiology of ET is unknown. However, germline mutations in

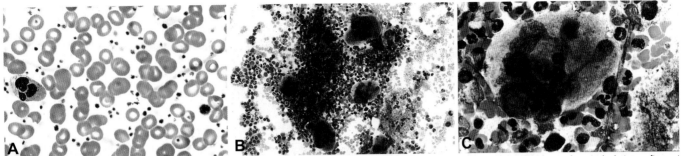

Fig. 2.24 Essential thrombocythaemia. **A** Peripheral blood smear. The major abnormality seen is marked thrombocytosis; the platelets show anisocytosis, but are often not remarkably atypical. **B** Bone marrow aspirate smear showing increased number and size of the megakaryocytes. **C** Bone marrow aspirate smear. Note the deeply lobulated megakaryocyte nuclei, as well as the large pools of platelets; aspirate smears fail to reveal the overall marrow architecture and distribution of the megakaryocytes, which can only be seen on biopsy.

JAK2 and mutations of the gelsolin gene (*GSN*) were recently reported in several pedigrees of hereditary thrombocytosis {1677,3457}.

Localization

The bone marrow and blood are the principal sites of involvement. The spleen does not show significant extramedullary haematopoiesis at the time of onset, but is a sequestration site for platelets {1217, 1563}.

Clinical features

More than half of all cases are asymptomatic at the time of diagnosis, discovered incidentally when an elevated platelet count is found on a routine peripheral blood count {254,1217,1378, 1563}. The other half present with some manifestation of vascular occlusion or haemorrhage {566,1096,1215,3088, 3933}. Microvascular occlusion can lead to transient ischaemic attacks, digital ischaemia with paraesthesias, and gangrene {566,3088}. Thrombosis of major arteries and veins can also occur, and ET can be a cause of splenic or hepatic vein thrombosis as seen in Budd–Chiari syndrome {1022,2012,3703}. Bleeding occurs most commonly from mucosal surfaces, such as in the gastrointestinal tract and upper airway passages {1096, 1215,1378}. In PVSG-defined ET, mild splenomegaly is present in approximately 50% of cases at diagnosis and hepatomegaly in 15–20% {1563,2791,3927}. When the WHO criteria, which exclude cases with thrombocytosis associated with prefibrotic/early primary myelofibrosis (pre-PMF), are used, minor palpable splenomegaly is seen in only 15–20% of ET cases {254,3917,3933,3977}. In three studies including almost 1500 WHO-defined cases of ET from various centres,

leukocytosis and erythrocytosis were unusual findings, as was an increased serum level of lactate dehydrogenase; leukoerythroblastosis and poikilocytosis were absent {254,3933,3977}.
Previously, the platelet count threshold for the diagnosis of ET was ≥600 × 10⁹/L {2791}. However, given that some patients experience haemorrhagic or thrombotic events at lower platelet counts {2265, 3331,3469}, several investigators have convincingly argued for a lower platelet count threshold for the diagnosis of ET, in order to avoid compromising the diagnosis in such cases. As a result, WHO has adopted the recommendation of a platelet count threshold of ≥450 × 10⁹/L, a value that exceeds the 95th percentile for

normal platelet counts (adjusted for sex and race) {2265,3452,3469,3931}. This threshold value has also been adopted by the British Committee for Standards in Haematology (BCSH) {1562}. Although this lowered threshold will encompass more cases of ET, it will also include more cases of conditions that mimic ET {257,1380}; therefore, it is essential that all diagnostic criteria for ET (see Table 2.12) are met in order to exclude other neoplastic and non-neoplastic causes of thrombocytosis {1380,3931,3932}. Bone marrow biopsy is particularly helpful in excluding other myeloid neoplasms associated with high platelet counts, such as myelodysplastic syndromes associated with isolated del(5q), myelodys-

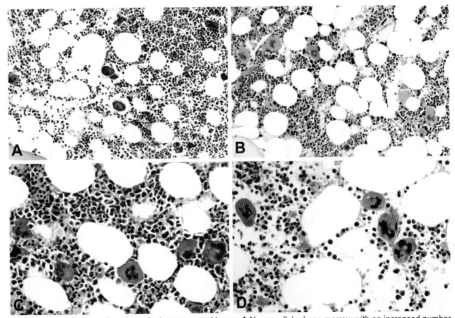

Fig. 2.25 Essential thrombocythaemia, bone marrow biopsy. **A** Normocellular bone marrow with an increased number of large to giant megakaryocytes. **B** There is no significant increase in erythropoiesis or granulopoiesis, as demonstrated by naphthol AS-D chloroacetate esterase (CAE) staining: granulocytic cells are stained red by the reaction product. **C** With periodic acid–Schiff (PAS) staining, the enlarged megakaryocytes demonstrate abundant amounts of mature cytoplasm and deeply lobulated and hyperlobulated (staghorn-like) nuclei. **D** The large to giant megakaryocytes may be arranged in small, loose clusters.

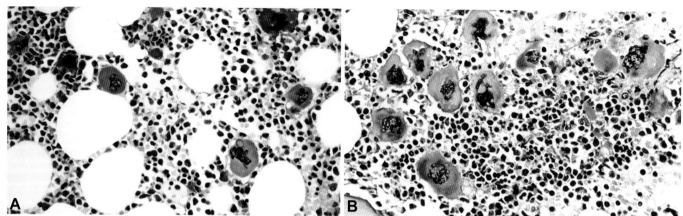

Fig. 2.26 A Essential thrombocythaemia, bone marrow biopsy. Large to giant megakaryocytes with deeply lobulated and conspicuously hypersegmented nuclei are randomly distributed in the marrow. **B** Prefibrotic/early primary myelofibrosis, bone marrow biopsy. Megakaryocytic abnormalities include abnormal nuclear:cytoplasmic ratios, abnormal chromatin clumping with hyperchromatic nuclei, plump lobulation of nuclei (cloud-like nuclei), and clustering.

plastic/myeloproliferative neoplasm with ring sideroblasts and thrombocytosis, and in particular pre-PMF. Although most WHO-defined ET cases harbour a phenotypic driver mutation in *JAK2* (present in 50–60% of cases), *CALR* (in ~30%), or *MPL* (in ~3%), about 12% of cases are triple-negative for these mutations. None of these mutations is specific for ET, but their presence does exclude reactive thrombocytosis {3920,3933}. Similarly, in vitro endogenous erythroid and/or megakaryocytic colony formation, although not specific for ET, also excludes reactive thrombocytosis {1011}.

Microscopy

The major abnormality seen in the peripheral blood is marked thrombocytosis. The platelets often display anisocytosis, ranging from tiny forms to atypical large or giant platelets. Bizarre shapes, pseudopods, and agranular platelets may be seen, but are not common. In WHO-defined ET, the white blood cell count and leukocyte differential count are usually normal, although a borderline elevation in the white blood cell count may occur {254,1378,3920,3933,3977}. The red blood cells are usually normocytic and normochromic, unless recurrent haemorrhage has caused iron deficiency, in which case they may be microcytic and hypochromic. Leukoerythroblastosis and teardrop-shaped red blood cells are not seen in ET {254,3977}.

Haematopoietic cellularity is normal in most cases {3975}, but a small proportion of cases show a hypercellular marrow (Table 2.04, p. 42) {3969,3972}. The most striking abnormality is a marked proliferation of megakaryocytes, with a predominance of large to giant forms displaying abundant, mature cytoplasm and deeply lobed and hypersegmented (staghorn-like) nuclei. The megakaryocytes are typically dispersed throughout the bone marrow, but may occur in loose clusters. Unlike in pre-PMF and overt primary myelofibrosis, bizarre, highly atypical megakaryocytes or large dense clusters are very rarely found in ET; if they are present, the diagnosis of ET should be reconsidered {1227,1366,3961,3966, 3977}. Proliferation of erythroid precursors is seen in some cases (most commonly when the patient has experienced recurrent major haemorrhages or has been pretreated with hydroxycarbamide), but granulocytic proliferation is highly unusual; if present, the increase in granulopoiesis is usually only slight. There is no increase in myeloblasts and no myelodysplasia. The network of reticulin fibres is usually normal, or is very rarely (in < 5% of cases) minimally increased (but never to more than WHO grade 1 {3975}) {254, 2105,3981}; infrequently, reticulin fibrosis may increase in sequential bone marrow biopsy examinations {2105,3981}. The finding of significant reticulin fibrosis or any collagen fibrosis at presentation excludes the diagnosis of ET {1227,1329, 1366,2105,3933,3966,3969}. Bone marrow aspirate smears also reveal markedly increased numbers of large megakaryocytes with hyperlobulated nuclei, as well as large sheets of platelets in the background. Emperipolesis of bone marrow elements is frequently observed in ET, but is not a specific finding. Stainable iron may be present in aspirated bone marrow specimens at diagnosis {2791}.

The morphological findings, i.e. the characteristic histological patterns in the bone marrow biopsy (Table 2.04, p. 42), are essential for distinguishing ET from other MPNs {1380} and myeloid disorders or reactive conditions that present with sustained thrombocytosis. The finding of even a low degree of combined granulocytic and erythroid proliferation should raise suspicion of the prodromal stage of polycythaemia vera {1364,2152,3972}, and the finding of granulocytic proliferation associated with bizarre, highly atypical megakaryocytes should raise suspicion of pre-PMF {1227,1366,2147,3962, 3984}. Significant dyserythropoiesis or dysgranulopoiesis suggests a diagnosis of myelodysplastic syndrome rather than ET. The large megakaryocytes with hypersegmented nuclei seen in ET contrast with the medium-sized non-lobated megakaryocytes seen in myelodysplastic syndrome with isolated del(5q) and with the small, dysplastic megakaryocytes seen in acute myeloid leukaemia or myelodysplastic syndrome with inv(3)(q21.3q26.2) or t(3;3)(q21.3;q26.2). Some cases of chronic myeloid leukaemia initially present with thrombocytosis without leukocytosis, and can mimic ET clinically. The large megakaryocytes of ET can be easily distinguished from the small (dwarf) megakaryocytes of chronic myeloid leukaemia, but cytogenetic and/or molecular genetic analysis to exclude *BCR-ABL1* fusion is recommended for all patients in whom the diagnosis of ET is considered {3350}.

Cell of origin

The postulated cell of origin is a haematopoietic stem cell.

Genetic profile

No molecular genetic or cytogenetic abnormality specific for ET is known. Approximately 50–60% of WHO-defined ET cases carry *JAK2* V617F or a functionally similar mutation, about 30% of cases have a mutation in *CALR* and 3% *MPL*, and about 12 % of cases are triple-negative for these mutations {3915,3920, 3933,3935}. A subset of triple-negative cases have been found to have gain-of-function mutations (e.g, *MPL* S204P and *MPL* Y591N) through whole-exome sequencing or other sensitive molecular techniques {517,2666}. This finding is consistent with the assumptions that *JAK2*/*CALR*/*MPL*-wildtype ET is not a homogeneous entity and that cases with polyclonal haematopoiesis probably constitute a hereditary disorder {2666}. These mutations are not specific for ET; they are found in polycythaemia vera and primary myelofibrosis as well. But none of these mutations have been reported in cases of reactive thrombocytosis {3920,3933}. Mutations similar to those described in MPNs {3915} have also been found at very low frequencies in elderly patients with no haematological malignancy {1326,1830,4386}. Very rarely, cases of ET acquire a *BCR-ABL1* rearrangement; however, the clinical significance of this is uncertain. Due to this additional phenotypic mutation, a morphological and haematological shift capable of producing a chronic myeloid leukaemia–like evolution may occur {1740}. An abnormal karyotype is found in only 5–10% of ET cases diagnosed according to the previous PVSG criteria {2791} and in 7.7% of WHO-defined cases {3920}. There is no consistent abnormality, but reported abnormalities include gain of chromosome 8, abnormalities of 9q, and del(20q) {1641,3045}. Isolated instances of del(5q) have also been reported in ET, and careful morphological examination is needed to distinguish such cases from myelodysplastic syndromes associated with this abnormality {3045}.

Prognosis and predictive factors

ET is an indolent disorder characterized by long symptom-free intervals interrupted by occasional life-threatening thromboembolic or haemorrhagic events {566, 1096,1215,1217,1378,1563,2791,3088, 3927}. After many years, a few patients with ET develop bone marrow fibrosis of grade 2–3 on a 0–3 scale {2148,3975}

Table 2.13 Diagnostic criteria for post–essential thrombocythaemia (ET) myelofibrosis {265}

Required criteria

1. Documentation of a previous diagnosis of WHO-defined ET
2. Bone marrow fibrosis of grade 2–3 on a
   0–3 scale {3975} or grade 3–4 on a
   0–4 scale {2146}

Additional criteria (2 are required)

1. Anaemia (i.e. below the reference range given age, sex, and altitude considerations) and a
   >2 g/dL decrease from baseline haemoglobin concentration
2. Leukoerythroblastosis
3. Increasing splenomegaly, defined as either an increase in palpable splenomegaly of
   >5 cm from baseline (distance from the left costal margin) or the development
   of a newly palpable splenomegaly
4. Elevated lactate dehydrogenase level (above the reference range)
5. Development of any 2 (or all 3) of the following constitutional symptoms:
   >10% weight loss in 6 months, night sweats, unexplained fever (>37.5 °C)

Reprinted by permission from Macmillan Publishers Ltd: Leukemia. Barosi G, Mesa RA, Thiele J, Cervantes F, Campbell PJ, Verstovsek S, et al. Proposed criteria for the diagnosis of post-polycythemia vera and post-essential thrombocythemia myelofibrosis: a consensus statement from the International Working Group for Myelofibrosis Research and Treatment. Leukemia. 2008;22:437-8. Copyright 2008.

or grade 3–4 on a 0–4 scale {2146}, associated with myeloid metaplasia (extramedullary haematopoiesis), but such progression is uncommon {254,612,717, 1217,1377,1378,1380,3511,3927}, occurring in only about 10% of cases in large, strictly WHO-defined cohorts {3920}. The diagnostic criteria for post-ET myelofibrosis are listed in Table 2.13. Strict adherence to these and other WHO criteria {265,3931,3932} is necessary to avoid diagnostic confusion associated with pre-PMF accompanied by thrombocytosis {263,1380}. Clear-cut differentiation of ET from pre-PMF is crucial, because these entities differ significantly in terms of complications and survival {11,254, 1086,1380,2150,3961,3977}. In large series of WHO-defined cases, the relative incidence rates of post-ET myelofibrosis were found to be approximately half the rates of post–polycythaemia vera myelofibrosis {254,3920}. Transformation of ET to the blast phase (i.e. acute myeloid leukaemia) or myelodysplastic syndrome occurs in <5% of cases, and is likely related to previous cytotoxic therapy {1217, 1563}; the risk of transformation is lower among strictly WHO-defined cases {254, 1378,3920}. Median survival times of 10–15 years are commonly reported. Because ET usually occurs late in middle age, life expectancy is near normal for many patients {254,717,1377,2150,3090, 4348}. However, most clinical studies are based on older diagnostic guidelines {2791}, which fail to differentiate clearly between pre-PMF with accompanying

thrombocytosis and ET according to the current WHO classification {263}. A substantial difference in overall prognosis has been reported depending on which classification system is applied {2150}. For patients with strictly WHO-defined ET, the observed and relative survival was similar to that of the general European population {254,2150}, and transformation to overt myelofibrosis and the blast phase appeared to be relatively rare {254,3933}. In contrast, the survival of patients with WHO-defined ET was found to be inferior to that of a sex- and age-matched United States population at one centre {3920}, whereas the observed rates of fibrotic and blast transformation were comparable with those found in a previous Italian study {254}. The rates of conversion of ET to overt polycythaemia vera in *JAK2*-mutated cases reported in some studies {540,3458} depend on the diagnostic criteria applied; when the WHO criteria are used, the incidence of transformation appears to be <5% {250}.

Chronic eosinophilic leukaemia, NOS

Bain B.J.
Horny H.-P.
Hasserjian R.P.
Orazi A.

Definition

Chronic eosinophilic leukaemia (CEL) not otherwise specified (NOS), is a myeloproliferative neoplasm (MPN) in which an autonomous, clonal proliferation of eosinophil precursors results in persistently increased numbers of eosinophils in the peripheral blood, bone marrow, and peripheral tissues, with eosinophilia being the dominant haematological abnormality. Organ damage occurs as a result of leukaemic infiltration or of the release of cytokines, enzymes, or other proteins by the eosinophils.

CEL, NOS excludes cases with a Philadelphia (Ph) chromosome; BCR-ABL1 fusion; rearrangement of PDGFRA, PDGFRB, or FGFR1; or PCM1-JAK2, ETV6-JAK2, or BCR-JAK2 fusion.

In CEL, NOS the eosinophil count is $\geq 1.5 \times 10^9$/L in the blood, and there are < 20% blasts in the peripheral blood and bone marrow. For a diagnosis of CEL, NOS to be made, there should be evidence for clonality of myeloid cells or an increase in myeloblasts in the peripheral blood or bone marrow. However, in many cases it is impossible to prove clonality; in such cases, providing there is no increase in blast cells, the diagnosis of idiopathic hypereosinophilic syndrome (HES) is made. It is clinically important to clearly distinguish between CEL, NOS and idiopathic HES. Idiopathic HES is defined as eosinophilia (eosinophil count $\geq 1.5 \times 10^9$/L) persisting for ≥ 6 months for which no underlying cause can be found, associated with signs of organ involvement and dysfunction {759,4291}; there is no evidence of eosinophil clonality. It is a diagnosis of exclusion, and may include some cases of true eosinophilic leukaemia that cannot currently be recognized, as well as cases of cytokine-driven eosinophilia due to the abnormal release of eosinophil growth factors (e.g. IL2, IL3, and IL5) for unknown reasons {226,759,3581,3759,4291}. If there is a similar unexplained hypereosinophilia but with no evidence of tissue damage, the designation 'idiopathic hypereosinophilia' is appropriate. As outlined in Table 2.14, diagnosis of CEL, NOS requires integration of clinical, laboratory, and molecular features.

ICD-O code   9964/3

Epidemiology

Due to the previous difficulty in distinguishing CEL from idiopathic HES, the true incidence of these rare diseases is unknown. CEL, NOS appears to be more common in men, with a reported median age of occurrence in the seventh decade of life {4249B,1606}. The epidemiological features of idiopathic cases of HES remain undefined.

Localization

CEL, NOS is a multisystemic disorder. The peripheral blood and bone marrow are always involved. Tissue infiltration by eosinophils and the release of cytokines

Table 2.14 Diagnostic criteria for chronic eosinophilic leukaemia, NOS

1. Eosinophilia (eosinophil count $\geq 1.5 \times 10^9$/L)

2. WHO criteria for BCR-ABL1–positive chronic myeloid leukaemia, polycythaemia vera, essential thrombocythaemia, primary myelofibrosis, chronic neutrophilic leukaemia, chronic myelomonocytic leukaemia and BCR-ABL1–negative atypical chronic myeloid leukaemia are not met

3. No rearrangement of PDGFRA, PDGFRB or FGFR1, and no PCM1-JAK2, ETV6-JAK2, or BCR-JAK2 fusion

4. Blast cells constitute < 20% of the cells in the peripheral blood and bone marrow, and inv(16)(p13.1q22), t(16;16)(p13.1;q22), t(8;21)(q22;q22.1), and other diagnostic features of acute myeloid leukaemia are absent

5. There is a clonal cytogenetic or molecular genetic abnormality[a]
   or
   Blast cells account for ≥ 2% of cells in the peripheral blood or ≥ 5% in the bone marrow

[a] Because some clonal molecular genetic abnormalities (e.g. mutations in TET2, ASXL1, and DNMT3A) can occur in a minority of elderly people in the absence of any apparent haematological abnormality, it is essential to exclude all possible causes of reactive eosinophilia before making this diagnosis solely on the basis of a molecular genetic abnormality in an elderly person.

Table 2.15 Diagnostic criteria for myeloproliferative neoplasm (MPN), unclassifiable see p.57

The diagnosis of myeloproliferative neoplasm (MPN), unclassifiable, requires that all 3 criteria are met.

1. Features of an MPN are present

2. WHO criteria for any other MPN, myelodysplastic syndrome[a], myelodysplastic/myeloproliferative[a] neoplasm, or BCR-ABL1–positive chronic myeloid leukaemia are not met

3. JAK2, CALR, or MPL mutation characteristically associated with MPN
   or
   Presence of another clonal marker[b]
   or
   Absence of a cause of reactive fibrosis[c]

[a] Effects of any previous treatment, severe comorbidity, and changes during the natural progression of the disease process must be excluded.

[b] In the absence of any of the 3 major clonal mutations, a search for other mutations associated with myeloid neoplasms (e.g. ASXL1, EZH2, TET2, IDH1, IDH2, SRSF2, and SF3B1 mutations) may be of help in confirming the clonal nature of a suspected MPN, unclassifiable.

[c] Bone marrow fibrosis secondary to infection, autoimmune disorder or another chronic inflammatory condition, hairy cell leukaemia or another lymphoid neoplasm, metastatic malignancy, or toxic (chronic) myelopathy.

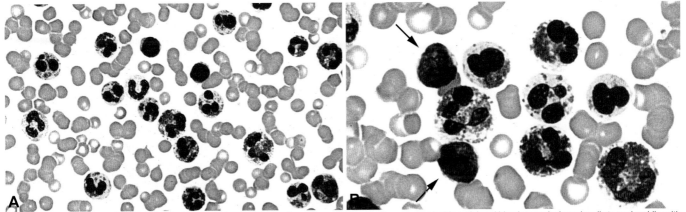

Fig. 2.27 Reactive eosinophilia in lymphoblastic leukaemia. **A** The elevation of the white blood cell count seen in this peripheral blood smear is due primarily to eosinophils, with only an occasional lymphoblast. **B** Lymphoblasts (arrows) are clearly appreciable in this blood smear.

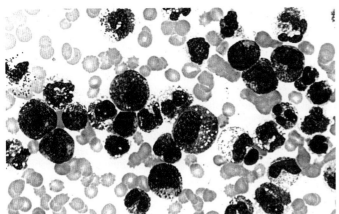

Fig. 2.28 Chronic eosinophilic leukaemia, NOS. Peripheral blood smear from a patient with a history of persistent eosinophilia. Immature and mature eosinophils are present. The cytogenetic analysis showed trisomy 10.

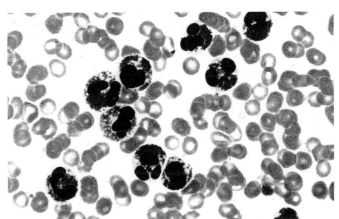

Fig. 2.29 Idiopathic hypereosinophilic syndrome. Blood smear from a patient with cardiac failure, leukocytosis, and hypereosinophilia.

and humoral factors from the eosinophil granules lead to tissue damage in a number of organs; the heart, lungs, central nervous system (CNS), skin, and gastrointestinal tract are commonly involved. Splenic and hepatic involvement is also common {1606}.

Clinical features

Eosinophilia is sometimes detected incidentally in patients who are otherwise asymptomatic. In other cases, patients experience constitutional symptoms such as weight loss, night sweats, fever, fatigue, cough, angio-oedema, muscle pain, pruritus, and diarrhoea. The most serious clinical findings relate to endomyocardial fibrosis, with ensuing restrictive cardiomegaly. Scarring of the mitral and tricuspid valves leads to valvular regurgitation and the formation of intracardiac thrombi, which can embolize to the brain or elsewhere. Cardiac failure can occur. Peripheral neuropathy, CNS dysfunction, pulmonary symptoms due to lung infiltra-

tion, and rheumatological findings are frequent manifestations {1606}.

Microscopy

In CEL, NOS the most striking feature in the peripheral blood is eosinophilia, mainly of mature eosinophils, with only small numbers of eosinophilic myelocytes and promyelocytes {2127}. There may be a range of eosinophil abnormalities, including sparse granulation (with clear areas of cytoplasm), cytoplasmic vacuolation, nuclear hypersegmentation or hyposegmentation, and increased size. Because these changes can be seen in both reactive and neoplastic eosinophilia, they are not very helpful in determining whether a case is likely to be CEL, NOS {226}. Occasional patients with CEL, NOS have cytologically normal eosinophils, but the absence of eosinophil dysplasia generally favours reactive eosinophilia {4249B}. Significant dysplasia in cells of other myeloid lineages supports the diagnosis of CEL, NOS

{4249B}. Neutrophilia often accompanies the eosinophilia, and some cases show mild monocytosis, but do not meet all the criteria for chronic myelomonocytic leukaemia. Mild basophilia has been reported. Blast cells may be present but account for <20% of the cells.

The bone marrow is hypercellular, due in part to eosinophilic proliferation {481, 1606,2127}. In most cases, eosinophil maturation is orderly (i.e. without a disproportionate increase in myeloblasts). Charcot–Leyden crystals are often present. Erythropoiesis and megakaryocytopoiesis are usually normal. Increased proportions of myeloblasts (≥2% in peripheral blood or 5–19% in bone marrow) support the diagnosis of CEL, NOS, as do dysplastic features in other cell lineages {4249B}. Marrow fibrosis is seen in about one third of cases, although severe fibrosis is rare {481,4249B}.

Any tissue can show eosinophilic infiltration, and Charcot–Leyden crystals are often present. Fibrosis is common, caused by the degranulation of the eosinophils and the resulting release of eosinophil basic proteins and eosinophil cationic proteins.

Cytochemistry

Cytochemical stains can be used to identify eosinophils but are not necessary for diagnosis. Partial degranulation can lead to eosinophils having reduced peroxidase content and can render automated leukocyte counts unreliable.

Differential diagnosis

Diagnosis requires positive evidence of the leukaemic nature of the condition and exclusion of myeloid neoplasms with rearrangement of *PDGFRA*, *PDGFRB* or *FGFR1*, or with *PCM1-JAK2*, *ETV6-JAK2*, or *BCR-JAK2* fusion. The diagnostic process often starts with exclusion of reactive eosinophilia. A detailed history, physical examination, blood count and examination of the blood smear are essential. Conditions to be excluded include parasitic infection, allergies, pulmonary diseases such as Löffler syndrome, cyclical eosinophilia, skin diseases such as angiolymphoid hyperplasia, collagen vascular disorders, and Kimura disease {226, 2043,3510}. In addition, a number of neoplastic disorders, such as T-cell lymphoma, Hodgkin lymphoma, systemic mastocytosis, lymphoblastic leukaemia and other MPNs can be associated with abnormal release of IL2, IL3, IL5, or granulocyte–macrophage colony-stimulating factor and a secondary eosinophilia that mimics CEL, NOS {226,2055,2063, 2609,2920,3501,3510,4402}; in systemic mastocytosis, there can also be eosinophils belonging to the neoplastic clone. The bone marrow should be carefully inspected for any process that could explain the eosinophilia as a secondary reaction, such as vasculitis, lymphoma, lymphoblastic leukaemia, systemic mastocytosis, or granulomatous disorders. Increased numbers of mast cells, which may be spindle-shaped, may indicate rearrangement of *PDGFRA* or *PDGFRB*. Some cases of persistent eosinophilia occur due to the abnormal release of cytokines by T cells that are immunophenotypically aberrant and that may be clonal {476,1607,2035,2255,3680}. When such a T-cell population is present, the case is considered to be neither CEL, NOS nor idiopathic HES; instead, the term 'lymphocytic variant of hypereosinophilic syndrome' is used. If the monocyte count is $\geq 1 \times 10^9$/L, the diagnosis of chronic myelomonocytic leukaemia with eosinophilia may be more appropriate. Similarly, if there are dysplastic features, > 10% neutrophil precursors in the peripheral blood and no monocytosis, the diagnosis of atypical chronic myeloid leukaemia, *BCR-ABL1*–negative, with eosinophilia should be considered.

Idiopathic HES can be diagnosed only in fully investigated patients and only when (1) there is an eosinophil count of $\geq 1.5 \times 10^9$/L persisting for ≥ 6 months; (2) reactive eosinophilia has been excluded by appropriate, thorough investigation; (3) acute myeloid leukaemia, MPN, myelodysplastic syndrome, myelodysplastic/myeloproliferative neoplasm and systemic mastocytosis have been excluded; (4) a cytokine-producing, immunophenotypically aberrant T-cell population has been excluded; and (5) there is tissue damage as a result of hypereosinophilia. If criteria 1–4 are met but there is no tissue damage, the appropriate diagnosis is idiopathic hypereosinophilia.

Patients in whom the diagnosis of idiopathic hypereosinophilia or idiopathic HES is made should be regularly monitored, because evidence may subsequently emerge that the condition is leukaemic in nature, and treatment may be necessary.

Immunophenotype

No specific immunophenotypic abnormality has been reported in CEL, NOS. However, immunophenotyping is relevant to the diagnosis of T lymphocyte–driven eosinophilia.

Cell of origin

The cell of origin is a haematopoietic stem cell, but the lineage potential of the affected cell may be variable. T-lymphoblastic transformation has been reported, so it appears that some cases arise from a pluripotent lymphoid–myeloid stem cell {1606}.

Genetic profile

No single or specific cytogenetic or molecular genetic abnormality has been identified in CEL, NOS. Cases with rearrangement of *PDGFRA*, *PDGFRB* or *FGFR1*, or with *PCM1-JAK2* or variants are specifically excluded. The presence of a Ph chromosome or *BCR-ABL1* fusion indicates one of the rare cases of chronic myeloid leukaemia with dominant eosinophilia, rather than CEL, NOS. Even when eosinophilia occurs in conjunction with a chromosomal abnormality that is usually myeloid neoplasm–associated, it may be difficult to determine whether the eosinophils are part of the clonal process, because reactive eosinophilia can occur in patients with myeloid neoplasms {1226}. However, the finding of a recurrent karyotypic abnormality that is usually observed in myeloid disorders (e.g. gain of chromosome 8, loss of chromosome 7, or isochromosome 17q) does support the diagnosis of CEL, NOS {226,3068}, as does the presence of a translocation. Occasional cases have a *JAK2* mutation, but mutations in *ASXL1*, *TET2* and *EZH2* appear to be more common {1872, 4249B}. Four patients with a somatic activating *KIT* M541L mutation, whose disease was responsive to low-dose imatinib, have been reported {1799}. Further studies to establish the frequency of this mutation are needed. X-linked polymorphism analysis of the *AR* (also called *HUMARA*) or *PGK* genes have been used in female patients to demonstrate clonality {652,2418}. In the appropriate context, the finding of somatic mutations in genes that are frequently mutated in other myeloid neoplasms can support the diagnosis of CEL, NOS. However, mutations in genes such as *TET2*, *ASXL1* and *DNMT3A* are sometimes detected by DNA sequencing in elderly people without neoplasms {1326,4386}, so their presence should not be considered definitive proof that eosinophilia results from a neoplastic rather than reactive process.

Prognosis and predictive factors

Survival is quite variable, but acute transformation is common and prognosis is generally poor {1606}. In one small series, the median survival time was 22.2 months {1606}. Response to imatinib is uncommon but has been reported {1606,1799}. Cytogenetic remission with interferon alfa has been reported in 3 cases with translocations with a 5q31-33 breakpoint {2407,2459,4404}; *PDGFRB* rearrangement was excluded in one of these cases {4404}. Marked splenomegaly, blasts in the blood or increased blasts in the bone marrow, cytogenetic abnormalities and dysplastic features in other myeloid lineages have been reported to be unfavourable prognostic findings {759,3581, 3759,4291}.

Myeloproliferative neoplasm, unclassifiable

Kvasnicka H.M.
Thiele J.
Orazi A.
Horny H.-P.
Bain B.J.

Definition

The designation of myeloproliferative neoplasm, unclassifiable (MPN-U) should be applied only to cases that have definite clinical, laboratory, molecular, and morphological features of a myeloproliferative neoplasm (MPN) but fail to meet the diagnostic criteria for any of the specific MPN entities, or that present with features that overlap between two or more of the MPN categories (Table 2.15, p.54). Most cases of MPN-U fall into one of three groups:

1. A subset of cases with so-called masked/pre-polycythaemic presentation of polycythaemia vera, prefibrotic/early primary myelofibrosis, or early-phase essential thrombocythaemia in which the characteristic features are not yet fully developed {1380,2147,2152} – a proportion of cases presenting with portal or splanchnic vein thrombosis that fail to meet the diagnostic criteria for any of the specific MPN entities may also be considered to belong in this group {1103, 1362};

2. Advanced-stage MPN, in which pronounced myelofibrosis, osteosclerosis, or transformation to a more aggressive stage with increased blast counts and/or myelodysplastic changes obscures the underlying disorder {404,405,2151,3968, 3978,3983}; or

3. Cases with convincing evidence of an MPN in which a coexisting neoplastic or inflammatory disorder obscures some of the usual diagnostic clinical and/or morphological features {2147}.

ICD-O code   9975/3

Epidemiology

The exact incidence of MPN-U is unknown, but some reports indicate that unclassifiable cases account for as many as 10–15% of all MPNs {3983}. The relative frequency varies significantly according to the experience of the diagnostician and the specific classification system and criteria used {1361,1361A, 1362,1363,2151,2348A,3978}. Careful evaluation of clinical, morphological, and molecular features reduces the frequency of unclassifiable cases to <5% {257, 1086,1361A,1799A,2147,2433}.

Localization

The blood and bone marrow are the major sites of involvement, but in advanced stages the spleen and liver (i.e. the major sites of extramedullary haematopoiesis) may be also affected.

Clinical features

The clinical features of MPN-U are similar to those of other MPNs. In early unclassifiable disease, organomegaly may be minimal or absent, but splenomegaly and hepatomegaly can be massive in advanced cases in which bone marrow specimens are characterized by marked myelofibrosis and/or increased numbers of blasts {3978,3983}. The haematological values are also variable, ranging from mild leukocytosis to moderate or marked thrombocytosis, with or without accompanying anaemia. Prominent cytopenia or myelodysplastic features should always prompt the definitive exclusion of MDS/MPN and myelodysplastic syndrome (MDS) {257,2147}. Discrepancies between morphological and clinical features are particularly common in cases presenting with otherwise unexplained portal or splanchnic vein thrombosis {1103,1362}.

Exclusionary criteria

The presence of *BCR-ABL1* fusion; rearrangement of *PDGFRA*, *PDGFRB*, or *FGFR1*; or *PCM1-JAK2* fusion excludes the diagnosis of MPN-U. This diagnosis is also inappropriate if clinical data sufficient for proper classification are not available, if the bone marrow specimen is of inadequate quality or size for accurate evaluation {2147,2151,2152,3978,3983}, or if the

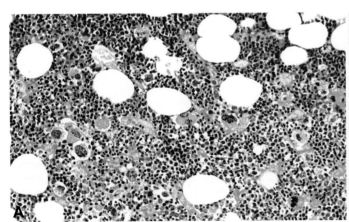 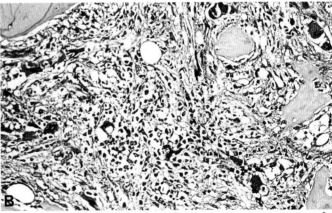

Fig.2.30 Myeloproliferative neoplasm, unclassifiable. **A** Early stage: a bone marrow biopsy specimen from a 50-year-old man with a platelet count of 500–1000 × 10⁹/L for many months and a haemoglobin concentration of 17 g/dL; the specimen shows hypercellularity, an increased number of enlarged mature-appearing megakaryocytes, a slightly increased number of erythroid precursors, and prominent sinuses filled with erythrocytes, suggesting the so-called masked presentation of polycythaemia vera; molecular testing revealed *JAK2* wild-type and *CALR* mutation. **B** Late fibrotic stage: a bone marrow biopsy specimen from a 65-year-old female with leukocytosis, pancytopenia, and marked splenomegaly; the specimen shows hypocellularity, fibrosis with osteosclerosis, and markedly atypical megakaryocytes; molecular testing revealed *JAK2* mutation.

patient has recently received cytotoxic or growth factor therapy that accounts for most of the ostensibly unclassifiable cases encountered in routine practice, particularly when myelodysplastic features are observed {1361}. There may be significant discrepancies between morphological and clinical features {1362}. It is often preferable to describe the morphological findings and to recommend additional clinical and laboratory procedures (e.g. adequate peripheral blood smears and bone marrow biopsy and aspirate specimens, as well as extended molecular testing) to further classify the process. When a diagnosis of MPN-U is made, the report should summarize the reason for the difficulty in reaching a more specific diagnosis, and if possible should specify which of the MPN subtypes can be excluded from consideration.

Differential diagnosis

If a case does not have the features of one of the well-defined entities, the possibility that it is not an MPN must be strongly considered {2147,2152}. A reactive bone marrow response to infection; an inflammatory response; the effects of toxins; and the results of administration of chemotherapy, growth factors, cytokines, or immunosuppressive agents can closely mimic MPN and must be definitively excluded {1363}. Furthermore, other haematopoietic and non-haematopoietic neoplasms, such as lymphoma or metastatic carcinoma, can infiltrate the marrow and cause reactive changes (including dense fibrosis and osteosclerosis) that can be misconstrued as MPN {3968}.

The detection of characteristic *JAK2*, *CALR*, or *MPL* driver mutations separates an MPN from reactive conditions, although not all cases of MPN-U express one of these major clonal markers {2019, 3924,3932}. In the absence of mutations in any of these genes, clonality should be confirmed whenever possible {2666}. It has been shown that non-canonical mutations of *MPL* and *JAK2* (i.e. those outside the exons usually investigated in routine diagnostic tests) are present in about 19% of triple-negative (i.e. apparently *JAK2/CALR/MPL*–wild-type) MPN cases {2666}; therefore, extended molecular testing can help to establish the diagnosis of an MPN. The identification of other mutations frequently associated with myeloid neoplasms (e.g. *ASXL1,*

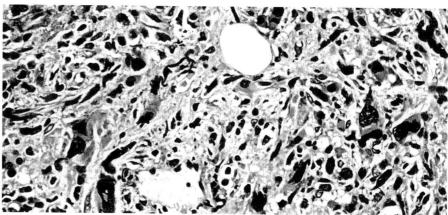

Fig. 2.31 Myeloproliferative neoplasm, unclassifiable, with features simulating myelodysplastic/myeloproliferative neoplasm, unclassifiable. Bone marrow biopsy shows severe dysmegakaryopoiesis: the dysplastic appearance of this case was therapy-related, a consequence of hydroxycarbamide administration for late-stage polycythaemia vera; molecular testing revealed mutations in *CALR* and *ASXL1*.

EZH2, *TET2*, *IDH1*, *IDH2*, *SRSF2*, and *SF3B1* mutations) can be of help in confirming the presence of clonal haematopoiesis {3924,3932}. However, acquired clonal mutations (including some of those mentioned above) may also occur in the haematopoietic cells of apparently healthy elderly individuals with no myeloid neoplasm {1326,1830,3772}. Therefore, caution is advised. Cytogenetic abnormalities occur in as many as 30% of cases {3920,3924} and can be useful in confirming clonality.

Cases with prominent cytopenia and/or significant accompanying myelodysplastic changes may be better categorized as myelodysplastic/myeloproliferative neoplasm (MDS/MPN) {994,1517,1748,2987}. The defining characteristics of each MPN must be considered with the understanding that (as with any biological process) variations do occur, and that the clinical and morphological manifestations can change over time as the disease progresses through various stages {257, 2147,2150,2151,2152}.

Microscopy

Many cases that are diagnosed as MPN-U constitute very early stage disease in which the differentiation between essential thrombocythaemia, primary myelofibrosis, and polycythaemia vera may be very difficult {2147,2151,2152}. In such cases, peripheral blood smears often reveal thrombocytosis and variable neutrophilia {2152}. The haemoglobin concentration may be normal, mildly decreased, or borderline increased {3966, 3969,3972}. Bone marrow biopsy specimens frequently show hypercellularity

and prominent megakaryocytic proliferation, with variable amounts of granulocytic and erythroid proliferation {2147,2152, 3978,3984,3985}. Careful application of the diagnostic guidelines recommended in this volume for each specific MPN, with close attention paid to the megakaryocyte morphology and histotopography, will enable the classification of most MPNs as a specific subtype {1361, 2433}; the remainder are best classified as MPN-U until careful follow-up or additional laboratory studies provide sufficient evidence for a more precise diagnosis {2147,2152}.

In late-stage disease, bone marrow specimens may show dense fibrosis and/or osteomyelosclerosis, indicating a terminal burnt-out stage; if no previous history or histology is available, it may be impossible to distinguish between the post-polycythaemic stage of polycythaemia vera (post–polycythaemia vera myelofibrosis) or, rarely, essential thrombocythaemia (post–essential thrombocythaemia myelofibrosis) and the overt fibrotic/osteosclerotic stage of primary myelofibrosis {407,3964,3968, 3978,3983}. Differential diagnosis with MDS (or MDS/MPN, unclassifiable) associated with severe bone marrow fibrosis may be challenging in cases with multilineage dysplasia, due to the overlapping clinical and morphological features {218, 941,942,2986}. In these cases, meticulous investigation with respect to splenomegaly, blood cell count, peripheral blood and bone marrow findings, presence or absence of MPN-associated mutations (in *JAK2*, *MPL*, or *CALR*), and karyotypic findings may facilitate diagnosis

{1261,2986}. Although chronic myeloid leukaemia may also be accompanied by marked myelofibrosis, the small size of the megakaryocytes indicates the correct diagnosis {3978,3983}, and cytogenetic and molecular genetic demonstration of the Philadelphia (Ph) chromosome or BCR-ABL1 fusion confirms the diagnosis of chronic myeloid leukaemia.

The presence of ≥ 10% blasts in the peripheral blood or bone marrow and/or the finding of significant myelodysplasia generally indicate a transition to a more aggressive, often terminal phase of the disease {404,405}. Cases initially diagnosed as MPN-U in which 10–19% blasts are found in the peripheral blood or bone marrow are considered to be in the accelerated phase. Blast percentages of ≥20% in the peripheral blood or bone marrow indicate the blast phase (i.e. acute leukaemic transformation) of previously diagnosed MPN-U. In most of these advanced-stage cases, fibrosis can cause dilution of bone marrow aspirates; therefore, immunohistochemical staining of the bone marrow biopsy sections for CD34 provides diagnostic value by demonstrating increased numbers and/or clusters or aggregates of blasts {3978,3983}. Prominent myelodysplastic features may appear during the natural progression of an MPN even without prior cytoreductive therapy {404}. However, if an initial, untreated case demonstrates significant myelodysplasia, the diagnostic alternatives of MDS/MPN or MDS, unclassifiable, should be considered {225, 994,1520,1748,2987,3919,3930}. In such cases, additional molecular testing and cytogenetic analysis may be necessary for better diagnostic characterization {1517,3930,4502}.

Cell of origin
The postulated cell of origin is a haematopoietic stem cell.

Genetic profile
There is no cytogenetic or molecular genetic finding specific for this group. There is no BCR-ABL1 fusion; no rearrangement of PDGFRA, PDGFRB, or FGFR1; and no PCM1-JAK2 fusion. The presence of a phenotypic driver mutation in JAK2, CALR, or MPL supports the diagnosis of an MPN. Cases that do not meet the clinical and/or morphological criteria for a specific MPN subtype or any other specific disease category are best categorized as MPN-U.

Prognosis and predictive factors
In patients with MPNs that are initially unclassifiable, follow-up studies performed at intervals of 6–12 months can often provide sufficient information for a more precise classification {257,2147, 2152,3978,3983}. In the early stages of disease, such patients have a prognosis similar to patients with the neoplasms into which their disease eventually evolves {2150}. Patients with advanced disease in whom the initial process is no longer recognizable due to bone marrow fibrosis or blastic infiltration are expected to have a poor prognosis {404,405}. Selective JAK1/JAK2 inhibitor therapy has been shown to rapidly reduce splenomegaly, markedly improve myelofibrosis-associated symptoms, and prolong overall survival in primary and secondary myelofibrosis (i.e. primary myelofibrosis, post–polycythaemia vera myelofibrosis, and post–essential thrombocythaemia myelofibrosis) {1798,1833,4316}. However, the same therapeutic approach was not found to be effective in MDS/MPN or MDS associated with bone marrow fibrosis. Therefore, the identification of MPNs {1261,2962}, even if they are unclassifiable, is of importance for clinical decision-making and overall prognosis {941,942}.

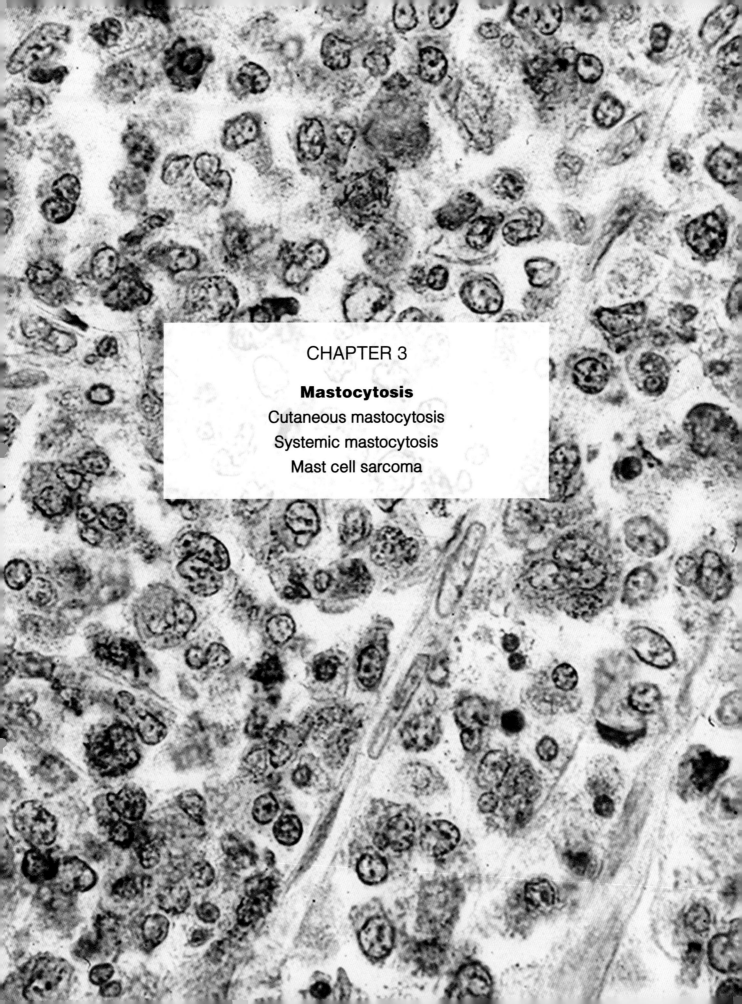

CHAPTER 3

Mastocytosis
Cutaneous mastocytosis
Systemic mastocytosis
Mast cell sarcoma

Mastocytosis

Horny H.-P.
Akin C.
Arber D.A.
Peterson L.C.
Tefferi A.

Metcalfe D.D.
Bennett J.M.
Bain B.J.
Escribano L.
Valent P.

Definition

Mastocytosis occurs due to a clonal, neoplastic proliferation of mast cells that accumulate in one or more organ systems. It is characterized by an abnormal mast cell infiltrate, which often contains multifocal compact clusters or cohesive aggregates. The disorder is heterogeneous, with manifestations ranging from skin lesions that can spontaneously regress to highly aggressive neoplasms associated with multiorgan failure and poor survival. Mastocytosis variants (Table 3.01) are recognized mainly by pathology investigations, distribution of the disease, and clinical manifestations. In cutaneous mastocytosis, the mast cell infiltrate remains confined to the skin, whereas systemic mastocytosis is characterized by the involvement of at least one extracutaneous organ, with or without evidence of skin lesions. Mastocytosis should be strictly distinguished from mast cell hyperplasia and mast cell activation states in which the morphological and molecular abnormalities that characterize the neoplastic proliferation of mast cells are absent. The diagnostic criteria for cutaneous and systemic mastocytosis are listed in Table 3.02.

ICD-O codes

Cutaneous mastocytosis	9740/1
Indolent systemic mastocytosis	9741/1
Systemic mastocytosis with an associated haematological neoplasm (AHN)	9741/3
Aggressive systemic mastocytosis (ASM)	9741/3
Mast cell leukaemia	9742/3
Mast cell sarcoma	9740/3

Epidemiology

Mastocytosis can occur at any age. Cutaneous mastocytosis is most common in children and can be present at birth. About 50% of affected children develop typical skin lesions before the age of 6 months. Cutaneous mastocytosis is much less common in adults than in children {576,1568,4105,4353}, and a slight male predominance has been

Table 3.01 Classification of mastocytosis variants

Cutaneous mastocytosis
  Urticaria pigmentosa / maculopapular cutaneous mastocytosis
  Diffuse cutaneous mastocytosis
  Mastocytoma of skin

Systemic mastocytosis
  Indolent systemic mastocytosis[a] (including the bone marrow mastocytosis subtype)
  Smouldering systemic mastocytosis[a]
  Systemic mastocytosis with an associated haematological neoplasm[b]
  Aggressive systemic mastocytosis[a]
  Mast cell leukaemia

Mast cell sarcoma

[a] The complete diagnosis of these variants requires information regarding B and C findings (Table 3.04, p. 66), all of which may not be available at the time of initial tissue diagnosis.
[b] This variant is equivalent to the previously described entity 'systemic mastocytosis with an associated clonal haematological non–mast cell lineage disease', and the terms can be used synonymously.

reported. Systemic mastocytosis is generally diagnosed after the second decade of life, and reported male-to-female ratios range from 1:1 to 1:1.5 {2646,3074}.

Localization

Approximately 80% of patients with mastocytosis have evidence of skin involvement {1568,3054}. In systemic mastocytosis, the bone marrow is almost always involved, so morphological and molecular analysis of a bone marrow biopsy specimen is strongly recommended in adults, to confirm or exclude the diagnosis of systemic mastocytosis {1698,1699,2268}. Rarely, the peripheral blood shows leukaemia due to significant numbers of circulating mast cells {1694}. Other organs that may be involved in systemic mastocytosis include the spleen, lymph nodes, liver, and gastrointestinal tract mucosa, but any tissue can be affected {1690,1692,1695,1698,2268, 3951,4107}. Skin lesions are more often observed in indolent systemic mastocytosis, whereas aggressive variants often present without skin lesions {3074, 4107}. However, patients with indolent systemic mastocytosis may also present without skin lesions; these patients may have isolated bone marrow mastocytosis, a rare subtype of indolent systemic mastocytosis.

Clinical features

There are three main forms of cutaneous mastocytosis, which constitute distinct clinicohistopathological entities: urticaria pigmentosa/maculopapular cutaneous mastocytosis, diffuse cutaneous mastocytosis and mastocytoma of skin. The lesions of all forms may urticate when stroked (Darier's sign), and most show intraepidermal accumulation of melanin pigment. The term 'urticaria pigmentosa' describes these two clinical features macroscopically. Blistering is usually seen in patients aged <3 years, and may be observed in all forms of paediatric cutaneous mastocytosis {1568, 4353}. However, blistering does not indicate a separate subtype of cutaneous mastocytosis.

The presenting symptoms of systemic mastocytosis have been grouped into four categories: constitutional symptoms (e.g. fatigue, weight loss, fever, diaphoresis), skin manifestations (e.g. pruritus, urticaria, dermatographism, flushing), mediator-related systemic events (e.g. abdominal pain, gastrointestinal distress, syncope, headache, hypotension, tachycardia, respiratory symptoms) and musculoskeletal symptoms (e.g. bone pain, osteopenia/osteoporosis, fractures, arthralgias, myalgias) {4107}. These disease manifestations can range from mild

Table 3.02 Diagnostic criteria for cutaneous and systemic mastocytosis

Cutaneous mastocytosis

Skin lesions demonstrating the typical findings of urticaria pigmentosa/maculopapular cutaneous mastocytosis, diffuse cutaneous mastocytosis or solitary mastocytoma, and typical histological infiltrates of mast cells in a multifocal or diffuse pattern in an adequate skin biopsy[a].

In addition, features/criteria sufficient to establish the diagnosis of systemic mastocytosis must be absent {1567,4105,4107}. There are three variants of cutaneous mastocytosis (see Table 3.01).

Systemic mastocytosis

The diagnosis of systemic mastocytosis can be made when the major criterion and at least 1 minor criterion are present, or when ≥ 3 minor criteria are present.

Major criterion

Multifocal dense infiltrates of mast cells (≥ 15 mast cells in aggregates) detected in sections of bone marrow and/or other extracutaneous organ(s)

Minor criteria

1. In biopsy sections of bone marrow or other extracutaneous organs, > 25% of the mast cells in the infiltrate are spindle-shaped or have atypical morphology or > 25% of all mast cells in bone marrow aspirate smears are immature or atypical.
2. Detection of an activating point mutation at codon 816 of *KIT* in the bone marrow, blood or another extracutaneous organ
3. Mast cells in bone marrow, blood or another extracutaneous organ express CD25, with or without CD2, in addition to normal mast cell markers[b].
4. Serum total tryptase is persistently > 20 ng/mL, unless there is an associated myeloid neoplasm, in which case this parameter is not valid.

[a] This criterion applies to both the dense focal and the diffuse mast cell infiltrates in the biopsy.
[b] CD25 is the more sensitive marker, by both flow cytometry and immunohistochemistry.

to life-threatening. Symptoms related to organ impairment (due to mast cell infiltrates) can also occur, in particular in patients with high-grade systemic mastocytosis, including aggressive systemic mastocytosis and mast cell leukaemia (Tables 3.03 and 3.04).

The physical findings at diagnosis of systemic mastocytosis may include splenomegaly (often minimal); lymphadenopathy and hepatomegaly are present less often {1690,1692,1695,2647}. Organomegaly is often absent in indolent systemic mastocytosis but is usually present (along with impaired organ function) in advanced systemic mastocytosis, including aggressive systemic mastocytosis and mast cell leukaemia. Severe systemic symptoms can occur in patients

with indolent systemic mastocytosis as a result of extensive generation and release of biochemical mediators such as histamine, eicosanoids, proteases and heparin. For example, gastrointestinal manifestations such as peptic ulcer disease and diarrhoea are more commonly attributed to the release of biologically active mediators than to infiltration of the gastrointestinal tract by excessive numbers of abnormal mast cells {1033,1853}. Patients with severe mediator-related symptoms occurring in temporal association with substantially increased serum tryptase levels may be diagnosed with mast cell activation syndrome (MCAS) {43,4103, 4104}. However, MCAS is not considered a subset of systemic mastocytosis. This is because MCAS occurs not only in the

setting of systemic mastocytosis but also in patients with other disorders, including IgE-dependent allergic reactions. In some patients with MCAS, the diagnostic criteria for systemic mastocytosis are not fulfilled but clonal mast cells with the *KIT* D816V mutation or aberrant surface CD25 are found; these patients are diagnosed with monoclonal MCAS. Patients with monoclonal MCAS and those with mediator-related symptoms and systemic mastocytosis are collectively designated as having primary (clonal) MCAS {4104}. The additional diagnosis of MCAS in the setting of systemic mastocytosis has clinical and therapeutic implications, and should therefore be included in the medical record in the same way as the presence or absence of B symptoms (i.e. fever, night sweats and weight loss) are documented in lymphomas.

The haematological abnormalities associated with systemic mastocytosis include anaemia, leukocytosis, eosinophilia (a common finding), neutropenia and thrombocytopenia {228,1694,2094, 3064}. Bone marrow failure occurs only in patients with aggressive or leukaemic disease variants. Significant numbers of circulating mast cells are rarely observed in systemic mastocytosis; when present, they suggest mast cell leukaemia {4107}. In as many as 30% of systemic mastocytosis cases, an associated haematological neoplasm is diagnosed before, simultaneously with, or after systemic mastocytosis. In principle, any defined myeloid or lymphoid malignancy can occur as an associated haematological neoplasm, but myeloid neoplasms predominate, with chronic myelomonocytic leukaemia and myelodysplastic/myeloproliferative neoplasm, unclassifiable being most common {1694,1696,1697, 3735,3751,3793}. In patients with systemic mastocytosis with an associated

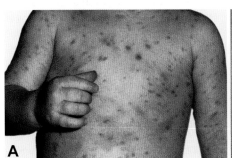 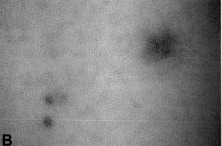 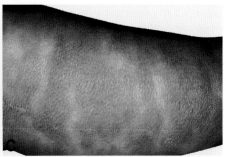

Fig. 3.01 Cutaneous mastocytosis. **A** Numerous typical macular and maculopapular pigmented lesions of urticaria pigmentosa in a young child. **B** The skin lesions of all forms of cutaneous mastocytosis may urticate when stroked (Darier's sign). A palpable wheal appears a few moments after the physical stimulation, due to the release of histamine from the mast cells. **C** Thickened, reddish, *peau chagrine* lesions characteristic of diffuse cutaneous mastocytosis, which occur almost exclusively in children.

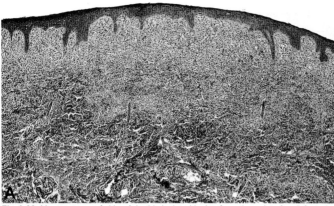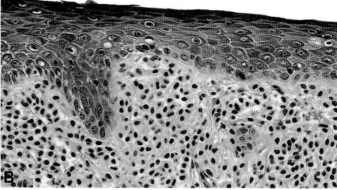

Fig. 3.02 Mastocytoma of skin. **A** In this isolated lesion from the wrist of an infant, the papillary dermis and reticular dermis are filled with mast cells. **B** At high magnification, the bland appearance of the mast cell infiltrate is apparent.

haematological neoplasm, the clinical symptoms, disease course and prognosis relate both to systemic mastocytosis and to the associated haematological disorder {2329,3751,4107}; in many cases, the clinical outcome is determined primarily by the associated haematological neoplasm {570,3928}. Therefore, both the type of systemic mastocytosis and the type of associated haematological neoplasm should be classified according to the WHO criteria in all cases.

Serum tryptase levels are used in the evaluation and monitoring of patients with mastocytosis. Serum total tryptase persistently > 20 ng/mL suggests systemic mastocytosis, and is a minor criterion for diagnosis (unless there is an associated myeloid neoplasm, in which case this parameter is not valid). In most patients with cutaneous mastocytosis, serum tryptase levels are normal to slightly elevated {3591,4107}.

Microscopy

The diagnosis of mastocytosis is usually based on the demonstration of multifocal clusters or cohesive aggregates/infiltrates of mast cells in adequate biopsy specimens (Table 3.02, p. 63). The histological pattern of the mast cell infiltrate can vary depending on the tissue sampled {1568, 1698,4107}. A diffuse interstitial infiltration pattern is defined as loosely scattered mast cells in the absence of compact aggregates. However, this pattern is also observed in reactive mast cell hyperplasia and in some myeloproliferative neoplasms, including cases in which elevated numbers of immature atypical mast cells are found but the criteria for systemic mastocytosis or mast cell leukaemia are not met {1696}. In patients with the

diffuse infiltration pattern, it is therefore impossible to establish the diagnosis of mastocytosis without additional studies, including the demonstration of an aberrant immunophenotype and/or detection of an activating point mutation in *KIT* {1698,1699,2122,3735,3736}. In contrast, the presence of multifocal compact mast cell infiltrates or a diffuse–compact mast cell infiltration pattern is highly compatible with the diagnosis of mastocytosis. However, additional immunohistochemical and molecular studies are strongly recommended even in these cases.

In tissue sections stained with haematoxylin and eosin, normal/reactive mast cells are usually loosely scattered throughout the sample and display round to oval nuclei with clumped chromatin, a low nuclear:cytoplasmic ratio, and absent or indistinct nucleoli. The mast cell cytoplasm is abundant and usually filled with small, faintly visible granules. Dense aggregates of mast cells are only very exceptionally detected in reactive states {2268,3074,4107}.

In smear preparations, mast cells are readily visible with Romanowsky staining as medium-sized round or oval cells with plentiful cytoplasm, containing densely packed metachromatic granules and round or oval nuclei. In normal/reactive states, mast cells are easily distinguished from basophils, which have segmented nuclei and larger and fewer granules. Enzyme cytochemistry shows that mast cells react strongly with naphthol AS-D chloroacetate esterase (CAE) but do not express myeloperoxidase. In mastocytosis, the cytology of mast cells varies, but abnormal cytological features (including marked spindling and hypogranularity) are almost always present {3750,4107}.

In high-grade mastocytosis lesions, cytological atypia is pronounced, and the occurrence of metachromatic blast cells is a typical feature of mast cell leukaemia {4107,4108}. The finding of frequent mast cells with bilobated or multilobated nuclei (called promastocytes) usually indicates an aggressive mast cell proliferation, although these cells may also be seen at lower frequency in other subtypes of the disease. Mitotic figures do occur in mast cells, but are infrequent even in the aggressive and leukaemic variants of systemic mastocytosis. In a few patients with systemic mastocytosis, the mast cells are mature and well granulated, without atypia or aberrant CD25 expression; such cases have been referred to as well-differentiated systemic mastocytosis. In most of these cases, no *KIT* mutation at codon 816 is found, and the mast cells usually respond to KIT tyrosine kinase inhibitors, including imatinib {42, 83}. However, well-differentiated morphology of mast cells can be present in any variant of systemic mastocytosis. Therefore, well-differentiated systemic mastocytosis is not considered a distinct category of systemic mastocytosis.

The number of mast cells can be assessed by conventional staining procedures, using Giemsa or toluidine blue staining to detect the metachromatic mast cell granules; CAE is also helpful {1698}. However, the most specific methods for identifying immature or atypical mast cells in tissue sections involve immunohistochemical staining for tryptase/chymase and KIT (CD117), and, for identifying neoplastic mast cells, CD25 or less commonly CD2. In a subset of cases, mast cells also express CD30 {2729,3734}. Aberrant expression of surface markers, including

CD2 and CD25, can also be detected by flow cytometry {1114}. The morphological and clinical features of the common forms of mastocytosis are described in the following sections on each variant.

Cutaneous mastocytosis

Definition
The diagnosis of cutaneous mastocytosis (CM) requires the demonstration of typical clinical findings and histological proof of abnormal mast cell infiltration of the dermis. In cutaneous mastocytosis, there is no evidence of systemic involvement in the bone marrow or any other organ. In addition, the diagnostic criteria for systemic mastocytosis are not fulfilled. However, patients with cutaneous mastocytosis may present with one or two of the minor diagnostic criteria for systemic mastocytosis, such as an elevated serum tryptase level or abnormal morphology of mast cells in the bone marrow (Table 3.02, p. 63).

Three major variants of cutaneous mastocytosis are recognized: urticaria pigmentosa/maculopapular cutaneous mastocytosis, diffuse cutaneous mastocytosis and mastocytoma of skin {4105,4107}.

ICD-O code   9740/1

Synonyms
Maculopapular cutaneous mastocytosis; diffuse cutaneous mastocytosis; solitary mastocytoma of skin; urticaria pigmentosa

Urticaria pigmentosa/maculopapular cutaneous mastocytosis
This is the most common form of cutaneous mastocytosis. In children, the lesions of urticaria pigmentosa tend to be larger, fewer, and more papular than the skin lesions seen in adults with systemic mastocytosis. Recent data suggest that monomorphic small lesions detected in early childhood are more likely to persist into adulthood than are larger polymorphic lesions {569,1567}. Histopathology typically reveals aggregates of spindle-shaped mast cells filling the papillary dermis and extending as sheets and aggregates into the reticular dermis, often in perivascular and periadnexal distribution {4353}. A subset of cases, usually occurring in young children, present as non-pigmented plaque-forming lesions.

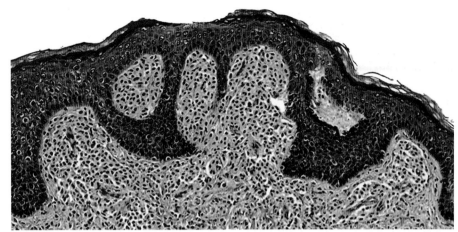

Fig. 3.03 Urticaria pigmentosa. In this typical skin lesion in a child, aggregates of mast cells fill the papillary dermis and extend as sheets into the reticular dermis.

In adults, the lesions are disseminated and they tend to be red or brownish red and macular or maculopapular. Histopathology of urticaria pigmentosa in adults typically reveals fewer mast cells than are seen in children. However, as mentioned above, cutaneous mastocytosis is very rare in adults; upon thorough bone marrow examination, most adult patients with skin lesions are found to have systemic mastocytosis. The number of lesional mast cells can sometimes overlap with the upper range of mast cell counts found in normal or inflamed skin. In some cases, examination of multiple biopsies and immunohistochemical analysis may be necessary to establish the diagnosis of cutaneous mastocytosis {4105,4353}. Various *KIT* mutations, including D816V, have been detected in lesional skin in childhood cutaneous mastocytosis.

Diffuse cutaneous mastocytosis
This clinically remarkable variant of cutaneous mastocytosis is much less common than urticaria pigmentosa and presents almost exclusively in childhood. The skin is diffusely thickened and may have a grain leather *(peau chagrine)* or orange peel *(peau d'orange)* appearance. There are no individual lesions. In patients with clinically less obvious infiltration of the skin, the biopsy usually shows a band-like infiltrate of mast cells in the papillary and upper reticular dermis. In massively infiltrated skin, the histology may be the same as that seen in mastocytoma of skin {1568,4353}.

Mastocytoma of skin
This variant typically occurs as a single lesion, almost exclusively in children, and without predilection for site {576,4353}. In some cases, two or three lesions occur. Histology shows sheets of mature-looking, highly metachromatic mast cells with abundant cytoplasm, which densely infiltrate the papillary and reticular dermis. These mast cell infiltrates may extend into the subcutaneous tissues. Cytological

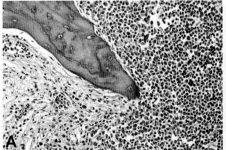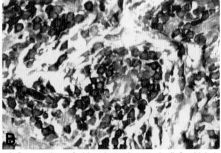

Fig. 3.04 Systemic mastocytosis, bone marrow biopsy. **A** One region of this photomicrograph (left side) is occupied by mast cells with fibrosis, whereas the adjacent area is hypercellular, with panmyelosis. In cases like this, it is important to consider the diagnosis of systemic mastocytosis with an associated haematological neoplasm. **B** Mast cells usually demonstrate metachromatic granules on Giemsa or toluidine blue staining. However, the most specific methods for identifying mast cells in tissue sections are immunohistochemical staining for tryptase/chymase and KIT (CD117), and for identifying neoplastic mast cells, CD2 and CD25.

Table 3.03 Diagnostic criteria for the variants of systemic mastocytosis

<table>
<tr><td>

Indolent systemic mastocytosis

Meets the general criteria for systemic mastocytosis

No C findings[a]

No evidence of an associated haematological neoplasm

Low mast cell burden

Skin lesions are almost invariably present

Bone marrow mastocytosis

As above (indolent systemic mastocytosis), but with bone marrow involvement and no skin lesions

Smouldering systemic mastocytosis

Meets the general criteria for systemic mastocytosis

≥2 B findings; no C findings[a]

No evidence of an associated haematological neoplasm

High mast cell burden

Does not meet the criteria for mast cell leukaemia

Systemic mastocytosis with an associated haematological neoplasm

Meets the general criteria for systemic mastocytosis

Meets the criteria for an associated haematological neoplasm (i.e. a myelodysplastic syndrome, myeloproliferative neoplasm, acute myeloid leukaemia, lymphoma or another haematological neoplasm classified as a distinct entity in the WHO classification)

Aggressive systemic mastocytosis

Meets the general criteria for systemic mastocytosis

≥1 C finding[a]

Does not meet the criteria for mast cell leukaemia

Skin lesions are usually absent.

Mast cell leukaemia

Meets the general criteria for systemic mastocytosis

Bone marrow biopsy shows diffuse infiltration (usually dense) by atypical, immature mast cells.
Bone marrow aspirate smears show ≥20% mast cells.
In classic cases, mast cells account for ≥10% of the peripheral blood white blood cells, but the aleukaemic variant (in which mast cells account for <10%) is more common.
Skin lesions are usually absent.

</td></tr>
</table>

[a] B and C findings indicate organ involvement without and with organ dysfunction, respectively; these findings are listed in Table 3.04.

Table 3.04 B ('burden of disease') and C ('cytoreduction-requiring') findings in systemic mastocytosis, which indicate organ involvement without and with organ dysfunction, respectively

B findings

1. High mast cell burden (shown on bone marrow biopsy): >30% infiltration of cellularity by mast cells (focal, dense aggregates) and serum total tryptase >200 ng/mL
2. Signs of dysplasia or myeloproliferation in non–mast cell lineage(s), but criteria are not met for definitive diagnosis of an associated haematological neoplasm, with normal or only slightly abnormal blood counts
3. Hepatomegaly without impairment of liver function, palpable splenomegaly without hypersplenism and/or lymphadenopathy on palpation or imaging

C findings

1. Bone marrow dysfunction caused by neoplastic mast cell infiltration, manifested by ≥1 cytopenia: absolute neutrophil count $< 1.0 \times 10^9$/L, haemoglobin level <10 g/dL, and/or platelet count $< 100 \times 10^9$/L
2. Palpable hepatomegaly with impairment of liver function, ascites and/or portal hypertension
3. Skeletal involvement, with large osteolytic lesions with or without pathological fractures (pathological fractures caused by osteoporosis do not qualify as a C finding)
4. Palpable splenomegaly with hypersplenism
5. Malabsorption with weight loss due to gastrointestinal mast cell infiltrates

---

atypia is absent, which enables the distinction of mastocytoma from an extremely rare mast cell sarcoma of the skin.

Systemic mastocytosis

Definition

Consensus criteria for the diagnosis of systemic mastocytosis have been established (Table 3.02, p. 63), and five variants are recognized: indolent systemic mastocytosis, smouldering systemic mastocytosis, systemic mastocytosis with an associated haematological neoplasm, aggressive systemic mastocytosis and mast cell leukaemia.

Table 3.03 summarizes the specific diagnostic criteria for each variant of systemic mastocytosis.

Indolent systemic mastocytosis

In indolent systemic mastocytosis (ISM), the mast cell burden is usually low and skin lesions are found in most patients. For cases that fulfil the criteria for indolent systemic mastocytosis and also present with one B finding (Table 3.04), the diagnosis remains indolent systemic mastocytosis. However, if two or more B findings are detected, the diagnosis changes to smouldering systemic mastocytosis. The KIT D816V mutation is present in the vast majority (>90%) of typical indolent systemic mastocytosis cases. If this mutation is not found but there remains high suspicion of systemic mastocytosis (e.g. in patients with well-differentiated mast cell morphology or advanced infiltration of the bone marrow), the KIT gene should be sequenced if possible, because other KIT mutations have been found in some patients.

ICD-O code   9741/1

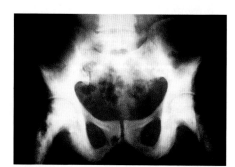

Fig. 3.05 Systemic mastocytosis. Skeletal lesions are common in systemic mastocytosis. This X-ray shows patchy osteosclerosis, osteoporosis and multiple lytic lesions in the femur.

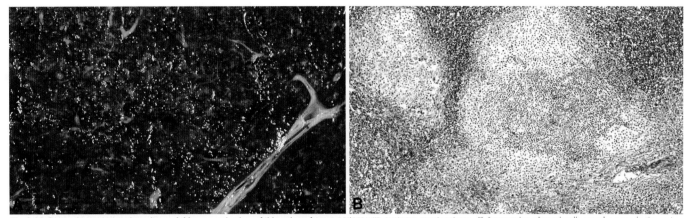

Fig. 3.06 Systemic mastocytosis, spleen. **A** Macroscopic view of this spleen from a patient with systemic mastocytosis. **B** Aggregates of mast cells may be seen in the red or white pulp, or in both. In this case, the mast cells have prominent, lightly stained cytoplasm and are seen in a perifollicular location.

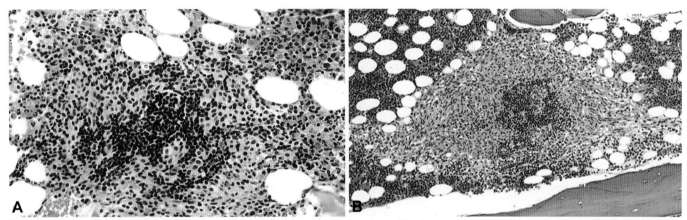

Fig. 3.07 Systemic mastocytosis, bone marrow biopsy. **A** The lesions often consist of a central core of lymphocytes surrounded by polygonal mast cells with pale, faintly granular cytoplasm, and with reactive eosinophils at the outer margin of the lesion. **B** The lesions are often well circumscribed; they may occur in paratrabecular or perivascular locations, or may be randomly distributed within the intertrabecular regions.

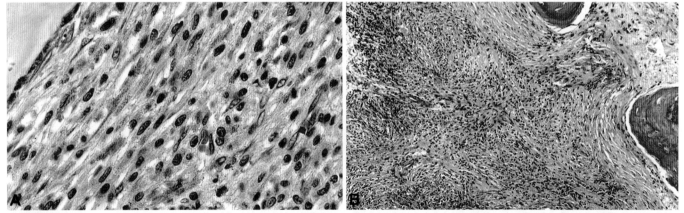

Fig. 3.08 Systemic mastocytosis, bone marrow biopsy. **A** Densely packed, spindled mast cells along a bone trabecula in paratrabecular infiltration of marrow. **B** The monomorphic, spindled mast cells are often accompanied by fibrosis and may replace large areas of the bone marrow biopsy specimen. Osteosclerosis often accompanies such lesions.

Bone marrow mastocytosis

In the bone marrow mastocytosis subtype of indolent systemic mastocytosis, the burden of neoplastic mast cells is usually low, and serum tryptase levels are often normal or nearly normal.

Smouldering systemic mastocytosis

In smouldering systemic mastocytosis, the mast cell burden is high, organomegaly is often found, and multilineage involvement is typically present. Although the clinical course is often stable for many years, progression to aggressive systemic mastocytosis or mast cell leukaemia

can occur. Skin lesions are found in most patients and the *KIT* D816V mutation is almost invariably present; unlike in typical indolent systemic mastocytosis, the mutation is usually detectable in several myeloid lineages and sometimes even in lymphocytes, reflecting multilineage involvement by the neoplastic process

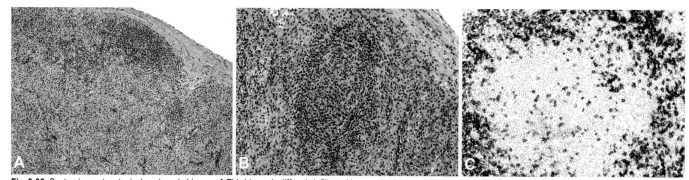

Fig. 3.09 Systemic mastocytosis, lymph node biopsy. **A** This biopsy is diffusely infiltrated by neoplastic mast cells; only a remnant of a normal follicle can be seen. **B** The infiltrate is often parafollicular in distribution; it is seen here as a monotonous population of cells with abundant, lightly staining cytoplasm. **C** Immunohistochemical staining for mast cell tryptase highlights the parafollicular distribution of the mast cell infiltrate.

despite a lack of morphological evidence of an associated haematological neoplasm.

Systemic mastocytosis with an associated haematological neoplasm

Systemic mastocytosis with an associated haematological neoplasm (AHN) fulfils the general criteria for systemic mastocytosis as well as the criteria for an AHN. In most cases, a myeloid disease of non–mast cell lineage is detected, such as a myelodysplastic syndrome, myeloproliferative neoplasm, myelodysplastic/myeloproliferative neoplasm or acute myeloid leukaemia {4107}. The AHN should usually be considered a secondary neoplasm with clinical and prognostic implications. The most commonly detected AHN is chronic myelomonocytic leukaemia. Lymphoid neoplasms, such as multiple myeloma and lymphoma, are rare. The activating *KIT* D816V mutation is found in most cases of systemic mastocytosis with an AHN, and in many cases is detectable not only in the systemic mastocytosis compartment but also in the AHN cells (e.g. acute myeloid leukaemia blasts or chronic myelomonocytic leukaemia monocytes). Depending on the type of AHN, additional mutations in other genes (e.g. *TET2*, *SRSF2*, *ASXL1*, *CBL*, *RUNX1* and the RAS family of oncogenes) may also be detected, and the accumulation of such mutations appears to be of prognostic significance.

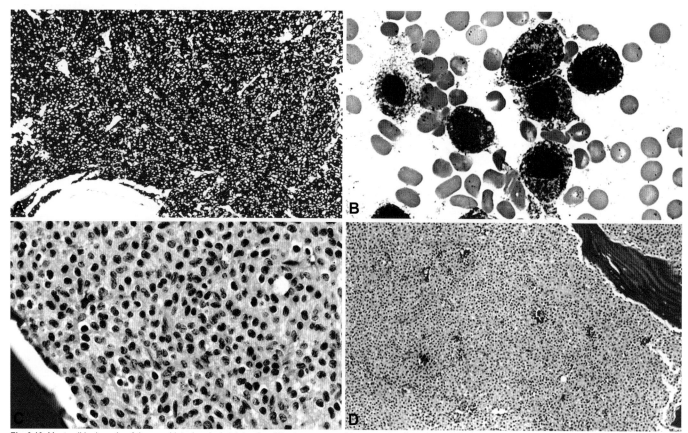

Fig. 3.10 Mast cell leukaemia. **A** Immunohistochemical staining for of the bone marrow biopsy mast cell tryptase. **B** Peripheral blood; note the bilobated nuclei and granulated cytoplasm often seen in this aggressive form of mastocytosis. **C** This image demonstrates the so-called clear-cell appearance and the folded, somewhat monocytoid nuclei that are typical of immature mast cells in mast cell leukaemia. **D** The bone marrow biopsy is diffusely infiltrated by the neoplastic mast cells.

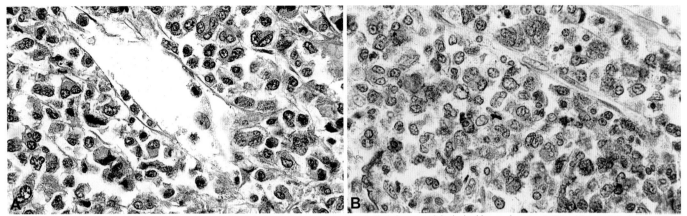

Fig. 3.11 Mast cell sarcoma. **A** This tumour is composed of poorly differentiated neoplastic cells that show no cytological evidence of mast cell differentiation. **B** On immunohistochemistry, the neoplastic cells stain for mast cell tryptase, which confirms the tumour's mast cell origin.

ICD-O code   9741/3

Synonyms

Systemic mastocytosis with an associated clonal haematological non–mast cell lineage disease (SH-AHNMD)

Aggressive systemic mastocytosis

In aggressive systemic mastocytosis (ASM), mast cells in bone marrow smears may be increased in number, but account for <20% of all nucleated bone marrow cells; cases in which the percentage of mast cells in bone marrow smears is >5% are diagnosed as ASM in transformation {4108}. In these cases, progression to mast cell leukaemia is common. Most patients with ASM have no skin lesions. One or more B findings (Table 3.04, p. 66) may be detected in patients with ASM, indicating a high burden of neoplastic cells. In a subset of patients, progressive lymphadenopathy and eosinophilia are found; these cases must be distinguished from myeloid/lymphoid neoplasms with *PDGFRA* rearrangements. The other major differential diagnoses are smouldering systemic mastocytosis and systemic mastocytosis with an associated haematological neoplasm. Most cases of ASM harbour the *KIT* D816V mutation. Additional mutations in other genes may also be found, but are more frequently identified in systemic mastocytosis with an associated haematological neoplasm.

ICD-O code   9741/3

Mast cell leukaemia

Mast cell leukaemia (MCL) is the leukaemic variant of systemic mastocytosis, in which bone marrow aspirate smears contain ≥ 20% mast cells {4107}. These mast cells are usually immature and atypical. Unlike in indolent systemic mastocytosis, the mast cells are often round rather than spindle-shaped. In classic mast cell leukaemia, mast cells account for ≥ 10% of the peripheral white blood cells, but the aleukaemic variant (the definition of which differs only in that the mast cells account for < 10% of peripheral blood white blood cells) is more common {4107, 4108}. In most patients with mast cell leukaemia, no skin lesions are detectable. Bone marrow biopsy shows a diffuse, dense infiltration with atypical, immature mast cells. C findings (Table 3.04, p. 66), indicative of organ damage caused by the malignant mast cell infiltration, are usually present at diagnosis {4107}, although rare cases present without them. Such cases, in which the mast cells are often mature and the clinical course less aggressive, constitute chronic mast cell leukaemia {4108}. In general, however, the prognosis of mast cell leukaemia is poor, with a survival of < 1 year in most patients. Unlike indolent systemic mastocytosis, mast cell leukaemia may harbour atypical *KIT* mutations, such as non-D816V codon 816 mutations or non–codon 816 mutations. Therefore, if a case of mast cell leukaemia is negative for the *KIT* D816V mutation, *KIT* should be sequenced if possible. Patients with mast cell leukaemia may also accumulate mutations in other genes, such as *TET2*, *SRSF2* and *CBL*.

ICD-O code   9742/3

Synonym

Systemic tissue mast cell disease

Mast cell sarcoma

Definition

Mast cell sarcoma (MCS) is an extremely rare entity characterized by localized destructive growth of highly atypical mast cells, which can be identified only through the application of appropriate immunohistochemical markers, such as antibodies specific for tryptase and KIT (CD117). Although the disease is initially localized, distant spread followed by a terminal phase resembling mast cell leukaemia occurs after a short interval of several months. Mast cell sarcomas have been reported occurring in the larynx, large bowel, meninges, bone and skin {745,1693, 2073,3461}.

ICD-O code   9740/3

Synonyms

Malignant mast cell tumour; malignant mastocytoma

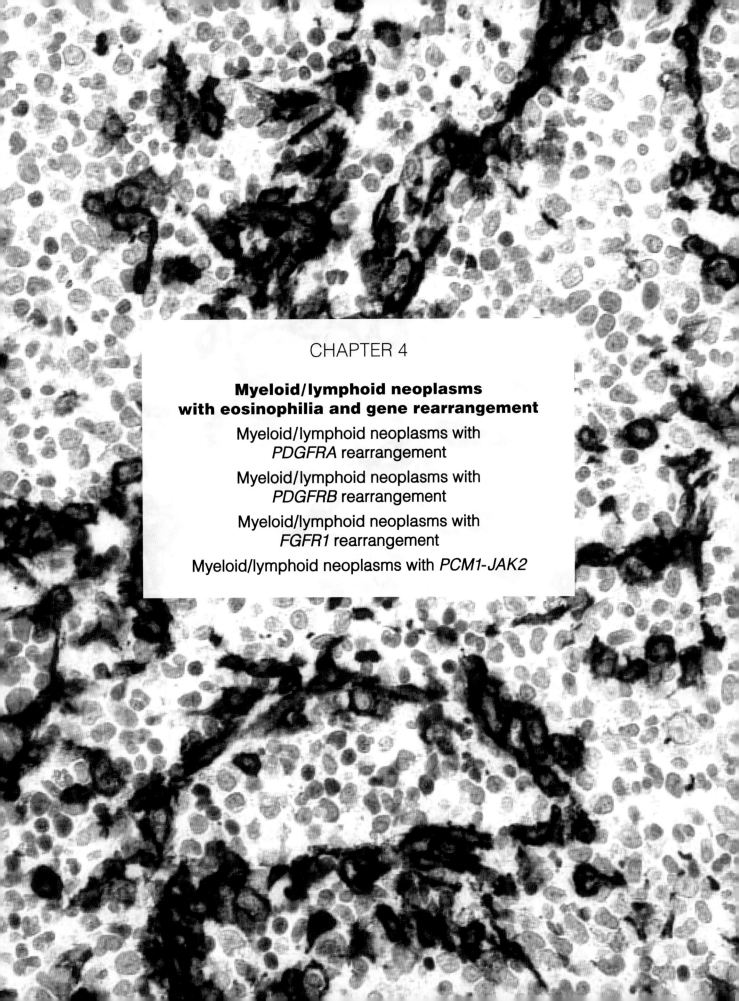

CHAPTER 4

Myeloid/lymphoid neoplasms with eosinophilia and gene rearrangement

Myeloid/lymphoid neoplasms with *PDGFRA* rearrangement

Myeloid/lymphoid neoplasms with *PDGFRB* rearrangement

Myeloid/lymphoid neoplasms with *FGFR1* rearrangement

Myeloid/lymphoid neoplasms with *PCM1-JAK2*

Myeloid / lymphoid neoplasms with eosinophilia and rearrangement of *PDGFRA, PDGFRB* or *FGFR1*, or with *PCM1-JAK2*

Bain B.J.
Horny H.-P.
Arber D.A.
Tefferi A.
Hasserjian R.P.

The category 'myeloid/lymphoid neoplasms with eosinophilia and rearrangement of *PDGFRA, PDGFRB* or *FGFR1*, or with *PCM1-JAK2*' contains three specific rare disease groups and a provisional entity. Within this category, some features are shared and others differ, but all the neoplasms result from the formation of a fusion gene, or (rarely) from a mutation, resulting in the expression of an aberrant tyrosine kinase. Eosinophilia is characteristic but not invariable. In at least some cases in each group, the cell of origin is a mutated pluripotent (lymphoid–myeloid) stem cell.

These disorders can present as chronic myeloproliferative neoplasms (MPNs), but the frequency of manifestation as lymphoid neoplasms or acute myeloid leukaemia varies. The clinical and haematological features are also influenced by the partner gene involved. *PDGFRA*-related disorders usually present as chronic eosinophilic leukaemia with prominent involvement of the mast cell lineage and sometimes the neutrophil lineage. Less often, they present as acute myeloid leukaemia or T-lymphoblastic leukaemia/lymphoma, with accompanying eosinophilia in either case. Uncommonly, there is B-lymphoblastic transformation {4050}. In the setting of *PDGFRB*-related disease, the features of the MPN are more variable, but are often those of chronic myelomonocytic leukaemia with eosinophilia. The proliferation of aberrant mast cells can also be a feature. Acute transformation is usually myeloid, but there have been reports of at least two cases of T-lymphoblastic transformation {726,2977} and one case of unspecified lymphoblastic transformation {2649}. In the setting of *FGFR1*-related disease, lymphomatous presentations are common, in particular T-lymphoblastic leukaemia/lymphoma with accompanying eosinophilia. Other presentations include chronic eosinophilic leukaemia, B-lymphoblastic leukaemia/lymphoma,

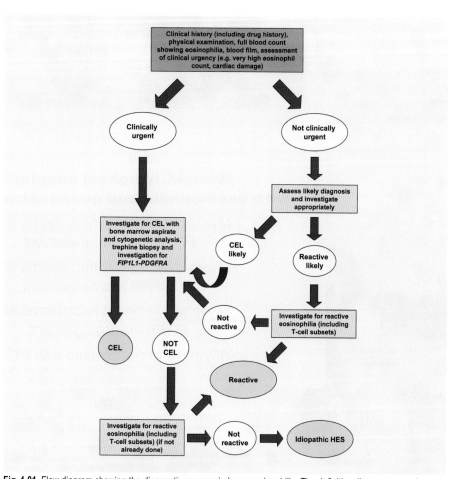

Fig. 4.01 Flow diagram showing the diagnostic process in hypereosinophilia. The definitive diagnoses are shown in blue. CEL, chronic eosinophilic leukaemia; HES, hypereosinophilic syndrome.

and acute myeloid leukaemia. *PCM1-JAK2*–related cases can undergo myeloblastic or B-lymphoblastic transformation {230}.

Recognizing these disorders is important, because the aberrant tyrosine kinase activity can make the disease responsive to tyrosine kinase inhibitors. This therapeutic approach has already proven successful for the treatment of cases of *PDGFRA*- and *PDGFRB*-related disease, which are responsive to imatinib and some related tyrosine kinase inhibitors, and to some extent for the treatment of *PCM1-JAK2*–related disease, which is

responsive to ruxolitinib. Related cases with *ETV6-JAK2* or *BCR-JAK2* may respond to JAK2 inhibitors. A similar specific therapy has not yet been developed for *FGFR1*-related disease. The relevant cytogenetic analysis and/or molecular genetic analysis should be carried out in all cases in which MPN with eosinophilia is suspected, as well as in cases presenting with an acute leukaemia or lymphoblastic lymphoma with eosinophilia. The identification of *PDGFRA*-related disease usually requires molecular genetic analysis (because most cases result from a cryptic deletion), whereas cytogenetic analysis can reveal the causative abnormality in cases related to *PDGFRB*, *FGFR1*, or *JAK2*.

Myeloid/lymphoid neoplasms with PDGFRA rearrangement

Definition
The most common myeloproliferative neoplasm associated with *PDGFRA* rearrangement is that associated with *FIP1L1-PDGFRA* gene fusion, which occurs as a result of a cryptic deletion at 4q12 {798} (see Table 4.01). These neoplasms generally present as chronic eosinophilic leukaemia (CEL), but can also present as acute myeloid leukaemia, T-lymphoblastic leukaemia/lymphoma, or both simultaneously {2650}. Acute transformation can follow presentation as CEL. Organ damage occurs as a result of leukaemic infiltration or the release of cytokines, enzymes or other proteins by eosinophils and possibly also by mast cells. The peripheral blood eosinophil count is usually markedly elevated, although it should be noted that, in some series of cases, investigation was limited to cases with eosinophilia. A small number of cases that lacked eosinophilia have been reported {1829,3450}. There is no Philadelphia (Ph) chromosome or *BCR-ABL1* fusion gene. Except when there is transformation to acute leukaemia, there are < 20% blasts in the peripheral blood and bone marrow.

Variants
Several possible molecular variants of *FIP1L1-PDGFRA*–associated CEL have been recognized in which other fusion genes incorporate part of *PDGFRA*. A male patient with imatinib-responsive CEL was found to have a *KIF5B-PDGFRA* fusion gene associated with a complex chromosomal abnormality involving chromosomes 3, 4 and 10 {3598}, and a female patient had a *CDK5RAP2-PDGFRA* fusion gene associated with ins(9;4) (q33;q12q25) {4235}. One case in a male patient with t(2;4)(p24;q12) and *STRN-PDGFRA* fusion {849} and another case in a male patient with t(4;12)(q12;p13.2) and an *ETV6-PDGFRA* fusion gene, both with the haematological features of CEL, responded to low-dose imatinib {849}. A case with *FIP1L1-PDGFRA* had the features of an atypical myeloproliferative neoplasm without eosinophilia {2900}.

Neoplasms with t(4;22)(q12;q11.2) and a *BCR-PDGFRA* fusion gene, at least 9 cases of which have been described, have disease characteristics intermediate between those of *FIP1L1-PDGFRA*–associated eosinophilic leukaemia and those of *BCR-ABL1*–positive chronic myeloid leukaemia; eosinophilia may or may not be prominent {298,1312,3471, 4050}. Accelerated phase, T-lymphoblastic transformation and B-lymphoblastic transformation {298,4050} have been reported. The disease is imatinib-sensitive {34/1,4050} and a tyrosine kinase inhibitor would normally be included in the treatment regime. One case has been reported of imatinib-sensitive CEL associated with t(4;10)(q12;q23.3) and *TNKS2-PDGFRA* {637}. CEL can also result from an activating point mutation in *PDGFRA* {1093}.

ICD-O code   9965/3

Synonyms
Myeloid and lymphoid neoplasms with *PDGFRA* rearrangement; myeloid and lymphoid neoplasms associated with *PDGFRA* rearrangement

Epidemiology
The *FIP1L1-PDGFRA* syndrome is rare. It is considerably more common in men than in women, with a male-to-female ratio of about 17:1. The peak incidence is between 25 and 55 years, with a me-

Table 4.01 Diagnostic criteria for myeloid/lymphoid neoplasms with eosinophilia associated with *FIP1L1-PDGFRA* or a variant fusion gene[a]

A myeloid or lymphoid neoplasm, usually with prominent eosinophilia
AND
The presence of *FIP1L1-PDGFRA* fusion gene or a variant fusion gene with rearrangement of *PDGFRA* or an activating mutation of *PDGFRA*[b]

[a] Cases presenting as a myeloproliferative neoplasm, acute myeloid leukaemia or lymphoblastic leukaemia/lymphoma with eosinophilia and *FIP1L1-PDGFRA* gene fusion are assigned to this category;
[b] If appropriate molecular analysis is not possible, this diagnosis should be suspected if there is a myeloproliferative neoplasm with no Philadelphia (Ph) chromosome and with the haematological features of chronic eosinophilic leukaemia associated with splenomegaly, marked elevation of serum vitamin B12, elevation of serum tryptase, and an increased number of bone marrow mast cells.

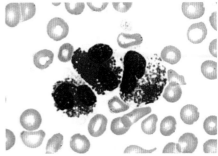

Fig. 4.02 *FIP1L1-PDGFRA*-related chronic eosinophilic leukaemia. Peripheral blood smear showing three moderately degranulated eosinophils (Romanowsky staining).

dian age at onset in the late 40s (range: 7–77 years) {233}.

Etiology
The cause is unknown, although several cases with *FIP1L1-PDGFRA* have occurred following cytotoxic chemotherapy {2946,3892}, as did a case with features resembling those of chronic myeloid leukaemia with a *BCR-PDGFRA* fusion gene {3471}.

Localization
CEL associated with *FIP1L1-PDGFRA* is a multisystem disorder. The peripheral blood and bone marrow are always involved. Tissue infiltration by eosinophils and the release of cytokines and humoral factors from the eosinophil granules result in tissue damage in a number of organs; the heart, lungs, central and peripheral nervous system, skin and gastrointestinal tract are commonly involved.

Clinical features
Patients usually present with fatigue or pruritus, or with respiratory, cardiac or gastrointestinal symptoms {798,2508, 4147}. Some patients are asymptomatic at diagnosis {1605}, but most have splenomegaly and some have hepatomegaly. The most serious clinical findings relate to endomyocardial fibrosis, with ensuing restrictive cardiomyopathy. Scarring of the mitral and/or tricuspid valves leads to valvular regurgitation and the formation of intracardiac thrombi, which may embolize. Venous thromboembolism and arterial thromboses can also occur. Pulmonary disease is restrictive and related to fibrosis; symptoms include dyspnoea and cough, and there may also be an obstructive element. Serum tryptase is elevated (> 12 ng/mL), usually to a lesser extent than in mast cell disease but with some overlap.

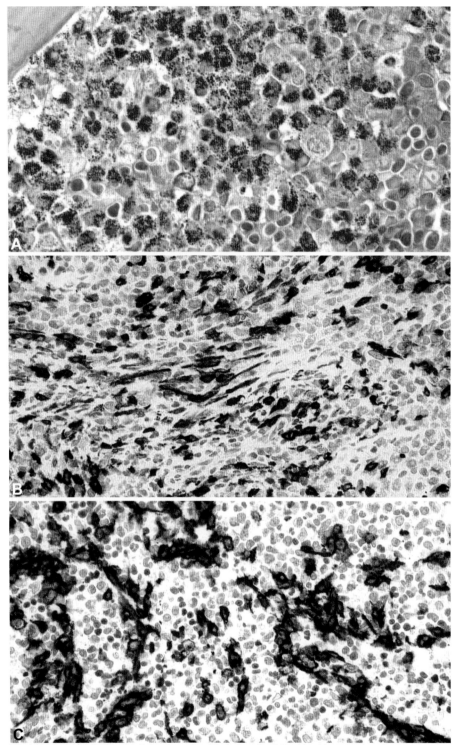

Fig. 4.03 *FIP1L1-PDGFRA*-related chronic eosinophilic leukaemia. **A** Trephine biopsy section showing abundant eosinophils and eosinophil precursors (Giemsa staining). **B** Trephine biopsy section showing abundant mast cells – many of which are spindle-shaped – forming small loose clusters (mast cell tryptase staining). **C** Trephine biopsy section showing CD25 expression in the mast cells.

promyelocytes. A range of eosinophil abnormalities can be present, including sparse granulation with clear areas of cytoplasm, cytoplasmic vacuolation, granules that are smaller than normal, immature granules that are purplish on Romanowsky staining, nuclear hyper- or hyposegmentation, and increased eosinophil size {798,4147}. However, these abnormalities can also be seen in cases of reactive eosinophilia {226} and in some cases of *FIP1L1-PDGFRA*–associated CEL the eosinophil morphology is close to normal. Only a minority of patients have any increase in the number of peripheral blast cells {4147}. Neutrophils may be increased, whereas basophil and monocyte counts are usually normal {3378}. Anaemia and thrombocytopenia are sometimes present.

Any tissue may show eosinophilic infiltration and Charcot–Leyden crystals may be present. The bone marrow is hypercellular, with markedly increased numbers of eosinophils and precursors. In most cases eosinophil maturation is orderly (without a disproportionate increase in blasts), but in some cases the proportion of blast cells is increased. There may be necrosis, particularly when the disease is becoming more acute {798}. The number of bone marrow mast cells seen on trephine biopsy is often increased {2045,3055}, and mast cell proliferation should be recognized as a feature of *FIP1L1-PDGFRA*–associated myeloproliferative neoplasm. The mast cells may be scattered, in loose non-cohesive clusters, or in cohesive clusters {2045,3055}. Many cases show a marked increase in spindle-shaped atypical mast cells, and in some cases the morphological features resemble those of systemic mastocytosis. Reticulin is increased {2045}.

Patients presenting with acute myeloid leukaemia or T-lymphoblastic leukaemia/lymphoma have been reported to have coexisting eosinophilia (i.e. peripheral blood counts of $1.4–17.2 \times 10^9$/L); in most cases, pre-existing eosinophilia was also documented {2650}.

Cytochemistry

Cytochemical stains are not necessary for diagnosis. The reduced granule content of the eosinophils can result in reduced peroxidase content and inaccurate automated eosinophil counts.

Serum vitamin B12 is markedly elevated {4147}. *FIP1L1-PDGFRA*–associated CEL is very responsive to imatinib; the FIP1L1-PDGFRA fusion protein is 100 times as sensitive as BCR-ABL1 {798}.

Microscopy

The most striking feature in the peripheral blood is eosinophilia. Most of the eosinophils are mature, with only small numbers of eosinophil myelocytes or

Immunophenotype

The eosinophils in this syndrome may show immunophenotypic evidence of activation, such as expression of CD23, CD25 and CD69 {2045}. The mast cells are usually CD2-negative and CD25-positive {2044}, but in some cases they are negative for both {2650} and in occasional cases they are positive for both {2650}. In comparison, the mast cells of systemic mastocytosis are CD25-positive in almost all cases and CD2-positive in about two thirds of cases.

Cell of origin

The cell of origin is a pluripotent haematopoietic stem cell that can give rise to eosinophils and (at least in some patients) neutrophils, monocytes, mast cells, T cells and B cells {3378}. The detection of the fusion gene in a given lineage does not necessarily correlate with morphological evidence of involvement of that lineage. For example, lymphocytosis is not typical, even in cases with apparent involvement of the B-cell or T-cell lineage {3378}. In chronic-phase disease, involvement is predominantly of eosinophils and to a lesser extent mast cells and neutrophils. Acute-phase disease can be myeloid, T-lymphoblastic {2650}, or (rarely) B-lymphoblastic {4050}.

Genetic profile

Cytogenetic findings are usually normal, with the *FIP1L1-PDGFRA* fusion gene resulting from a cryptic del(4)(q12). In some patients, there is a chromosomal rearrangement with a 4q12 breakpoint, such as t(1;4)(q44;q12) {798} or t(4;10) (q12;p11.1-p11.2) {3907}. In other patients, there is an unrelated cytogenetic abnormality (e.g. trisomy 8), which is likely to represent disease evolution. The fusion gene can be detected by reverse transcriptase-polymerase chain reaction (RT-PCR), with nested RT-PCR often being required {798}. The causative deletion can also be detected by FISH analysis, often using a probe for the *CHIC2* gene (which is uniformly deleted) or using a break-apart probe that encompasses *FIP1L1* and *PDGFRA*. Because most patients do not have increased blast cells or any abnormality on conventional cytogenetic analysis, it is usually the detection of the *FIP1L1-PDGFRA* fusion gene that enables the definitive diagnosis of this neoplasm. Cytogenetic abnormalities appear to be

more common when evolution to acute myeloid leukaemia has occurred {2650}.

Prognosis and predictive factors

Because *FIP1L1-PDGFRA*–associated CEL and its responsiveness to imatinib were not recognized until 2003 {798}, the long-term prognosis is still unknown. However, the prognosis appears to be favourable if cardiac damage has not yet occurred and imatinib treatment is available. Imatinib resistance can develop (e.g. as a result of a T674I mutation, which is equivalent to the T315I mutation that can occur in the *BCR-ABL1* gene) {798,1461}. Alternative tyrosine kinase inhibitors such as midostaurin (PKC412) and sorafenib may be effective in these patients {800,2326,3806}. Patients presenting with acute myeloid leukaemia or T-lymphoblastic leukaemia can achieve sustained complete molecular remission with imatinib {2650}.

Myeloid/lymphoid neoplasms with *PDGFRB* rearrangement

Definition

A distinct type of myeloid neoplasm occurs in association with rearrangement of *PDGFRB* at 5q32 (see Table 4.02). Usually there is t(5;12)(q32;p13.2) with formation of an *ETV6-PDGFRB* fusion gene {1398,1980}. In uncommon variants, other translocations with a 5q32 breakpoint lead to the formation of other fusion genes, also incorporating part of *PDGFRB* (see Table 4.03, p. 77). However, fusion genes typically associated only with *BCR-ABL1*–like B-lymphoblastic leukaemia are specifically excluded from this category; these include *EBF1-PDGFRB*, *SSBP2-PDGFRB*, *TNIP1-PDGFRB*, *ZEB2-PDGFRB* and *ATF7IP-PDGFRB* {2059,3370}. Cases with *ETV6-PDGFRB* that present as *BCR-ABL1*–like B-lymphoblastic leukaemia may be more appropriately assigned to that category. In cases with t(5;12) and in the variant translocations, there is synthesis of an aberrant, constitutively activated tyrosine kinase. The haematological features are most often those of chronic myelomonocytic leukaemia (usually with eosinophilia), but some cases have been characterized as atypical chronic myeloid leukaemia, *BCR-ABL1*–negative (usually with eosinophilia), chronic eosinophilic leukaemia

Table 4.02 Diagnostic criteria for myeloid/lymphoid neoplasms associated with *ETV6-PDGFRB* or other rearrangement of *PDGFRB* [a]

A myeloid or lymphoid neoplasm, often with prominent eosinophilia and sometimes with neutrophilia or monocytosis

AND

Presence of t(5;12)(q32;p13.2) or a variant translocation[a,b] or demonstration of *ETV6-PDGFRB* fusion gene or other rearrangement of *PDGFRB* [b]

[a] Cases with fusion genes typically associated only with *BCR-ABL1*–like B lymphoblastic leukaemia are specifically excluded (see text);
[b] Because t(5;12)(q32;p13.2) does not always result in *ETV6-PDGFRB* fusion, molecular confirmation is highly desirable; if molecular analysis is not possible, this diagnosis should be suspected if there is a myeloproliferative neoplasm associated with eosinophilia, with no Philadelphia (Ph) chromosome and with a translocation with a 5q32 breakpoint.

or myeloproliferative neoplasm (MPN) with eosinophilia {233,3776}. Single cases have been reported of acute myeloid leukaemia, probably superimposed on primary myelofibrosis {4013}, and of juvenile myelomonocytic leukaemia {2728}, the latter associated with a variant fusion gene. Eosinophilia is typical but not invariable {3776}. Acute transformation can occur, often in a relatively short period of time. MPNs with *PDGFRB* rearrangement are sensitive to tyrosine kinase inhibitors such as imatinib {123}.

Variants

A number of molecular variants of MPNs with *ETV6-PDGFRB* fusion have been reported {233,3776}. In addition, a patient who developed eosinophilia at relapse of acute myeloid leukaemia was found to have acquired t(5;14)(q32;q32.1), with a *TRIP11-PDGFRB* fusion gene. Other patients have rearrangement of *PDGFRB* with an unknown partner gene. Complex rearrangements appear to be common (e.g. a small inversion as well as translocation) {3776}. Because of the therapeutic implications of *PDGFRB* rearrangement, FISH (break-apart FISH with a *PDGFRB* probe) is indicated in all patients with a presumptive diagnosis of MPN with a 5q31-33 breakpoint, in particular if there is eosinophilia. However, FISH analysis does not always demonstrate rearrangement of *PDGFRB*, even when such rearrangement is detectable on Southern blot analysis {3776}. Molecular analysis

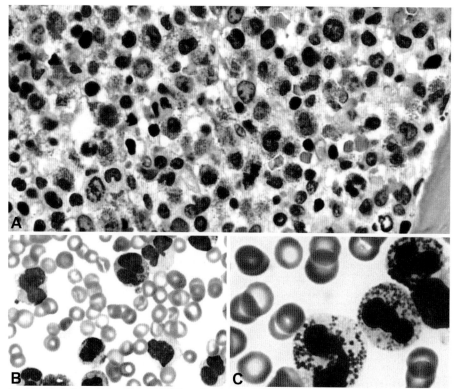

Fig. 4.04 Myeloid neoplasm with eosinophilia and rearrangement of *PDGFRB*. **A** Bone marrow trephine biopsy section from a patient with t(5;12) shows a marked increase in eosinophils. **B** Peripheral blood smear from a patient with t(5;12) shows numerous abnormal eosinophils, at lower (**B**) and higher (**C**) magnification. Eosinophils accounted for 40% of the leukocytes.

is not indicated when no 5q31-33 break-point is found by conventional cytogenetic analysis, because almost all cases reported to date in which 20 metaphases were available for examination have had a cytogenetically detectable abnormality.

ICD-O code   9966/3

Synonyms
Chronic myelomonocytic leukaemia with eosinophilia associated with t(5;12); myeloid neoplasms with *PDGFRB* rearrangement; myeloid neoplasms associated with *PDGFRB* rearrangement

Epidemiology
This neoplasm is considerably more common in men than in women (male-to-female ratio: 2:1) and occurs over a wide age range (8–72 years), with peak incidence in middle-aged adults and a median age of onset in the late 40s {3776}.

Localization
MPN associated with t(5;12)(q32;p13.2) is a multisystem disorder. The peripheral blood and bone marrow are always involved. The spleen is enlarged in most cases. Tissue infiltration by eosinophils and the release of cytokines, humoral factors or granule contents by eosinophils can contribute to tissue damage in several organs.

Clinical features
Most patients have splenomegaly and some have hepatomegaly. Some patients have skin infiltration and some have cardiac damage leading to cardiac failure. Serum tryptase may be mildly or moderately elevated. The vast majority of patients who have been treated with imatinib have been found to be responsive.

Microscopy
The white blood cell count is increased. There may be anaemia and thrombocytopenia. There is a variable increase in neutrophils, eosinophils, monocytes and eosinophil and neutrophil precursors. Rarely, there is a marked increase in basophils {4236}.
The bone marrow is hypercellular as a result of active granulopoiesis (neutrophilic and eosinophilic). Bone marrow trephine biopsy may show an increase in mast cells, which may be spindle-shaped

{858,4236}. Bone marrow reticulin may also be increased {4236}. In chronic-phase disease, blast cells account for <20% of the cells in the peripheral blood and bone marrow.

Cytochemistry
The eosinophils, neutrophils and monocytes show the cytochemical reactions expected for cells of these lineages.

Immunophenotype
Immunophenotypic analysis of the mast cells has shown expression of CD2 and CD25, which is also found in most cases of mast cell disease {4236}.

Cell of origin
The postulated cell of origin is a pluripotent haematopoietic stem cell that can give rise to neutrophils, monocytes, eosinophils, probably mast cells and (in some patients) B-cell lineage lymphoblasts.

Genetic profile
Cytogenetic analysis usually shows t(5;12)(q32;p13.2), with the translocation resulting in *ETV6-PDGFRB* gene fusion {1398} (previously called *TEL-PDGFRB*). In one patient, *ETV6-PDGFRB* fusion resulted from a four-way translocation: t(1;12;5;12)(p36;p13.2;q32;q24) {835}; in another, the fusion occurred in association with ins(2;12)(p21;q13q22) and del(5q) {883}. The 5q breakpoint is sometimes assigned to 5q31 and sometimes to 5q33, although the gene map locus of *PDGFRB* is 5q32.
Not all translocations characterized as t(5;12)(q31-33;p12) lead to *ETV6-PDGFRB* fusion. Cases without a fusion gene are not assigned to this category of MPN and, importantly, are not likely to respond to imatinib; in such cases, an alternative leukaemogenic mechanism is upregulation of interleukin 3 (IL3) {799}. Therefore, RT-PCR using primers suitable for all known breakpoints is recommended for confirmation of *ETV6-PDGFRB* {850}, but if molecular analysis is not available, a trial of imatinib is justified in patients with an MPN associated with t(5;12). Due to the large number of potential partner genes, molecular analysis to demonstrate variant fusion genes is only feasible after a translocation has been shown by cytogenetic analysis. If subsequent monitoring of treatment response is planned, the fusion

Table 4.03 Variant translocation–associated myeloid/lymphoid neoplasms with *PDGFRB* rearrangement [a]. Modified from Bain BJ and Fletcher SH {233}

Translocation	Fusion gene	Haematological diagnosis
t(1;3;5)(p36;p22.2;q32)	WDR48-PDGFRB	CEL
der(1)t(1;5)(p34;q32), der(5)t(1;5)(p34;q15), der(11)ins(11;5)(p13;q15q32)	CAPRIN1-PDGFRB	CEL
t(1;5)(q21.3;q32)	TPM3-PDGFRB	
t(1;5)(q21.2;q32)	PDE4DIP-PDGFRB	MDS/MPN with eosinophilia
t(2;5)(p16.2;q32)	SPTBN1-PDGFRB	
t(4;5;5)(q21.2;q31;q32)	PRKG2-PDGFRB	Chronic basophilic leukaemia
t(3;5)(p22.2;q32)	GOLGA4-PDGFRB	CEL or aCML with eosinophilia
Cryptic interstitial deletion of 5q	TNIP1-PDGFRB	CEL with thrombocytosis
t(5;7)(q32;q11.2)	HIP1-PDGFRB	CMML with eosinophilia
t(5;7)(q32;p14.1)	HECW1-PDGFRB	JMML
t(5;9)(q32;p24.3)	KANK1-PDGFRB	Essential thrombocythaemia without eosinophilia
t(5;10)(q32;q21.2)	CCDC6-PDGFRB	aCML with eosinophilia or MPN with eosinophilia
Uninformative	SART3-PDGFRB	MPN with eosinophilia and myelofibrosis
t(5;12)(q32;q24.1)	GIT2-PDGFRB	CEL
t(5;12)(q32;p13.3)	ERC1-PDGFRB	AML without eosinophilia
t(5;12)(q32;q13.1)	BIN2-PDGFRB	aCML with eosinophilia
t(5;14)(q32;q22.1)	NIN-PDGFRB	Ph-negative CML (13% eosinophils)
t(5;14)(q32;q32.1)	CCDC88C-PDGFRB	CMML with eosinophilia
t(5;15)(q32;q15.3)	TP53BP1-PDGFRB	Ph-negative CML with prominent eosinophilia
t(5;16)(q32;p13.1)	NDE1-PDGFRB	CMML
t(5;17)(q32;p13.2)	RABEP1-PDGFRB	CMML
t(5;17)(q32;p11.2)	SPECC1-PDGFRB	JMML
t(5;17)(q32;q11.2)	MYO18A-PDGFRB	MPN with eosinophilia
t(5;17)(q32;q21.3)	COL1A1-PDGFRB	MDS or MPN with eosinophilia
t(5;20)(q32;p11.2)	DTD1-PDGFRB	CEL

aCML, atypical chronic myeloid leukaemia, *BCR-ABL1*–negative; AML, acute myeloid leukaemia; CEL, chronic eosinophilic leukaemia; CML, chronic myeloid leukaemia; CMML, chronic myelomonocytic leukaemia; JMML, juvenile myelomonocytic leukaemia; MDS, myelodysplastic syndrome; MDS/MPN, myelodysplastic myeloproliferative neoplasm; MPN, myeloproliferative neoplasm; Ph, Philadelphia chromosome.

[a] Cases with fusion genes typically associated only with *BCR-ABL1*–like B-lymphoblastic leukaemia are specifically excluded (see text).

gene should be characterized at diagnosis by RT-PCR or RNA sequencing.

Prognosis and predictive factors

Before the introduction of imatinib therapy, the median survival was <2 years. Reliable survival data are not yet available for imatinib-treated patients, but in a small series (10 cases) the median survival was 65 months {883}. Median survival is likely to improve as patients are increasingly identified and started on appropriate treatment at the time of diagnosis rather than after cardiac damage or transformation has already occurred.

Myeloid/lymphoid neoplasms with *FGFR1* rearrangement

Definition

Haematological neoplasms with *FGFR1* rearrangement are heterogeneous. They are derived from a pluripotent haematopoietic stem cell; however, in different patients or at different stages of the disease the neoplastic cells may be precursor cells or mature cells. Cases can present as a myeloproliferative neoplasm or (in transformation) as acute myeloid leukaemia, T- or B-lymphoblastic leukaemia/lymphoma or mixed-phenotype acute leukaemia (see Table 4.04, p. 78). In one reported case, there was coexisting atypical chronic myeloid leukaemia, *BCR-ABL1*–negative, with t(8;19)(p11.2;q13.1) and *KIT* D816V–positive systemic mastocytosis {1051}. Such cases, which are rare, can be classified as systemic mastocytosis with an associated haematological neoplasm.

ICD-O code   9967/3

Synonyms

8p11 myeloproliferative syndrome; 8p11 stem cell syndrome; 8p11 stem cell leukaemia/lymphoma syndrome; haematopoietic stem cell neoplasm with *FGFR1* abnormalities; myeloid and lymphoid neoplasms with *FGFR1* abnormalities

Epidemiology

This neoplasm occurs across a wide age range (3–84 years), but most patients are young, with a median age at onset of about 32 years {2424}. Unlike in myeloid/lymphoid neoplasms with *PDGFRA* or *PDGFRB* rearrangement, there is only a moderate male predominance, with a male-to-female ratio of 1.5:1.

Localization

The tissues primarily involved are the bone marrow, peripheral blood, lymph nodes, liver and spleen. Lymphadenopathy occurs as a result of infiltration by either lymphoblasts or myeloid cells.

Clinical features

Some cases present as lymphoma with mainly lymph node involvement or with a mediastinal mass; others present with myeloproliferative features, such as splenomegaly and hypermetabolism, or with features of acute myeloid leukaemia or myeloid sarcoma {15,1760,2424,

Table 4.04 Diagnostic criteria for myeloid/lymphoid neoplasms with FGFR1 rearrangement

A myeloproliferative or myelodysplastic/myeloproliferative neoplasm with prominent eosinophilia and sometimes with neutrophilia or monocytosis

OR

Acute myeloid leukaemia, T- or B-lymphoblastic leukaemia/lymphoma, or mixed-phenotype acute leukaemia (usually associated with peripheral blood or bone marrow eosinophilia)

AND

The presence of t(8;13)(p11.2;q12) or a variant translocation leading to FGFR1 rearrangement, demonstrated in myeloid cells, lymphoblasts or both

4167}. Systemic symptoms such as fever, weight loss and night sweats are often present {233}.

Microscopy

Cases can present as chronic eosinophilic leukaemia, acute myeloid leukaemia, T-lymphoblastic leukaemia/lymphoma, or (least often) B-lymphoblastic leukaemia/lymphoma or mixed-phenotype acute leukaemia. In cases that present with chronic eosinophilic leukaemia, there may be subsequent transformation to acute myeloid leukaemia (including myeloid sarcoma), T- or B-lymphoblastic leukaemia/lymphoma, or mixed-phenotype acute leukaemia. Lymphoblastic lymphoma appears to be more common in patients with t(8;13) than in those with variant translocations {2424}. Patients who present in the chronic phase usually have eosinophilia and neutrophilia and occasionally have monocytosis. Those who present in acute transformation are also often found to have eosinophilia. Overall, about 90% of patients have peripheral blood or bone marrow eosinophilia {2424}. The eosinophils belong to the neoplastic clone, as do the lymphoblasts and myeloblasts in cases in acute transformation. Basophilia is not typical, but may be more common in cases with BCR-FGFR1 fusion {3429}, and has also been observed in association with t(1;8) (q31.1;p11.2) and TPR-FGFR1 {2298}. An association with polycythaemia vera has been reported in 3 cases with t(6;8)/FGFR1OP-FGFR1 fusion {3217, 4207}.

T-lymphoblastic leukaemia/lymphoma characteristically shows eosinophilic infiltration within the lymphoma, which can be a clue to this diagnosis.

Cases should be classified as leukaemia/lymphoma associated with FGFR1 rearrangement, followed by further details of the specific presentation; for example, 'leukaemia/lymphoma associated with FGFR1 rearrangement/chronic eosinophilic leukaemia, T-lymphoblastic leukaemia/lymphoma' or 'leukaemia/lymphoma associated with FGFR1 rearrangement/myeloid sarcoma'.

Cytochemistry

The neutrophil alkaline phosphatase score is often low, but cytochemistry is not diagnostically useful {2298}.

Immunophenotype

Immunophenotypic analysis is not useful in chronic phase disease, but is important in demonstrating the lineage in B- or T-lymphoblastic leukaemia/lymphoma and in acute myeloid transformation.

Cell of origin

A pluripotent lymphoid–myeloid haematopoietic stem cell

Table 4.05 Cytogenetics (chromosomal rearrangements) and molecular genetics (fusion genes) reported in myeloid/lymphoid neoplasms with FGFR1 rearrangement[a]. Modified from Bain BJ and Fletcher SH {233}, Macdonald D et al. {2424}

Cytogenetics	Molecular genetics
t(8;13)(p11.2;q12.1)	ZMYM2-FGFR1
t(8;9)(p11.2;q33.2)	CNTRL-FGFR1
t(6;8)(q27;p11.2)	FGFR1OP-FGFR1
t(8;22)(p11.2;q11.2)	BCR-FGFR1
t(7;8)(q33;p11.2)	TRIM24-FGFR1
t(8;17)(p11.2;q11.2)	MYO18A-FGFR1
t(8;19)(p11.2;q13.3)	HERVK-FGFR1
ins(12;8)(p11.2;p11.2p22)	FGFR1OP2-FGFR1
t(1;8)(q31.1;p11.2)	TPR-FGFR1
t(2;8)(q13;p11.2)	RANBP2-FGFR1
t(2;8)(q37.3;p11.2)	LRRFIP1-FGFR1
t(7;8)(q22.1;p11.2)	CUX1-FGFR1
t(8;12)(p11.2;q15)	CPSF6-FGFR1

[a] FGFR1 rearrangement has also been found in association with t(8;12)(p11.2;q15) and t(8;17)(p11.2;q25), but the suspected involvement of FGFR1 in t(8;11)(p11.1-p11.2;p15) was not confirmed.

Genetic profile

A variety of translocations with an 8p11 breakpoint can underlie this syndrome. Secondary cytogenetic abnormalities (most commonly trisomy 21) also occur. Depending on the partner chromosome, a variety of fusion genes incorporating part of FGFR1 can be formed. All such fusion genes encode an aberrant tyrosine kinase (see Table 4.05).

Prognosis and predictive factors

Due to the high incidence of transformation, the prognosis is poor, even for patients presenting in the chronic phase. There is no established tyrosine kinase inhibitor therapy for myeloproliferative neoplasms with FGFR1 rearrangement, although midostaurin (PKC412) was effective in one case {673}. Interferon has induced a cytogenetic response in several cases {2424,2532A}. Until a specific therapy has been developed, haematopoietic stem cell transplantation should be considered even for patients who present in the chronic phase.

Myeloid/lymphoid neoplasms with PCM1-JAK2

Definition

Myeloid and lymphoid neoplasms associated with t(8;9)(p22;p24.1) {3799} and PCM1-JAK2 {3337} share characteristic features that justify the recognition of this group as a provisional entity {230}.

The haematological features may be those characteristic of a myeloproliferative neoplasm (e.g. chronic eosinophilic leukaemia or primary myelofibrosis) or those characteristic of a myelodysplastic/myeloproliferative neoplasm (e.g. atypical chronic myeloid leukaemia, BCR-ABL1–negative), often with eosinophilia. Acute myeloid transformation can occur; in addition, one patient presented with B-lymphoblastic leukaemia {3337}, two patients experienced B-lymphoblastic transformation {1656,3108} and one patient presented with T-lymphoblastic lymphoma {25}. Another patient developed a constellation of T-cell lineage neoplasms {1084}.

Variants

Cases with translocations resulting in a fusion gene between JAK2 and an alternative partner – specifically, t(9;12) (p24.1;p13.2) resulting in ETV6-JAK2 and t(9;22)(p24.1;q11.2) resulting in *BCR-JAK2* – may be considered variants of this provisional entity {230}. Both of these groups of disorders are more heterogeneous than are cases with *PCM1-JAK2*. Among the small number of reported cases with *ETV6-JAK2*, B- and T-lymphoblastic leukaemia/lymphoma have been common, but myeloid neoplasms (including myelodysplastic syndromes) have also been reported; eosinophilia has not been commonly observed {230}. Cases of B-lymphoblastic leukaemia/lymphoma associated with *ETV6-JAK2* may have the features of *BCR-ABL1*–like lymphoblastic leukaemia {3370}. Most of the few reported cases with *BCR-JAK2* have been myeloid neoplasms (most commonly atypical chronic myeloid leukaemia, *BCR-ABL1*–negative), but there have also been 3 reported cases of B-lymphoblastic leukaemia/lymphoma {230,3370}, which may also have the features of *BCR-ABL1*–like lymphoblastic leukaemia {3370}.

ICD-O code   9968/3

Epidemiology
There is a marked male predominance, with a male-to-female ratio of 27:5, and a wide age range (12–75 years), with a median age of 47 years {230}.

Localization
The peripheral blood and bone marrow are involved.

Clinical features
Patients often have hepatosplenomegaly.

Microscopy
The haematological features often include eosinophilia, and neutrophil precursors may be present in the peripheral blood. Some cases have the haematological features of chronic eosinophilic leukaemia. Monocytosis is uncommon, and an increase in basophils is only occasionally observed. There may be dyserythropoiesis (which is often prominent) and dysgranulopoiesis. Erythropoiesis may be considerably increased.

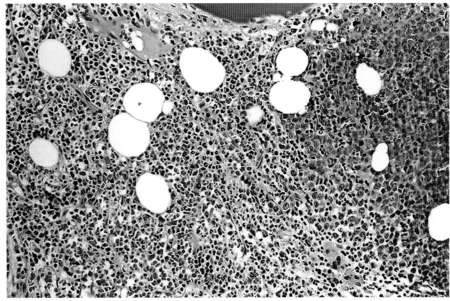

Fig. 4.05 Myeloid/lymphoid neoplasm with *PCM1-JAK2*. Trephine biopsy section. Hypercellular bone marrow with increased granulopoiesis and numerous eosinophilic forms, associated with a sheet-like proliferation of proerythroblasts (at far right).

There may be sheets of proerythroblasts, as seen in acute leukaemia. There have been reports of several cases with features similar to those of primary myelofibrosis, and other patients have shown bone marrow fibrosis.

Immunophenotype
Immunophenotypic analysis is useful in characterizing any lymphoid component and in cases with acute myeloid transformation.

Cell of origin
For *PCM1-JAK2*–related cases, the postulated cell of origin is a pluripotent haematopoietic stem cell that can give rise to neutrophils, eosinophils, and T- and B-lineage cells. Cases with variant fusion genes are also thought to arise from a pluripotent haematopoietic stem cell.

Genetic profile
More than 30 cases with t(8;9)(p22;p24.1) and resulting *PCM1-JAK2* fusion have been reported {230}. To date, smaller numbers of cases with other fusion genes involving *JAK2* have been reported: 8 cases with t(9;12)(p24.1;p13.2) and

ETV6-JAK2 and 11 cases with t(9;22) (p24.1;q11.2) and *BCR-JAK2* {230}; some of these cases are *BCR-ABL1*–like B-lymphoblastic leukaemia/lymphoma and may be best categorized with other cases of *BCR-ABL1*–like B-lymphoblastic leukaemia/lymphoma.

Prognosis and predictive factors
Survival is highly variable; for patients presenting in the chronic phase, it ranges from a matter of days to many years. The prognosis is also quite variable for cases presenting as acute leukaemia or with acute transformation, ranging from a few weeks to >5 years (or longer when haematopoietic stem cell transplantation is possible). Other than acute phase disease, no predictive factors are known.

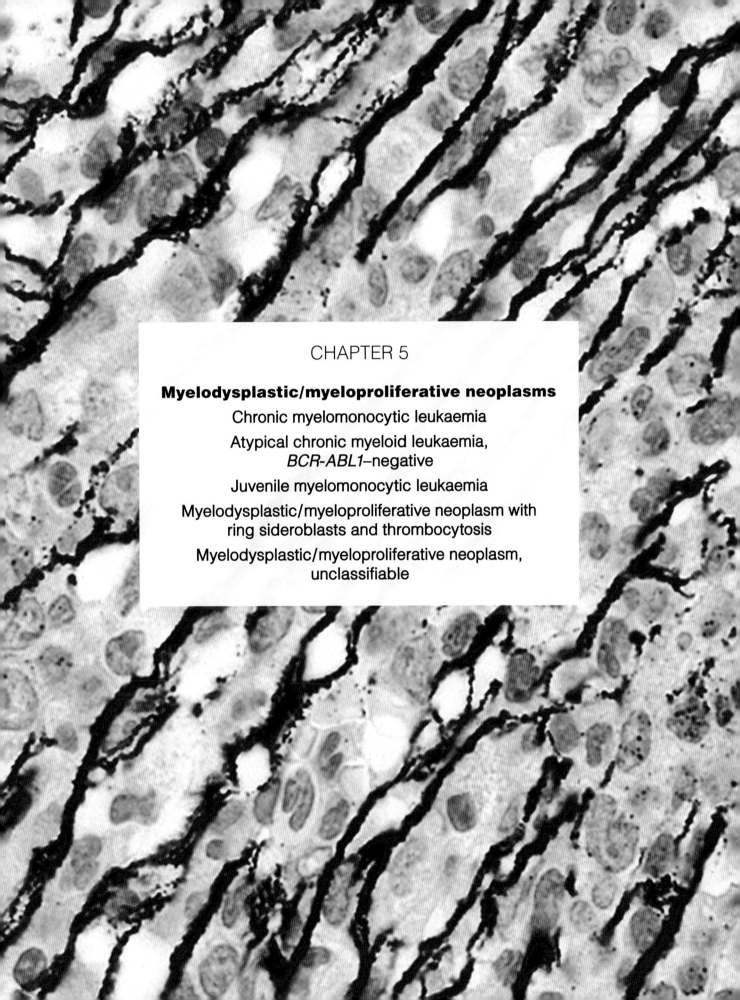

CHAPTER 5

Myelodysplastic/myeloproliferative neoplasms

Chronic myelomonocytic leukaemia

Atypical chronic myeloid leukaemia,
BCR-ABL1–negative

Juvenile myelomonocytic leukaemia

Myelodysplastic/myeloproliferative neoplasm with
ring sideroblasts and thrombocytosis

Myelodysplastic/myeloproliferative neoplasm,
unclassifiable

Chronic myelomonocytic leukaemia

Orazi A.
Bennett J.M.
Germing U.
Brunning R.D.

Bain B.J.
Cazzola M.
Foucar K.
Thiele J.

Definition

Chronic myelomonocytic leukaemia (CMML) is a clonal haematopoietic malignancy with features of both a myeloproliferative neoplasm (MPN) and a myelodysplastic syndrome (MDS). The diagnostic criteria for this entity are listed in Table 5.01.

On the basis of the percentage of blasts and promonocytes in the blood and bone marrow (see *Microscopy*), CMML cases can be further divided into three subcategories: CMML-0, CMML-1 and CMML-2. The clinical, haematological, and morphological features of CMML are heterogeneous, varying along a spectrum from predominantly myelodysplastic to mainly myeloproliferative in nature. Unlike *BCR-ABL1*–negative MPN, the *JAK2* V617F mutation is uncommon in CMML {1863, 3775}.

Rarely, cases previously diagnosed as MDS or MPN show evolution to a CMML-like phenotype {404,4245}; because this evolution constitutes disease progression, such cases should not be classified as CMML. Therapy-related CMML is discussed separately (see *Therapy-related myeloid neoplasms*, p. 153).

ICD-O codes

Chronic myelomonocytic leukaemia
9945/3
Chronic myelomonocytic leukaemia-0
9945/3
Chronic myelomonocytic leukaemia-1
9945/3
Chronic myelomonocytic leukaemia-2
9945/3

Synonyms

Chronic myelomonocytic leukaemia, type I; chronic myelomonocytic leukaemia, type II; chronic myelomonocytic leukaemia in transformation (obsolete); chronic myelomonocytic leukaemia, NOS

Epidemiology

There are few reliable incidence data for CMML; in some epidemiological surveys, CMML has been grouped with chronic myeloid leukaemias and in others it has been considered an MDS subtype. In one study, in which CMML accounted for 31% of the cases of MDS, the annual incidence of MDS was estimated to be approximately 12.8 cases per 100 000 population {4327}. An epidemiological report on a well-defined population, with centralized morphology review, reported a much lower age-standardized annual incidence (0.41 cases per 100 000 population) and a crude prevalence of 1.05–1.94 cases per 100 000 population {2854}. This incidence rate was confirmed by a recent study that found an annual incidence in 2008–2010 of 0.4 cases per 100 000 population {999}; in this study, the annual incidence of CMML was highest in patients aged >80 years (3.8 cases per 100 000 population) and higher in males (0.5 cases per 100 000 males; 95% CI: 0.4–0.6) than in females (0.2 cases per 100 000 females; 95% CI: 0.2–0.3). The median patient age at diagnosis is 65–75 years, with a male-to-female ratio of 1.5–3:1 {1334,3719,3805}.

Etiology

The etiology of CMML is unknown. Occupational and environmental carcinogens and ionizing irradiation are possible causes in some cases {196,3686}. Therapy-related CMML also exists {3872} (see *Therapy-related myeloid neoplasms*, p. 153).

Localization

The blood and bone marrow are always involved. The spleen, liver, skin and lymph nodes are the most common sites of extramedullary leukaemic infiltration {1334,4206}, but other organs can also be involved {3819}.

Clinical features

Half or more of all cases present with an increased white blood cell (WBC) count. In the remaining cases, the WBC count is normal or slightly decreased (with variable neutropenia), and the disease resembles MDS. Although once consid-

Table 5.01 Diagnostic criteria for chronic myelomonocytic leukaemia (CMML)

1. Persistent peripheral blood monocytosis ($\geq 1 \times 10^9$/L) with monocytes accounting for $\geq 10\%$ of the leukocytes
2. WHO criteria for *BCR-ABL1*–positive chronic myeloid leukaemia, primary myelofibrosis, polycythaemia vera and essential thrombocythaemia[a] are not met
3. No rearrangement of *PDGFRA*, *PDGFRB* or *FGFR1* and no *PCM1-JAK2* (which should be specifically excluded in cases with eosinophilia)
4. Blasts[b] constitute < 20% of the cells in the peripheral blood and bone marrow
5. Dysplasia involving ≥ 1 myeloid lineages

   or

   If myelodysplasia is absent or minimal, criteria 1–4 are met and:
   - an acquired, clonal cytogenetic or molecular genetic abnormality is present in haematopoietic cells[c]

     or
   - the monocytosis has persisted for ≥ 3 months and all other causes of monocytosis (e.g. malignancy, infection, and inflammation) have been excluded

---

[a] Myeloproliferative neoplasms (MPN) can be associated with monocytosis or it can develop during the course of the disease; such cases can mimic CMML. In these rare instances, a documented history of MPN excludes CMML, whereas the presence of MPN features in the bone marrow and/or MPN-associated mutations (in *JAK2, CALR or MPL*) tends to support MPN with monocytosis rather than CMML.

[b] Blasts and blast equivalents include myeloblasts, monoblasts and promonocytes. Promonocytes are monocytic precursors with abundant light-grey or slightly basophilic cytoplasm with a few scattered fine lilac-coloured granules, finely distributed stippled nuclear chromatin, variably prominent nucleoli and delicate nuclear folding or creasing. Abnormal monocytes, which can be present in both the peripheral blood and the bone marrow, are excluded from the blast count (see *Introduction and overview of the classification of myeloid neoplasms*, Fig. 1.04, p. 18).

[c] In the appropriate clinical context, mutations in genes often associated with CMML (e.g. *TET2, SRSF2, ASXL1* and *SETBP1*) support the diagnosis. However, some of these mutations can be age-related or present in other neoplasms; therefore, these genetic findings must be interpreted with caution.

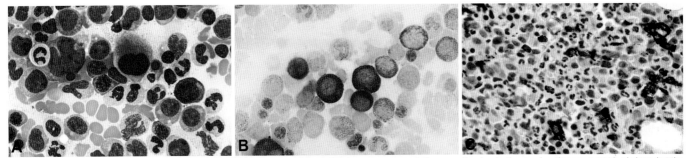

Fig. 5.01 Chronic myelomonocytic leukaemia-1. **A** With Wright-Giemsa staining in this bone marrow aspirate smear, the dysplastic granulocytic component is obvious, but the monocytic component is more difficult to identify. **B** The monocytic component can be highlighted with special staining: naphthol AS-D chloroacetate esterase (CAE) reaction combined with alpha-naphthyl butyrate esterase stains monocytes brown, neutrophils blue and myelomonooytic cells a mixture of blue and brown. **C** CD163 immunostaining of a bone marrow biopsy section shows positivity in scattered monocytic cells and strong staining of the bone marrow macrophages. Immunohistochemistry can be used to identify monocytes in tissue sections, but is less sensitive than cytochemistry applied to bone marrow aspirate smears.

ered to be controversial, the subdivision of CMML into dysplastic (WBC count < 13 × 10⁹/L) and proliferative (WBC count ≥ 13 × 10⁹/L) groups appears to be justified {620,3349,3587,3827}. The incidence of constitutional symptoms (e.g. weight loss, fever, and night sweats) is higher with the proliferative type, whereas consequences of haematopoietic insufficiency (e.g. fatigue, infection, and bleeding due to thrombocytopenia) are more common with the dysplastic type {1334,3719,3805}. Splenomegaly and hepatomegaly can be present in either type, but are more frequent (occurring in as many as 50% of cases) in patients with leukocytosis {1334}. In rare cases, life-threatening hyperleukocytosis can occur {197}.

Microscopy

Peripheral blood monocytosis is the hallmark of CMML. By definition, the monocyte count is always ≥ 1 × 10⁹/L; it is usually 2–5 × 10⁹/L, but can exceed 80 × 10⁹/L {2517,2653}. Monocytes should account for ≥ 10% of the leukocytes {339}. In general, the monocytes are mature and have unremarkable morphology, but they can exhibit unusual nuclear segmentation or chromatin patterns and abnormal granulation {2092}. Those with abnormal granulation are best termed abnormal monocytes, a designation used to describe monocytes that are immature but have denser chromatin, more nuclear convolutions and folds, and more abundant greyish cytoplasm than do promonocytes and monoblasts (see *Introduction and overview of the classification of myeloid neoplasms,* Fig. 1.04, p. 18). Blasts and promonocytes may also be seen, but if they account for ≥20% of the leukocytes,

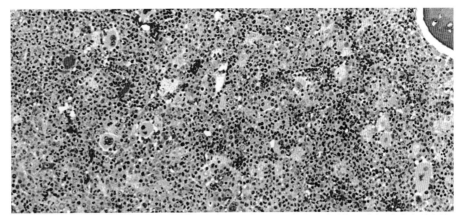

Fig. 5.02 Chronic myelomonocytic leukaemia-1. The degree of leukocytosis, neutrophilia and dysplasia is variable. Often, the granulocytic component is most obvious in the biopsy specimen, and monocytes may not be readily appreciable. This specimen shows hypercellular bone marrow with prominent granulocytic and megakaryocytic proliferation.

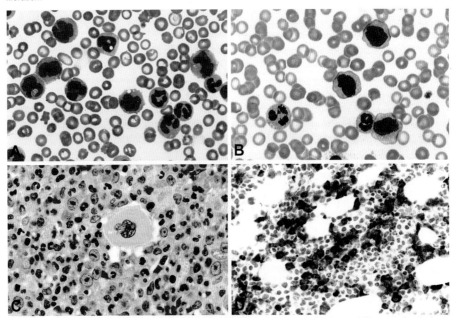

Fig. 5.03 Chronic myelomonocytic leukaemia-1. The degree of leukocytosis, neutrophilia and dysplasia is variable. **A** The white blood cell count in this case is elevated, with minimal dysplasia in the neutrophil series. **B** The white blood cell count in this case is normal, with absolute monocytosis, neutropenia and dysgranulopoiesis. **C** In this biopsy section, monocytes (with their characteristic folded nuclei and delicate nuclear chromatin) can be seen among the granulocytes. **D** Bone marrow biopsy section immunostain shows that the monocytic cells in this case are strongly positive for CD14.

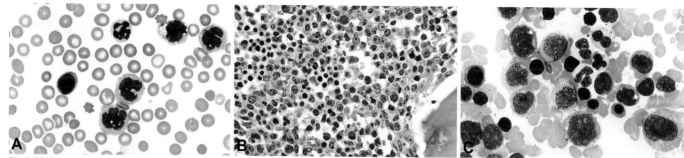

Fig. 5.04 Chronic myelomonocytic leukaemia-2. **A** Blood smear from a newly diagnosed patient shows occasional blasts and atypical monocytes. **B** Bone marrow biopsy specimen from the same patient illustrates the shift towards immaturity of the marrow cells, which is usually readily appreciable. **C** In this bone marrow aspirate smear, blasts and promonocytes account for 12% of the marrow cells.

the diagnosis is acute myeloid leukaemia (AML; acute myelomonocytic leukaemia or acute monocytic leukaemia) rather than CMML. Other changes in the blood are variable. The WBC count may be normal or slightly decreased with neutropenia, but in half or more of all cases it is increased due to both monocytosis and neutrophilia {1334,2517,2978}. Neutrophil precursors (promyelocytes and myelocytes) usually account for < 10% of the leukocytes {339}. Dysgranulopoiesis, including the formation of neutrophils with hyposegmented or abnormally segmented nuclei or abnormal cytoplasmic granulation, is present in most cases, but may be less prominent in patients with leukocytosis than in those with a normal or low WBC count {2092,2517}. In some cases, it may be difficult to distinguish between hypogranular neutrophils and dysplastic monocytes. Mild basophilia is sometimes present. Eosinophils are usually normal or slightly increased in number, but in some cases eosinophilia is striking. CMML with eosinophilia can be diagnosed when the criteria for CMML are met and the eosinophil count in the peripheral blood is ≥ 1.5 × 10⁹/L. Patients with this diagnosis

may have complications related to the degranulation of the eosinophils. These hypereosinophilic cases of CMML can closely resemble cases of myeloid neoplasms with eosinophilia associated with specific genetic abnormalities, which are classified and discussed separately from CMML (see *Myeloid/lymphoid neoplasms with PDGFRB rearrangement*, p. 75). Mild anaemia, often normocytic but sometimes macrocytic, is common. Platelet counts vary, but moderate thrombocytopenia is often present. Atypical, large platelets and nucleated red blood cell precursors may be seen {1338,2517}. The bone marrow is hypercellular in > 75% of cases, but normocellular specimens are also seen {2653,2985,3805}. Hypocellularity is very rare. One recent study on the histological assessment of marrow found that < 5% of CMML cases were hypocellular and 84% were hypercellular {3554}.

Granulocytic proliferation is often the most striking finding in the bone marrow, but an increase in erythroid precursors may also be seen {339,2653}. Monocytic proliferation is invariably present, but can be difficult to recognize in the

biopsy or on marrow aspirate smears. Cytochemical and immunohistochemical studies that facilitate the identification of monocytes and their precursors are strongly recommended when the diagnosis of CMML is suspected {2985, 2987}. Dysgranulopoiesis, similar to that in the blood, is present in the bone marrow of most patients with CMML. Dyserythropoiesis (e.g. megaloblastoid changes, other abnormal nuclear features and ring sideroblasts) may also be observed, but is usually mild {1334,2517, 2653}. Micromegakaryocytes and/or megakaryocytes with hyposegmented nuclei are found in as many as 80% of cases {1338,2517,2653}.

Unlike in chronic myeloid leukaemia, pseudo-Gaucher cells are usually absent. A mild to moderate increase in the number of reticulin fibres is seen in the bone marrow in nearly 30% of cases {2538}. Careful attention to morphological features and other disease-specific clinicopathological findings may be needed to distinguish CMML from MPN associated with monocytosis {404,1097}. The presence of one of the characteristic MPN driver mutations (in *JAK2*, *CALR* or

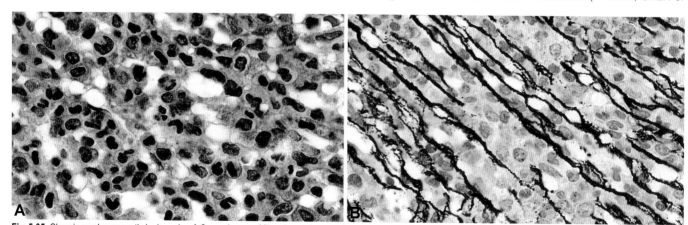

Fig. 5.05 Chronic myelomonocytic leukaemia. **A** Some degree of fibrosis may be seen in as many as 30% of cases; this bone marrow biopsy specimen shows streaming of cells suggestive of underlying reticulin fibrosis, the presence of which was confirmed by reticulin silver staining (**B**).

MPL) is helpful for identifying MPN associated with monocytosis.

Nodules composed of mature plasmacytoid dendritic cells in the bone marrow biopsy have been reported in 20% of cases {2985}. The cells have round nuclei, finely dispersed chromatin, inconspicuous nucleoli, and a rim of eosinophilic cytoplasm. The cytoplasmic membrane is usually distinct with well-defined cytoplasmic borders, imparting a cohesive appearance to the infiltrating cells. Apoptotic bodies, often within starry-sky histiocytes, are frequently present. The relationship of the plasmacytoid dendritic cell proliferation to the leukaemic cells was previously uncertain {216,1127,1555, 1691}, but there is now evidence that the proliferation is neoplastic in nature and is clonally related to the associated CMML {1126}.

The splenic enlargement seen in CMML is usually due to infiltration of the red pulp by leukaemic cells. Lymphadenopathy is uncommon, but when it occurs it may indicate transformation to a more acute phase, and the lymph node may show diffuse infiltration by myeloid blasts. There is sometimes lymph node (and less commonly splenic) involvement by a diffuse infiltration of plasmacytoid dendritic cells. In some cases, generalized lymphadenopathy due to tumoural proliferations of plasmacytoid dendritic cells is the presenting manifestation of CMML. Blast cells and promonocytes usually account for <5% of the peripheral blood leukocytes and <10% of the nucleated marrow cells at the time of diagnosis. A higher proportion may indicate poor prognosis or higher risk of rapid transformation to acute leukaemia {1180,1339, 1442,3805,3922,4365}. The previously

used category of CMML-1 (defined by blasts including promonocytes accounting for <5% of the leukocytes in the peripheral blood and <10% in the bone marrow) has now been split into two new categories: CMML-0 and CMML-1. It is currently recommended {2978,3587, 3805} that CMML be subdivided into three categories, defined by the percentage of blasts and promonocytes in the peripheral blood and bone marrow:

CMML-0: <2% blasts in the blood and <5% in the bone marrow; no Auer rods.

CMML-1: 2–4% blasts in the blood or 5–9% in the bone marrow; <5% blasts in the blood, <10% blasts in the bone marrow, and no Auer rods.

CMML-2: 5–19% blasts in the blood, 10–19% in the bone marrow or Auer rods are present; <20% blasts in the bone marrow and blood.

Cytochemistry

Cytochemical studies are strongly recommended whenever the diagnosis of CMML is considered {2985}. Alpha-naphthyl butyrate esterase or alpha-naphthyl acetate esterase (with fluoride inhibition) staining of blood and bone marrow aspirate smears, alone or in combination with naphthol AS-D chloroacetate esterase (CAE) staining, is extremely useful for assessing the monocytic component, and in some cases may facilitate distinguishing monocytes from monoblasts and promonocytes (blast equivalents) and from non-monocytic cells.

Immunophenotype

The blood and marrow cells usually express typical myelomonocytic antigens (e.g. CD33 and CD13) and variably express CD14, CD68 and CD64 {1993,

2482,3640,4364}. The blood and marrow monocytes often have aberrant phenotypes, with two or more aberrant features shown by flow cytometric analysis {4396}. Decreased CD14 expression may reflect relative monocyte immaturity {3618}. Other aberrant characteristics include: overexpression of CD56; aberrant expression of CD2; and decreased expression of HLA-DR, CD13, CD11c, CD15, CD16, CD64 and CD36 {2554, 3618,3714,4396}. An increased proportion of CD14+/CD16– monocytes has recently been described {3618}. Maturing myeloid cells may also have aberrant immunophenotypic features, and neutrophils may show aberrant light-scattering properties. An increased proportion of CD34+ cells and an emerging blast population with an aberrant immunophenotype have been associated with early transformation to acute leukaemia {1063, 4365,4396}.

For the identification of monocytic cells, immunohistochemistry on tissue sections is less sensitive than cytochemistry or flow cytometry. The most reliable marker is CD14 {3257}. CD68R and CD163 can also be helpful {2985}. Lysozyme used in conjunction with cytochemistry for CAE can facilitate the identification of monocytic cells, which are lysozyme positive but CAE negative (in contrast to the granulocyte precursor cells, which are positive for both). An increased proportion of CD34+ cells detected by immunohistochemistry has been associated with transformation to acute leukaemia {2985}.

The mature plasmacytoid dendritic cells associated with CMML have a characteristic immunophenotype. They are positive for antigens normally expressed

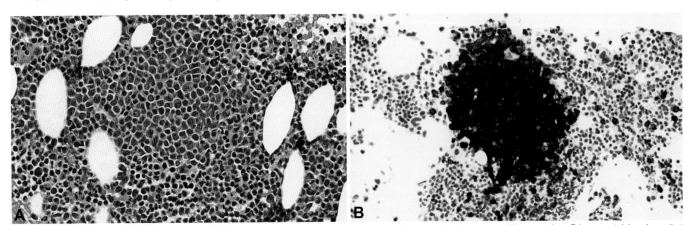

Fig. 5.06 Chronic myelomonocytic leukaemia-1. **A** Nodules composed of mature plasmacytoid dendritic cells in the bone marrow biopsy section. **B** Immunostaining shows that these cells strongly express CD123.

by reactive cells of this lineage, such as CD123, CD2AP, CD4, CD43, CD45RA, CD68/CD68R, CD303, BCL11A and granzyme B {406,870,2497}. Rarely, they also express some of the following antigens: CD2, CD5, CD7, CD10, CD13, CD14, CD15 and CD33 and, very rarely, CD56. TIA1 and perforin are usually negative. The Ki-67 (MIB1) proliferation index is usually low.

Cell of origin

A haematopoietic stem cell

Genetic profile

Clonal cytogenetic abnormalities are found in 20–40% of CMML cases, but none is specific {1182,1334,3105,3805, 3826,3896,3922}. The most common recurrent abnormalities include gain of chromosome 8 and loss of chromosome 7 or del(7q). In a large study of 414 patients with CMML, 73% of the patients had a normal karyotype, 7% had trisomy 8, 4% had loss of Y chromosome, 3% had a complex karyotype, 1.5% had an abnormality of chromosome 7 and 10% had another aberration {3826}. Some myeloid neoplasms with isolated isochromosome 17q have haematological features of CMML {1220,1912,2594}, whereas others are better diagnosed as myelodysplastic/myeloproliferative neoplasm, unclassifiable {1912,1913}. Abnormalities of 11q23.3 are uncommon in CMML and suggest an alternate diagnosis of acute leukaemia. Several of the prognostic systems for CMML currently in use include cytogenetic features {3827,3896}.

Myeloid neoplasms with eosinophilia associated with t(5;12)(q32;p13.2) and ETV6-PDGFRB fusion were formerly included in the CMML category, but are now considered to be a distinct entity (see Myeloid/lymphoid neoplasms with PDGFRB rearrangement, p. 75). Cases of chronic myeloid leukaemia that express the p190 BCR-ABL1 isoform can mimic CMML. Therefore, even if t(9;22)(q34.1;q11.2) is not detected by conventional karyotyping, PCR analysis for the presence of p210 and p190 and/or FISH analysis for the BCR-ABL1 fusion gene must be performed.

Many patients with CMML harbour somatic mutations, most frequently in ASXL1 (found in 40% of cases), TET2 (in 58%), SRSF2 (in 46%), RUNX1 (in 15%), NRAS (in 11%) and CBL (in 10%); many other genes can also be mutated (in < 10% of cases) {1795,2779}. Studies that confirmed the frequency of mutations in TET2, SRSF2, SETBP1 and ASXL1 {1170, 2611,3100} have shown that at least one of these four genes is mutated in most CMML cases. Recently proposed prognostic models include mutation analysis {3025,3100,3105,4264}. NPM1 mutations are uncommon in CMML (occurring in < 5% of cases); if they are found, the alternative diagnosis of AML with monocytic differentiation associated with NPM1 mutation should be carefully excluded. Confirmed cases of CMML with NPM1 mutation (in particular cases with a high mutation burden) appear to have a high probability of progressing to AML and may require aggressive clinical intervention {3129}.

Prognosis and predictive factors

The reported survival times of patients with CMML range from 1 month to > 100 months; the median survival time in most series is 20–40 months {198,1180, 1334,1336,1442,3587,3719,3805,3922, 4365}. Progression to AML occurs in 15–30% of cases. Clinical and haematological parameters including lactate dehydrogenase level, splenomegaly, anaemia, thrombocytopenia and lymphocytosis {2978} have been reported as important factors for predicting the course of the disease. However, in virtually all studies, the percentage of blood and bone marrow blasts is the most important factor determining survival, together with karyotype, WBC count, and haematopoietic function {816,1180,1334,1339,1442,3719, 3805,3922,4365}. These factors are included in a CMML-specific prognostic scoring system {3827}. Somatic ASXL1 mutation has also been incorporated in a clinical prognostic scoring system {1795}. AML as transformation of CMML is an aggressive disease that belongs in the group of AML with myelodysplasia-related changes; the blasts often exhibit morphological features of acute myelomonocytic leukaemia or acute monocytic leukaemia, i.e. French–American–British (FAB) classification M4 or M5 {827}.

Atypical chronic myeloid leukaemia, BCR-ABL1–negative

Orazi A.
Bennett J.M.
Bain B.J.
Brunning R.D.
Thiele J.

Definition

Atypical chronic myeloid leukaemia, BCR-ABL1–negative (aCML) is a leukaemic disorder with myelodysplastic as well as myeloproliferative features present at the time of initial diagnosis (Table 5.02). It is characterized by principal involvement of the neutrophil lineage, with leukocytosis resulting from an increase of morphologically dysplastic neutrophils and their precursors. However, multilineage dysplasia is common, and reflects the stem-cell origin of this entity. The neoplastic cells do not have BCR-ABL1 fusion; rearrangement of PDGFRA, PDGFRB or FGFR1, or PCM1-JAK2. Therapy-related cases with features of aCML are discussed separately (see *Therapy-related myeloid neoplasms*, p. 153).

ICD-O code   9876/3

Synonyms
Atypical chronic myeloid leukaemia, Philadelphia chromosome–negative (Ph1–); atypical chronic myeloid leukaemia, BCR/ABL1-negative

Epidemiology
The exact incidence of aCML is unknown, but it is estimated that there are only 1–2 aCML cases for every 100 cases of BCR-ABL1–positive chronic myeloid leukaemia {2987,4248}. Patients with aCML tend to be elderly. In the few series reported to date, the median patient age at diagnosis is in the seventh or eighth decade of life, although the disease has also

Table 5.02 Diagnostic criteria for atypical chronic myeloid leukaemia, BCR-ABL1–negative (aCML)

- Peripheral blood leukocytosis $\geq 13 \times 10^9$/L, due to increased numbers of neutrophils and their precursors (i.e. promyelocytes, myelocytes and metamyelocytes), with neutrophil precursors constituting $\geq 10\%$ of the leukocytes
- Dysgranulopoiesis, which may include abnormal chromatin clumping
- No or minimal absolute basophilia; basophils constitute < 2% of the peripheral blood leukocytes
- No or minimal absolute monocytosis; monocytes constitute < 10% of the peripheral blood leukocytes
- Hypercellular bone marrow with granulocytic proliferation and granulocytic dysplasia, with or without dysplasia in the erythroid and megakaryocytic lineages
- < 20% blasts in the blood and bone marrow
- No evidence of PDGFRA, PDGFRB or FGFR1 rearrangement, or of PCM1-JAK2
- WHO criteria for BCR-ABL1–positive chronic myeloid leukaemia, primary myelofibrosis, polycythaemia vera, or essential thrombocythaemia[a] are not met

[a] Myeloproliferative neoplasms (MPNs), in particular those in accelerated phase and/or in post–polycythaemia vera or post–essential thrombocythaemia myelofibrosis, if neutrophilic, may simulate aCML. A history of MPN, the presence of MPN features in the bone marrow, and/or MPN-associated mutations (in JAK2, CALR or MPL) tend to exclude the diagnosis of aCML; conversely, the diagnosis is supported by the presence of SETBP1 and/or ETNK1 mutations. CSF3R mutation is uncommon and, if detected, should prompt careful morphological review to exclude an alternative diagnosis of chronic neutrophilic leukaemia or another myeloid neoplasm.

been reported in teenagers {447,1621, 2143,2517,4248}. The reported male-to-female ratio varies, but in larger series it is approximately 1:1 {447,1621,2143,2517, 4248}.

Localization
The peripheral blood and bone marrow are always involved; splenic and hepatic involvement is also common.

Clinical features
There are only a few reports of the clinical features of aCML. Patients usually have symptoms related to anaemia or some-times to thrombocytopenia; for other patients, the primary symptoms are related to splenomegaly {447,1621,2143,2517}.

Microscopy
The white blood cell count is always $\geq 13 \times 10^9$/L {339}, but median values of $24–96 \times 10^9$/L have been reported, and some patients have white blood cell counts of $> 300 \times 10^9$/L {447,1621,2143, 2517,4248}. Blasts are usually < 5% and always < 20% of peripheral blood leukocytes. Neutrophil precursors (promyelocytes, myelocytes, and metamyelocytes) constitute $\geq 10\%$ of the leukocytes. The absolute monocyte count may be

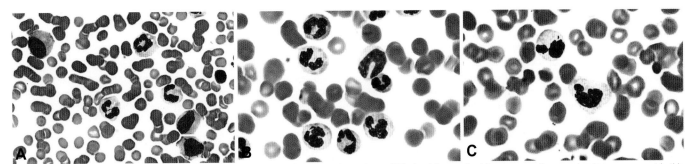

Fig. 5.07 Atypical chronic myeloid leukaemia, BCR-ABL1–negative. **A** The diagnosis requires $\geq 10\%$ circulating neutrophil precursors; three myelocytes are apparent in this peripheral blood microscopic field. **B** The white blood cell count is elevated, with dysplastic neutrophils. **C** Marked granulocytic dysplasia and immature granulocytes. Cytogenetic studies revealed a gain of chromosome 8, but no Philadelphia (Ph) chromosome. No BCR-ABL1 fusion gene was detected by FISH.

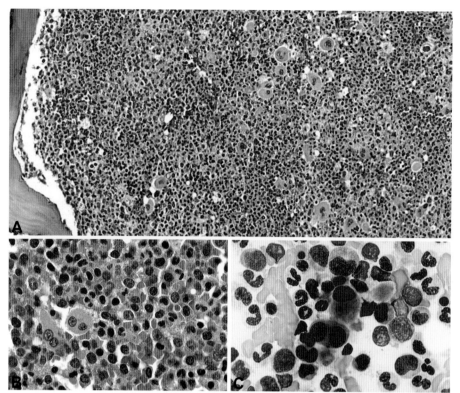

Fig. 5.08 Atypical chronic myeloid leukaemia, *BCR-ABL1*–negative. **A** The bone marrow biopsy shows hypercellularity, due to granulocytic proliferation. **B** Note the increased number of megakaryocytes, with small, abnormal forms. From the biopsy alone, the morphology would be difficult to differentiate from that of *BCR-ABL1*–positive chronic myeloid leukaemia. **C** Dysplasia in the granulocytic and megakaryocytic lineages is evident on the bone marrow aspirate smear.

increased, but the percentage of peripheral blood monocytes is < 10%. Basophilia may be observed but is not prominent {339,447,1621,2517,4248}. One of the major features that characterize aCML is dysgranulopoiesis, which may be pronounced. Acquired Pelger–Huët anomaly or other nuclear abnormalities, such as hypersegmentation with abnormally clumped nuclear chromatin or bizarrely segmented nuclei, abnormal cytoplasmic granularity (usually hypogranularity) and multiple nuclear projections, may be observed in the neutrophils. Moderate anaemia is common, and the red blood cells may show changes indicative of dyserythropoiesis. The platelet count is variable, but thrombocytopenia is common {339,1621,2517}. Careful morphological examination of the peripheral blood is crucial for distinguishing this entity from chronic neutrophilic leukaemia {4248}, which lacks dysplastic features in the neutrophils and has < 10% circulating immature myeloid cells. There are also differences in the frequency of associated mutations (see *Genetic profile*).

The bone marrow is hypercellular due to an increase of neutrophils and their pre-cursors. The myeloid-to-erythroid ratio is usually > 10:1, reflecting the increased granulopoiesis and the decreased erythropoiesis, but in some cases erythroid precursors account for > 30% of the marrow cells. Dyserythropoiesis is present in about 40% of cases {339,447,4248}. Dysgranulopoiesis is invariably present, and the changes in the neutrophil lineage observed in the bone marrow are similar to those in the blood. Megakaryopoiesis is usually quantitatively normal or increased, but is sometimes decreased; there is often evidence of dysmegakaryopoiesis, including micromegakaryocytes and small megakaryocytes with hypolobated nuclei {447,1621}. Blasts may be moderately increased in number, but are always < 20%; large sheets or clusters of blasts are not present. Marrow fibrosis (usually mild) is seen in some cases at the time of diagnosis; in others, it appears later in the course of the disease.

Variant
Most cases reported as the syndrome of abnormal chromatin clumping can in fact be considered a variant of aCML {460, 1178,1766}. These cases are character-ized in the peripheral blood and bone marrow by a high percentage of neutrophils and precursors that exhibit exaggerated clumping of the nuclear chromatin.

Cytochemistry
No specific cytochemical abnormalities have been reported to date, although the use of esterase stains or immunohistochemistry to exclude a significant monocytic component can facilitate the exclusion of chronic myelomonocytic leukaemia. Neutrophil alkaline phosphatase scoring is rarely done; the scores can be low, normal, or high, and are therefore not useful for distinguishing this entity from *BCR-ABL1*–positive chronic myeloid leukaemia {2143,2517}.

Immunophenotype
No specific immunophenotypic characteristics have been reported to date. Like esterase cytochemistry, immunohistochemistry for CD14 or CD68R on biopsy sections may facilitate the identification of monocytes; the finding of significant marrow monocytosis should call into question a diagnosis of aCML. In some cases with decreased megakaryocytes, CD61 or CD42b immunohistochemistry may facilitate the identification of dysmegakaryopoiesis. CD34 can facilitate the identification of blasts.

Cell of origin
A bone marrow haematopoietic stem cell

Genetic profile
Karyotypic abnormalities are reported in as many as 80% of cases. The most common abnormalities are gain of chromosome 8 and del(20q), but abnormalities of chromosomes 13, 14, 17, 19 and 12 are also common {447,1621,2517}. Rarely, cases is which the neoplastic cells have an isolated isochromosome 17q have features of aCML, although most fulfil the criteria for chronic myelomonocytic leukaemia {2594}. There is no *BCR-ABL1* fusion. Cases with rearrangement of *PDGFRA*, *PDGFRB* or *FGFR1*, or with *PCM1-JAK2*, are also specifically excluded. In the past, some cases of t(8;9)(p22;p24) with *PCM1-JAK2* fusion were diagnosed as aCML {436,3337}, but such cases are now grouped with other eosinophilic neoplasms associated with specific chromosomal rearrangements, and are discussed separately (see *Myeloid/lymphoid neoplasms with PCM1-*

JAK2, p. 78). *JAK2* V617F mutation has only rarely been reported in patients with aCML {1184,2288,4248}; therefore, the typical myeloproliferative neoplasm–associated mutations (in *JAK2*, *CALR* and *MPL*) tend to exclude the diagnosis of aCML {1184}. Recent data indicate that *SETBP1* and *ETNK1* mutations are relatively common in aCML {1286,2610,2779, 3167}, whereas *CSF3R* mutation is present in < 10% of cases {2779}. Because this mutation is found in a considerably larger proportion of chronic neutrophilic leukaemia cases {1414,2588,3057,3918}, it is helpful in distinguishing between the two neoplasms.

Prognosis and predictive factors
Patients with aCML fare poorly. Among the small numbers of patients included in reported series to date, the median survival time is 14–29 months {447,1621, 2143,4248}. Age > 65 years, female sex, white blood cell count > 50×10^9/L, thrombocytopenia and haemoglobin level < 10 g/dL have been reported to be adverse prognostic findings {447, 1621}. However, patients who receive a bone marrow transplant may have an improved outcome {2077}. In 30–40% of patients, aCML evolves to acute myeloid leukaemia {4248}; most of the remaining patients die of marrow failure {447,2143}.

Juvenile myelomonocytic leukaemia

Baumann I.
Bennett J.M.
Niemeyer C.M.
Thiele J.

Definition
Juvenile myelomonocytic leukaemia (JMML) is a clonal haematopoietic disorder of childhood characterized by a proliferation principally of the granulocytic and monocytic lineages. Blasts and promonocytes account for < 20% of the white blood cells in the peripheral blood and bone marrow. Erythroid and megakaryocytic abnormalities are often present {88,507,2662}. *BCR-ABL1* fusion is absent, whereas mutations involving genes of the RAS pathway are characteristic. The diagnostic criteria are listed in Table 5.03.

ICD-O code   9946/3

Synonym
Juvenile chronic myelomonocytic leukaemia

Epidemiology
The annual incidence of JMML is estimated to be approximately 0.13 cases per 100 000 children aged 0–14 years. It accounts for < 2–3% of all leukaemias in children, but for 20–30% of all cases of myelodysplastic and myeloproliferative diseases in patients aged < 14 years {1585,3092}. Patient age at diagnosis ranges from 1 month to early adolescence, but 75% of cases occur in children aged < 3 years {2415,2872}. Boys are affected nearly twice as frequently as girls. Approximately 15% of cases occur in infants with Noonan syndrome–like disorder (which is caused by a *CBL* mutation) {2381}, and 10% occur in children with neurofibromatosis type 1 (NF1) {2872}.

Etiology
The cause of JMML is unknown. Rare cases have been reported in identical twins {3093}. The association between NF1 and JMML has long been established {581,2872,3804}. In children with NF1 (unlike in adults with the disorder), the risk of developing myeloid malignancy (mainly JMML) is reported to be 200–500 times that in the general paediatric population {2872}. Occasionally, infants with Noonan syndrome develop a JMML-like disorder, which resolves

Table 5.03 Diagnostic criteria for juvenile myelomonocytic leukaemia; modified from Locatelli F and Niemeyer CM {2377}

Clinical and haematological criteria (all 4 criteria are required)
- Peripheral blood monocyte count ≥ 1 × 10^9/L
- Blast percentage in peripheral blood and bone marrow of < 20%
- Splenomegaly
- No Philadelphia (Ph) chromosome or *BCR-ABL1* fusion

Genetic criteria (any 1 criterion is sufficient)
- Somatic mutation[a] in *PTPN11, KRAS* or *NRAS*
- Clinical diagnosis of neurofibromatosis type 1 or *NF1* mutation
- Germline *CBL* mutation and loss of heterozygosity of *CBL*[b]

Other criteria
Cases that do not meet any of the genetic criteria above must meet the following criteria in addition to the clinical and haematological criteria above:
- Monosomy 7 or any other chromosomal abnormality
  or
- ≥ 2 of the following:
  - Increased haemoglobin F for age
  - Myeloid or erythroid precursors on peripheral blood smear
  - Granulocyte-macrophage colony-stimulating factor (also called CSF2) hypersensitivity in colony assay
  - Hyperphosphorylation of STAT5

---
[a] If a mutation is found in *PTPN11, KRAS* or *NRAS* it is essential to consider that it might be a germline mutation and the diagnosis of transient abnormal myelopoiesis of Noonan syndrome must be considered.
[b] Occasional cases have heterozygous splice-site mutations.

without treatment in some cases and behaves more aggressively in others {217}. These children carry germline mutations in *PTPN11* (the gene encoding the protein tyrosine phosphatase SHP2 {3906}) or *KRAS* {3586}.

Localization

The peripheral blood and bone marrow always show evidence of myelomonocytic proliferation. Leukaemic infiltration of the liver and spleen is found in virtually all cases. The lymph nodes, skin, respiratory system, and gut are other common sites of involvement, although any tissue can be infiltrated {2415,2872}.

Clinical features

Most patients present with constitutional symptoms or evidence of infection {2415, 2872}. There is generally marked hepatosplenomegaly. Occasionally, spleen size is normal at diagnosis but rapidly increases thereafter. About half of all patients have lymphadenopathy, and leukaemic infiltrates may give rise to markedly enlarged tonsils. Dry cough, tachypnoea and interstitial infiltrates on chest X-ray are signs of pulmonary infiltration. Gut infiltration may predispose patients to diarrhoea and gastrointestinal infections. Signs of bleeding are common, and about a quarter of all patients have skin rashes (eczematous eruptions or indurations with central clearing). Café-au-lait spots might be indicative of an underlying germline condition such as NF1 or Noonan syndrome–like disorder {2528, 2874}. JMML rarely involves the central nervous system (CNS), although a small number of patients with CNS myeloid sarcoma and ocular infiltrates have been described {2872}.

A notable feature of many JMML cases is markedly increased synthesis of haemoglobin F, particularly in cases with a

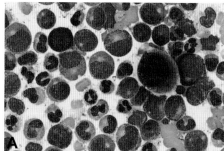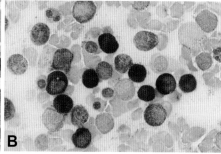

Fig. 5.09 Juvenile myelomonocytic leukaemia. **A** The bone marrow aspirate smear usually reflects the changes noted in the blood, but the monocyte component may be difficult to distinguish from other marrow cells in Wright–Giemsa–stained preparations. **B** Combined alpha-naphthyl butyrate esterase and naphthol AS-D chloroacetate esterase (CAE) reaction identifies the granulocytic (blue) and monocytic (brown) components; a few cells contain both blue and brown reaction products.

normal karyotype {2872}. Other features include polyclonal hypergammaglobulinaemia and the presence of autoantibodies {2872}. In vitro hypersensitivity of JMML myeloid progenitors to granulocyte–macrophage colony-stimulating factor (also called CSF2) {1100} is a hallmark of the disease, and served as an important diagnostic tool before the discovery of the five canonical RAS pathway mutations (in *PTPN11*, *NRAS*, *KRAS*, *NF1* and *CBL*), which now allow molecular diagnosis in approximately 85% of all JMML cases, greatly facilitating the diagnosis. In RAS pathway mutation–negative cases, disorders with a clinical and haematological picture mimicking that of JMML, such as infection {2481}, Wiskott–Aldrich syndrome (eczema–thrombocytopenia–immunodeficiency syndrome) {4436} and malignant infantile osteopetrosis {3811}, must be excluded.

Microscopy

The peripheral blood is the most important specimen for diagnosis. It typically shows leukocytosis and thrombocytopenia, and often anaemia {2415,2872}. The median reported white blood cell counts are 25–30 × 10⁹/L. The leuko-

cytosis consists mainly of neutrophils, with some immature cells (e.g. promyelocytes and myelocytes) and monocytes. Blasts (including promonocytes) usually account for < 5% of the white blood cells, and always < 20%. Eosinophilia and basophilia are observed in a minority of cases. Nucleated red blood cells are often seen. Red blood cell changes include macrocytosis (particularly in patients with monosomy 7), but normocytic red blood cells are more common; microcytosis due to iron deficiency or acquired thalassaemia phenotype {1680} may be seen as well. Platelet counts vary, but thrombocytopenia is typical and may be severe {2415,2872,3093}.

Bone marrow findings alone are not diagnostic. The bone marrow aspirate and biopsy are hypercellular with granulocytic proliferation, although in some patients erythroid precursors may predominate {2872,3093}. Monocytes in the bone marrow are often less prominent than in the peripheral blood, generally accounting for 5–10% of the bone marrow cells. Blasts (including promonocytes) account for < 20% of the bone marrow cells, and Auer rods are never present. Dysplasia is usually minimal; however, dysgranu-

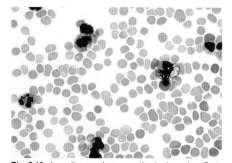

Fig. 5.10 Juvenile myelomonocytic leukaemia. Peripheral blood smear showing abnormal monocytes with cytoplasmic vacuoles and two normoblasts.

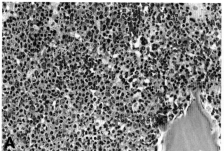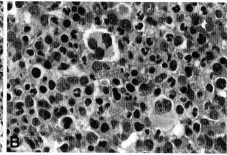

Fig. 5.11 Juvenile myelomonocytic leukaemia. **A** The bone marrow biopsy specimen is hypercellular, with granulocytic proliferation and a decreased number of megakaryocytes. **B** Although the megakaryocytes in this specific case are reduced in number, they appear morphologically normal; blasts are not substantially increased in number.

lopoiesis (including pseudo–Pelger–Huët neutrophils and hypogranularity) may be noted in some cases, and erythroid precursors may be enlarged. Megakaryocytes are often reduced in number, but marked megakaryocytic dysplasia is unusual {2872,3093}.

Leukaemic infiltrates are common in the skin, where myelomonocytic cells infiltrate the papillary and reticular dermis. In the lung, leukaemic cells spread from the capillaries of the alveolar septa into alveoli; in the spleen, they infiltrate the red pulp and have a predilection for trabecular and central arteries; in the liver, the sinusoids and portal tracts are infiltrated.

Cytochemistry

No specific cytochemical abnormalities have been reported. In bone marrow aspirate smears, cytochemical staining for alpha-naphthyl acetate esterase or alpha-naphthyl butyrate esterase, alone or in combination with staining for naphthol AS-D chloroacetate esterase (CAE), may be helpful in identifying the monocytic component. Neutrophil alkaline phosphatase scores are reported to be elevated in about 50% of cases, but this test is not helpful in establishing the diagnosis {2415}.

Immunophenotype

No specific immunophenotypic abnormalities have been reported in JMML. In extramedullary tissues, the monocytic component is best identified using immunohistochemical techniques that detect lysozyme and CD68R. However, individual cases may show infiltration almost exclusively by MPO-positive granulopoietic precursor cells. Flow cytometry, which enables simultaneous analysis of cell phenotype and cell signalling, shows that JMML cells exhibit an aberrant response of phospho-STAT5A to subsaturating doses of granulocyte–macrophage colony-stimulating factor {1578,2090}.

Cell of origin

A haematopoietic stem cell

Genetic profile

Karyotyping studies reveal monosomy 7 in about 25% of patients, other abnormalities in 10% and a normal karyotype in 65% {2872}. The Philadelphia (Ph) chromosome and the *BCR-ABL1* fusion gene are absent.

JMML occurs, at least in part, due to

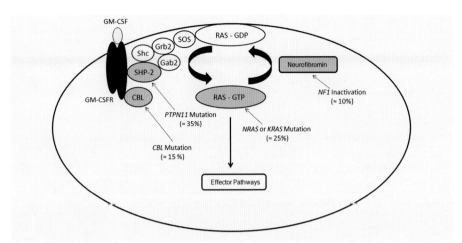

Fig. 5.12 Juvenile myelomonocytic leukaemia (JMML): molecular lesions in RAS signalling proteins. Granulocyte–macrophage colony-stimulating factor (GM-CSF; also called CSF2) normally binds to its receptor, induces heterodimerization, and assembles a complex of signalling molecules and adapters that include SHC1 and GRB2. These proteins, in turn, recruit GAB2, SHP2 (encoded by *PTPN11*) and SOS1, which catalyse guanine nucleotide exchange on RAS and increase intracellular levels of GTP-bound RAS (RAS-GTP). Once activated, RAS-GTP interacts with several downstream effectors. The GTPase-activating protein RASA1 (also called p120GAP) and neurofibromin bind to RAS-GTP and accelerate its conversion to RAS-GDP. Hypersensitivity to GM-CSF is a cellular hallmark of JMML that results from a number of distinct mechanisms. Mutations in *PTPN11* increase SHP2 phosphatase activity and increase RAS signalling. Similarly, cancer-associated amino acid substitutions in *KRAS* and *NRAS* result in mutant RAS proteins that accumulate in the active, GTP-bound conformation. Inactivation of the *NF1* tumour suppressor gene deregulates RAS signalling through loss of neurofibromin (reviewed by Niemeyer CM {2871}). Finally, CBL acts as a GM-CSF receptor responsive protein that targets SRC for ubiquitin-mediated destruction upon GM-CSF stimulation. Loss of negative regulation by SRC results in hyperactive GM-CSF {497}. Modified from Niemeyer CM {2871}.

aberrant signal transduction of the RAS signalling pathway. As many as 85% of patients harbour driving molecular alteration in one of five particular genes (*PTPN11*, *NRAS*, *KRAS*, *CBL* and *NF1*), which encode proteins that when mutated are predicted to activate RAS effector pathways. Heterozygous somatic gain-of-function mutations in *PTPN11* are the most frequent alterations, occurring in approximately 35% of patients {2382, 3906}. Typical oncogenic heterozygous somatic *NRAS* and *KRAS* mutations in codons 12, 13, and 61 account for 20–25% of JMML cases {3484,3801,3906}. Approximately 15% of children with JMML harbour germline *CBL* mutations {2874, 3131}, commonly missense alterations in the linker region or ring finger domain (exons 8 and 9), with JMML cells showing duplication of the mutant *CBL* through acquired uniparental disomy {587,2381, 2788}. Occasionally, heterozygous germline splice-site *CBL* mutations are noted in CBL-associated JMML {2381,2528, 3817}. Germline mutations in *NF1* are present in approximately 10% of children with JMML {587,2872,3484}. Because the *NF1* gene product (neurofibromin) is a negative modulator of RAS function, loss of heterozygosity (LOH) with loss of

the normal *NF1* allele in leukaemic cells is associated with RAS hyperactivity. Despite the central role of RAS pathway mutation, a small subset (approximately 15%) of cases remain RAS pathway mutation negative {3484,3801}. JMML is characterized by a paucity of additional genetic abnormalities {3484}. Secondary abnormalities (in addition to the canonical RAS pathway mutation) are present in fewer than half of all cases, and include second hits in one of the other RAS pathway genes (so-called RAS double mutants) as well as mutations in *SETBP1*, *JAK3*, *SH2B3*, the genes of the polycomb repressor complex, and *ASXL1* {587,3484,3801}. Secondary mutations are often subclonal and may be involved in disease progression rather than initiation of leukaemia {587,3484,3802}.

Genetic susceptibility

The RASopathies constitute a class of autosomal dominant developmental disorders caused by germline mutations in genes that encode components of the RAS pathway. These disorders' major features include facial dysmorphism, cardiac defects, reduced growth, variable cognitive deficits, ectodermal and skeletal anomalies, and susceptibility to

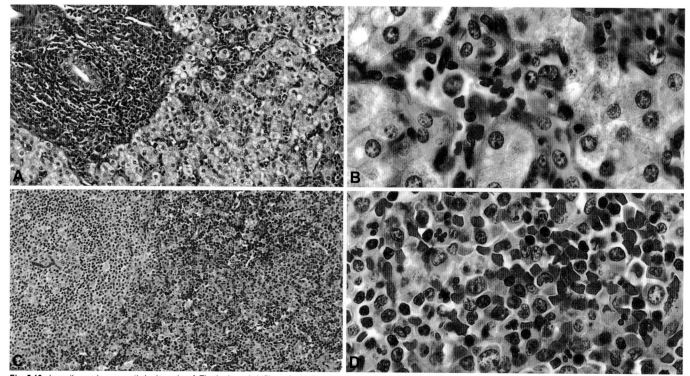

Fig. 5.13 Juvenile myelomonocytic leukaemia. **A** The leukaemic infiltrate in the liver is in the portal regions as well as in hepatic sinusoids. **B** The hepatic sinusoids are filled with the leukaemic infiltrate. **C** The leukaemic infiltrate in the red pulp of the spleen encroaches on the germinal centre. **D** The infiltrate in the splenic red pulp consists of immature and mature neutrophils and monocytes.

malignancies (including JMML) {2102, 2871,3316}.

NF1, the first syndrome found to be associated with a germline mutation in the RAS pathway, can manifest in early childhood with café-au-lait spots, JMML, plexiform neurofibromas, optic pathway tumours, and bone lesions {3314}. In children with NF1, the risk of developing JMML is estimated to be 200–350 times the risk in children without the syndrome {3804}. For about half of the patients with JMML and NF1, a positive family history is known. In most affected children, the clinical diagnosis of NF1 can be made at the time of leukaemic presentation; JMML may be the first manifestation of NF1 in some of these infants {3801}. Patients with Noonan syndrome–like disorder exhibit a variable Noonan syndrome–like phenotype, with a high frequency of neurological features and pigmented skin lesions {2528,2874,3817}. Susceptibility for JMML in children with germline *CBL* mutation is high, although the small number of patients precludes more precise risk estimation {2528}.

Noonan syndrome is the most common RASopathy, with an incidence of 1 case per 1000–2500 births {3317}. It is characterized by a typical facial appearance,

heart defects, and a variety of abnormalities in other organs. Heterozygous germline mutations in *PTPN11*, *SOS1*, *RAF1*, *KRAS*, *NRAS* and other components of the RAS pathway {811} are recognized, with *PTPN11* mutations accounting for about half of the cases {3317}. As many as 10% of children with Noonan syndrome develop a transient myeloproliferative disorder in early infancy {217, 2871}. The vast majority of patients with Noonan syndrome/myeloproliferative disorder harbour germline *PTPN11* mutations predicted to result in a weaker gain-of-function effect than the somatic *PTPN11* mutations found in children with JMML {2103}. The abnormal myelopoiesis in Noonan syndrome/myeloproliferative disorder is benign in most infants, but about 10% of these children acquire clonal chromosomal abnormalities and develop JMML {217,2871}.

Prognosis and predictive factors

JMML with somatic *PTPN11* mutation or occurring in children with NF1 is invariably rapidly fatal if left untreated. The median survival time without allogeneic haematopoietic stem cell transplantation is about 1 year. Low platelet count, patient age > 2 years at diagnosis and high

haemoglobin F levels at diagnosis are the main clinical predictors of short survival {2872,3093}.

JMML with *KRAS* or *NRAS* mutation generally has an aggressive course, with early haematopoietic stem cell transplantation needed. In a few infants with *KRAS* or *NRAS* alterations, long-term survival in the absence of therapy has been observed; these children had low haemoglobin F levels, normal or moderately decreased platelet counts, and no subclonal mutations {2377,3801}. There are similarities between JMML with *KRAS* or *NRAS* mutation and RAS-associated autoimmune leukoproliferative disorder (RALD) {530}. JMML and RALD show overlapping clinical and laboratory features (with the exception of the leukopenia seen in RALD). However, long-term follow-up suggests that RALD has an indolent clinical course, unlike most cases of JMML with RAS mutations {530}.

Most children with JMML and germline *CBL* mutations experience spontaneous regression of JMML with persistence of uniparental disomy of the *CBL* locus in haematopoietic cells. Occasionally, secondary genetic alterations occur that result in an aggressive clinical course.

Myelodysplastic / myeloproliferative neoplasm with ring sideroblasts and thrombocytosis

Orazi A.
Hasserjian R.P.
Cazzola M.
Thiele J.
Malcovati L.

Definition

Myelodysplastic/myeloproliferative neoplasm (MDS/MPN) with ring sideroblasts and thrombocytosis (MDS/MPN-RS-T) is a subtype of MDS/MPN characterized by the presence of thrombocytosis ($\geq 450 \times 10^9$/L) and < 1% blasts in the peripheral blood and associated with ring sideroblasts accounting for $\geq 15\%$ of erythroblasts, dyserythropoiesis and < 5% blasts in the bone marrow {1499, 1890,3104,3862}.

In the original 4th edition of the WHO classification, refractory anaemia with ring sideroblasts associated with marked thrombocytosis (RARS-T) was proposed as a provisional entity to encompass cases with the clinical and morphological features of myelodysplastic syndrome with ring sideroblasts (MDS-RS) but also with thrombocytosis associated with abnormal megakaryocytes similar to those seen in BCR-ABL1–negative myeloproliferative neoplasms {1499,1890}. More recently, MDS/MPN-RS-T has become a well-characterized, distinct MDS/MPN overlap entity, particularly following the discovery of a strong association with SF3B1 mutations, which are often concurrent with the JAK2 V617F mutation and less commonly with MPL or CALR mutation {409,594,1310,2461, 2464,3103,3339,3344,3569,3575,3773, 3862,4249}.

Cases that fulfil the diagnostic criteria for MDS with isolated del(5q) or that have t(3;3)(q21.3;q26.2) or inv(3)(q21.3q26.2) cytogenetic abnormalities are excluded from this category, as are cases with a BCR-ABL1 fusion gene. If there has been a prior diagnosis of an MPN without ring sideroblasts, or if there is evidence that the ring sideroblasts might be a consequence of therapy or might reflect disease progression of a case that meets the criteria for another well-defined MPN, this designation should not be used. It is unclear how to best categorize the rare cases that initially present as MDS-RS and later evolve to MDS/MPN-RS-T upon acquisition of a JAK2 V617F mutation {2461} or other MPN-associated muta-

tions. By convention, these cases would be considered to constitute disease progression of MDS, and would therefore be excluded from the MDS/MPN category (see Table 5.04); however, given the lack of prognostic difference, it might be most appropriate to group these cases with the rest of the cases of MDS/MPN-RS-T. Therapy-related cases with features of MDS/MPN-RS-T are diagnosed as therapy-related myeloid neoplasms and are discussed separately (see *Therapy-related myeloid neoplasms*, p. 153).

ICD-O code   9982/3

Synonym

Refractory anaemia with ring sideroblasts associated with marked thrombocytosis

Epidemiology

A median patient age at the time of diagnosis of 74 years has been reported, which is higher than that observed in MPN such as essential thrombocythaemia. A slight female prevalence has been consistently reported across studies {462,463}.

Localization

The peripheral blood and bone marrow are always involved. Splenomegaly has been reported in about 40% of cases, and hepatomegaly can also occur {3861}.

Clinical features

The clinical features of MDS/MPN-RS-T greatly overlap those seen in MDS-RS and the BCR-ABL1–negative MPN categories, in particular essential thrombocythaemia. Anaemia is always present, but at the time of clinical presentation, patients with MDS/MPN-RS-T tend to have higher haemoglobin levels, white blood cell (WBC) counts, and platelet counts than do patients with MDS-RS, with similar mean corpuscular volumes. In contrast, patients with MDS/MPN-RS-T have lower haemoglobin levels, WBC counts, and platelet counts, but higher mean corpuscular volumes than do patients with essential thrombocythaemia {463}.

Microscopy

The peripheral blood typically shows normochromic macrocytic or normocytic anaemia. The red blood cells in the blood smear may show anisocytosis, often with a dimorphic pattern. Circulating blasts are absent or rare (accounting for < 1% of the cells). Thrombocytosis ($\geq 450 \times 10^9$/L) is one of the defining features. The platelets often display anisocytosis, ranging from tiny forms to atypical large or giant platelets. Bizarrely shaped or agranular platelets may be seen, but are uncommon. The WBC count and leukocyte differential count are usually normal, although a borderline elevation in the WBC count can occur.

Table 5.04 Diagnostic criteria for myelodysplastic/myeloproliferative neoplasm with ring sideroblasts and thrombocytosis

- Anaemia associated with erythroid-lineage dysplasia, with or without multilineage dysplasia; $\geq 15\%$ ring sideroblasts[a], < 1% blasts in the peripheral blood and < 5% blasts in the bone marrow
- Persistent thrombocytosis, with platelet count $\geq 450 \times 10^9$/L
- SF3B1 mutation or, in the absence of SF3B1 mutation, no history of recent cytotoxic or growth factor therapy that could explain the myelodysplastic/myeloproliferative features[b]
- No BCR-ABL1 fusion; no rearrangement of PDGFRA, PDGFRB or FGFR1; no PCM1-JAK2 and no t(3;3)(q21.3;q26.2), inv(3)(q21.3q26.2), or del(5q)[c]
- No history of myeloproliferative neoplasm, myelodysplastic syndrome (except myelodysplastic syndrome with ring sideroblasts), or other myelodysplastic/myeloproliferative neoplasm

---

[a] $\geq 15\%$ ring sideroblasts is a required criterion even if SF3B1 mutation is detected.
[b] The diagnosis of myelodysplastic/myeloproliferative neoplasm with ring sideroblasts and thrombocytosis is strongly supported by the presence of SF3B1 mutation together with a JAK2 V617F, CALR or MPL mutation.
[c] In a case that otherwise meets the diagnostic criteria for myelodysplastic syndrome with isolated del(5q).

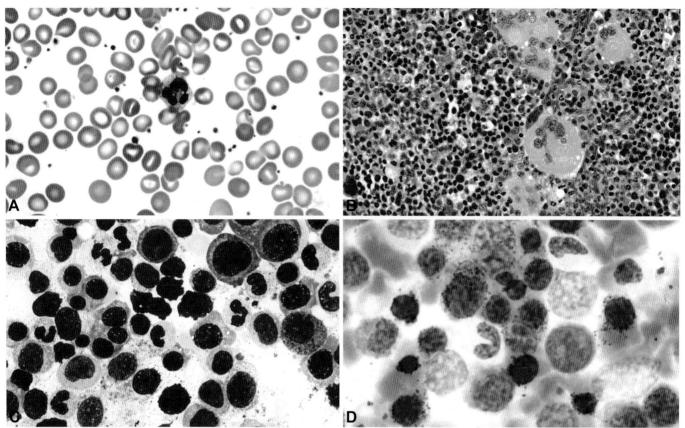

Fig. 5.14 Myelodysplastic/myeloproliferative neoplasm with ring sideroblasts and thrombocytosis, in a 62-year-old man who presented with severe anaemia and a platelet count of 850 × 10⁹/L. **A** The blood smear shows abnormal red blood cells and thrombocytosis. **B** Marked erythroid proliferation and essential thrombocythaemia–like megakaryocytes are apparent in the bone marrow biopsy section. **C** The bone marrow aspirate smear shows mild dyserythropoiesis. **D** Iron (Prussian blue) staining of the marrow aspirate highlights marked erythroid proliferation, in which most of the erythroid precursors are ring sideroblasts.

The bone marrow shows increased erythropoiesis due to ineffective erythroid proliferation, with megaloblastoid and/or other dyserythropoietic features of the erythroid precursors associated with ≥ 15% ring sideroblasts present on iron staining. Multilineage dysplasia, similar to that seen in MDS-RS and multilineage dysplasia, occurs in some cases {3569, 3570}. Megakaryocytes are increased and usually have morphological features similar to those observed in the *BCR-ABL1*–negative MPN. A proportion of patients have marrow fibrosis {3569,3570}.

Cell of origin
A haematopoietic stem cell

Genetic profile
Cytogenetic abnormalities have been reported in about 10% of patients {2461}. Many cases (60–90%) harbour the *SF3B1* mutation {2460}. The mutant allele burden is comparable to that seen in other WHO categories with ring side-

roblasts. The *SF3B1* mutation is often (in > 60% of cases) found in association with the *JAK2* V617F mutation, and much less commonly (in < 10% of cases) in association with the *CALR* or *MPL* W515 mutation. The presence of these MPN-associated mutations may account for the proliferative aspects of MDS/MPN-RS-T and would seem to confirm its true hybrid nature {2461,2464,3103,3570,4202}. Therefore, although studies for *SF3B1*, *JAK2* V617F, *CALR* and *MPL* W515 mutations are not required for the diagnosis of MDS/MPN-RS-T, the presence of these mutations supports the diagnosis and appears to have prognostic significance.

Prognosis and predictive factors
A median overall survival of 76–128 months has been reported in patients with MDS/MPN-RS-T {462,463}. A retrospective study including a total of 200 cases from 16 centres in six European countries showed that sex- and age-standardized survival in patients with

MDS/MPN-RS-T is significantly shorter than that of patients with essential thrombocythaemia, but longer than that of patients with MDS-RS and single lineage dysplasia (P < 0.001) {463,4249}.
Patient age, *JAK2* V617F and *SF3B1* mutation have been reported as independent prognostic factors. In one study of MDS/MPN-RS-T, *SF3B1* mutation was associated with a significantly longer median overall survival (6.9 years with *SF3B1* mutation vs 3.3 years with *SF3B1* wildtype, P = 0.003); *JAK2* V617F mutation was also associated with a more favourable outcome compared with *JAK2* wildtype (P = 0.019) {462}.
The existing scientific literature does not support any therapy specific for patients with MDS/MPN-RS-T; the treatments available for MDS and MPN are typically adopted for these patients, depending on the clinical picture {2460}.

Myelodysplastic / myeloproliferative neoplasm, unclassifiable

Orazi A.
Bennett J.M.
Bain B.J.
Baumann I.

Thiele J.
Bueso-Ramos C.
Malcovati L.

Definition

Myelodysplastic/myeloproliferative neoplasm (MDS/MPN), unclassifiable (MDS/MPN-U) meets the criteria for the MDS/MPN category in that at the time of initial presentation, it has clinical, laboratory and morphological features that overlap with both myelodysplastic syndrome (MDS) and myeloproliferative neoplasm (MPN) categories {1748,2987, 4152} (Table 5.05). Cases diagnosed as MDS/MPN-U do not meet the criteria for chronic myelomonocytic leukaemia, juvenile myelomonocytic leukaemia, BCR-ABL1–negative atypical chronic myeloid leukaemia, or MDS/MPN with ring sideroblasts and thrombocytosis (MDS/MPN-RS-T). The removal of MDS/MPN-RS-T from the category of MDS/MPN-U is a change from the original 4th edition of the WHO classification. The finding of BCR-ABL1 fusion; rearrangement of PDGFRA, PDGFRB, or FGFR1; or PCM1-JAK2 also rules out the diagnosis of MDS/MPN-U. Therapy-related cases with features of MDS/MPN-U are discussed separately (see Therapy-related myeloid neoplasms, p. 153).

The designation MDS/MPN-U must not be used for cases in which a previously well-defined MPN has developed dysplastic features in association with progression to a more aggressive phase. However, the MDS/MPN-U category may include some cases in which the chronic phase of an MPN was not previously detected, and that therefore initially present in an advanced phase, with myelodysplastic features. If the underlying MPN in such cases cannot be identified, the designation of MDS/MPN-U is appropriate.

If a patient has recently received any growth factor or other therapy capable of producing peripheral blood and/or bone marrow changes simulating MDS/MPN, clinical and laboratory follow-up is essential to determine whether the observed anomalies are persistent or a consequence of such treatments.

ICD-O code   9975/3

Table 5.05 Diagnostic criteria for myelodysplastic/myeloproliferative neoplasm, unclassifiable

Myeloid neoplasm with mixed myeloproliferative and myelodysplastic features at onset, not meeting the WHO criteria for any other myelodysplastic/myeloproliferative neoplasm, myelodysplastic syndrome or myeloproliferative neoplasm

- < 20% blasts in the peripheral blood and bone marrow
- Clinical and morphological features of one of the categories of myelodysplastic syndrome[a]
- Clinical and morphological myeloproliferative features manifesting as a platelet count of ≥ 450 × 10^9/L associated with bone marrow megakaryocytic proliferation and/or a white blood cell count of ≥ 13 × 10^9/L[a]
- No history of recent cytotoxic or growth factor therapy that could explain the myelodysplastic/myeloproliferative features
- No PDGFRA, PDGFRB, or FGFR1 rearrangement and no PCM1-JAK2

[a] Cases that meet criteria for myelodysplastic syndrome with isolated del(5q) are excluded irrespective of the presence of thrombocytosis or leukocytosis.

Synonyms

Chronic myelodysplastic/myeloproliferative disease (no longer used); mixed myeloproliferative/myelodysplastic syndrome, unclassifiable; overlap syndrome, unclassifiable

Localization

The bone marrow and peripheral blood are always involved. The spleen, liver, and other extramedullary tissues may be involved.

Clinical features

The clinical features of MDS/MPN-U overlap with those of entities in the MDS and MPN categories {227,2857,4152}.

Microscopy

MDS/MPN-U is characterized by ineffective and/or dysplastic proliferation of one or more myeloid lineages and simultaneously by effective proliferation (with or without dysplasia) of another myeloid lineage or lineages. Laboratory features usually include anaemia of variable severity, with or without macrocytosis. There is evidence of effective proliferation in one or more lineages: either thrombocytosis (platelet count ≥ 450 × 10^9/L) or leukocytosis (white blood cell count ≥ 13 × 10^9/L). In a recent study, the median white blood cell count was lower in MDS/MPN-U (19.4 × 10^9/L) than in atypical chronic myeloid leukaemia, BCR-ABL1–negative, (40.8 × 10^9/L)

{4248}. Neutrophils may show dysplastic features, but dysgranulopoiesis is seen in only about 50% of cases {4248}. There may be giant or hypogranular platelets. Dysmegakaryopoiesis with megakaryocytes resembling those seen in MDS is found in more than half of cases. In the remaining cases, there is a mixture of MDS-like and MPN-like megakaryocytes or (rarely) a predominance of MPN-like megakaryocytes. Dysmegakaryopoiesis is absent in < 10% of cases {4248}. Blasts account for < 20% of leukocytes in the peripheral blood and < 20% of nucleated cells in the bone marrow. The bone marrow biopsy specimen is hypercellular and may show proliferation in any or all of the myeloid lineages; however, significant (≥ 10%) dysplastic features are simultaneously present in at least one cell line. Although cases of MDS/MPN-RS-T are classified separately, rare cases of MDS/MPN with ≥ 15% ring sideroblasts and ≥ 1% peripheral blood blasts or ≥ 5% bone marrow blasts belong in the MDS/MPN-U group.

Cytochemistry

The cytochemical findings may be similar to those seen in MDS or MPN.

Immunophenotype

The immunophenotype may be similar to that of MDS or MPN.

Cell of origin

The postulated cell of origin is a haematopoietic stem cell.

Genetic profile

There are no cytogenetic or molecular genetic findings specific for this group. The Philadelphia (Ph) chromosome and the *BCR-ABL1* fusion gene should always be excluded prior to making the diagnosis of MDS/MPN-U. Cases with re-arrangements of *PDGFRA*, *PDGFRB*, or *FGFR1* or with *PCM1-JAK2*, are excluded from this category as well.

The appropriate categorization of cases associated with isolated isochromosome 17q is uncertain. A proportion of cases meet the criteria for chronic myelomonocytic leukaemia, *BCR-ABL1*–negative atypical chronic myeloid leukaemia, MPN in accelerated or blast phase, MDS or acute myeloid leukaemia, but other cases may be appropriately categorized as MDS/MPN-U {1220,1912,2594}.

Relatively high frequencies of *TET2*, *NRAS*, *RUNX1*, *CBL*, *SETBP1* and *ASXL1* mutations have been reported in several studies {2610,4248,4502}. In diagnostically difficult cases, the presence of one or more of these mutations in the appropriate clinicopathological context may help to confirm a suspected diagnosis. *SF3B1* mutation should prompt careful exclusion of MDS/MPN-RS-T, including rare instances of disease progression from MDS with ring sideroblasts. Although cases that meet the criteria for MDS with isolated del(5q) are excluded, a small proportion of such cases with a combined del(5q) and *JAK2* V617F mutation have been reported to have proliferative features in the bone marrow associated with higher median platelet counts {1759}. However, it is unclear whether their clinical presentation or prognosis is any different from that of the MDS with isolated del(5q) and wildtype *JAK2* {3101,3717}. Until more evidence is published, it is recommended that cases with combined del(5q) and *JAK2* V617F mu-

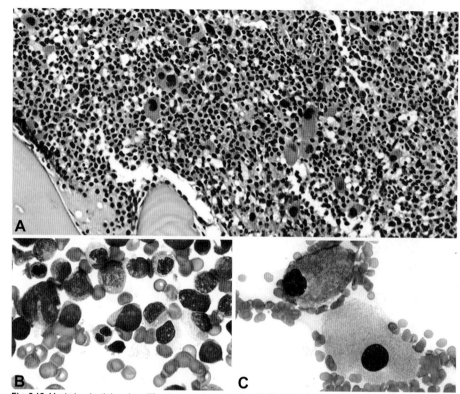

Fig. 5.15 Myelodysplastic/myeloproliferative neoplasm, unclassifiable. A case associated with isolated isochromosome 17q. **A** Bone marrow core biopsy showing hypercellularity with increased dysplastic megakaryocytes and increased immature cells. **B** Bone marrow aspirate smear showing increased blasts and dysplastic granulocytes with pseudo–Pelger–Huët nuclei (Wright-Giemsa). **C** Bone marrow aspirate showing dysplastic non-lobated megakaryocytes (Wright-Giemsa).

tation be classified as MDS with isolated del(5q) rather than included in the MDS/MPN-U category.

Cases with MDS/MPN features that harbour one of the types of driver mutations seen in classic MPN (i.e. *JAK2*, *MPL* or *CALR* mutations) most likely constitute MPN with features of disease progression. However, if a chronic phase has not been previously detected or cannot be documented and therefore the underlying MPN cannot be confirmed, then the designation of MDS/MPN-U is justified.

Prognosis and predictive factors

There is very limited information available about this rare subgroup. In a recent study, patients with MDS/MPN-U had a median overall survival of 21.8 months and leukaemia-free survival of 18.9 months {4248}. Prognosis is variable, with its uncertainty further compounded by inadequate representation of the subgroup in commonly used prognostic scoring systems, including the International Prognostic Scoring System (IPSS) and Revised IPSS (IPSS-R) {4011}. As with other MDS/MPN overlap disorders, the treatment for patients with MDS/MPN-U is based on therapies used for MDS or MPN and is guided by symptoms and/or cytopenias {4011}. Growth factors (erythropoiesis- and granulopoiesis-stimulating agents) can alleviate cytopenias, whereas leukocytosis can be managed with cytoreductive therapies.

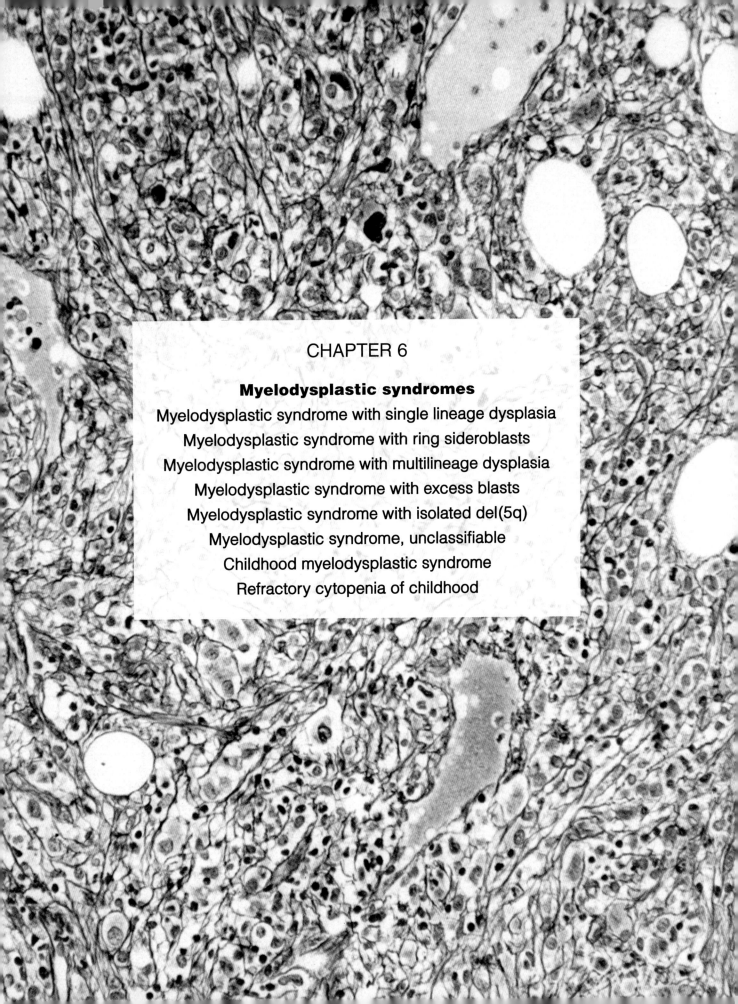

CHAPTER 6

Myelodysplastic syndromes
Myelodysplastic syndrome with single lineage dysplasia
Myelodysplastic syndrome with ring sideroblasts
Myelodysplastic syndrome with multilineage dysplasia
Myelodysplastic syndrome with excess blasts
Myelodysplastic syndrome with isolated del(5q)
Myelodysplastic syndrome, unclassifiable
Childhood myelodysplastic syndrome
Refractory cytopenia of childhood

Myelodysplastic syndromes: Overview

Hasserjian R.P.
Orazi A.
Brunning R.D.
Germing U.
Le Beau M.M.
Porwit A.

Baumann I.
Hellström-
  Lindberg E.
List A.F.
Cazzola M.
Foucar K.

Definition

The myelodysplastic syndromes (MDS) are a group of clonal haematopoietic stem cell diseases characterized by cytopenia, dysplasia in one or more of the major myeloid lineages, ineffective haematopoiesis, recurrent genetic abnormalities and increased risk of developing acute myeloid leukaemia (AML) {340, 592,4151}. There is an increased degree of apoptosis within the bone marrow progenitors, which contributes to the cytopenias {439}. Cytopenia in at least one haematopoietic lineage is required for a diagnosis of MDS. The recommended thresholds for cytopenias established in the original International Prognostic Scoring System (IPSS) for risk stratification (haemoglobin concentration < 10 g/dL, platelet count < 100 × 10^9/L, and absolute neutrophil count < 1.8 × 10^9/L {1442,1442A}), have traditionally been used to define cytopenias for MDS diagnosis and most MDS patients will have a cytopenia below at least one of these thresholds. However, a diagnosis of MDS may still be made in patients with milder degrees of anaemia (haemoglobin < 13 g/dL in men or < 12 g/dL in women) or thrombocytopenia (platelets < 150 x 10^9/L) if definitive morphologic and/or cytogenetic findings are present {1444A,4179}. In determining whether a patient is cytopenic, it is important to be cognizant of each laboratory's lower reference range and to take into account conditional variants of these values, such as due to ethnicity and sex. These are particularly important considerations in patients with a borderline low neutrophil count {229}. Persistent neutrophilia, monocytosis, erythrocytosis or thrombocytosis in a patient with cytopenias and dysplastic morphology generally warrants classification as a myelodysplastic/myeloproliferative neoplasm (MDS/MPN) or myeloproliferative neoplasm rather than MDS. However, thrombocytosis (platelet count ≥450 × 10^9/L) is allowed in MDS with isolated del(5q) or with inv(3) (q21.3q26.2) or t(3;3)(q21.3;q26.2).

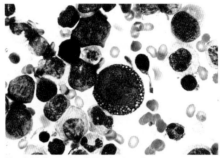

Fig. 6.01 Parvovirus B19 infection. Bone marrow smear shows marked erythroid hypoplasia, with occasional giant erythroblasts with dispersed chromatin and fine cytoplasmic vacuoles.

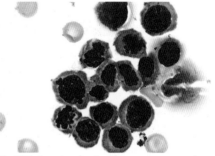

Fig. 6.02 Arsenic poisoning. Bone marrow smear from a 47-year-old man with pancytopenia being chronically exposed to arsenic; there is marked dyserythropoiesis.

The morphological hallmark of MDS is dysplasia in one or more myeloid lineages. Dysplasia may be accompanied by an increase in myeloblasts in the peripheral blood and/or bone marrow, but the blast percentage is always < 20%, which is the requisite threshold recommended for the diagnosis of AML. It is important to recognize that the threshold of 20% blasts distinguishing AML from MDS does not reflect a therapeutic mandate to treat cases with ≥20% blasts as acute leukaemia. Recurrent cytogenetic abnormalities are present in 40–50% of cases, whereas acquired somatic gene mutations are seen in the vast majority of MDS cases at diagnosis.

The MDS category encompasses several distinct subtypes, which are defined by the number of cytopenias at presentation, the number of myeloid lineages manifesting dysplasia, the presence of ring sideroblasts, and the blast percentages in the blood and bone marrow. In the current classification, only one cytogenetic abnormality, del(5q), is used in the definition of a specific MDS subtype. Mutation of one gene, *SF3B1*, is closely associated with MDS with ring sideroblasts as well as with one of the MDS/MPN subtypes: MDS/MPN with ring sideroblasts and thrombocytosis.

Although progression to AML is the natural course in many cases of MDS, the percentage of patients who progress varies substantially across the subtypes, with a higher probability of progression in subtypes with increased myeloblasts

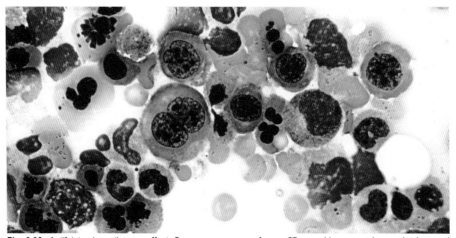

Fig. 6.03 Antifolate chemotherapy effect. Bone marrow smear from a 57-year-old woman who received several chemotherapeutic agents for breast carcinoma, including folic acid antagonists, showing transient marked dyserythropoiesis and megaloblastic changes.

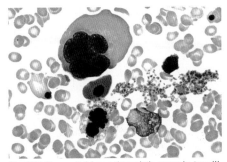

Fig. 6.04 Congenital dyserythropoietic anaemia, type III. Bone marrow smear shows marked dyserythropoiesis.

{1340,2467}. Most subtypes are characterized by progressive bone marrow failure, but the biological course of some subtypes is prolonged and indolent, with a very low incidence of evolution to AML {2462,4179}.

Epidemiology
MDS occurs principally in older adults (median patient age: 70 years), with a male predominance. The annual incidence is 3–5 cases per 100 000 population overall (non–age-corrected) and is at least 20 cases per 100 000 individuals aged >70 years. Due to underreporting of MDS in most cancer registries, the true annual incidence in patients aged >65 years may be closer to 75 cases per 100 000 population {199,777,1342}. Approximately 10 000 new cases of MDS are diagnosed annually in the USA, according to 2003–2004 data from the Surveillance, Epidemiology, and End Results (SEER) Program and the North American Association of Central Cancer Registries (NAACCR), but estimates based on Medicare claims for the same time period are as high as 45 000 cases diagnosed in individuals aged >65 years annually {1394,2421,3397}. Therapy-related myeloid neoplasms are discussed separately (see *Therapy-related myeloid neoplasms*, p. 153). MDS affecting children is rare and has unique characteristics and diagnostic criteria that differ from those of MDS in adults; therefore, childhood cases are also discussed separately (p. 116).

Etiology
Primary or de novo MDS occurs without a known history of chemotherapy or radiation exposure. Possible etiologies for primary MDS include benzene exposure (at levels well above the minimum allowed by most government agencies), cigarette smoking (at least in part also due to benzene in cigarette smoke), exposure to agricultural chemicals or solvents, and family history of haematopoietic neoplasms {3815}. Some inherited haematological disorders, such as Fanconi anaemia, dyskeratosis congenita, Shwachman–Diamond syndrome and Diamond–Blackfan anaemia, are also associated with an increased risk of MDS; familial syndromes predisposing to MDS and AML are discussed separately (see *Myeloid neoplasms with germline predisposition*, p. 121). Acquired aplastic anaemia is also associated with increased risk of development of MDS {222}.

Clinical features
The majority of patients present with symptoms related to cytopenia. Most patients are anaemic, whereas neutropenia and/or thrombocytopenia are less common; about one third of patients are dependent on red blood cell transfusions at diagnosis {1444,2511}. Organomegaly is infrequently observed.

Microscopy
The morphological classification of MDS is principally based on the percentage of blasts in the bone marrow and peripheral blood, the type and degree of dysplasia, and the percentage of ring sideroblasts (Table 6.01, p. 101). The myeloid lineages affected by cytopenias are not necessarily those that manifest dysplasia {1338, 2423,4179}. To determine blast percentage in the bone marrow and blood, a 500-cell differential count of all nucleated cells in a smear or trephine biopsy imprint is recommended for the bone marrow and a 200-leukocyte differential count for the peripheral blood. In patients with severe cytopenia, buffy coat smears of peripheral blood may facilitate the differential count. An accurate blast count in the peripheral blood is important, because patients with higher blast percentages in the blood than in the bone marrow (seen in ~13% of MDS cases) appear to have more aggressive disease {89}. The blast count in myeloid neoplasms is expressed as a percentage of all nucleated cells (always including nucleated erythroid cells) in the bone marrow and as a percentage of the leukocytes (excluding nucleated erythroid cells) in the peripheral blood.

The number of dysplastic lineages (i.e. single lineage vs multilineage dysplasia) is relevant for distinguishing between the types of MDS (see Table 6.01, p. 101) and may be important for predicting disease behaviour {947,4179}. Assessment of the degree of dysplasia may be problematic, depending on the quality of the smear preparations and the stain. Poor-quality smears may result in misinterpretation of the presence or absence of dysplasia, particularly in assessing neutrophil granulation. Given the critical importance of recognizing dysplasia, the need for high-quality slide preparations for the diagnosis of MDS cannot be overemphasized. Slides for the assessment of dysplasia should be made from freshly obtained specimens; specimens exposed to anticoagulants for >2 hours are unsatisfactory. It should be noted that the determination of whether significant dysplasia is present (particularly in the erythroid lineage) and the distinction between single lineage and multilineage dysplasia have been found in some studies to be subject to significant interobserver variability {1233,3622}. This interobserver variability is more problematic for cases in which the degree of dysplasia is near the requisite 10% threshold, and some authors have reported individual lineage dysplasia exceeding the 10% threshold in non-cytopenic controls {947,3067, 3297}; consequently, it is essential to apply strict criteria for dysplasia and to evaluate high-quality and well-stained material.

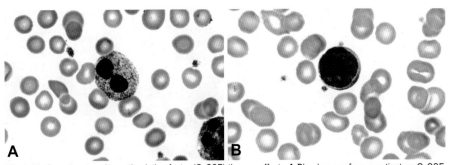

Fig. 6.05 Granulocyte colony-stimulating factor (G-CSF) therapy effect. **A** Blood smear from a patient on G-CSF, showing a neutrophil with a bilobed nucleus and increased azurophilic granulation and a myeloblast (**B**).

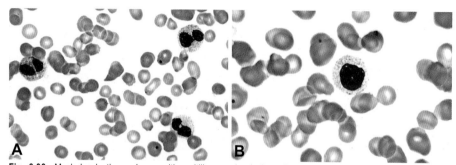

Fig. 6.06 Myelodysplastic syndrome with multilineage dysplasia and a complex karyotype including del(17p). Dysgranulopoiesis is evident on these blood smears, showing three neutrophils with bilobed nuclei (pseudo–Pelger–Huët anomaly) (**A**) and a neutrophil with a non-segmented nucleus (**B**).

As a general precaution, no patient should be diagnosed with MDS if the clinical and drug history is unknown, and no case of MDS should be reclassified while the patient is on growth factor therapy, including erythropoietin. Certain drugs, infections, metabolic deficiencies and immune disorders can cause both cytopenias and morphological dysplasia; these possible secondary etiologies must be carefully considered prior to rendering a diagnosis of MDS (see *Differential diagnosis*). Unexplained, persistent cytopenia in the absence of dysplasia should not be interpreted as MDS unless certain specific cytogenetic abnormalities are present (see *Genetic profile* below and Table 6.03, p. 104). Persistent cytopenia without dysplasia and without one of the specific cytogenetic abnormalities should be diagnosed as idiopathic cytopenia of undetermined significance, and the patient's haematological and cytogenetic status should be carefully monitored {4106,4336}. Patients with MDS-associated clonal gene mutations identified in haematopoietic cells but without significant dysplasia on bone marrow examination should not be diag-

nosed with MDS either; this condition has been termed 'clonal haematopoiesis of indeterminate potential' {3772}.

Cases of MDS without an increase in blasts are recognized as manifesting either single lineage dysplasia or multilineage dysplasia. In most cases of MDS with single lineage dysplasia, the dysplasia is confined to the erythroid lineage. Single lineage dysplasia can also affect the granulocytic lineage or megakaryocytes, but this is much less common than dysplasia isolated to erythroid cells {450,2423}. In MDS with multilineage dysplasia, significant dysplastic features are recognized in two or more lineages. The recommended requisite percentage of erythroid and granulocytic cells manifesting dysplasia to be considered significant is ≥10% {3404}. Significant megakaryocyte dysplasia is defined as ≥10% dysplastic megakaryocytes based on evaluation of ≥30 megakaryocytes in smears or sections; however, some studies suggest that a 30–40% threshold for megakaryocyte dysplasia may provide greater specificity {947,1309,2567}. Micromegakaryocytes and multinucleated megakaryocytes with separated nuclei

are the most reliable dysplastic findings in the megakaryocyte series {947,2567, 4179}.

Characteristics of dysplasia
Dyserythropoiesis manifests principally as nuclear alterations, including budding, internuclear bridging, karyorrhexis and multinuclearity. Megaloblastoid changes are often present in MDS, but alone they are insufficiently specific to firmly establish dyserythropoiesis. Cytoplasmic features include formation of ring sideroblasts, vacuolization and aberrant periodic acid–Schiff (PAS) positivity (either diffuse or granular). Dysgranulopoiesis is characterized primarily by nuclear hyposegmentation (pseudo–Pelger–Huët anomaly) or hypersegmentation, cytoplasmic hypogranularity, pseudo–Chédiak–Higashi granules and small size {1387}. Megakaryocyte dysplasia is characterized by micromegakaryocytes, non-lobated nuclei in megakaryocytes of all sizes, and multiple widely separated nuclei {1388}; however, the finding of multiple widely separated nuclei is of limited specificity for MDS, unless the nuclei are rounded and roughly similar in size. Megakaryocytic dysplasia is readily apparent in bone marrow sections, and both biopsy and aspirate specimens should be evaluated. The morphological manifestations of dysplasia in each lineage are summarized in Table 6.02. Auer rods are considered to be evidence of MDS with excess blasts regardless of the blast percentage. Cases of MDS with <5% blasts in the bone marrow and <1% in the peripheral blood may rarely have Auer rods, and such cases are associated with an adverse prognosis {4328}.

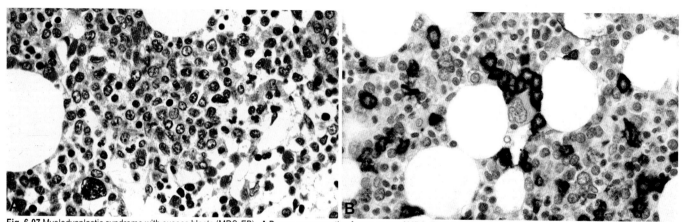

Fig. 6.07 Myelodysplastic syndrome with excess blasts (MDS-EB). **A** Bone marrow section from a case of MDS-EB-1 containing a focus of immature myeloid precursors. **B** Bone marrow biopsy from a case of MDS-EB-2 showing a focus of immature cells, most of which stain positively for CD34.

Table 6.01 Diagnostic criteria for myelodysplastic syndrome (MDS) entities

Entity name	Number of dysplastic lineages	Number of cytopenias[a]	Ring sideroblasts as percentage of marrow erythroid elements	Bone marrow (BM) and peripheral blood (PB) blasts	Cytogenetics by conventional karyotype analysis
MDS-SLD	1	1–2	< 15% / < 5%[b]	BM < 5%, PB < 1%, no Auer rods	Any, unless fulfils all criteria for MDS with isolated del(5q)
MDS-MLD	2–3	1–3	< 15% / < 5%[b]	BM < 5%, PB < 1%, no Auer rods	Any, unless fulfils all criteria for MDS with isolated del(5q)
MDS-RS					
MDS-RS-SLD	1	1–2	≥ 15% / ≥ 5%[b]	BM < 5%, PB < 1%, no Auer rods	Any, unless fulfils all criteria for MDS with isolated del(5q)
MDS-RS-MLD	2–3	1–3	≥ 15% / ≥ 5%[b]	BM < 5%, PB < 1%, no Auer rods	Any, unless fulfils all criteria for MDS with isolated del(5q)
MDS with isolated del(5q)	1–3	1–2	None or any	BM < 5%, PB < 1%, no Auer rods	del(5q) alone or with 1 additional abnormality, except loss of chromosome 7 or del(7q)
MDS-EB					
MDS-EB-1	1–3	1–3	None or any	BM 5–9% or PB 2–4%, BM < 10% and PB < 5%, no Auer rods	Any
MDS-EB-2	1–3	1–3	None or any	BM 10–19% or PB 5–19% or Auer rods, BM and PB < 20%	Any
MDS-U					
with 1% blood blasts	1–3	1–3	None or any	BM < 5%, PB = 1%[c], no Auer rods	Any
with SLD and pancytopenia	1	3	None or any	BM < 5%, PB < 1%, no Auer rods	Any
based on defining cytogenetic abnormality	0	1–3	< 15%[d]	BM < 5%, PB < 1%, no Auer rods	MDS-defining abnormality[e]

MDS-EB, MDS with excess blasts; MDS-MLD, MDS with multilineage dysplasia; MDS-RS, MDS with ring sideroblasts; MDS-RS-MLD, MDS with ring sideroblasts and multilineage dysplasia; MDS-RS-SLD, MDS with ring sideroblasts and single lineage dysplasia; MDS-SLD, MDS with single lineage dysplasia; MDS-U, MDS, unclassifiable; SLD, single lineage dysplasia.

[a] Cytopenias defined as haemoglobin concentration < 10 g/dL, platelet count < 100 × 10^9/L and absolute neutrophil count < 1.8 × 10^9/L, although MDS can present with mild anaemia or thrombocytopenia above these levels; PB monocytes must be < 1 × 10^9/L.

[b] If *SF3B1* mutation is present.

[c] 1% PB blasts must be recorded on ≥ 2 separate occasions.

[d] Cases with ≥ 15% ring sideroblasts by definition have significant erythroid dysplasia and are classified as MDS-RS-SLD.

[e] See Table 6.03, p. 104.

Differential diagnosis

A major difficulty in the diagnosis of MDS is the determination of whether the presence of morphological dysplasia and cytopenia is due to a clonal disorder or is the result of another factor. Dysplasia, even if prominent, is not in itself definitive evidence of a clonal process. Some dysplastic features, such as micromegakaryocytes, are strongly associated with MDS {947}, but several nutritional, toxic and other factors can also cause myelodysplastic changes in any of the haematopoietic lineages. These factors include vitamin B12 and folic acid deficiency, essential element deficiencies (such as copper deficiency), exposure to heavy metals (in particular arsenic, lead and toxic levels of zinc) and exposure to several commonly used drugs and biological agents {439}. Isoniazole treatment in the absence of vitamin B6 supplementation causes ring sideroblast formation. The antibiotic cotrimoxazole and the immunosuppressants tacrolimus and mycophenolate mofetil can cause marked neutrophil hyposegmentation, often indistinguishable from the changes seen in MDS. In some patients on multiple drugs or with multiple comorbidities, it may be difficult to identify the cause of dysplastic changes {1991,3867}. Dysplastic changes can also be encountered in otherwise

Table 6.02 Morphological manifestations of dysplasia

Dyserythropoiesis
Nuclear
Nuclear budding
Internuclear bridging
Karyorrhexis
Multinuclearity
Megaloblastoid changes
Cytoplasmic
Ring sideroblasts
Vacuolization
Periodic acid–Schiff (PAS) positivity

Dysgranulopoiesis
Small or unusually large size
Nuclear hyposegmentation
(pseudo–Pelger–Huët)
Nuclear hypersegmentation
Decreased granules; agranularity
Pseudo–Chédiak–Higashi granules
Döhle bodies
Auer rods

Dysmegakaryopoiesis
Micromegakaryocytes
Nuclear hypolobation
Multinucleation (normal megakaryocytes are uninuclear with lobated nuclei)

normal marrow {3067}, such as in individuals with the hereditary autosomal dominant Pelger–Huët anomaly resulting from mutations in the *LBR* gene (encoding lamin B receptor) {1658}. Therefore, it is extremely important to correlate the morphological findings with the clinical presentation and any pertinent family history. Congenital haematological disorders such as congenital dyserythropoietic anaemia must also be considered as a possible cause of isolated dyserythropoiesis. Parvovirus B19 infection may be associated with erythroblastopenia with giant pronormoblasts; the immunosuppressive agent mycophenolate mofetil may also be associated with erythroblastopenia. Chemotherapeutic agents may result in transient marked dysplasia of all

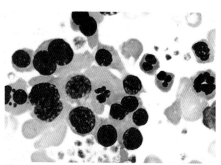

Fig. 6.08 Myelodysplastic syndrome with multilineage dysplasia and complex cytogenetic abnormalities, including del(17p) and del(5q). Dyserythropoiesis is evident on this bone marrow smear from an adult male patient.

myeloid lineages. Granulocyte colony-stimulating factor therapy causes morphological alterations in the neutrophils, including a substantial left shift, marked hypergranularity and nuclear hyposegmentation {3572}. Additionally, blasts (usually < 5%) may be observed transiently in the peripheral blood; the bone marrow blast percentage is generally normal in such cases, but is transiently increased in some cases. Hypothyroidism, infections, autoimmune disorders, paroxysmal nocturnal haemoglobinuria and bone marrow lymphomatous involvement (in particular large granular lymphocytic leukaemia and hairy cell leukaemia) may clinically mimic MDS.

Given all these possibilities, it is extremely important to be aware of the clinical history (including exposure to drugs or chemicals) and to always consider non-clonal disorders as possible etiologies of morphological dysplasia in haematopoietic cells, particularly in cases with no increase in blasts. Haematological follow-up over a period of several months, possibly including repeated bone marrow sampling, may be necessary for difficult cases.

Microscopy

The value of bone marrow biopsy in MDS is well established {2981}. It increases the diagnostic accuracy compared with examination of the aspirate smear alone and provides additional information about blast percentage and distribution within the marrow space {4180}. Bone marrow cellularity, megakaryocyte morphology and stromal fibrosis are important features revealed by the biopsy. The bone marrow in MDS is usually hypercellular and less commonly normocellular or hypocellular for age; cytopenias result from ineffective haematopoiesis despite the typically increased cellularity. Histologically, aggressive MDS subtypes can be characterized by the presence of aggregates (3–5 cells) or clusters (> 5 cells) of immature myeloid cells in bone marrow biopsies, usually localized in the central portion of the bone marrow away from the vascular structures and endosteal surfaces of the bone trabeculae (so-called abnormal localization of immature precursors) {942}. Immunohistochemistry with an antibody to CD34 (an antigen expressed in the blasts in most MDS cases) can be used to confirm the blast nature of immature myeloid cells in the biopsy

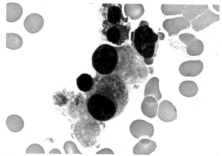

Fig. 6.09 Dysplastic megakaryocytes. Bone marrow aspirate smear from a 37-year-old man with pancytopenia, showing hypolobated megakaryocytes and micromegakaryocytes.

sections {3724,3895A}. Immunohistochemical analysis with CD34 is especially useful for assessing blast percentage in cases of MDS with fibrosis or a hypocellular marrow, in which blast percentages are often underestimated in the smear preparations. CD34 is positive in megakaryocytes in some cases of MDS, but may also stain megakaryocytes in megaloblastic anaemia {1761}. KIT (CD117) staining can be informative in MDS cases with CD34-negative blasts. However, KIT is expressed not only by myeloblasts but also by proerythroblasts, promyelocytes and mast cells. Megakaryocyte markers (e.g. CD42b and CD61) can facilitate identification of small megakaryocytes and micromegakaryocytes, although apoptotic megakaryocytes may superficially mimic micromegakaryocytes in the immunostained sections. Immunostaining for p53 can be useful {2983,2988}, because it correlates well with *TP53* mutation status and has important prognostic significance {769,3472}.

Hypoplastic myelodysplastic syndrome
In approximately 10% of MDS cases, the bone marrow is hypocellular for age. These cases have been referred to as hypoplastic MDS. This group does not constitute a specific MDS subtype in this classification. It can present with or without increased bone marrow blasts; some studies have suggested that hypocellularity may be an independent favourable prognostic variable in MDS {1723,4453}. Hypocellularity in MDS may lead to difficulties in the differential diagnosis with aplastic anaemia {1445,2982}; significant dysplasia (most often micromegakaryocytes), increased blasts identified by CD34 staining of bone marrow biopsy sections, and an abnormal karyotype (excluding trisomy 8, which may be seen

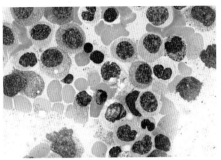

Fig. 6.10 Myelodysplastic syndrome with multilineage dysplasia. Dysgranulopoiesis is present in the bone marrow aspirate smear, including hypogranular neutrophils with pseudo–Pelger–Huët anomaly.

in some cases of aplastic anaemia) are helpful in this distinction {342,945,947}. MDS-associated somatic mutations have been reported to occur in as many as one third of patients with aplastic anaemia {4440}. Immunosuppressive therapies used to treat aplastic anaemia have been used with some degree of success in this MDS subgroup {439,2334,3698,4447, 4448}. When considering the diagnosis of hypoplastic MDS, it is important to exclude acute marrow injury due to a toxin, infection or an autoimmune disorder.

Myelodysplastic syndrome with fibrosis
Significant degrees of myelofibrosis (i.e. corresponding to grade 2 or 3 of the WHO grading scheme) {3975} are observed in 10–15% of MDS cases, and these cases have been referred to as MDS with fibrosis (MDS-F) {2201}. Significant fibrosis does not define a specific MDS subtype in this classification. However, many of the cases with fibrosis have an excess of blasts, and significant fibrosis is associated with an aggressive clinical course in MDS, independent of the blast count {942,1261}. MDS-F cases with excess blasts may erroneously be diagnosed as low-grade MDS based only on the blast count determined from the bone marrow aspirate, which is usually diluted with peripheral blood. In this fibrotic group, as in other cases of MDS with inadequate aspirates, accurate blast determination requires a bone marrow biopsy, and immunohistochemical studies for CD34 may prove invaluable. Unlike the myeloproliferative neoplasm entity primary myelofibrosis, MDS-F is usually not associated with splenomegaly, leukoerythroblastosis or intrasinusoidal haematopoiesis and typically exhibits MDS-type megakaryocyte morphology (i.e. micromegakaryocytes), other dysplastic

changes and often increased blasts as revealed by CD34 immunostaining {947}.

Immunophenotype
The immunophenotypic abnormalities that have been described in MDS haematopoietic cells compared with normal haematopoiesis are abnormal quantity and aberrant phenotypes of progenitor cells; aberrant immunophenotypic profiles of maturing granulocytic, erythroid and monocytic cells; and a decrease of haematogones {63,1856,2555,2935, 3895}. Abnormal myeloid maturation patterns include asynchrony of CD15 and CD16 on granulocytes; altered expression of CD13 in relation to CD11b or CD16; and aberrant expression of CD56 and/or CD7 on progenitors, granulocytes or monocytes. Decreased side-scatter of granulocytes can also be seen. In erythroid cells, an increased coefficient of variation and decreased intensity of CD71 or CD36 expression are highly associated with MDS {2563}. There is generally good correlation between the percentage of blasts as determined by morphological examination of the bone marrow aspirate smear or touch imprint, immunohistochemistry of the bone marrow biopsy section and flow cytometry (CD34+ cells) {1994}. However, in some cases there may be significant discordance due to marrow fibrosis or haemodiluted samples; therefore, percentages of CD34+ cells as determined by flow cytometry cannot replace the morphological differential count. Nevertheless, the finding of CD34+ myeloid progenitors accounting for > 2% of nucleated cells has been reported to be of adverse prognostic significance in MDS {2555A,2556}.
Flow cytometry findings alone are not sufficient to establish a primary diagnosis of MDS in the absence of definitive morphological and/or cytogenetic findings. A series of consensus guidelines has been published by the European LeukemiaNet (ELN) MDS working group regarding the use of flow cytometry in the diagnostic work-up of patients with MDS {3223, 4117,4118,4305}, including a summary of the reported aberrations associated with MDS and how to report the results {2463, 3223,4119}. Aberrant findings in at least three tested features and at least two cell compartments have been reported to be highly associated with an MDS or MDS/MPN diagnosis in several studies {3221,3223,4063,4119}. More limited

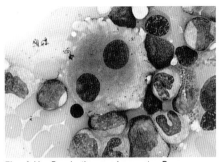

Fig. 6.11 Dysplastic megakaryocyte. Bone marrow smear from a case of myelodysplastic syndrome with single lineage dysplasia shows a binucleated megakaryocyte with separated round nuclei.

screening panels have also been applied {4,259,945,1856,2933,3287}, but may be less sensitive and less specific than larger panels.

Cell of origin
The postulated cell of origin is a haematopoietic stem cell.

Genetic profile
Cytogenetic studies play a major role in the evaluation of patients with MDS in regard to prognosis, determination of clonality {1442,3551,2971} and recognition of cytogenetic correlates with morphological and clinical features. MDS with isolated del(5q), i.e. either with a del(5q) alone or with one additional abnormality other than loss of chromosome 7 or del(7q), is a specific MDS subtype in this classification. It occurs more often in women and is characterized by megakaryocytes with non-lobated or hypolobated nuclei, macrocytic anaemia, normal or increased platelet count, and a favourable clinical course. Loss of 17p is associated with MDS or AML with pseudo–Pelger–Huët anomaly, small vacuolated neutrophils, *TP53* mutation and an unfavourable clinical course; it is most common in therapy-related MDS {2187}. Complex karyotypes (≥3 abnormalities) typically include abnormalities of chromosomes 5 and/or 7, such as del(5q) or t(5q), loss of chromosome 7, and del(7q); these are generally associated with an unfavourable clinical course. Several other cytogenetic findings appear to be associated with characteristic morphological abnormalities; for example, isolated del(20q) is associated with dysmegakaryopoiesis and thrombocytopenia, and inv(3)(q21.3q26.2) or t(3;3)(q21.3;q26.2) is associated with abnormal megakaryocytes and may be associated with thrombocytosis. {446,1500,2142,3392}.

Certain clonal cytogenetic abnormalities that often occur in MDS, i.e. loss of Y chromosome, gain of chromosome 8, and del(20q), have also been described in non-neoplastic conditions; when these occur as a sole abnormality in the absence of defining morphological criteria, they are not considered definitive evidence of MDS. In cases with refractory, unexplained cytopenia but no morphological evidence of dysplasia or increased blasts, the other cytogenetic abnormalities listed in Table 6.03 are considered presumptive evidence of MDS, and such cases are included in the category of MDS, unclassifiable. It is recommended that these patients be followed carefully for emerging morphological evidence of a more specific MDS subtype. The presence of MDS-type cytogenetic abnormalities may be used to support a diagnosis of MDS-EB in rare cases associated with excess blasts without clear-cut evidence of dysplasia.

In addition to recurrent cytogenetic abnormalities identified by conventional karyotyping, which are present in about 50% of MDS cases, recurrent somatic mutations in more than 50 genes have been identified in 80–90% of MDS cases. The genes found to be mutated in at least 5% of MDS cases are listed in Table 6.04. The most commonly mutated genes in MDS encode proteins that control RNA splicing (*SF3B1*, *SRSF2*, *U2AF1* and *ZRSR2* in aggregate mutated in >50% of cases) or epigenetic regulation of gene expression via DNA methylation (*TET2*, *DNMT3A*, *IDH1* and *IDH2*) or histone modification (*ASXL1* and *EZH2*). Other commonly mutated genes are those encoding transcription factors (*RUNX1*, *NRAS*, *BCOR*), signalling proteins (*CBL*), the tumour suppressor p53 (*TP53*), and the cohesin complex (*STAG2*), which controls the cohesion of sister chromatids {1513,3050}. As with cytogenetic abnormalities, specific mutations have been associated with specific morphological features in MDS. For example, *SF3B1* mutation is associated with ring sideroblasts and mutations in *ASXL1*, *RUNX1*, *TP53* and *SRSF2* are associated with severe granulocytic dysplasia {947}.

The mutational landscape of MDS is complex and dynamic. Multiple mutations can be present (most often in a spliceosome gene plus an epigenetic regulator); distinct mutation profiles can

Table 6.03 Recurrent chromosomal abnormalities and their frequencies in myelodysplastic syndrome (MDS) at diagnosis

Chromosomal abnormality	Frequency	
	MDS overall	Therapy-related MDS
Unbalanced		
Gain of chromosome 8[a]	10%	
Loss of chromosome 7 or del(7q)	10%	50%
del(5q) or t(5q)	10%	40%
del(20q)[a]	5–8%	
Loss of Y chromosome[a]	5%	
Isochromosome 17q or t(17p)	3–5%	25–30%
Loss of chromosome 13 or del(13q)	3%	
del(11q)	3%	
del(12p) or t(12p)	3%	
del(9q)	1–2%	
idic(X)(q13)	1–2%	
Balanced		
t(11;16)(q23.3;p13.3)		3%
t(3;21)(q26.2;q22.1)		2%
t(1;3)(p36.3;q21.2)	1%	
t(2;11)(p21;q23.3)	1%	
inv(3)(q21.3q26.2) / t(3;3)(q21.3;q26.2)	1%	
t(6;9)(p23;q34.1)	1%	

[a] As a sole cytogenetic abnormality in the absence of morphological criteria, gain of chromosome 8, del(20q) and loss of Y chromosome are not considered definitive evidence of MDS; in the setting of persistent cytopenia of undetermined origin, the other abnormalities shown in this table are considered presumptive evidence of MDS, even in the absence of definitive morphological features.

be present in two or more subclones; and the relative proportions of these subclones can shift over the course of treatment and disease progression {4232}. Acquired clonal mutations identical to those seen in MDS (affecting genes such as *ASXL1*, *TP53*, *JAK2*, *SF3B1*, *TET2* and *DNMT3A*) can also occur in the haematopoietic cells of apparently healthy older individuals without MDS {1326,1830,3772}. Therefore, MDS-associated somatic mutations alone are not considered diagnostic of MDS in this classification, even in patients with unexplained cytopenia. Rare cases of familial MDS are associated with germline mutations, which can be investigated by sequencing non-MDS tissue (e.g. normal lymphocytes). These cases and their associated mutations are discussed separately (see *Myeloid neoplasms with germline predisposition*, p. 121). In the current classification, *SF3B1* mutation is the only genetic abnormality that influences MDS subtype assignment, as part of the diagnostic criteria for MDS with ring sideroblasts.

Prognosis and predictive factors

The subtypes of MDS included in this classification can be generally categorized into three risk groups on the basis of survival time and incidence of evolution to AML. The low-risk group contains MDS with single lineage dysplasia, MDS with ring sideroblasts and single lineage dysplasia, and MDS with isolated del(5q). The intermediate-risk group contains MDS with multilineage dysplasia and MDS with ring sideroblasts and multilineage dysplasia. The high-risk group consists of MDS with excess blasts. The category of MDS, unclassifiable, encompasses cases with heterogeneous clinical behaviour. Patients with bicytopenia despite single lineage dysplasia have been reported to have shorter survival times than patients with one cytopenia; conversely, patients with one cytopenia and multilineage dysplasia have longer survival times than patients with bicytopenia {4179}.

The importance of cytogenetic features as prognostic indicators in MDS was codified by the International MDS Risk Analysis Workshop in 1997 {1442}, and this cytogenetic risk categorization was updated in 2012 {3551}. The current Comprehensive Cytogenetic Scoring System (CCSS) for MDS contains five prognostic subgroups (Table 6.05). The original IPSS risk stratification scheme for MDS {1442} was also updated in 2012. The Revised IPSS (IPSS-R) {1444} incorporates the percentage of bone marrow blasts, CCSS cytogenetic risk group, and degree of cytopenia in each lineage to predict survival and risk of evolution to AML (Table 6.06). The blast percentage thresholds used in the IPSS-R differ from those in the current WHO classification, and include a 0–2% blast category that is not included in this classification; therefore, it is important to note the actual

Table 6.04 Common gene mutations in myelodysplastic syndromes (i.e. found in at least 5% of cases) {311,312,1513,3050,3988,4478}

Gene mutated	Pathway	Frequency	Prognostic impact
SF3B1 [a]	RNA splicing	20–30%	Favourable
TET2 [a]	DNA methylation	20–30%	See footnote [b]
ASXL1 [a]	Histone modification	15–20%	Adverse
SRSF2 [a]	RNA splicing	~15%	Adverse
DNMT3A [a]	DNA methylation	~10%	Adverse
RUNX1	Transcription factor	~10%	Adverse
U2AF1 [a]	RNA splicing	5–10%	Adverse
TP53 [a]	Tumour suppressor	5–10%	Adverse
EZH2	Histone modification	5–10%	Adverse
ZRSR2	RNA splicing	5–10%	See footnote [b]
STAG2	Cohesin complex	5–7%	Adverse
IDH1/IDH2	DNA methylation	~5%	See footnote [b]
CBL [a]	Signalling	~5%	Adverse
NRAS	Transcription factor	~5%	Adverse
BCOR [a]	Transcription factor	~5%	Adverse

[a] These genes are also reported to be mutated in clonal haematopoietic cells in a subset of healthy individuals (clonal haematopoiesis of indeterminate potential).
[b] Either neutral prognostic impact or conflicting data.

Table 6.05 The Comprehensive Cytogenetic Scoring System (CCSS) for myelodysplastic syndromes. From: Schanz J, et al. {3551}

Prognostic subgroup	Defining cytogenetic abnormalities
Very good	Loss of Y chromosome
	del(11q)
Good	Normal
	del(5q)
	del(12p)
	del(20q)
	Double, including del(5q)
Intermediate	del(7q)
	Gain of chromosome 8
	Gain of chromosome 19
	Isochromosome 17q
	Single or double abnormalities not specified in other subgroups
	Two or more independent non-complex clones
Poor	Loss of chromosome 7
	inv(3), t(3q) or del(3q)
	Double including loss of chromosome 7 or del(7q)
	Complex (3 abnormalities)
Very poor	Complex (> 3 abnormalities)

bone marrow blast percentage in all MDS diagnoses, so that the IPSS-R can be applied. Five IPSS-R risk groups are defined, on the basis of the total score of the parameters listed in Table 6.06: very low, low, intermediate, high and very high. The IPSS-R is significantly better at predicting survival and evolution to AML than the original IPSS {4219}. Consideration of patient age further improves

survival prediction in the IPSS-R {1444}. Another risk-stratification scheme used to predict outcome in MDS is the WHO Classification–based Prognostic Scoring System (WPSS), which incorporates additional variables of transfusion requirement and morphological dysplasia (single lineage vs multilineage) that are not included in the IPSS-R. The WPSS may be particularly useful when applied to

lower-risk cases and at time points after the initial diagnosis {2462}.
Accumulating data indicate that both number and type of individual gene mutations are strongly associated with disease outcome in MDS. The addition of mutation data improves the ability of existing risk-stratification schemes such as the IPSS to predict prognosis in MDS {311,312}. Many commonly mutated

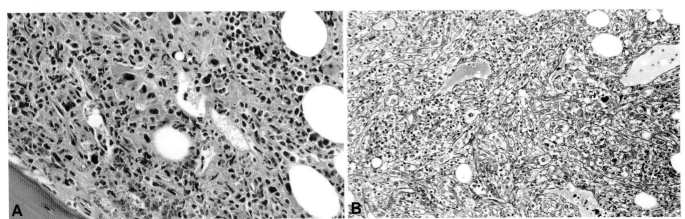

Fig. 6.12 Myelodysplastic syndrome with fibrosis (MDS-F). **A** Bone marrow biopsy from a case of MDS with excess blasts and fibrosis shows several micromegakaryocytes. **B** Reticulin of a marrow biopsy from a case of MDS with fibrosis reveals a marked increase in reticulin fibres.

genes have been associated with an unfavourable prognosis in MDS; whereas mutation in *SF3B1* is associated with a more favourable prognosis (Table 6.04, p. 105). Certain mutations may also be associated with responses to specific therapies. For example, *TET2* and *DNMT3A* mutations appeared to affect the therapeutic response of patients with MDS to hypomethylating agents in one study {4041}, and *TP53* mutation in MDS with del(5q) may predict a poorer response to lenalidomide {2474}. *TP53* mutation in MDS is associated with very aggressive disease, and predicts shorter survival in patients undergoing stem cell transplantation {769,313}. Sensitive sequencing techniques should optimally be applied in MDS mutation analysis for prognosis, because even small subclones present at the initial diagnosis may show mutations in relevant genes, such as *TP53*, and can later expand to confer therapeutic resistance {1894,4232}.

Table 6.06 The Revised International Prognostic Scoring System (IPSS-R) score values for myelodysplastic syndromes. From: Greenberg PL, et al. {1444}

Prognostic variable	Score values						
	0	0.5	1	1.5	2	3	4
Karyotype (CCSS group [a])	Very good	—	Good	—	Intermediate	Poor	Very poor
Bone marrow blast percentage	≤2%	—	>2% to <5%	—	5–10%	>10%	—
Haemoglobin concentration (g/dL)	≥10	—	8 to <10	<8	—	—	—
Platelets (× 10^9/L)	≥100	50 to <100	<50	—	—	—	—
Absolute neutrophil count (× 10^9/L)	≥0.8	<0.8	—	—	—	—	—

Five risk groups are defined, on the basis of the total score of the parameters listed above:
Very low: ≤1.5
Low: >1.5 to 3
Intermediate: >3 to 4.5
High: >4.5 to 6
Very high: >6

— Indicates not applicable

[a] The Comprehensive Cytogenetic Scoring System (CCSS) group definitions are listed in Table 6.05, p. 105.

Myelodysplastic syndromes

Myelodysplastic syndrome with single lineage dysplasia

Brunning R.D.
Hasserjian R.P.
Porwit A.
Bennett J.M.
Orazi A.
Thiele J.
Hellström-
   Lindberg E.
List A.F.

Definition

The category of myelodysplastic syndrome (MDS) with single lineage dysplasia (MDS-SLD) encompasses the MDS cases that present with unexplained cytopenia or bicytopenia, with ≥10% dysplastic cells in one myeloid lineage. Most patients present with persistent unexplained anaemia or bicytopenia; some present with persistent unexplained neutropenia or thrombocytopenia {2423}.

In the 2008 edition of this classification, MDS-SLD was called refractory cytopenia with unilineage dysplasia, and was divided into three subtypes: refractory anaemia, refractory neutropenia and refractory thrombocytopenia. This subclassification has been controversial; some studies have demonstrated no clear correlation between lineage cytopenia and lineage dysplasia and no significant differences in survival between the three subtypes {1503,2423,2568,4179}. However, other studies have found some survival differences {449,2511}. Given these conflicting findings and the inconsistencies between lineage cytopenia and lineage dysplasia, we recommend that cases of MDS presenting with single lineage cytopenia or bicytopenia and unilineage dysplasia be classified as MDS-SLD, without additional subclassification.

The presenting lineage dysplasia and cytopenias(s) should be noted in the diagnostic conclusion. The defining feature of this type of MDS is ≥10% dysplastic cells in one myeloid lineage. Cases with erythroid dysplasia only and ≥15% ring sideroblasts (or ≥5% ring sideroblasts in the presence of *SF3B1* mutation) are classified as MDS with ring sideroblasts and single lineage dysplasia (MDS-RS-SLD). If *SF3B1* mutation status is unknown, it is recommended that cases with 5–14% ring sideroblasts and single lineage dysplasia be classified as MDS-SLD. As in the 2008 classification, it is recommended that cases with single lineage dysplasia and pancytopenia be categorized as MDS, unclassifiable.

As noted in the *Overview* section (p. 98), the recommended thresholds for defining cytopenias are haemoglobin concentration < 10 g/dL, absolute neutrophil count < 1.8 × 10^9/L and platelet count < 100 × 10^9/L, as per the risk stratification guidelines of the original International Prognostic Scoring System (IPSS) {1442,1444}. Ethnicity and sex should be taken into consideration when assessing cytopenias. Presentation with milder cytopenias above the IPSS levels does not exclude a diagnosis of MDS if definitive morphological and/or cytogenetic evidence of MDS is present. The type of cytopenia may correspond to the type of lineage dysplasia (e.g. anaemia and erythroid dysplasia), or there may be discordance between the cytopenia and the dysplastic lineage. If there is no clonal cytogenetic abnormality, it is recommended that the patient be observed for ≥6 months before a definitive diagnosis of MDS-SLD is established, unless more definitive morphological and/or cytogenetic evidence emerges during the observation period.

All potential non-clonal causes of the dysplasia must be excluded before the diagnosis of MDS is established {1503}, including drug and toxin exposure, growth factor therapy, viral infections, immunological disorders, congenital disorders, vitamin deficiencies and essential element deficiencies (e.g. copper deficiency) {1449}. Excessive zinc supplementation has also been reported to be associated with severe cytopenia and dysplastic changes {1778}.

The presence of blasts in the peripheral blood essentially excludes a diagnosis of MDS-SLD, although in an occasional case a rare blast may be identified; cases with the characteristics of MDS-SLD and 1% blasts in the peripheral blood on two successive evaluations and <5% blasts in the bone marrow should be categorized as MDS, unclassifiable, due to the more aggressive clinical course reported for such cases {2423}. The number of these patients is very low; they should be carefully monitored for increasing bone marrow blast percentage and, if appropriate, reclassified. Cases in which there are 2–4% blasts in the peripheral blood and <5% blasts in the bone marrow should be classified as MDS with excess blasts 1 if other criteria for MDS are present.

MDS-SLD should not be equated with idiopathic cytopenia of undetermined significance, which lacks the minimal morphological criteria requisite for a diagnosis of MDS {4336}. Given the evidence of MDS-associated mutations in healthy older individuals, referred to as clonal haematopoiesis of indeterminate

potential, the presence of mutations alone, even in a patient with cytopenia, is not sufficient for a diagnosis of MDS-SLD in the absence of ≥10% dysplastic cells in one myeloid lineage {3772}.

Differential diagnosis

The major features of MDS-SLD are cytopenia and ≥10% dysplastic cells in one myeloid cell line. As emphasized in the *Overview* section (p. 98), it is essential to exclude all possible non-clonal etiologies for the abnormalities. In the age group in which MDS-SLD most commonly occurs, this can be particularly problematic because of the frequency of anaemia due to a number of comorbid conditions, including nutritional deficiencies, impaired renal function, inflammatory responses and non-haematopoietic neoplasms.

In patients presenting with anaemia, the evaluation should include a detailed clinical history and laboratory studies, with particular emphasis on possible vitamin B12 or folic acid deficiency. Less common causes (e.g. paroxysmal nocturnal haemoglobinuria) must also be excluded. The possibility of toxic exposure should always be considered. Arsenic poisoning, either accidental or intentional, may cause cytopenias with substantially dysplastic features.

Persistent unexplained neutropenia and thrombocytopenia as specific entities are much less common. Detailed evaluation should exclude the possibility of familial occurrence and comorbid conditions such as immune disorders, T-cell large granular lymphocytic leukaemia, viral infections and medications {1503}. Cytogenetic studies will facilitate the diagnosis in some cases with insufficient or borderline dysplasia.

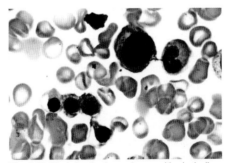

Fig. 6.13 Myelodysplastic syndrome with single lineage dysplasia. Bone marrow smear shows dyserythropoiesis. The nuclei of two polychromatic erythroid precursors in the upper right are connected by a thin chromatin strand (internuclear bridging); the two cells are unequal in size and the nucleus on the right is lobed.

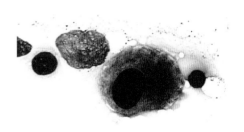

Fig. 6.14 Myelodysplastic syndrome with single lineage dysplasia. Bone marrow smear from a 27-year-old man shows a dysplastic megakaryocyte. There is asynchronous nuclear–cytoplasmic maturation, with well-granulated cytoplasm and a non-lobated immature nucleus.

Persistent cytopenias without morphological evidence of dysplasia or MDS-defining cytogenetic abnormalities should not be diagnosed as MDS-SLD. The designation of idiopathic cytopenia of undetermined significance may be appropriate in such cases, but the use of the term is not equivalent to a diagnosis of MDS {4336}.

The distinction of MDS-SLD from other types of MDS is based on the criteria for the various types outlined in the *Overview* section (p. 98). The most difficult distinction is with MDS with multilineage dysplasia (MDS-MLD); this distinction is based on the presence of dysplastic changes in ≥10% of two or three myeloid lineages in MDS-MLD. MDS-RS-SLD is also characterized by unilineage dysplasia and is distinguished from MDS-SLD by the presence of ≥15% ring sideroblasts, or ≥5% ring sideroblasts if *SF3B1* mutation is present.

ICD-O code   9980/3

Synonyms

Refractory neutropenia (no longer recommended); refractory cytopenia with unilineage dysplasia; refractory anaemia (no longer recommended); refractory thrombocytopenia (no longer recommended)

Epidemiology

MDS-SLD accounts for 7–20% of all cases of MDS {947,1338,1341,2467}. It is primarily a disease of older adults; the median patient age at onset is 65–70 years. There is no significant sex predilection. The vast majority of cases present with refractory anaemia or bicytopenia. Presentations with persistent unexplained isolated neutropenia or thrombocytopenia are uncommon and extreme caution should be used in making a diagnosis of MDS-SLD in these settings {1503,2423}. The frequency of MDS-SLD appears to be higher in the Japanese population than in Germans {2566}.

Localization
The peripheral blood and bone marrow are the principal sites of involvement.

Clinical features
The presenting symptoms are generally related to the type of cytopenia. The cytopenias are unresponsive to haematinic therapy but may respond to growth factors {1707}.

Microscopy
In the peripheral blood, the red blood cells are usually normochromic and normocytic or normochromic and macrocytic. Unusually, there is anisochromasia or dimorphism with populations of both normochromic and hypochromic red blood cells; this finding is more common in MDS with ring sideroblasts. Anisocytosis and poikilocytosis range from absent to marked.

As noted, circulating blasts are rarely seen, and if present, account for < 1% of the peripheral blood leukocytes. The presence of any blasts should call into question the diagnosis of MDS-SLD; as previously stated, the presence of 1% blasts on two successive examinations warrants categorization of the case as MDS, unclassifiable.

In cases of MDS-SLD with dyserythropoiesis, the erythroid precursors in the bone marrow can vary from markedly decreased to markedly increased. Dyserythropoiesis varies in degree, but is always present in ≥ 10% of the nucleated erythroid precursors. There may be a shift to more immature cells. The primary manifestation of dyserythropoiesis is in the nucleus. There may be nuclear budding, internuclear chromatin bridging, multinuclearity, megaloblastoid changes or karyorrhexis. Megaloblastoid nuclear changes are best evaluated in the polychromatic and orthochromatic stages of development because of the normally fine chromatin pattern in the nuclei of proerythroblasts and basophilic erythroblasts. Dysplastic cytoplasmic features include impaired haemoglobinization, vacuolization, and periodic acid–Schiff (PAS) positivity (either diffuse or granular). Ring sideroblasts may be present,

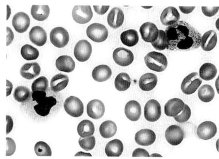

Fig. 6.15 Myelodysplastic syndrome with single lineage dysplasia. Peripheral blood smear from a 56-year-old man shows granulocytic dysplasia. The neutrophil in the upper right is normal-appearing, with well-granulated cytoplasm and a normally segmented nucleus. The neutrophil in the lower left is dysplastic, with moderately hypogranular cytoplasm and occasional Döhle bodies; the nucleus shows retarded segmentation. Approximately half of the neutrophils were dysplastic.

but account for < 15% of the erythroid precursors. If the proportion of ring sideroblasts is ≥5% but < 15% and there is *SF3B1* mutation, the case should be classified as MDS-RS-SLD. If the *SF3B1* mutation status is unknown, the case should be classified as MDS-SLD.

Neutrophil dysplasia can manifest as small size, dense chromatin, variable degrees of nuclear hyposegmentation, pseudo–Pelger–Huët changes, and abnormalities of granulation (either agranularity or hypogranularity). Less commonly, large granules resembling those found in Chédiak–Higashi syndrome may be seen. Nuclear hypersegmentation may also be noted.

The principal manifestations of megakaryocytic dysplasia include hypolobated or bilobed nuclei, multiple separated nuclei, and micromegakaryocytes; micromegakaryocytes are considered to be the most reliable and reproducible evidence of megakaryocytic dysplasia {1338,2568,4179}. Megakaryocytic dysplasia may be more apparent in bone marrow sections than smears, and its conspicuousness is increased by immunohistochemical reactions and PAS stain. The assessment of megakaryocytic dysplasia should be based on examination of ≥30 megakaryocytes. A threshold of ≥10% dysplastic megakaryocytes is recommended for the diagnosis of megakaryocytic dysplasia. However, some experts have found thresholds of 30–40% dysplastic megakaryocytes to be more reliable for distinguishing normal from dysplastic bone marrow {1338, 2568,947}. The bone marrow is typically

normocellular or hypercellular; hypocellularity is observed in a subset of cases {1338,2566}.

Immunophenotype
The immunophenotyping principles described in the *Overview* section (p. 98) should be followed. In MDS-SLD with erythroid dysplasia, aberrant immunophenotypic features of erythropoietic precursors can be found by flow cytometry analysis {944,1994,3223}. In a fraction of these cases, flow cytometry also detects aberrant immunophenotypic features in the myelomonocytic compartment or in precursors {259,946,1994, 3223}. These patients should be reassessed and closely observed for development of multilineage dysplasia {3223}.

Cell of origin
A haematopoietic stem cell

Genetic profile
Cytogenetic abnormalities may be observed in as many as 50% of cases {1341,2423}. Several acquired clonal chromosomal abnormalities may be observed, but although useful for establishing a diagnosis of MDS, they are not specific. The abnormalities generally associated with MDS-SLD include del(20q), gain of chromosome 8, and abnormalities of chromosomes 5 and 7; del(20q) has been reported in patients with MDS-SLD (as well as MDS-MLD) presenting with thrombocytopenia {446, 1500,3526}. This finding may be useful in distinguishing MDS from immune-mediated thrombocytopenia.

Somatic driver mutations have been identified in 60–70% of cases of MDS-SLD. The underlying mutations affect a haematopoietic stem cell and are present in all lineages despite the limitation of dysplastic findings to one lineage {4354}. *TET2* and *ASXL1* appear to be the most commonly mutated genes in MDS-SLD {1513}. However, mutations in other DNA methylation genes, splicing factors, RAS pathway genes, cohesin complex genes and *RUNX1* are less common than in MDS-MLD and MDS with excess blasts {2465}. *SF3B1* mutation is rare. Cases with features of MDS-SLD, an *SF3B1* mutation, and < 5% ring sideroblasts should be diagnosed as MDS-SLD, whereas cases with features of MDS-SLD, an *SF3B1* mutation, and ≥5% ring sideroblasts should be diagnosed as MDS-RS-SLD. In the absence of diagnostic dysplasia or a defining cytogenetic abnormality, somatic mutations or copy number abnormalities are not sufficient to establish a diagnosis of MDS-SLD in a patient with cytopenia, and are considered to be within the spectrum of clonal haematopoiesis of indeterminate potential {3772}.

Prognosis and predictive factors

The clinical course is usually protracted. The median overall survival of patients with MDS-SLD is approximately 66 months, and the rate of progression to acute myeloid leukaemia at 5 years is 10% {1341,2423,2467}. In one study, the median survival of patients aged ≥70 years with MDS-SLD was not significantly different from that of the non-affected population {2467}. Approximately 90–95% of patients with MDS-SLD have a low or intermediate 1 IPSS risk score {1442,2423}. A similar percentage of patients have a very low or low WHO Classification–based Prognostic Scoring System (WPSS) risk score {948,2423,2467}. Approximately 85% of patients have good or very good cytogenetic profiles. Most patients with MDS-SLD presenting with thrombocytopenia have low IPSS risk scores, and 90% of the patients live more than 2 years {3526}. However, one study reported shorter survival for patients presenting with thrombocytopenia as a result of haemorrhagic complications {450}.

Myelodysplastic syndrome with ring sideroblasts

Hasserjian R.P.
Gattermann N.
Bennett J.M.
Brunning R.D.
Malcovati L.
Thiele J.

Definition

Myelodysplastic syndrome (MDS) with ring sideroblasts (MDS-RS) is an MDS characterized by cytopenias, morphological dysplasia and ring sideroblasts usually constituting ≥15% of the bone marrow erythroid precursors; secondary causes of ring sideroblasts must be excluded. There is associated SF3B1 mutation in most cases, and in the presence of such mutation, the diagnosis can be made with ≥5% marrow ring sideroblasts. Myeloblasts account for <5% of the nucleated bone marrow cells and <1% of peripheral blood leukocytes. Auer rods are absent, and the diagnostic criteria for MDS with isolated del(5q) are not fulfilled. Two categories of MDS-RS are recognized. In MDS with ring sideroblasts and single lineage dysplasia (MDS-RS-SLD), patients present with anaemia, and dysplasia is limited to the erythroid lineage. In MDS with ring sideroblasts and multilineage dysplasia (MDS-RS-MLD), patients present with any number of cytopenias, and significant dysplasia is present in two or three haematopoietic lineages.

ICD-O codes

Myelodysplastic syndrome with ring
  sideroblasts and single lineage
  dysplasia   9982/3
Myelodysplastic syndrome with
  ring sideroblasts and
  multilineage dysplasia   9993/3

Synonyms

Refractory anaemia with ring sideroblasts; refractory cytopenia with multilineage dysplasia and ring sideroblasts

Epidemiology

MDS-RS-SLD accounts for 3–11% of all MDS cases. It occurs primarily in older individuals, with a median patient age of 60–73 years, and has a similar frequency in males and females {448,1341,2467}. MDS-RS-MLD appears to be more common, accounting for about 13% of MDS cases, and has an age distribution similar to that of MDS-RS-SLD {1341}.

Etiology

Ring sideroblasts are erythroid precursors with abnormal accumulation of iron within mitochondria, including some iron deposited as mitochondrial ferritin {591, 1425}. Stem cells from patients with MDS-RS display poor erythroid colony formation in vitro and manifest abnormal iron deposition at a very early stage of erythroid development {761,3936}, as well as deregulated expression of genes encoding mitochondrial and iron metabolism {930,1344}. MDS-RS is closely associated with heterozygous mutations in SF3B1, which encodes a core component of the U2 snRNP spliceosome that is critical for RNA splicing; less often, other genes that control RNA splicing are mutated in MDS-RS {3049,4433}. Recent data suggest that haploinsufficiency of SF3B1 is associated with a globally altered and distinct gene expression profile {1344}. The effects include altered splicing of the mitochondrial iron transporter gene ABCB7 and other mitochondrial metabolism genes, which may lead to the ineffective erythropoiesis and ring sideroblasts that characterize MDS-RS {1019,2881,4201}. However, data have been conflicting as to the association of SF3B1 haploinsufficiency with an MDS-RS disease phenotype in mouse models {4201,4203,4239}.

Localization

The peripheral blood and bone marrow are the principal sites of involvement. The liver and spleen may show evidence of iron overload.

Clinical features

The presenting symptoms are usually related to anaemia; a minority of patients with MDS-RS-SLD may additionally have thrombocytopenia or neutropenia, whereas bicytopenia occurs in a higher proportion of patients with MDS-RS-MLD {1341}. There may be symptoms related to progressive iron overload. Most patients with MDS-RS-SLD (64% and 34%, respectively) fall into the low or very low Revised International Prognostic Scoring System (IPSS-R) risk groups, whereas patients with MDS-RS-MLD more frequently have a higher IPSS-R risk score {3104}.

Microscopy

Patients typically present with normochromic macrocytic or normochromic normocytic anaemia. The red blood cells in the peripheral blood smear may show a dimorphic pattern, with a major population of normochromic red blood cells and a minor population of hypochromic cells. Blasts in the peripheral blood are absent or very rare (accounting for <1% of the leukocytes).

In MDS-RS-SLD, the bone marrow aspirate smear shows an increase in erythroid precursors with erythroid lineage dysplasia, including nuclear segmentation and megaloblastoid features. Granulocytes and megakaryocytes show no significant dysplasia (<10% dysplastic forms). Haemosiderin-laden macrophages are often abundant. Myeloblasts constitute <5% of the nucleated bone marrow cells. On iron-

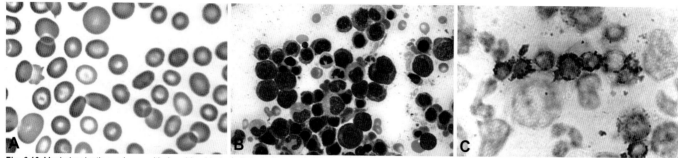

Fig. 6.16 Myelodysplastic syndrome with ring sideroblasts and single lineage dysplasia. **A** Blood smear with dimorphic red blood cells and macrocytes. **B** Bone marrow aspirate smear showing marked erythroid proliferation, with a dysplastic binucleated form. **C** Iron stain of bone marrow aspirate showing numerous ring sideroblasts.

stained aspirate smears, ≥ 15% (or ≥5% if *SF3B1* mutation has been documented) of the red blood cell precursors are ring sideroblasts, as defined by ≥5 iron granules encircling one third or more of the nucleus {2778}. The bone marrow biopsy specimen is normocellular to markedly hypercellular, usually with marked erythroid proliferation. Megakaryocytes are normal in number and morphology. In MDS-RS-MLD, in addition to ring sideroblasts and erythroid lineage dysplasia, there is significant dysplasia (≥ 10% dysplastic forms) in one or two non-erythroid lineages. Aside from the presence of ring sideroblasts, the morphological features of MDS-RS-MLD are generally similar to those of MDS with multilineage dysplasia.

Ring sideroblasts are often observed in other types of MDS and can also be seen in other myeloid neoplasms, including acute myeloid leukaemia {1333, 1891}. For example, cases of MDS with ring sideroblasts that have excess blasts in the peripheral blood or bone marrow are classified as MDS with excess blasts, and cases that fulfil the criteria for MDS with isolated del(5q) should be classified as such, even if ring sideroblasts and/or *SF3B1* mutation are present.

Non-neoplastic causes of ring sideroblasts, including alcohol, toxins (e.g. lead and benzene), drugs (e.g. isoniazid), copper deficiency (which may be induced by zinc administration), and congenital sideroblastic anaemia must be excluded {55}. Unlike in MDS-RS, patients with congenital sideroblastic anaemia tend to present at a much younger age and with microcytic (rather than macrocytic) anaemia {2940}.

Immunophenotype

In MDS-RS, aberrant immunophenotypic features of erythropoietic precursors may be found by flow cytometry analysis {944}.

Cell of origin

A haematopoietic stem cell

Genetic profile

Mutation in the spliceosome gene *SF3B1* is frequent in MDS-RS, being present in 80–90% of MDS-RS-SLD cases and 30–70% of MDS-RS-MLD cases {593,2464,3104}. Mutations in other splicing factor genes (e.g. *SRSF2*, *U2AF1* and *ZRSR2*) are present in < 10% of MDS-RS cases and are mutually exclusive with the *SF3B1* mutation {2464,4433}. Additional mutations in *TET2* and *DNMT3A*, genes affecting DNA methylation, are associated with *SF3B1* mutation and are more frequent in MDS-RS-MLD than in MDS-RS-SLD {2464}. In cases with multiple mutations, *SF3B1* mutation tends to be present at the highest allele burden and is stable during disease progression, suggesting that it is an early event in the disease pathogenesis {593, 1513,2337,4354}.

A diagnosis of MDS-RS can be made if ring sideroblasts constitute ≥5% of erythroid cells provided an *SF3B1* mutation is present. Cases of MDS-RS with < 15% ring sideroblasts tend to have a lower *SF3B1* mutant allele burden than do cases with ≥ 15% ring sideroblasts, but they appear to have a similar prognosis {2466, 3099}.

Clonal chromosomal abnormalities are seen in 5–20% of cases of MDS-RS-SLD; when present, they typically involve a single chromosome {448,1333,1335}. Cytogenetic abnormalities are seen in about half of MDS-RS-MLD cases and more often include high-risk abnormalities such as loss of chromosome 7 {1341,2467,2940}.

Prognosis and predictive factors

Approximately 1–2% of cases of MDS-RS-SLD evolve to acute myeloid leukaemia. The reported median overall survival is 69 to 108 months {943,1335}. Overall survival is 28 months in MDS-RS-MLD (similar to that in MDS with multilineage dysplasia), and approximately 8% of cas-

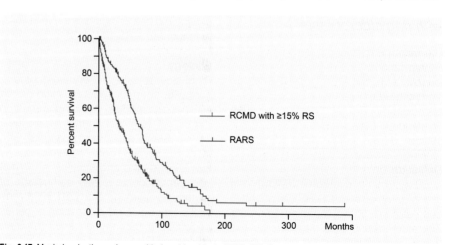

Fig. 6.17 Myelodysplastic syndrome with ring sideroblasts (MDS-RS). Survival curves based on long-term follow-up of 167 patients with MDS-RS with single lineage dysplasia and >15% ring sideroblasts (formerly called refractory anaemia with ring sideroblasts, RARS) and 318 patients with MDS-RS with multilineage dysplasia (formerly called refractory cytopenia with multilineage dysplasia, RCMD) with ≥ 15% ring sideroblasts (RS), showing inferior survival of patients with MDS-RS with multilineage dysplasia (*P* = 0.00005); data from the Düsseldorf MDS registry.

es progress to acute myeloid leukaemia {448,1335,1341}. In MDS-RS, adverse prognostic features include poor-risk karyotype, the presence of multilineage dysplasia (MDS-RS-MLD), thrombocytopenia and absence of *SF3B1* mutation; however, data are conflicting as to whether the influence of *SF3B1* mutation on prognosis is independent of multilineage dysplasia {845,2464,3103}. Among *SF3B1*-mutant MDS-RS cases, *RUNX1* mutation appears to be associated with shorter survival {2464}.

Myelodysplastic syndrome with multilineage dysplasia

Brunning R.D.
Bennett J.M.
Matutes E.
Orazi A.
Cazzola M.
Vardiman J.W.
Thiele J.
Hasserjian R.P.

Definition

Myelodysplastic syndrome (MDS) with multilineage dysplasia (MDS-MLD), called refractory cytopenia with multilineage dysplasia in the 2008 edition of this classification, is an MDS characterized by one or more cytopenias and dysplastic changes in two or more of the myeloid lineages (erythroid, granulocytic, and megakaryocytic) {3404}.

ICD-O code   9985/3

Synonym

Refractory cytopenia with multilineage dysplasia

The blast percentage is < 1% in the peripheral blood and < 5% in the bone marrow. Auer rods are absent, and the monocyte count in the peripheral blood is < 1 × 10⁹/L. The recommended values for defining cytopenias are those suggested in the International Prognostic Scoring System (IPSS): haemoglobin concentration < 10 g/dL, platelet count < 100 × 10⁹/L and absolute neutrophil count < 1.8 × 10⁹/L {1442,1442A}. Ethnicity and sex should be taken into consideration when assessing cytopenias. Milder cytopenias in excess of these thresholds do not exclude a diagnosis of MDS if definitive morphological and/or cytogenetic findings are consistent with the diagnosis.

The thresholds for dysplasia are ≥ 10% in each of the affected cell lineages. For assessing dysplasia, it is recommended that 200 erythroid precursors and 200 neutrophils and precursors be evaluated in bone marrow smear and/or trephine biopsy imprint preparations. Neutrophil dysplasia may also be evaluated in peripheral blood smears. At least 30 megakaryocytes should be evaluated for dysplasia in bone marrow smears, imprint preparations or sections. In particular, the presence of micromegakaryocytes should be noted, because this is considered by most experts to be the most significant feature of megakaryocytic dysplasia. Some experts have found thresholds for megakaryocytic dysplasia of 30–40% to be more reliable for distinguishing normal marrow from dysplastic marrow {1338, 2567,4179}. In some cases, dysplastic megakaryocytes may be more readily identified in sections than on smears, in particular with immunohistochemistry using antibodies such as anti-CD61.

The presence of 1% blasts in the peripheral blood excludes a diagnosis of MDS-MLD; cases that otherwise fulfil the criteria for MDS-MLD but have 1% blasts in the blood on two separate occasions should be diagnosed as MDS, unclassifiable, because of the more aggressive course associated with this finding. Cases with multilineage dysplasia, 2–4% blasts in the peripheral blood, and no Auer rods should be classified as MDS with excess blasts 1, even with < 5% bone

marrow blasts. Cases that otherwise have the features of MDS-MLD and have 5–19% blasts in the peripheral blood and/or Auer rods should be classified as MDS with excess blasts 2, even with < 5% bone marrow blasts. Cases with multilineage dysplasia and ≥ 15% ring sideroblasts (or ≥ 5% ring sideroblasts and *SF3B1* mutation) should be classified as MDS with ring sideroblasts and multilineage dysplasia (MDS-RS-MLD). Cases with multilineage dysplasia and ≥ 5% but < 15% ring sideroblasts with unknown *SF3B1* mutation status should be classified as MDS-MLD.

Epidemiology

MDS-MLD occurs in older individuals; the median patient age is 67–70 years. There is a higher incidence in males. The peak incidence in males is 70–74 years and in females is 75–79 years {1338, 1341,2423,2467}. MDS-MLD accounts for about 30% of all cases of MDS and 48% of cases of MDS without excess blasts. Combined, MDS-MLD and MDS-RS-MLD account for approximately 65% of all cases of MDS without excess blasts {2423}.

Etiology

The etiology of de novo MDS-MLD is unknown. Exposure to toxic environmental factors probably increases risk. Given that the vast majority of cases occur in older individuals, haematopoietic stem cell mutations (which occur with ageing) may underlie the age-associated risk {1326,1830}.

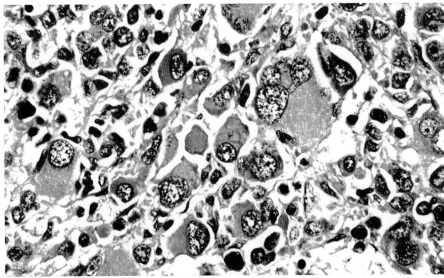

Fig. 6.18 Myelodysplastic syndrome with multilineage dysplasia and complex cytogenetic abnormalities. Bone marrow section from a 37-year-old man with pancytopenia showing markedly increased megakaryocytes, many with dysplastic features.

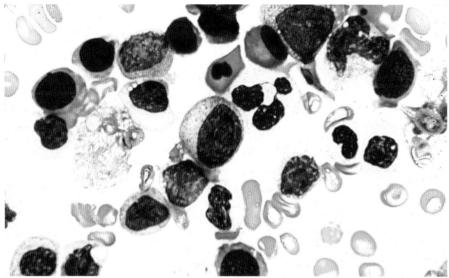

Fig. 6.19 Myelodysplastic syndrome with multilineage dysplasia. Bone marrow smear shows evidence of dysplasia in both the erythroid precursors and the neutrophils; the mature neutrophils are small and have hyposegmented nuclei.

Localization
The blood and bone marrow are involved.

Clinical features
Patients usually present with evidence of bone marrow failure. In most patients, there is unicytopenia or bicytopenia. Some patients present with pancytopenia or milder cytopenias above the threshold levels in the IPSS {2423}.

Microscopy
The erythrocytes frequently show anisopoikilocytosis with macrocytosis. The major dysplastic changes in neutrophils are nuclear clumping and hyposegmentation or lack of lobation (pseudo–Pelger–Huët anomaly) and cytoplasmic hypogranularity or agranularity. Infrequently, abnormal granular clumping resembling the findings in Chédiak–Higashi syndrome is present. Blasts are not usually identified in the peripheral blood; however, the presence of < 1% peripheral blood blasts with < 5% blasts in the bone marrow does not alter the classification, because the prognosis for cases with rare (<1%) circulating blasts is essentially the same as that for cases without this finding {2423}.
The bone marrow is usually normocellular or hypercellular, but is hypocellular in a small subset of cases {2423}. The erythroid precursors are usually increased in number; uncommonly there is erythroid hypoplasia. Erythroid precursors may show cytoplasmic vacuoles and marked nuclear irregularity, including internu-clear chromatin bridging, multilobation, nuclear budding, multinucleation and megaloblastoid nuclei. The latter are better evaluated in the polychromatic and orthochromatic erythroblasts, due to the fine nuclear chromatin pattern normally present in proerythroblasts and early basophilic erythroblasts. The cytoplasmic vacuoles are usually poorly defined and dissimilar to the sharply demarcated vacuoles observed in copper deficiency or alcoholism. The vacuoles may give a positive periodic acid–Schiff (PAS) reaction; there may also be diffuse cytoplasmic PAS positivity. Variable numbers of ring sideroblasts may be identified, but they must account for < 15% of the erythroblasts. If ≥ 15% ring sideroblasts or ≥ 5% ring sideroblasts and *SF3B1* mutation are present, the case should be classified as MDS-RS-MLD. The percentage of neutrophils and precursors in the bone marrow varies; a relative increase in granulocytes is present in approximately 25% of cases {2423}. There may be a left shift in maturation. Neutrophil dysplasia is characterized principally by nuclear cytoplasmic asynchrony, hypogranulation, and/or nuclear hyposegmentation with marked clumping of the nuclear chromatin (pseudo–Pelger–Huët nuclei). Nuclear hyposegmentation may occur as two clumped nuclear lobes connected by a thin chromatin strand (pince-nez type) or non-lobated nuclei with markedly clumped chromatin. Myeloblasts account for < 5% of the bone marrow cells. Megakaryocyte abnormalities that may be observed include non-lobated or hypolo-bated nuclei, binucleation or multinucleation, and micromegakaryocytes. A micro-megakaryocyte is a megakaryocyte that is approximately the size of a promye-locyte or smaller, with a non-lobated or bi-lobated nucleus; this morphological finding is considered by most experts to be the most reliable and reproducible dysplastic feature in the megakaryocyte series {1341,2567,4179}. In some cases, bone marrow sections may be more reliable than smears for evaluating mega-karyocyte dysplasia, in particular with the addition of immunohistochemical reactions with appropriate antibodies such as CD61 and CD41. PAS staining may also be helpful. Several studies have documented the various morphological abnormalities that constitute evidence of dysplasia {947,1341,2567,4179}.
In a study of marrow fibrosis in patients with MDS, 16% of cases classified as MDS-MLD had a significant degree of marrow fibrosis {491}. In general, marrow fibrosis in MDS correlated with multilineage dysplasia, more severe thrombocytopenia, higher probability of clonal karyotype, higher percentage of blasts in the peripheral blood and shorter survival than for patients without fibrosis {491}.

Immunophenotype
Flow cytometry usually reveals immunophenotypic abnormalities in various cell populations, including aberrations in the immature progenitor compartment and abnormal maturation in granulopoiesis, the monocytic compartment and erythropoiesis {3221,3223,4119}. Immunophenotypic abnormalities in the progenitor compartment are reported to be of prognostic significance and can be used to guide therapy and for followup {64,4304}. CD34+ cells are typically < 5%, but the blast percentage determination for classification purposes should be based on a microscopic differential of the aspirate smear, not on the flow cytometry blast percentage. Details concerning the overall use of flow cytometry analysis in MDS are given in the *Overview* section (p. 98).

Cell of origin
A haematopoietic stem cell

Genetic profile
Clonal cytogenetic abnormalities, including trisomy 8, monosomy 7, del(7q),

del(5q) or t(5q), and del(20q), as well as complex karyotypes, are found in as many as 50% of patients with MDS-MLD {2423}. Whole-genome sequencing has shown that more than half of all cases of MDS-MLD carry mutations in genes that are also mutated in MDS with excess blasts and acute myeloid leukaemia. These include genes from the cohesin family (*STAG2*), chromatin modifiers (*ASXL1*), spliceosome genes (*SRSF2*), transcription factors (*RUNX1*), signalling molecules (*CBL*), tumour suppressors (*TP53*) and DNA modifiers (*TET2*) {1513, 3050,4392}. Mutations in *SF3B1* are present in a minority (1–5%) of patients with 0–1% ring sideroblasts and as high as 15% of cases with 3–9% ring sideroblasts {2464}; cases with ≥5% ring sideroblasts should be classified as MDS-RS-MLD if *SF3B1* mutation is present.

Prognosis and predictive factors
The clinical course varies {948,2423, 2462,2467}. Prognostic factors relate to the karyotype and the degree of cytopenia and dysplasia. In a very large study, approximately 40% of patients with MDS-MLD or MDS-RS-MLD had low IPSS risk scores, and approximately 50% had an intermediate 1 risk score {2423}. Approximately 50% had a low WHO Classification–based Prognostic Scoring System (WPSS) risk score, 20% had an intermediate risk score, and 20% had a high risk score; no patients had a very low risk score. Approximately 75% were in the good karyotype risk group, 17% were in the poor risk group, and 8% were in the intermediate risk group {948, 2423,2462}. Although gene mutations may have a prognostic impact on overall survival and progression-free survival for MDS in general, there is no definitive evidence that mutations influence the prognosis within the MDS-MLD group specifically {4392}.

In a database of 1010 patients with MDS-MLD, the frequency of acute leukaemia evolution was approximately 15% at 2 years and 28% at 5 years and the median overall survival was 36 months (data from the Düsseldorf MDS registry, September 2015). Patients with complex karyotypes have survivals similar to those of patients with MDS with excess blasts {2423}.

Myelodysplastic syndrome with excess blasts

Orazi A.
Brunning R.D.
Hasserjian R.P.
Germing U.
Thiele J.

Definition
Myelodysplastic syndrome (MDS) with excess blasts (MDS-EB) is an MDS characterized by 5–19% myeloblasts in the bone marrow or 2–19% blasts in the peripheral blood (but < 20% blasts in both bone marrow and blood). Two subcategories, with differences in survival and incidence of evolution to acute myeloid leukaemia (AML), have been defined. MDS with excess blasts 1 (MDS-EB-1) is defined by 5–9% blasts in the bone marrow or 2–4% blasts in the peripheral blood (but < 10% blasts in the bone marrow and < 5% blasts in the blood), and MDS with excess blasts 2 (MDS-EB-2) is defined by 10–19% blasts in the bone marrow or 5–19% blasts in the peripheral blood {1442}. The presence of Auer rods in blasts designates any MDS case as MDS-EB-2 irrespective of the blast percentage {1340}.

ICD-O code   9983/3

Synonym
Refractory anaemia with excess blasts

Epidemiology
This disease affects primarily individuals aged > 50 years. It accounts for approximately 40% of all cases of MDS.

Etiology
The etiology is unknown. Exposure to environmental toxins, including pesticides, petroleum derivatives, and some heavy metals, increases risk, as does cigarette smoking {3816}.

Localization
The blood and bone marrow are affected.

Clinical features
Most patients initially present with clinical features related to cytopenias, including anaemia, thrombocytopenia, and neutropenia.

Microscopy
Peripheral blood smears frequently show

abnormalities in all three myeloid cell lines, including anisopoikilocytosis and macrocytosis; large, giant or hypogranular platelets; and abnormal cytoplasmic granularity and nuclear segmentation of the neutrophils. Pseudo–Pelger–Huët nuclei and hypogranulated forms are usually detected. Blasts are commonly present.

The bone marrow is usually hypercellular. The degree of dysplasia varies. Erythropoiesis may be increased, with megaloblastoid changes. The erythroid precursors may show dyserythropoiesis, including the presence of abnormally lobated nuclei and internuclear bridging. Granulopoiesis is variable in quantity and usually shows dysplasia, which is characterized primarily by neutrophils with nuclear hyposegmentation (pseudo–Pelger–Huët nuclei) or hypersegmented nuclei, cytoplasmic hypogranularity, and/or pseudo–Chédiak–Higashi granules. Megakaryopoiesis is variable in quantity but is frequently normal to increased. Dysmegakaryopoiesis is almost invariably present and is usually characterized by abnormal forms that are predominantly small, including micromegakaryocytes {3987}. However, megakaryocytes of all sizes, as well as forms with multiple widely separated nuclei, can also occur. The megakaryocytes may show a tendency to

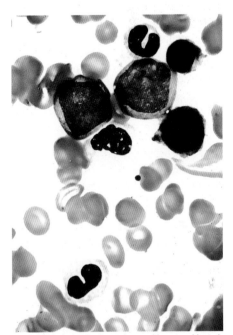

Fig. 6.20 Myelodysplastic syndrome with excess blasts 1. On the bone marrow aspirate smear, the mature neutrophils in this case show nuclear hyposegmentation (pseudo–Pelger–Huët nuclei) and cytoplasmic hypogranularity.

cluster. The bone marrow biopsy specimen shows alteration of the normal histotopography. Both erythroid precursors and megakaryocytes are frequently dislocated towards the paratrabecular areas, which are normally predominantly occupied by granulopoietic cells. The blasts in MDS-EB often tend to form cell clusters or aggregates, which are usually located away from bone trabeculae and vascular structures, a histological finding referred to as abnormal localization of immature precursors. Immunohistochemical staining for CD34 may be particularly helpful in the identification of this finding. In many cases of MDS-EB, aberrant CD34 expression may also be seen in megakaryocytes. Small CD34+ megakaryocytes should not be counted as blasts.

In a minority of cases the bone marrow is normocellular or hypocellular. In hypocellular cases, the bone marrow biopsy can be very useful in documenting the presence of an excess of blasts, in particular in cases with suboptimal aspirate smears such as those often associated with hypocellular and/or fibrotic marrow.

Myelodysplastic syndrome with excess blasts and erythroid predominance

In the 2008 WHO classification, the category of erythroid/myeloid-type acute erythroid leukaemia (erythroleukaemia) encompassed cases of myeloid neoplasms in which maturing erythroblasts accounted for ≥50% of marrow cells and myeloblasts accounted for ≥20% of non-erythroid nucleated marrow cells. Such cases are now classified according to the blast percentage of all marrow cells, irrespective of the marrow erythroid percentage, and most (those with 5–19% blood or bone marrow blasts) are now categorized as MDS-EB. The significance of the erythroid predominance in such cases is uncertain, and the bone marrow erythroid percentage may fluctuate with exogenous factors such as metabolic deficiencies and therapy {4246}. High-risk karyotype and the presence of TP53, RUNX1, or ASXL1 mutations are associated with poor prognosis in MDS-EB with erythroid predominance {1475,1592}. NPM1 mutations, which are relatively uncommon in this group {4506}, may define a subset with a relatively favourable prognosis when treated with intensive chemotherapy {1475}.

Myelodysplastic syndrome with excess blasts and fibrosis

In about 15% of cases of MDS, the bone marrow shows a significant degree of reticulin fibrosis (grade 2 or 3 according to the WHO grading system). Such cases have been termed MDS with fibrosis (MDS-F) {2201,2538}, and most belong to the MDS-EB category (MDS-EB-F). The presence of fibrosis is an independent prognostic parameter in MDS {942, 1261}. Marrow fibrosis can also be seen in cases of therapy-related myeloid neoplasms, myeloproliferative neoplasms, lymphoid neoplasms and various reactive conditions, including infections and autoimmune disorders {4182}. These conditions must be ruled out. Bone marrow smears are often inadequate. The presence of excess of blasts in cases of MDS-EB-F can usually be confirmed by immunohistochemistry, in particular for CD34. A characteristic finding in MDS-F is an increased number of megakaryocytes with a high degree of dysplasia, including small forms and micromegakaryocytes {2201}. MDS-EB-F may overlap morphologically with acute panmyelosis with myelofibrosis; however, acute panmyelosis with myelofibrosis is distinguished by its abrupt onset with fever and bone pain, as well as by its higher blast count {2991,3986}.

Immunophenotype

In MDS-EB, flow cytometry often shows increased numbers of cells positive for the precursor cell–associated antigens CD34 and/or KIT (CD117). These cells are usually positive for CD38, HLA-DR and the myeloid-associated antigens CD13 and/or CD33. Asynchronous expression of the granulocytic maturation antigens CD15, CD11b and/or CD65 can be seen in the blast population. Aberrant expression of CD7 on blast cells is seen in 20% of cases, and CD56 is present in 10% of cases; expression of other lymphoid markers is rare {2936,3724}. Expression of CD7 has been reported to correlate with worse prognosis {2936}.

In tissue sections, CD34 immunohistochemistry can be used to confirm the presence of an increased number of blasts; it highlights their arrangement into clusters or aggregates, a characteristic finding seen in most cases of MDS-EB {942,2201,3724}. Antibodies such as CD61 and CD42b can facilitate the identification of micromegakaryocytes and

other small dysplastic megakaryocytes, which are often particularly numerous in MDS-EB-F {2201,3987}.

Cell of origin

A haematopoietic stem cell

Genetic profile

A variable percentage (30–50%) of cases of MDS-EB have clonal cytogenetic abnormalities, including gain of chromosome 8, del(5q) or t(5q), loss of chromosome 7, del(7q), and del(20q). Complex karyotypes may also be observed {1341}. Mutations affecting mRNA splicing genes are common in MDS-EB. SRSF2 mutations are present in both the MDS-EB-1 and MDS-EB-2 subtypes. Splicing mutations are mutually exclusive and less likely to occur in patients with complex cytogenetics or TP53 mutations {209, 864}. Other mutations relatively common in MDS-EB include mutations in IDH1 and IDH2 {3098}, ASXL1 and CBL {3380}, as well as mutations in RUNX1, cohesin complex family genes and RAS pathway genes {2465}.

Excess blasts appear to define a distinct disease phenotype that is independent of mutation status, underscoring the importance of blast count for risk-stratifying MDS, irrespective of the mutation profile {2465}. Both FLT3 and NPM1 mutations are found primarily in AML and occur very rarely in MDS-EB {880,3380}; when present, these mutations are associated with more rapid progression to AML {234}. Therefore, an alternative diagnosis of AML must be excluded in such cases by careful verification of the bone marrow and blood blast counts and close clinical follow-up.

Prognosis and predictive factors

MDS-EB is usually characterized by progressive bone marrow failure, with increasing cytopenias. Approximately 25% of cases of MDS-EB-1 and 33% of cases of MDS-EB-2 progress to AML; the remainder of patients succumb to the sequelae of bone marrow failure. The median survival times are approximately 16 months for MDS-EB-1 and 9 months for MDS-EB-2 {1341,3818}. Patients with MDS-EB-2 with 5–19% blasts in the peripheral blood have a median survival of 3–8 months {89}, whereas patients with MDS-EB-2 based only on the presence of Auer rods have a median survival of about 12 months {4328}.

Myelodysplastic syndrome with isolated del(5q)

Hasserjian R.P.
Le Beau M.M.
List A.F.
Bennett J.M.
Brunning R.D.
Thiele J.

Definition

Myelodysplastic syndrome (MDS) with isolated del(5q) is an MDS characterized by anaemia (with or without other cytopenias and/or thrombocytosis) and in which the cytogenetic abnormality del(5q) occurs either in isolation or with one other cytogenetic abnormality, other than monosomy 7 or del(7q). Myeloblasts constitute < 5% of the nucleated bone marrow cells and < 1% of the peripheral blood leukocytes. Auer rods are absent.

ICD-O code   9986/3

Synonyms

Myelodysplastic syndrome with 5q deletion; 5q minus syndrome

Epidemiology

MDS with isolated del(5q) occurs more often in women, with a median age of 67 years.

Etiology

The presumed etiology is loss of a tumour suppressor gene or genes in the minimally deleted region (5q33.1) {433, 2370}. Haploinsufficiency of *RPS14*, which encodes a ribosomal structural protein, appears to contribute to the disease phenotype, possibly through p53

pathway activation {261,1078A,3574A}. Haploinsufficiency of miR-145 and miR-146a in the deleted region may contribute to the megakaryocyte abnormalities and thrombocytosis {3767}. Haploinsufficiency of *CSNK1A1* (encoding casein kinase 1A1) leading to WNT/beta-catenin pathway deregulation has been implicated in proliferation of the del(5q) clone {3574}. Haploinsufficiency of additional genes on 5q, such as *APC* (another WNT pathway regulator) and *EGR1*, may also contribute to disease pathogenesis {1885}.

Localization

The blood and bone marrow are affected.

Clinical features

The most common symptoms are related to anaemia, which is often severe and usually macrocytic. Thrombocytosis is present in one third to one half of cases, whereas thrombocytopenia is uncommon {1358,2561}. Pancytopenia is rare {2423}; it is recommended that cases otherwise fulfilling the criteria for MDS with isolated del(5q), but with pancytopenia (haemoglobin concentration < 10 g/dL, absolute neutrophil count < 1.8 × 10^9/L and platelet count < 100 × 10^9/L) be categorized as MDS, unclassifiable, because their clinical behaviour is uncertain.

Microscopy

The bone marrow is usually hypercellular or normocellular and frequently exhibits erythroid hypoplasia {4263}. Megakaryocytes are increased in number and are normal to slightly decreased in size, with conspicuously non-lobated and hypolobated nuclei. In contrast, dysplasia in the erythroid lineage is less pronounced

{434,1358}. Significant granulocytic dysplasia is uncommon. The blast percentage is < 5% in the bone marrow and < 1% in the peripheral blood. Ring sideroblasts may be present and do not exclude the diagnosis of MDS with isolated del(5q), provided the other criteria are fulfilled.

Cell of origin

The cell of origin is a haematopoietic stem cell. FISH analysis has demonstrated the presence of the del(5q) abnormality in differentiating erythroid, myeloid and megakaryocytic cells, but generally not in mature lymphoid cells {96,376}. The del(5q) abnormality is the dominant clone in most cases and is present in the stem cell compartment, consistent with an early or initiating event in disease pathogenesis {4354}.

Genetic profile

The defining cytogenetic abnormality involves an interstitial deletion of chromosome 5; the size of the deletion and the breakpoints vary, but bands q31-q33 are invariably deleted. Cases with one additional cytogenetic abnormality, with the exception of monosomy 7 or del(7q), have similar outcome as cases in which del(5q) is the sole abnormality, and are included in this category {1337,2473,3551}.

A small subset of patients with isolated del(5q) show concomitant *JAK2* V617F or *MPL* W515L mutation, which does not appear to alter the disease phenotype or prognosis {1759,3101}; in some of these cases, the *JAK2* mutation and del(5q) have been found in different clones {3717}. A subset of cases have *SF3B1* mutation {2464,2466}.

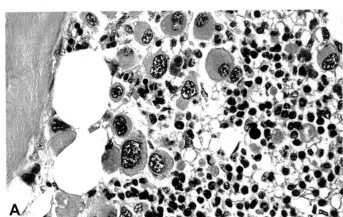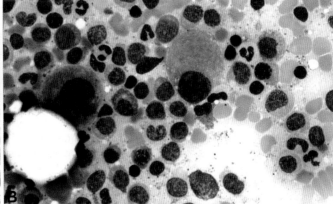

Fig. 6.21 Myelodysplastic syndrome with isolated del(5q). **A** Bone marrow section showing numerous megakaryocytes of various sizes, several with non-lobated nuclei. **B** Bone marrow aspirate smear showing two megakaryocytes with non-lobated, rounded nuclei.

Prognosis and predictive factors

This disease is associated with a median survival of 66–145 months, with transformation to acute myeloid leukaemia occurring in < 10% of cases {1358,2473, 3101}. Cases with del(5q) associated with loss of chromosome 7, del(7q), two or more additional chromosomal abnormalities, or excess blasts have an inferior survival and are excluded from this diagnosis. Significant granulocytic dysplasia has been associated with additional cytogenetic abnormalities and an inferior prognosis {671,1350}.

The thalidomide analogue lenalidomide has been shown to benefit patients with MDS with isolated del(5q) or del(5q) with additional cytogenetic abnormalities, most likely by targeting casein kinase 1A1 for ubiquitin-mediated degradation. It has been reported that transfusion independence was achieved in two thirds of patients and was closely linked to suppression of the abnormal clone {1359,2361}. TP53 mutation is present in a significant subset of cases, and is associated with increased risk of leukaemic transformation, inferior response to lenalidomide, and shorter survival {1894,2129A,2474}. Therefore, in MDS with isolated del(5q), it is recommended that TP53 mutation status be determined by sequencing or p53 immunohistochemistry to identify high-risk cases {3472}.

Myelodysplastic syndrome, unclassifiable

Orazi A.
Brunning R.D.
Baumann I.
Hasserjian R.P.
Germing U.

Definition

The category of myelodysplastic syndrome (MDS), unclassifiable (MDS-U) encompasses the cases of MDS that initially lack appropriate findings for classification into any other MDS category.

ICD-O code   9989/3

Synonyms

Myelodysplastic syndrome, NOS; preleukaemia (obsolete); preleukaemic syndrome (obsolete)

Epidemiology

The exact incidence is unknown. In one study of 2032 patients, MDS-U accounted for 6.3% of cases of MDS with a bone marrow blast count of < 5% {2423}. A higher incidence of MDS-U has been reported among Japanese patients, in particular those with single lineage dysplasia and pancytopenia {1746,2566}.

Localization

The peripheral blood and bone marrow are the principal sites of involvement.

Clinical features

Patients present with symptoms similar to those seen in the other MDS.

Microscopy

There are no specific morphological findings. The diagnosis of MDS-U can be made in any of the following settings:
1. There are findings that would otherwise suggest classification as MDS with single lineage dysplasia, MDS with multilineage dysplasia, MDS with ring sideroblasts and single lineage dysplasia, MDS with ring sideroblasts and multilineage dysplasia, or MDS with isolated del(5q), but with 1% blasts in the peripheral blood measured on at least two separate occasions {2052}.
2. There are findings that would otherwise suggest classification as MDS with single lineage dysplasia, MDS with ring sideroblasts and single lineage dysplasia, or MDS with isolated del(5q) associated with pancytopenia. In contrast, pancytopenia is allowed in both MDS with multilineage dysplasia and MDS with ring sideroblasts and multilineage dysplasia.
3. There is persistent cytopenia with < 2% blasts in the blood and < 5% in the bone marrow, no significant (< 10%) unequivocal dysplasia (Table 6.02, p. 102) in any myeloid lineage, and the presence of a cytogenetic abnormality considered presumptive evidence of MDS (Table 6.03, p. 104) {3774}. Patients with MDS-U should be carefully followed for evidence of disease evolution to a more specific MDS type.

Cell of origin

A haematopoietic stem cell

Genetic profile

See Table 6.03 (p. 104).

Prognosis and predictive factors

If characteristics of a specific subtype of MDS develop later in the course of the disease, the case should be reclassified accordingly.

In a recent study, cases otherwise meeting the criteria for MDS with single lineage dysplasia, but with 1% blasts in the peripheral blood or with pancytopenia, were shown to have a prognosis similar to that of MDS with multilineage dysplasia cases {2423}. In that study, patients with MDS-U and 1% peripheral blood blasts had a median survival of 35 months and a 14% 5-year cumulative risk of acute myeloid leukaemia progression, whereas patients with MDS-U and pancytopenia had a median survival of 30 months and an 18% 5-year cumulative risk of acute myeloid leukaemia progression {2423}. The prognosis for MDS-U defined by cytogenetic abnormalities is unknown.

Childhood myelodysplastic syndrome

Baumann I.
Niemeyer C.M.
Bennett J.M.

Myelodysplastic syndrome (MDS) is very uncommon in children, accounting for < 5% of all haematopoietic neoplasms in patients aged less than 14 years {1586, 2873}. Some cases of MDS in children are secondary to cytotoxic therapy, inherited bone marrow failure disorders, or acquired severe aplastic anaemia. Other cases are generally categorized as primary MDS, but it is reasonable to assume that most of these are in fact secondary to a known or as-yet-unknown genetic predisposition (see Myeloid neoplasms with germline predisposition, p. 121). GATA2 germline mutation is present in 7% of all primary MDS cases in children, but absent in children with secondary MDS {4342}. The pre-leukaemic and leukaemic phase of myeloid leukaemia associated with Down syndrome is a unique disease entity of early childhood characterized by acquired GATA1 mutations (see Myeloid proliferations associated with Down syndrome, p. 169), but little is known about the pathophysiology of MDS in older children with Down syndrome {3369}. Many of the morphological, immunophenotypic and genetic features observed in MDS in adults are also seen in childhood forms of the disease, but there are some significant differences reported, particularly in patients who do not have increased blasts in their peripheral blood or bone marrow. For example, MDS with ring sideroblasts and MDS with isolated del(5q) are exceedingly rare in children {2873}. Isolated anaemia, which is the major presenting manifestation of lower-grade MDS affecting adults, is uncommon in children, who are more likely to present with neutropenia and thrombocytopenia {1587,1940}. In addition, hypocellularity of the bone marrow is more commonly observed in childhood MDS than in older patients. Therefore, some childhood cases do not readily fit into the typical lower-grade MDS categories. To address these differences, a provisional entity, refractory cytopenia of childhood, is recognized and defined below. For childhood cases of MDS with 2–19% blasts in the peripheral blood or 5–19% blasts in the bone marrow, the same criteria should be applied as for adult cases of MDS with excess blasts. Unlike in adult MDS, there are no data indicating that a distinction between MDS with excess blasts 1 and MDS with excess blasts 2 is of prognostic relevance in children {2009,3808}. Children with MDS with excess blasts generally have relatively stable peripheral blood counts for weeks or months. Some cases diagnosed in children as acute myeloid leukaemia with 20–29% blasts in the peripheral blood and/or bone marrow that have myelodysplasia-related changes, including cases with myelodysplasia-related cytogenetic abnormalities (see *Acute myeloid leukaemia with myelodysplasia-related changes*, p. 150) may also be slowly progressive disease. These cases, categorized by the French–American–British (FAB) classification as refractory anaemia with excess blasts in transformation, may lack the clinical features of acute leukaemia and may behave more like MDS than acute myeloid leukaemia {1587}; therefore, follow-up peripheral blood and bone marrow studies are often necessary to determine the pace of the disease in such cases. Children who present with a peripheral blood and/or bone marrow disorder associated with one of the core-binding factor rearrangements – t(8;21)(q22;q22.1); *RUNX1-RUNX1T1*; inv(16)(p13.1q22); *CBFB-MYH11,* or t(16;16)(p13.1;q22); *CBFB-MYH11* – or with *PML-RARA* rearrangement should be consid-

ered to have acute myeloid leukaemia regardless of the blast count. The mutational landscape differs between adult and paediatric MDS. In children, most of the somatic mutations identified alter genes of the RAS pathway, transcription factors and epigenetic modifiers {2096}.

Refractory cytopenia of childhood

Definition
Refractory cytopenia of childhood (RCC) is a provisional MDS entity characterized by persistent cytopenia, with < 5% blasts in the bone marrow and < 2% blasts in the peripheral blood {1587}. Although the presence of dysplasia is required for the diagnosis, the cytological finding of dysplasia constitutes only one aspect of the morphological diagnosis of RCC. The evaluation of an adequate bone marrow trephine biopsy specimen is essential for diagnosis. About 80% of children with RCC show considerable hypocellularity of the bone marrow {2873}. Therefore, it may be very challenging to differentiate hypocellular RCC from other bone marrow failure disorders, in particular acquired aplastic anaemia and inherited bone marrow failure disorders.

ICD-O code   9985/3

Epidemiology
RCC is the most common subtype of MDS in childhood, accounting for about 50% of all cases {3092,3246}. It is diag-

nosed in all age groups and affects boys and girls with equal frequency {1940}.

Etiology
The etiology is unknown in most cases. In some cases, it is related to an underlying germline mutation.

Localization
The blood and bone marrow are always affected. Generally, the spleen, liver and lymph nodes are not sites of initial manifestation.

Clinical features
The most common symptoms are malaise, bleeding, fever and infection {1940}. Lymphadenopathy secondary to local or systemic infection may be present, but hepatosplenomegaly is generally not a feature of RCC. In as many as 20% of patients, no clinical signs or symptoms are reported {1940}. Congenital abnormalities of different organ systems may be present.
Three quarters of patients have a platelet count < 150 × 10⁹/L, and anaemia with a haemoglobin concentration of < 10 g/dL is noted in about half of all affected children {1940}. Age-specific macrocytosis of red blood cells is seen in most patients. The white blood cell count is generally decreased, with severe neutropenia noted in about 25% of cases {1940}.

Microscopy
The classic picture of RCC is a peripheral blood smear that shows anisopoikilocy-

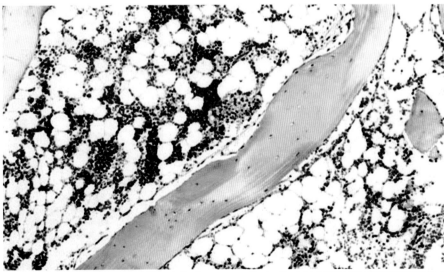

Fig. 6.22 Refractory cytopenia of childhood. The bone marrow biopsy shows hypoplasia and patchy distribution of haematopoiesis, in particular erythropoiesis.

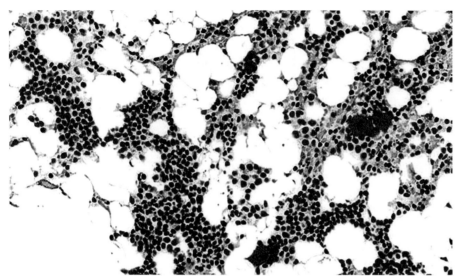

Fig. 6.23 Refractory cytopenia of childhood. On bone marrow biopsy, CD61 immunohistochemistry shows dysplasia of megakaryocytes, with small, non-lobated nuclei or separated nuclei.

tosis and macrocytosis. Anisochromasia and polychromasia may be present. Platelets often display anisocytosis, and giant platelets can occasionally be detected. Neutropenia, with pseudo–Pelger–Huët nuclei and/or hypogranularity or agranularity of neutrophil cytoplasm, may be noted. Blasts are absent or account for < 2% of the white blood cells.

On bone marrow aspirate smears, dysplastic changes should be present in two myeloid cell lineages or account for at least 10% in one cell line (Table 6.07). Erythroid abnormalities include nuclear budding, multinuclearity, karyorrhexis, internuclear bridging, cytoplasmic granules and megaloblastoid changes. Cells of the granulocytic lineage may exhibit nuclear hyposegmentation (with pseudo–Pelger–Huët nuclei), hypogranularity or agranularity of the cytoplasm, macrocytic (giant) bands and asynchronous nuclear–cytoplasmic maturation. Myeloblasts account for < 5% of the bone

marrow cells. Megakaryocytes are usually absent or very few. The detection of micromegakaryocytes is a strong indicator of RCC. Ring sideroblasts are not found. In cases of RCC with normocellular or hypercellular bone marrow, there is a slight to moderate increase in erythropoiesis, with accumulation of immature precursor cells (mainly proerythroblasts). Increased numbers of mitoses are present, indicating ineffective erythropoiesis. Granulopoiesis appears slightly to moderately decreased and cells of the granulocytic lineage are often loosely scattered. Blasts account for < 5% of the bone marrow cells. Megakaryocytes may be normal, decreased or increased in number, and display dysplasia with small non-lobated nuclei, abnormally separated nuclear lobes, and (infrequently) characteristic micromegakaryocytes. There is no increase in reticulin fibres.

About 80% of patients with RCC show a marked decrease of bone marrow

cellularity, as low as 5–10% of the normal value {2873}. The morphological findings in these cases are similar to those observed in normocellular or hypercellular cases. Immature erythroid precursors form one or several islands consisting of ≥20 cells. This patchy pattern of erythropoiesis is usually accompanied by sparsely distributed granulopoiesis. Megakaryocytes are significantly decreased or absent. Although micromegakaryocytes may be rare or not always found, they should be searched for carefully because they are important for establishing the diagnosis. Immunohistochemistry to identify micromegakaryocytes is obligatory. Multiple sections prepared from the biopsy may facilitate the identification of megakaryocytes and erythroid aggregates. Fatty tissue between the areas of haematopoiesis can mimic aplastic anaemia (Table 6.08). Therefore, at least two biopsies ≥2 weeks apart or two biopsies from two different locations of the pelvis are recommended to facilitate the detection of representative bone marrow spaces containing foci of erythropoiesis.

Differential diagnosis
In children, a variety of non-haematological disorders (e.g. viral infections, nutritional deficiencies and metabolic diseases) can give rise to secondary dysplastic morphology mimicking RCC (Table 6.09). In the absence of a cytogenetic marker, the clinical course in cases suspected of RCC must be carefully evaluated before a clear-cut diagnosis can be made. The haematological differential diagnosis includes acquired aplastic anaemia, inherited bone marrow failure diseases, and paroxysmal nocturnal haemoglobinuria. Unlike RCC, acquired aplastic anaemia presents with adipocytosis of the bone marrow spaces or with sparsely scattered

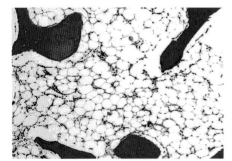

Fig. 6.24 Aplastic anaemia. Bone marrow biopsy shows adipocytosis of bone marrow spaces; the few scattered cells are mainly lymphocytes, plasma cells, macrophages, mast cells and occasional mature myeloid cells.

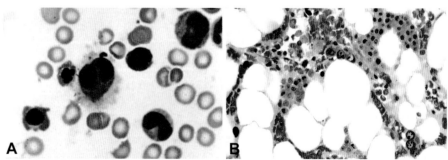

Fig. 6.25 Refractory cytopenia of childhood (RCC). **A** Bone marrow aspirate smear showing abnormal nuclear segmentation of an erythropoietic precursor cell and a small megakaryocyte with a bilobed nucleus. **B** Bone marrow biopsy showing a cluster of proerythroblasts without maturation.

myeloid cells. There are no significant erythroid islands, no increased immature erythroblasts, and no granulocytic or megakaryocytic dysplasia, in particular no micromegakaryocytes (Table 6.08). Contrary to what is sometimes reported in adults with aplastic anaemia, acquired aplastic anaemia in children does not have megaloblastoid features at presentation. The vast majority of cases of RCC and severe aplastic anaemia can be reliably differentiated by histomorphological means alone {296}, and flow cytometry can be a relevant addition {3}. However, after immunosuppressive therapy, the histological pattern of acquired aplastic anaemia can no longer be distinguished from that observed in RCC. The inherited bone marrow failure disorders (e.g. Fanconi anaemia, dyskeratosis congenita, Shwachman–Diamond syndrome, and amegakaryocytic thrombocytopenia or pancytopenia with radioulnar synostosis) as well as some DNA repair deficiency disorders (e.g. LIG4 syndrome) show morphological features overlapping those of RCC {1942,4437,4481}. These entities must be excluded by medical history, physical examination and the appropriate laboratory and molecular studies before a definite diagnosis of RCC can be made. The clinical picture of paroxysmal nocturnal haemoglobinuria is rare in childhood, although paroxysmal nocturnal haemoglobinuria clones in the absence of haemolysis or thrombosis may be observed in children with RCC {5}. The association between RCC with two or more dysplastic lineages and MDS with multilineage dysplasia has not been fully investigated {4418}. It is currently recommended that cases that would otherwise fulfil the criteria for MDS with multilineage dysplasia be considered as RCC until further studies clarify whether the number of lineages involved is an important prognostic discriminator in childhood MDS.

Immunophenotype

Micromegakaryocytes can easily be missed in H&E–stained bone marrow trephine biopsy sections, but are more readily apparent with immunostaining for platelet glycoproteins such as CD61 (also called glycoprotein IIIa), CD41 (also called glycoprotein IIb/IIIa) or von Willebrand factor. Myeloblasts are <5% of the bone marrow cells; detection of ≥5% blast cells that are positive for myeloperoxidase (MPO), lysozyme, and/or

Table 6.07 Minimal diagnostic criteria for refractory cytopenia of childhood. The criteria of dysplasia must be fulfilled in ≥ 10% of cells in ≥ 1 lineage; in some cases, lesser degrees of dysplasia are present in 2 or 3 lineages.

Specimen	Erythropoiesis	Granulopoiesis	Megakaryopoiesis
Bone marrow aspirate	Dysplastic changes[a] and/or megaloblastoid changes	Dysplastic changes[b] in granulocytic precursors and neutrophils; <5% blasts	Unequivocal micromegakaryocytes; other dysplastic changes[c] in variable numbers
Bone marrow biopsy	A few clusters of ≥ 20 erythroid precursors. Arrest in maturation, with increased number of proerythroblasts. Increased number of mitoses.	No minimal diagnostic criteria	Unequivocal micromegakaryocytes; immunohistochemistry is obligatory (CD61, CD41); other dysplastic changes[c] in variable numbers
Peripheral blood		Dysplastic changes[b] in neutrophils	

[a] Erythroid dysplasia: abnormal nuclear segmentation, multinucleated cells, nuclear bridges.
[b] Granulocytic dysplasia: pseudo–Pelger–Huët cells, hypogranularity or agranularity, giant bands (in cases with severe neutropenia, this criterion may not be fulfilled).
[c] Megakaryocytic dysplasia: variable size with separated nuclei or round nuclei; the absence of megakaryocytes does not rule out refractory cytopenia of childhood.

Table 6.08 Comparison of the morphological criteria for hypoplastic refractory cytopenia of childhood and aplastic anaemia in children

Criterion	Refractory cytopenia of childhood		Aplastic anaemia in children	
	Bone marrow biopsy	*Bone marrow aspirate cytology*	*Bone marrow biopsy*	*Bone marrow aspirate cytology*
Erythropoiesis	Patchy distribution Left shift Increased mitosis	Nuclear segmentation Multinuclearity Megaloblastoid changes	Absent or single small focus; < 10 cells with maturation	Absent or very few cells, without dysplasia or megaloblastoid change
Granulopoiesis	Marked decrease Left shift	Pseudo–Pelger–Huët anomaly Agranularity of cytoplasm Hypogranularity of cytoplasm Nuclear–cytoplasmic maturation defects	Absent or markedly decreased, with very few small foci with maturation	Few maturing cells, with no dysplasia
Megakaryopoiesis	Marked decrease or aplasia Dysplastic changes Micromegakaryocytes	Micromegakaryocytes Multiple separated nuclei Small round nuclei	Absent or very few non-dysplastic megakaryocytes	Absent or few non-dysplastic megakaryocytes
Lymphocytes	May be increased focally or dispersed	May be increased	May be increased focally or dispersed	May be increased
CD34+ precursor cells	No increase		No increase	
KIT+ (CD117+) precursor cells	No increase		No increase	
KIT+ (CD117+) mast cells	Slightly increased		Slightly increased	

Table 6.09 Disorders that can present with morphological features indistinguishable from those of refractory cytopenia of childhood

- Infection (e.g. cytomegalovirus, herpesviruses, parvovirus B19, visceral leishmaniasis)

- Vitamin deficiency (e.g. deficiency of vitamin B12, folate, vitamin E)

- Metabolic disorders (e.g. mevalonate kinase deficiency)

- Rheumatological disease

- Systemic lupus erythematosus

- Autoimmune lymphoproliferative disorders (e.g. FAS deficiency)

- Mitochondrial DNA deletions (e.g. Pearson syndrome)

- Inherited bone marrow failure disorders (e.g. Fanconi anaemia, dyskeratosis congenita, Shwachman–Diamond syndrome, amegakaryocytic thrombocytopenia, thrombocytopenia with absent radii, radioulnar synostosis, Seckel syndrome)

- Paroxysmal nocturnal haemoglobinuria

- Acquired aplastic anaemia during haematological recovery during or after immunosuppression

KIT (CD117) may indicate progression to higher-grade MDS. CD34 staining is useful for identifying myeloblasts, but an increase of haematogones positive for CD34 and CD79a should be excluded. Clusters of myeloblasts are not seen in RCC. In most cases, flow cytometric immunophenotyping indicates a greatly reduced myeloid compartment, but not as severely reduced as in children with aplastic anaemia {3}.

Cell of origin
A haematopoietic stem cell with multi-lineage potential

Genetic profile
The genetic changes that predispose individuals to MDS in childhood remain largely obscure. The presumed underlying mechanism may also give rise to subtle phenotypic abnormalities noted in many children with MDS. *GATA2* deficiency was identified as germline predisposition in 5% of consecutively diagnosed children with RCC and can be associated with monosomy 7 or trisomy 8 {4342}. Monosomy 7 is the most common cytogenetic abnormality in RCC {1504,1940,2749,2873}. In one study, patients with normocellular or hypercellular bone marrow showed a normal karyotype, monosomy 7 or other aberrations in 61%, 19% and 12% of cases, respectively {2873}. In hypocellular RCC, the incidence of monosomy 7 and other aberrations is approximately 20%.

Prognosis and predictive factors
Karyotype is the most important factor predicting progression to advanced MDS. Patients with monosomy 7 have a significantly higher probability of progression than do patients with other chromosomal abnormalities or a normal karyotype {1940}. Spontaneous disappearance of cytopenia with monosomy 7 and del (7q) has been reported in some infants, but remains a rare event {3065}. Unlike with monosomy 7, patients with trisomy 8 or a normal karyotype may experience a long, stable course of disease. Currently, haematopoietic stem cell transplantation is the only curative therapy available, and is the treatment of choice for patients with monosomy 7 or complex karyotypes early in the course of their disease. Given the low rate of transplant-related mortality, haematopoietic stem cell transplantation can also be recommended for patients with other karyotypes if a suitable donor is available {3807}.

An expectant approach, with careful observation, is reasonable in the absence of transfusion requirement, severe cytopenia and infections {1579}. Because early bone marrow failure can be mediated at least in part by T-cell immunosuppression of haematopoiesis, and because T-cell receptor V beta skewing with expansion of effector cytotoxic T cells is noted in approximately 40% of RCC cases, immunosuppressive therapy can be an effective therapeutic strategy in select patients {1580,4438}; however, the long-term risk of relapse or clonal evolution remains.

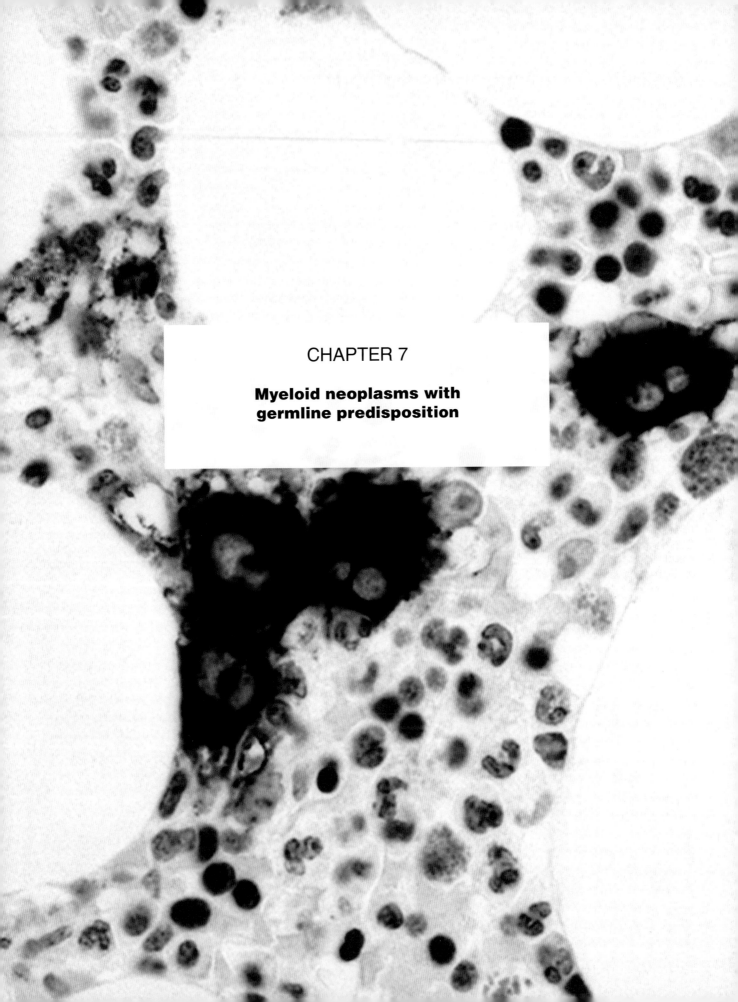

CHAPTER 7

Myeloid neoplasms with germline predisposition

Myeloid neoplasms with germline predisposition

Peterson L.C.
Bloomfield C.D.
Niemeyer C.M.
Döhner H.
Godley L.A.

Definition

Myelodysplastic syndromes (MDSs) and acute myeloid leukaemia (AML) present primarily as sporadic diseases and typically occur in older adults. However, it has become increasingly apparent that some cases of myeloid neoplasms, in particular MDS and AML, occur in association with inherited or de novo germline mutations characterized by specific genetic and clinical findings. The most established of these disorders are those that occur in the setting of well-defined inherited syndromes that exhibit additional non-haematological findings and often present in childhood, such as the bone marrow failure syndromes (including Fanconi anaemia) and the telomere biology disorders (e.g. dyskeratosis congenita, see Table 7.01) {2866,3613, 3800}. However, we have become increasingly aware of additional autosomal dominant disorders with predisposition to MDS/AML. Some patients with these disorders initially present with a myeloid neoplasm, whereas others have a pre-existing disorder or organ dysfunction. Some of the first cases to be described were AML with germline-mutated *CEBPA* and MDS/AML with germline mutations in *RUNX1* and a pre-existing familial platelet disorder, but the list of these disorders is expanding (Table 7.01) {854, 1390,3015,4301}. Myeloid neoplasms associated with predisposing mutations are generally considered to be rare, but as recognition grows, they may be found to be more common than is currently realized. Because the hereditary basis for these neoplasms is only beginning to be understood, it is likely that more disorders will be identified and that many of the currently recognized disorders will become more clearly defined.

The recognition and diagnosis of myeloid malignancies that arise from a germline mutation is critical for the proper clinical management and long-term follow-up of affected individuals. Even if a patient has not developed malignancy, the presence of additional organ dysfunction and abnormalities in platelet number and function warrant clinical management. For example, patients with germline *RUNX1*, *ANKRD26*, or *ETV6* mutations can bleed out of proportion to their platelet counts and may require anticipatory transfusion of normal platelets prior to invasive procedures or childbirth. Individuals in these families benefit greatly from genetic counselling from counsellors with training in familial haematopoietic disorders. Because the clinical management of patients with malignant myeloid disorders often involves allogeneic haematopoietic stem cell transplantation, careful donor selection is critical in these families, to avoid re-introduction of the deleterious mutation. Inadvertent use of affected donor stem cells has resulted in poor or failed stem cell engraftment, poor graft function, and donor-derived leukaemias. Therefore, it is critical to distinguish myeloid neoplasms that arise as a consequence of germline predisposition from those that arise spontaneously or are secondary to environmental or chemical exposures.

This chapter discusses the major myeloid neoplasms with germline predisposition. The discussion focuses on myeloid neoplasms, but lymphoid neoplasms and solid tumours also occasionally occur in these same pedigrees, and are mentioned when relevant. There is increasing evidence to support germline mutations with predisposition to lymphoblastic leukaemia {1734,3134,3630}; this is discussed in the sections on T- and B-lymphoblastic leukaemias/lymphomas. The familial myeloid neoplasms included in this chapter are categorized into three groups (Table 7.01). The first group includes myeloid neoplasms associated with germline mutations of *CEBPA* or *DDX41*, with a clinical picture dominated by either MDS or AML and with no other significant organ dysfunction or pre-existing disorder. The second group consists of myeloid neoplasms associated with germline mutations of *RUNX1*, *ANKRD26*, or *ETV6* in which affected patients have a pre-existing platelet disorder. The third category includes myeloid neoplasms with predisposing mutations

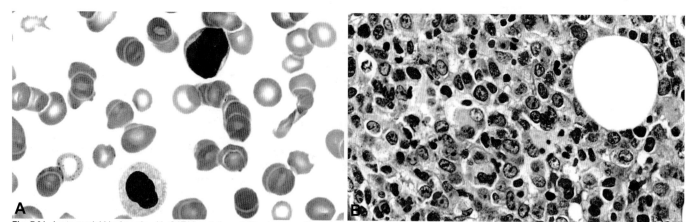

Fig. 7.01 Acute myeloid leukaemia with *GATA2* mutation. **A** Blood smear with a circulating myeloblast and a dysplastic neutrophil **B** Bone marrow biopsy showing increased blasts and dysplastic megakaryocytes.

in which affected patients frequently exhibit additional non-haematological phenotypic abnormalities; the entities in this group are neoplasms with germline *GATA2* mutation, the telomere biology disorders, and the inherited bone marrow failure disorders that often present in childhood (Table 7.01). Myeloid proliferations associated with Down syndrome, neurofibromatosis, and Noonan syndrome are also germline predisposition disorders, but are discussed elsewhere in this volume.

Synonyms
Familial myeloid neoplasms; familial myelodysplastic syndromes / acute leukaemias

Epidemiology
The frequency of myeloid neoplasms associated with genetic predisposition is unknown, but they are considered rare. Some germline mutations are associated with pre-existing non-neoplastic haematological disorders or organ dysfunction that may present during childhood or in young adults. The neoplasms can present in any age group, often in children and young adults but also in older individuals, depending on the specific gene mutation.

Etiology
The etiology of these neoplasms is related to the underlying germline mutations. In some instances, the development of the myeloid neoplasm has been found to be associated with additional molecular and / or cytogenetic events.

Clinical features
There are no clinical features specific to myeloid neoplasms with a predisposing germline mutation. However, many of the germline mutations are associated with non-neoplastic haematological disorders, organ dysfunction, or inherited syndromic disorders that correlate with the specific gene involved and often manifest before the myeloid neoplasm develops.

Recognition of the presence of a germline predisposition syndrome requires familiarity with the currently defined syndromes and their clinical features. Guidelines recommend conducting a complete family history in the context of a comprehensive medical history and physical examination of all patients diagnosed with a

Table 7.01 Classification of myeloid neoplasms with germline predisposition

Myeloid neoplasms with germline predisposition without a pre-existing disorder or organ dysfunction

Acute myeloid leukaemia with germline *CEBPA* mutation
Myeloid neoplasms with germline *DDX41* mutation[a]

Myeloid neoplasms with germline predisposition and pre-existing platelet disorders

Myeloid neoplasms with germline *RUNX1* mutation[a]
Myeloid neoplasms with germline *ANKRD26* mutation[a]
Myeloid neoplasms with germline *ETV6* mutation[a]

Myeloid neoplasms with germline predisposition and other organ dysfunction

Myeloid neoplasms with germline *GATA2* mutation
Myeloid neoplasms associated with bone marrow failure syndromes[b]
Myeloid neoplasms associated with telomere biology disorders[b]
Juvenile myelomonocytic leukaemia associated with neurofibromatosis, Noonan syndrome, or Noonan syndrome–like disorders[c]
Myeloid neoplasms associated with Down syndrome[a,d]

[a] Lymphoid neoplasms have also been reported.
[b] See Table 7.03 (p. 127) for specific genes.
[c] See *Juvenile myelomonocytic leukaemia*, p. 89.
[d] See *Myeloid proliferations associated with Down syndrome*, p. 169.

haematological malignancy. It is particularly important to include detailed questioning about personal and family history including bleeding history as described in Table 7.02; documentation may be facilitated by genetic counselling with a counsellor familiar with inherited haematological malignancies {757}.

Microscopy and immunophenotype
The morphology of the neoplasm depends on its subtype (MDS or AML). In many instances, the morphology has not been defined in detail or the number of cases described is limited. There is no known morphological finding specific for any neoplasm with an underlying germline mutation, but some findings (e.g. bone marrow hypocellularity, dysplasia, and the presence of Auer rods) characteristic of certain mutations are described here. The neoplasms have a myeloid immunophenotype. Some of these disorders exhibit distinctive blood and bone marrow morphology at baseline, before the development of overt neoplasia. The presence of a genetic predisposition does not in itself place a case into the category of a myeloid neoplasm until the appearance of standard diagnostic features of MDS, AML, or other myeloid malignancy. In general, the diagnostic criteria for the germline predisposition disorders are the same as those for sporadic cases; however, the diagnosis of MDS may be challenging in some cases. For example, some cases

exhibit early dysplastic features that are stable and may not progress to MDS or AML for decades. These include the familial disorders in which dysmegakaryopoiesis accompanies thrombocytopenia secondary to germline *ANKRD26* or *ETV6* mutations. It is recommended that these cases not be considered neoplastic unless additional signs of neoplasia develop (e.g. increased blasts, increasing marrow cellularity in the presence of persisting cytopenias, increasing cytopenias, and / or the presence of additional cytogenetic or molecular genetic abnormalities to suggest progression to MDS/AML). Diagnosis of the childhood syndromic disorders can also be challenging. For example, patients with Fanconi anaemia often have a clinical course with fluctuating clonal haematopoiesis that can be difficult to distinguish from overt MDS {78,79}. Close collaboration of pathologists and clinicians with clinical geneticists and / or certified genetic counsellors is essential for addressing these challenges.

Another challenge is that the genetic predisposition may not be known or identified at the time of diagnosis of the first myeloid neoplasm within a family, which is often classified as a sporadic neoplasm. When the germline mutation becomes known, the diagnosis can be modified. For example, after a germline mutation is identified, a diagnosis of AML could be modified to AML with germline *CEBPA* mutation. Similarly, myeloid neoplasms

Table 7.02 Individuals in whom the possibility of a myeloid neoplasm with germline predisposition should be considered. From: Churpek JE, et al. {757}

Any patient presenting with myelodysplastic syndrome (MDS) or acute leukaemia, i.e. acute myeloid leukaemia (AML) or lymphoblastic leukaemia, with any of the following:
- A personal history of multiple cancers
- Thrombocytopenia, bleeding propensity, or macrocytosis preceding the diagnosis of MDS/AML by several years
- A first- or second-degree relative with a haematological neoplasm
- A first- or second-degree relative with a solid tumour consistent with germline predisposition; i.e. sarcoma, early-onset breast cancer (at patient age < 50 years), or brain tumours
- Abnormal nails or skin pigmentation, oral leukoplakia, idiopathic pulmonary fibrosis, unexplained liver disease, lymphoedema, atypical infections, immune deficiencies, congenital limb anomalies, or short stature (in the patient or a first- or second-degree relative)
Any healthy potential haematopoietic stem cell donor who is planning to donate for a family member with a haematological malignancy with any of the conditions listed above or who fails to mobilize stem cells well using standard protocols

occurring in association with the syndromic disorders often presenting in childhood should be classified according to the genetic abnormality (e.g. AML with germline *SBDS* mutation). If the affected gene has not been determined in a given patient, the neoplasm can be classified as AML associated with Shwachman–Diamond syndrome.

Genetic profile

Each of these neoplasms exhibits a specific germline predisposition mutation (described below) identified by molecular genetic testing (including gene sequencing). Routine cytogenetic analysis may be normal or may reveal non-defining karyotypic alterations. Because many of the genes that are mutated in the germline can also be mutated as acquired events in MDS/AML, it is critical to perform germline testing on constitutional DNA. Growth of skin fibroblasts is the gold standard for obtaining germline DNA, but DNA from nails or hair can also be used. Because blood and bone marrow are both affected by haematological tumours, they should be used cautiously as a source of germline DNA. Saliva and buccal swabs are often contaminated with blood cells and should not be considered to be purely germline material. Once true germline DNA is obtained, it can be sent for molecular genetic testing. Panel-based testing for all known predisposition genes and testing for individual genes is available at academic and commercial laboratories (for availability details, consult https://www.genetests.org). Because many individuals and families have unique familial mutations, many variants are initially classified as variants of uncertain significance and require functional testing to determine whether they are deleterious.

The results of molecular testing of myeloid neoplasms must be interpreted carefully, with these syndromes in mind. Standard testing for prognostication of AML includes *CEBPA* mutation testing; in about 10% of cases with biallelic *CEBPA* mutations, one of the mutations is a germline event. Because many mutations in familial syndromes can also be acquired events, panel-based mutation tests must be interpreted with caution. For example, if a *RUNX1* or *ETV6* mutation is found by mutation testing of affected blood and/or bone marrow, consideration should be given as to whether the mutation is actually germline.

Genetic susceptibility

When a patient's personal or family history suggests familial predisposition to myeloid malignancies, clinical testing for mutations known to confer increased risk of development of myeloid malignancies is often negative, suggesting that additional predisposition alleles exist and await discovery. Therefore, the number of recognized germline predisposition syndromes is likely to increase. For example, recently described germline mutations of *SRP72* {1390,2033} and germline duplications of *ATG2B* and *GSKIP* {3496} may emerge as myeloid neoplasm predisposition syndromes as more information becomes available.

Myeloid neoplasms with germline predisposition without a pre-existing disorder or organ dysfunction

Acute myeloid leukaemia with germline *CEBPA* mutation

This familial AML syndrome is due to the inheritance of a single copy of mutated *CEBPA*, which encodes a granulocyte differentiation factor on chromosome band 19q13.1 {3708}. The AML is associated with biallelic *CEBPA* mutations, with the germline mutation usually found in the 5' end of the gene and a somatic mutation at the 3' end of the other allele acquired at the time of progression to AML {3015,3023}. Acquired *GATA2* mutations are also common in this setting {1430}.

This disorder appears to have near-complete penetrance for development of AML {3015,3792}, but the prevalence is unknown. Both monoallelic and biallelic mutations occur in sporadic AML, but only biallelic mutations are associated with a good prognosis {3023,3908}. In the current WHO classification, only cases with biallelic *CEBPA* mutations are recognized as a specific subtype of AML. Because some of these cases may constitute AML with genetic predisposition, the identification of biallelic *CEBPA* mutations within leukaemic cells should prompt evaluation for germline inheritance of one of the alleles.

Patients with AML with germline mutations of *CEBPA* typically present with AML as children or young adults; in one report of 10 affected families, 24 patients with AML presented at a median age of 24.5 years (range: 1.75–46 years) {3909}. AML is the primary presenting feature, with no preceding blood count abnormalities. The familial forms have morphological and immunophenotypic features similar to those of sporadic AML with *CEBPA* mutations, including a predominance of AML with or without maturation, the presence of Auer rods, frequent aberrant CD7 expression in the blast population, and a normal karyotype {3015,3708}. Overall, AML with germline *CEBPA* mutation has a favourable prognosis. In one series, the 10-year overall survival rate was 67%, although multiple relapses were reported {3909}. The somatic *CEBPA* mutations were found to be unstable throughout the disease course, with different mutations identified at recurrence, suggesting that apparent relapses may in fact represent novel, independent clones rather than being true relapses {3909}.

Myeloid neoplasms with germline *DDX41* mutation

This is a recently described autosomal dominant familial MDS/AML syndrome {3208} characterized by inherited mutations in the gene on chromosome 5 encoding the DEAD box RNA helicase DDX41. As with *CEBPA*, there is a significant subset of cases in which the *DDX41* mutation is biallelic, with one mutation being germline. The prevalence of this germline *DDX41* mutation is unknown. However, *DDX41* mutations have been found in about 1.5% of myeloid neoplasms, and half of these patients had germline mutations {114,2291, 3208}. Although the number of described pedigrees with MDS/AML with germline *DDX41* mutation is limited, this disorder appears to be associated with long latency (with a mean patient age of 62 years at haematological malignancy onset) and development of high-grade myeloid neoplasms. The neoplasms reported are mainly MDS – MDS with multilineage dysplasia, MDS with excess blasts, and MDS with isolated del(5q) – and AML. Chronic myeloid leukaemia, chronic myelomonocytic leukaemia (CMML), and Hodgkin and non-Hodgkin lymphomas have also been reported. The penetrance of the disease is not fully established, but appears to be high. Patients with germline *DDX41* mutation who develop MDS/AML usually present with leukopenia (with or without other cytopenias or macrocytosis), hypocellular bone marrow with prominent erythroid dysplasia, and a normal karyotype, often leading to erythroleukaemia. The prognosis is generally poor. Early data suggest that patients may respond to lenalidomide, but this observation is based on a limited number of patients {3208}.

Myeloid neoplasms with germline predisposition and pre-existing platelet disorders

Myeloid neoplasms with germline *RUNX1* mutation

Familial platelet disorder with predisposition to AML is an autosomal dominant syndrome characterized by abnormalities in platelet number and function and enhanced risk of developing MDS/AML at a young age {2866,3015}. Patients with this disorder have germline monoallelic mutations in *RUNX1*, a gene on chromosome band 21q22 encoding one subunit of the core binding transcription factor that regulates expression of several genes essential for haematopoiesis. Somatic *RUNX1* alterations also occur in sporadic myeloid neoplasms, including participation as a partner in the *RUNX1-RUNX1T1* fusion associated with t(8;21) (q22;q22.1) in AML and in the newly recognized WHO provisional entity AML with mutated *RUNX1*. The prevalence of germline *RUNX1* mutations has not been determined.

The clinical presentation is variable, even within the same family. Most affected individuals have a mild to moderate bleeding tendency, usually evident from childhood, but some have no bleeding history. Platelet counts are normal or mildly reduced, with normal platelet morphology and variable degrees of platelet dysfunction. Most patients exhibit impaired platelet aggregation with collagen and epinephrine, as well as a dense granule storage pool deficiency {3015,3729}.

Distinct families with germline *RUNX1* mutations exhibit varying risks of development of myeloid neoplasms, with 11–100% (median: 44%) of family members affected. The median patient age at onset of MDS/AML is 33 years, younger than for sporadic MDS/AML {4301}. MDS and AML are the most common haematological neoplasms with germline *RUNX1* mutations, but CMML, T-lymphoblastic leukaemia/lymphoma, and (rarely) B-cell neoplasms (including hairy cell leukaemia) have also been reported {1390}. There are limited data on the morphology of MDS and AML, but the AMLs are reported to typically be AML with or without maturation, and Auer rods are common {3014}. Anticipation appears to occur in many of the reported pedigrees, with children sometimes presenting before family members of older generations. Long-term data on the outcomes of patients treated for myeloid neoplasms with germline *RUNX1* mutation are limited, making the determination of prognosis difficult {1390}.

The causative germline *RUNX1* mutations include nonsense mutations, frameshift mutations, duplications, deletions, and missense mutations. Some of the mutations appear to act by haploinsufficiency and have dominant negative effects. Progression to MDS/AML likely requires additional mutations, which may account for some of the variation in penetrance of MDS/AML as well as the variable neoplasm phenotypes that develop {4301}. Acquisition of a mutation of the second *RUNX1* allele appears to be a common second hit, but it is not required {3235}. Other additional acquired abnormalities, including a *CBL* mutation in an individual who developed CMML and a mutation of *ASXL1* in addition to loss of *NF1* in a case of T lymphoblastic leukaemia, have also been reported {1390,4038,4301}. For cases suspected to harbour *RUNX1* mutations in which standard sequencing fails to reveal a point mutation, it is recommended that germline testing include testing for gene deletions, duplications, and rearrangements {1390}.

Myeloid neoplasms with germline *ANKRD26* mutation

Thrombocytopenia 2 (germline *ANKRD26* mutation) is an autosomal dominant disorder characterized by moderate thrombocytopenia and increased risk of developing MDS/AML. This disorder is characterized by germline mutations in *ANKRD26*, located on chromosome band 10p12.1 {2894}. Most such mutations occur within the 5' untranslated region of the gene and disrupt the assembly of RUNX1 and FLI1 on the *ANKRD26* promoter, ultimately resulting in increased gene transcription and signalling through the MPL pathway. This leads to impaired proplatelet formation by megakaryocytes. It has been shown that inhibition of EPHB2/MAPK (also called ERK) reverses the proplatelet defect in vitro, which implicates the MAPK pathway in the pathogenesis of the thrombocytopenia 2 platelet defect {1390}. Notably, one missense mutation (D158G) has been identified within a family {45}.

The incidence of this disorder is unknown, but more than 20 affected families have been reported. Platelet count is variable, but the thrombocytopenia is usually moderate, with normal platelet size and volume. Most patients have glycoprotein Ia and alpha-granule deficiency, whereas in vitro platelet aggregation studies are often normal. Thrombopoietin levels in these patients are elevated. Bleeding tendencies in affected patients are usually mild.

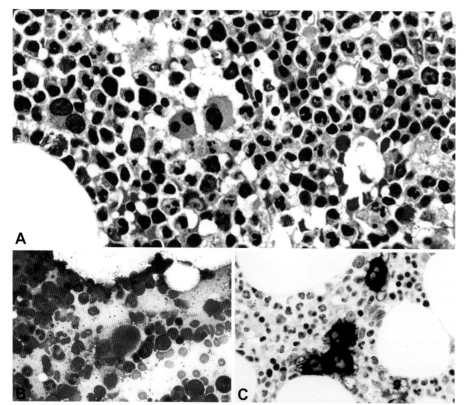

Fig. 7.02 Thrombocytopenia associated with germline *ANKRD26* mutation. **A** Bone marrow biopsy showing small hyposegmented and binucleated megakaryocytes; there is no definitive evidence for a myelodysplastic syndrome or acute leukaemia. **B** Bone marrow aspirate showing a small binucleated megakaryocyte. **C** Immunostaining for CD61 highlights the small hyposegmented megakaryocytes in the bone marrow biopsy.

Evidence of dysmegakaryopoiesis has been observed in the small number of patients without leukaemia who have undergone bone marrow biopsies: megakaryocytes are increased in number and small, have hyposegmented nuclei or two nuclei, and include micromegakaryocytes. A small subset of patients have elevated haemoglobin concentrations and leukocyte counts {2894}.

Although the number of reported families with this disorder is limited, the prevalence of the development of myeloid neoplasms in these families is estimated to be approximately 30 times higher than that in the general population. Most of the reported cases are AML or MDS, but the number of reported cases is low {2893}. A smaller number of patients had chronic myeloid leukaemia, CMML {3132}, or chronic lymphocytic leukaemia {2894}.

Myeloid neoplasms with germline *ETV6* mutation

Thrombocytopenia 5 (germline *ETV6* mutation) is a recently described disorder characterized by autosomal dominant familial thrombocytopenia and haematological neoplasms. Affected patients have variable thrombocytopenia with normal-sized platelets, and a mild to moderate bleeding tendency, occasionally presenting in infancy. The limited number of bone marrow biopsies from affected individuals without leukaemia have shown small hyposegmented megakaryocytes. Mild dyserythropoiesis has also been reported. The haematological malignancies reported in these individuals are diverse, including MDS, AML, CMML, B lymphoblastic leukaemia, and plasma cell myeloma. Non-haematological neoplasms, including colorectal adenocarcinoma, have been also reported in these families. The missense mutations identified to date have a dominant negative effect, resulting in disrupted nuclear localization of the ETV6 transcription factor and reduced expression of platelet-associated genes {2887,4024,4480}.

Myeloid neoplasms with germline predisposition associated with other organ dysfunction

Myeloid neoplasms with germline *GATA2* mutation

Germline *GATA2* gene mutations were originally identified as four separate syndromes:
- MonoMAC syndrome, characterized by monocytopenia and non-tuberculous mycobacterial infection {1715,4197}
- Dendritic cell, monocyte, B- and NK-lymphoid (DCML) deficiency with vulnerability to viral infections {375,977, 1518}
- Familial MDS/AML {1293,1518}
- Emberger syndrome, characterized by primary lymphoedema, warts and a predisposition to MDS/AML {2490,3002}

GATA2 mutations were also recognized in a minority of cases of congenital neutropenia and aplastic anaemia. Considering the overlapping features present in these disorders, they are now recognized as a single genetic disorder with protean manifestations {784,978,1292, 3755}.

GATA2 is a zinc-finger transcription factor regulating haematopoiesis, autoimmunity, and inflammatory and developmental processes. Germline *GATA2* mutations have been identified in both coding and non-coding regions; they are monoallelic and broadly classified as missense, null, and regulatory mutations. Germline *GATA2* mutations result in loss of function of the mutated allele, resulting in haploinsufficiency {3755}. No significant association between genotype and clinical manifestations has been identified, with the exception of lymphoedema and severe infections that are seen preferentially in patients with null mutations {1289}. *GATA2* haploinsufficiency is diagnosed by full gene sequencing and large rearrangement testing. The incidence of *GATA2* haploinsufficiency is unknown.

The clinical presentation of germline *GATA2* mutation is heterogeneous. In a study of 57 *GATA2*-mutated cases, the median patient age at presentation was 20 years (range: 5 months to 78 years), with 64% of cases presenting with infection, 21% with MDS/AML, and 9% with lymphoedema {3755}. A small subset of cases present with AML, but many

Table 7.03 Selected bone marrow failure syndromes and telomere biology disorders with germline predisposition to myeloid neoplasms[a] {206,1390,2471,3613,3658,3800,4301}

Syndrome	Inheritance patterns and genes	Characteristic haematological neoplasms	Risk of myeloid neoplasm	Other phenotypic findings	Diagnostic testing
Fanconi anaemia	AR: *FANCA* XLR: *FANCB, FANCC, BRCA2 (FANCD1), FANCD2, FANCE, FANCF, FANCG, FANCI, BRIP1 (FANCJ), FANCL, FANCM, PALB2 (FANCN), RAD51C, SLX4 (BTBD12)*	MDS, AML	MDS: 7% AML: 9%	Bone marrow failure, low birth weight, short stature, radial anomalies, congenital heart disease, microphthalmia, ear anomalies, deafness, renal malformations, hypogonadism, café-au-lait spots, solid tumours	Screening: chromosomal breakage analysis Gene sequencing for relevant mutations
Severe congenital neutropenia	AD: *ELANE, CSF3R, GFI1* AR: *HAX1, G6PC3* XLR: *WAS*	MDS, AML	21–40%	*HAX1*: neurodevelopmental *G6PC3*: cardiac and other	Gene sequencing for relevant mutations
Shwachman–Diamond syndrome	AR: *SBDS*	MDS, AML, ALL	5–24%	Preceding isolated neutropenia, pancreatic insufficiency, short stature, skeletal abnormalities including metaphyseal dysostosis	Gene sequencing for *SBDS* mutations
Diamond–Blackfan anaemia	AD: *RPS19, RPS17, RPS24, RPL35A, RPL5, RPL11, RPS7, RPS26, RPS10* XLR: *GATA1*	MDS, AML, ALL	5%	Small stature, congenital anomalies (e.g. craniofacial, cardiac, skeletal, genitourinary)	Screening: elevated erythrocyte adenosine deaminase and haemoglobin F Gene sequencing for relevant mutations
Telomere biology disorders including dyskeratosis congenita and syndromes due to *TERC* or *TERT* mutation	XLR: *DKC1* AD: *TERT, TERC, TINF2, RTEL1* AR: *NOP10, NHP2, WRAP53, RTEL1, TERT, CTC1*	MDS, AML	2–30%	Nail dystrophy, abnormal skin and pigmentation, oral leukoplakia, pulmonary fibrosis, hepatic fibrosis, squamous cell carcinoma	Telomere length measurement by flow-FISH If abnormal, gene sequencing for relevant mutations

AD, autosomal dominant; ALL, lymphoblastic leukaemia/lymphoma; AML, acute myeloid leukaemia; AR, autosomal recessive; CMML, chronic myelomonocytic leukaemia; MDS, myelodysplastic syndrome; XLR, X-linked recessive.

[a] Because phenotypes are variable, some cases may show additional features or lack the key features listed.

patients develop MDS with a high risk of evolution to AML or development of CMML {3755}. Concurrent *ASXL1* mutations have been reported in many patients with monosomy 7, some of whom have a germline *GATA2* mutation {514,2656,4303}. MDS/AML develops in approximately 70% of affected individuals, at a median patient age of 29 years {2656}.

The clinical history of immunodeficiency associated with reduced monocytes, B cells, and NK cells; lymphoedema; and/or other clinical manifestations of *GATA2* mutation may point to the diagnosis. However, some patients with germline *GATA2* mutation present with MDS/AML without these clues. In MDS in children and adolescents, *GATA2* mutation accounts for 15% of advanced MDS cases and 7% of all MDS cases {4342}. It is highly prevalent among patients with monosomy 7, with 37% of such patients harbouring *GATA2* germline mutations,

and peak incidence in adolescence. In most children with germline *GATA2* mutation, MDS appears to be sporadic, without a family history of myeloid leukaemia or other *GATA2*-related symptoms {4342}. *GATA2*-mutant MDS can be heralded by anaemia, neutropenia, or thrombocytopenia. Characteristic morphological features are bone marrow hypocellularity and multilineage dysplasia (most prominent in the megakaryocyte lineage), including micromegakaryocytes and megakaryocytes with separated and peripheralized nuclear lobes. Increased reticulin fibrosis is also a feature. Flow cytometric immunophenotyping shows abnormal granulocytic maturation, mono-cytopenia, and reduced numbers of bone marrow NK cells and B cells. Plasma cells are present, but are often abnormal (e.g. CD56+). Increased T-cell large granular lymphocyte populations are common {531}. The most common cytogenetic abnormalities are monosomy 7 and trisomy 8. Based on the limited numbers of cases reported in the literature, affected patients appear to have a poor prognosis. However, improved clinical outcomes have been reported with haematopoietic stem cell transplantation in patients with MDS {4303}.

Myeloid neoplasms with germline predisposition associated with inherited bone failure syndromes and telomere biology disorders

The remaining cases of familial MDS/AML associated with other organ dysfunction include the well-known classic disorders often diagnosed in childhood and known as the inherited bone marrow failure syndromes and telomere biology disorders. The main features of these disorders are listed in Table 7.03 (p. 127), and the reader is referred to excellent reviews of this topic {1390,2866, 3613,3800}. It should be noted that the phenotypes of these disorders are highly variable; in some cases key findings may be absent, and patients may not be diagnosed until adulthood {3658}. The inherited bone marrow failure syndromes are a heterogeneous group of disorders including Fanconi anaemia, Shwachman–Diamond syndrome, Diamond–Blackfan anaemia, and severe congenital neutropenia {1390,3613}. Although lymphoblastic leukaemias have been described in these syndromes, MDS and AML are the most common haematological neoplasms {2471}. Patients are typically diagnosed in childhood due to bone marrow failure or systemic manifestations such as limb abnormalities in Fanconi anaemia or pancreatic dysfunction in Shwachman–Diamond syndrome, but some cases may not be recognized until adulthood {3658}. One of the classic disorders in this group, Fanconi anaemia, lacks the characteristic physical features of short stature and radial anomalies in about 25% of cases. Because there is a 600- to 800-fold increased risk of MDS/AML, development of a haematological malignancy may be the presenting feature of the disease {4301}. Also within the spectrum of inherited bone marrow failure syndromes are the telomere biology disorders associated with abnormal telomere maintenance and predisposition to MDS and AML. Dyskeratosis congenita is a prototypical disorder in this group, with the classic triad of nail dystrophy, abnormal reticular skin pigmentation, and oral leukoplakia, and a high risk of developing MDS/AML. Telomere biology disorders result from mutations in one of several genes, and inheritance patterns are diverse (Table 7.03, p. 127). The clinical presentations of telomere biology disorders are heterogeneous, and not all patients exhibit the classic features. The involvement of at least two genes (*TERC*, which encodes the telomerase RNA components, and *TERT*, which encodes the telomerase reverse transcriptase component) can cause clinical presentations that completely lack the characteristic mucocutaneous findings. These disorders predispose patients not only to MDS/AML, but also to a variety of solid tumours {1390}.

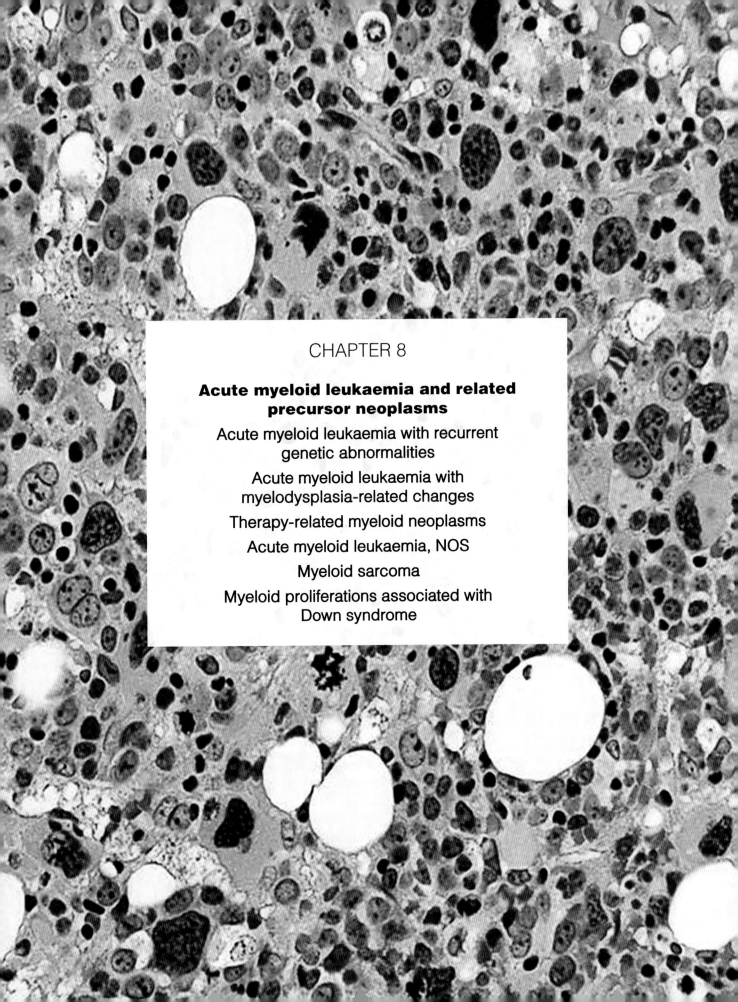

CHAPTER 8

Acute myeloid leukaemia and related precursor neoplasms

Acute myeloid leukaemia with recurrent genetic abnormalities

Acute myeloid leukaemia with myelodysplasia-related changes

Therapy-related myeloid neoplasms

Acute myeloid leukaemia, NOS

Myeloid sarcoma

Myeloid proliferations associated with Down syndrome

Acute myeloid leukaemia with recurrent genetic abnormalities

Arber D.A.
Brunning R.D.
Le Beau M.M.
Falini B.
Vardiman J.W.

Porwit A.
Thiele J.
Foucar K.
Döhner H.
Bloomfield C.D.

Introduction

Acute myeloid leukaemia with balanced translocations/inversions

The recurrent genetic abnormalities in acute myeloid leukaemia (AML) are associated with distinctive clinicopathological features and have prognostic significance. Those most commonly identified are balanced abnormalities: t(8;21)(q22;q22.1), inv(16)(p13.1q22) or t(16;16)(p13.1;q22), t(15;17)(q24.1;q21.2), and t(9;11)(p21.3;q23.3) {511,1236,1465, 1466,3701}. Most of these structural chromosomal rearrangements create a fusion gene encoding a chimeric protein that is required, but usually not sufficient, for leukaemogenesis {3746}. Many of these disease groups have characteristic morphological and immunophenotypic features {126}. Many other balanced translocations and inversions also recur in AML, but are uncommon. Several of these occur more commonly in paediatric patients, and are summarized in Table 8.01.

AML with t(8;21)(q22;q22.1), AML with inv(16)(p13.1q22) or t(16;16)(p13.1;q22), and acute promyelocytic leukaemia with PML-RARA are considered to be acute leukaemias without regard to blast cell count. It is controversial whether all cases with t(9;11)(p21.3;q23.3), t(6;9) (p23;q34.1), inv(3)(q21.3q26.2), t(3;3) (q21.3;q26.2), or t(1;22)(p13.3;q13.1) as well as AML with the BCR-ABL1 fusion should be categorized as AML when the blast cell count is < 20%. Therapy-related myeloid neoplasms may also have the balanced translocations and inversions described in this section, but these should be diagnosed as therapy-related myeloid neoplasms, with the associated genetic abnormality noted.

Acute myeloid leukaemia with gene mutations

It is now understood that, in addition to translocations and inversions, gene mutations are also common in AML {9,545, 1074,3095,3651}. The Cancer Genome Atlas (TCGA) Research Network evalua-

tion of 200 AML cases found an average of 13 mutations per case of AML, with at least 23 recurrent mutations identified {545}. These discoveries and others have identified at least eight distinct categories of mutations in AML, which are discussed in more detail in Chapter 1 (Introduction and overview of the classification of the myeloid neoplasms, p. 15). The current WHO classification recognizes AML with mutated NPM1 and AML with biallelic mutation of CEBPA as specific AML classification categories (entities), and AML with mutated RUNX1 as a provisional entity. However, many other mutations also occur in AML, and some that have prognostic significance, such as FLT3 internal tandem duplication (FLT3-ITD) and KIT mutations, may be mutated in specific AML types.

Next-generation sequencing panels are now available to screen for a large number of mutations in AML. Table 8.02 (p. 146) summarizes the more common gene mutations in AML. It is beyond the scope of this classification to discuss each prognostically significant mutation in AML individually, and the significance of some mutations is still unclear. Some combinations of gene mutations (e.g. NPM1 mutation and FLT3-ITD in normal-karyotype AML) appear to cluster within certain disease categories {9,545}; the prognostic significance of these mutations and combinations of mutations is discussed within the various sections throughout this volume.

Acute myeloid leukaemia with t(8;21)(q22;q22.1); RUNX1-RUNX1T1

Definition

Acute myeloid leukaemia (AML) with t(8;21)(q22;q22.1) resulting in RUNX1-RUNX1T1 is an AML showing predominantly neutrophilic maturation. The bone marrow and peripheral blood show large myeloblasts with abundant basophilic cytoplasm, often containing azurophilic granules. This type of AML is associated

with a high rate of complete remission and favourable long-term outcome.

ICD-O code   9896/3

Synonyms

Acute myeloid leukaemia, t(8;21) (q22;q22); acute myeloid leukaemia, AML1(CBF-alpha)/ETO; acute myeloid leukaemia with t(8;21)(q22;q22), RUNX1-RUNX1T1

Epidemiology

The t(8;21)(q22;q22.1) is found in 1–5% of cases of AML, usually in younger patients and in cases with features of AML with granulocytic maturation.

Clinical features

Tumour manifestations, such as myeloid sarcoma, may be present at presentation. In such cases the initial bone marrow aspiration may show a low number of blast cells.

Microscopy

The common morphological features include the presence of large blasts with abundant basophilic cytoplasm, often containing numerous azurophilic granules and perinuclear clearing (hofs). In many cases, a few blasts show very large granules (pseudo–Chédiak–Higashi granules), suggesting abnormal fusion. Auer rods are frequently found and appear as a single long and sharp rod with tapered ends; they may be detected in mature neutrophils. In addition to the large blast cells, some smaller blasts, predominantly in the peripheral blood, may be found. Promyelocytes, myelocytes, and mature neutrophils with variable dysplasia are present in the bone marrow. These cells may show abnormal nuclear segmentation (e.g. pseudo–Pelger–Huët nuclei) and/or cytoplasmic staining abnormalities, including homogeneous pink cytoplasm in neutrophils. However, dysplasia of other cell lines is uncommon; erythroblasts and megakaryocytes usually have normal morphology. A monocytic component is usually minimal or absent. Eosino-

Table 8.01 Chromosomal translocations with higher prevalence in paediatric acute myeloid leukaemia than in adult cases

Chromosomal translocations					
Translocation	Gene fusions	Frequency in children and adults, respectively	Age group predilection	Comments and Prognosis	References
t(1;22)(p13.3;q13.1)	RBM15-MKL1	0.8% 0%	Infants	Acute megakaryoblastic leukaemia (FAB M7) Intermediate	{2422,2637}
t(7;12)(q36.3;p13.2)	MNX1-ETV6	0.8% <0.5%	Infants	Gain of chromosome 19 considered secondary abnormality Adverse	{364A,1559,1641A, 4208A}
t(8;16)(p11.2;p13.3)	KAT6A-CREBBP	0.5% <0.5%	Infants and children	Can spontaneously remit in infancy Intermediate prognosis in later childhood	{776A}
t(6;9)(p23;q34.1)	DEK-NUP214	1.7% 1%	Older children; rare in infants	Adverse 65% with FLT3-ITD	{3502A,3905}
11q23.3	KMT2A translocated	25% 5–10%	Infants (50%)	Prognosis dependent on the partner gene	{1177A,2104A}
t(9;11)(p21.3;q23.3)	KMT2A-MLLT3	9.5% 2%	Children	Intermediate	{239C}
t(10;11)(p12;q23.3)	KMT2A-MLLT10	3.5% 1%	Children	Includes subtle and cryptic KMT2A rearrangements Adverse	{239C}
t(6;11)(q27;q23.3)	KMT2A-AFDN	2% <0.5%	Children	Adverse	{239C}
t(1;11)(q21;q23.3)	KMT2A-MLLT11	1% <0.5%	Children	Favourable	{239C}
Cryptic chromosomal translocations					
t(5;11)(q35.3;p15.5)	NUP98-NSD1	7% 3% (16% of FLT3-ITD cases)	Older children and young adults	Adverse 80% with FLT3-ITD In combination associated with induction failure	{908A,1668A,3002A}
inv(16)(p13.3q24.3)	CBFA2T3-GLIS2	3% 0%	Infants (10%) FAB M7 (20%)	Adverse	{1477A,2538A,3585A}
t(11;12)(p15.5;p13.5)	NUP98-KDM5A	3% 0%	Children aged <5 years AML, NOS, acute megakaryoblastic leukaemia (10%)	Intermediate	{908A,3905A}

FAB, French–American–British classification; FLT3-ITD, FLT3 internal tandem duplication.
Data tabulated by Betsy Hirsch, Susana Raimondi, Soheil Meschinchi, Nyla Heerema and Andrew J. Carroll.

phil precursors are frequently increased, but they do not exhibit the cytological or cytochemical abnormalities characteristic of AML with inv(16)(p13.1q22) or t(16;16)(p13.1;q22); basophils and/or mast cells are sometimes present in excess. Concurrent systemic mastocytosis is reported in some cases; mast cell infiltrates may be masked by the acute leukaemia infiltration of the bone marrow at diagnosis {1868}. Rare cases with a bone marrow blast percentage <20% occur; these should be classified as AML rather than myelodysplastic syndrome.

Immunophenotype

Most cases of AML with t(8;21) display a characteristic immunophenotype, with a subpopulation of blast cells showing high-intensity expression of CD34, HLA-DR, MPO, and CD13, but relatively weak expression of CD33 {2002,3224}. There

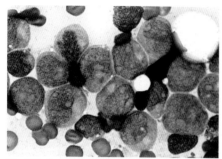

Fig. 8.01 Acute myeloid leukaemia with t(8;21) (q22;q22.1). Bone marrow blasts showing abundant granular cytoplasm with perinuclear clearing and large orange-pink granules/globules in some blasts.

are usually signs of neutrophilic differentiation, with subpopulations of cells showing neutrophilic maturation demonstrated by CD15 and/or CD65 expression. Populations of blasts showing maturation asynchrony (e.g. coexpressing CD34 and CD15) are sometimes present. These leukaemias frequently express the lymphoid markers CD19 and PAX5, and may express cytoplasmic CD79a {1738, 2034,3996}. In t(8;21) AML, PAX5 is not directly activated by RUNX1-RUNX1T1, but expression requires constitutive MAPK signalling {3322}. Some cases are TdT-positive, but TdT expression is generally weak. CD56 is expressed in a fraction of cases and may have adverse prognostic significance {221,1777}. The adverse prognostic significance of CD56 may be due to higher CD56 expression in cases with *KIT* mutations {894}.

Postulated normal counterpart

A haematopoietic progenitor cell with the potential to differentiate along granulocytic and monocytic lineages

Genetic profile

The genes for both heterodimeric components of core-binding factor (CBF), *RUNX1* (also called *AML1* and *CBFA*) and *CBFB*, are involved in rearrangements associated with acute leukaemias {3746}. The t(8;21)(q22;q22.1) involves *RUNX1*, which encodes the alpha subunit of CBF, and *RUNX1T1* (*ETO*) {1032,2321, 3149}. The *RUNX1-RUNX1T1* fusion transcript is consistently detected in patients with t(8;21)(q22;q22.1) AML. The CBF transcription factor is essential for haematopoiesis; transformation by *RUNX1-RUNX1T1* likely results from transcriptional repression of normal *RUNX1* target genes via aberrant recruitment of nuclear transcriptional co-repressor complexes.

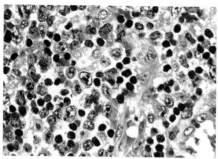

Fig. 8.02 Myeloid sarcoma with t(8;21)(q22;q22.1). Biopsy of an orbital mass from a child with acute myeloid leukaemia with t(8;21)(q22;q22.1); eosinophil precursors are scattered within the predominant blast population.

More than 70% of cases show additional chromosome abnormalities, such as loss of a sex chromosome or del(9q) with loss of 9q22. *KIT* mutations occur in 20–30% of cases {3078}. Secondary cooperating mutations of *KRAS* or *NRAS* are common, occurring in 30% of paediatric and 10–20% of adult CBF-associated leukaemias {1392,3077}. *ASXL1* mutations occur in approximately 10% of patients, mostly adults; *ASXL2* mutations occur in 20–25% of patients of all ages {2657}.

Prognosis and predictive factors

AML with t(8;21)(q22;q22.1) is usually associated with a high rate of complete remission and long-term disease-free survival when treated with intensive consolidation therapy (e.g. high-dose cytarabine) {393,1466}. Some factors appear to adversely affect prognosis, including the presence of *KIT* mutations in adults and CD56 expression {221,3078}. Therapeutic trials investigating mutant *KIT* in this AML type are under way.

Acute myeloid leukaemia with inv(16)(p13.1q22) or t(16;16) (p13.1;q22); CBFB-MYH11

Definition

Acute myeloid leukaemia (AML) with inv(16)(p13.1q22) or t(16;16)(p13.1;q22) resulting in *CBFB-MYH11* is an AML that usually shows monocytic and granulocytic differentiation and characteristically an abnormal eosinophil component in the bone marrow {2236,2513,3746}.

ICD-O code   9871/3

Synonyms

Acute myeloid leukaemia, t(16;16) (p13;q11); acute myeloid leukaemia,

CBF-beta/MYH11; acute myelomonocytic leukaemia with abnormal eosinophils; French–American–British (FAB) classification M4Eo; acute myeloid leukaemia, inv(16)(p13q22)

Epidemiology

Either inv(16)(p13.1q22) or t(16;16) (p13.1;q22) is found in 5–8% of younger patients with AML; the frequency is lower in older adults.

Clinical features

Myeloid sarcoma may be present at initial diagnosis or at relapse and may constitute the only evidence of relapse in some patients. The white blood cell count at diagnosis is significantly higher in AML with inv(16)(p13.1q22) or t(16;16) (p13.1;q22) than in cases with t(8;21) (q22;q22.1) {2502,3559}.

Microscopy

In AML with inv(16)(p13.1q22) or t(16;16) (p13.1;q22), in addition to the usual morphological features of acute myelomonocytic leukaemia, the bone marrow shows a variable number of eosinophils (usually increased, but sometimes <5%) at all stages of maturation, without significant maturation arrest. The most striking abnormalities involve the immature eosinophilic granules, mainly evident at the late promyelocyte and myelocyte stages. The abnormalities are usually not present at later stages of eosinophil maturation. The eosinophilic granules are often larger than those normally present in immature eosinophils, are purple-violet in colour, and in some cells are so dense that they obscure the cell morphology. The mature eosinophils occasionally show nuclear hyposegmentation. Auer rods may be observed in myeloblasts. Neutrophils in the bone marrow are usually sparse, with a decreased number of

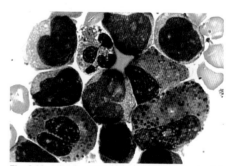

Fig. 8.03 Acute myeloid leukaemia with inv(16) (p13.1q22). Abnormal eosinophils, one with large basophilic coloured granules, are present.

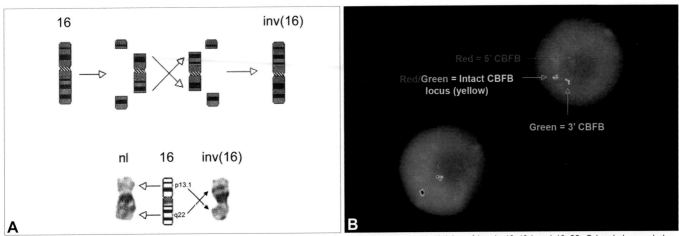

Fig. 8.04 Acute myeloid leukaemia with inv(16)(p13.1q22). **A** The inversion results from the breakage and rejoining of bands 16p13.1 and 16q22; G-banded normal chromosome 16 (nl) and inv(16) are shown. **B** Dual-colour *FISH*, with the 5' region of *CBFB* labelled in red and the 3' region in green; in a normal chromosome 16, the 5' and 3' regions are contiguous, resulting in a single yellow or overlapping red/green signals; the inv(16) splits the *CBFB* locus, resulting in separate red and green signals; both interphase cells have one normal chromosome 16 and one inv(16).

mature neutrophils. The peripheral blood is not different from that in other cases of acute myelomonocytic leukaemia; eosinophils are not usually increased, but an occasional case has been reported with abnormal and increased eosinophils in the peripheral blood. Most cases with inv(16)(p13.1q22) have abnormal eosinophils, but in some cases they are rare and difficult to find. Occasional cases with this genetic abnormality lack eosinophilia, show only granulocytic maturation without a monocytic component, or show only monocytic differentiation. In some cases, the blast percentage is at the 20% threshold or occasionally lower. Cases with inv(16)(p13.1q22) or t(16;16) (p13.1;q22) and <20% bone marrow blasts should be diagnosed as AML.

Cytochemistry
The naphthol AS-D chloroacetate esterase (CAE) reaction, which is normally negative in eosinophils, is characteristically faintly positive in the abnormal eosinophils. Such a reaction is not seen in eosinophils of AML with t(8;21)(q22;q22.1). At least 3% of the blasts show MPO reactivity. The monoblasts and promonocytes usually show non-specific esterase reactivity, although it may be weaker than expected or even absent in some cases.

Immunophenotype
Most of these leukaemias are characterized by a complex immunophenotype, with the presence of multiple blast populations: immature blasts with high CD34 and KIT (CD117) expression and populations differentiating towards the granulocytic lineage (positive for CD13, CD33, CD15, CD65, and MPO) and the monocytic lineage (positive for CD14, CD4, CD11b, CD11c, CD64, CD36, and lysozyme). Maturation asynchrony is often seen. Coexpression of CD2 with myeloid markers has been frequently documented, but it is not specific for this diagnosis.

Postulated normal counterpart
A haematopoietic progenitor cell with the potential to differentiate along granulocytic and monocytic lineages

Genetic profile
The inv(16)(p13.1q22) found in the vast majority of this subtype and the less common t(16;16)(p13.1;q22) both result in the fusion of *CBFB* at 16q22 to *MYH11* at 16p13.1 {3650}. *MYH11* codes for a smooth muscle myosin heavy chain {871}. *CBFB* codes for the beta subunit of core-binding factor (CBFB), a heterodimeric transcription factor known to bind the enhancers of the T-cell receptor, cytokine genes, and other genes. The CBFB subunit heterodimerizes with RUNX1 (*CBFA2*), the gene product of *RUNX1*, which is one of the genes involved in AML with t(8;21) (q22;q22.1). Occasionally, cytological features of AML with abnormal eosinophils may be present without karyotypic evidence of a chromosome 16 abnormality, but with *CBFB-MYH11* nevertheless demonstrated by molecular genetic studies {2775,3432}. By conventional cytogenetic analysis, inv(16)(p13.1q22) is a subtle rearrangement that may be overlooked when metaphase prepara-

tions are suboptimal. Therefore FISH and RT-PCR methods may be necessary at diagnosis to document the genetic alteration. Secondary cytogenetic abnormalities occur in approximately 40% of cases, with gains of chromosomes 22 and 8 (each occurring in 10–15% of cases), del(7q), and gain of chromosome 21 (in ~5% of cases) most commonly observed {2502}. Trisomy 22 is fairly specific for inv(16)(p13.1q22) cases, being rarely detected with other primary aberrations in AML, whereas gain of chromosome 8 is commonly seen in patients with other primary aberrations. Rare cases of AML and chronic myeloid leukaemia with both inv(16)(p13.1q22) and t(9;22) (q34.1;q11.2) have been reported, and this finding in chronic myeloid leukaemia is usually associated with the accelerated or blast phase of the disease {4379}. Secondary gene mutations are very common in this AML type; present in >90% of cases. Mutations of *KIT* (most commonly in exons 8 and 17) occur in 30–40% of cases {3078}. Mutations of *NRAS* (in 45% of cases), *KRAS* (in 13%), and *FLT3* (in 14%) have also been reported {3076}. *ASXL2* mutations, although common in AML with t(8;21), are uncommon in AML with inv(16) or t(16;16) {2657}.

Prognosis and predictive factors
Like AML with t(8;21)(q22;q22.1), AML with inv(16)(p13.1q22) or t(16;16) (p13.1;q22) is associated with a high rate of complete remission and favourable overall survival when treated with intensive consolidation therapy (e.g. high-dose cytarabine) {1466,2772}.

Adult patients with *KIT* mutations (in particular mutations involving exon 8) have a higher risk of relapse and worse survival {935,3078}, but the prognostic implications of *KIT* mutation in AML with inv(16) or t(16;16) do not appear to be as significant as in AML with t(8;21). Patients with gain of chromosome 22 as a secondary abnormality have been reported to have an improved outcome {2502,3559}. Older age, elevated white blood cell count, *FLT3* mutations (especially tyrosine kinase domain mutation, *FLT3*-TKD), and trisomy 8 are associated with a worse outcome {3076,3077}. Clinical therapeutic trials investigating mutant *KIT* and *FLT3* in this AML type are under way.

Acute promyelocytic leukaemia with PML-RARA

Definition
Acute promyelocytic leukaemia (APL) with *PML-RARA* is an acute myeloid leukaemia (AML) in which abnormal promyelocytes predominate. Both hypergranular (so-called typical) APL and microgranular (hypogranular) types exist.

ICD-O code   9866/3

Synonyms
Acute promyelocytic leukaemia, t(15;17)(q24.1;q21.2), *PML-RARA*; acute myeloid leukaemia, t(15;17)(q24.1;q21.1), *PML-RARA*; acute promyelocytic leukaemia, NOS; French–American–British (FAB) classification M3; acute myeloid leukaemia, *PML/RAR-alpha*; acute promyelocytic leukaemia, *PML-RAR-alpha*

Epidemiology
APL accounts for 5–8% of AML cases in younger patients, with a lower relative frequency in elderly patients {3766}. The disease can occur at any age, but most patients are middle-aged adults. The annual incidence rate is 0.08 cases per 100 000 population {3113}.

Clinical features
Both hypergranular and microgranular APL are frequently associated with disseminated intravascular coagulation and increased fibrinolysis {454,3519}. Coagulopathy is associated with significant early death rates in APL patients {3282}. In microgranular APL, unlike hypergranular APL, the leukocyte count is very high, with a short doubling time.

Microscopy
The nuclear size and shape in the abnormal promyelocytes of hypergranular APL are irregular and greatly variable; the abnormal promyelocyte nuclei are often kidney-shaped or bilobed. The cytoplasm is marked by densely packed or even coalescent large granules, staining bright pink, red, or purple on Romanowsky staining. The cytoplasmic granules may be so large and/or numerous that they totally obscure the nuclear–cytoplasmic margin. In some cells, the cytoplasm is filled with fine dust-like granules. Characteristic cells containing bundles of Auer rods randomly distributed within the cytoplasm are present in most cases. Myeloblasts with single Auer rods may also be observed. Auer rods in hypergranular APL are usually larger than those in other types of AML, and they may have a characteristic morphology at the ultrastructural level, with a hexagonal arrangement of tubular structures with a specific periodicity of approximately 250 nm, in contrast to the 6–20 laminar periodicity of Auer rods in other types of AML. Only occasional obvious leukaemic promyelocytes may be observed in the peripheral blood, especially in hypergranular APL, in which the white blood cell count is often very low.

Cases of microgranular (hypogranular) APL are characterized by distinct morphological features such as an apparent paucity or absence of granules, and predominantly bilobed nuclei {1397}. The hypogranular appearance of the cytoplasm is due to the submicroscopic size of the azurophilic granules. This may cause confusion with acute monocytic leukaemia on Romanowsky-stained preparations; however, a small number of abnormal promyelocytes with clearly visible granules and/or bundles of Auer rods can be identified in many cases. The leukocyte count is frequently markedly elevated in the microgranular variant of APL, with numerous abnormal microgranular promyelocytes, in contrast to hypergranular APL. Abnormal promyelocytes with deeply basophilic cytoplasm have been described mainly in the relapse phase in patients who have been previously treated with tretinoin. The bone marrow is usually hypercellular. The abnormal promyelocytes have relatively abundant cytoplasm with numerous granules; occasionally, Auer rods may be identified in well-prepared specimens. The nuclei are often convoluted.

Cytochemistry
The MPO reaction is always strongly positive in all the leukaemic promyelocytes, with the reaction product covering the entire cytoplasm and often the nucleus. The non-specific esterase reaction is weakly positive in approximately 25% of cases. In cases of microgranular (hypogranular) APL, the MPO reaction is strongly positive in the leukaemic cells, contrasting with the weak or negative reaction in monocytes.

Immunophenotype
APL with *PML-RARA* (hypergranular variant) is characterized by low or absent expression of HLA-DR, CD34, and the leukocyte integrins CD11a, CD11b, and CD18. It shows homogeneous bright expression of CD33 and heterogeneous expression of CD13. Most cases show expression of KIT (CD117), although this is sometimes weak. The granulocytic dif-

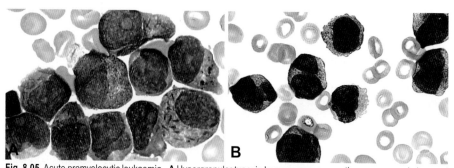

Fig. 8.05 Acute promyelocytic leukaemia. **A** Hypergranular type; in bone marrow smear, there are several abnormal promyelocytes, with intense azurophilic granulation; bundles of numerous Auer rods are seen in some of the promyelocytes. **B** Microgranular variant; in peripheral blood smear, there are several abnormal promyelocytes with lobed, almost cerebriform nuclei; the cytoplasm contains numerous small azurophilic granules; other cells appear sparsely granular.

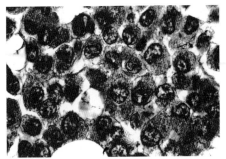

Fig. 8.06 Acute promyelocytic leukaemia. Bone marrow biopsy shows abnormal promyelocytes with abundant hypergranulated cytoplasm; the nuclei are generally round to oval; several of the nuclei are irregular and invaginated.

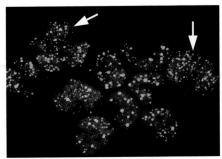

Fig. 8.07 Acute promyelocytic leukaemia. PML antibody shows a characteristic nuclear multigranular pattern with nucleolar exclusion.

ferentiation markers CD15 and CD65 are negative or only weakly expressed {3028, 4490}, and CD64 expression is common. In cases with microgranular morphology or the bcr3 transcript of the *PML-RARA* fusion gene, there is frequently expression of CD34 and CD2 by at least some cells {1123}. CD11c can also be expressed in some cells. CD2 expression in APL has been associated with *FLT3*-ITD {3881}. Expression of CD11b and CD11c can be upregulated after tretinoin treatment {1687}. Approximately 10% of APL cases express CD56, which has been associated with a worse outcome {451,2704}. On immunocytochemistry, antibodies against the PML gene product show a characteristic nuclear multigranular pattern with nucleolar exclusion, in contrast to the speckled, relatively large nuclear bodies seen in normal promyelocytes or the blasts in other types of AML {1142}.

Postulated normal counterpart

A myeloid progenitor cell with the poten-tial to differentiate along a granulocytic lineage

Genetic profile

The sensitivity of APL cells to tretinoin (also called all-trans retinoic acid) has led to the discovery that the *RARA* gene on 17q21.2 fuses with a nuclear regula-tory factor gene on 15q24.1 (*PML*), giving rise to a *PML-RARA* fusion gene product {871,911,2618}. Rare cases of APL lack-ing the classic t(15;17)(q24.1;q21.2) on routine cytogenetic studies have been described with complex variant trans-locations involving chromosomes 15 and 17, with an additional chromosome or with submicroscopic insertion of *RARA* into *PML* leading to the expres-sion of the *PML-RARA* transcript; the cases with submicroscopic insertion of *RARA* into *PML* are considered to have cryptic or masked t(15;17)(q24.1;q21.2) and are included in the category of AML/ APL with *PML-RARA*. Morphological analysis shows no differences between the t(15;17)(q24.1;q21.2)-positive group and *PML-RARA*–positive cases without t(15;17)(q24.1;q21.2). Secondary cytoge-netic abnormalities are noted in about 40% of cases, with gain of chromo-some 8 being the most frequent (present in 10–15% of cases). Mutations involving *FLT3*, including *FLT3*-ITD and *FLT3* tyros-ine kinase domain (*FLT3*-TKD) mutation, occur in 30–40% of APL. *FLT3*-ITD muta-tions are most common and are associ-ated with a higher white blood cell count, microgranular morphology, and involve-ment of the bcr3 breakpoint of PML {451, 529}.

Variant RARA translocations in acute leukaemia

A subset of cases, often with morpho-logical features resembling those of APL, show variant translocations involving *RARA*. The variant fusion partners in-clude *ZBTB16* (previously called *PLZF*) at 11q23.2, *NUMA1* at 11q13.4, *NPM1* at 5q35.1, and *STAT5B* at 17q21.2 {4464}. Some cases with variant translocations were initially reported as having APL morphology {3482}. However, the sub-group of cases with t(11;17)(q23.2;q21.2) resulting in *ZBTB16-RARA* shows some morphological differences, with a pre-dominance of cells with regular nuclei, many granules, usually an absence of Auer rods, an increased number of pel-geroid neutrophils, and strong MPO ac-tivity {3482}. The initial cases of APL as-sociated with t(5;17)(q35.1;q21.2) had a predominant population of hypergranular promyelocytes and a minor population of hypogranular promyelocytes; Auer rods

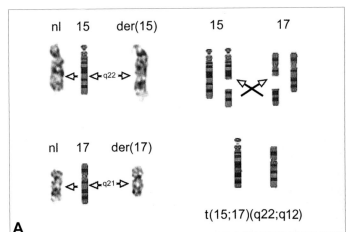

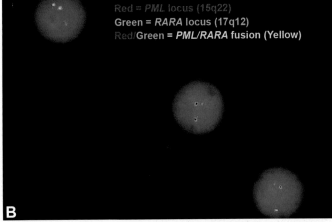

Red = *PML* locus (15q22)
Green = *RARA* locus (17q12)
Red/Green = *PML/RARA* fusion (Yellow)

t(15;17)(q22;q12)

Fig. 8.08 Acute promyelocytic leukaemia with t(15;17)(q24.1;q21.2). **A** The translocation results from the breakage and rejoining of bands 15q22 and 17q12; G-banded normal (nl) chromosomes 15 and 17 and the derivatives der(15) and der(17) are shown. **B** Dual-colour FISH with probes for *PML* (15q22) and *RARA* (17q12) demonstrates the presence of a *PML-RARA* fusion resulting from the 15;17 translocation; each of the three interphase cells has a separate red (*PML*) signal, a separate green (*RARA*) signal, and a yellow or overlapping red/green signal, consistent with the presence of *PML-RARA* fusion.

were not identified by light microscopy {812}. Some APL variants, including those with *ZBTB16-RARA* and *STAT5B-RARA* fusions, are resistant to tretinoin {2618}. APL with t(5;17)(q35.1;q21.2) appears to respond to tretinoin {2618}. Cases with these variant translocations should be diagnosed as APL with a variant *RARA* translocation.

Prognosis and predictive factors
APL has a particular sensitivity to treatment with tretinoin and arsenic trioxide, which act as differentiating agents {574, 3641,3885}. The prognosis for APL treated optimally with tretinoin and an anthracycline was more favourable than that for any other AML cytogenetic subtype. More recently, however, the combination of tretinoin and arsenic trioxide therapy has become the standard therapeutic approach for most patients with an excellent outcome, with anthracycline added for high-risk patients {505,1116,2376}. Previously reported adverse prognostic factors include hyperleukocytosis, CD56 expression, *FLT3*-ITD mutation, and older patient age {451,879,2704,3113}, but the significance of these features with current therapy is unclear.

Acute myeloid leukaemia with t(9;11)(p21.3;q23.3); KMT2A-MLLT3

Definition
Acute myeloid leukaemia (AML) with t(9;11)(p21.3;q23.3) resulting in *KMT2A-MLLT3* fusion is usually associated with monocytic features.

ICD-O code   9897/3

Synonym
Acute myeloid leukaemia with t(9;11)(p22;q23) resulting in *KMT2A-MLLT3*

Epidemiology
The t(9;11)(p21.3;q23.3) can occur at any age, but is more common in children; it is present in 9–12% of paediatric and 2% of adult AML cases {511,1236}.

Clinical features
Patients may present with disseminated intravascular coagulation. They may have extramedullary myeloid sarcoma and/or tissue infiltration (gingiva, skin).

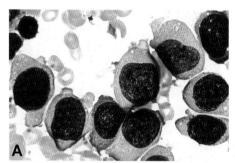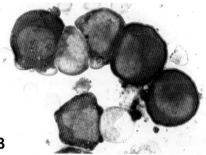

Fig. 8.09 Acute myeloid leukaemia (monoblastic) with t(9;11)(p21.3;q23.3). **A** Bone marrow smear shows several monoblasts, some with very abundant cytoplasm; fine MPO-negative azurophilic granules are present. **B** Non-specific esterase reaction shows intensely positive monoblasts.

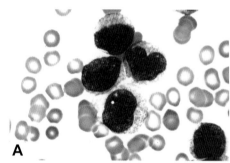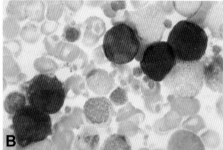

Fig. 8.10 Acute myeloid leukaemia (monocytic) with t(9;11)(p21.3;q23.3). **A** Bone marrow smear shows several monoblasts and promonocytes with very pale cytoplasm containing numerous fine azurophilic granules; the promonocytes have delicate nuclear folds. **B** Non-specific esterase staining shows that the promonocytes are intensely reactive.

Microscopy
Cytochemistry
Monoblasts and promonocytes usually show strongly positive non-specific esterase reactions. The monoblasts often lack MPO reactivity.

Immunophenotype
Cases of AML with t(9;11)(p21.3;q23.3) in children are associated with strong expression of CD33, CD65, CD4, and HLA-DR, whereas expression of CD13, CD34, and CD14 is usually low {837}. Most AML cases with 11q23.3 abnormalities express the NG2 homologue encoded by *CSPG4*, a chondroitin sulfate molecule reacting with the anti-7.1 monoclonal antibody {4380}. Most adult AML cases with 11q23.3 abnormalities express some markers of monocytic differentiation, including CD14, CD4, CD11b, CD11c, CD64, CD36, and lysozyme, whereas variable expression of markers of immaturity, such as CD34, KIT (CD117), and CD56 has been reported {2783}.

Postulated normal counterpart
A haematopoietic progenitor cell of probable haematopoietic stem cell or granulocyte–macrophage progenitor origin {2120}

Genetic profile
Molecular studies have identified a human homologue of the Drosophila trithorax gene designated *KMT2A* (previously called *MLL* and *HRX*) that results in a fusion gene in translocations involving 11q23.3 {203}. The KMT2A protein is a histone methyltransferase that assembles in protein complexes that regulate gene transcription via chromatin remodelling. The t(9;11)(p21.3;q23.3), involving *MLLT3* (AF9), is the most common *KMT2A* translocation in AML and appears to define a distinct entity. Secondary cytogenetic abnormalities are common with t(9;11)(p21.3;q23.3), with gain of chromosome 8 most frequently observed (usually *MECOM*-negative), but do not appear to influence survival {511,2773}. Overexpression of *MECOM* (also called *EVI1*) is reported in 40% of cases of AML with t(9;11) {1482}. There is evidence that *MECOM*-positive *KMT2A*-rearranged AMLs differ genetically, molecularly, morphologically, and immunophenotypically from *MECOM*-negative *KMT2A*-rearranged leukaemias {381,1482}.

Variant KMT2A translocations in acute leukaemia

More than 120 different translocations involving *KMT2A* (previously called *MLL*) have been described in adult and paediatric acute leukaemia, with 79 translocation partner genes now characterized {2651, 3653}. Translocations involving *AFF1* (*MLLT2*, *AF4*), resulting predominantly in lymphoblastic leukaemia, and *MLLT3* (*AF9*), resulting predominantly in AML, are the most common. Other *KMT2A* translocations that commonly result in AML have *MLLT1* (*ENL*), *MLLT10* (*AF10*), *AFDN* (*MLLT4*, *AF6*), or *ELL* as partner genes. Other than the *KMT2A-ELL* fusion resulting from t(11;19)(q23.3;p13.1), which is strongly associated with AML, these fusions occur predominantly in AML but can also be seen in lymphoblastic leukaemia. Some *KMT2A* translocations in AML are subtle; FISH or other molecular studies may be necessary to identify these variant translocations {3653}. *MECOM* overexpression is common in this group of AMLs, with the highest expression associated with an *AFDN* (*MLLT4*) translocation {1482}. AML cases with these fusions usually have myelomonocytic or monoblastic morphological and immunophenotypic features. In the past, all of these translocations were encompassed by the category of AML with 11q23.3 abnormalities, but the diagnosis should now include the specific abnormality and should be limited to cases of *de novo* AML and with 11q23.3 balanced translocations involving *KMT2A*. For example, a case of AML with *KMT2A-MLLT1* fusion should be diagnosed as AML with t(11;19)(q23.3;p13.3).

AML that is associated with prior therapy and has a *KMT2A* translocation, such as t(2;11)(p21;q23.3), should be classified as therapy-related myeloid neoplasm with *KMT2A* rearrangement. Similarly, AML with myelodysplasia-related changes and a *KMT2A* translocation, such as t(11;16)(q23.3;p13.3), should be diagnosed as AML with myelodysplasia-related changes.

Prognosis and predictive factors

AML with t(9;11)(p21.3;q23.3) has an intermediate survival, superior to that of AML with other 11q23.3 translocations {2773,3448}. Overexpression of *MECOM* has been reported to be associated with a poor prognosis {1482}. Cases with t(9;11) and <20% blasts are not currently

classified as AML (although this is controversial), but they may be treated as such if clinically appropriate.

Acute myeloid leukaemia with t(6;9)(p23;q34.1); DEK-NUP214

Definition

Acute myeloid leukaemia (AML) with t(6;9)(p23;q34.1) resulting in *DEK-NUP214* is an AML with ≥20% peripheral blood or bone marrow blasts with or without monocytic features. It is often associated with basophilia and multilineage dysplasia {3116,3700}.

ICD-O code   9865/3

Epidemiology

The t(6;9)(p23;q34.1) is detected in 0.7–1.8% of AML cases, and occurs in both children and adults, with a median patient age of 13 years in childhood and 35–44 years in studies of younger adults {511,1464,3700,3701,3905}.

Clinical features

AML with t(6;9)(p23;q34.1) usually presents with anaemia and thrombocytopenia, and often with pancytopenia. In adults, the presenting white blood cell count is generally lower than in other AML types, with a median white blood cell count of 12 × 10⁹/L {3700}.

Microscopy

The bone marrow blasts of AML with t(6;9)(p23;q34.1) may have morphological and cytochemical features similar to those of many subtypes of AML (other than acute promyelocytic leukaemia and acute megakaryoblastic leukaemia), most commonly AML with maturation and acute myelomonocytic leukaemia {76, 3020,3700}. Auer rods are present in approximately one third of cases. Therefore, there are no features specific to the blast cell population in this entity. Marrow and peripheral blood basophilia, defined as ≥2% basophils, is generally uncommon in AML, but is seen in 44–62% of cases of AML with t(6;9)(p23;q34.1). Most cases show evidence of granulocytic and erythroid dysplasia. Ring sideroblasts are present in some cases.

Cytochemistry

Blasts are positive for MPO and can

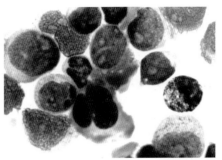

Fig. 8.11 Acute myeloid leukaemia with t(6;9)(p23;q34.1). The blasts are admixed with dysplastic erythroid precursors and scattered basophils (centre, right).

be positive or negative for non-specific esterase.

Immunophenotype

The blasts have a non-specific myeloid immunophenotype, with consistent expression of MPO, CD9, CD13, CD33, CD38, CD123, and HLA-DR {76,707, 2191,3020,3700}. Most cases also express KIT (CD117), CD34, and CD15; some cases express the monocyte-associated marker CD64; and approximately half are TdT-positive. Other lymphoid antigen expression is uncommon. Basophils can be seen as separate clusters of cells positive for CD123, CD33, and CD38 but negative for HLA-DR.

Postulated normal counterpart

A haematopoietic progenitor cell with multilineage potential

Genetic profile

The t(6;9)(p23;q34.1) results in a fusion of *DEK* on chromosome 6 with *NUP214* (also called *CAN*) on chromosome 9. The resulting nucleoporin fusion protein acts as an aberrant transcription factor and alters nuclear transport by binding to soluble transport factors {3544}. The t(6;9) is the sole clonal karyotypic abnormality in the vast majority of cases, but some patients have t(6;9)(p23;q34.1) in association with a complex karyotype {3700}. *FLT3*-ITD mutations are very common in AML with t(6;9)(p23;q34.1), occurring in 69% of paediatric and 78% of adult cases {3020,3700,3905}. *FLT3*-TKD mutation appears to be uncommon in this entity.

Prognosis and predictive factors

In both adults and children, AML with t(6;9)(p23;q34.1) has a generally poor prognosis. Elevated white blood cell counts are most predictive of shorter overall survival, and increased bone marrow blasts are associated with shorter disease-free survival. The limited data suggest that allogeneic haematopoietic stem cell transplantation may be associated with better overall survival versus no stem cell transplantation {3700}. Despite the high frequency of *FLT3*-ITD, this genetic event does not appear to negatively impact survival in paediatric patients {3905}. Cases with t(6;9)(p23;q34.1) and < 20% blasts are not currently classified as AML (although this is controversial), but they may be treated as such if clinically appropriate. Given the very high frequency of *FLT3*-ITD, patients may benefit from therapy with FLT3 inhibitors.

Acute myeloid leukaemia with inv(3)(q21.3q26.2) or t(3;3)(q21.3;q26.2); GATA2, MECOM

Definition

Acute myeloid leukaemia (AML) with inv(3)(q21.3q26.2) or t(3;3)(q21.3;q26.2) resulting in deregulated *MECOM* (also called *EVI1*) and *GATA2* expression is an AML with ≥ 20% peripheral blood or bone marrow blasts. It is often associated with normal or elevated platelet counts and has increased dysplastic megakaryocytes with unilobed or bilobed nuclei and multilineage dysplasia in the bone marrow {386,3608,3844}.

ICD-O code   9869/3

Epidemiology

AML with inv(3)(q21.3q26.2) or t(3;3) (q21.3;q26.2) accounts for 1–2% of all AML {511,3701}. It occurs most commonly in adults, with no sex predilection.

Clinical features

Patients most commonly present with anaemia and a normal platelet count, but marked thrombocythaemia occurs in 7–22% of cases {1462,3608}. Some patients present with hepatosplenomegaly, but lymphadenopathy is uncommon {3608,3644,3948}.

Microscopy

Peripheral blood changes may include hypogranular neutrophils with a pseudo–Pelger–Huët anomaly, with or without associated peripheral blasts. Red blood cell

abnormalities are usually mild, without teardrop cells. Giant and hypogranular platelets are common, and bare megakaryocyte nuclei may be present {386}. The bone marrow blasts of AML with inv(3)(q21.3q26.2) or t(3;3)(q21.3;q26.2) have variable morphological and cytochemical features; the morphologies of AML without maturation, acute myelomonocytic leukaemia, and acute megakaryoblastic leukaemia are most common {1228,3608}. Multilineage dysplasia of non-blast bone marrow elements is a frequent finding, with dysplastic megakaryocytes being most common {1228,1852, 3608}. Megakaryocytes may be normal or increased in number with many small non-lobated or bilobed forms, but other dysplastic megakaryocytic forms may also occur. Dysplasia of maturing erythroid cells and neutrophils is also common. Marrow eosinophils, basophils, and/or mast cells may be increased. The bone marrow biopsy shows increased small non-lobated or bilobed megakaryocytes and sometimes other dysplastic forms. Bone marrow cellularity is variable, with some cases presenting as hypocellular AML. Marrow fibrosis is also variable.

Immunophenotype

Flow cytometry studies show blasts that are positive for CD34, CD33, CD13, KIT (CD117), and HLA-DR; most are CD38-positive, with aberrant CD7 expression frequently observed {2606}. High CD34 expression is more common with inv(3) than with t(3;3) {3323}. A subset of cases may express megakaryocytic markers such as CD41 and CD61. Aberrant expression of lymphoid markers other than CD7 appears to be uncommon {3644}.

Postulated normal counterpart

A haematopoietic progenitor cell with multilineage potential

Genetic profile

A variety of abnormalities of the long arm of chromosome 3 occur in myeloid malignancies, with inv(3)(q21.3q26.2) and t(3;3)(q21.3;q26.2) being the most common {2410}. The abnormalities involve the oncogene *MECOM* at 3q26.2. The inv(3) or t(3;3) repositions a distal *GATA2* enhancer to activate *MECOM* expression, and simultaneously confers *GATA2* haploinsufficiency {1480,4413}. *MECOM* overexpression is not limited to leukaemias with inv(3)(q21.3q26.2)

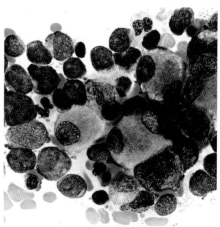

Fig. 8.12 Acute myeloid leukaemia with inv(3) (q21.3q26.2). Bone marrow aspirate shows increased blasts and atypical, non-lobated megakaryocytes.

or t(3;3)(q21.3;q26.2) {2186}. Other cytogenetic aberrations involving 3q26.2, such as t(3;21)(q26.2;q22.1), resulting in a *MECOM-RUNX1* fusion and usually seen in therapy-related disease, are not included in this disease category.

Secondary karyotypic abnormalities are common with inv(3)(q21.3q26.2) and t(3;3)(q21.3;q26.2); monosomy 7 is most frequent, occurring in more than half of all cases, followed by 5q deletions and complex karyotypes {2410,3608}. Secondary gene mutations are found in virtually all cases of AML with inv(3) or t(3;3). Mutations of genes activating RAS/receptor tyrosine kinase signalling pathways are reported in 98% of cases, with the most common of these mutations affecting *NRAS* (mutated in 27% of cases), *PTPN11* (in 20%), *FLT3* (in 13%), *KRAS* (in 11%), *NF1* (in 9%), *CBL* (in 7%), and *KIT* (in 2%). Other commonly mutated genes are *GATA2* (mutated in 15% of cases), *RUNX1* (in 12%), and *SF3B1* (in 27%, often with *GATA2*) {1481,2907}.

Patients with *BCR-ABL1*–positive chronic myeloid leukaemia may acquire inv(3) (q21.3q26.2) or t(3;3)(q21.3;q26.2), and such a finding indicates an accelerated or blast phase of disease. Cases with both t(9;22)(q34.1;q11.2) and inv(3) (q21.3q26.2) or t(3;3)(q21.3;q26.2) at presentation are best considered an aggressive phase of chronic myeloid leukaemia, rather than AML with inv(3) or t(3;3).

Prognosis and predictive factors

AML with inv(3)(q21.3q26.2) or t(3;3) (q21.3;q26.2) is an aggressive disease with short survival {1228,2410,3338, 3392,3608}. The outcomes for patients with <20% or ≥20% blasts are similarly poor. Cases with inv(3)(q21.3q26.2) or t(3;3)(q21.3;q26.2) and <20% blasts are not currently classified as AML (although this is controversial), but they may be treated as such if clinically appropriate. Complex karyotype and additional monosomy 7, regardless of blast percentage, are associated with an even worse prognosis in this already poor-prognosis disease {2410,3392}.

Acute myeloid leukaemia (megakaryoblastic) with t(1;22) (p13.3;q13.1); RBM15-MKL1

Definition
Acute myeloid leukaemia (AML) with t(1;22)(p13.3;q13.1) resulting in *RBM15-MKL1* fusion is an AML generally showing maturation in the megakaryocyte lineage.

ICD-O code
9911/3

Epidemiology
The t(1;22)(p13.3;q13.1) is an uncommon abnormality in AML, occurring in <1% of all cases. It occurs most commonly in infants without trisomy 21 (Down syndrome), with a female predominance. Some cases are congenital {232}.

Clinical features
Most of the balanced translocations and inversions discussed in this chapter are more common in adult AML than in paediatric cases. However, AML with t(1;22) (p13.3;q13.1) is a *de novo* AML restricted to infants and young children (aged ≤ 3 years), with most cases occurring in the first 6 months of life (median patient age: 4 months). The vast majority of cases present with marked organomegaly, most commonly hepatosplenomegaly. Patients also have anaemia and usually have thrombocytopenia and a moderately elevated white blood cell count.

Microscopy
The peripheral blood and bone marrow blasts of AML with t(1;22)(p13.3;q13.1) are similar to those of acute megakaryoblastic leukaemia (one of the subtypes of AML, NOS). Small and large megakaryoblasts may be present and they may be admixed with more morphologically undifferentiated blast cells with a high N:C ratio, resembling lymphoblasts. The megakaryoblasts are usually

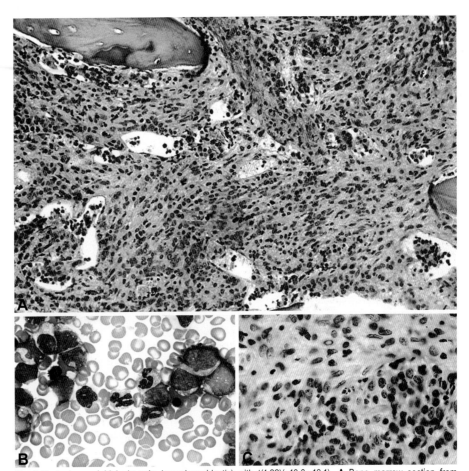

Fig. 8.13 Acute myeloid leukaemia (megakaryoblastic) with t(1;22)(p13.3;q13.1). **A** Bone marrow section from a 3.5-month-old child shows extensive replacement of marrow by blast cells in areas arranged into clusters and aggregates surrounded by fibrotic stroma. **B** Bone marrow smear contains a heteromorphic population of blasts. **C** High magnification of the specimen shows blasts without differentiating features.

medium-sized to large blasts (12–18 µm) with a round, slightly irregular, or indented nucleus with fine reticular chromatin and 1–3 nucleoli. The cytoplasm is basophilic, often agranular, and may show distinct blebs or pseudopod formation. Micromegakaryocytes are common, but dysplastic features of granulocytic and erythroid cells are not usually present.

The bone marrow is usually normocellular to hypercellular, with reticulin and collagenous fibrosis usually present. Due to the often dense fibrosis, the pattern of bone marrow infiltration may mimic that of a metastatic tumour {357,567}. The presence of fibrosis may cause difficulties in establishing the presence of ≥20% blast cells in the bone marrow based on the aspirate; correlation with bone marrow biopsy findings may be crucial.

Cytochemistry
Cytochemical staining for Sudan Black B and MPO is consistently negative in the megakaryoblasts.

Immunophenotype
The megakaryoblasts express one or more of the platelet glycoproteins: CD41 (glycoprotein IIb/IIIa), CD61 (glycoprotein IIIa), and CD42b (glycoprotein Ib). The myeloid-associated markers CD13 and CD33 may also be positive. CD34, CD45, and HLA-DR are often negative; CD36 is characteristically positive but not specific. Blasts are negative with MPO antibodies. Lymphoid markers and TdT are not expressed. Cytoplasmic expression of CD41 or CD61 is more specific and sensitive than is surface staining.

Postulated normal counterpart
A myeloid progenitor cell with predominant megakaryocytic differentiation

Genetic profile
Cases should show karyotypic evidence of t(1;22)(p13.3;q13.1) or molecular genetic evidence of *RBM15-MKL1* fusion. In most cases, t(1;22)(p13.3;q13.1) is the sole karyotypic abnormality. This translo-

cation results in a fusion of *RBM15* (also called *OTT*) and *MKL1* (also called *MAL*) {2422}. *RBM15* encodes RNA recognition motifs and a split-end (spen) paralogue and orthologue C-terminal (SPOC) domain; *MKL1* encodes a DNA-binding motif involved in chromatin organization. The fusion gene may modulate chromatin organization, HOX-induced differentiation, and extracellular signalling pathways {2637}.

Prognosis and predictive factors

Despite some earlier reports suggesting that patients with AML with t(1;22) (p13.3;q13.1) respond well to intensive AML chemotherapy, with long disease-free survival {357,1050}, most studies have shown this to be a high-risk disease compared with paediatric acute megakaryocytic leukaemia without t(1;22) {357, 567,1756A,3593}. In cases with t(1;22) (p13.3;q13.1) and < 20% blasts on aspirate smears, the aspirate smears should be correlated with the biopsy to exclude bone marrow fibrosis as a cause of a falsely low blast cell count. If this is excluded, the patient must be monitored closely for development of more-definitive evidence of AML, such as the presence of extramedullary disease or myeloid sarcoma.

Acute myeloid leukaemia with BCR-ABL1

Definition

Acute myeloid leukaemia (AML) with *BCR-ABL1* (a provisional entity in the current classification) is a *de novo* AML in which patients show no evidence (either before or after therapy) of chronic myeloid leukaemia (CML). Cases that meet the criteria for mixed-phenotype acute leukaemia, therapy-related myeloid neoplasms, or other AML types with recurrent genetic abnormalities are excluded from this category.

ICD-O code   9912/3

Epidemiology

AML with *BCR-ABL1* accounts for < 1% of all AMLs and < 1% of all *BCR-ABL1*–positive acute and chronic leukaemias. It occurs primarily in adults, with a possible male predominance {2082,3029,3740}.

Clinical features

Patients most commonly present with leukocytosis with a blast predominance and variable presence of anaemia and thrombocytopenia. Compared with patients with myeloid blast transformation of CML, patients with AML with *BCR-ABL1* have less frequent splenomegaly and lower peripheral blood basophilia (usually < 2% basophils) {2082,3740}.

Microscopy

The morphological features of AML with *BCR-ABL1* are non-specific; they demonstrate the presence of bone marrow and peripheral blood myeloblasts, with features ranging from those of minimal differentiation to those of granulocytic maturation. Average bone marrow cellularity is reported to be less than that typically seen in blast transformation of CML (80% versus 95–100% in blast crisis), and dwarf megakaryocytes are reported to be less common in AML with *BCR-ABL1* than in blast transformation of CML. The non-blast cell myeloid-to-erythroid ratio is reported to be relatively normal compared with the more elevated ratio associated with blast transformation of CML {2082,3029,3740}.

Immunophenotype

The limited number of immunophenotypic studies of AML with *BCR-ABL1* have demonstrated expression of myeloid antigens (CD13 and CD33) and CD34. Aberrant expression of CD19, CD7, and TdT appears to be common. However, cases meeting the criteria for a mixed phenotype should be diagnosed as mixed-phenotype acute leukaemia with *BCR-ABL1* {3029,3740}.

Postulated normal counterpart

A haematopoietic progenitor cell with multilineage potential

Genetic profile

All cases demonstrate t(9;22) (q34.1;q11.2) or molecular genetic evidence of *BCR-ABL1* fusion. Most cases demonstrate the p210 fusion, with b2a2 and b3a2 fusions being next most common. A minority of reported cases have demonstrated p190 transcripts. In most cases, cytogenetic abnormalities, such as loss of chromosome 7, gain of chromosome 8, and complex karyotypes, are present in addition to t(9;22)(q34.1;q11.2) {2082,3029,3740}.

AML-associated mutations, in particular *NPM1* and *FLT3*-ITD, have been reported to be restricted to AML with *BCR-ABL1*, not occurring in blast transformation of CML, but these mutations are relatively infrequent {2082}. A recent study reported frequent loss of *IKZF1* and *CDKN2A* in AML with *BCR-ABL1*, as well as cryptic deletions within the IGH and TRG genes. These deletions are also reported in B-lymphoblastic leukaemia with *BCR-ABL1*, but they do not appear to occur in myeloid blast transformation of CML; if these results are confirmed, such testing may be a useful means of distinguishing between these disorders in the future {2801}.

Although some recurrent genetic abnormalities, in particular inv(16)(p13.1q22), have been reported to be acquired in CML at the time of blast transformation {4379}, these and other additional genetic abnormalities are reported to occur in *de novo* AML with *BCR-ABL1*. These genetic abnormalities include *CEBPA* and *NPM1* mutations, inv(16)(p13.1q22), and inv(3) (q21.3q26.2) {520,1533,2082,3421}, all of which, if present at diagnosis, define entities in the category of AML with recurrent genetic abnormalities, which would take precedence over a diagnosis of AML with *BCR-ABL1*. Late acquisition of *BCR-ABL1* fusion in a pre-existing AML has also been reported, and is not considered sufficient for a diagnosis of AML with *BCR-ABL1* {3273,3629,4401}. However, despite the ultimate classification of the disorder, therapy targeting the *BCR-ABL1* fusion is indicated in cases with this acquired abnormality.

Prognosis and predictive factors

AML with *BCR-ABL1* appears to be an aggressive disease, with poor response to traditional AML therapy or tyrosine kinase inhibitor therapy alone {3029,3740}. Recent reports suggest improved survival with tyrosine kinase inhibitor therapy followed by allogeneic haematopoietic cell transplantation {368,520,1171}.

Acute myeloid leukaemia with gene mutations

Acute myeloid leukaemia with mutated NPM1

Definition

Acute myeloid leukaemia (AML) with mutated *NPM1* carries mutations that usually involve exon 12 of *NPM1*. Aberrant cytoplasmic expression of NPM1 is a surrogate marker of such mutations {1149}. This AML type frequently has myelomonocytic or monocytic features and typically presents *de novo* in adults with a normal karyotype.

ICD-O code   9877/3

Synonym

Acute myeloid leukaemia with cytoplasmic nucleophosmin

Epidemiology

NPM1 mutation is one of the most common recurrent genetic lesions in AML {470,1075,1149,1150,3958,4185}, and is relatively specific for AML; it occurs in 2–8% of childhood cases and 27%–35% of adult cases overall, as well as in 45–64% of adult cases with a normal karyotype {470,590,749,1149,3958,4185}. There is a female predominance.

Clinical features

Patients with AML with mutated *NPM1* often have anaemia and thrombocytopenia, and often have higher white blood cell and platelet counts than seen with other AML types {1075}. Cases may show extramedullary involvement; the most frequently affected sites are gingiva, lymph nodes, and skin.

Microscopy

There is a strong association between

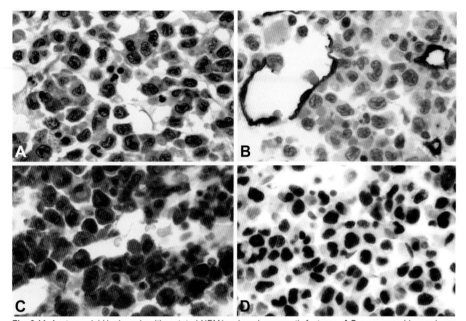

Fig. 8.14 Acute myeloid leukaemia with mutated *NPM1* and myelomonocytic features. **A** Bone marrow biopsy shows complete replacement by large blasts with abundant cytoplasm and folded nuclei. **B** and **C** Leukaemic cells are CD34-negative (B) and show aberrant cytoplasmic expression of NPM1 (C). **D** Expression of nucleolin (also called C23) is restricted to the nucleus.

both acute myelomonocytic and acute monocytic leukaemia and *NPM1* mutation {1149,1150}; notably, 80–90% of acute monocytic leukaemias show *NPM1* mutation. However, *NPM1* mutations are also detected in AML with and without maturation and in pure erythroid leukaemia.

The diagnosis relies on the identification of the genetic lesion by molecular techniques and/or immunohistochemical detection in paraffin sections of aberrant cytoplasmic expression of NPM1 {1150}. Immunostaining with anti-NPM1 antibodies reveals involvement of two or more bone marrow lineages (myeloid, monocytic, erythroid, megakaryocytic) in the vast majority of cases {3083}. The variability of bone marrow cell types showing *NPM1* mutation accounts for the wide morphological spectrum of this leukaemia. Multilineage dysplasia, as seen in many cases of AML with myelodysplasia-related changes (AML-MRC), is observed in almost a quarter of cases of *de novo* AML with mutated *NPM1*. These cases usually have a normal karyotype, and the blast cells are CD34-negative. The bone marrow is usually markedly hypercellular. In the setting of *NPM1* mutation, this type of dysplasia does not result in a worse prognosis, and its presence does not eliminate a diagnosis of AML with mutated *NPM1* {975,1145}.

Immunophenotype

AML with mutated *NPM1* is characterized by high CD33 expression and variable (often low) CD13 expression. KIT (CD117), CD123, and CD110 expression are common {2889}. HLA-DR is often negative. Two major subgroups of

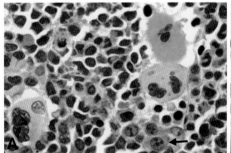
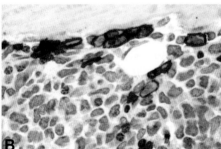
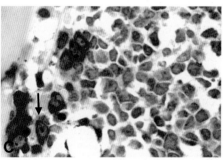

Fig. 8.15 Multilineage involvement in acute myeloid leukaemia with mutated *NPM1*. **A** Bone marrow biopsy shows massive replacement by myeloid blasts with maturation; there are also megakaryocytes and occasional immature erythroid cells (arrow). **B** Bone marrow biopsy of a minimally differentiated case shows occasional immature glycophorin-positive erythroid cells. **C** Myeloid blasts and immature erythroid cells (arrow) show cytoplasmic expression of NPM1.

AML with mutated *NPM1* have been described: one with an immature myeloid immunophenotypic profile and one with a monocytic (CD36+, CD64+, CD14+) immunophenotypic profile {2375}. CD34 is negative in most cases but CD34+ cases do occur and have been associated with an adverse prognosis {669,866}. A very small fraction of cells with the immunophenotype of leukaemic stem cells (CD34+, CD38−, CD123+) is detectable by flow cytometry in most patients with AML with mutated *NPM1* {2515}. The presence of a CD34+/CD25+/CD123+/CD99+ population is reportedly associated with *FLT3*-ITD mutations {105}.

On paraffin sections, immunohistochemical staining for NPM1 shows the characteristic aberrant expression of the protein in the cytoplasm of leukaemic cells {1149}. In contrast, positivity for another major nucleolar protein, nucleolin (also called C23), is restricted to the nucleus of leukaemic cells. Immunohistochemical detection of cytoplasmic NPM1 is predictive of *NPM1* mutations {1146}, because the mutations cause critical changes (i.e. loss of the nucleolar localization signal and addition of a nuclear export signal) in the structure of native NPM1 protein (characteristically located in the nucleolus), leading to its increased export from the nucleus and aberrant accumulation in the cytoplasm {1140}.

Postulated normal counterpart
A haematopoietic progenitor cell

Genetic profile
AML with mutated *NPM1* is usually associated with a normal karyotype; however, 5–15% of cases show chromosomal aberrations {1149,1150,1511}, including gain of chromosome 8 and del(9q) {3958}. In most AMLs, del(9q) is considered a myelodysplasia-associated abnormality, and was previously used to define AML-MRC. However, this does not appear to be true when *NPM1* is mutated, and such cases should be diagnosed as AML with mutated *NPM1* {1511}. Other myelodysplasia-associated cytogenetic abnormalities seen in AML-MRC are uncommon when *NPM1* is mutated {1511}, and such rare cases should continue to be diagnosed as AML-MRC. *NPM1* mutations are usually mutually exclusive of the other AMLs with recurrent genetic abnormalities {1148}. Secondary mutations are common in AML with mutated *NPM1*

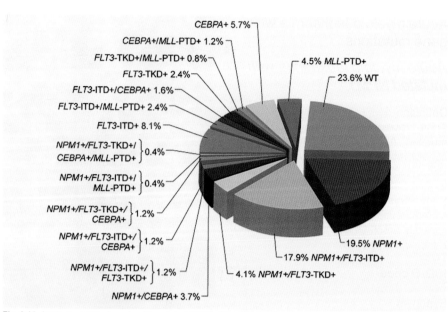

Fig. 8.16 Acute myeloid leukaemia with mutated *NPM1*. Pie chart showing the frequencies (in 246 patients) of *NPM1* mutations, *CEBPA* mutations (both biallelic and monoallelic), *FLT3* internal tandem duplication (*FLT3*-ITD), FLT3 tyrosine kinase domain (*FLT3*-TKD) mutation, and *KMT2A* (previously called MLL) partial tandem duplication (*MLL*-PTD); the size of each slice indicates the percentage of patients harbouring ≥ 1 of the mutations indicated; WT indicates patients with only wildtype alleles of the genes tested. From Mrózek K et al. {2774} and adapted from Döhner K et al. {1075}.

and most frequently involve *FLT3* and *DNMT3A*, but mutations of *IDH1*, *KRAS*, *NRAS*, and cohesin complex genes are also relatively common {545,1149}. Although *NPM1* mutation is a class-defining lesion, it is frequently a later event in leukaemogenesis, commonly secondary to mutations in epigenetic modifiers such as *DNMT3A*, *TET2*, *IDH1*, and *IDH2* {809, 2126,3665}. *NPM1* mutations appear to precede *FLT3*-ITD {749,3958}. AML with mutated *NPM1* shows a distinct gene expression profile (characterized by upregulation of HOX genes {54,4185}) that differs from that of other AML types, including AML with *KMT2A* rearrangement {2782}. AML with mutated *NPM1* is also characterized by a unique microRNA signature {1304}.

Prognosis and predictive factors
AML with mutated *NPM1* typically shows a good response to induction therapy {1149}. Cases with a normal karyotype, in the absence of *FLT3*-ITD mutation, have a characteristically favourable prognosis {470,1075,3560,3577,3958, 4185}. Younger patients with a normal karyotype and no *FLT3*-ITD have a prognosis comparable to that of patients with AML with t(8;21)(q22;q22.1) or AML with inv(16)(p13.1q22) or t(16;16)(p13.1;q22), and may be exempted from allogeneic haematopoietic cell transplantation in

first complete remission {1075}. At least in younger adult patients, the coexistence of *FLT3*-ITD mutations is associated with a poorer prognosis, but these patients still appear to have a better prognosis than do patients with AML with *FLT3*-ITD and wildtype *NPM1*, especially when the allelic ratio of *FLT3*-ITD is low {1278, 3233,3561}. The negative prognostic impact of a concomitant *FLT3*-ITD mutation in older patients (in particular those aged ≥70 years) with AML with mutated *NPM1* is less clear {310}. Co-occurrence of *NPM1*, *FLT3*-ITD, and *DNMT3A* mutations has been associated with a particularly poor outcome {2380}. It is unknown whether a *NPM1*-mutated, *FLT3*-ITD–negative genotype also confers a favourable prognosis in the rare cases of AML with a chromosomal aberration.

Acute myeloid leukaemia with biallelic mutation of CEBPA

Definition
Acute myeloid leukaemia (AML) with biallelic mutation of *CEBPA* usually meets the criteria for AML with maturation or AML without maturation, but some cases show myelomonocytic or monoblastic features. This leukaemia usually presents *de novo*.

ICD-O code   9878/3

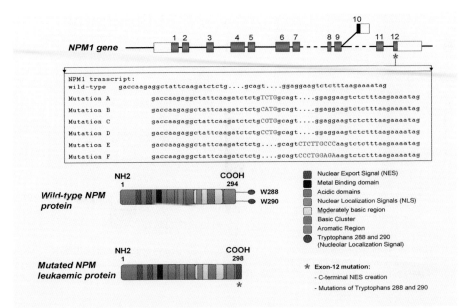

Fig. 8.17 Acute myeloid leukaemia with mutated *NPM1*. Mutations usually occur at exon 12 of the *NPM1* gene; the first-identified *NPM1* mutations (mutations A to F) are shown {1149}; mutation A is the most frequent, accounting for 70–80% of cases; all mutations result in common changes at the C-terminus (COOH) of the wildtype NPM1 (NPM) protein; these changes (asterisk) consist of replacement of tryptophan(s) at positions 288 and 290 and creation of a new nuclear export signal (NES) motif; both changes are responsible for the increased nuclear export and aberrant cytoplasmic accumulation of mutant NPM1.

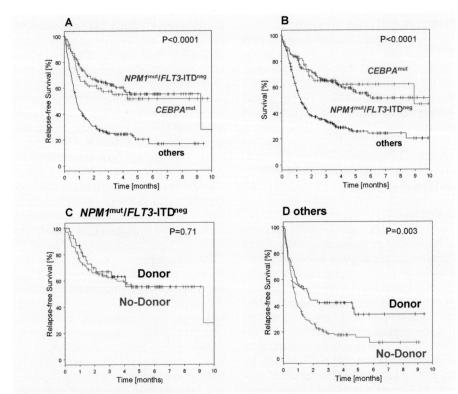

Fig. 8.18 Prognosis of acute myeloid leukaemia (AML) according to *NPM1*, *FLT3*, and *CEBPA* mutations. The genotypes *NPM1*^mut/*FLT3*-ITD^neg and *CEBPA*^mut are favourable prognostic markers (**A** and **B**). For univariate donor versus no-donor analysis on relapse-free survival for AML with normal karyotype in first complete remission, according to genotype, the donor group was defined by the availability of an HLA-matched related donor. As evidenced by the results of this analysis in cases with the favourable genotype *NPM1*^mut/*FLT3*-ITD^neg (**C**) and those with the adverse genotypes *FLT3*-ITD^pos and *NPM1*^wt/*CEBPA*^wt/*FLT3*-ITD^neg (**D**), only cases with adverse genotypes (**D**) benefit from allogeneic stem cell transplantation. From Schlenk R F et al. {3560}.

ITD, internal tandem duplication; mut, mutant; neg, negative; pos, positive; wt, wildtype.

Epidemiology

Biallelic mutations of *CEBPA* are reported in 4–9% of children and young adults with AML {1429,1668,1705,3022,4368}, with a frequency in normal-karyotype AML similar to the overall incidence {1052,3908}. However, the frequency in older patients is probably lower.

Clinical features

AML with biallelic mutation of *CEBPA* tends to be associated with higher haemoglobin levels, lower platelet counts, and lower lactate dehydrogenase levels than does *CEBPA*-wildtype AML {1052, 1705,3908}. It may also be associated with a lower frequency of lymphadenopathy and myeloid sarcoma {372,1260}. The diagnosis of AML with biallelic mutation of *CEBPA* (especially in younger patients) should raise concern and prompt investigation for the possibility of a germline mutation with predisposition to develop AML (see *Myeloid neoplasms with germline predisposition*, p. 121).

Microscopy

AML with biallelic mutation of *CEBPA* has no distinctive morphological features, but the vast majority of cases have features of AML either with or without maturation {1052,1429,1668}.

Multilineage dysplasia is reportedly present in 26% of cases of *de novo* AML with mutated CEBPA (similar to in AML with mutated *NPM1*), with no adverse prognostic significance {211}. Therefore, in the setting of biallelic *CEBPA* mutations, this type of dysplasia no longer excludes a case from this category.

Immunophenotype

In earlier studies that did not distinguish between single and double mutations in *CEBPA*, leukaemic blasts were reported to usually express one or more of the myeloid-associated antigens (CD13, CD33, CD65, CD11b, and CD15). There was usually expression of HLA-DR and CD34 by most blasts. CD7 was present in 50–73% of cases, whereas expression of CD56 or other lymphoid antigens was uncommon {372,1776,2341}. In contrast, cases with biallelic mutation of *CEBPA* are reported to have a higher frequency of HLA-DR, CD7, and CD15 expression and a lower frequency of CD56 expression than are cases with a single mutation {1705,2341}. Monocytic markers such as CD14 and CD64 are usually absent.

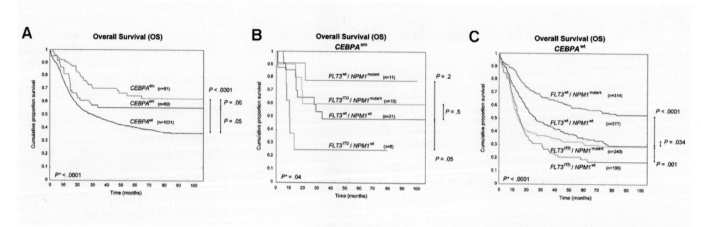

Fig. 8.19 Significance of *CEPBA* mutation type in acute myeloid leukaemia. **A** Kaplan–Meier overall survival curves for cases with *CEBPA* double mutations (*CEBPA*^dm), single mutations (*CEBPA*^sm) and wildtype (*CEBPA*^wt). **B and C**. Kaplan–Meier overall survival curves for *CEBPA*^sm cases (**B**) and *CEBPA*^wt cases (**C**) with four genotypes: *FLT3* internal tandem duplication (*FLT3*-ITD) and mutant *NPM1* (*FLT3*^ITD/*NPM1*^mutant), *FLT3*-ITD and wildtype *NPM1* (*FLT3*^ITD/*NPM1*^wt), wildtype *FLT3* and mutant *NPM1* (*FLT3*^wt/*NPM1*^mutant), and wildtype *FLT3* and *NPM1* (*FLT3*^wt/*NPM1*^wt) {3908}.
*P value by global log-rank test.

Postulated normal counterpart
A haematopoietic progenitor cell

Genetic profile
The favourable prognosis associated with *CEBPA* mutation in AML is now known to be related to biallelic mutations only; therefore, biallelic mutation is now required for assignment to this category {1429,1668,1705,3022,4368}. The biallelic mutation is associated with a specific gene expression profile that is not associated with the single mutation {3908, 4368}. More than 70% of cases of AML with biallelic mutation of *CEBPA* have a normal karyotype. *FLT3*-ITD mutations are found in 5–9% of cases {1052,3562, 3908}. *GATA2* zinc finger 1 mutations are also associated with biallelic *CEBPA* mutation, and occur in approximately 39% of cases {1450}.

A subset of cases of AML with biallelic mutation of *CEBPA* have an abnormal karyotype. Similarly to in AML with mutated *NPM1*, del(9q) is common among this group and does not appear to influence prognosis {3562}. Therefore, detection of biallelic mutation of *CEBPA* and del(9q) should not place a case into the category of AML with myelodysplasia-related changes. Other myelodysplasia-related cytogenetic abnormalities are less common, although del(11q) in association with biallelic *CEBPA* mutation has been reported {3562}. Until more data are available, such rare cases should continue to be diagnosed as AML with myelodysplasia-related changes.

Patients with biallelic *CEBPA* mutations should be evaluated for a familial syndrome (see *Myeloid neoplasms with germline predisposition*, p. 121).

Prognosis and predictive factors
AML with biallelic mutation of *CEBPA* is associated with a favourable prognosis, similar to that of AML with inv(16)(p13.1q22) or t(8;21)(q22;q22.1). The influence of *FLT3*-ITD and *GATA2* mutations on prognosis in this group is currently unclear.

Acute myeloid leukaemia with mutated RUNX1

Definition
Acute myeloid leukaemia (AML) with mutated *RUNX1* (a provisional entity in the current classification) is a *de novo* leukaemia with ≥20% bone marrow or peripheral blood blast cells that may have morphological features of most AML, NOS, categories and has a higher frequency among cases with minimal differentiation. The diagnosis of AML with mutated *RUNX1* should not be made for cases that fulfil the criteria for other specific AML subtypes in the categories of AML with recurrent genetic abnormalities, therapy-related myeloid neoplasms, or AML with myelodysplasia-related changes.

ICD-O code   9879/3

Epidemiology
RUNX1 mutations are reported to occur in 4–16% of AML cases. Most studies find a higher frequency in older adults (aged >60 years). One study reported a male predominance {3897}, but most have not identified a sex predilection {192,1274, 2627,3236,3576,3897}. *RUNX1* mutations in AML and myelodysplastic syndrome (MDS) are associated with radiation exposure {1546} and prior alkylating agent chemotherapy {751,1546}; cases associated with alkylating agent chemotherapy are also associated with monosomy 7 or del(7q). Such cases are considered to be therapy-related AML rather than *de novo* disease. Patients with Fanconi anaemia or congenital neutropenia who develop AML or MDS also frequently carry *RUNX1* mutations {3261,3694}.

Clinical features
Patients with AML with mutated *RUNX1* may have lower haemoglobin and lactate dehydrogenase levels and lower white blood cell and peripheral blood blast cell counts than patients with wildtype *RUNX1* {2627,3897}. Cases with a history of prior therapy (in particular radiation therapy), MDS, or a myelodysplastic/myeloproliferative neoplasm may also harbour *RUNX1* mutations {1546,2050}, but are excluded from this category.

Microscopy
There are no morphological features specific for AML with mutated *RUNX1*. Although 15–65% of cases of minimally

differentiated AML demonstrate this mutation, most reported cases have other morphological features, including AML with maturation and AML with monocytic or myelomonocytic features {1274,3576, 3897}.

Immunophenotype
The leukaemic blasts usually express CD13, CD34, and HLA-DR, with variable expression of CD33, monocytic markers, and MPO {3576,3897}.

Postulated normal counterpart
A haematopoietic progenitor cell with multilineage potential

Genetic profile
Most RUNX1 mutations are monoallelic, involving the runt homology domain (RHD), spanning exons 3–5, and the transactivation domain (TAD), spanning exons 6–8; they are most commonly frameshift or missense mutations {1274, 2627,3576,3897}. Mutations may occur with karyotypic abnormalities, most commonly trisomies 8 and 13 {976, 1274,3576}. Cases with myelodysplasia-related cytogenetic abnormalities should be classified as AML with myelodysplasia-related changes. The recurrent cytogenetic abnormalities described in this chapter for other specific WHO categories are not commonly associated with RUNX1 mutation, and the presence of such abnormalities takes diagnostic precedence over this provisional entity. Cooperating mutations are common with RUNX1 mutation, commonly involving ASXL1, KMT2A partial tandem duplication (KMT2A-PTD), FLT3-ITD, IDH1 R132, and IDH2 R140 and R172; however, some of these mutations do not appear to be increased versus in RUNX1-wildtype cases. Studies in MDS with mutated RUNX1 find a characteristic mutation signature involving SRSF2, EZH2, STAG2, and ASXL1 {1513,3050}, which appears to be similar in AML with mutated RUNX1. Mutations of NPM1, CEBPA, and JAK2 are uncommon in this group {1274,2627, 3576,3897}. Cases with both RUNX1 and NPM1 or RUNX1 and biallelic CEBPA mutations should be classified as AML with mutated NPM1 or AML with biallelic mutation of CEBPA, respectively.

A subset of these patients have germline mutations of RUNX1; when RUNX1 mutation is detected, germline studies should be performed or careful family histories obtained. Affected family members may have autosomal dominant thrombocytopenia and dense granule platelet storage pool deficiency, as well as an increased risk of development of AML or MDS (see Myeloid neoplasms with germline predisposition, p. 121) {1291,1390}.

Prognosis and predictive factors
In some studies, RUNX1 mutations in AML have been associated with worse overall survival in multivariate analysis {1274,2627,3576,3897}. The combination of RUNX1 and ASXL1 mutations is reported to be associated with an adverse prognosis {3079}. It is unclear whether other cooperating mutations influence the prognosis of this disease group. Improved survival in patients treated with allogeneic haematopoietic cell transplantation has been reported {1274,3897}.

Table 8.02 Molecular genetic alterations affecting clinical outcome of patients with acute myeloid leukaemia in specific cytogenetic groups

Molecular genetic alteration	Cytogenetic group	Prognostic significance[a]
KIT mutation	t(8;21)(q22;q22.1)	Significantly shorter DFS {3063A}, RFS {408A}, EFS {408A,2016A,3576B}, and OS {408A,523A,2016A,3063A,3095,3576B} and higher CIR {3078} and RI {523A} for patients with KIT mutation (especially in exon 17) than for patients with wildtype KIT
		In series from the USA {3207A} and Taiwan, China {3653A}, no significant difference in CRR {3207A}, DFS {3207A}, EFS {3653A}, RR {3207A,3653A}, or OS {3207A,3653A} between paediatric patients with and without KIT mutation; in a Japanese study, significantly shorter DFS and OS and higher RR for paediatric patients with KIT mutation (especially in exon 17) than for those with wildtype KIT {3657A}
KIT mutation	inv(16)(p13.1q22)/t(16;16)(p13.1;q22)	In most studies, no significant difference in RI {523A}, RFS {408A}, PFS {1876A}, EFS {408A}, or OS {408A,523A,1876A,3076,3095} between patients with and without KIT mutation, or in EFS {2016A} or OS {2016A} between patients with and without KIT mutation in exon 17 at codon D816
		In single studies, shorter RFS {3076} for patients with KIT mutation (especially in exon 8), higher RR {564A} for patients with exon 8 KIT mutation, and higher CIR and shorter OS {3078} for patients with exon 17 KIT mutation than for patients with wildtype KIT
		In paediatric studies, no significant difference in CRR {3207A}, DFS {3207A}, EFS {3653A}, RR {3207A,3653A}, or OS {3207A,3653A} between patients with and without KIT mutation
FLT3-ITD	Normal karyotype	Significantly shorter DFS {372,4307A,4307C}, CRD {345A,1259A}, and OS {345A,372,1259A,4307C} for patients with FLT3-ITD than for patients without FLT3-ITD
		No significant difference in CRR between patients with and without FLT3-ITD {345A,372,4307A,4307C}
FLT3-ITD with no expression of wildtype FLT3	Normal karyotype	Significantly shorter DFS and OS for patients with FLT3-ITD and no expression of wildtype FLT3 than for patients without FLT3-ITD {4307A}
FLT3-ITD	Various abnormal and normal karyotypes combined	Among younger patients (aged <60 years), significantly shorter OS for patients with FLT3-ITD than for patients without FLT3-ITD {3095}
FLT3-ITD mutant level	Various abnormal and normal karyotypes combined	Increasingly worse RR and OS (but not CRR) with increasing FLT3-ITD mutant level (i.e. the proportion of total FLT3 alleles accounted for by FLT3-ITD) in a comparison of mutant levels in 4 subsets of patients: without FLT3-ITD, with low (1–24%) FLT3-ITD mutant level, with intermediate (25–50%) mutant level, and with high (>50%) mutant level {1278}
Biallelic CEBPA mutation	Normal karyotype	Significantly higher CRR {3908} and DFS {1705} and longer RFS {3908}, EFS {3908}, and OS {1052,1705,3908} for patients with double CEBPA mutation than for patients with wildtype CEBPA
Biallelic CEBPA mutation	Various abnormal and normal karyotypes combined	Significantly longer DFS {1705,3022}, EFS {4368}, and OS {1429,1705,3022,4368} for patients with double CEBPA mutation than for patients with wildtype CEBPA or single CEBPA mutation
Single CEBPA mutation	Normal karyotype	Significantly lower CRR {3908} and shorter DFS {1705} and OS {1705} for patients with single CEBPA mutation than for patients with double CEBPA mutation
NPM1 mutation	Normal karyotype	In some studies, significantly higher CRR {3577} and longer DFS {3958}, RFS {1075}, and EFS {3577} for patients with NPM1 mutation than for patients with wildtype NPM1; in other studies, no significant difference in CRR {258A,408C}, RFS {258A,408C,3577}, or EFS {258A,408C} between patients with and without NPM1 mutation
		No consistently observed significant difference in OS between patients with and without NPM1 mutation {258A,408C,1075,3577,3958}
		Among older patients (aged ≥60 years), significantly better CRR, DFS, and OS for patients with NPM1 mutation than for patients with wildtype NPM1 {310}
NPM1 mutation & FLT3-ITD	Normal karyotype	Significantly better CRR {3560}, EFS {3577}, RFS {1075,3560}, DFS {3958}, and OS {1075,3560,3577,3958} for patients with NPM1 mutation without FLT3-ITD than for patients with NPM1 mutation and FLT3-ITD or with wildtype NPM1 with or without FLT3-ITD
RUNX1 mutation	Normal karyotype	Significantly lower CRR {2627}; higher resistant disease rate {1274}; and shorter DFS {2627,3897}, EFS {1274,2627,3576}, and OS {2627,3576,3897} for patients with RUNX1 mutation than for patients with wildtype RUNX1

Molecular genetic alteration	Cytogenetic group	Prognostic significance[a]
RUNX1 mutation	Various abnormal and normal karyotypes combined	Significantly lower CRR {3897}; higher resistant disease rate {1274}; and shorter DFS {3897}, RFS {1274}, EFS {1274}, and OS {1274,3897} for patients with RUNX1 mutation than for patients with wildtype RUNX1
RUNX1 mutation	Non-complex karyotype (i.e. 1 or 2 abnormalities and a normal karyotype combined)	Significantly shorter EFS and OS for patients with RUNX1 mutation than for patients with wildtype RUNX1 {3576}
KMT2A-PTD	Normal karyotype	No difference in CRR, DFS, or OS between patients with and without KMT2A-PTD, either among younger patients (aged < 60 years) receiving intensive treatment including autologous stem cell transplantation {4307D} or among older patients (aged ≥ 60 years) {4307B} In earlier studies, significantly worse CRD (but not CRR or OS) {526A,1075A} and higher RR or risk of death during CR {3560} for patients with KMT2A-PTD than for patients without KMT2A-PTD
KMT2A-PTD	Various abnormal and normal karyotypes combined	Among younger patients (aged < 60 years), significantly shorter OS for patients with KMT2A-PTD than for patients without KMT2A-PTD {3095}
WT1 mutation	Normal karyotype	Significantly lower CRR {4197A}; higher resistant disease rates {4197A}, RR {3343B}, and CIR {4197A}; and shorter DFS {3078A}, RFS {4197A}, EFS {2104B}, and OS {3078A} for patients with WT1 mutation than for patients with wildtype WT1 Among younger patients (aged ≤ 60 years), significantly worse CRR, RFS, and OS for patients with WT1 mutation and FLT3-ITD than for patients with WT1 mutation without FLT3-ITD {1274B} In studies in Europe {1668B} and the USA {1646A}, significantly worse CRR {1668B}, EFS {1646A,1668B}, and OS {1646A,1668B} for paediatric patients with WT1 mutation than for those with wildtype WT1; in a Japanese study {3513A}, no significant difference in DFS or OS
WT1 mutation	Various abnormal and normal karyotypes combined	Significantly worse RR and OS for patients with WT1 mutation than for patients with wildtype WT1 {3343B}; no significant difference in EFS {2104B} In studies in Europe {1668B} and the USA {1646A}, significantly worse resistant disease rates {1668B}, CIR {1668B}, EFS {1646A,1668B}, and OS {1646A,1668B} for paediatric patients with WT1 mutation than for those with wildtype WT1; in a Japanese study {3513A}, no significant difference in DFS or OS
TET2 mutation	Normal karyotype	No significant difference in CRR {864A,1274A,2648C}, DFS {2648C}, RFS {864A,1274A}, EFS {1274A,2648C}, or OS {864A,1274A,2648C,4290A} between patients with and without TET2 mutation Significantly worse CRR {2648C}, DFS {2648C}, RR {4290A}, EFS {2648C,4290A}, and OS {2648C} for patients with TET2 mutations classified in the ELN favourable genetic group[c] (but not those in the intermediate-I group[c]) than for patients with wildtype TET2; one study {1274A}, reported higher CRR for younger patients (aged ≤ 60 years) with TET2 mutations classified in the ELN intermediate-I genetic group[c] (but not those in the favourable group[c]) than for those with wildtype TET2 Significantly worse RR {4290A}, EFS {4290A}, and OS {3998A} for patients with TET2 and NPM1 mutation without FLT3-ITD than for patients with wildtype TET2; similarly, TET2 mutation was associated with shorter RFS and OS in younger patients (aged ≤ 60 years) with FLT3-ITD {864A} and with shorter OS in patients with NPM1 mutation {3998A}
TET2 mutation	Various abnormal and normal karyotypes combined	Among younger patients (aged ≤ 60 years), no significant difference in CRR, RFS, EFS, or OS between patients with and without TET2 mutation {1274A}
ASXL1 mutation	Normal karyotype	Significantly worse CRR {2648A}, DFS {2648A}, EFS {2648A,3576A}, and OS {2648A,3576A} for patients with ASXL1 mutation than for patients with wildtype ASXL1 Among older patients (aged ≥ 60 years), significantly worse CRR, DFS, EFS, and OS for patients with ASXL1 mutation classified in the ELN favourable genetic group[c] (but not those in the intermediate-I genetic group[c]) than for patients with wildtype ASXL1 {2648A}
ASXL1 mutation	Various abnormal and normal karyotypes combined	Significantly worse CRR {748A,3079,3232A}, RFS {3079}, and OS {748A,3079, 3095,3232A} for patients with ASXL1 mutation than for patients with wildtype ASXL1
ASXL1 mutation	Intermediate-risk karyotype[b]	Significantly shorter EFS and OS for patients with ASXL1 mutation than for patients with wildtype ASXL1 {3576A}

Molecular genetic alteration	Cytogenetic group	Prognostic significance[a]
DNMT3A mutation	Normal karyotype	In some studies, significantly worse CRR {3987A}, DFS {2501E}, EFS {3343A}, and OS {3343A,3987A} for patients with DNMT3A mutation (R882 or non-R882) than for patients with wildtype DNMT3A; in other studies, no difference in CRR {1274C}, RFS {1274C,3987A}, EFS {1274C}, or OS {1274C}

Among younger patients (aged ≤60 years) with NPM1 mutation, significantly shorter EFS and OS for patients with DNMT3A mutation (mainly R882) than for patients with wildtype DNMT3A {3343A}

Among younger patients (aged ≤60 years), significantly shorter RFS and OS for patients with DNMT3A mutation (mainly R882) classified in the ELN intermediate-I genetic groupc than for patients with wildtype DNMT3A; no difference in outcome between patients with and without DNMT3A mutation classified in the favourable genetic groupc {1274C}

Among younger patients (aged ≤60 years) with either NPM1 mutation without FLT3-ITD or biallelic CEBPA mutation, significantly shorter EFS and OS for patients with DNMT3A mutation than for patients with wildtype DNMT3A {3343A} |
DNMT3A R882 mutation	Normal karyotype	Among older patients (aged ≥60 years), significantly shorter DFS and OS for patients with DNMT3A R882 mutation than for patients with wildtype DNMT3A {2501E}
Non-R882 DNMT3A mutation	Normal karyotype	Among younger patients (aged <60 years), significantly shorter DFS for patients with non-R882 DNMT3A mutation than for patients with wildtype DNMT3A {2501E}
DNMT3A mutation	Various abnormal and normal karyotypes combined	Among younger patients (aged ≤60 years), significantly higher CRR but no significant difference in RFS, EFS, or OS for patients with DNMT3A mutation (R882 and non-R882 combined) than for patients with wildtype DNMT3A {1274C}
IDH1 mutation	Normal karyotype	No significant difference in CRR {408B,2501D}, DFS {2501D}, RR {408B}, or OS {408B,2501D} between patients with IDH1 mutation and patients with wildtype IDH1 and IDH2
IDH1 R132 mutation	Normal karyotype	Among patients with NPM1 mutation without FLT3-ITD, significantly shorter DFS for patients with IDH1 R132 mutation than for patients with wildtype IDH1 and IDH2 {2501D}

Among patients with NPM1 or CEBPA mutation without FLT3-ITD, significantly higher RR and shorter OS for patients with IDH1 R132 mutation than for patients with wildtype IDH1 {408B} |
IDH2 mutation	Normal karyotype	No significant difference in CRR, RFS, or OS between patients with and without IDH2 mutation (mostly R140); this was also true in a subset of patients with NPM1 mutation without FLT3-ITD {3987B}
IDH2 R172 mutation	Normal karyotype	Significantly worse CRR {408B,2501D}, RR {408B}, and OS {408B} for patients with IDH2 R172 mutation than for patients with wildtype IDH2
IDH2 R140 mutation	Normal karyotype	No significant difference in CRR, DFS, or OS between patients with IDH2 R140 mutation and patients with wildtype IDH1 and IDH2 {2501D}
IDH2 R140Q mutation	Various abnormal and normal karyotypes combined	Among younger patients (aged <60 years), significantly longer OS for patients with IDH2 R140Q mutation than for patients with wildtype IDH2 {3095}
IDH1 and IDH2 mutations combined	Normal karyotype	Significantly shorter DFS and OS for patients with IDH1 or IDH2 mutation than for patients with wildtype IDH1 and IDH2 {2889A}

Among younger patients (aged ≤60 years), no significant difference in CRR, RFS, or OS between patients with IDH1 or IDH2 mutation and patients with wildtype IDH1 and IDH2; but in a subset of patients with NPM1 mutation without FLT3-ITD, significantly shorter RFS for patients with IDH1 or IDH2 mutation than for patients with wildtype IDH1 and IDH2 {3078B} |
IDH1 and IDH2 mutations combined	Various abnormal and normal karyotypes combined	Among younger patients (aged ≤60 years), no significant difference in CRR, RFS, or OS between patients with IDH1 mutation or with either IDH1 or IDH2 mutation and patients with wildtype IDH1 and IDH2 {3078B}
TP53 alteration (mutation or loss)	Complex karyotype (≥3 abnormalities)[d]	Significantly shorter RFS, EFS, and OS for patients with TP53 alteration than for patients with wildtype TP53 {3462A}
TP53 mutation	Complex karyotype (≥5 abnormalities)	No significant difference in CRR, DFS, or OS between patients with and without TP53 mutation {439A}
TP53 mutation	Abnormalities of chromosome 5, 7, or 17 and/or complex karyotype (≥5 abnormalities)	Significantly shorter OS for patients with TP53 mutation than for patients with wildtype TP53 {439A}

Molecular genetic alteration	Cytogenetic group	Prognostic significance[a]
BAALC expression	Normal karyotype	Significantly worse CRR {239B,3594C}, primary resistant disease rates {239B}, DFS {239A,372,3594C}, EFS {239A}, RR {239B}, CIR {239B}, and OS {239A,239B,372,3594C} for patients with high BAALC expression in blood than for patients with low expression No significant difference in CIR or EFS between paediatric patients with high and low BAALC expression, whereas OS was significantly shorter for patients with high expression in univariate but not multivariate analysis {1620A}
BAALC expression	Various abnormal and normal karyotypes combined	No significant difference in CIR {1620A}, EFS {1620A}, or OS {1620A,3763A} between paediatric patients with high and low BAALC expression; in one study {3763A}, high expression was associated with significantly shorter EFS
ERG expression	Normal karyotype	Significantly worse CRR {2501C,2648B}, DFS {2648B}, EFS {2501C}, CIR {2501A}, and OS {2501A,2648B,3594C} for patients with high ERG expression in blood {2501A,2501C} or bone marrow {2648B} than for patients with low expression No significant difference in CIR, EFS, or OS between paediatric patients with high and low ERG expression {1620A}
ERG expression	Various abnormal and normal karyotypes combined	No significant difference in CIR, EFS, or OS between paediatric patients with high and low ERG expression {1620A}
MN1 expression	Normal karyotype	Significantly lower CRR {2217A,3594B}; higher RR {1631A}; and shorter RFS {1631A}, EFS {3594B}, and OS {1631A,2217A} for patients with high MN1 expression than for patients with low expression
DNMT3B expression	Normal karyotype	Among older patients (aged ≥ 60 years), significantly lower CRR and shorter DFS and OS for patients with high DNMT3B expression than for patients with low expression {2870A}
SPARC expression	Normal karyotype	Among younger patients (aged < 60 years), significantly lower CRR and shorter DFS and OS for patients with high SPARC expression than for patients with low expression {50A}
MECOM expression	Normal karyotype	Among younger patients (aged ≤ 60 years), significantly shorter EFS for patients with high MECOM (EVI1) expression than for patients with low expression {1479A}
MECOM expression	Various abnormal and normal karyotypes combined	Among younger patients (aged ≤ 60 years), significantly lower CRR and shorter RFS and EFS for patients with high MECOM (EVI1) expression than for patients with low expression {1479A}
MECOM expression	Intermediate-risk karyotype[b]	Among younger patients (aged ≤ 60 years), significantly shorter RFS and EFS for patients with high MECOM (EVI1) expression than for patients with low expression {1479A}
MIR181A expression	Normal karyotype	Among younger patients (aged < 60 years), significantly better CRR and OS for patients with high MIR181A expression than for patients with low expression {3594A}
MIR3151 expression	Normal karyotype	Among older patients (aged ≥ 60 years), significantly shorter DFS and OS for patients with high MIR3151 expression than for patients with low expression {1085A}
MIR3151 expression	Intermediate-risk karyotype[b]	Significantly shorter DFS and OS and higher CIR for patients with high MIR3151 expression than for patients with low expression {974B}
MIR155 expression	Normal karyotype	Significantly lower CRR and shorter DFS and OS for patients with high MIR155 expression than for patients with low expression {2501B}

CIR, cumulative incidence of relapse; CR, complete remission; CRD, complete remission duration; CRR, complete remission rate; DFS, disease-free survival; EFS, event-free survival; ELN, European LeukemiaNet; FLT3-ITD, FLT3 internal tandem duplication; KMT2A-PTD, KMT2A (MLL) partial tandem duplication; OS, overall survival; PFS, progression-free survival; RFS, relapse-free survival; RI, relapse incidence; RR, risk of relapse.

[a] The data presented pertain to adult patients, unless otherwise indicated.

[b] According to the refined UK Medical Research Council criteria {1464}.

[c] Cytogenetically normal patients classified in the ELN favourable genetic group have mutated CEBPA and/or mutated NPM1 without FLT3-ITD, whereas patients classified in the intermediate-I genetic group have wildtype CEBPA and either wildtype NPM1 (with or without FLT3-ITD) or mutated NPM1 with FLT3-ITD.

[d] Complex karyotype is defined by ELN as ≥ 3 chromosome abnormalities in the absence of the WHO-designated recurring translocations or inversions, i.e. t(8;21), inv(16) or t(16;16), t(15;17), t(9;11), t(v;11)(v;q23.3), t(6;9), inv(3), or t(3;3). Table prepared by Krzysztof Mrózek.

Acute myeloid leukaemia with myelodysplasia-related changes

Arber D.A.
Brunning R.D.
Orazi A.
Bain B.J.

Porwit A.
Le Beau M.M.
Greenberg P.L.

Definition

Acute myeloid leukaemia with myelodysplasia-related changes (AML-MRC) is an acute leukaemia with ≥20% peripheral blood or bone marrow blasts with morphological features of myelodysplasia, or occurring in patients with a prior history of a myelodysplastic syndrome (MDS) or myelodysplastic/myeloproliferative neoplasm (MDS/MPN), with MDS-related cytogenetic abnormalities; the specific genetic abnormalities characteristic of acute myeloid leukaemia (AML) with recurrent genetic abnormalities are absent. Patients should not have a history of prior cytotoxic or radiation therapy for an unrelated disease. Therefore, there are three possible reasons for classifying a case as this subtype (Table 8.03): AML arising from previous MDS or MDS/MPN, AML with an MDS-related cytogenetic abnormality and AML with multilineage dysplasia. A given case may be classified as this subtype for one, two or all three of these reasons.

ICD-O code   9895/3

Synonyms

Acute myeloid leukaemia with multilineage dysplasia; acute myeloid leukaemia with prior myelodysplastic syndrome

Epidemiology

AML-MRC occurs mainly in elderly patients, and is rare in children {1595,2261}. Although the definitions of multilineage dysplasia in the literature vary, this category appears to account for 24 to 35% of all cases of AML {132,885,1514,2682, 4276,4416}.

Clinical features

AML-MRC often presents with severe pancytopenia. Some cases with 20–29% blasts, especially cases arising from MDS or in childhood, may be slowly progressive. Such cases, with relatively stable peripheral blood counts for weeks or months, are categorized by the French–American–British (FAB) classification as refractory anaemia with excess blasts in

Table 8.03 Diagnostic criteria for acute myeloid leukaemia with myelodysplasia-related changes (AML-MRC)

The diagnosis of AML-MRC requires that the following 3 criteria are met.
1 ≥20% blood or marrow blasts

2 Any of the following:
    - History of myelodysplastic syndrome or myelodysplastic/myeloproliferative neoplasm
    - Myelodysplastic syndrome–related cytogenetic abnormality (Table 8.04)
    - Multilineage dysplasia[a]

3 Absence of both of the following:
    - Prior cytotoxic or radiation therapy for an unrelated disease
    - Recurrent cytogenetic abnormality as described in *Acute myeloid leukaemia with recurrent genetic abnormalities* (p. 130)

[a] Multilineage dysplasia alone is insufficient for a diagnosis of AML-MRC in a *de novo* case of AML with mutated *NPM1* or biallelic mutation of *CEBPA* (see text for details).

transformation, and may have clinical behaviour more similar to that of MDS than that of AML {1590}. Some authors recommended categorizing such cases as a favourable prognostic subtype of AML {1590}. However, this recommendation is controversial. The National Comprehensive Cancer Network (NCCN) Clinical Practice Guidelines for Myelodysplastic Syndromes, which endorse using the WHO classification system, recommend that cases with 20–29% marrow blasts and a stable clinical course for ≥2 months be considered as either MDS or AML, in order for such cases to be eligible for treatment as either entity {1443}. Several important findings support this recommendation: (1) patients with 20–29% marrow blasts have previously been included in and benefited from major therapeutic trials for MDS {1183,1796}; (2) survival and disease evolution were similar in the MDS patient groups with 10–19% and 20–29% marrow blasts {1444}; and (3) molecular and cytogenetic features have been reported to be similar between these two patient groups {210}. Molecular genetic factors (rather than strictly morphological or historical factors) have helped refine the diagnosis of MDS-type AML; a set of gene mutations defines a subset of *de novo* AML cases, including those that evolved from MDS, with clinical features and therapeutic responses highly specific for MDS {2351}.

Microscopy

Most cases in this category of AML have morphological evidence of multilineage dysplasia, which must be assessed on well-stained smears of peripheral blood and bone marrow. For an AML to be classified as having myelodysplasia-related changes based on morphology, dysplasia must be present in ≥50% of the cells in at least two haematopoietic cell lines. Dysgranulopoiesis is characterized by neutrophils with hypogranular cytoplasm, hyposegmented nuclei (pseudo–Pelger–Huët anomaly) or bizarrely segmented nuclei. In some cases, these features can be more readily identified on peripheral blood than bone marrow smears. Dyserythropoiesis is characterized by megaloblastosis, karyorrhexis, and nuclear irregularity, fragmentation or multinucleation. Ring sideroblasts, cytoplasmic vacuoles and periodic acid–Schiff (PAS) positivity are additional features of dyserythropoiesis. Dysmegakaryopoiesis is characterized by micromegakaryocytes and normal-sized or large megakaryocytes with non-lobated or multiple nuclei. Dysplastic megakaryocytes may be more readily appreciated in sections than on smears {132,1270}.

Some cases lack sufficient non-blast bone marrow elements to adequately assess for multilineage dysplasia; others have sufficient non-blast cells but do not meet the criteria described above for

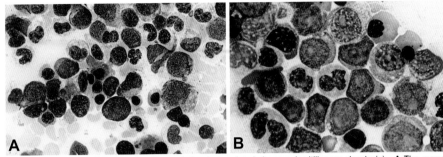

Fig. 8.20 Acute myeloid leukaemia with myelodysplasia-related changes (multilineage dysplasia). **A** The marrow aspirate shows numerous agranular blasts admixed with hypogranular neutrophils with clumped nuclear chromatin and erythroid precursors with irregular nuclear contours; a small, hypolobated megakaryocyte is present at the bottom of the field. **B** The marrow aspirate shows numerous agranular blasts admixed with hypogranular neutrophils with clumped nuclear chromatin and erythroid precursors with irregular nuclear contours.

a morphological diagnosis of AML with multilineage dysplasia. These cases are diagnosed as AML-MRC on the basis of detection of MDS-related cytogenetic abnormalities and/or a history of MDS or MDS/MPN.

Differential diagnosis

The principal differential diagnoses are MDS with excess blasts, pure erythroid leukaemia, acute megakaryoblastic leukaemia and the other categories of AML, not otherwise specified (NOS). Careful blast cell counts, adherence to the diagnostic criteria for morphological dysplasia and evaluation for MDS-related cytogenetic abnormalities should resolve most cases, with this category taking priority over the purely morphological categories of AML, NOS. For example, a case with ≥ 20% bone marrow megakaryoblasts and multilineage dysplasia should be considered AML-MRC (megakaryoblastic type) if AML with t(1;22)(p13.3;q13.1) and myeloid proliferations associated with Down syndrome are excluded.

Immunophenotype

Immunophenotyping results are variable due to the heterogeneity of the underlying genetic changes, but an increase in CD14 expression on blasts cells has been reported {4276} and is related to a poor prognosis {739}. An increased frequency of CD11b expression has been noted in patients with high-risk and monosomal karyotypes {677,1889,2309}. Decreased expression of HLA-DR, KIT (CD117), FLT3 (CD135) and CD38 and increased expression of lactoferrin are reported to be associated with the presence of multilineage dysplasia {2658}. In cases with aberrations of chromosomes 5 and 7, a high incidence

of CD34, TdT, and CD7 expression has been reported {4172}. In cases with antecedent MDS, CD34+ cells frequently constitute only a subpopulation of blasts and may have a stem-cell immunophenotype, with low expression of CD38 and/ or HLA-DR. An increase in the fraction of cells with this stem-cell immunophenotype has been correlated with high-risk cytogenetics and poor outcome {3415}. Blasts often express panmyeloid markers (CD13, CD33), but aberrantly high or low expression of these markers is common. There is frequently aberrant expression of CD56 and/or CD7 {2934, 2936}. The maturing myeloid cells may show patterns of antigen expression differing from those seen in normal myeloid development, and there may be alterations in the light-scattering properties of maturing cells (in particular neutrophils), similar to those described in MDS (see *Myelodysplastic syndromes: Overview*, p. 98). There is an increased incidence of expression of the multidrug resistance glycoprotein ABCB1 (also called MDR1) in the blast cells {2141,2260,2261}.

Postulated normal counterpart

A multipotent haematopoietic stem cell

Genetic profile

The chromosome abnormalities are similar to those found in MDS; they often involve gain or loss of major segments of certain chromosomes, with complex karyotypes, loss of chromosome 7/del(7q), del(5q) and unbalanced translocations involving 5q being most common {2261, 2772,2929}. Additional abnormalities that are considered sufficient to include a case in this category are listed in Table 8.04. Although trisomy 8 and del(20q) are also common in MDS, these findings

are not considered to be disease-specific and are not by themselves sufficient to classify a case as AML-MRC. Similarly, loss of Y chromosome is a non-specific finding in older men and should not be considered sufficient cytogenetic evidence of this disease category.

Balanced translocations are less common in this disorder, but when they occur they often involve 5q32-33. The presence of t(3;5)(q25.3;q35.1) is associated with multilineage dysplasia and a younger patient age at presentation compared with most other cases in this disease group {127}. In addition, AML with inv(3) (q21.3q26.2) or t(3;3)(q21.3;q26.2) and AML with t(6;9)(p23;q34.1) may show evidence of multilineage dysplasia, but these are recognized as distinct entities within the AML with recurrent genetic abnormalities group, and should be classified as such. However, cases with the specific 11q23.3 rearrangements t(11;16) (q23.3;p13.3) and t(2;11)(p21;q23.3), if not associated with prior cytotoxic therapy, should be classified in this group rather than as AML with a variant translocation of 11q23.3.

Cases of AML with multilineage dysplasia may carry *NPM1* and/or *FLT3* mutations, or mutations of *CEBPA* {4237}. Most *NPM1*-mutated or *CEBPA*-double-mutated cases have a normal karyotype and no history of prior MDS {3664} and have a prognosis similar to that of cases

Table 8.04 Cytogenetic abnormalities sufficient for the diagnosis of acute myeloid leukaemia with myelodysplasia-related changes when ≥ 20% peripheral blood or bone marrow blasts are present and prior therapy has been excluded

Complex karyotype (≥ 3 abnormalities)

Unbalanced abnormalities

Loss of chromosome 7 or del(7q)
del(5q) or t(5q)
Isochromosome 17q or i(17p)
Loss of chromosome 13 or del(13q)
del(11q)
del(12p) or t(12p)
idic(X)(q13)

Balanced abnormalities

t(11;16)(q23.3;p13.3)
t(3;21)(q26.2;q22.1)
t(1;3)(p36.3;q21.2)
t(2;11)(p21;q23.3)
t(5;12)(q32;p13.2)
t(5;7)(q32;q11.2)
t(5;17)(q32;p13.2)
t(5;10)(q32;q21)
t(3;5)(q25.3;q35.1)

without multilineage dysplasia {211,1145}. Therefore, such cases are now considered to be AML with mutated *NPM1* or AML with biallelic mutation of *CEBPA*, respectively, rather than AML-MRC. In the absence of *NPM1* mutation or biallelic *CEBPA* mutation, the presence of multilineage dysplasia in the absence of prior MDS or an MDS-related cytogenetic abnormality appears to remain a significantly poor prognostic indicator in adults {975,3442,4276}. However, the presence of an MDS-associated karyotypic abnormality takes diagnostic precedence over the detection of an *NPM1* mutation or biallelic *CEBPA* mutation for classification purposes. Although del(9q) was previously accepted as an MDS-related cytogenetic abnormality, its presence as a sole abnormality in patients with mutation of *NPM1* or biallelic mutation of *CEBPA* does not appear to have prognostic significance {1511,3562}, and it is no longer considered diagnostic of AML-MRC. However, the other MDS-related cytogenetic abnormalities are very uncommon in association with *NPM1* or biallelic *CEBPA* mutation, and are diagnostic of AML-MRC even when these mutations are present.

NPM1 mutation and biallelic mutation of *CEBPA* are fairly uncommon in AML-MRC, but other mutations are reported with variable frequency. These include a variety of MDS-related mutations, such as mutation of *U2AF1* and mutations of *ASXL1* and *TP53*, which are more frequent in this entity than in AML, NOS. *TP53* mutations are almost always associated with a complex karyotype, but may suggest an even worse prognosis in this generally poor prognostic group {963,964,2943}.

Prognosis and predictive factors

AML-MRC generally has a poor prognosis, with a lower rate of complete remission than in other AML subtypes {132, 1270,2682,4276,4416}. Although there

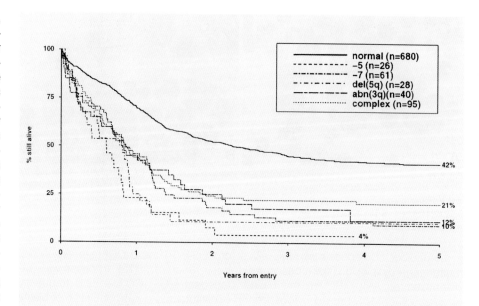

Fig. 8.21 Overall survival curves for cases of acute myeloid leukaemia (AML) with adverse cytogenetic findings (irrespective of the presence of additional abnormalities) in the Medical Research Council (MRC) AML 10 trial. The group with normal karyotype is included for comparison. Reproduced from Grimwade D et al. {1466}

are no overall prognostic differences between cases with and without prior MDS {132}, cases with prior MDS and relatively low blast counts may constitute less clinically aggressive disease. Some cases with prior MDS and 20–29% bone marrow blasts, considered refractory anaemia with excess blasts in transformation in the FAB classification, may behave in a manner more similar to MDS than to other AMLs {1590}. These cases, as well as cases with myelodysplasia and slightly less than 20% blasts, require regular monitoring of peripheral blood counts and bone marrow morphology for changes suggesting disease progression to overt AML.

Although AML-MRC is generally associated with a poor prognosis, several studies have not found morphology to be a significant parameter when using multivariable analysis that also incorporates the results of cytogenetics, with high-risk cytogenetic abnormalities being more significantly associated with prognosis

{1514,4237,4416}. Therefore, multilineage dysplasia should be considered a possible indicator of high-risk cytogenetic abnormalities. In the absence of karyotype abnormalities diagnostic of AML-MRC or a history of MDS or MDS/MPN, investigation for mutation of *NPM1* and biallelic mutation of *CEBPA* is essential to exclude these specific AML disease groups that have a more favourable prognosis. In the absence of *CEBPA* double mutation or *NPM1* mutation, the detection of multilineage dysplasia still appears to confer a poor prognosis, although not as poor as the prognosis for cases with high-risk cytogenetic abnormalities {975, 3442,4276}. The increasing use of gene mutation panels may be of value in this group to evaluate for other gene mutations with prognostic significance. In one study, *ASXL1* mutations were reported in almost half of such cases, and they may be associated with a worse prognosis {963,964}.

Therapy-related myeloid neoplasms

Vardiman J.W.
Arber D.A.
Brunning R.D.
Larson R.A.

Matutes E.
Baumann I.
Kvasnicka H.M.

Definition

Therapy-related myeloid neoplasms (t-MNs) include therapy-related cases of acute myeloid leukaemia (t-AML), myelodysplastic syndromes (t-MDS), and myelodysplastic/myeloproliferative neoplasms (t-MDS/MPN) that occur as a late complication of cytotoxic chemotherapy and/or radiation therapy administered for a prior neoplastic or non-neoplastic disorder. Although cases may be diagnosed morphologically as t-MDS, t-MDS/MPN, or t-AML according to the number of blasts in the blood and/or bone marrow, these t-MNs are best considered together as a unique clinical syndrome distinguished by prior iatrogenic exposure to mutagenic agents {756,2221,3435, 3709}. Excluded from this category are progression of myeloproliferative neoplasms (MPNs) and evolution of primary MDS or primary MDS/MPN to AML (so-called 'secondary' AML); in each of these latter cases evolution to AML is part of the natural history of the primary disease and it may be impossible to distinguish natural progression from therapy-induced changes.

ICD-O code   9920/3

Synonyms

Therapy-related acute myeloid leukaemia, alkylating agent–related; therapy-related acute myeloid leukaemia, epipodophyllotoxin-related; therapy-related acute myeloid leukaemia, NOS

Epidemiology

t-MNs account for 10–20% of all cases of AML, MDS and MDS/MPN {1420,1976, 2757}. The incidence of t-MN among patients treated with cytotoxic agents varies depending on the underlying disease and the treatment strategy. Most patients have been treated for a previous malignancy; of these, recently reported data suggest that about 70% have been treated for a solid tumour and 30% for a haematological neoplasm, with breast cancer and non-Hodgkin lymphoma accounting for the largest numbers of cases, respectively, within these two subgroups. However, 5–20% of all cases of t-MN occur following therapy for a non-neoplastic disorder {1211,1976,2757}, and a similar proportion of cases occur following high-dose chemotherapy and autologous haematopoietic cell transplantation for a previously treated, non-myeloid neoplasm {367,756,1211,1976, 3709}. Any age group can be affected, but the risk associated with alkylating agents or radiation therapy generally increases with age, whereas the risk associated with topoisomerase II inhibitors is similar across all ages {3709}. The incidence increases with increasing age proportionate to the increased prevalence of cancer in older adults. As the number of cancer survivors increases due to improved outcomes for the primary malignancy, the incidence of t-MN is expected to increase.

Etiology

Therapy-related neoplasms are thought to be the consequence of mutation events or other changes in haematopoietic stem cells and/or the bone marrow microenvironment induced by cytotoxic therapy or via the selection of a myeloid clone with a mutator phenotype that has a markedly elevated risk for mutation events {367, 1813,2351,4360}. The fact that only a small proportion of patients treated with identical protocols develop t-MN suggests that some individuals may have a heritable predisposition due to mutations in DNA damage–sensing or repair genes (e.g. BRCA1/2 or TP53) or polymorphisms in genes that affect drug metabolism, drug transport or DNA-repair mechanisms {69,758,1489,2224,2356}. However, for most cases the underlying pathogenesis remains uncertain.

The cytotoxic agents commonly implicated in t-MN are listed in Table 8.05. Other therapies, such as hydroxycarbamide (hydroxyurea), radioisotopes, L-asparaginase, purine analogues and mycophenolate mofetil, have also been suggested to be leukaemogenic, but their primary role in t-MN, if any, is unclear. Adjunctive use of haematopoietic growth factors during chemotherapy reportedly increases the risk {756}. Characteristic clinical, morphological, and genetic features are often related to the therapy previously received, although the common use of multiple classes of agents concurrently and combined modality therapy (i.e. chemotherapy plus radiation therapy) result in overlapping features {1976,3709}.

Table 8.05 Cytotoxic agents implicated in therapy-related myeloid neoplasms

Alkylating agents
Melphalan, cyclophosphamide, nitrogen mustard, chlorambucil, busulfan, carboplatin, cisplatin, dacarbazine, procarbazine, carmustine, mitomycin C, thiotepa, lomustine

Ionizing radiation therapy[a]
Large fields containing active bone marrow

Topoisomerase II inhibitors[b]
Etoposide, teniposide, doxorubicin, daunorubicin, mitoxantrone, amsacrine, actinomycin

Others
Antimetabolites:
thiopurines, mycophenolate mofetil, fludarabine

Antitubulin agents (usually in combination with other agents):
vincristine, vinblastine, vindesine, paclitaxel, docetaxel

[a] The incidence of therapy-related acute myeloid leukaemia due to the genetic effects of modern limited-field radiation therapy is unknown {2824};
[b] Topoisomerase II inhibitors may also be associated with therapy-related lymphoblastic leukaemia.

Localization

The blood and bone marrow are the principal sites of involvement, but initial presentation as an extramedullary myeloid sarcoma has also been reported {369, 3122}.

Clinical features

Two subsets of t-MNs are generally recognized clinically {1976,2221,3119, 3435,3709}. The more common occurs 5–10 years after exposure to alkylating agents and/or ionizing radiation. These cases often present with an MDS with marrow failure and one or more cytopenias, although a minority present with t-MDS/MPN or overt t-AML. This subset is commonly associated with unbalanced loss of genetic material, often involving chromosomes 5 and/or 7, as well as complex karyotypes and mutations or loss of *TP53*. The second t-MN subset accounts for 20–30% of cases, has a shorter latent period (1–5 years), and follows treatment with agents that interact with DNA topoisomerase II (topoisomerase II inhibitors). Most cases in this subset do not have a myelodysplastic phase but present with overt acute leukaemia, often associated with a balanced chromosomal translocation. Although it may be useful to consider t-MN cases as being either alkylating agent/radiation–related or topoisomerase II inhibitor–related, many patients have received multiple types of therapy, and the boundaries between these two categories are therefore not always clear {1976}. Most cases of t-MN present within 10 years of the most recent exposure, and the origin of AML in cases with very long latent periods may be unrelated to therapy {1420}.

Microscopy

Most patients present with an MDS or

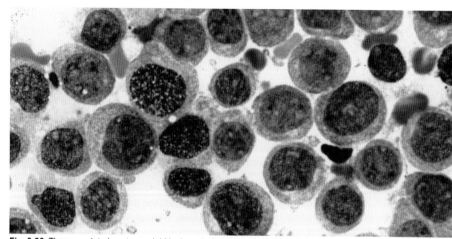

Fig. 8.22 Therapy-related acute myeloid leukaemia (t-AML) with t(9;11)(p21.3;q23.3). This patient developed t-AML < 1 year following initiation of therapy for osteosarcoma, which included both alkylating agents and topoisomerase II inhibitors.

acute leukaemia associated with multilineage dysplasia {130,2654,3709,4154, 4479}. There is commonly an elicited history of prior therapy with alkylating agents and/or radiation therapy, and cytogenetic studies often reveal abnormalities of chromosomes 5 and/or 7 or a complex karyotype, often associated with mutated *TP53* {2351,3253,3652}. The peripheral blood shows one or more cytopenias. Anaemia is almost always present and red blood cell morphology is usually characterized by macrocytosis and poikilocytosis. Dysplastic changes in the neutrophils include abnormal nuclear segmentation and hypogranular cytoplasm. Basophilia is frequently present. The bone marrow may be hypercellular, normocellular, or hypocellular, and reticulin fibrosis is common {852,2654}. Dysgranulopoiesis and dyserythropoiesis are usually present. Most cases show dysplastic megakaryocytes with nonlobated or hypolobated nuclei or widely separated nuclear lobes. Cases presenting with myelodysplasia and cytopenias

may be designated as t-MDS or t-AML depending on the blast percentage, but whether the percentage of blasts is prognostically significant in this group with MDS-related features is unclear {208, 1211,2124,3686,4479}. About half of the cases that present with a myelodysplastic phase have < 5% bone marrow blasts, but they often exhibit poor-risk cytogenetics {2654,3686}. The diagnosis of t-MDS, t-AML, or t-MDS/MPN should include the associated cytogenetic abnormalities.

In 20–30% of cases, the first manifestation of a t-MN is overt acute leukaemia without a preceding myelodysplastic phase {2654,3435,3709}. These cases often occur following topoisomerase II inhibitor therapy, and most are associated with recurrent balanced chromosomal translocations, which frequently involve 11q23.3 (*KMT2A*, previously called *MLL*) or 21q22.1 (*RUNX1*) and have a morphology resembling that of *de novo* acute leukaemia associated with these same chromosomal abnormalities, although a few such cases present as MDS or

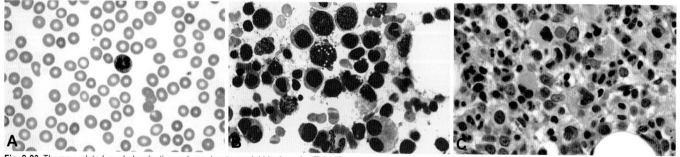

Fig. 8.23 Therapy-related myelodysplastic syndrome/acute myeloid leukaemia. This 42-year-old man was treated with ABVD chemotherapy (i.e. doxorubicin, bleomycin, vinblastine, and dacarbazine) for classic Hodgkin lymphoma, then relapsed 16 months later and was given salvage chemotherapy and radiotherapy; 2 years later, he presented with pancytopenia in the peripheral blood (**A**) and a bone marrow aspirate (**B**) and bone marrow biopsy (**C**) showed increased blasts and multilineage dysplasia. The karyotype was complex and included loss of chromosomes 5 and 7.

have myelodysplastic features as well {130,852,3435}. Many of these cases have monoblastic or myelomonocytic morphology, but cases morphologically and cytogenetically identical to those observed in any of the subtypes of *de novo* AML with recurrent cytogenetic abnormalities have been described, including therapy-related acute promyelocytic leukaemia with *PML-RARA*. Such cases should be designated t-AML with the appropriate cytogenetic abnormality; for example, t-AML with t(9;11)(p21.3;q23.3) {94,392,2223}.

Immunophenotype

There are no specific immunophenotypic findings in t-MN. Immunophenotyping studies of t-MNs reflect the heterogeneity of the underlying morphology and show changes similar to their *de novo* counterparts {130,2984}. Blasts are generally CD34 positive {2984} and express pan-myeloid antigens such as CD13, CD33, and MPO, although MPO expression has been reported to be downregulated in the neoplastic cells of some patients with t-MN {3252,4153}. The maturing myeloid cells may show patterns of antigen expression that differ from that seen in normal myeloid development, and there may be alterations in the light-scattering properties of maturing cells (in particular neutrophils) when studied by flow cytometry. Immunohistochemical staining of p53-positive cells in bone marrow biopsies has been demonstrated to correlate well with *TP53* mutations and with a poor prognosis {769,2983}.

Cell of origin

An abnormal haematopoietic stem cell

Genetic profile

The leukaemic cells of >90% of patients with t-MN show an abnormal karyotype {1211,2587,3435,3709}. The cytogenetic abnormalities often correlate with the latent period between the initial therapy and the onset of the leukaemic disorder, as well as with the particular cytotoxic agent(s). Approximately 70% of patients harbour unbalanced chromosomal aberrations, most commonly partial loss of 5q or t(5q), loss of chromosome 7, or a deletion of 7q. Loss of 5q is often associated with one or more additional chromosomal abnormalities in a complex karyotype, such as del(13q), del(20q), del(11q), del(3p), loss of 17p or chromosome 17, loss of chromosome 18 or 21, or gain of chromosome 8. As many as 80% of patients with del(5q) have mutations or loss of *TP53* as a result of abnormalities of 17p. These changes are usually associated with a long latent period, a preceding myelodysplastic phase or t-AML with myelodysplastic features, and alkylating agent and/or radiation therapy. The other 20–30% of patients have balanced translocations that involve rearrangements of 11q23.3, including t(9;11)(p21.3;q23.3) and t(11;19)(q23.3;p13.1); 21q22.1, as well as t(8;21)(q22;q22.1) and t(3;21) (q26.2;q22.1) and other abnormalities, such as t(15;17)(q24.1;q21.1) and inv(16) (p13.1q22). These translocations are generally associated with a short latent period, most often present as t-AML without a preceding myelodysplastic phase, and are associated with prior topoisomerase II inhibitor therapy or radiation therapy alone. A small proportion of patients with t-MN have an apparently normal karyotype. Mutation analyses have shown that mutations of *TP53* occur in as many as 50% of t-MN cases (substantially more commonly than in *de novo* AML or MDS) and are associated with worse survival. Other genes reported to be most frequently mutated are *TET2*, *PTPN11*, *IDH1/2*, *NRAS*, and *FLT3*, but their clinical significance, if any, is not yet clear {367,2958,3652,4360}.

Prognosis and predictive factors

The prognosis of t-MN is generally poor, although it is strongly influenced by the associated karyotypic abnormality as well as the comorbidity of the underlying malignancy or illness for which the cytotoxic therapy was administered {1211, 1976,3119,3709}. Overall 5-year survival rates of <10% are commonly reported. Cases associated with abnormalities of chromosomes 5 and/or 7, *TP53* mutations, and a complex karyotype have a particularly poor outcome, with a median survival time of <1 year, regardless of presentation as overt t-AML or as t-MDS {769,1211,1976,1995,3709}. Cases with balanced chromosomal translocations generally have a better prognosis; however, such cases, except those with t(15;17) and inv(16) or t(16;16), have shorter median survival times than do their de novo counterparts. Patients with therapy-related acute promyelocytic leukaemia (APL) with *PML-RARA* should be managed with the same degree of urgency as de novo APL. {94,2222,2223,3119}. Occasional cases assigned to the category of t-MN on the basis of the medical history may in fact constitute coincidental disease, and would consequently be expected to behave like *de novo* disease.

Acute myeloid leukaemia, NOS

Arber D.A.
Brunning R.D.
Orazi A.
Porwit A.

Peterson L.C.
Thiele J.
Le Beau M.M.
Hasserjian R.P.

Introduction

The category of acute myeloid leukaemia (AML), NOS, encompasses the cases that do not fulfil the criteria for inclusion in one of the previously described groups (i.e. AML with recurrent genetic abnormalities, myelodysplasia-related changes or therapy-related AML). With the possible exception of pure erythroid leukaemia, the subgroups of AML, NOS, are not prognostically significant {132, 3886} when AML with mutated *NPM1* and *CEBPA* are excluded {4233}. Most of the subgroups are nevertheless retained in this classification, because they define criteria for the diagnosis of AML across a diverse morphological spectrum and include the specific diagnostic criteria for pure erythroid leukaemia. Mutation analysis and cytogenetic studies are required before a case can be placed into this category, and such studies offer key prognostic information that appears to be independent of the morphological subtypes. Cytochemical studies are often useful in the subtyping of AML, NOS, but they are not considered essential for diagnosis, given the lack of prognostic significance of the subgroups.

The primary basis for subclassification within this category is the morphological and cytochemical/immunophenotypic features of the leukaemic cells, which indicate the major lineages involved and their degree of maturation. The defining criterion for AML is the presence of ≥20% myeloid blasts in the peripheral blood or bone marrow; the promonocytes in AML with monocytic differentiation are considered blast equivalents. The classification of pure erythroid leukaemia is unique and is based on the percentage of abnormal, immature erythroblasts; by definition, such cases cannot be classified as AML with myelodysplasia-related changes because they have <20% myeloid blasts, but they should be classified as therapy-related myeloid neoplasms or AML with recurrent genetic abnormalities if they fulfil the criteria for one of those entities. The previously recognized subtype of acute erythroid leukaemia termed erythro-leukaemia (erythroid/myeloid type), has been eliminated from AML, NOS; cases with myeloblasts accounting for <20% of total bone marrow and peripheral blood cells are now classified as myelodysplastic syndrome, whereas cases with ≥20% myeloblasts continue to be classified according to standard AML criteria.

It is recommended that the blast percentage in the bone marrow be determined from a 500-cell differential count using an appropriate Romanowsky stain (e.g. Wright-Giemsa stain). In the peripheral blood, the differential should include 200 leukocytes; if there is marked leukopenia, buffy coat films can be used. If an aspirate film is not obtainable due to bone marrow fibrosis and if the blasts express CD34, immunohistochemical detection of CD34 on biopsy sections may enable the diagnosis of AML if the 20% blast threshold is met. The major criteria required for this diagnosis are based on examination of bone marrow aspirates, peripheral blood smear, and bone marrow biopsy sections. The recommendations for classification apply only to specimens obtained prior to chemotherapy. Please note that the epidemiological data cited for each AML, NOS, subtype have been gathered from studies using the prior French–American–British (FAB) classification. The current limited use of the FAB diagnostic approach has prevented accrual of more recent epidemiological data for the morphological subtypes of AML, NOS.

ICD-O code   9861/3

Synonyms

Acute non-lymphocytic leukaemia; acute granulocytic leukaemia; acute myelogenous leukaemia; acute myelocytic leukaemia

Acute myeloid leukaemia with minimal differentiation

Definition

Acute myeloid leukaemia (AML) with minimal differentiation is an AML with no morphological or cytochemical evidence of myeloid differentiation. The myeloid nature of the blasts is demonstrated by immunological markers, which are essential for distinguishing this entity from lymphoblastic leukaemia. AML with minimal differentiation does not fulfil the criteria for inclusion in any of the previously described groups (i.e. AML with recurrent genetic abnormalities, AML with myelodysplasia-related changes, or therapy-related AML).

ICD-O code   9872/3

Synonyms

Acute myeloblastic leukaemia; French–American–British (FAB) classification M0

Epidemiology

AML with minimal differentiation accounts for <5% of AML cases. It can occur at

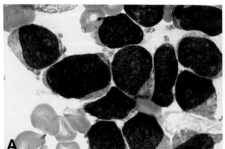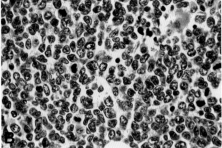

Fig. 8.24 Acute myeloid leukaemia with minimal differentiation. **A** Bone marrow smear shows blasts that vary in size, amount of cytoplasm, and prominence of nucleoli; there are no features of differentiation. **B** Bone marrow section shows that marrow is completely replaced by blasts with no features of differentiation.

any age, but most patients are either infants or older adults.

Clinical features
Patients present with evidence of bone marrow failure, with anaemia, thrombocytopenia, and neutropenia. Some patients present with leukocytosis and numerous circulating blasts.

Microscopy
The blasts are usually medium-sized, with dispersed nuclear chromatin and round or slightly indented nuclei with one or two nucleoli. The cytoplasm is agranular, with a variable degree of basophilia. Less frequently, the blasts are small, with more-condensed chromatin, inconspicuous nucleoli, and scant cytoplasm resembling that of lymphoblasts. Cytochemical staining for/with MPO, Sudan Black B, and naphthol AS-D chloroacetate esterase (CAE) is negative (i.e. < 3% of blasts are positive); alpha-naphthyl acetate esterase and alpha-naphthyl butyrate esterase are either negative or show a non-specific weak or focal reaction distinct from that of monocytic cells {330,1903,3430}. Sensitive ultrastructural studies may reveal MPO and CAE activity in small cytoplasmic granules, endoplasmic reticulum, the Golgi region, and/or nuclear membranes. In some unusual cases, there is a residual normal population of maturing neutrophils; these cases may resemble AML with maturation, but are distinguished by the absence of MPO or Sudan Black B positivity in the blasts and the absence of Auer rods. The bone marrow is usually markedly hypercellular, with poorly differentiated blasts.

Differential diagnosis
The differential diagnosis includes lymphoblastic leukaemia, acute megakaryoblastic leukaemia, mixed-phenotype acute leukaemia, acute undifferentiated leukaemia, and (more rarely), the leukaemic phase of large cell lymphoma. Immunophenotyping is essential for distinguishing these conditions.

Immunophenotype
Most cases express early haematopoietic-associated antigens (e.g. CD34, CD38, and HLA-DR) and lack antigens associated with myeloid and monocytic maturation, such as CD11b, CD15, CD14, and CD65. Blast cells express at least two myeloid-associated markers, usually CD13 and KIT (CD117), and approximately 60% of cases express CD33. CD38 and/or HLA-DR expression may be decreased. There are no signs of monocytic differentiation, such as coexpression of CD64 and CD36. Blasts are negative for the B-cell and T-cell cytoplasmic lymphoid markers cCD3, cCD79a, and cCD22. MPO is negative by cytochemistry, but may be positive in some blasts by flow cytometry or immunohistochemistry. Nuclear TdT is positive in approximately 50% of cases and has been suggested to be of favourable prognostic significance {3096}. CD7 expression has been reported in approximately 40% of cases, but expression of other lymphoid-associated membrane markers is rare. Expression of a single, relatively non-specific myeloid-associated antigen (e.g. CD13 or CD33), especially on only some blasts and along with other markers of primitive cells (e.g. CD7, CD34, and HLA-DR) is more typical of acute undifferentiated leukaemia than of AML with minimal differentiation.

Cell of origin
A haematopoietic stem cell

Genetic profile
No unique chromosomal abnormality has been identified in AML with minimal differentiation. The most common abnormalities reported are complex karyotypes and unbalanced abnormalities, such as del(5q) or t(5q), loss of chromosome 7 or del(7q), gain of chromosome 8, and del(11q), but the presence of some of these abnormalities would place the case in the category of AML with myelodysplasia-related changes. Mutations of *RUNX1* (also called *AML1*) occur in 27% of cases, and 16–22% of cases have *FLT3* mutations, but *de novo* cases with *RUNX1* mutations are now classified as the provisional entity of AML with mutated *RUNX1*.

Acute myeloid leukaemia without maturation

Definition
Acute myeloid leukaemia (AML) without maturation is characterized by a high percentage of bone marrow blasts without significant evidence of maturation to more mature neutrophils; maturing cells of the granulocytic lineage constitute < 10% of the nucleated bone marrow

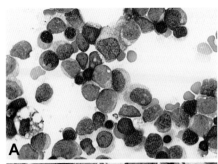
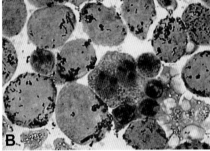

Fig. 8.25 Acute myeloid leukaemia without maturation. **A** On bone marrow smear, the cells are predominantly myeloblasts; occasional myeloblasts contain azurophilic granules or Auer rods; there is no evidence of maturation beyond the myeloblast stage. **B** MPO reaction reveals numerous myeloblasts with strong peroxidase reactivity; there are several peroxidase-negative erythroid precursors in the centre.

cells. The myeloid nature of the blasts is demonstrated by positivity for MPO or Sudan Black B staining (in ≥3% of blasts) and/or the presence of Auer rods. AML without maturation does not fulfil the criteria for inclusion in any of the previously described groups (i.e. AML with recurrent genetic abnormalities, AML with myelodysplasia-related changes, or therapy-related AML).

ICD-O code   9873/3

Synonym
French–American–British (FAB) classification M1

Epidemiology
AML without maturation accounts for 5–10% of AML cases. It can occur at any age, but most patients are adults; the median patient age is about 46 years.

Clinical features
Patients usually present with evidence of bone marrow failure, with anaemia, thrombocytopenia, and neutropenia. There may be leukocytosis with markedly increased blasts.

Microscopy

Some cases are characterized by myeloblasts with azurophilic granules and/or Auer rods. In other cases, the blasts resemble lymphoblasts and lack azurophilic granules. Bone marrow biopsy sections are usually markedly hypercellular, although normocellular or hypocellular cases also occur.

Cytochemistry

MPO and Sudan Black B positivity is present in a variable proportion of blasts, but always ≥3%.

Differential diagnosis

The differential diagnosis includes lymphoblastic leukaemia in cases with blast cells lacking granules or that have a low percentage of MPO-positive blasts, and AML with maturation in cases with a higher percentage of MPO-positive blasts.

Immunophenotype

AML without maturation usually presents with a population of blasts expressing MPO and one or more myeloid-associated antigens, such as CD13, CD33, and KIT (CD117). CD34 and HLA-DR are positive in approximately 70% of cases. There is generally no expression of markers associated with granulocytic maturation (e.g. CD15 and CD65) or monocytic markers (e.g. CD14 and CD64). CD11b is expressed in some cases. Blasts are negative for the B-cell and T-cell cytoplasmic lymphoid markers cCD3, cCD79a, and cCD22. CD7 is found in about 30% of cases, and expression of other lymphoid-associated membrane markers (e.g. CD2, CD4, CD19, and CD56) has been described in 10–20% of cases.

Cell of origin

The postulated cell or origin is a haematopoietic stem cell.

Genetic profile

There is no demonstrated association between AML without maturation and specific recurrent chromosomal abnormalities.

Acute myeloid leukaemia with maturation

Definition

Acute myeloid leukaemia (AML) with maturation is characterized by the presence of ≥20% blasts in the bone marrow or peripheral blood and evidence of maturation (with ≥10% of maturing cells of granulocytic lineage) in the bone marrow; cells of monocyte lineage constitute <20% of bone marrow cells. AML with maturation does not fulfil the criteria for inclusion in any of the previously described groups (i.e. AML with recurrent genetic abnormalities, AML with myelodysplasia-related changes, or therapy-related AML).

ICD-O code   9874/3

Synonym

French–American–British (FAB) classification M2, NOS

Epidemiology

AML with maturation accounts for approximately 10% of AML cases {132}. It occurs in all age groups; 20% of patients are aged <25 years and 40% are aged ≥60 years {3766}.

Clinical features

Patients often present with symptoms related to anaemia, thrombocytopenia, and neutropenia. The white blood cell count is variable, as is the number of blasts.

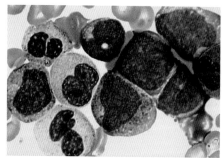

Fig. 8.26 Acute myeloid leukaemia with maturation. On bone marrow smear, in addition to the myeloblasts, there are several more-mature neutrophils; one has a pseudo–Pelger–Huët nucleus.

Microscopy

Blasts with and without azurophilic granulation are present. Auer rods are frequently present. Promyelocytes, myelocytes, and mature neutrophils constitute ≥10% of bone marrow cells; variable degrees of dysplasia are frequently present, but ≤50% of cells in two lineages are dysplastic. Eosinophil precursors are frequently increased, but do not exhibit the cytological or cytochemical abnormalities characteristic of the abnormal eosinophils in acute myelomonocytic leukaemia associated with inv(16)(p13.1q22) or t(16;16)(p13.1;q22). Basophils and/or mast cells are sometimes increased. Bone marrow biopsy sections usually show hypercellularity.

Differential diagnosis

The differential diagnosis includes myelodysplastic syndrome with excess blasts (for cases with a low blast percentage), AML without maturation (when the blast percentage is high), and acute myelomonocytic leukaemia (for cases with increased numbers of monocytes). AML with t(8;21)(q22;q22.1) usually has histological features of AML with maturation, but should be classified according to its genetic abnormality.

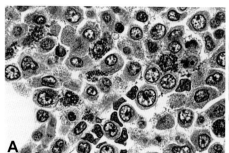
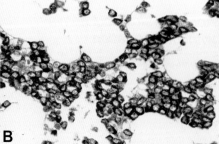
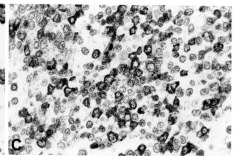

Fig. 8.27 Acute myeloid leukaemia with maturation. **A** Bone marrow biopsy reveals myeloblasts with abundant cytoplasm and azurophilic granules; occasional blasts contain an Auer rod and scattered eosinophils are present. There are numerous blasts with intense MPO activity (**B**) and lysozyme positivity (C).

Immunophenotype

Leukaemic blasts in AML with maturation usually express one or more of the myeloid-associated antigens CD13, CD33, CD65, CD11b, and CD15. Flow cytometric analysis reveals patterns associated with granulocytic differentiation. There is often expression of HLA-DR, CD34, and/or KIT (CD117), which may be present only in some blasts. Monocytic markers such as CD14, CD36, and CD64 are usually absent. CD7 is expressed in 20–30% of cases; expression of CD56, CD2, CD19, and CD4 is uncommon (seen in ~10% of cases) and may be found only in the most immature blasts.

Cell of origin

The postulated cell of origin is a haematopoietic stem cell.

Genetic profile

There is no demonstrated association between AML with maturation and specific recurrent chromosomal abnormalities.

Acute myelomonocytic leukaemia

Definition

Acute myelomonocytic leukaemia is an acute leukaemia characterized by the proliferation of both neutrophil and monocyte precursors. The peripheral blood or bone marrow has ≥20% blasts (including promonocytes); neutrophils and their precursors and monocytes and their precursors each constitute ≥20% of bone marrow cells. This conventional minimal limit of 20% monocytes and their precursors distinguishes acute myelomonocytic leukaemia from cases of acute myeloid leukaemia (AML) with or without maturation, in which some monocytes may be present. A high number of monocytic cells

may be present in the peripheral blood. Acute myelomonocytic leukaemia does not fulfil the criteria for inclusion in any of the previously described groups (i.e. AML with recurrent genetic abnormalities, AML with myelodysplasia-related changes, or therapy-related AML).

ICD-O code   9867/3

Synonym

French–American–British (FAB) classification M4

Epidemiology

Acute myelomonocytic leukaemia accounts for 5–10% of AML cases. It occurs in all age groups, but is more common in older individuals; the median patient age is 50 years. The male-to-female ratio is 1.4:1 {3766}.

Clinical features

Patients typically present with anaemia, thrombocytopenia, fever, and fatigue. The white blood cell count may be high, with numerous blasts and promonocytes.

Microscopy

The monoblasts are large cells with abundant cytoplasm that can be moderately to intensely basophilic and may show pseudopod formation. Scattered fine azurophilic granules, vacuoles, and Auer rods may be present. The monoblasts usually have round nuclei with delicate lacy chromatin and one or more large prominent nucleoli. Promonocytes have a more irregular and delicately convoluted nuclear configuration; the cytoplasm is usually less basophilic and sometimes more obviously granulated, with occasional large azurophilic granules and vacuoles. Monocytes and promonocytes are not always readily distinguishable from maturing myeloid cells in routinely

stained bone marrow smears; cytochemistry may be useful in such cases. The peripheral blood typically shows an increase in monocytes, which are often more mature than those in the bone marrow. The monocytic component may be more evident in the peripheral blood than in the bone marrow.

Cytochemistry

At least 3% of the blasts should show MPO positivity. The monoblasts, promonocytes, and monocytes are typically positive for non-specific esterase, although reactivity can be weak or absent in some cases. If the cells meet the morphological criteria for monocytes, absence of non-specific esterase does not exclude this diagnosis. Double staining for non-specific esterase and naphthol AS-D chloroacetate esterase (CAE) or MPO may reveal dual-positive cells.

Differential diagnosis

The major differential diagnoses include AML with maturation, acute monocytic leukaemia, and chronic myelomonocytic leukaemia. Distinction from the other AML types is based on the cytochemical findings and percentage of monocytic cells. The differential diagnosis with chronic myelomonocytic leukaemia is critical; it relies on the proper identification of blasts and promonocytes, which may be increased only in the bone marrow. In some cases, reliance on peripheral blood only may lead to a misdiagnosis of chronic myelomonocytic leukaemia instead of AML.

Immunophenotype

Acute myelomonocytic leukaemia generally shows several populations of blasts variably expressing the myeloid antigens CD13, CD33, CD65, and CD15. One of the blast populations is usually also posi-

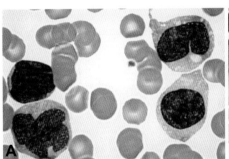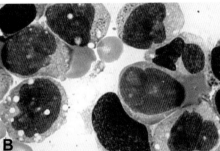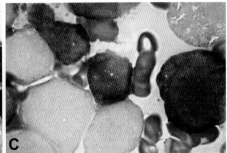

Fig. 8.28 Acute myelomonocytic leukaemia. **A** Blood smear shows a myeloblast, a monoblast, and promonocytes. **B** Bone marrow smear shows myeloblasts and several more-mature monocytes, including promonocytes. **C** Non-specific esterase reaction on a bone marrow smear reveals several positive cells; the non-reacting cells are predominantly myeloblasts and neutrophil precursors.

tive for some markers characteristic of monocytic differentiation, such as CD14, CD64, CD11b, CD11c, CD4, CD36, CD68 (PGM1), CD163, and lysozyme. Coexpression of CD15, CD36, and strong CD64 is characteristic of monocytic differentiation. There is often also a population of immature blasts that express CD34 and/or KIT (CD117). Most cases are positive for HLA-DR and approximately 30% for CD7; expression of other lymphoid-associated markers is rare.

Cell of origin
The postulated cell of origin is a haematopoietic stem cell.

Genetic profile
Myeloid-associated, non-specific cytogenetic abnormalities (e.g. gain of chromosome 8) are present in most cases.

Acute monoblastic and monocytic leukaemia

Definition
Acute monoblastic leukaemia and acute monocytic leukaemia are myeloid leukaemias in which the peripheral blood or bone marrow has ≥20% blasts (including promonocytes) and in which ≥80% of the leukaemic cells are of monocytic lineage, including monoblasts, promonocytes, and monocytes; a minor neutrophil component (<20%) may be present. Acute monoblastic leukaemia and acute monocytic leukaemia are distinguished by the relative proportions of monoblasts and promonocytes. In acute monoblastic leukaemia, most (≥80%) of the monocytic cells are monoblasts. In acute monocytic leukaemia, most of the monocytic cells are promonocytes or monocytes. Acute monoblastic and monocytic leukaemia does not fulfil the criteria for inclusion in

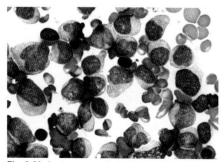

Fig. 8.29 Acute monocytic leukaemia. Bone marrow aspirate smears show a mixture of blasts and promyelocytes; most of the leukaemic cells are promonocytes.

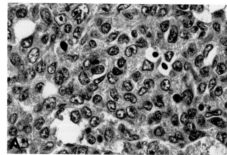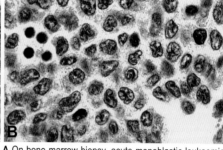

Fig. 8.30 Acute monoblastic and monocytic leukaemia. **A** On bone marrow biopsy, acute monoblastic leukaemia shows complete replacement of the marrow by a population of large blasts with abundant cytoplasm; the nuclei are generally round to oval; occasional nuclei are distorted. **B** On bone marrow section of acute monocytic leukaemia, the nuclear folds in the promonocytes are prominent.

any of the previously described groups; i.e. acute myeloid leukaemia (AML) with recurrent genetic abnormalities, AML with myelodysplasia-related changes, or therapy-related AML.

ICD-O code   9891/3

Synonyms
Acute monocytic leukaemia; acute monoblastic leukaemia; French–American–British (FAB) classification M5; monoblastic leukaemia, NOS

Epidemiology
Acute monoblastic leukaemia accounts for <5% of cases of AML. It can occur at any age, but is most common in young individuals. Extramedullary lesions can occur.
Acute monocytic leukaemia accounts for <5% of cases of AML. It is more common in adults; the median patient age is 49 years {3766}. The male-to-female ratio is 1.8:1.

Clinical features
Patients commonly present with bleeding disorders. Extramedullary masses, cutaneous and gingival infiltration, and CNS involvement are common.

Microscopy
The monoblasts are large cells with abundant cytoplasm that can be moderately to intensely basophilic and may show pseudopod formation. Scattered fine azurophilic granules and vacuoles may be present. The monoblasts usually have round nuclei with delicate lacy chromatin and one or more large prominent nucleoli. Promonocytes have a more irregular and delicately convoluted nuclear configuration; the cytoplasm is usually less basophilic and sometimes more

obviously granulated, with occasional large azurophilic granules and vacuoles. Auer rods are rare; when present, they are usually in cells identifiable as myeloblasts. Haemophagocytosis (erythrophagocytosis) may be observed and is often associated with t(8;16)(p11.2;p13.3) {972,1512,3768}. Haemophagocytosis with associated t(8;16)(p11.2;p13.3) may also be observed in acute myelomonocytic leukaemia and some cases of AML with maturation. The bone marrow in acute monoblastic leukaemia is usually hypercellular, with a predominant population of large, poorly differentiated blasts with abundant cytoplasm. Nucleoli may be prominent. The promonocytes in acute monocytic leukaemia show nuclear segmentation. The extramedullary lesion may be composed predominantly of monoblasts or promonocytes or an admixture of two cell types.

Cytochemistry
In most cases, the monoblasts and promonocytes show intense non-specific esterase activity. In as many as 10–20% of cases of acute monoblastic leukaemia, the non-specific esterase reaction is negative or only very weakly positive. In cases in which non-specific esterase is negative, immunophenotyping may be necessary for establishing monocytic differentiation. Monoblasts are typically MPO-negative; promonocytes may show some scattered MPO positivity.

Differential diagnosis
The major differential diagnoses of acute monoblastic leukaemia include AML without maturation, AML with minimal differentiation, AML with t(9;11)(p21.3;q23.3), and acute megakaryoblastic leukaemia. Extramedullary myeloid (monoblastic) sarcoma may be confused with malig-

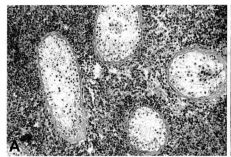
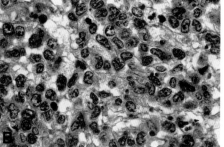

Fig. 8.31 Acute monocytic leukaemia, testicular infiltration. **A and B** The monocytic cells have relatively abundant cytoplasm and very dispersed chromatin.

nant lymphoma or soft tissue sarcomas. Occasional cases resemble prolymphocytic leukaemia; they are readily distinguished by immunophenotyping and cytochemistry. The major differential diagnoses of acute monocytic leukaemia include chronic myelomonocytic leukaemia, acute myelomonocytic leukaemia, and microgranular acute promyelocytic leukaemia. These can be distinguished by careful examination of well-stained smears. The differential diagnosis with chronic myelomonocytic leukaemia is critical; it relies on the proper identification of promonocytes and their inclusion as blast equivalents. The abnormal promyelocytes in acute promyelocytic leukaemia show intense MPO and naphthol AS-D chloroacetate esterase (CAE) positivity, whereas the monocytes are weakly reactive or negative.

Immunophenotype

Flow cytometry shows that these leukaemias variably express the myeloid antigens CD13, CD33 (often very bright), CD15, and CD65. There is generally expression of at least two markers characteristic of monocytic differentiation, such as CD14, CD4, CD11b, CD11c, CD64 (bright), CD68, CD36 (bright), and lysozyme. CD34 is positive in only 30% of cases, whereas KIT (CD117) is more often expressed. Most cases are positive for HLA-DR. MPO can be expressed in acute monocytic leukaemia and less often in monoblastic leukaemia. Aberrant expression of CD7 and/or CD56 is found in 25–40% of cases. By immunohistochemistry in paraffin-embedded bone marrow biopsy specimens and in extramedullary myeloid (monoblastic) sarcomas, MPO and CAE are typically negative but can be weakly positive. Lysozyme is often positive, but is also expressed in AML lacking monocytic differentiation. CD68 (PGM1) and CD163 are often positive.

Cell of origin

The postulated cell of origin is a haematopoietic stem cell.

Genetic profile

Myeloid-associated, non-specific cytogenetic abnormalities are present in most cases. The t(8;16)(p11.2;p13.3) can be associated with acute monocytic leukaemia or acute myelomonocytic leukaemia and in most cases is associated with haemophagocytosis (in particular erythrophagocytosis) by leukaemic cells and with coagulopathy {972,3768}.

Pure erythroid leukaemia

Definition

Pure erythroid leukaemia is a neoplastic proliferation of immature cells (undifferentiated or proerythroblastic in appearance) committed exclusively to the erythroid lineage (>80% of the bone marrow cells are erythroid, with ≥30% proerythroblasts), with no evidence of a significant myeloblastic component {2095,2281,2371}.

Cases previously classified as erythroleukaemia (erythroid/myeloid type) on the basis of counting myeloblasts as a percentage of non-erythroid cells when erythroid precursor cells constituted ≥50% of the marrow cells are now classified on the basis of the total bone marrow or peripheral blood blast cell count. Such cases are classified as myelodysplastic syndrome with excess blasts if blasts constitute <20% of all marrow or blood cells, and usually as acute myeloid leukaemia (AML) with myelodysplasia-related changes if blasts constitute ≥20% of the cells, irrespective of the erythroid precursor cell count.

ICD-O code   9840/3

Synonyms

Acute myeloid leukaemia, M6 type; acute erythroid leukaemia; erythroleukaemia; pure erythroid leukaemia (M6B); erythroleukaemia; French–American–British (FAB) classification M6; erythraemic myelosis, NOS; acute erythraemia; Di Guglielmo disease; acute erythraemic myelosis

Epidemiology

Pure erythroid leukaemia is extremely rare. It can occur at any age, including in childhood. It can occur de novo, but more often occurs as progression of a prior myelodysplastic syndrome or as therapy-related disease {2371,4247}. Therapy-related cases should be diagnosed as therapy-related myeloid neoplasms.

Clinical features

The clinical features are not unique, but profound anaemia and circulating erythroblasts are common.

Microscopy

Pure erythroid leukaemia is characterized by the presence of medium-sized to large erythroblasts, usually with round nuclei, fine chromatin, and one or more nucleoli (proerythroblasts); the cytoplasm is deeply basophilic and agranular and frequently contains vacuoles, which often give a positive periodic acid–Schiff (PAS) reaction. Occasionally, the blasts are smaller, with scanty cytoplasm, and can resemble the lymphoblasts of lymphoblastic leukaemia. The cells are negative for MPO and Sudan Black B staining; they show reactivity with alpha-naphthyl acetate esterase, acid phosphatase, and PAS (with PAS, usually in a block-like staining pattern). In bone marrow biopsy sections of pure erythroid leukaemia, the cells appear undifferentiated and

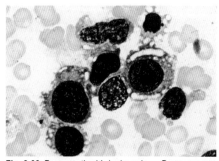

Fig. 8.32 Pure erythroid leukaemia. Bone marrow smear with numerous very immature erythroid precursors; these cells have cytoplasmic vacuoles, which occasionally coalesce.

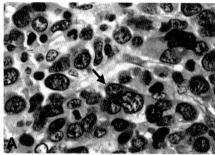

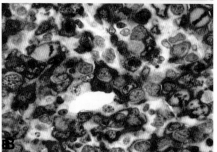

Fig. 8.33 Pure erythroid leukaemia. **A** Bone marrow section shows a predominant population of very immature erythroid precursors, some of which are multilobed (arrow). **B** The immature erythroid precursors and mitotic figures show positivity for glycophorin A.

are arranged in a sheet-like pattern. An intrasinusoidal growth pattern is seen in some cases {4247}. Due to haemodilution, erythroblasts may constitute <80% of the cells on an aspirate film; in such cases, the diagnosis of pure erythroid leukaemia can be made if the neoplastic erythroblasts occur in sheets and constitute >80% of the cells in the trephine biopsy sample {4247}. Proerythroblasts should constitute ≥30% of the cells in either the aspirate or the biopsy samples {2095}. Background dysmegakaryopoiesis is common, whereas dysgranulopoiesis is infrequent; ring sideroblasts are often present {2371}.

Differential diagnosis
Pure erythroid leukaemia without morphological evidence of erythroid maturation can be difficult to distinguish from other types of AML (in particular acute megakaryoblastic leukaemia). It can also be difficult to distinguish from lymphoblastic leukaemia, lymphoma, and (occasionally) metastatic tumours. Distinction from megakaryoblastic leukaemia is the most difficult; if the immunophenotype is characteristic of erythroid precursors, a diagnosis can be established, but some cases are ambiguous and there may be cases with concurrent erythroid and megakaryocytic differentiation {2942,4247}. Erythroid leukaemia with some morphological evidence of maturation must be distinguished from reactive erythroid hyperplasia, including hyperplasia secondary to erythroid growth factor administration or megaloblastic anaemia. Pure erythroid leukaemia should not be diagnosed as AML with myelodysplasia-related changes, even if there is a history of prior myeloid neoplasm, significant dysplasia of two lineages, or a defining cytogenetic abnormality: the diagnosis of AML with myelodysplasia-related changes requires ≥20% myeloblasts, whereas the neoplastic cells in pure erythroid leukaemia are erythroblasts.

Immunophenotype
The erythroblasts usually express glycophorin and haemoglobin A, as well as the less lineage-specific marker CD71. However, glycophorin and/or haemoglobin can be negative in the presence of poorly differentiated erythroblasts. E-cadherin, which stains early erythroid forms, is positive in the vast majority of cases and is specific for erythroid differentiation {2371,2942}. The blasts are often positive for KIT (CD117) and usually negative for HLA-DR and CD34. CD36 is positive in most cases, but is not specific for erythroblasts and can be expressed by monocytes and megakaryocytes.

Antigens associated with megakaryocytes (i.e. CD41 and CD61) are typically negative, but may be partially expressed in some cases.

Cell of origin
The postulated cell of origin is a haematopoietic stem cell.

Genetic profile
No specific chromosome abnormality is described in this type of AML. Complex karyotypes with multiple structural abnormalities are present in almost all cases, with del(5q) or t(5q), and loss of chromosome 7 / del(7q), being most common {2281,2371}.

Prognosis and predictive factors
Pure erythroid leukaemia is usually associated with a rapid clinical course; the median survival is only 3 months {2371}.

Acute megakaryoblastic leukaemia

Definition
Acute megakaryoblastic leukaemia is an acute leukaemia with ≥20% blasts, of which ≥50% are of megakaryocyte lineage; however, this category excludes cases of acute myeloid leukaemia with myelodysplasia-related changes (AML-MRC), therapy-related acute myeloid leukaemia (AML), and AML with recurrent genetic abnormalities, such as AML associated with t(1;22)(p13.3;q13.1), inv(3)(q21.3q26.2), or t(3;3)(q21.3;q26.2). Acute megakaryoblastic leukaemia occurring in a patient with Down syndrome should be classified as myeloid leukaemia associated with Down syndrome.

ICD-O code   9910/3

Synonyms
Megakaryocytic leukaemia; French–American–British (FAB) classification M7

Epidemiology
Acute megakaryoblastic leukaemia is an uncommon disease, accounting for <5% of cases of AML. It occurs in both adults and children.

Clinical features
Patients present with cytopenias (often thrombocytopenia), although some may have thrombocytosis. Dysplastic features

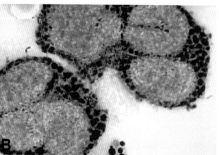

Fig. 8.34 Pure erythroid leukaemia. **A** Bone marrow smear shows four abnormal proerythroblasts; the erythroblasts are large, with finely dispersed chromatin, prominent nucleoli, and cytoplasmic vacuoles, some of which are coalescent. **B** The cytoplasm of the proerythroblasts shows intense globular periodic acid–Schiff (PAS) staining.

in the neutrophils, erythroid precursors, platelets, and megakaryocytes may be present, but the criteria for AML-MRC are not met. An association between acute megakaryoblastic leukaemia and mediastinal germ cell tumours has been observed in young adult males {2865}.

Microscopy

The megakaryoblasts are usually medium-sized to large blasts (12–18 μm) with a round, slightly irregular, or indented nucleus with fine reticular chromatin and 1–3 nucleoli. The cytoplasm is basophilic, often agranular, and may show distinct blebs or pseudopod formation. In some cases, the blasts are predominantly small with a high N:C ratio, resembling lymphoblasts; large and small blasts may be present in the same patient. Occasionally, the blasts occur in small clusters. Circulating micromegakaryocytes, megakaryoblast fragments, dysplastic large platelets, and hypogranular neutrophils may be present. Micromegakaryocytes should not be counted as blasts. In some patients, because of extensive bone marrow fibrosis resulting in so-called dry tap, the percentage of bone marrow blasts is estimated from the bone marrow biopsy. Imprints of the biopsy may also be useful. Although acute megakaryoblastic leukaemia can be associated with extensive fibrosis, this is not an invariable finding. The histopathology of the biopsy specimen varies; some cases have a uniform population of poorly differentiated blasts and others have a mixture of poorly differentiated blasts and maturing dysplastic megakaryocytes. Various degrees of reticulin fibrosis can be present.

Cytochemistry

Cytochemical staining with/for Sudan Black B, naphthol AS-D chloroacetate

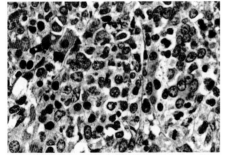

Fig. 8.35 Acute megakaryoblastic leukaemia. Bone marrow biopsy section showing virtually complete replacement by a population of blasts; one micromegakaryocyte can be seen.

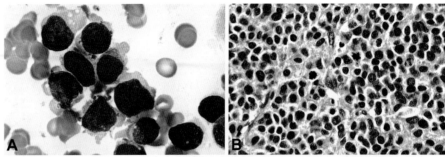

Fig. 8.36 Acute megakaryoblastic leukaemia. Bone marrow smear (**A**) and bone marrow section (**B**) from a 22-month-old child, with complete replacement by poorly differentiated blasts.

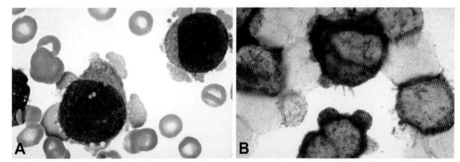

Fig. 8.37 Acute megakaryoblastic leukaemia **A** Bone marrow smear shows two megakaryoblasts, which are large cells with cytoplasmic pseudopod formation; portions of the cytoplasm are zoned, with granular basophilic areas and clear cytoplasm; nucleoli are unusually prominent. **B** The cytoplasm of the megakaryoblasts is intensely reactive with antibody to CD61 (platelet glycoprotein IIIa).

esterase (CAE), and MPO is consistently negative in the megakaryoblasts; the blasts may give a positive periodic acid–Schiff (PAS) reaction, show reactivity for acid phosphatase, and show punctate or focal non-specific esterase reactivity.

Differential diagnosis

The differential diagnosis includes minimally differentiated AML, AML-MRC, acute panmyelosis with myelofibrosis, lymphoblastic leukaemia, pure erythroid leukaemia, blastic transformation of chronic myeloid leukaemia, and the blast phase of any other myeloproliferative neoplasm. In blastic transformation of chronic myeloid leukaemia and the blast phase of any other myeloproliferative neoplasm, there is usually a history of a chronic phase, and splenomegaly is an almost invariable finding. Some metastatic tumours in the bone marrow, in particular in children (e.g. alveolar rhabdomyosarcoma), may resemble acute megakaryoblastic leukaemia. In general, acute megakaryoblastic leukaemia constitutes a proliferation predominantly of megakaryoblasts, whereas acute panmyelosis is characterized by a trilineage proliferation of granulocytes, megakaryocytes, and erythroid precursors. In some cases, the distinction between acute

megakaryoblastic leukaemia, acute panmyelosis with fibrosis, and AML-MRC can be problematic. In such cases, careful immunohistochemical analysis of bone marrow biopsy can be particularly helpful {2991}.

Immunophenotype

The megakaryoblasts express one or more of the platelet glycoproteins: CD41 (glycoprotein IIb/IIIa), CD61 (glycoprotein IIIa), and CD42b (glycoprotein Ib). The myeloid-associated markers CD13 and CD33 may be positive. CD34, the panleukocyte marker CD45, and HLA-DR are often negative, especially in children; CD36 is characteristically positive but not specific. Blasts are negative with MPO antibody and with other markers of granulocytic differentiation. Lymphoid markers and TdT are not expressed, but there may be aberrant expression of CD7. Cytoplasmic expression of CD41 or CD61 is more specific and sensitive than is surface staining, due to possible adherence of platelets to blast cells, which can be misinterpreted as positive staining on flow cytometry. In cases with fibrosis, immunophenotyping on bone marrow trephine biopsy sections is particularly important for diagnosis. Megakaryocytes (and in some cases megakaryoblasts)

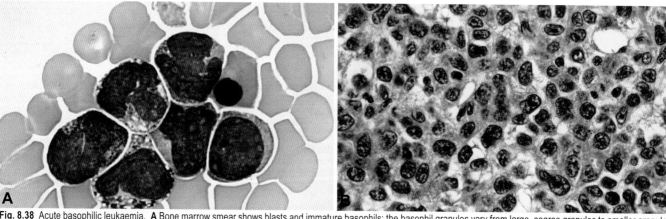

Fig. 8.38 Acute basophilic leukaemia. **A** Bone marrow smear shows blasts and immature basophils; the basophil granules vary from large, coarse granules to smaller granules. **B** Bone marrow trephine biopsy shows poorly differentiated blasts.

can be recognized by a positive reaction with antibodies to von Willebrand factor, the platelet glycoproteins (CD61 and CD42b), and linker for activation of T cells (LAT); the detection of platelet glycoproteins is most lineage-specific, but detection is highly dependent on the procedures used for fixation and decalcification.

Cell of origin
The postulated cell of origin is a haematopoietic stem cell.

Genetic profile
There is no unique chromosomal abnormality associated with acute megakaryoblastic leukaemia in adults. Complex karyotypes typical of myelodysplastic syndrome, inv(3)(q21.3q26.2), and t(3;3)(q21.3q26.2) can all be associated with megakaryoblastic/ megakaryocytic differentiation {873,2964}, but such cases should be assigned to other categories of AML (see *Acute myeloid leukaemia with recurrent genetic abnormalities*, p. 130).
In young males with mediastinal germ cell tumours and acute megakaryoblastic leukaemia, several cytogenetic abnormalities have been observed; of these, isochromosome 12p is particularly characteristic {633,2990}.

Prognosis and predictive factors
The prognosis of this category of acute megakaryoblastic leukaemia is usually poorer than that of other AML types, AML (megakaryoblastic) with t(1;22)(p13.3;q13.1) {1050,2964}, and acute megakaryoblastic leukaemia in Down syndrome.

Acute basophilic leukaemia

Definition
Acute basophilic leukaemia is an acute myeloid leukaemia (AML) in which the primary differentiation is to basophils. Acute basophilic leukaemia does not fulfil the criteria for inclusion in any of the previously described groups (i.e. AML with recurrent genetic abnormalities, AML with myelodysplasia-related changes, or therapy-related AML).

ICD-O code   9870/3

Synonym
Basophilic leukaemia (no longer used)

Epidemiology
Acute basophilic leukaemia is a very rare disease, with a relatively small number of reported cases. It accounts for < % of cases of AML.

Clinical features
As with other acute leukaemias, patients present with features related to bone marrow failure and may or may not have circulating blasts. Cutaneous involvement, organomegaly, lytic lesions, and symptoms related to hyperhistaminaemia may be present.

Microscopy
The circulating peripheral blood and bone marrow blasts are medium-sized, with a high N:C ratio; an oval, round, or irregular nucleus characterized by dispersed chromatin, and 1–3 prominent nucleoli. The cytoplasm is moderately basophilic and contains a variable number of coarse basophilic granules that are positive with metachromatic staining; there

may be vacuolation of the cytoplasm. Immature forms can be seen, but mature basophils are usually sparse. Dysplastic features in the erythroid precursors may be present. Electron microscopy shows that the granules have features characteristic of basophil precursors; they contain an electron-dense particulate substance, are internally bisected (e.g. have a theta character), or contain crystalline material arranged in a pattern of scrolls or lamellae (which is more typical of mast cells) {3148}. The most characteristic cytochemical reaction is metachromatic staining with toluidine blue. The blasts usually show a diffuse pattern of staining with acid phosphatase, and in some cases show periodic acid–Schiff (PAS) positivity in large blocks; the blasts are often negative for naphthol AS-D chloroacetate esterase (CAE), Sudan Black B staining, MPO, and non-specific esterase. The lack of CAE reactivity can be helpful in distinguishing blasts of acute basophilic leukaemia from mast cells {1360}. Bone marrow biopsy shows diffuse replacement by blast cells.

Differential diagnosis
The differential diagnosis includes the blast phase of a myeloproliferative neoplasm; other AML subtypes with basophilia, such as AML with t(6;9)(p23;q34.1); AML with *BCR-ABL1;* mast cell leukaemia; and (more rarely) a subtype of lymphoblastic leukaemia with prominent coarse granules. The clinical features and cytogenetic pattern distinguish cases presenting *de novo* from those resulting from transformation of chronic myeloid leukaemia and from other AML subtypes with basophilia. Immunological markers distinguish between

granular lymphoblastic leukaemia and acute basophilic leukaemia; cytochemistry and immunophenotyping distinguish acute basophilic leukaemia from other leukaemias.

Immunophenotype

Leukaemic blasts express myeloid markers such as CD13 and CD33; are usually positive for CD123, CD203c, and CD11b; and are negative for other monocytic markers and KIT (CD117) {3761}. Blasts may express CD34. Unlike normal basophils, they may be positive for HLA-DR but are negative for KIT. Immunophenotypic detection of abnormal mast cells expressing KIT, mast cell tryptase, and CD25 distinguishes mast cell leukaemia from acute basophilic leukaemia. Blasts usually express CD9. Some cases are positive for membrane CD22 and/or TdT. Other membrane and cytoplasmic lymphoid-associated markers are usually negative {2322,3762}.

Genetic profile

No consistent chromosomal abnormality has been identified, but a recurrent t(X;6)(p11.2;q23.3) resulting in *MYB-GATA1* appears to occur in male infants with acute basophilic leukaemia {872, 3260}. Other cytogenetic abnormalities reported in acute basophilic leukaemia include t(3;6)(q21;p21) and abnormalities involving 12p {1710,1711}. AML with t(6;9)(p23;q34.1) is specifically excluded, as are cases associated with *BCR-ABL1*.

Prognosis and predictive factors

There is little information on survival with this rare type of acute leukaemia. The cases observed have generally been associated with a poor prognosis.

Acute panmyelosis with myelofibrosis

Definition

Acute panmyelosis with myelofibrosis (APMF) is an acute panmyeloid proliferation with increased blasts (≥20% of cells in the bone marrow or peripheral blood) and accompanying fibrosis of the bone marrow {307,2991,3831}. APMF does not fulfil the criteria for inclusion in any of the previously described groups; i.e. acute myeloid leukaemia (AML) with recurrent genetic abnormalities, acute myeloid leukaemia with myelodysplasia-related

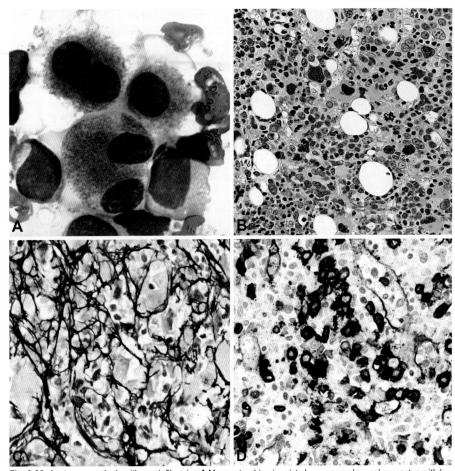

Fig. 8.39 Acute panmyelosis with myelofibrosis. **A** Marrow trephine imprint shows several megakaryocytes with hyposegmented nuclei and blast forms. **B** The marrow is markedly hypercellular, with increased fibrosis and a heterogeneous mixture of cells that include numerous dysplastic megakaryocytes. **C** Reticulin staining shows marked marrow fibrosis. **D** Immunohistochemistry for CD34 shows an increase in blast cells.

changes, or therapy-related acute myeloid leukaemia.

ICD-O code   9931/3

Synonyms

Acute panmyelosis, NOS; acute (malignant) myelofibrosis; acute (malignant) myelosclerosis, NOS; malignant myelosclerosis; acute myelofibrosis; acute myelosclerosis, NOS

Epidemiology

APMF is a very rare form of AML. It occurs *de novo* and is primarily a disease of adults, but has also been reported in children.

Clinical features

Patients are acutely sick at presentation, with severe constitutional symptoms including weakness and fatigue. Fever and bone pain are also common. Pancytopenia is always present. There is no or only minimal splenomegaly. The clinical evolution is usually rapidly progressive {3986}.

Microscopy

The peripheral blood shows pancytopenia, which is usually marked. The red blood cells show no or minimal anisopoikilocytosis and variable macrocytosis; rare erythroblasts can be seen, but teardrop-shaped cells (dacryocytes) are not observed. Occasional neutrophil precursors, including blasts, may be seen. Dysplastic changes in myeloid cells are frequent, but the criteria for AML with myelodysplasia-related changes are not met. Abnormal platelets may be noted. Bone marrow aspiration is frequently unsuccessful; either no bone marrow can be obtained or the specimen is suboptimal. Bone marrow biopsy supplemented with immunohistochemistry is required for diagnosis {3837,3986}. The bone marrow is hypercellular and shows, within a diffusely fibrotic stroma, increased erythroid precursors, increased granulocyte precursors, and increased megakaryocytes; i.e. there is panmyelosis, which is variable in terms of the relative proportion of each component. Characteristic findings include foci of blasts associated with conspicuously dysplastic megakaryocytes predominately of small size with eosinophilic cytoplasm showing variable degrees of cytological atypia, including the presence of hyposegmented or non-lobated nuclei with dispersed chromatin. Micromegakaryocytes may be present but should not be counted as blasts. The visibility of the small megakaryocytes may be improved with periodic acid–Schiff (PAS) staining and immunohistochemistry {3986}. The overall frequency of blasts in APMF marrows is variable; based on bone marrow biopsy, a median value of 22.5% was found in one study {2991}. Most cases have a range of 20–25%. The degree of marrow fibrosis is variable. In most patients, reticulin staining shows markedly increased fibrosis with coarse fibres; diffuse collagenous fibrosis is less common.

Differential diagnosis
The major differential diagnosis of APMF includes other types of AML with associated bone marrow fibrosis, including acute megakaryoblastic leukaemia {2991}. Usually less problematic is the distinction from primary myelofibrosis, post–polycythaemia vera myelofibrosis, post–essential thrombocythaemia myelofibrosis, and other neoplasms that can be encountered in a myelofibrotic bone marrow such as metastatic malignancies with a desmoplastic stromal reaction. It can be difficult to distinguish APMF from AML (especially cases with myelodysplasia-related changes and myelofibrosis) or acute megakaryoblastic leukaemia with myelofibrosis, particularly if no specimen suitable for cytogenetic analysis can be obtained.

If the proliferative process is predominantly of one cell type (i.e. myeloblasts) and there is associated myelofibrosis, the case should be classified as AML with a specific subtype (e.g. myelodysplasia-related) and designated with the qualifying phrase 'with myelofibrosis'. Acute megakaryoblastic leukaemia is associated with the presence of ≥20% blasts, of which ≥50% are megakaryoblasts. Usually they do not express CD34. In contrast, the blasts of APMF are myeloid and poorly differentiated, express CD34, do not express megakaryocytic markers, and are associated with a panmyelotic proliferative process that involves all of the major bone marrow cell lines {2991}.

Another difficult distinction is from cases of myelodysplastic syndrome (MDS) with excess blasts associated with marrow fibrosis, which can share most of the morphological findings seen in APMF. However, bone marrow biopsy supplemented by immunohistochemistry reveals more blasts in APMF than in MDS with excess blasts. Clinically, APMF can be distinguished from MDS by its more-abrupt onset with fever and bone pain. APMF is distinguished from primary myelofibrosis by its more numerous blast cells, and the megakaryocytes in primary myelofibrosis show distinctive cytological characteristics. The presence of a metastatic malignancy or (rarely) a lymphoid disorder can be excluded by studies with appropriate antibodies.

Immunophenotype
If the bone marrow specimen obtained for immunological markers is adequate or if circulating blasts are present, the cells show phenotypic heterogeneity, with varying degrees of expression of myeloid-associated antigens. The blasts usually express the progenitor/early precursor marker CD34 and one or more myeloid-associated antigens: CD13, CD33, and KIT (CD117) {2991,3837,3986}. MPO is usually negative in the blasts. In some

cases, some of the immature cells express erythroid antigens. Immunohistochemistry can facilitate determination of the relative proportions of the various myeloid components in the biopsy specimen, and is generally used to confirm the multilineage nature of the proliferation. This is usually done using a panel of antibodies that includes MPO, lysozyme, megakaryocytic markers (e.g. CD61, CD42b, CD41, and von Willebrand factor), and erythroid markers (e.g. CD71, glycophorin, and haemoglobin A). These confirm the presence of panmyelosis and allow exclusion of specific unilineage-predominant proliferations, such as acute megakaryoblastic leukaemia.

Cell of origin
The postulated cell of origin is a haematopoietic stem cell. The fibroblastic proliferation is secondary.

Genetic profile
If the specimen obtained for cytogenetic analysis is adequate, the results are usually abnormal. The presence of a complex karyotype, frequently involving chromosomes 5 and/or 7, such as del(5q) or t(5q), or loss of chromosome 7 or del(7q) {3986} should result in a diagnosis of AML with myelodysplasia-related changes, rather than acute panmyelosis, as should the presence of any other MDS-related cytogenetic abnormality.

Prognosis and predictive factors
The disease is usually associated with poor response to chemotherapy and survival times of only a few months {2991, 3837}.

Myeloid sarcoma

Pileri S.A.
Orazi A.
Falini B.

Definition

A myeloid sarcoma is a tumour mass consisting of myeloid blasts, with or without maturation, occurring at an anatomical site other than the bone marrow. Infiltration of any site of the body by myeloid blasts in a patient with leukaemia is not classified as myeloid sarcoma unless it presents with tumour masses in which the tissue architecture is effaced.

ICD-O code   9930/3

Synonyms

Granulocytic sarcoma; chloroma; extramedullary myeloid tumour

Epidemiology

There is a predilection for males and older individuals, with a male-to-female of 1.2:1 and a median patient age of 56 years (range: 1 month to 89 years) {1144,3177}. Myeloid sarcoma has been the subject of >2000 case reports indexed in PubMed, but only a few comprehensive studies have been conducted {60,238,1144, 2768,2846,3177,3423,4049,4424}, which reflects both the rarity of the neoplasm and the difficulties encountered in its treatment.

Etiology

The etiology of myeloid sarcoma is the same as that of acute myeloid leukaemia (AML) and other myeloid neoplasms, such as myelodysplastic syndrome (MDS) and myeloproliferative neoplasm (MPN). Although most cases of myeloid sarcoma occur as de novo neoplasms, some may be therapy-related.

Localization

Almost any site in the body can be involved; the most frequently affected are the skin, lymph nodes, gastrointestinal tract, bone, soft tissue, and testes {1144, 3177}. In < 10% of cases, myeloid sarcoma presents at multiple anatomical sites {1144,3177}.

Clinical features

Myeloid sarcoma occurs in the absence of an underlying AML or other myeloid neoplasm in about one quarter of cases; its detection should be considered equivalent of a diagnosis of AML. It may precede or coincide with AML or constitute acute blastic transformation of MDSs, myelodysplastic/myeloproliferative neoplasms (MDS/MPNs), or MPNs {1144, 3177}.

Isolated myeloid sarcoma occurs in 8–20% of patients who have undergone allogeneic stem cell transplantation {3177}; the reasons for this are unclear, but might be related to graft-versus-leukaemia surveillance or the biology of high-risk AML treated with transplantation.

Myeloid sarcoma can be the initial manifestation of relapse in a patient with previously diagnosed AML, regardless of blood or bone marrow findings {3177}.

Myeloid sarcoma can also be associated with a simultaneous or previously treated non-Hodgkin lymphoma (e.g. follicular lymphoma; mycosis fungoides; or peripheral T-cell lymphoma, NOS), or with a previous history of non-haematopoietic tumour (e.g. germ cell tumour, prostatic carcinoma, endometrial carcinoma, breast cancer, or intestinal adenocarcinoma) {3177}; in the setting of such a history, myeloid sarcoma might be secondary to prior chemotherapy {3177}.

Microscopy

Myeloid sarcoma most commonly consists of myeloblasts with or without features of promyelocytic or neutrophilic maturation. In a significant proportion of cases, it displays myelomonocytic or pure monoblastic morphology {1144, 3177}. Tumours predominantly composed of erythroid precursors or megakaryoblasts are rare and have been reported more often in conjunction with blast transformation of MPN {3177}. Architecturally, at extranodal sites neoplastic cells frequently mimic metastatic carcinoma by forming cohesive nests and/or single files surrounded by fibrotic septa. In the lymph node, they can either infiltrate the paracortex surrounding reactive follicles or grow diffusely, often extending into the perinodal fat.

Cytochemistry

On imprints, cytochemical stains for MPO, naphthol AS-D chloroacetate esterase (CAE), and non-specific esterase may enable differentiation of granulocytic-lineage forms (positive for MPO and CAE) and monoblastic forms (positive for non-specific esterase). In addition, CAE reaction can be applied to routine sections, although the results may depend on fixation and decalcifying agents.

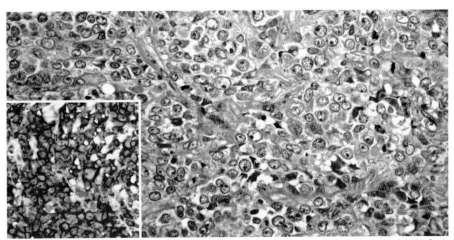

Fig. 8.40 Myeloid sarcoma. The tumour consists of blasts with scant cytoplasm and round-oval nuclei with finely dispersed chromatin and minute but distinct nucleoli. Mitotic figures are numerous. Neoplastic cells strongly express MPO (inset).

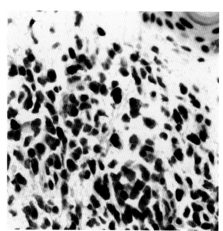

Fig. 8.41 Myeloid sarcoma. On skin biopsy with staining for NPM1, leukaemic cells infiltrating the derma show, in addition to the expected nuclear positivity, aberrant cytoplasmic expression of NPM1, which indicates the presence of *NPM1* mutation; cells of the overlying epidermis show a nuclear-restricted positivity for NPM1.

Differential diagnosis

The major differential diagnosis is with malignant lymphoma. The diagnosis of myeloid sarcoma is validated by the results of cytochemical and/or immunophenotypic analyses. These allow the distinction of myeloid sarcoma from B- and T-lymphoblastic leukaemia/lymphoma, Burkitt lymphoma, diffuse large B-cell lymphoma, small round cell tumours (in particular in children), and blastic plasmacytoid dendritic cell neoplasm {3177}. Myeloid sarcoma must be distinguished from non-effacing extramedullary blastic proliferations, which can occur in AML or in conjunction with acute transformation of MPN, MDS, or MDS/MPN, as well as from extramedullary haematopoiesis following the administration of growth factors that can produce pseudotumoural masses in virtually every part of the body {2915,3177}. Nodular accumulations of mature haematopoietic cells can occur in advanced-stage MPN. Although they may clinically mimic myeloid sarcoma, the often trilineage haematopoiesis and the lack of a significant blast component confirm a diagnosis of extramedullary haematopoiesis (myeloid metaplasia) and exclude myeloid sarcoma {3177, 3232}.

Immunophenotype

On immunohistochemistry in paraffin sections, tumours with a more immature myeloid profile express CD33, CD34, CD68 (KP1 but not PGM1), and KIT (CD117). Staining for TdT, MPO, and CD45 is inconsistent {1144,2039,3177,4424}. Promyelo-

cytic cases lack CD34 and TdT but express MPO and CD15. Myelomonocytic tumours are homogeneously positive for CD68/KP1, with MPO and CD68/PGM1 (or CD163) confined to distinct subpopulations, which are CD34-negative. The monoblastic variant expresses CD68/PGM1 and CD163 but lacks MPO and CD34. CD14 and KLF4 are also useful markers {2915}. The rare erythroid cases show strong positivity for glycophorin A and C, as well as haemoglobin and CD71. Megakaryoblastic myeloid sarcoma expresses CD61, linker for activation of T cells (LAT), and von Willebrand factor. CD99 staining is positive in more than half of all cases, with no association with a specific subtype. About 20% of myeloid sarcomas show variable degrees of CD56 expression, irrespective of their myeloid, myelomonocytic, or monoblastic profile. Foci of plasmacytoid dendritic cell differentiation (CD123+, CD303+, but CD56−) are occasionally detected, more often in cases with inv(16) {4424}. About 16% of tumours stain for NPM1 at the nuclear and cytoplasmic level; this indicates the presence of *NPM1* mutations {1144}. Exceptionally, aberrant antigenic expressions (cytokeratins, B-cell or T-cell markers, or CD30) are observed {2295, 3177}. Cases that meet the criteria for mixed-phenotype acute leukaemia are not classified as myeloid sarcoma. Flow cytometric analysis on cell suspensions reveals positivity for CD13, CD33, KIT, and MPO in tumours with myeloid differentiation, and for CD14, CD163, and CD11c in monoblastic tumours.

Postulated normal counterpart

A haematopoietic stem cell

Genetic profile

By FISH and/or cytogenetics, chromosomal aberrations are detected in about 55% of cases. They include monosomy 7; trisomy 8; *KMT2A* rearrangement; inv(16); trisomy 4; monosomy 16; loss of 16q, 5q, or 20q; and trisomy 11 {3177}. About 16% of cases carry NPM1 mutations, as evidenced by aberrant cytoplasmic *NPM1* expression {1144,1149}. Such cases frequently have myelomonocytic or monoblastic morphology, CD34 negativity, normal karyotype, and mutual exclusivity with MDS or MPN {1144,1149}. Interestingly, next-generation sequencing studies show a much higher (>50%) prevalence of *NPM1* mutations in AML

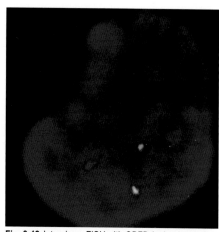

Fig. 8.42 Interphase FISH with *CBFB* dual-colour break-apart rearrangement probe shows splitting of the gene: one red and one green signal appear separately in the nucleus, and the normal *CBFB* allele appears as a fused red/green signal.

involving the skin, and 75% of these cases have monocytic features {2419}. The t(8;21)(q22;q22.1) observed in paediatric series seems to be less frequent in adulthood {516,3177,3596}. Inv(16) or amplification of *CBFB* has been linked to breast, uterus, or intestinal involvement and possible foci of plasmacytoid dendritic cell differentiation {60,2475,3177}. Trisomy 8 and *KMT2A-MLLT3* fusion seem to have a higher incidence in myeloid sarcoma involving the skin or breasts {60,3177,4373}. In one series, *FLT3* internal tandem duplication (*FLT3*-ITD) was observed in <15% of cases {111}.

Prognosis and predictive factors

Clinical behaviour and response to therapy do not seem to be influenced by age, sex, anatomical site(s) involved, type of presentation (with or without clinical history of AML, MDS, MDS/MPN, or MPN), therapy-relatedness, histological features, immunophenotype, or cytogenetic findings {3177}. Radiotherapy or surgery is sometimes used upfront in patients who need debulking or rapid symptom relief {238,4424}. Patients who undergo allogeneic or autologous bone marrow transplantation seem to have a higher probability of prolonged survival or cure {452,3177}; in one study, the 5-year overall survival rate among 51 patients with myeloid sarcoma treated with allogeneic bone marrow transplantation was 47% {706}.

Myeloid proliferations associated with Down syndrome

Arber D.A.
Baumann I.
Niemeyer C.M.
Brunning R.D.
Porwit A.

Individuals with Down syndrome have an increased risk of leukaemia {1229,4269}. This increased risk is variously estimated at 10- to 100-fold and extends into adulthood. The incidence ratio of lymphoblastic leukaemia to acute myeloid leukaemia (AML) in children aged <4 years with Down syndrome is 1.0:1.2, whereas the ratio in the same age group of children without Down syndrome is 4:1. There is an approximately 150-fold increase in AML in children aged <5 years with Down syndrome; acute megakaryoblastic leukaemia accounts for 70% of cases of AML in children aged <4 years with Down syndrome, versus only 3–6% in children without Down syndrome.

The acute megakaryoblastic leukaemia that occurs in children with Down syndrome has unique morphological, immunophenotypic, molecular genetic, and clinical characteristics that distinguish it from other forms of acute megakaryoblastic leukaemia, including *GATA1* mutations {1447,2216,2438,3437}. These features serve as the rationale for the recognition of this form of leukaemia as a distinct type in the WHO classification. In addition, approximately 10% of neonates with Down syndrome manifest a haematological disorder referred to as transient abnormal myelopoiesis (or transient myeloproliferative disorder), which may be morphologically indistinguishable from the predominant form of AML in children with Down syndrome {456,2544}. This disorder resolves spontaneously over

a period of several weeks to 3 months. In 20–30% of cases, non-remitting acute megakaryoblastic leukaemia subsequently develops within 1–3 years.

The aforementioned disorders, which occur in specific age groups in individuals with Down syndrome, have received the most attention, but other forms of acute leukaemia (both lymphoblastic leukaemia and AML) also affect individuals with Down syndrome. Such cases should not automatically be classified as myeloid leukaemia associated with Down syndrome; if they meet the diagnostic criteria for leukaemic disorders not associated with Down syndrome, they should be classified as such. The overall increased risk of leukaemia reported for individuals with Down syndrome applies for all types of leukaemias, not just those included in this category. To ensure that appropriate therapy is administered, the same approach for characterizing specific types of leukaemia (including careful morphological, immunophenotypic, cytogenetic, and molecular evaluation) must be used regardless of whether a patient has Down syndrome {4466}.

Transient abnormal myelopoiesis associated with Down syndrome

Definition
Transient abnormal myelopoiesis (TAM) associated with Down syndrome is a

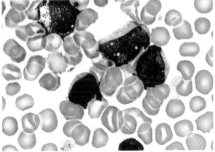

Fig. 8.43 Myeloid sarcoma. Transient abnormal myelopoiesis (TAM) associated with Down syndrome. Blood smear from a 1-day-old infant with Down syndrome and TAM; the peripheral blood contained 55% blasts; cytogenetic analysis showed trisomy 21 as the sole abnormality; the process resolved spontaneously over a period of 4 weeks.

unique disorder of newborns with Down syndrome that presents with clinical and morphological findings indistinguishable from those of acute myeloid leukaemia. The blasts have morphological and immunological features of megakaryocytic lineage.

ICD-O code   9898/1

Epidemiology
TAM is diagnosed in approximately 10% of newborns with Down syndrome, but the true incidence may be higher because a subset of patients are asymptomatic. It uncommonly occurs in phenotypically normal neonates with trisomy 21 mosaicism, and is extremely rare in neonates without chromosome 21 abnormalities {3441,3555}.

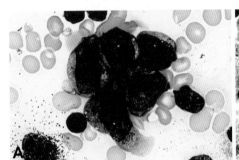
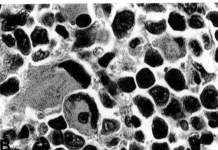
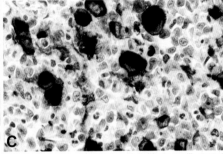

Fig. 8.44 Myeloid leukaemia associated with Down syndrome in a 2-year-old child. **A** The peripheral blood and bone marrow smears contained multiple blasts, as illustrated in this bone marrow smear; many of the blasts contained numerous coarse basophilic, coloured granules, which were MPO-negative; cytogenetic study showed trisomy 8 in addition to trisomy 21. **B** Bone marrow trephine biopsy from the same patient shows numerous blasts and occasional megakaryocytes, including one with a unilobed nucleus. **C** Numerous cells are immunohistochemically reactive for CD61, including obvious megakaryocytes and several smaller cells.

Clinical features

TAM associated with Down syndrome is usually diagnosed at the age of 3–7 days, but some patients are asymptomatic and diagnosed later {3437,3438}. At presentation, thrombocytopenia is most common; other cytopenias are less frequently encountered. There may be a marked leukocytosis and the percentage of blasts in the peripheral blood may exceed the blast percentage in the bone marrow. Hepatosplenomegaly is often present. Less common clinical features include jaundice, ascites, respiratory distress, bleeding, and pericardial or pleural effusions. Rarely, clinical complications include skin rash, cardiopulmonary failure, hyperviscosity, splenic necrosis, renal failure, hydrops fetalis, and progressive hepatic fibrosis {1009,3438}. In most patients, the process undergoes spontaneous remission within the first 3 months of life; a few children experience life-threatening or fatal clinical complications.

Microscopy

The morphological and immunophenotypic features of TAM are similar to those seen in most cases of acute myeloid leukaemia associated with Down syndrome {2363}. Peripheral blood and bone marrow blasts often have basophilic cytoplasm with coarse basophilic granules and cytoplasmic blebbing suggestive of megakaryoblasts. Some patients have peripheral blood basophilia; erythroid and megakaryocytic dysplasia is often present in the bone marrow {456}.

Immunophenotype

The blasts in TAM have a characteristic megakaryoblastic immunophenotype {441,1939,2217}. In most cases, they are positive for CD34, KIT (CD117), CD13, CD33, HLA-DR, CD4 (dim), CD41, CD42, CD110 (TPOR), IL3R, CD36, CD61, and CD71, often with aberrant expression of CD7 and CD56. The blasts are negative for MPO, CD15, CD14, CD11a, and glycophorin A. Immunohistochemistry with CD41, CD42b, and CD61 may be particularly useful for identifying blasts of megakaryocytic lineage in bone marrow biopsies.

Postulated normal counterpart

A haematopoietic stem cell

Genetic profile

In addition to trisomy 21, acquired *GATA1* mutations are present in blast cells of TAM {1447,1644,4222}. The mutation results in a truncated protein that appears to promote megakaryocytic proliferation {1923,4012}. Gene array studies have suggested differences in expression between myeloid leukaemia associated with Down syndrome and TAM {435, 2327,2596}, and mutation studies have shown acquisition of additional mutations in cases that progress to acute leukaemia {4434}.

Prognosis and predictive factors

Although the disorder is characterized by a high rate of spontaneous remission, non-transient acute myeloid leukaemia develops 1–3 years later in 20–30% of these children {4500}. Indications for chemotherapy in TAM are not firmly established, but treatment for life-threatening hepatic, renal, or cardiac failure is sometimes necessary {3438}.

Myeloid leukaemia associated with Down syndrome

Definition

Among individuals with Down syndrome, the incidence rate of acute leukaemia during the first 5 years of life is 50 times the rate among individuals without Down syndrome. In Down syndrome, most cases of acute myeloid leukaemia (AML) are acute megakaryoblastic leukaemia, which accounts for ≥50% of all cases of acute leukaemia in Down syndrome

beyond the neonatal period. AML often follows a prolonged myelodysplastic syndrome (MDS)-like phase {2216}. In individuals with Down syndrome, there are no biological differences between MDS and overt AML; therefore, a comparable diagnostic differentiation algorithm is not relevant and would have no prognostic or therapeutic implications. Because this type of disease is unique to children with Down syndrome, the term 'myeloid leukaemia associated with Down syndrome' encompasses both MDS and AML.

ICD-O code   9898/3

Synonym

Acute myeloid leukaemia associated with Down syndrome

Epidemiology

The vast majority of children with myeloid leukaemia associated with Down syndrome are aged <5 years. About 1–2% of children with Down syndrome develop AML during the first 5 years of life. Children with Down syndrome account for about 20% of all paediatric patients with AML/MDS {456,1009,1587}. Myeloid leukaemia associated with Down syndrome occurs in 20–30% of children with a history of transient abnormal myelopoiesis (TAM), and the leukaemia usually occurs 1–3 years after TAM.

Localization

The blood and bone marrow are the principal sites of involvement. Extramedullary involvement, mainly of the spleen and liver, is almost always present as well.

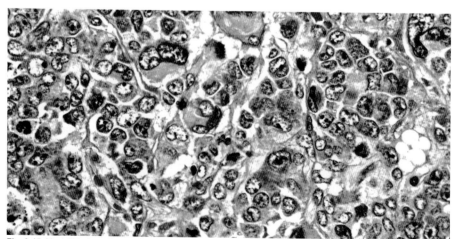

Fig. 8.45 Myeloid leukaemia associated with Down syndrome. Section of an abdominal lymph node from a child with Down syndrome and acute megakaryoblastic leukaemia; the node is completely replaced by blasts and occasional megakaryocytes, some of which are dysplastic.

Clinical features

The disorder manifests predominantly in the first 3 years of life. The clinical course in children with <20% blast cells in the bone marrow appears to be relatively indolent, initially presenting with a period of thrombocytopenia. A preleukaemic phase comparable to refractory cytopenia of childhood generally precedes MDS with excess blasts or overt leukaemia.

Microscopy

In the preleukaemic phase, which can last for several months, the disease has the features of refractory cytopenia of childhood lacking a significant increase of blasts. Erythroid cells are macrocytic. Dysplastic features may be more pronounced than in primary refractory cytopenia.

In cases of AML, blasts and occasionally erythroid precursors are usually present in the peripheral blood. Erythrocytes often show considerable anisopoikilocytosis, and dacryocytes can be observed. The platelet count is usually decreased, and giant platelets may be observed.

In the bone marrow aspirate, the morphology of the leukaemic blasts shows distinctive features, with round to slightly irregular nuclei and a moderate amount of basophilic cytoplasm; cytoplasmic blebs may be present. The cytoplasm of a variable number of blasts contains coarse granules resembling basophilic granules. The granules are generally MPO-negative. Erythroid precursors often show megaloblastic changes and dysplastic forms, including binucleated or trinucleated cells and nuclear fragments. Dysgranulopoiesis may be present.

The bone marrow core may show a dense network of reticulin fibres, making adequate bone marrow aspiration difficult or impossible. Erythropoiesis may be increased in cases with a low blast percentage, and decreases with disease progression. Maturing cells of neutrophil lineage are usually decreased. In cases with a dense blast cell infiltrate, rare dysplastic megakaryocytes may be seen. In other cases, megakaryocytes may be markedly increased, with clusters of dysplastic small forms and micromegakaryocytes.

Immunophenotype

Leukaemic blasts in acute megakaryocytic leukaemia associated with Down syndrome have an immunophenotype similar to that of blasts in TAM {1939, 2217}. In most cases, the blasts are positive for KIT (CD117), CD13, CD33, CD11b, CD7, CD4, CD42, CD110 (TPOR), IL3R, CD36, CD41, CD61, and CD71, and are negative for MPO, CD15, CD14, and glycophorin A {4243}. But unlike in TAM, CD34 is negative in 50% of cases, and approximately 30% of cases are negative for CD56 and CD41. Leukaemic blasts in other types of AML associated with Down syndrome have phenotypes corresponding to the particular AML category.

Antibodies to CD41, CD42b, and CD61 may be particularly useful for identifying cells of megakaryocytic lineage in immunohistochemical preparations.

Postulated normal counterpart

A haematopoietic stem cell

Genetic profile

In addition to trisomy 21, somatic mutations of the gene encoding the transcription factor GATA1 are considered pathognomonic of TAM associated with Down syndrome or MDS/AML-associated with Down syndrome {1447,1644,2438}. Children aged >5 years with myeloid leukaemia may not have GATA1 mutations, and such cases should be considered conventional MDS or AML. Trisomy 8 is a common cytogenetic abnormality in myeloid leukaemia associated with Down syndrome, occurring in 13–44% of patients {1587,1609}. Monosomy 7 is very rare in myeloid leukaemia associated with Down syndrome.

Although GATA1 mutations are present in both TAM and myeloid leukaemia associated with Down syndrome, myeloid leukaemias in this setting appear to arise from a GATA1-mutant TAM clone that has acquired additional mutations. Implicated additional mutations include mutations of CTCF, EZH2, KANSL1, JAK2, JAK3, MPL, SH2B3, and RAS pathway genes {1923,2895,3529,4434}.

Prognosis and predictive factors

The clinical outcome for young children with Down syndrome and myeloid leukaemia with GATA1 mutations is unique; these cases are associated with a better response to chemotherapy and a very favourable prognosis compared with that AML in children without Down syndrome {2216}. The children should be treated using Down syndrome–specific protocols. Myeloid leukaemia in older children with Down syndrome with GATA1 mutation has a poorer prognosis, comparable to that of AML in patients without Down syndrome {1287}.

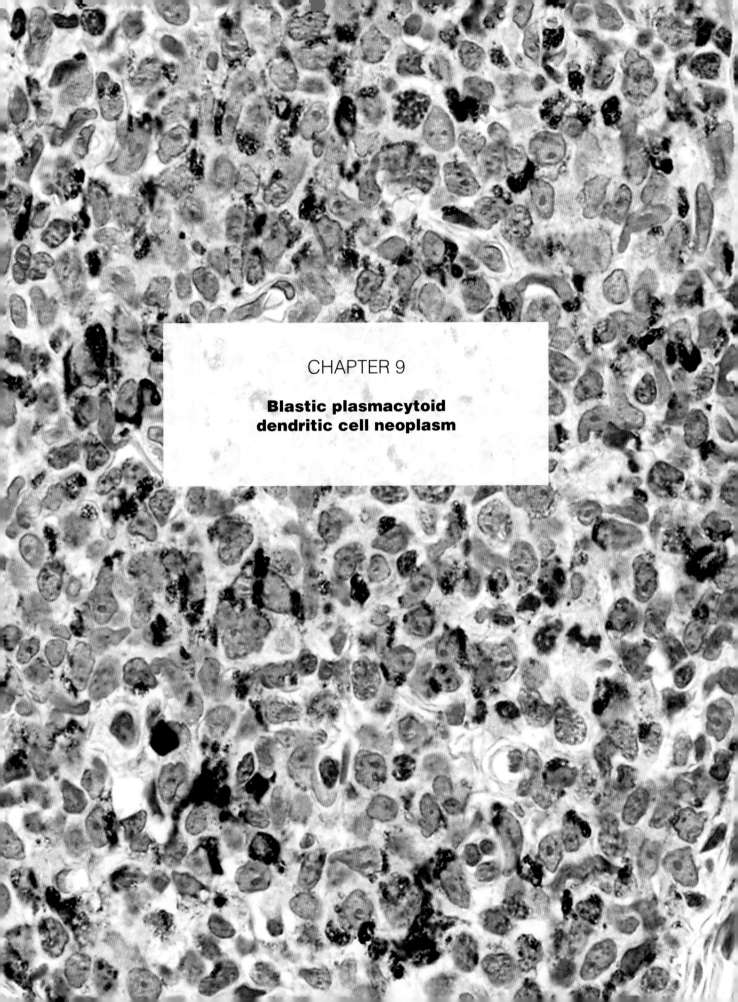

CHAPTER 9

Blastic plasmacytoid dendritic cell neoplasm

Blastic plasmacytoid dendritic cell neoplasm

Facchetti F.
Petrella T.
Pileri S.A.

Definition

Blastic plasmacytoid dendritic cell neoplasm (BPDCN) is a clinically aggressive tumour derived from the precursors of plasmacytoid dendritic cells (PDCs, also called professional type I interferon–producing cells or plasmacytoid monocytes), with a high frequency of cutaneous and bone marrow involvement and leukaemic dissemination.

ICD-O code   9727/3

Synonyms

Blastic NK-cell lymphoma (obsolete); agranular CD4+ NK leukaemia (obsolete); blastic NK leukaemia/lymphoma (obsolete); agranular CD4+ CD56+ haematodermic neoplasm/tumour

Epidemiology

This rare form of haematological neoplasm has no known racial or ethnic predilection. The male-to-female ratio is 3.3:1. Most patients are elderly, with a mean/median patient age at diagnosis of 61–67 years, but this neoplasm can occur at any age, including in children {1209,1812}.

Etiology

There are currently no clues to the etiology of BPDCN, but its association with myelodysplastic syndrome (MDS) in some cases may suggest a related pathogenesis. There is no association with EBV.

Localization

The disease tends to involve multiple sites, most commonly the skin (involved in 64–100% of cases), followed by the bone marrow and peripheral blood (in 60–90%) and lymph node (in 40–50%) {2525,3151}.

Clinical features

Skin manifestations are the most frequent clinical presentation of typical cases of BPDCN, and the diagnosis is made on skin biopsy. Patients usually present with asymptomatic solitary or multiple lesions. Three types of presentation are most commonly observed: an isolated (one or few) purplish nodule type (accounting for two thirds of cases), an isolated (one or few) bruise-like papule type, and a disseminated type with purplish nodules and/or papules and/or macules {820, 1887}. Isolated nodules are preferentially found on the head and lower limbs and can be > 10 cm in diameter. The isolated bruise-like papule type is clinically very challenging. The disseminated type is the most characteristic clinical presentation. In some patients lacking skin involvement and with leukaemic presentation, the diagnosis is made based on peripheral blood or bone marrow analyses. Regional lymphadenopathy at presentation is common (seen in 20% of cases). Peripheral blood and bone marrow involvement can be minimal at presentation, but invariably develops with progression of disease. Oral mucosal infiltration may be seen. Cytopenias (especially thrombocytopenia) can occur at diagnosis and in a minority of cases is severe, indicating bone marrow failure {1209}. Following initial response to chemotherapy, relapses invariably occur, involving skin alone or skin and other sites, including soft tissue and the CNS. In most cases, a fulminant leukaemic phase ultimately develops {1209}. About 10–20% of cases of BPDCN are associated with or develop into other myeloid neoplasms, most commonly chronic myelomonocytic leukaemia, but also MDS or acute myeloid leukaemia (AML) {1209,1618,2004,3151, 3332,4206}.

BPDCN must be distinguished from mature plasmacytoid dendritic cell proliferation (MPDCP), in which PDCs are morphologically mature and CD56-negative. This condition may be associated with cutaneous lesions (rash, macules

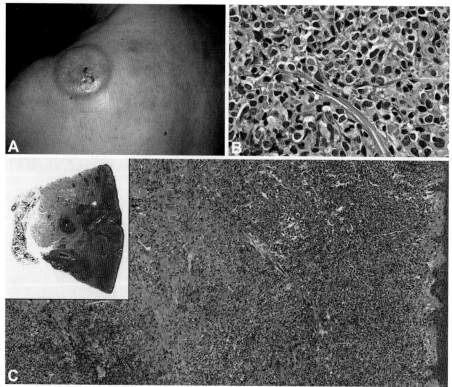

Fig. 9.01 Blastic plasmacytoid dendritic cell neoplasm. **A** Skin tumour and plaques. **B** The neoplastic cells are medium-sized, with fine chromatin and scanty cytoplasm, reminiscent of undifferentiated blasts. **C** Massive dermal infiltrate diffusely involves the dermis and extends into subcutaneous fat, but spares the epidermis.

or papules, and rarely nodules) together with lymph node and/or bone marrow infiltration. MPDCP is invariably associated with a myeloid disorder (most commonly chronic myelomonocytic leukaemia, MDS, or AML) {869,3155,4191,4206}.

Microscopy

BPDCN is characterized by a diffuse, monomorphous infiltrate of medium-sized blast cells resembling either lymphoblasts or myeloblasts. Nuclei have irregular contours, fine chromatin, and one to several small nucleoli. The cytoplasm is usually scant and appears greyish-blue and agranular on Giemsa staining. Mitoses are variable in number, and the Ki-67 proliferation index is 20–80%; angioinvasion and coagulative necrosis are absent {820,1887,2004,3182}.

In cutaneous infiltrates, the dermis is usually massively involved, with extension to the subcutaneous fat; the epidermis and adnexa are spared, with rare exceptions {820}. Lymph nodes are diffusely involved in the interfollicular areas and medulla, whereas B cell follicles are often spared. Bone marrow biopsy shows either a mild interstitial infiltrate (detectable only by immunophenotyping) or massive replacement; residual haematopoietic tissue may exhibit dysplastic features, especially in megakaryocytes {3151}. On peripheral blood and bone marrow smears, tumour cells may show cytoplasmic microvacuoles localized along the cell membrane and pseudopodia; granules and crystals are absent {1209}.

Cytochemistry

The neoplastic cells in BPDCN are negative with alpha-naphthyl butyrate esterase, naphthol AS-D chloroacetate esterase (CAE), and MPO cytochemical reactions {300,1209,2004,3332}.

Immunophenotype

The tumour cells express CD4, CD43, CD45RA, and CD56, as well as the PDC-associated antigens CD123 (IL3 alpha-chain receptor), CD303, TCL1A, CD2AP, and SPIB and the type I interferon–dependent molecule MX1 {107,406,1618, 1887,2497,2702,3151,3152,3157,3182, 3248,3332}. Recently, the TCF4 (E2-2) transcription factor, which is essential to drive PDCs development, was found to represent a faithful diagnostic marker for BPDCN {605B}. In about 8% of cases, CD4 or CD56 is negative, which

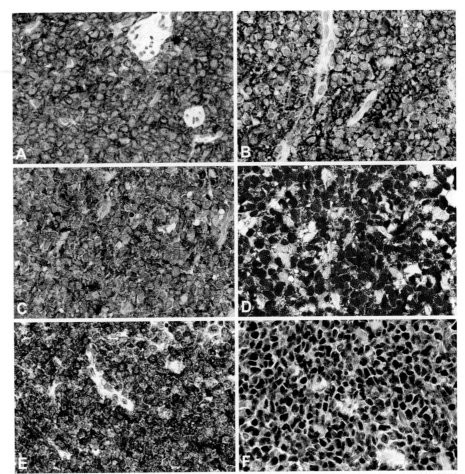

Fig. 9.02 Blastic plasmacytoid dendritic cell neoplasm. The neoplastic cells show immunoreactivity for CD4 (**A**), CD56 (**B**), CD123 (**C**), TCL1A (**D**), CD303 (**E**), BCL11A (**F**).

does not rule out the diagnosis if other PDC-associated antigens (in particular CD123, TCL1A, or CD303) are expressed {53,406,1887}. Tumours that have some immunophenotypic features of BPDCN may be better classified as one of the subtypes of acute leukaemia of ambiguous lineage. CD68 (an antigen typically expressed strongly on normal PDCs) is detected in 50–80% of cases, in the form of small cytoplasmic dots {3151, 3157}. Of the lymphoid and myeloid-associated antigens, CD7 and CD33 are relatively commonly expressed; some cases show expression of CD2, CD5, CD36, CD38, and CD79a, whereas CD3, CD13, CD16, CD19, CD20, linker for activation of T cells (LAT), lysozyme, and MPO are negative. Granzyme B, which is found in normal PDCs, has also been demonstrated on flow cytometry immunophenotyping and mRNA analysis in BPDCN {663,1410}, but it is typically negative on tissue sections, as are other cytotoxic molecules such as perforin

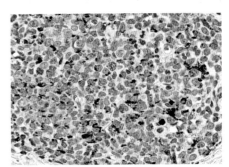

Fig 9.03 Blastic plasmacytoid dendritic cell neoplasm. The neoplastic cells show immunoreactivity for CD68 in the form of small perinuclear dots.

and TIA1. In addition to CD56, BPDCN may also express other antigens that are usually negative in normal PDCs, such as BCL6, IRF4, and BCL2 {820} (with BCL2 potentially acting against tumour cell apoptosis {3520}). In addition, S100 protein is expressed in 25–30% of all cases {1887}, and even more frequently in paediatric cases {1847,1849}; the zonal distribution of this antigen and its variable expression in tumour cells may reflect divergent subclones with maturation

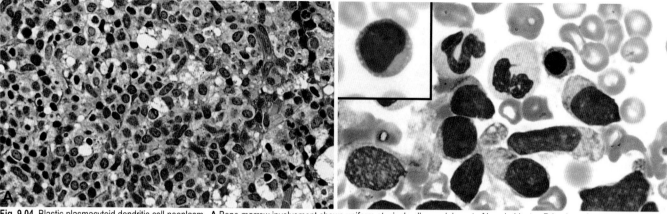

Fig. 9.04 Blastic plasmacytoid dendritic cell neoplasm. **A** Bone marrow involvement shows uniform atypical cells, reminiscent of lymphoblasts. **B** Leukaemic cells in bone marrow aspirate and blood (inset); the blasts show finely dispersed chromatin and abundant cytoplasm that contains microvacuoles (inset).

along the dendritic cell pathway {1847, 1887}. TdT is positive in about one third of cases, with expression in 10–80% of the cells {985,1887,2497,2546,3152,3153}. Occasional cases express KIT (CD117). CD34 is negative on sections {663,820, 1977,3151,3153,4065}, but has been found by flow immunophenotyping in 17% of cases, all invariably associated with other-lineage CD34+ blasts {2525}. EBV antigens and EBV-encoded small RNA (EBER) are negative.

The identification of BPDCN by flow cytometry benefits from gate and intensity evaluation criteria {663,1209,1303, 1410,4058,4065}. BPDCN is characterized by high levels of CD123 and weak expression of CD45 (blast gate); in addition, CD36, CD304, and LILRB4 (also called ILT3), but not CD141, are expressed {4058,4065}. The absence of lineage-associated antigens, together with positivity for CD4, CD45RA, CD56, and CD123, is considered a unique phenotype virtually pathognomonic of BPDCN {4058}; CD303 positivity has the highest diagnostic score within a panel of markers used for BPDCN identification {1303}. Subgroups of tumours may be identified on the basis of mutually exclusive expression of antigens, such as TdT/CD303 {1846}, TdT/S100 {1887}, and CD34/KIT/CD56 {2525}. These subgroups may correspond to diverse levels of maturation and may be associated with different clinical presentations {2525}, but their prognostic significance remains unclear. Among the antigens generally overexpressed by BPDCN blasts, CD123 could serve as a therapeutic target of engineered monoclonal antibodies {108,506, 1248,2877}.

Because other haematological neoplasms

can share morphological and immunophenotypic features with BPDCN (especially AML with monocytic differentiation, which can express CD4, CD56, and CD123 {987,3157,4206}), extensive immunohistochemical and/or genetic analysis is necessary before a definitive diagnosis of BPDCN can be made. BPDCNs must also be distinguished from MPDCPs associated with other myeloid neoplasms, which are predominantly found in lymph nodes, skin, and bone marrow. MPDCPs consist of nodules or irregular aggregates composed of cells morphologically similar to normal PDCs; these nodules can be very numerous, are sometimes confluent, and may show prominent apoptosis. The PDCs in these nodules generally have the same phenotype as their normal counterparts, although in occasional cases aberrant single or multiple antigen expression (e.g. of CD2, CD5, CD7, CD10, CD13, CD14, CD15, and/or CD33) has been reported {333,869,2497,4191,4206}. Most importantly, CD56 is negative in most cases, or shows only focal and weak reactivity {1130,4206}. The PDCs in MPDCP have a low Ki-67 proliferation index (< 10%) and lack TdT. Their neoplastic nature and relatedness with the associated myeloid neoplasm have been evidenced by the demonstration of identical clonal chromosomal abnormalities in the two cellular components {684,3177,4191}.

Cell of origin/normal counterpart

The cell of origin is a haematopoietic stem cell; the normal counterpart is the precursor of PDCs.
Data on antigen {663,664,1410,1618,1812, 1846,3152,3157} and chemokine receptor expression {329}, in vitro functional

assays {329,664}, gene expression profiling {987,3520}, and the tumour-derived cell lines {2437,2828} all point towards derivation from the precursors of a special subset of dendritic cells: PDCs {597, 1476,3739}. In humans, these cells are distinguished by their production of large amounts of type I interferon {598}; they have been known by many names, such as lymphoblasts, T-cell–associated plasma cells, plasmacytoid T cells, and plasmacytoid monocytes {1129}.

Recent gene expression profiling studies have revealed that the neoplastic cells show a gene expression signature similar to that of resting normal PDCs and closer to that of myeloid than of lymphoid precursors {3520}. The immunophenotypic heterogeneity with regard to TdT and the association with myeloid disorders suggest a multilineage potential for some cases.

Furthermore, recent data obtained by TCF4 (E2-2) ChIP-seq data and gene expression changes following TCF4 knockdown revealed the similarity between normal PDCs, BPDCN cell lines and primary BPDCN, distinguishing BPDCN from AML lines {605B}.

Genetic profile

T-cell and B-cell receptor gene mutations are usually germline {3151,3332}, except in a few cases that show T-cell receptor gamma rearrangement, possibly due to clonal bystander T cells {53,3151}. Two thirds of patients with BPDCN have an abnormal karyotype. Specific chromosomal aberrations are lacking, but complex karyotypes are common; six major recurrent chromosomal abnormalities have been recognized, involving 5q21 or 5q34 (seen in 72% of cases), 12p13 (in 64%), 13q13-21 (in 64%), 6q23-qter (in 50%), 15q (in 43%), and loss of chromosome 9 (in 28%) {2278,3153,3332}. Genomic abnormalities mainly involve tumour suppressor genes or genes related to the G1/S transition {53,987, 1840,2278,3153,3332,4312}; the most recurrent being deletions of CDKN2A {2409,3795}. Array-based comparative genomic hybridization shows recurrent deletions of regions on chromosomes 4 (4q34), 9 (9p11-p13 and 9q12-q34), and 13 (13q12-q31), with diminished expression of tumour suppressor genes (RB1, LATS2), whereas elevated expression of the products of the oncogenes HES6, RUNX2, and FLT3 is not associated with genomic amplification {987}.

Gene expression analysis of BPDCN reveals a unique signature, distinct from those of myeloid and lymphoid acute leukaemias {987,3520}; this proves that BPDCN originates from the myeloid lineage; in particular, from resting PDCs {3520}. Compared with normal PDCs, BPDCN shows increased expression of genes involved in Notch signalling {987} and BCL2, as well as aberrant activation of the NF-kappaB pathway, which is a potential therapeutic target {3520}.

TET2 is the most commonly mutated gene in BPDCN {53,1840,2629}, suggesting that it may play a role in tumour pathogenesis. Conflicting data on NPM1 mutations have been obtained; the mutations were absent in two series of BPDCN {1128,3795} and present in 20% of cases in another series {2629}, although the finding of their presence requires further confirmation and functional validation. In one study, recurrent somatic mutations were detected in ASXL1, the RAS family of genes, and the newly identified genes IKZF3 and ZEB2; in addition, somatic mutations affecting genes involved in DNA methylation and chromatin remodelling were detected in half of all cases {2629}. Importantly, the same mutations have been previously observed in MDS and AML, further supporting the myeloid nature of BPDCN. More recently, targeted ultra-deep sequencing has revealed mutations in NRAS (present in 27.3% of cases); ATM (in 21.2%); MET, KRAS, IDH2, and KIT (in 9.1% each); APC and RB1 (in 6.1% each); and VHL, BRAF, MLH1, TP53, and RET (in 3% each) {3795}.

Prognosis and predictive factors

The clinical course is aggressive, with a median survival of 10.0–19.8 months, irrespective of the initial pattern of disease. Most cases (80–90%) show an initial response to multiagent chemotherapy, but relapses with subsequent resistance to drugs are regularly observed {820,1812, 1888,3026,3151}.

Age has an adverse impact on prognosis {315,3839}, and long-term survival has been reported in 36% of paediatric patients {1847}. Among biological parameters, high marrow or peripheral blood blastosis {3839}, low TdT expression {1846,3839}, positivity for CD303 (also called CLEC4C or BDCA2) {1846}, low Ki-67 proliferation index {1887}, CDKN2A/B deletions {2409}, and mutations in DNA methylation pathway genes {2629} have been associated with shorter survival. Lymphoblastic leukaemia–oriented induction treatment seemed to be more effective than AML-oriented therapy in both children {1847} and adults {3026}, which might be due to the deregulation of several genes in common with lymphoblastic leukaemia, resulting in higher sensitivity to drugs included in lymphoma/lymphoblastic leukaemia–tailored regimens {3520}. In patients in first complete remission, allogeneic haematopoietic stem cell transplantation has been recommended as the best way to achieve long-term survival {861,1604,3400}, even in elderly patients (with reduced-intensity conditioning) {984}.

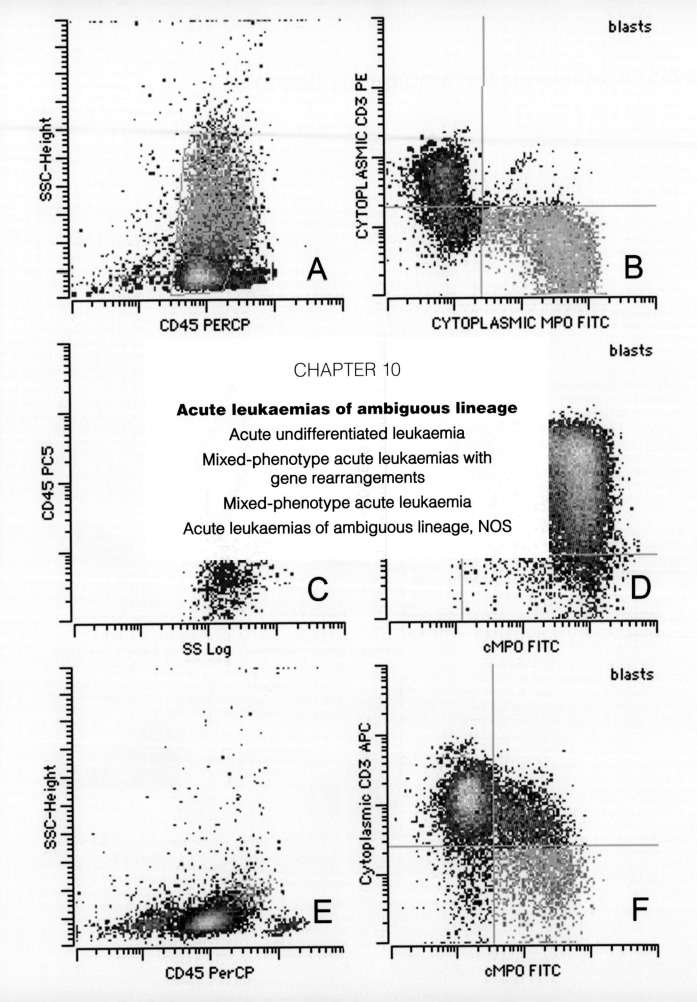

CHAPTER 10

Acute leukaemias of ambiguous lineage

Acute undifferentiated leukaemia

Mixed-phenotype acute leukaemias with gene rearrangements

Mixed-phenotype acute leukaemia

Acute leukaemias of ambiguous lineage, NOS

Acute leukaemias of ambiguous lineage

Borowitz M.J.
Béné M.-C.
Harris N.L.
Porwit A.
Matutes E.
Arber D.A.

Definition

Acute leukaemias of ambiguous lineage are leukaemias that show no clear evidence of differentiation along a single lineage. They include acute undifferentiated leukaemias, which show no lineage-specific antigens, and mixed-phenotype acute leukaemias (MPALs), which have blasts that express antigens of more than one lineage to such a degree that it is not possible to assign the leukaemia to any one lineage with certainty. MPALs can contain distinct blast populations each of a different lineage, one population with multiple antigens of different lineages on the same cells, or a combination. The ambiguity of antigen expression most often involves myeloid antigens coexisting with either T-cell or B-cell antigens, but rare cases of ambiguity of assignment between B-cell and T-cell lineages also occur. Leukaemia with well-defined lineage engagement but expressing one or more antigens associated with a different lineage should be considered acute leukaemia with aberrant antigen expression rather than MPAL.

Epidemiology

Ambiguous-lineage leukaemias are rare, accounting for <4% of all acute leukaemia cases. Many cases that have been reported as undifferentiated leukaemia can in fact be demonstrated to be leukaemias of unusual lineages, and many cases that have been reported as biphenotypic acute leukaemias may in fact be acute lymphoid or myeloid leukaemias with cross-lineage antigen expression; therefore, the true frequency of ambiguous-lineage leukaemias may be even lower than reported. These leukaemias occur in both children and adults, but more frequently in adults, although some subtypes of MPAL may be more common in children {2013,3013}.

Terminology

Historically, there has been confusion regarding the terminology and definitions of all ambiguous-lineage leukaemias and in particular the MPALs. The term 'acute bilineage (or bilineal) leukaemia' has been applied to MPALs containing separate populations of blasts of more than one lineage. The term 'biphenotypic leukaemia' has typically been reserved for MPALs containing a single population of blasts coexpressing antigens of more than one lineage {1539,2257,2578,3830}, but is sometimes used more broadly to also encompass bilineage leukaemias.

In this volume, the term 'mixed-phenotype acute leukaemia' is applied to this group in general; the more specific terms 'B/myeloid leukaemia' and 'T/myeloid leukaemia', as defined below, refer to leukaemias containing the two lineages specified, irrespective of whether one or more than one population of blasts is seen.

Some well-defined myeloid leukaemia entities have immunophenotypic features that might suggest that they be classified as B/myeloid or T/myeloid leukaemia. However, the MPAL group, as defined in this volume, excludes cases that can be classified (either by genetic or clinical features) in another category, such as cases with the recurrent genetic abnormalities t(8;21), inv(16), or *PML-RARA* fusion, which are associated with acute myeloid leukaemia (AML); cases with t(8;21) express multiple B-cell markers

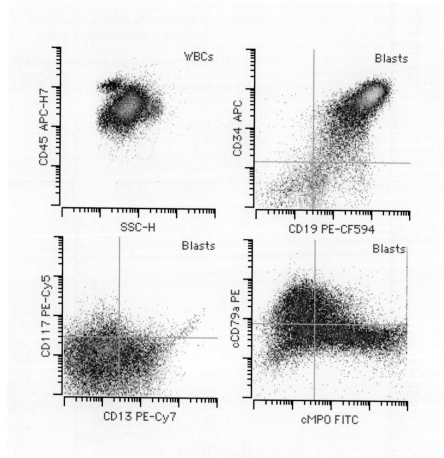

Fig. 10.01 B/myeloid mixed-phenotype acute leukaemia. Flow cytometry reveals a dominant, relatively homogeneous blast population (red) with bright CD34 and CD19, and little to no expression of myeloid antigens CD117 and CD13. The CD79a vs MPO plot is more heterogeneous, with the brighter CD79a (i.e. more lymphoid) population expressing little or no MPO, and the MPO-positive cells lacking CD79a. Courtesy Dr B. Wood.

especially frequently {3996}. Cases of leukaemia with *FGFR1* rearrangements are not considered to be T/myeloid leukaemias either. All cases of chronic myeloid leukaemia in blast crisis, AML with myelodysplasia-related changes, and therapy-related AML should be classified primarily as such, with a secondary notation that they have a mixed phenotype if applicable.

General approach to diagnosis

The diagnosis of ambiguous-lineage leukaemias relies on immunophenotyping. Flow cytometry is the preferred method for establishing the diagnosis, especially when a diagnosis of MPAL requires demonstrating coexpression of lymphoid and myeloid differentiation antigens on the same cell. Cases in which the diagnosis requires demonstration of two distinct leukaemic populations with different phenotypes can also be established by immunohistochemistry in tissue sections, or with cytochemical stains for MPO on smears coupled with flow cytometry to detect a leukaemic B-cell or T-cell lymphoid population. The hallmark of MPAL is that the combination of antigens expressed on the blast population or populations does not allow classification into a single lineage. There are several scenarios in which this can occur.

In the most straightforward scenario, there are two (or more) distinct populations of leukaemic cells: one (or more) of which would independently fulfil the immunophenotypic criteria for AML and one (or more) the criteria for T- and/or B-lymphoblastic leukaemia (ALL); the specific antigens associated with these diagnoses are described in the respective sections devoted to these diseases. However, although abnormal blasts must constitute ≥20% of all nucleated cells overall, this need not be true of each distinct population. Cases like these would previously have been considered bilineage leukaemia.

In the second scenario, there is a dominant single population of blasts that expresses combinations of antigens that alone would be considered specific for more than one lineage. There are also hybrid cases in which this dominant population is accompanied by one or more minor populations with a different immunophenotype. In this setting, the criteria for classifying a leukaemia are more stringent (Table 10.01), and there

Table 10.01 Requirements for assigning more than one lineage to a single blast population.

Myeloid lineage
MPO (by flow cytometry, immunohistochemistry, or cytochemistry)
or
Monocytic differentiation (≥ 2 of the following: non-specific esterase, CD11c, CD14, CD64, lysozyme)
T-cell lineage
Cytoplasmic CD3 (by flow cytometry with antibodies to CD3 epsilon chain. Immunohistochemistry using polyclonal anti-CD3 antibody may detect CD3 zeta chain, which is not T-cell–specific)
or
Surface CD3 (rare in mixed-phenotype acute leukaemias)
B-cell lineage (multiple antigens required)
Strong CD19 with ≥ 1 of the following strongly expressed: CD79a, cytoplasmic CD22, CD10
or
Weak CD19 with ≥ 2 of the following strongly expressed: CD79a, cytoplasmic CD22, CD10

are several caveats as to how the expression of lineage-specific markers should be interpreted to achieve a diagnosis of MPAL.

T-cell component of mixed-phenotype acute leukaemia

The T-cell component of an MPAL is characterized by strong expression of cCD3, usually in the absence of surface CD3. For cCD3 to be T-cell–specific, it must be expressed strongly. Expression of cCD3 is best determined by flow cytometry, using relatively bright fluorophores such as phycoerythrin or allophycocyanin. Although cCD3 expression is commonly heterogeneous, the brightest cCD3-positive blasts should reach the intensity of the normal residual T cells present in the sample. Some cases of demonstrable T-ALL have cCD3 that is dimmer than this, but brighter expression is required to establish a diagnosis of MPAL. T-cell lineage can also be demonstrated by immunohistochemistry for CD3 expression in blasts on bone marrow biopsies, but the polyvalent T-cell antibodies used in immunohistochemistry can also react with CD3 zeta chains that can be present in the cytoplasm of activated NK cells, and are therefore not absolutely T-cell–specific.

B-cell component of mixed-phenotype acute leukaemia

The B-cell component of an MPAL is characterized by surface expression of CD19 together with CD10, or in the absence of CD10, together with cCD79a,

CD22, or PAX5 (with PAX5 typically detected by immunohistochemistry). As with cCD3 and T-cell lineage, bright CD19 expression at a level comparable to that of normal B cells has considerable specificity for the B-cell lineage, and is almost always expressed together with one or more of the other markers noted above; caution is required if CD19 is the only marker seen. If the expression of CD19 is dimmer, the presence of at least two other markers is required. CD19 can even be negative with three other B-cell markers present, but this is exceptionally rare.

Myeloid component of mixed-phenotype acute leukaemia

The single most specific hallmark of the myeloid component of an MPAL is MPO in the blast cytoplasm. In cases in which the myeloid component is monocytic, MPO can be negative and unequivocal evidence of monoblastic differentiation would be considered acceptable, including diffuse positivity for non-specific esterase or expression of more than one monocytic marker, such as CD11c, CD14, CD36, CD64, or lysozyme. However, despite the generally high specificity associated with MPO, using it as the sole diagnostic criterion for MPAL has been problematic, in part due to technical factors associated with its measurement. Several anti-MPO antibodies have been shown to react with B-lymphoblastic leukaemia/lymphoma on flow cytometry {2277,2815} or immunohistochemistry {131}, and MPO staining on flow cytometry can appear positive but actually constitute non-specific staining. Small numbers of cases of otherwise typical B-ALL have also been identified in which MPO is definitively positive by flow cytometry; the clinical significance of this is still uncertain. Therefore, a diagnosis of MPAL may not be appropriate for cases that otherwise have a typical precursor B-cell lymphoid phenotype with only a single blast population present; these should not be considered MPAL if weak MPO expression by flow cytometry is the only evidence of myeloid differentiation. Additional criteria that can be helpful for diagnosis include cytochemical positivity for MPO, expression of myeloid antigens such as KIT (CD117) {2890}, and very bright CD13 and CD33. However, the most recognizable feature of MPAL is that nearly all cases display a particular pattern of heterogeneity of antigen expression: in appropriate dual-parameter displays, populations that are relatively bright for lymphoid markers show lower-level expression of myeloid antigens, and vice versa (Figure 10.01). In such cases, the subset of blasts expressing a more myeloid pattern may be larger by forward scatter than the subset of those showing a lymphoid pattern. Caution should be exercised when making a diagnosis of MPAL if such heterogeneity cannot be demonstrated.

A recent report discussed a variety of cases of MPAL submitted to a session of the Society for Hematopathology/European Association for Haematopathology Workshop that focused on acute leukaemias of ambiguous origin {3222}.

Other considerations

MPAL cases with a single population of blasts at diagnosis (so-called biphenotypic leukaemia) can change over time to (or can relapse as) a leukaemia containing separate blast populations (so called bilineage leukaemia), and vice versa. Following therapy, persistent disease or relapse can also occur as pure ALL or AML. Some cases of what has been termed lineage switch {3047,3326} may reflect this phenomenon.

A variety of genetic lesions have been reported in ambiguous lineage leukaemias, especially in MPAL; two such lesions, t(9;22)(q34.1;q11.2) resulting in BCR-ABL1 and translocations associated with KMT2A (previously called MLL), occur frequently enough and are associated with such distinctive features that

they are considered to define separate entities.

Acute undifferentiated leukaemia

Definition

Acute undifferentiated leukaemia expresses no markers considered to be specific for either lymphoid or myeloid lineage. Before categorizing a leukaemia as undifferentiated, it is necessary to perform immunophenotyping with a comprehensive panel of monoclonal antibodies in order to exclude leukaemias of unusual lineages, such as those derived from plasmacytoid dendritic cell precursors, NK-cell precursors, basophils, or even non-haematopoietic tumours.

ICD-O code 9801/3

Synonyms

Blast cell leukaemia; stem cell leukaemia; stem cell acute leukaemia; undifferentiated leukaemia

Epidemiology

These leukaemias are very rare. Their precise frequency is unknown.

Localization

Acute undifferentiated leukaemia affects the bone marrow and blood. Due to the small number of cases reported to date, it is unknown whether there is any predilection for other sites.

Microscopy

The blasts have no morphological features of myeloid differentiation. They are negative for MPO and esterase.

Immunophenotype

These leukaemias typically express no more than one membrane marker for any given lineage. By definition, they lack the T-cell and myeloid markers cCD3 and MPO and do not express B-cell markers such as cCD22, cCD79a, or strong CD19. They also lack the specific features of cells of other lineages, such as megakaryocytes or plasmacytoid dendritic cells. Blasts often express HLA-DR, CD34, and/or CD38 and may be positive for TdT. CD7, although often considered a T-cell antigen, is expressed weakly on some CD34+ haematopoietic progenitors and may be similarly expressed in these leukaemias.

Postulated normal counterpart

A haematopoietic stem cell

Genetic profile

The limited data available suggest that genes associated with poor prognosis in acute myeloid leukaemia (such as BAALC, ERG, and MN1) are often expressed. To date, there have been no reports of cases showing the genetic mutations commonly seen in lymphoblastic leukaemia or acute myeloid leukaemia, including FLT3, WT1, rearrangements of KMT2A (previously called MLL), or BCR-ABL1 {1599}.

Prognosis and predictive factors

The limited data suggest that these leukaemias have a very poor prognosis {1599}.

Mixed-phenotype acute leukaemia with t(9;22)(q34.1;q11.2); BCR-ABL1

Definition

Mixed-phenotype acute leukaemia (MPAL) with t(9;22)(q34.1;q11.2) fulfils the criteria for MPAL and has blasts with t(9;22) and/or BCR-ABL1 rearrangement. Some patients with chronic myeloid leukaemia (CML) develop or even present with a mixed blast phase that would fulfil the criteria for MPAL; however, this diagnosis should not be made in patients known to have had CML.

ICD-O code 9806/3

Synonym

Mixed-phenotype acute leukaemia with t(9;22)(q34;q11.2)

Epidemiology

Although t(9;22)(q34.1;q11.2) is the most common recurrent genetic abnormality seen in MPAL, this leukaemia is rare, probably accounting for < 1% of all acute leukaemia. It occurs in both children and adults, but is more common in adults {560,2013}.

Clinical features

Patients present similarly to other patients with acute leukaemia. Although there are not enough data to be certain, it is likely that patients with MPAL with t(9;22)(q34.1;q11.2) present with high white

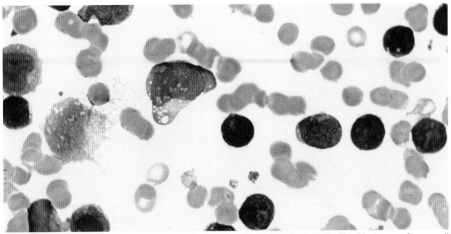

Fig. 10.02 B/myeloid mixed-phenotype acute leukaemia with t(9;22)(q34.1;q11.2). The blasts vary from small lymphoid-appearing blasts to large blasts with dispersed chromatin, prominent nucleoli, and a moderate amount of pale cytoplasm.

blood cell counts, similar to patients with Philadelphia (Ph) chromosome–positive lymphoblastic leukaemia.

Microscopy

Many cases show a dimorphic blast population, with some blasts resembling lymphoblasts and others myeloblasts, although other cases have no distinguishing features. Cases generally do not show significant myeloid maturation; caution should be exercised when making this diagnosis in a case of myeloid leukaemia with maturation that also expresses lymphoid markers, because such a pattern can also be seen in the blast phase of CML.

Immunophenotype

The great majority of cases have blasts that meet the criteria for B-cell and myeloid lineage, as described above, although some cases have T-cell and myeloid blasts. Triphenotypic cases have also rarely been reported.

Postulated normal counterpart

The postulated normal counterpart is a multipotent haematopoietic stem cell. There is no evidence that this leukaemia derives from a different cell than do other cases of Ph chromosome–positive acute leukaemia.

Genetic profile

All cases have either t(9;22) detected by conventional karyotyping or the *BCR-ABL1* translocation detected by FISH or PCR. The p190 fusion transcript is more common than the p210 transcript {4256}. If the p210 transcript is present, CML in a

mixed blast crisis should be considered in the differential diagnosis, especially if there are two distinct lymphoid and myeloid blast populations. Many cases have additional cytogenetic abnormalities, and complex karyotypes are common.

Prognosis and predictive factors

This type of leukaemia has a poor prognosis, which appears to be worse than that of other MPALs {2013}, in particular in adults {2583}.

It is unclear whether the prognosis is worse than that of Ph chromosome–positive lymphoblastic leukaemia. Some data suggest that treatment with tyrosine kinase inhibitors may improve outcome as is seen in lymphoblastic leukaemia with *BCR-ABL1* {1973,3659}. There are no known biological factors that predict whether patients with this leukaemia will do better or worse with therapy.

Mixed-phenotype acute leukaemia with t(v;11q23.3); KMT2A-rearranged

Definition

Mixed-phenotype acute leukaemia (MPAL) with t(v;11q23.3) fulfils the criteria for MPAL and has blasts with a translocation involving *KMT2A* (previously called *MLL*). Many cases of lymphoblastic leukaemia (ALL) with *KMT2A* translocations express myeloid-associated antigens, but such cases should not be considered MPAL unless they fulfil the specific criteria noted above.

ICD-O code   9807/3

Synonyms
Mixed-phenotype acute leukaemia, t(v;11q23), *MLL* rearranged; mixed-phenotype acute leukaemia with *MLL* rearrangement

Epidemiology

This rare leukaemia is more common in children than in adults. Like ALL and acute myeloid leukaemia with *KMT2A* rearrangements, this leukaemia is relatively more common in infancy {2013,3013}.

Clinical features

Patients present similarly to other patients with acute leukaemia. As with other acute leukaemias with *KMT2A* translocations, high white blood cell counts are common.

Microscopy

These leukaemias typically show a dimorphic blast population, with some blasts clearly resembling monoblasts and others resembling lymphoblasts. However, some cases have no distinguishing features and appear only as undifferentiated blast cells. Cases in which the entire blast population appears monoblastic are more likely to be acute myeloid leukaemia with a *KMT2A* translocation, but this diagnosis requires flow cytometry to exclude the presence of a small lymphoblastic population.

Immunophenotype

In most cases, it is possible to recognize a lymphoblast population with a CD19+, CD10–, pro-B (B-cell precursor, B-1) immunophenotype, frequently positive for CD15. Expression of other B-cell markers, such as CD22 and CD79a, is often weak. Cases also fulfil the criteria for myeloid lineage as defined above, most commonly via demonstration of a separate population of myeloid (usually monoblastic) leukaemic cells {3013,4279}. Co-expression of MPO on lymphoid blasts is rare. Because *KMT2A* translocations can also produce T-ALL, it is theoretically possible that T/myeloid leukaemias with t(v;11q23.3) could occur, although no such cases have been reported.

Genetic profile

All cases have rearrangements of *KMT2A*, with the most common partner gene being *AFF1* (*AF4*) on chromosome 4 band q21.3 {560,3013}. Translocations t(9;11) and t(11;19) have also been reported. The rearrangement may be detected by standard karyotyping, by FISH with a *KMT2A* break-apart probe, or (less commonly) by PCR. Cases with deletions of chromosome 11q23.3 detected by karyotyping should not be considered part of this category. The *KMT2A* translocation may be the only lesion present or there may be secondary cytogenetic or molecular abnormalities, but no additional genetic lesions common to multiple cases have been described.

Prognosis and predictive factors

This leukaemia has a poor prognosis {2013,4279}. Patients with B/myeloid leukaemia with *KMT2A* translocations are often treated differently than are patients diagnosed with ALL with *KMT2A* translocations, but there is no evidence that this is necessary or beneficial.

Mixed-phenotype acute leukaemia, B/myeloid, not otherwise specified

Definition

B/myeloid mixed-phenotype acute leukaemia (MPAL), not otherwise specified (NOS), fulfils the criteria for B/myeloid leukaemia as described above, but does not fulfil the criteria for any of the genetically defined subgroups.

ICD-O code   9808/3

Epidemiology

This is a rare leukaemia, probably accounting for about 1% of all leukaemia cases. It occurs in both children and adults, but more commonly in adults.

Microscopy

Most cases either have blasts with no distinguishing features – morphologically resembling lymphoblastic leukaemia (ALL) – or have a dimorphic population with some blasts resembling lymphoblasts and others myeloblasts.

Immunophenotype

The blasts meet the criteria for both B-cell and myeloid lineage assignment as listed above. MPO-positive myeloblasts and monoblasts commonly also express other myeloid-associated markers, including CD13, CD33, and KIT (CD117). Expression of more mature B-cell markers, such as CD20, is rare, occurring most

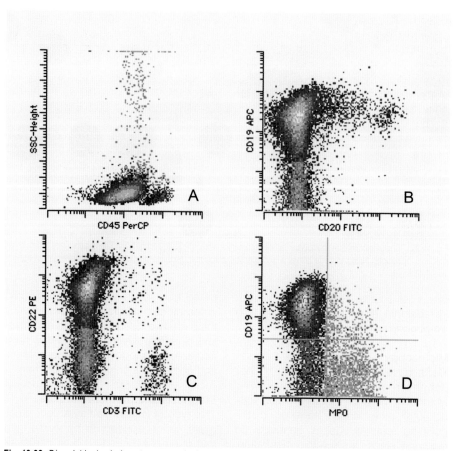

Fig. 10.03 B/myeloid mixed-phenotype acute leukaemia, NOS: flow cytometry histograms. **A** Side scatter (SSC) versus CD45 histogram showing a major population of dim CD45+ blasts; B-cell lymphoblasts are blue, residual normal B-cells red, and MPO+ cells (both blasts and residual normal cells) green. **B and C** The B-cell markers CD19 and CD22 are strongly expressed on the B-cell lymphoid blasts, at levels comparable to those seen on the residual normal B-cells (in red). **D** Most of the B-cell blasts lack MPO and many of the non–B-cell blasts are MPO+; there is also a small population of blasts coexpressing CD19 and MPO.

commonly when a separate population of B-cell lineage blasts is present {4279}.

Postulated normal counterpart

The postulated normal counterpart is a multipotent haematopoietic stem cell. There is growing evidence of a possible relationship between B-cell and myeloid development, suggesting the involvement of either a common precursor or a precursor of one lineage that has reactivated a differentiation programme of the other {1974,2193}.

Genetic profile

Most cases have clonal cytogenetic abnormalities. Many different lesions have been demonstrated, although none commonly enough to suggest specificity for this group of leukaemias. The lesions that have been seen in more than a single case include del(6p), 12p11.2 abnormalities, del(5q), structural abnormalities of chromosome 7, and numerical abnor-

malities including near-tetraploidy {560, 3013}. Complex karyotypes are common {2487,2583}. Gene expression profile studies suggest a signature intermediate between that of ALL and that of acute myeloid leukaemia in most cases {3447}. Mutations frequently found in either acute myeloid or ALLs have also been reported in MPAL, including mutations of *ASXL1, TET1/2, IDH1, IDH2, DNMT3A, NOTCH1,* and *ETV6,* and deletion of *IKZF1* {4414}. There are as yet insufficient data in the literature and too few reported cases to determine whether any genetic entities can be defined other than those discussed above, involving *BCR-ABL1* and *KMT2A.*

Prognosis and predictive factors

B/myeloid MPAL, NOS, is generally considered a poor-prognosis leukaemia, although data on outcome of these cases versus other MPALs are limited. In children, outcome is worse than that of ALL {923,1343,2402,3447}; in adults, outcome appears to be better than that of acute myeloid leukaemia and no different than that of other ALLs {923,3646,4275}. Many cases that meet the criteria for B/myeloid MPAL, NOS, have one or more of the unfavourable genetic lesions noted above; it has been suggested that this accounts for their poor prognosis {2013}. Whether adverse cytogenetic features entirely explain the poor outcome has not been definitively established {2257, 4279}. Patients with B/myeloid MPAL, NOS, have not been treated uniformly. Various combinations and sequential administration of myeloid-directed and lymphoid-directed therapies have been tried {2583,3447,4347}, and some patients may respond to one or the other.

Mixed-phenotype acute leukaemia, T/myeloid, not otherwise specified

Definition
T/myeloid mixed-phenotype acute leukaemia (MPAL), not otherwise specified

(NOS), fulfils the criteria for both T-cell and myeloid lineage as described above, but its blasts lack the above-described genetic abnormalities.

ICD-O code   9809/3

Epidemiology
This is a rare leukaemia, probably accounting for < 1% of all leukaemia cases. It can occur in both children and adults. It may be more frequent in children than is B/myeloid MPAL.

Microscopy
Most cases either have blasts with no distinguishing features (morphologically resembling lymphoblastic leukaemia) or have a dimorphic population with some blasts resembling lymphoblasts and others myeloblasts.

Immunophenotype
The blasts meet the criteria for both T-cell and myeloid lineage assignment as listed above. MPO-positive myeloblasts and monoblasts commonly also express

other myeloid-associated markers, including CD13, CD33, and KIT (CD117). In addition to cCD3, the T-cell component frequently also expresses other T-cell markers, including CD7, CD5, and CD2. Expression of surface CD3 can occur when a separate population of T-cell lineage blasts is present {4279}.

Postulated normal counterpart
The postulated normal counterpart is a multipotent haematopoietic stem cell. There is growing evidence of a possible relationship between T-cell and myeloid development, suggesting the involvement of either a common precursor or a lymphoid precursor that has reactivated a myeloid differentiation programme {1974,2193}.

Genetic profile
Most cases have clonal chromosomal abnormalities, although none is frequent enough to suggest specificity for this group of leukaemias. There are insufficient data in the literature to determine whether B/myeloid and T/myeloid MPALs have different frequencies of various

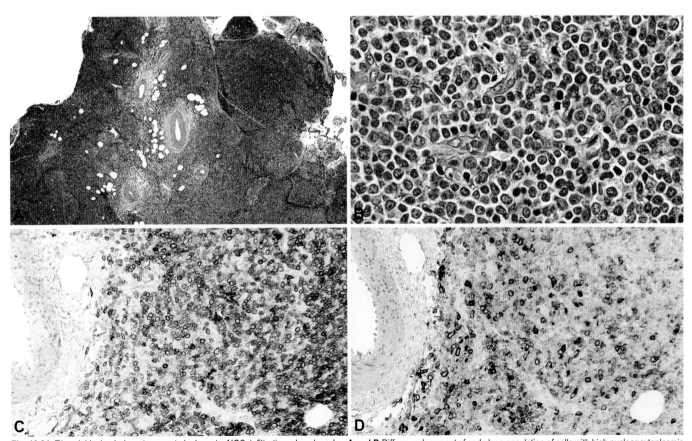

Fig. 10.04 T/myeloid mixed-phenotype acute leukaemia, NOS, infiltrating a lymph node. **A and B** Diffuse replacement of node by a population of cells with high nuclear:cytoplasmic ratios and fine chromatin, histologically indistinguishable from lymphoblastic leukaemia/lymphoma. **C** Immunoperoxidase staining for CD3 stains most of the blast cells. **D** Immunoperoxidase staining for MPO shows distinct staining of a subpopulation of cells with round nuclei; this indicates that they are part of the neoplasm rather than infiltrating granulocytes.

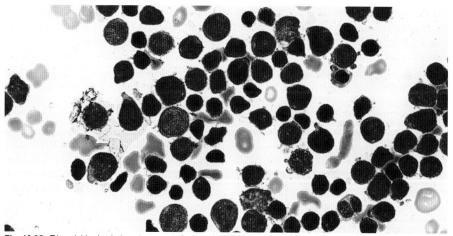

Fig. 10.05 T/myeloid mixed-phenotype acute leukaemia, NOS. There is a dimorphic population of blasts, with many small lymphoblasts. Larger blasts also have a high nuclear:cytoplasmic ratio, fine chromatin and inconspicuous nucleoli.

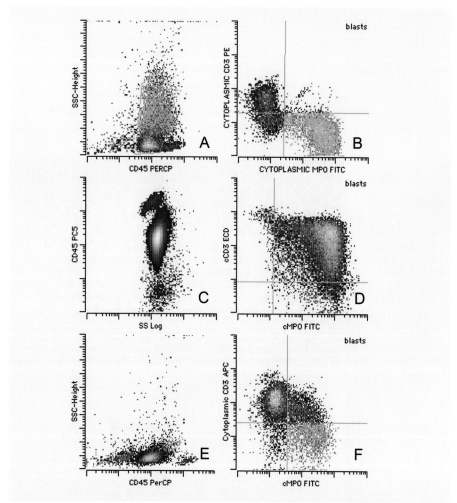

Fig. 10.06 T/myeloid mixed-phenotype acute leukaemia, NOS: flow cytometry in several cases, with gating on all cells (**A,C,E**) and on blasts (**B,D,F**), and with normal T-cells superimposed in violet. **A and B** So-called bilineage leukaemia, with two separate populations of T-cell (blue) and myeloid (green) blasts; the side scatter (SSC) versus CD45 histogram shows that (**A**) the myeloid and T-cell populations have distinct light-scattering profiles. **B** The cCD3 expression on the T-cell blasts is comparable in intensity to that on the residual normal T-cells. **C and D** So-called biphenotypic leukaemia, with a single population of blasts (red) coexpressing cCD3 and MPO; there is a wide range of cCD3 expression intensity, but the brightest blasts are about as bright as the normal T-cells. **E and F** Leukaemia in which both coexpression (red) and separate populations of T-cell (blue) and myeloid (green) blasts can be seen; neither the term 'biphenotypic' nor the term 'bilineage' readily fits this case.

genetic lesions, once the t(9;22) and *KMT2A* rearrangements have been accounted for.

Prognosis and predictive factors

T/myeloid MPAL, NOS is generally considered a poor-prognosis leukaemia, although data on outcome of these cases versus other MPALs are limited {923, 1343,2402,3447}. Patients with T/myeloid MPAL, NOS have not been treated uniformly. Various combinations and sequential administration of myeloid-directed and lymphoid-directed therapies have been tried {3447,4347}, and some patients may respond to one or the other.

Mixed-phenotype acute leukaemia, not otherwise specified, rare types

Definition

In some documented cases of leukaemia, the leukaemic blasts show clear-cut evidence of both T-cell and B-cell lineage commitment as defined above. This is a very rare phenomenon, with a frequency that is likely even lower than has typically been reported in the literature {2583}. As strictly applied, the European Group for the Immunological Characterization of Leukemias (EGIL) criteria for biphenotypic leukaemia (i.e. scores >2 in more than one lineage), which assign a 2-point value to CD79a expression {331, 332} may overestimate the incidence of B-/T-leukaemia, because CD79a can be detected in T-lymphoblastic leukaemia with some antibodies {1584}. For the purpose of assigning B-cell lineage to a case of T-lymphoblastic leukaemia, CD79a and CD10 should not be considered evidence of B-cell differentiation. There have also been a few cases with evidence of trilineage (B-cell, T-cell, and myeloid lineage) assignment. Overall, there are too few cases with these characteristics for any specific statements to be made about clinical features, genetic lesions, or prognosis.

To date, there have been no reports of mixed B- or T-cell and megakaryocytic or mixed B- or T-cell and erythroid leukaemias. It has been postulated that erythroid and megakaryocytic lineages are the earliest to branch off from the pluripotent haematopoietic stem cell, leaving progenitor cells with T-cell, B-cell, and myeloid potential {1803}; therefore, neoplasms of these combinations of lineages are not expected to occur. If they do occur, it is possible that the definitions provided in this volume might not detect all cases, because such leukaemias would not be expected to express MPO.

Acute leukaemias of ambiguous lineage, not otherwise specified

Definition
Acute leukaemias of ambiguous lineage, not otherwise specified (NOS), express combinations of markers that do not allow for their classification as either acute undifferentiated leukaemia or mixed-phenotype acute leukaemia as defined above, and definitive classification along a single lineage is difficult.

Epidemiology
These are rare leukaemias, but there are no specific data on their frequency. They occur in both children and adults.

Immunophenotype
There is no unique immunophenotype that defines this class of leukaemias. Acute leukaemias of ambiguous lineage, NOS include cases that express T-cell–associated markers such as CD7 and CD5 but lack more specific markers such as cCD3, along with myeloid-associated antigens such as CD33 and CD13 without MPO. Care should be taken not to misinterpret a case as ambiguous based on the expression of antigens with limited lineage specificity, especially when the antigens are expressed only dimly. For example, a leukaemia expressing CD13, CD33 and KIT (CD117) along with CD7 and dim CD19 is more properly classified as acute myeloid leukaemia with aberrant antigen expression. With more-extended panels containing newer, less commonly used markers, such leukaemias might be able to be classified more specifically.

Cell of origin
The postulated cell of origin is a multipotent haematopoietic stem cell.

Genetic profile
Like other leukaemias in this category, most cases of acute leukaemia of ambiguous lineage, NOS, have clonal chromosomal abnormalities, although none is frequent enough to suggest specificity for this group of leukaemias.

Prognosis and predictive factors
These leukaemias are generally considered to have a poor prognosis, although data on outcome of these cases versus other ambiguous-lineage leukaemias are limited. Patients with this type of leukaemia are most often treated with myeloid-directed therapy, but definitive data justifying this approach have not been published.

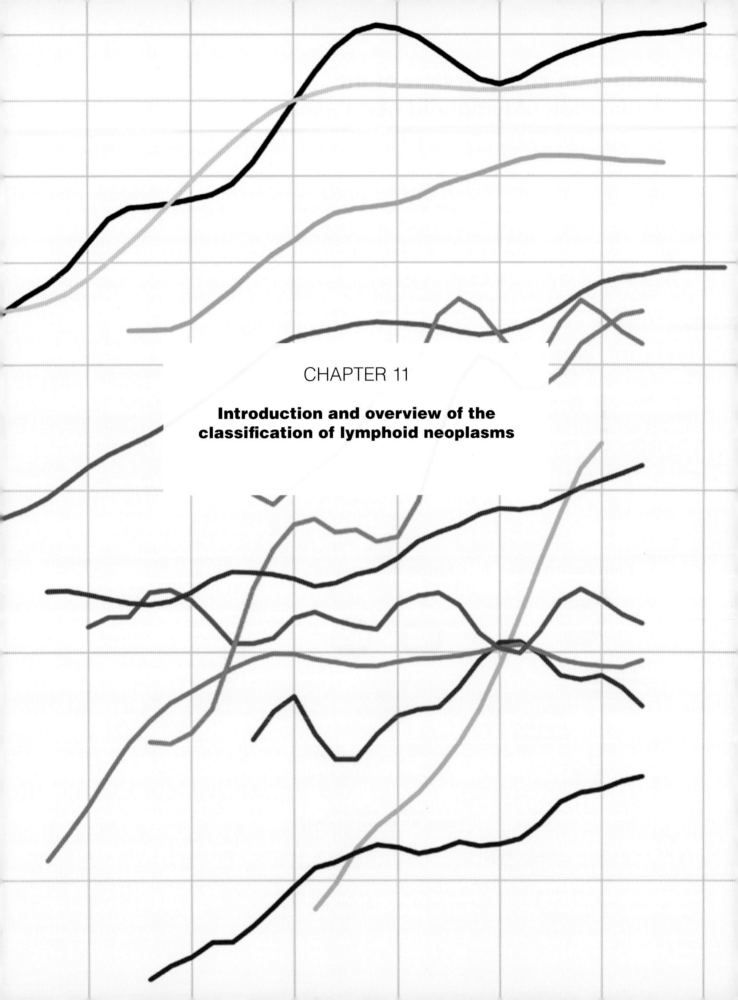

CHAPTER 11

**Introduction and overview of the
classification of lymphoid neoplasms**

Introduction and overview of the classification of lymphoid neoplasms

Jaffe E.S.
Campo E.
Harris N.L.
Pileri S.A.
Stein H.
Swerdlow S.H.

Definition

B-cell and T/NK-cell neoplasms are clonal tumours of mature and immature B cells, T cells, or NK cells at various stages of differentiation. Because NK cells are closely related to and share some immunophenotypic and functional properties with T cells, these two classes of neoplasms are considered together.

In many respects, B-cell and T-cell neoplasms appear to recapitulate stages of normal B-cell or T-cell differentiation, so to some extent they can be classified according to the corresponding normal stage. However, some common B-cell neoplasms (e.g. hairy cell leukaemia) do not clearly correspond to a normal B-cell differentiation stage. Some neoplasms exhibit lineage heterogeneity, or even more rarely, lineage plasticity {1819, 2431}. Therefore, the normal counterpart of the neoplastic cell cannot be the sole basis for classification.

Pathobiology of lymphoid neoplasms and the normal immune system

The immune system has two major subsystems, which differ in the nature of their targets and types of immune response: the innate and adaptive immune systems. The innate immune system provides a first line of defence, a primitive response. The cells of the innate immune system include NK cells, CD3+ CD56+ T cells (NK-like T cells), and gamma delta T cells. These cells play a role in barrier immunity involving mucosal and cutaneous defences. They do not need to encounter antigens in the context of major histocompatibility complex (MHC) molecules, and therefore do not require antigen-presenting cells in order to initiate an immune response.

The adaptive immune system provides a more sophisticated type of immune response; two key features are antigen specificity and memory. This contrasts with the innate immune response, which is non-specific and does not require or result in immunological memory.

B-cell lymphomas: Lymphocyte differentiation and function

B-cell neoplasms tend to mimic various stages of normal B-cell differentiation, and this resemblance to normal cell stages is a major basis for their classification and nomenclature.

Normal B-cell differentiation begins with B lymphoblasts, which undergo IGH VDJ gene rearrangement and differentiate into mature surface immunoglobulin (sIg)-positive (IgM+ IgD+) naïve B cells via pre-B cells with cytoplasmic mu heavy chains and immature IgM+ B cells. Naïve B cells, which are often CD5-positive, are small resting lymphocytes that circulate in the peripheral blood and also occupy primary lymphoid follicles and follicle mantle zones (so-called recirculating B cells) {1758,2032}. Many cases of mantle cell lymphoma are thought to correspond to CD5+ naïve B cells {1733}, but somatically mutated variants also exist {1187}.

Upon encountering antigen that fits their sIg receptors, naïve B cells undergo transformation, proliferate, and ultimately mature into antibody-secreting plasma cells and memory B cells. Transformed cells derived from naïve B cells that have encountered antigen may mature directly into plasma cells that produce the early IgM antibody response to antigen. T-cell–independent maturation can take place outside the germinal centre {721}. Other antigen-exposed B cells migrate into the centre of a primary follicle, proliferate, and fill the follicular dendritic cell meshwork, forming a germinal centre {2374, 2427}. Germinal centre centroblasts express low levels of sIg and switch off expression of BCL2; therefore, they and their progeny are susceptible to apoptosis {3329}. Centroblasts express CD10 as well as BCL6, a nuclear transcription factor also expressed by centrocytes. BCL6 is not expressed in naïve B cells and is switched off in memory B cells and plasma cells {3483,3199}. More recently de-

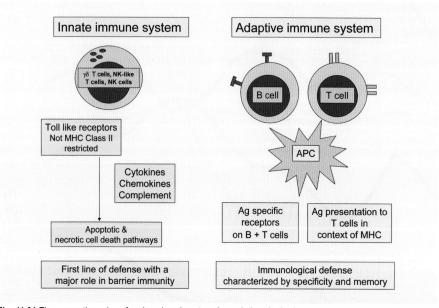

Fig. 11.01 The respective roles of various lymphocyte subpopulations in the immune system's two main arms: the innate and adaptive immune systems. In the innate immune system, which lacks specificity and memory, NK cells, NK-like T cells, and gamma delta T cells, along with other cells including granulocytes and macrophages, function as a first line of defence. These cells have cytotoxic granules (shown in red) containing perforin and granzymes. In the adaptive immune system, B cells and T cells recognize pathogens through specific receptors: immunoglobulins and the T-cell receptor complex, respectively. Antigen (Ag) presentation to T cells takes place via antigen-presenting cells (APCs) in the context of the appropriate major histocompatibility complex (MHC) class II molecule. Modified from Jaffe ES {1816}.

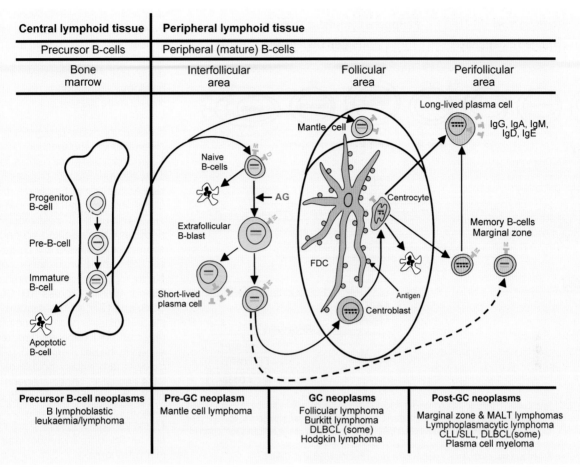

Central lymphoid tissue	Peripheral lymphoid tissue		
Precursor B-cells	Peripheral (mature) B-cells		
Bone marrow	Interfollicular area	Follicular area	Perifollicular area

Precursor B-cell neoplasms
B lymphoblastic leukaemia/lymphoma

Pre-GC neoplasm
Mantle cell lymphoma

GC neoplasms
Follicular lymphoma
Burkitt lymphoma
DLBCL (some)
Hodgkin lymphoma

Post-GC neoplasms
Marginal zone & MALT lymphomas
Lymphoplasmacytic lymphoma
CLL/SLL, DLBCL(some)
Plasma cell myeloma

Fig. 11.02 Normal B-cell differentiation and its relationship to major B-cell neoplasms. B-cell neoplasms correspond to various stages of normal B-cell maturation, although the normal cell counterparts are unknown in some instances. Precursor B cells, which mature in the bone marrow, may undergo apoptosis or develop into mature naïve B cells, which, following exposure to antigen (AG) and blast transformation, may develop into short-lived plasma cells or enter the germinal centre (GC), where somatic hypermutation and heavy-chain class switching occur. Centroblasts, the transformed cells of the GC, either undergo apoptosis or develop into centrocytes. Post-GC cells include both long-lived plasma cells and memory/marginal-zone B cells. Most B cells are activated within the GC, but T-cell–independent activation can take place outside the GC and probably also leads to memory-type B cells. Monocytoid B cells, many of which lack somatic hypermutation, are not illustrated. The red bars indicate IGH gene rearrangement and the blue bars IG light chain gene rearrangement; the black insertions in red and blue bars indicate somatic hypermutation {3848}.
CLL/SLL, chronic lymphocytic leukaemia / small lymphocytic lymphoma; D, surface IgD; DLBCL, diffuse large B-cell lymphoma; FDC, follicular dendritic cell; M, surface IgM; MALT, mucosa-associated lymphoid tissue.

scribed germinal centre markers include LMO2 and HGAL. LMO2 is expressed in haematopoietic precursors in the bone marrow, but appears to be specific for germinal centre B cells in normal reactive lymphoid tissues {2840}; it lacks this specificity in lymphoid neoplasms {35}. HGAL (also called GCET2) is expressed in germinal centre B cells and germinal centre–derived malignancies {3043}.

In the germinal centre, somatic hypermutation occurs in the IGV genes; these mutations can result in a non-functional gene or a gene that produces antibody with lower or higher affinity for antigen. Also in the germinal centre, some cells switch from IgM production to IgG or IgA production. Through these mechanisms, the germinal centre reaction gives rise to the higher-affinity IgG or IgA antibodies

of the late primary or secondary immune response {2428}. *BCL6* also undergoes somatic mutation in the germinal centre, but at a lower frequency than do the IG genes {3084}. Ongoing IGV gene mutation with intraclonal diversity is a hallmark of germinal centre cells, and both IGV gene and *BCL6* mutations serve as markers of cells that have been through the germinal centre. Most diffuse large B-cell lymphomas (DLBCLs) are composed of cells that at least in part resemble centroblasts and have mutated IGV genes, consistent with a derivation from cells that have been exposed to the germinal centre. Burkitt lymphoma cells are BCL6-positive and have mutated IGH genes, and are therefore also thought to correspond to a germinal centre blast cell. Both Burkitt lymphoma and DLBCL

correspond to proliferating cells and are clinically aggressive tumours.

Centroblasts mature to centrocytes, and these cells are seen predominantly in the light zone of the germinal centre. Centrocytes express sIg that has an altered antibody-combining site compared with that of their progenitors, due to both somatic mutations and heavy-chain class switching. Centrocytes with mutations that result in increased affinity are rescued from apoptosis and re-express BCL2 {2427}. Through interaction with surface molecules on follicular dendritic cells and T cells (e.g. CD23 and CD40 ligand), centrocytes switch off BCL6 expression {584,3199} and differentiate into either memory B cells or plasma cells {2427}. BCL6 and IRF4 (also called MUM1) are reciprocally expressed, with

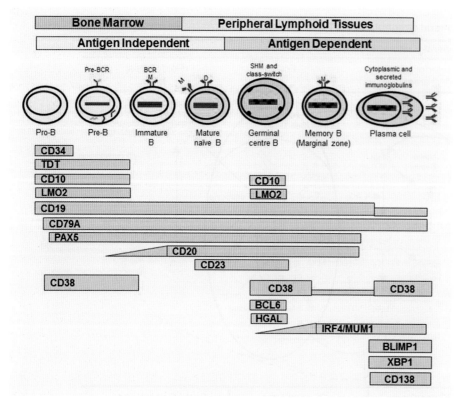

Fig. 11.03 B-cell differentiation. B cells go through various stages of differentiation as they mature from pro-B cells to plasma cells. The antigen-dependent phase of differentiation usually begins in the germinal centre, where B cells encounter antigen. Red bar in nucleus indicates heavy chain gene rearrangement; blue bar indicates light chain re-arrangement; black boxes connote somatic hypermutation. Cells coloured in yellow have not encountered antigen, as opposed to antigen-dependent stages shown in violet. Modified from Swerdlow SH et al. {3848}.
BCR, B-cell receptor; D, surface IgD; M, surface IgM; SHM, somatic hypermutation.

IRF4 being positive in late centrocytes and plasma cells {1141,3483}. IRF4 plays a critical role in downregulating BCL6 expression {3483}. Recent studies indicate that MYC plays an important role in germinal centre formation {1020}. MYC is upregulated upon interaction of naïve B cells with antigen and T cells by the action of BCL6, and is essential for germinal centre formation. In normal reactive lymph nodes, staining for MYC highlights a population of centrocytes in the light zone of the germinal centre, and is repressed in the dark zone. However, MYC is re-induced in a subset of light-zone B cells (centrocyes), allowing re-entry into the dark zone and maintenance of the germinal centre reaction {1020}. Follicular lymphomas are tumours of germinal centre B cells (centrocytes and centroblasts) in which the germinal centre cells fail to undergo apoptosis, in most cases due to a chromosomal rearrangement, t(14;18), that prevents the normal switching off of BCL2 expression. Centrocytes usually predominate over centroblasts, and these neoplasms tend to be indolent.

Post–germinal centre memory B cells circulate in the peripheral blood and account for at least some of the cells in the follicular marginal zones of lymph nodes, spleen, and mucosa-associated lymphoid tissue (MALT). Marginal-zone B cells of this compartment typically express pan–B-cell antigens and surface IgM (with only low levels of IgD), and lack both CD5 and CD10 {3749,4124}. Plasma cells produced in the germinal centre enter the peripheral blood and home to the bone marrow. They contain predominantly IgG or IgA; they lack sIg and CD20 but express IRF4, CD79a, CD38, and CD138. Both memory B cells and long-lived plasma cells have mutated IGV genes, but do not continue to undergo mutation. Post–germinal centre B cells retain the ability to home to tissues in which they have undergone antigen stimulation, probably through surface integrin expression, so that B cells that arise in MALT tend to return there, whereas B cells that arise in the lymph nodes home to nodal sites and bone marrow {508}. Marginal zone lymphomas of the MALT type, splenic type,

and nodal type correspond to post–germinal centre memory B cells of marginal zone type that derive from and proliferate specifically in extranodal, splenic, and nodal tissues, respectively. Plasma cell myeloma corresponds to a bone marrow–homing plasma cell.

T-cell lymphomas: Lymphocyte differentiation and function
T lymphocytes arise from a bone marrow precursor that undergoes maturation and acquisition of function in the thymus gland. Antigen-specific T cells mature in the thymic cortex. T cells recognizing self peptides are eliminated via apoptosis, in a process mediated by cortical epithelial cells and thymic nurse cells. Cortical thymocytes have an immature T-cell phenotype and express TdT, CD1a, CD3, CD5, and CD7. CD3 is first expressed in the cytoplasm, prior to complete T-cell receptor (TR) gene rearrangement and export to the cell membrane. Cortical thymocytes are initially double-negative for CD4 and CD8. These antigens are coexpressed in maturing thymocytes; more-mature T cells express only CD4 or CD8. These various stages of T-cell maturation are reflected in T-lymphoblastic leukaemia/lymphoma.
Medullary thymocytes have a phenotype similar to that of mature T cells of the peripheral lymphoid organs. There are two classes of T cells: alpha beta T cells and gamma delta T cells {3850}. This distinction is based on the structure of the T-cell receptor. The alpha beta and gamma delta chains are each composed of a variable portion and a constant portion. They are both associated with the CD3 complex, which contains gamma, delta, and epsilon chains. NK cells do not have a complete T-cell receptor complex; activated NK cells express the epsilon and zeta chains of CD3 in the cytoplasm. They express CD2, CD7, and sometimes CD8, but not surface CD3. They also typically express CD16 and CD56, variably express CD57, and contain cytoplasmic cytotoxic granule proteins. NK cells kill their targets through antibody-dependent cell-mediated cytotoxicity or a second mechanism involving killer activation receptors and inhibitory killer-cell immunoglobulin-like receptors. Because NK cells do not rearrange the TR genes, antibodies to the various killer-cell immunoglobulin-like receptors can be used for analysis of clonality in NK-cell proliferations.

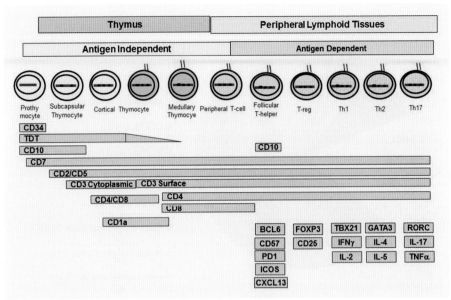

Fig. 11.04 T-cell differentiation. T cells mature in the thymus gland and then leave to occupy peripheral lymphoid tissues. T-cell receptor (TR) genes are shown schematically with a solid red bar indicating absence of rearrangement. The black boxes in the red bars reflect the rearrangements of the TR genes. The double red lines on the cell membrane represent the expressed T-cell receptor complex. Antigen dependent maturation leads to the different T-cell subsets, also illustrated in Fig. 11.05. The phenotypes of several key T-cell subsets are illustrated: T follicular helper (TFH), T regulatory (T-reg), T helper 1 (Th1), T helper 2 (Th2), and T helper 17 (Th17). Modified and updated from {3848}.

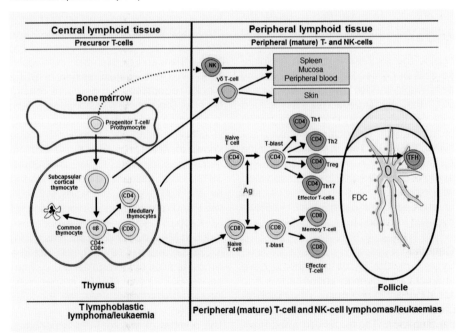

Fig. 11.05 T-cell differentiation. T-cell neoplasms correspond to various stages of normal T-cell maturation. Mature T cells include alpha beta and gamma delta T cells, both of which mature in the thymus gland. Recently recognized T-cell subsets include the various types of CD4+ effector T cells, including T helper 1 (Th1), T helper 2 (Th2), T regulatory (Treg), T helper 17 (Th17), and T follicular helper (TFH) cells. Modified and updated from {3848}. Ag, antigen; FDC, follicular dendritic cell.

Toll-like receptors play a role in cell–cell interactions and signalling. They play a critical role in the recognition of infectious agents, initiating signalling through NF-kappaB. They function most prominently in innate immune responses, but they also play a role in the adaptive immune system {2284}.

The lymphomas of the innate immune system are predominantly extranodal in presentation, mirroring the distribution of the functional components of this system. It is interesting that many T-cell and NK-cell lymphomas observed commonly in the paediatric and young-adult age groups are derived from cells of the innate immune system {1816}. Lymphoid neoplasms derived from innate lymphoid cells include aggressive NK-cell leukaemia, systemic EBV-positive T-cell lymphoma of childhood, hepatosplenic gamma delta T-cell lymphoma, and gamma delta T-cell lymphomas often arising in cutaneous and mucosal sites.

Gamma delta T cells usually lack expression of CD4 and CD8, as well as CD5. A subpopulation expresses CD8. Gamma delta T cells account for <5% of all normal T cells and have a restricted distribution, being found mainly in the splenic red pulp, intestinal epithelium, and other epithelial sites. These sites are more commonly affected by gamma delta T-cell lymphomas, which are otherwise relatively rare {150,1299,3850}. Gamma delta T cells have a restricted range of antigen recognition, and serve as a first line of defence against bacterial peptides, such as heat shock proteins {3850}. They are often involved in responses to mycobacterial infections and in mucosal immunity.

The T cells of the adaptive immune system, which are heterogeneous and functionally complex, include naïve, effector (regulatory and cytotoxic), and memory T cells. T-cell lymphomas of the adaptive immune system present primarily in adults and are mainly nodal in origin, in contrast with the extranodal T-cell lymphomas of the innate immune system {1816}. CD4+ T cells are primarily regulatory, acting via cytokine production; based on their cytokine secretion profiles, CD4+ T cells are divided into two major types: T helper 1 (Th1) cells and T helper 2 (Th2) cells. Th1 cells secrete IL2 and interferon gamma, but not IL4, IL5, or IL6. In contrast, Th2 cells secrete IL4, IL5, IL6, and IL10 {3850}. Th1 cells provide help mainly to other T cells and to macrophages, whereas Th2 cells provide help mainly to B cells, in the production of antibodies {1758A}. CD4+ T cells can act both to help and to suppress immune responses, and consist of multiple subpopulations only recently recognized. For example, T regulatory (Treg) cells have diverse functions, including suppressing immune responses to cancer and limiting inflammatory responses in tissues {2403,4350}. Recent studies have identified transcription factors, TBX21 (also known as T-BET) and GATA3, that are overexpressed in Th1 and Th2 lymphocytes, respectively {1775}, and that also appear to delineate subsets of peripheral T-cell lymphomas (PTCLs) {1775,4253}. T helper 17 (Th17) cells are a more recently identified subset of CD4+ effector T cells. They are characterized by expression of the IL17 family of cytokines and play a role in immune-mediated inflammatory diseases and in other conditions {3834}.

Much has been learned about a unique CD4+ T-cell subset found in the normal germinal centre. These cells, called T follicular helper (TFH) cells, provide help to B cells in the context of the germinal centre reaction {1067,1469,2993}. They have a unique phenotype, expressing the germinal centre markers BCL6 and CD10, which are also normally found on germinal centre B cells. TFH cells also express CD4, CD57, and CD279/PD1 and produce the chemokine CXCL13 and its receptor CXCR5. CXCL13 causes induction and proliferation of follicular dendritic cells; it also facilitates the migration of B cells and T cells expressing CXCR5 into the germinal centre. Increased expression of CXCL13 in angioimmunoblastic T-cell lymphoma (AITL) is a finding that helps to link many of its clinical and pathological features {1067,1469, 2993}. Notably, AITL is associated with polyclonal hypergammaglobulinaemia and expansion and proliferation of both B cells and CD21+ follicular dendritic cells within the lymph node. Some other nodal PTCLs display a TFH-cell phenotype and share many genetic features with AITL {178}. However, a TFH-cell phenotype is also seen in a very different disease: primary cutaneous CD4+ small/medium T-cell lymphoproliferative disorder.

A CD4+ T cell with very different properties is the Treg cell, which functions to shut off and suppress immune responses {3715}. This cell is thought to play an important role in preventing autoimmunity. Treg cells express high-density CD25 and the transcription factor FOXP3, in combination with CD4. Adult T-cell leukaemia/lymphoma (ATLL) has been linked to Treg cells on the basis of expression of both CD25 and FOXP3, and this finding helps to explain the marked immunosuppression associated with ATLL {1948,3398}.

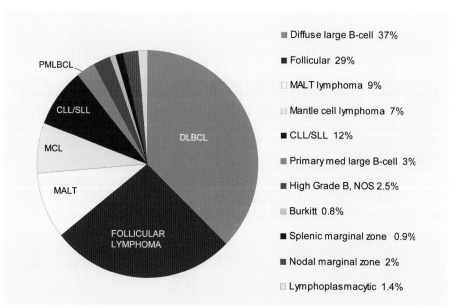

- Diffuse large B-cell 37%
- Follicular 29%
- MALT lymphoma 9%
- Mantle cell lymphoma 7%
- CLL/SLL 12%
- Primary med large B-cell 3%
- High Grade B, NOS 2.5%
- Burkitt 0.8%
- Splenic marginal zone 0.9%
- Nodal marginal zone 2%
- Lymphoplasmacytic 1.4%

Fig. 11.06 Relative frequencies of B-cell lymphoma subtypes in adults. There are significant differences in the relative frequencies across geographical regions. However, diffuse large B-cell lymphoma (DLBCL) and follicular lymphoma are the most common subtypes on a worldwide basis, but varying in some geographical regions and among some ethnic groups. Note that these estimates underestimate the incidence of chronic lymphocytic leukaemia / small lymphocytic lymphoma (CLL/SLL), because only patients presenting clinically with lymphoma were included. Data from the Non-Hodgkin's Lymphoma Classification Project {1}.
MCL, mantle cell lymphoma; PMLBCL, primary mediastinal large B-cell lymphoma.

Recent studies have tried to relate the pathological or clinical manifestations of T-cell lymphomas to cytokine or chemokine expression by the neoplastic cells or by accompanying accessory cells within the lymph node. For example, the hypercalcaemia associated with ATLL has been linked to secretion of factors with osteoclast-activating activity {2896A}. The haemophagocytic syndrome seen in some T-cell and NK-cell malignancies has been associated with secretion of both cytokines and chemokines, in the setting of defective cytolytic function {1834,2011,2970 }.

Genetics

Several mature B-cell neoplasms have characteristic genetic abnormalities that are important in determining their biological features and can be useful in differential diagnosis. These genetic abnormalities include t(11;14)(q13;q32) in mantle cell lymphoma, t(14;18)(q32;q21) in follicular lymphoma, t(8;14)(q24;q32) and variants in Burkitt lymphoma, and t(11;18)(q21;q21) in MALT lymphoma {889,1933, 2286}. The t(11;14) translocation is seen in both mantle cell lymphoma and some cases of plasma cell myeloma, but there are minor differences in the translocation, involving different portions of the IGH gene {350}. The most common paradigm

for translocations involving an IGH gene on 14q32 is that a cellular proto-oncogene comes under the influence of the IGH enhancer. For example, in follicular lymphoma, the overexpression of BCL2 blocks apoptosis in germinal centre B cells. The t(11;18) translocation, which is common in MALT lymphoma, results in a fusion gene, in which *BIRC3* (also known as *API2*) is fused to the C-terminal sequences of *MALT1* {982,2406,3341, 3812}. The chimeric protein encoded by the fusion gene promotes cell survival and proliferation via activation of NF-kappaB {2406}. Other translocations found in MALT lymphoma, such as t(1;14) (p22;q32) and t(14;18)(q32;q21), act in a similar fashion by deregulating the oncogenes *BCL10* and *MALT1*, respectively, through juxtaposition next to the IGH enhancer.

The number of mature T-cell lymphomas with recurrent genetic aberrations has increased significantly in recent years with the introduction of next-generation sequencing and mutation analysis. ALK-positive anaplastic large cell lymphoma was the first T-cell lymphoma to be linked to a specific aberration: translocations involving the *ALK* gene on chromosome 2p23. *ALK* is fused to a variety of partner genes, most often *NPM1*, as a consequence of t(2;5)(p23.2-23.1;q35.1) {1136,

Table 11.01 Immunophenotypic features of common mature B-cell neoplasms; the symbols indicate the proportion of cases in which each marker listed is positive. Modified and updated from Swerdlow SH, et al. {3848}.

Neoplasm	sIg, cIg	CD5	CD10	CD23	CD43	CD103	BCL6	IRF4/MUM1	Cyclin D1	ANXA1
CLL/SLL	+, −/+	+	−	+	+	−	−	+ (PCs)	−	−
LPL	+/−, +	− [c]	−	−	−/+	−	−	+ [a]	−	−
SMZL	+, −/+	−	−	−	−	−	−	−	−	−
HCL	+, −	−	−	−	−	+	−	−	+/−	+
PCM	−, +	−	−/+	−	−/+	−	−	+	−/+	−
MALT lymphoma	+, +/−	− [c]	−	−	−/+	−	−	+ [a]	−	−
FL	+, −	− [c]	+/−	−/+	−	−	+	−/+ [b]	−	
MCL	+, −	+	−	−	+	−	−	−	+	−
DLBCL	+/−, −/+	− [c]	−/+ [d]	n/a	−/+	n/a	+/− [d]	+/− [e]	−	−
BL	+, −	−	+	−	−/+	n/a	+	−/+	−	−

> 90% (+), > 50% (+/−), < 50% (−/+), or < 10% (−)

ANXA1, annexin A1; BL, Burkitt lymphoma; cIg, cytoplasmic immunoglobulin; CLL/SLL, chronic lymphocytic leukaemia / small lymphocytic lymphoma; DLBCL, diffuse large B-cell lymphoma; FL, follicular lymphoma; HCL, hairy cell leukaemia; LPL, lymphoplasmacytic lymphoma; MCL, mantle cell lymphoma; n/a, not applicable; PC, proliferation centre; PCM, plasma cell myeloma; sIg, surface immunoglobulin; SMZL, splenic marginal zone lymphoma.

[a] The plasma cell components of LPL and MALT lymphoma are IRF4+.
[b] Some grade 3A and 3B FLs are IRF4+.
[c] Some DLBCLs are CD5+. Other B-cell neoplasms can sometimes be CD5+, including LPL, MALT and FL.
[d] DLBCLs of germinal centre B-cell type express CD10 and BCL6.
[e] DLBCLs of activated B-cell type are typically IRF4+

1815,2199}. Hepatosplenic T-cell lymphoma of gamma delta origin has mutations in *STAT5B* in approximately 35% of cases {2869}, and the same mutation is recurrent in gamma delta T-cell lymphomas involving the gastrointestinal tract and skin {2160}. The JAK/STAT pathway is implicated in many forms of T-cell lymphoma, including anaplastic large cell lymphoma (both ALK-positive and ALK-negative) and monomorphic epitheliotropic intestinal T-cell lymphoma {836, 2807}.

Other genetic tools have also been applied in the study of mature lymphoid neoplasms. These include comparative genomic hybridization and more sensitive techniques of array-based copy-number profiling, both of which can identify areas of deletion or amplification within the genome. Gene expression microarrays can interrogate the expression of thousands of genes at the RNA level, helping to elucidate pathways of activation and transformation {877,878,884,1208,1775, 2719,3409,3538}. Most recently, studies have begun to explore changes at the epigenetic level that control the expression of multiple genes {2352, 3528}.

Principles of classification

The classification of lymphoid neoplasms is based on all available information to define disease entities {1557}. Having sufficient tissue for this multiparameter approach is critical. Great caution is advised when core needle biopsies are used for the primary diagnosis of lymphoma; fine-needle aspiration is generally inadequate for this purpose. Morphology and immunophenotype are sufficient for the diagnosis of most lymphoid neoplasms. However, no one antigenic marker is specific for any neoplasm, and a combination of morphological features and a panel of antigenic markers are necessary for correct diagnosis. Most B-cell lymphomas have characteristic immunophenotypic profiles that are very helpful in diagnosis. However, immune profiling is somewhat less helpful in the subclassification of T-cell lymphomas.

Although certain antigens are commonly associated with specific disease entities, these associations are not entirely disease-specific. For example, CD30 is a universal feature of anaplastic large cell lymphoma, but can also be expressed in other T-cell and B-cell lymphomas and in classic Hodgkin lymphoma (CHL). Similarly, CD56 is a characteristic feature of nasal NK/T-cell lymphoma, but it can also be found in other T-cell lymphomas, in plasma cell neoplasms, and in non-lymphoid cells such as in blastic plasmacytoid dendritic cell neoplasms {173, 315,746,987,4357}. Within a given disease entity, variation in immunophenotypic features can be seen. For example, most hepatosplenic T-cell lymphomas are of the gamma delta T-cell phenotype, but some cases are of alpha beta T-cell derivation. Likewise, some follicular lymphomas are CD10-negative. An aberrant immunophenotype may suggest or help to confirm a diagnosis of malignancy {1815}.

Although lineage is a defining feature of most lymphoid malignancies, in recent years there has been an increasing appreciation of lineage plasticity within the haematopoietic system. Lineage switch or demonstration of multiple lineages is most often encountered in immature haematolymphoid neoplasms, but also can be seen rarely in mature lymphomas {772,1172,1536}.

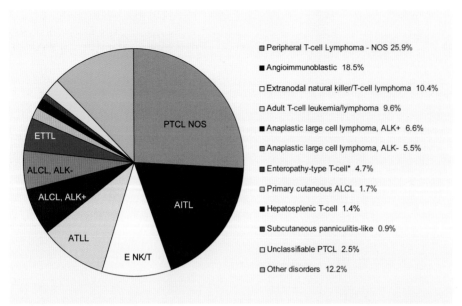

Legend:
- □ Peripheral T-cell Lymphoma - NOS 25.9%
- ■ Angioimmunoblastic 18.5%
- □ Extranodal natural killer/T-cell lymphoma 10.4%
- □ Adult T-cell leukemia/lymphoma 9.6%
- ■ Anaplastic large cell lymphoma, ALK+ 6.6%
- ■ Anaplastic large cell lymphoma, ALK- 5.5%
- ■ Enteropathy-type T-cell* 4.7%
- □ Primary cutaneous ALCL 1.7%
- ■ Hepatosplenic T-cell 1.4%
- ■ Subcutaneous panniculitis-like 0.9%
- □ Unclassifiable PTCL 2.5%
- □ Other disorders 12.2%

Fig. 11.07 Relative frequencies of mature T-cell lymphoma subtypes in an adult patient population. There are significant differences in the relative frequencies across geographical regions. However, peripheral T-cell lymphoma (PTCL), NOS, and angioimmunoblastic T-cell lymphoma (AITL) are two of the most common subtypes globally. Note that the category of enteropathy-type T-cell lymphoma (ETTL) used in this study is not equivalent to the category of enteropathy-associated T-cell lymphoma (EATL) as defined in this volume. The ETTL category was used largely as a generic category for most T-cell lymphomas involving the intestine, including EATL and more recently defined monomorphic epitheliotropic intestinal T-cell lymphomas. Data from the International T-Cell Lymphoma Project {4217}.
ALCL, anaplastic large cell lymphoma; ATLL, adult T-cell leukaemia/lymphoma; E NK/T, extranodal NK/T-cell lymphoma.

Genetic features are playing an increasingly important role in the classification of lymphoid malignancies. However, the molecular pathogenesis of many forms of lymphoma remains unknown. Genetic studies, in particular PCR studies of IG and TR genes and FISH, are valuable diagnostic tools for the determination of clonality in B-cell and T-cell proliferations (aiding in the differential diagnosis with reactive hyperplasia) and for the identification of translocations associated with some disease entities. The identification of the *MYD88* L265P mutation in most cases of lymphoplasmacytic lymphoma but only rarely in marginal zone lymphoma has provided new tools for diagnosis {1527}. Similarly, mutations in *BRAF* are recurrent in certain histiocytic and dendritic cell proliferations, such as Langerhans cell histiocytosis {215} and Erdheim–Chester disease {1102}, but are nearly ubiquitous in hairy cell leukaemia {3997,3998}.

The WHO classification emphasizes the importance of knowledge of clinical features, both for accurate diagnosis and for the definition of some diseases, such as extranodal marginal zone lymphoma of MALT (MALT lymphoma) versus nodal or splenic marginal zone lymphoma,

primary mediastinal large B-cell lymphoma (PMLBCL) versus DLBCL, and most mature T-cell and NK-cell neoplasms. The diagnosis of lymphoid neoplasms should not take place in a vacuum, but rather within the context of a complete clinical history.

Lymphoid malignancies range in their clinical behaviour from indolent to aggressive. Within any given entity, a range in clinical behaviour can also be seen, and histological or clinical progression is often encountered during a patient's clinical course. For these reasons, the WHO classification does not attempt to stratify lymphoid malignancies in terms of histologic grade or clinical aggressiveness. Both morphology and immunophenotype often change over time, as the lymphoid neoplasm undergoes clonal evolution with the acquisition of additional genetic changes. Transformation can arise by divergent evolution from a common precursor, or by more-direct linear transformation, and examples of both patterns have been shown {1434}. In addition, evolution over time does not necessarily lead to the development of a more aggressive lymphoma. For example, patients with DLBCL can relapse with a more indolent clonally related follicular lymphoma.

Some of these clonal evolutions can be unexpected and not obviously connected, such as the development of a plasmacytoma in a patient with CHL {1824}. Traditionally, CHLs have been considered separately from the so-called non-Hodgkin lymphomas. However, with the recognition that CHL is of B-cell lineage, greater overlap has been recognized between CHL and many other forms of B-cell malignancies. This revised 4th edition of the WHO classification acknowledges these grey zones and provides for the identification of cases that bridge the gap between these various forms of lymphoma {4047}. The borders are further blurred by conditions such as nodular lymphocyte predominant Hodgkin lymphoma, which manifests many clinical and biological characteristics of Hodgkin and non-Hodgkin lymphomas.

Epidemiology
Precursor lymphoid neoplasms, including B-lymphoblastic leukaemia/lymphoma and T-lymphoblastic leukaemia/lymphoma, are primarily diseases of children. About 75% of cases occur in children aged <6 years. Approximately 85% of cases presenting as lymphoblastic leukaemia are of precursor B-cell type, whereas lymphoblastic malignancies of precursor T-cell type more often present as lymphoma, with mediastinal masses. A male predominance is seen in lymphoblastic malignancies of both B-cell and T-cell lineages.

According to the *World Cancer Report 2014* {205}, there were 566 000 new cases of lymphoma and about 305 000 deaths due to lymphoma in 2012. Mature B-cell neoplasms constitute >90% of lymphoid neoplasms worldwide {1,148} and account for approximately 4% of all new cancer cases each year. They are more common in developed countries, in particular in North America, Australia, New Zealand, and northern and western Europe. Globally, the incidence is greatest in Israel, followed by Lebanon, Australia, and the USA. The incidence of lymphomas, in particular B-cell lymphomas, has increased worldwide, but may be plateauing over the past decade. The International Lymphoma Epidemiology (InterLymph) Consortium is examining factors associated with increased lymphoma incidence using a case–control study methodology {2758}.

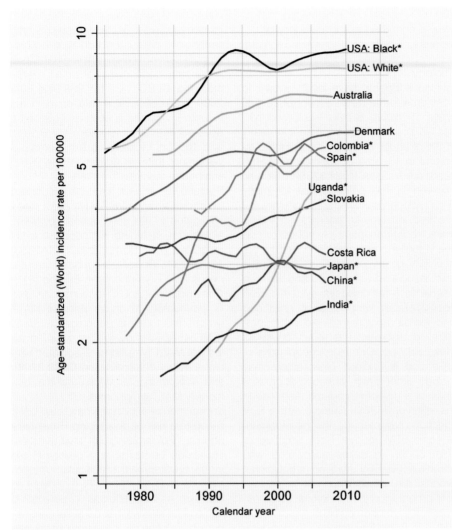

Fig. 11.08 Age-standardized incidence rates (per 100 000 men per year) of lymphoma among men in selected populations, 1975–2011. Data from Stewart BW and Wild CP {205}.

The most common lymphoma types are follicular lymphoma and DLBCL, which together make up >60% of all lymphomas other than Hodgkin lymphoma and plasma cell myeloma {1,95}. The individual B-cell neoplasms vary in their relative frequency in various parts of the world. Follicular lymphoma is more common in the USA (where it accounts for 35% of non-Hodgkin lymphomas) and western Europe, and is uncommon in South America, eastern Europe, Africa, and Asia. Burkitt lymphoma is endemic in equatorial Africa, where it is the most common childhood malignancy, but it accounts for only 1–2% of lymphomas in the USA and western Europe. The median patient age for all types of mature B-cell neoplasms is in the sixth or seventh decade of life, but PMLBCL has a median patient age of about 35 years. Of the mature B-cell lymphomas, only Burkitt lymphoma and DLBCL occur with any significant frequency in children. Most types have a male predominance (with 52–55% of cases occurring in males), but mantle cell lymphoma has a striking male predominance (with 74% of the cases occurring in males), whereas females account for 58% of follicular lymphoma cases and 66% of PMLBCL cases. PMLBCL and nodular sclerosis CHL have similar clinical profiles at presentation, most commonly affecting adolescent and young-adult females. It was their shared clinical features that first prompted consideration that these lymphomas might be related {3412,3538,4047}.

One known major risk factor for mature B-cell neoplasia appears to be an abnormality of the immune system, either immunodeficiency or autoimmune disease.

Although evidence of immune system abnormality is absent in most patients with mature B-cell neoplasms, immunodeficient patients have a markedly increased incidence of B-cell neoplasia, in particular DLBCL and Burkitt lymphoma {345, 547,2819}. Major forms of immunodeficiency include HIV infection, iatrogenic immunosuppression to prevent allograft rejection or graft-versus-host disease, and primary immune deficiencies. Some autoimmune diseases are also associated with an increased risk of lymphoma {4252}; for example, patients with Sjögren syndrome or Hashimoto thyroiditis have a particularly high risk of developing B-cell lymphomas {1953,1959}.

Mutations in genes controlling lymphocyte apoptosis have been linked to increased risk of both autoimmune diseases and lymphomas (mainly B-cell types). Patients with autoimmune lymphoproliferative syndrome (which can be caused by germline mutations in *FAS*) have an increased risk of B-cell lymphomas and Hodgkin lymphoma {3810}. Somatically acquired *FAS* mutations have also been reported in some sporadic B-cell lymphomas, most commonly marginal zone lymphomas {1483}. Genome-wide association studies have identified a substantial number of SNPs that are associated with increased risk of lymphoma {603}. Many of these polymorphisms involve immunoregulatory genes {604,2206,4251}.

Mature T-cell and NK-cell neoplasms are relatively uncommon. In a large international study that evaluated lymphoma cases from the USA, Europe, Asia, and South Africa, T-cell and NK-cell neoplasms accounted for only 12% of all non-Hodgkin lymphomas {1}. The most common mature T-cell lymphomas are PTCL, NOS (accounting for 25.9% of cases) and AITL (accounting for 18.5%) {4217}.

T-cell and NK-cell lymphomas show substantial variations in incidence across geographical regions and racial populations. In general, T-cell lymphomas are relatively more common in Asia {4217}, due to both a higher incidence of some subtypes and a lower relative frequency of some B-cell lymphomas, such as follicular lymphoma. In Japan, one of the main risk factors for T-cell lymphoma is HTLV-1 infection. In endemic regions of south-western Japan, the seroprevalence of HTLV-1 is 8–10%. The cumulative lifetime risk for the development of ATLL is 6.9% for seropositive males and 2.9% for seropositive females {3869}. Other regions with relatively high seroprevalence of HTLV-1 include the Caribbean basin, where Black populations are primarily affected, over other racial groups {1818, 2287}. Differences in viral strain may also affect the incidence of the disease {796, 3869}.

Another major factor influencing the incidence of T-cell and NK-cell lymphomas is racial predisposition. EBV-associated NK-cell and T-cell neoplasms, including extranodal NK/T-cell lymphoma, nasal type (ENKTL), aggressive NK-cell leukaemia, and paediatric EBV-positive T-cell and NK-cell lymphomas, are much more common among Asians than in other populations {640,780,1814,2058}. In Hong Kong SAR, China, ENKTL is one of the more common subtypes, accounting for 8% of cases. By contrast, in Europe and North America it accounts for < 1% of all lymphomas. Other populations at increased risk for this disease are individuals of Native American descent in Central and South America and Mexico {275,780,3266,3269}, who are genetically related to Asians {3280A}. Enteropathy-associated T-cell lymphoma is most common in individuals of Welsh and Irish descent, who share HLA haplotypes that confer an increased risk of gliadin allergy and susceptibility to gluten-sensitive enteropathy {937}.

PTCLs with a gamma delta phenotype occur with increased frequency in the setting of immune suppression (in particular following organ transplantation), a finding that is not well understood {1301,2842}. The risk appears to be increased by the combination of two factors: immunosuppression and chronic antigenic stimulation. Hepatosplenic T-cell lymphomas are most common, but primary cutaneous and mucosa-associated T-cell lymphomas have also been reported {150}. Recent data from the SEER programme indicate a modest increase in the annual incidence of T-cell neoplasms in the USA: to 2.6 cases per 100 000 population, with the greatest increase occurring in the category of cutaneous T-cell lymphoma {839,2759}.

Etiology

Infectious agents have been shown to contribute to the development of several types of mature B-cell, T-cell, and NK-cell lymphomas. EBV is present in nearly 100% of endemic Burkitt lymphoma cases and in 15–35% of sporadic and HIV-associated cases {1531,3238}; it is also involved in the pathogenesis of many B-cell lymphomas arising in immunosuppressed or elderly patients, including many post-transplant lymphoproliferative disorders, plasmablastic lymphoma, and EBV-positive DLBCL, NOS. EBV is also associated with ENKTL and with two paediatric T-cell diseases: systemic EBV-positive T-cell lymphoma of childhood and hydroa vacciniforme–like lymphoproliferative disorder. The exact cause of these EBV-positive T-cell neoplasms of childhood is unclear. Risk factors may include either a high viral load at presentation or a defective immune response to the infection {3269}. Chronic active EBV infection may precede the development of some EBV-positive T-cell lymphomas {1918,3269}. In cases associated with chronic active EBV infection, a polyclonal process may be seen early in the course, with progression to monoclonal EBV-positive T-cell lymphoma {1918}.

HHV8 is found in primary effusion lymphoma, multicentric Castleman disease, and HHV8-positive DLBCL, NOS, all of which are mainly seen in HIV-infected patients {623,1046}, but the virus has also been implicated in germinotropic lymphoproliferative disease not associated with HIV. HTLV-1 is the causative agent of ATLL, and is clonally integrated into the genome of transformed T cells {796}. In this condition, like in HHV8-associated disorders, a spectrum of clinical behaviours is seen, although most cases of ATLL are aggressive.

Hepatitis C virus has been implicated in some cases of lymphoplasmacytic lymphoma associated with type II cryoglobulinaemia, splenic marginal zone lymphoma, nodal marginal zone lymphoma, and DLBCL {32,168,909,912,1884, 2589,3229,4503}. The role of the virus in tumour initiation is unclear; however, it does not directly infect neoplastic B cells, and appears to influence lymphoma development through activation of a B-cell immune response.

Bacteria, or at least immune responses to bacterial antigens, have also been implicated in the pathogenesis of MALT lymphoma, including *Helicobacter pylori* in gastric MALT lymphoma {1741,2853, 4366,4367}; *Borrelia burgdorferi* in cutaneous MALT lymphoma in Europe {611}; *Chlamydia psittaci*, *C. pneumoniae*, and *C. trachomatis* in ocular adnexal MALT lymphomas in some geographical areas {658,3454}; *Campylobacter jejuni* in intestinal MALT lymphoma associated with alpha heavy chain disease {3239,3298}; and *Achromobacter xylosoxidans* in pulmonary MALT lymphomas {20}.

Environmental exposures have also been linked to a risk of developing B-cell lymphoma. Epidemiological studies have implicated herbicide and pesticide use in the development of follicular lymphoma and DLBCL {787,1566}. Exposure to hair dyes was identified as a risk factor in some older studies, but potential carcinogens have been removed from newer dye formulations {4485}.

Conclusion

The multiparameter approach to classification adopted by the WHO classification has been validated in international studies. It is highly reproducible and improves the interpretation of clinical and translational studies. Accurate and precise classification of disease entities also facilitates the determination of the molecular basis of lymphoid neoplasms in the basic science laboratory {1,1815,2759}.

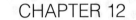

CHAPTER 12

Precursor lymphoid neoplasms

B-lymphoblastic leukaemia/lymphoma, NOS

B-lymphoblastic leukaemia/lymphoma with
recurrent genetic abnormalities

T-lymphoblastic leukaemia/lymphoma

NK-lymphoblastic leukaemia/lymphoma

B-lymphoblastic leukaemia / lymphoma, not otherwise specified (NOS)

Borowitz M.J.
Chan J.K.C.
Downing J.R.
Le Beau M.M.
Arber D.A.

Definition

B-lymphoblastic leukaemia/lymphoma (B-ALL/LBL) is a neoplasm of precursor lymphoid cells committed to the B-cell lineage, typically composed of small to medium-sized blast cells with scant cytoplasm, moderately condensed to dispersed chromatin, and inconspicuous nucleoli, involving bone marrow and blood (B-ALL) and occasionally presenting with primary involvement of nodal or extranodal sites (B-LBL). By convention, the term lymphoma is used when the process is confined to a mass lesion with no or minimal evidence of blood and marrow involvement. With extensive marrow and blood involvement, the appropriate term is B-ALL. If a patient presents with a mass lesion and lymphoblasts in the marrow, the distinction between leukaemia and lymphoma is arbitrary {2792}. In many treatment protocols, a value of >25% marrow blasts is used to define leukaemia. Unlike with myeloid leukaemias, there is no agreed-upon lower limit for the proportion of blasts required to establish a diagnosis of lymphoblastic leukaemia (ALL). In general, the diagnosis should be avoided when there are <20% blasts. Presentations of ALL with low blast counts are uncommon; there is no compelling evidence that failure to treat a patient when there are <20% marrow lymphoblasts has an adverse effect on outcome.

Exclusionary criteria

The term B-ALL should not be used to indicate Burkitt leukaemia/lymphoma. Furthermore, some cases of B-ALL/LBL have specific recurrent genetic abnormalities that are associated with distinctive clinical and phenotypic properties, have important prognostic implications, or demonstrate other evidence that they are mutually exclusive of other entities. These cases should not be classified as B-ALL/LBL, NOS, but rather according to their genetic abnormalities. There are currently nine genetically defined B-ALL/LBLs, which are further described in section *B-lymphoblastic leukaemia/*

lymphoma with recurrent genetic abnormalities (p. 203).

ICD-O code   9811/3

Synonyms

Pro-B lymphoblastic leukaemia; common precursor B-lymphoblastic leukaemia; pre-B lymphoblastic leukaemia; pre-pre-B lymphoblastic leukaemia; common lymphoblastic leukaemia; precursor B-cell lymphoblastic lymphoma; precursor B-cell lymphoblastic leukaemia, NOS; B-cell acute lymphoblastic leukaemia

Epidemiology

ALL is primarily a disease of children; 75% of cases occur in children aged <6 years. The estimated annual incidence worldwide is 1–4.75 cases per 100 000 population {3327}. The estimated number of new cases in the USA is approximately

6000 per year {1603}, with approximately 80–85% being of precursor B-cell phenotype {1501,3358}.

B-LBL constitutes about 10% of lymphoblastic lymphomas (LBLs); the remainder are of T-cell lineage {419}. In one literature review, approximately 64% of 98 reported cases were in patients aged <18 years {2448}. One report indicated a male predominance {2345}.

Etiology

The etiology of B-ALL/LBL is unknown. There is an increased risk of B-ALL in children with Down syndrome and other constitutional genetic disorders {4494}. Genome-wide association studies have shown increased risk of B-ALL associated with certain single nucleotide polymorphisms (SNPs) of genes including *GATA3*, *ARID5B*, *IKZF1*, *CEBPE*, and *CDKN2A/B* {3051,3133}. However, true familial ALL is rare, with some kindreds

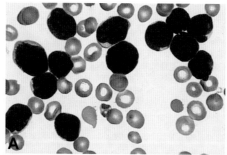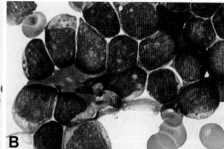

Fig. 12.01 B-lymphoblastic leukaemia. **A** Bone marrow smears showing several lymphoblasts with a high nuclear:cytoplasmic ratio and variably condensed nuclear chromatin. **B** B-cell lymphoblasts containing numerous coarse azurophilic granules.

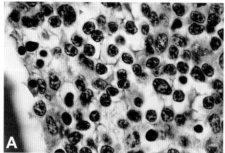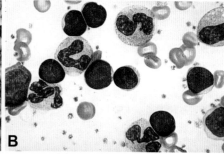

Fig. 12.02 Benign B-cell precursors (haematogones) in bone marrow. **A** Increased haematogones in bone marrow biopsy section may resemble lymphoblasts. **B** Bone marrow aspirate smear with increased haematogones, from an 8-year-old boy, shows lymphoid cells with a high nuclear:cytoplasmic ratio and homogeneous nuclear chromatin; nucleoli are not observed or are indistinct. These cells resemble the lymphoblasts in lymphoblastic leukaemia of childhood.

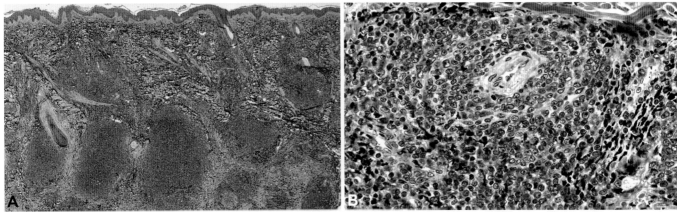

Fig. 12.03 B-lymphoblastic lymphoma in skin. **A** Neoplastic cells diffusely infiltrate the dermis but spare the epidermis. **B** Higher magnification of the same case shows lymphoblasts surrounding a blood vessel.

described having mutations in *PAX5* {3630}, *ETV6* {4435}, and *TP53* {3226}. *TP53* mutation, as discussed below, shows a specific association with low hypodiploid B-ALL {1929}. Some translocations associated with ALL have been detected in neonatal specimens long before the onset of leukaemia, and monozygotic twins with concordant leukaemia frequently share genetic abnormalities {1428,2731}. However, these findings are thought to reflect somatic mutations occurring in one twin and shared via in utero circulation rather than constitutional genetic lesions.

Localization

By definition, the bone marrow is involved in all cases classified as B-ALL, and the peripheral blood is usually involved. Extramedullary involvement is common, with particular predilection for the central nervous system (CNS), lymph nodes, spleen, liver, and testes. The most frequent sites of involvement in B-LBL are the skin, soft tissue, bone, and lymph nodes {354, 2345,2448}. Mediastinal masses are uncommon {354,2448,3506}.

Clinical features

Most patients with B-ALL present with evidence and consequences of bone marrow failure: thrombocytopenia, anaemia, and/or neutropenia. The leukocyte count may be decreased, normal, or markedly elevated. Lymphadenopathy, hepatomegaly, and splenomegaly are frequent. Bone pain and arthralgias may be prominent symptoms. Patients presenting with B-LBL are usually asymptomatic, and most have limited-stage disease. Head and neck presentations are particularly common, especially in

children. Marrow and blood involvement may be present, but by definition the proportion of lymphoblasts in the marrow is < 25% {2345,2448}.

Microscopy

In smear and imprint preparations, the lymphoblasts in B-ALL/LBL vary from small blasts with scant cytoplasm, condensed nuclear chromatin, and indistinct nucleoli to larger cells with moderate amounts of light-blue to bluish-grey cytoplasm (occasionally vacuolated), dispersed nuclear chromatin, and multiple variably prominent nucleoli. The nuclei are round or show convolutions. Coarse azurophilic granules are present in some lymphoblasts in approximately 10% of cases. In some cases, the lymphoblasts have cytoplasmic pseudopods (hand-mirror cells). Normal B-cell precursors (haematogones) can mimic lymphoblasts, but they typically have even higher nuclear:cytoplasmic ratios, more-homogeneous chromatin, and no discernible nucleoli.

In bone marrow biopsies, the lymphoblasts in B-ALL are relatively uniform in appearance, with round to oval, indented, or convoluted nuclei. Nucleoli range from inconspicuous to prominent. The chromatin is finely dispersed. The number of mitotic figures varies. LBL is generally characterized by a diffuse or (less commonly) paracortical pattern of involvement of lymph node. A single-file pattern of infiltration of soft tissue is common. Mitotic figures are usually numerous, and in some cases there may be a focal so-called starry-sky pattern. The morphological features of B-lymphoblastic and T-lymphoblastic proliferations are indistinguishable.

Cytochemistry

Cytochemistry seldom contributes to the diagnosis of ALL. Lymphoblasts are negative for MPO. Granules, if present, may stain light grey with Sudan Black B but are less intense than myeloblasts. Lymphoblasts may show periodic acid–Schiff (PAS) positivity, usually in the form of coarse granules. They may react with nonspecific esterase, with a multifocal punctate or Golgi region pattern that shows variable inhibition with sodium fluoride.

Immunophenotype

The lymphoblasts in B-ALL/LBL are almost always positive for the B-cell markers CD19, cCD79a, and cCD22; although none of these by itself is specific, their positivity in combination or at high intensity strongly supports the diagnosis. The lymphoblasts are positive for CD10, surface CD22, CD24, PAX5, and TdT in most cases, whereas CD20 and CD34 expression is variable; CD45 may be absent and if present is nearly always more dimly expressed than on mature B cells. The myeloid-associated antigens CD13 and CD33 may be expressed and the presence of these myeloid markers

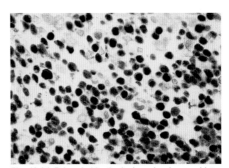

Fig. 12.04 B-lymphoblastic leukaemia. Immunohistochemical demonstration of nuclear TdT in a bone marrow biopsy.

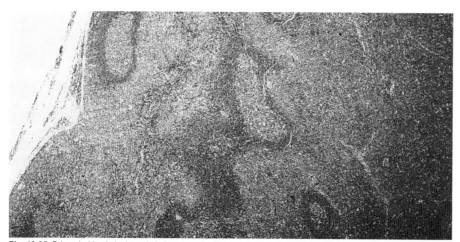

Fig. 12.05 B-lymphoblastic leukaemia in lymph node. The neoplastic cells infiltrate diffusely, sparing normal follicles.

does not exclude the diagnosis of precursor B-ALL. In tissue sections, CD79a and PAX5 are most frequently used to demonstrate B-cell differentiation, but CD79a is positive in many cases of T-ALL and is not specific {1584}. PAX5 is generally considered the most sensitive and specific marker for B-cell lineage in tissue sections {4028}, but it is also positive in acute myeloid leukaemia with t(8;21)(q22;q22.1) resulting in *RUNX1-RUNX1T1* and rarely in other acute myeloid leukaemias {4102}. MPO can sometimes be detected, most commonly by immunohistochemistry but also sometimes by flow cytometry, and should not automatically exclude the diagnosis, but MPO immunoreactivity most often indicates either acute myeloid leukaemia or B/myeloid acute leukaemia {131}.

The degree of differentiation of precursor B-lineage lymphoblasts has clinical and genetic correlates. In the earliest stage (so-called early precursor B-ALL or pro-B ALL), the blasts express CD19, cCD79a, cCD22, and nuclear TdT. In the intermediate stage (so-called common B-ALL), the blasts express CD10. The most mature precursor B-cell differentiation stages include pre-B ALL, wherein the blasts express cytoplasmic mu chain, and occasional cases with surface heavy chain without light chain may be seen in so-called transitional pre-B ALL. Clonal surface immunoglobulin light chain is characteristically absent, although its presence does not exclude the possibility of B-ALL/LBL {2844}. Although both B-ALL and normal B-cell precursors (haematogones) express CD10, their im-

munophenotypes nearly always differ. Haematogones show a continuum of expression of markers of B-cell maturation, including surface immunoglobulin light chain, and display a reproducible pattern of acquisition and loss of normal antigens {2600}. In contrast, B-ALL shows patterns that differ from normal, with either overexpression or underexpression of many markers, including CD10, CD45, CD38, CD58, and TdT {537,674,2408,4280}. These differences can be very useful in the evaluation of follow-up marrow specimens for minimal residual disease.

Postulated normal counterpart
Either a haematopoietic stem cell or a B-cell progenitor

Genetic profile
Antigen receptor genes
Nearly all cases of B-ALL have clonal rearrangements of IGH. In addition, T-cell receptor (TR) gene rearrangements may be seen in a substantial proportion of cases (as many as 70%) {4126}. Therefore, IGH and TR gene rearrangements are not helpful for lineage assignment.

Cytogenetic abnormalities and oncogenes
Cytogenetic abnormalities are seen in most cases of B-ALL/LBL; in many cases, they define specific entities with unique phenotypic and prognostic features (see following section). Additional cytogenetic lesions that are not associated with the entities in the category of B-ALL with recurrent genetic abnormalities include del(6q), del(9p), and del(12p),

but these do not have an impact on prognosis. However, it is likely that some genetic lesions are prognostically important, although there is not yet sufficient evidence to considering these as distinct entities. For example, the very rare ALL with t(17;19)(q22;p13.3) resulting in *TCF3-HLF* is associated with a very poor prognosis, but there are too few cases to include this in the classification.

A very large number of recurrent genetic alterations occur in B-ALL, detected either as copy-number alterations or as specific mutations. Many of these, such as alterations of *PAX5*, are seen in most subtypes of B-ALL and are likely fundamental to the pathogenesis of the disease. Mutations in other genes, such as the RAS family of oncogenes and *IKZF1*, are seen in a more restricted distribution. Although they are not strictly part of the definition of genetic entities, they do tend to be associated with particular types.

Prognosis and predictive factors
B-ALL has a good prognosis in children, but a less favourable prognosis in adults. The overall complete remission rate is >95% in children, versus 60–85% in adults. Approximately 80% of children with B-ALL appear to be cured, versus <50% of adults. More-intensive therapy improves cure rates, and there is some evidence that, at least in younger adults, therapy with more-intensive so-called paediatric-type regimens is associated with better outcome {408,1521}.

Infancy, older patient age, higher white blood cell count, slow response to initial therapy as assessed by morphological examination of blood and/or bone marrow, and the presence of minimal residual disease after therapy are all associated with adverse prognosis {380,572,829, 3589,3679,4129}. The presence of CNS disease at diagnosis is associated with adverse outcome and requires specific therapy {764}. The important effect of genetic lesions is discussed in the sections below.

The prognosis of B-LBL is also relatively favourable, and like that of B-ALL, it appears to be better in children than in adults {2448}.

B-lymphoblastic leukaemia/lymphoma with recurrent genetic abnormalities

Borowitz M.J.
Chan J.K.C.
Downing J.R.
Le Beau M.M.
Arber D.A.

Definition

B-lymphoblastic leukaemia/lymphoma (B-ALL/LBL) with recurrent genetic abnormalities is a group of diseases characterized by recurrent genetic abnormalities, including balanced translocations and abnormalities involving chromosome number. Many chromosomal abnormalities that are non-randomly associated with B-ALL are not included as separate entities in this section. Although the inclusion or exclusion of a given genetic entity is somewhat arbitrary, those included have been chosen because they are associated with distinctive clinical or phenotypic properties, have important prognostic implications, demonstrate other evidence that they are biologically distinct, and are generally mutually exclusive with other entities.

B-lymphoblastic leukaemia/lymphoma with t(9;22)(q34.1;q11.2); BCR-ABL1

Definition

B-lymphoblastic leukaemia/lymphoma (B-ALL/LBL) with t(9;22)(q34.1;q11.2) is a neoplasm of lymphoblasts committed to the B-cell lineage in which the blasts harbour a translocation between *BCR* on chromosome 22 and the *ABL1* oncogene on chromosome 9.

ICD-O code   9812/3

Epidemiology

B-ALL with *BCR-ABL1* is relatively more common in adults than in children, accounting for about 25% of adult ALL but only 2–4% of childhood cases.

Clinical features

The presenting features are generally similar to those seen in patients with other B-ALLs. Most children with B-ALL with *BCR-ABL1* are considered to have high-risk on the basis of age and white blood cell count, but there are otherwise no

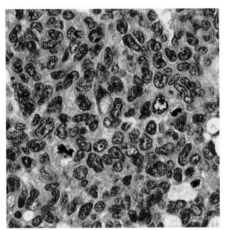

Fig. 12.06 B-lymphoblastic leukaemia with t(9;22) (q34.1;q11.2); *BCR-ABL1*. This bone marrow from an adult is completely replaced by lymphoblasts. Mitotic figures are numerous.

characteristic clinical findings. Although patients with B-ALL with *BCR-ABL1* may have organ involvement, lymphomatous presentations are rare.

Microscopy

There are no unique morphological or cytochemical features that distinguish this entity from other types of ALL.

Immunophenotype

B-ALL with *BCR-ABL1* is typically positive for CD10, CD19, and TdT. There is frequent expression of myeloid-associated antigens CD13 and CD33 {1712}; KIT (CD117) is typically not expressed. CD25 is highly associated with B-ALL with *BCR-ABL1*, at least in adults {3030}. Rare cases of ALL with *BCR-ABL1* have a T-cell precursor phenotype.

Cell of origin

There is some evidence that the cell of origin of B-ALL with *BCR-ABL1* is more immature than that of other B-ALL cases {773}.

Genetic profile

The t(9;22) translocation results from fusion of *BCR* at 22q11.2 and the cytoplasmic tyrosine kinase gene *ABL1* at 9q34.1, with production of a BCR-ABL1 fusion protein. In most childhood cases of ALL

with t(9;22), a p190 BCR-ABL1 fusion protein is produced. In adults, about half of all cases produce the p210 fusion protein that is characteristic of *BCR-ABL1*–positive chronic myeloid leukaemia, and the remainder produce the p190 transcript. No definite clinical differences have been attributed to these two gene products. The t(9;22) may be associated with other genetic abnormalities, including (in rare cases) abnormalities that might otherwise cause a case to be placed in one of the other categories discussed below. It is generally believed that the clinical features in such cases are governed by the presence of the t(9;22).

Prognosis and predictive factors

Historically, in both children and adults, B-ALL with *BCR-ABL1* has been considered to have the worst prognosis of the major cytogenetic subtypes of ALL. Its higher frequency in adult ALL explains in part the relatively poor outcome of adults with ALL. In children, favourable clinical features including younger age, lower white blood cell count, and response to therapy are associated with somewhat better outcome {146}. Therapy with tyrosine kinase inhibitors has had a significantly favourable effect on outcome {3588}.

B-lymphoblastic leukaemia/lymphoma with t(v;11q23.3); KMT2A-rearranged

Definition

B-lymphoblastic leukaemia/lymphoma (B-ALL/LBL) with t(v;11q23.3) is a neoplasm of lymphoblasts committed to the B-cell lineage in which the blasts harbour a translocation between *KMT2A* (also called *MLL*) at band 11q23.3 and any of a large number of fusion partners. Leukaemias that have deletions of 11q23.3 without *KMT2A* rearrangement are not included in this group.

ICD-O code   9813/3

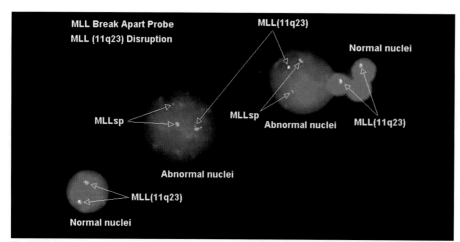

Fig. 12.07 B-lymphoblastic leukaemia/lymphoma with t(v;11q23.3); *KMT2A*-rearranged. FISH study using a break-apart probe for *KMT2A* (previously called *MLL*); the normal *KMT2A* gene [MLL(11q23)] appears as juxtaposed red and green signals or sometimes a yellow signal; the translocation is demonstrated by separation of the red and green probes (MLLsp).

Synonym

B-lymphoblastic leukaemia/lymphoma with t(v;11q23); *MLL*-rearranged

Epidemiology

B-ALL with *KMT2A* rearrangement is the most common leukaemia in infants aged < 1 year. It is less common in older children and then becomes increasingly common with age into adulthood.

Etiology

Although the specific etiology of leukaemia with *KMT2A* translocations is unknown, this rearrangement may occur in utero, with a short latency between the translocation and development of disease. Evidence for this includes the fact that these leukaemias are frequent in very young infants, as well as the fact that this translocation has been identified in neonatal blood spots of patients who subsequently develop leukaemia {1277}.

Clinical features

Patients with this leukaemia typically present with very high white blood cell counts: frequently $> 100 \times 10^9$/L. There is also a high frequency of CNS involvement at diagnosis. Although organ involvement may be seen, pure lymphomatous presentations are not typical.

Microscopy

There are no unique morphological or cytochemical features that distinguish this entity from other types of ALL. In some cases of leukaemias with *KMT2A* rearrangement, it may be possible to recognize distinct lymphoblastic and mono-

blastic populations, a finding that can be confirmed by immunophenotyping; such cases should be considered B/myeloid leukaemias.

Immunophenotype

Cases of B-ALL with *KMT2A* rearrangements, especially t(4;11), typically have a CD19+, CD10−, CD24−, pro-B immunophenotype, and are also positive for CD15 {1712,3066}. The NG2 homologue encoded by *CSPG4* is also characteristically expressed and is relatively specific.

Genetic profile

The *KMT2A* gene on chromosome 11q23.3 is a promiscuous oncogene, with > 100 fusion partners. Translocations involving this gene can be detected by standard karyotyping studies or by FISH with a break-apart probe directed against the *KMT2A* gene. PCR can be used to identify major translocation partners, but a negative PCR result cannot exclude an alternative fusion partner. The most common partner gene is *AFF1* (*AF4*) on chromosome 4q21. Other common partner genes include *MLLT1* (*ENL*) on chromosome 19p13.3 and *MLLT3* (*AF9*) on chromosome 9p21.3. *KMT2A-MLLT1* fusions are also common in T-ALL, whereas fusions between *KMT2A* and *MLLT3* are more typically associated with acute myeloid leukaemia. Leukaemias with *KMT2A* rearrangement are frequently associated with overexpression of *FLT3* {149}. In contrast to nearly all other categories of B-ALL, B-ALL with *KMT2A* rearrangement in infants has very few associated additional mutations,

with frequencies among the lowest of all cancers {99}; when mutations occur, they typically involve RAS pathways {1039}.

Prognosis and predictive factors

Leukaemias with the *KMT2A-AFF1* translocation have a poor prognosis. There is some controversy as to whether leukaemias with translocations other than the *KMT2A-AFF1* translocation have as poor a prognosis as those with *KMT2A-AFF1*. Infants with *KMT2A* rearrangement, in particular those aged < 6 months, have a particularly poor prognosis {1039}.

B-lymphoblastic leukaemia/lymphoma with t(12;21)(p13.2;q22.1); ETV6-RUNX1

Definition

B-lymphoblastic leukaemia/lymphoma (B-ALL/LBL) with t(12;21)(p13.2;q22.1) is a neoplasm of lymphoblasts committed to the B-cell lineage in which the blasts harbour a translocation between *ETV6* (also called *TEL*) on chromosome 12 and *RUNX1* (also called *AML1*) on chromosome 21.

ICD-O code   9814/3

Synonym

B acute lymphoblastic leukaemia/lymphoma with t(12;21)(p13;q22), *TEL/AML1* (*ETV6-RUNX1*)

Epidemiology

This leukaemia is not seen in infants, but is common in children, accounting for about 25% of cases of B-ALL in that age group. It decreases in frequency with age to the point that it is rare in adulthood.

Clinical features

The presenting features are generally similar to those seen in patients with other ALLs.

Microscopy

There are no unique morphological or cytochemical features that distinguish this entity from other types of ALL.

Immunophenotype

Blasts have a CD19+, CD10+ phenotype and are most often CD34 positive; other phenotypic features, including near or

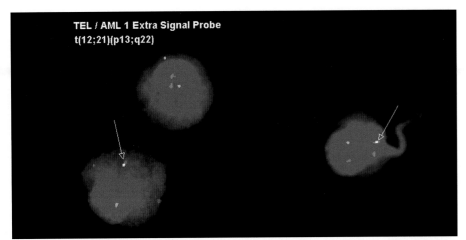

TEL / AML 1 Extra Signal Probe
t(12;21)(p13;q22)

Fig. 12.08 B-lymphoblastic leukaemia/lymphoma with t(12;21)(p13.2;q22.1); *ETV6-RUNX1*. FISH study using probes against *RUNX1 (AML1)* (red) and *ETV6 (TEL)* (green). The normal genes appear as isolated red or green signals, and the fusion gene (arrows) appears as a yellow signal.

complete absence of CD9, CD20, and CD66c {421,914,1712}, are relatively specific. Myeloid-associated antigens, especially CD13, are frequently expressed {283}.

Cell of origin
This leukaemia appears to derive from a B-cell progenitor rather than a haemato-poietic stem cell {580}.

Genetic profile
The *ETV6-RUNX1* translocation results in the production of a fusion protein that probably acts in a dominant negative fashion to interfere with normal function of the transcription factor RUNX1. This leukaemia appears to have a unique gene

expression signature {4423}. The *ETV6-RUNX1* translocation is considered to be an early lesion in leukaemogenesis, as evidenced by studies of neonatal blood spots that have shown the presence of the translocation in children who develop leukaemia many years later {4311}. There is evidence that the translocation is necessary but not sufficient for the development of leukaemia {4311}.

Prognosis and predictive factors
B-ALL with the *ETV6-RUNX1* translocation has a very favourable prognosis, with cure seen in >90% of children, especially if they have other favourable risk factors. Relapses often occur much later than do those of other types of ALL. Because this

translocation appears to occur as an early event, it has been suggested that some late relapses in fact derive from persistent so-called preleukaemic clones that harbour the translocation and undergo additional genetic events after the first leukaemic clone has been eliminated {1234}. Children with this leukaemia who also have adverse prognostic factors, such as age > 10 years or high white blood cell count, do not have as good a prognosis, but may still fare better as a group than other ALL patients with the same adverse factors.

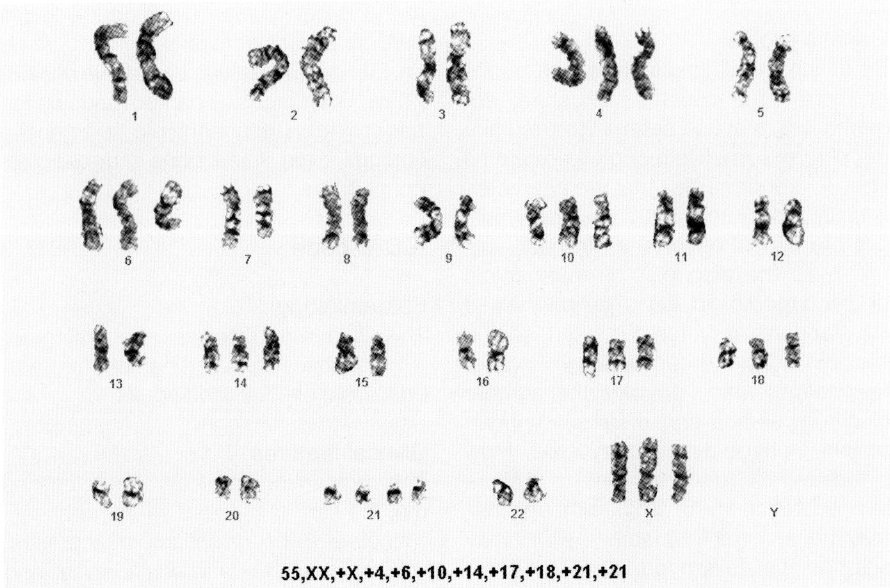

B-lymphoblastic leukaemia/lymphoma with hyperdiploidy

Definition
B-lymphoblastic leukaemia/lymphoma (B-ALL/LBL) with hyperdiploidy is a neoplasm of lymphoblasts committed to the B-cell lineage whose blasts contain >50 chromosomes (usually <66), typically without translocations or other structural alterations. There is controversy as to whether the specific chromosomal additions, rather than the specific number of chromosomes, should be part of the definition {1554,3284,3835}.

ICD-O code   9815/3

Synonyms
Hyperdiploid acute lymphoblastic leukaemia; high hyperdiploid acute lymphoblastic leukaemia; acute lymphoblastic leukaemia with favourable trisomies

Epidemiology
This leukaemia is common in children, accounting for about 25% of cases of B-ALL in this age group. It is not seen in infants, and decreases in frequency among older children. It is uncommon in adulthood, accounting for about 7–8% of cases of B-ALL in adults {2771}.

Clinical features
The presenting features are generally similar to those seen in patients with other ALLs.

Microscopy
There are no unique morphological or cytochemical features that distinguish this entity from other types of ALL.

55,XX,+X,+4,+6,+10,+14,+17,+18,+21,+21

Fig. 12.09 B-lymphoblastic leukaemia with hyperdiploidy. G-banded karyotype showing 55 chromosomes, including trisomies of chromosomes 4, 10, and 17 and tetrasomy 21. There are no structural abnormalities.

Immunophenotype

Blasts are positive for CD19 and CD10, and express other markers typical of B-ALL. Most cases are CD34 positive, and CD45 is often absent {1712}. Patients with T-ALL with hyperdiploidy should not be considered part of this group, although most such patients have near-tetraploid karyotypes.

Genetic profile

Hyperdiploid B-ALL contains a numerical increase in chromosomes, usually without structural abnormalities. Extra copies of chromosomes are non-random: chromosomes 21, X, 14, and 4 are the most common, and chromosomes 1, 2, and 3 are the least often seen {1598}. Hyperdiploid B-ALL can be detected by conventional karyotyping, FISH, or flow cytometric DNA index {2523}. Some cases that appear to be hyperdiploid ALL by conventional karyotyping may in fact be hypodiploid ALL that has undergone endoreduplication, doubling the number of chromosomes. The specific chromosomes that appear as trisomies may be more important to prognosis than the actual number of chromosomes, with simultaneous trisomies of chromosomes 4 and 10 carrying the best prognosis {3835}.

Prognosis and predictive factors

Hyperdiploid B-ALL has a very favourable prognosis, with cure seen in >90% of children overall, and even more commonly among children with a favourable risk profile. Adverse factors such as advanced patient age and high white blood cell count may adversely affect the prognosis, but these patients may not fare as badly as others without this favourable genetic abnormality. Too few adult cases have been studied to determine the prognosis in adulthood.

B-lymphoblastic leukaemia/lymphoma with hypodiploidy

Definition

B-lymphoblastic leukaemia/lymphoma (B-ALL/LBL) with hypodiploidy is a neoplasm of lymphoblasts committed to the B-cell lineage whose blasts contain <46 chromosomes. Hypodiploid ALL is divided into three (or sometimes four)

subtypes: (1) near-haploid ALL (with 23–29 chromosomes), (2) low hypodiploid ALL (with 33–39 chromosomes), and (3) high hypodiploid ALL (with 40–43 chromosomes). A fourth category, near-diploid ALL (with 44–45 chromosomes), is often not included in definitions of hypodiploid ALL, at least for treatment purposes, because such cases do not share the poor prognostic features of the other three categories {2802}.

ICD-O code   9816/3

Epidemiology

Hypodiploid ALL accounts for about 5% of ALL cases overall, but when the definition is restricted to cases with <45 chromosomes, the figure is closer to 1%. Hypodiploid ALL occurs in both children and adults, although near-haploid ALL (23–29 chromosomes) appears to be limited to childhood.

Clinical features

The presenting features are generally similar to those seen in patients with other ALLs.

Microscopy

There are no unique morphological or cytochemical features that distinguish this entity from other types of ALL.

Immunophenotype

Blasts have a B-cell precursor phenotype (typically CD19+, CD10+), but there are no other distinctive phenotypic features.

Genetic profile

By definition, all cases show loss of one or more chromosomes. Structural abnormalities may be seen in the remaining chromosomes, although there are no specific abnormalities that are characteristically associated. Structural abnormalities are almost never seen in near-haploid ALL. The diagnosis of near-haploid or low hypodiploid ALL may be missed by standard karyotyping, because the hypodiploid clone can undergo endoreduplication, which doubles the number of chromosomes and results in a near-diploid or hyperdiploid karyotype. Flow cytometry can generally detect a clone with a DNA index of <1.0, although this may be a minor population. FISH may also identify cells hypodiploid for chromosomes, and this diagnosis should be suspected when there is a discrepancy

between a karyotype and FISH results with respect to the number of chromosomes present.

The various classes of hypodiploid ALL are associated with distinctive genetic lesions {1929}. Near-haploid ALL often has RAS or receptor tyrosine kinase mutations. Low hypodiploid ALL is the most distinctive class: the great majority of cases show loss-of-function mutations in *TP53* and/or *RB1*. Some of the *TP53* mutations are germline, suggesting a form of Li–Fraumeni syndrome. These genetic lesions do not occur in high hypodiploid ALL, which is not associated with any specific gene alterations.

Prognosis and predictive factors

Hypodiploid ALL has a poor prognosis, with near-haploid ALL having the worst prognosis in some studies {1560,2802}. There is some evidence that patients may fare poorly even if they do not have minimal residual disease following therapy, which is in contrast to other types of ALL.

B-lymphoblastic leukaemia/lymphoma with t(5;14)(q31.1;q32.1); IGH/IL3

Definition

B-lymphoblastic leukaemia/lymphoma (B-ALL/LBL) with t(5;14)(q31.1;q32.1) is a neoplasm of lymphoblasts committed to the B-cell lineage in which the blasts harbour a translocation between *IL3* and an IGH gene, resulting in variable eosinophilia. This diagnosis can be made on the basis of immunophenotypic and genetic findings even if the bone marrow blast count is low.

ICD-O code   9817/3

Epidemiology

This is a rare disease, accounting for <1% of cases of ALL. It has been reported in both children and adults.

Clinical features

The presenting clinical characteristics may be similar to those seen in patients with other ALLs, or patients may present with an asymptomatic eosinophilia, and blasts may be deceptively absent in the peripheral blood.

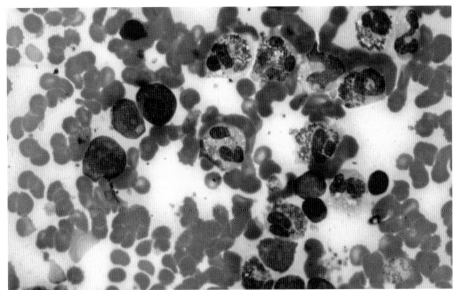

Fig. 12.10 B-lymphoblastic leukaemia with t(5;14)(q31.1;q32.1); IGH/IL3. Bone marrow smear showing a population of typical lymphoblasts along with numerous mature eosinophils. The granule distribution in some of the eosinophils is unusual, but this is not a consistent factor.

Microscopy

Blasts in this neoplasm have the typical morphology of lymphoblasts, but the striking finding is an increase in circulating eosinophils. This is a reactive population and not part of the leukaemic clone.

Immunophenotype

Blasts have a CD19+, CD10+ phenotype. The finding of even small numbers of blasts with this phenotype in a patient with eosinophilia strongly suggests this diagnosis.

Genetic profile

The unique characteristics of this neoplasm derive from a functional rearrangement between the *IL3* gene on chromosome 5 and an IGH gene on chromosome 14, resulting in constitutive overexpression of IL3 {1463}. Other than eosinophilia, the functional consequences of this rearrangement are not well understood. The abnormality is typically detected by conventional karyotyping; it can also be detected by FISH, although appropriate probes are not widely available.

Prognosis and predictive factors

The prognosis is not considered to be different from that of other types of ALL, although there are too few cases to be certain. Blast percentage at diagnosis is not known to be a predictive factor.

B-lymphoblastic leukaemia/lymphoma with t(1;19)(q23;p13.3); TCF3-PBX1

Definition

B-lymphoblastic leukaemia/lymphoma (B-ALL/LBL) with t(1;19)(q23;p13.3) is a neoplasm of lymphoblasts committed to the B-cell lineage in which the blasts harbour a translocation between *TCF3* (also known as *E2A*) on chromosome 19 and *PBX1* on chromosome 1.

ICD-O code   9818/3

Epidemiology

This leukaemia is relatively common in children, accounting for about 6% of cases of B-ALL. It is less common in adults.

Clinical features

The presenting features are generally similar to those seen in patients with other ALLs.

Microscopy

There are no unique morphological or cytochemical features that distinguish this entity from other types of ALL.

Immunophenotype

Blasts typically have a pre-B phenotype, with positivity for CD19, CD10, and cytoplasmic mu heavy chain, although not all cases of pre-B ALL have the t(1;19).

This diagnosis can be suspected even when cytoplasmic mu is not determined, because these leukaemias typically show strong expression of CD9 and lack CD34, or show very limited CD34 expression on only a minor subset of leukaemic cells {420}.

Genetic profile

The *TCF3-PBX1* translocation results in the production of a fusion protein that has an oncogenic role as a transcriptional activator, and also likely interferes with the normal function of the transcription factors coded by *TCF3* and *PBX1* {2243}. The functional fusion gene resides on chromosome 19, and there may be loss of the derivative chromosome 1 in some cases, resulting in an unbalanced translocation. Gene expression profiling studies have identified a signature unique to this lesion {4423}. An alternative *TCF3* translocation, t(17;19), occurs in rare cases of ALL involving the *HLF* gene on chromosome 17 and is associated with a dismal prognosis. Therefore, demonstration of a *TCF3* rearrangement by itself is not a diagnostic criterion for this leukaemia.

A subset of B-ALL cases, most commonly hyperdiploid B-ALLs, have a karyotypically identical t(1;19) that involves neither *TCF3* nor *PBX1*, and should not be confused with this entity.

Prognosis and predictive factors

In early studies, B-ALL with *TCF3-PBX1* was associated with a poor prognosis, but this is now readily overcome with modern intensive therapy. However, there may be an increased relative risk of CNS relapse in these patients {1850}. Many treatment protocols no longer require identification of this genetic lesion; the importance of identifying it as a distinct entity is controversial, although the findings of unique immunophenotypic and genetic features support its inclusion as a distinct entity.

B-lymphoblastic leukaemia/lymphoma, BCR-ABL1–like

Definition
BCR-ABL1–like B-lymphoblastic leukaemia/lymphoma (B-ALL/LBL) is a neoplasm of lymphoblasts committed to the B-cell lineage that lack the BCR-ABL1 translocation but show a pattern of gene expression very similar to that seen in ALL with BCR-ABL1. Leukaemias with these properties frequently have translocations involving other tyrosine kinases, or alternatively have translocations involving CRLF2 or (less commonly) re-arrangements leading to truncation and activation of the erythropoietin receptor (EPOR). From a practical standpoint, it is difficult to identify these leukaemias without complex laboratory analysis, and it is also difficult to screen cases of B-ALL to determine which cases would need such analysis; however, diagnostic technology in this area is progressing rapidly. Because of the clinical importance of identifying these cases, BCR-ABL1–like B-ALL/LBL has been included as a provisional entity.

ICD-O code   9819/3

Epidemiology
This leukaemia is relatively common, occurring in 10–25% of patients with ALL; the frequency is lowest in children with United States National Cancer Institute (NCI) standard-risk ALL and progressively higher in children with high-risk ALL, adolescents, and adults. Children with Down syndrome have a very high frequency of B-ALL with CRLF2 translocations. The frequency of certain genomic lesions varies with ethnicity; IGH/CRLF2 translocations are more common in Hispanics and in individuals with Native American genetic ancestry {1577}.

Etiology
No details are known about the etiology of this leukaemia, but it has been shown that certain inherited GATA3 variants confer an increased risk of this entity {3133}.

Clinical features
The presenting clinical features are generally similar to those seen in patients with other ALLs, although patients tend to have high white blood cell counts at presentation.

Microscopy
There are no unique morphological or cytochemical features that distinguish this entity from other types of ALL.

Immunophenotype
Blasts typically have a CD19+, CD10+ phenotype. The subset of cases with CRLF2 translocations show very high levels of surface expression of the protein product by flow cytometry; this can be a useful screen for translocations, because cases without elevated expression essentially never show a CRLF2 translocation. There are no specific immunophenotypic features associated with translocations involving EPOR or tyrosine kinases.

Genetic profile
BCR-ABL1–like B-ALLs were originally identified by their distinctive gene expression profile, although different groups' algorithms do not always identify the same patients {398}. BCR-ABL1–like leukaemias show various types of chromosomal rearrangements, involving many different genes and various partners {3370}. Cases with CRLF2 rearrangements, which account for about half of cases overall, often show an interstitial deletion of the PAR1 gene family on Xp22.3 and Yp11.3, which juxtaposes CRLF2 to the promoter of the P2RY8 gene. An alternative translocation involves IGH. IGH translocation can also involve EPOR. The tyrosine kinase–type translocations have been reported to involve ABL1 with partners other than BCR, as well as other kinases, including ABL2, PDGFRB, NTRK3, TYK2, CSF1R, and JAK2. More than 30 partner genes have been described. Kinase translocations only rarely coexist with CRLF2 rearrangements. Some of these translocations can be detected by standard karyotype analysis, but many are cryptic, in particular those involving an interstitial deletion of CRLF2. Many cases of BCR-ABL1–like ALL also show deletions or mutations in other genes known to be important to leukaemogenesis, including IKZF1 and CDKN2A/B, although IKZF1 in particular is not specific enough for this group of diseases to be part of the definition {398}. About half of the cases of CRLF2-rearranged ALL have mutations in JAK2 or JAK1.

Prognosis and predictive factors
Overall, patients with BCR-ABL1–like ALL have a poor prognosis {397,398};

however, these patients also have a higher risk of being positive for minimal residual disease, and determining the extent to which the outcome is impacted by minimal residual disease status is difficult {3371}. CRLF2 translocations have specifically been associated with poor prognosis in several studies, but there is some controversy as to whether this is true only in certain subgroups of patients {1111,1577,3038,4125}.

Many of the small number of children who are primarily resistant to induction chemotherapy have a translocation targeting PDGFRB, most often with EBF1 as the partner. These patients have shown dramatic responses to ABL-class tyrosine kinase inhibitors such as imatinib and dasatinib {4306}. Clinical trials are being developed to test the hypothesis that treatment of all patients with ABL-class fusions with tyrosine kinase inhibitors will greatly improve their poor outcome. Patients with JAK mutations or translocations may be candidates for treatment with JAK inhibitors, although the effectiveness of such treatment has not yet been proven.

B-lymphoblastic leukaemia/lymphoma with iAMP21

Definition
B-lymphoblastic leukaemia/lymphoma (B-ALL/LBL) with iAMP21 is a neoplasm of lymphoblasts committed to the B-cell lineage characterized by amplification of a portion of chromosome 21, typically detected by FISH with a probe for RUNX1 that reveals ≥5 copies of the gene (or ≥3 extra copies on a single abnormal chromosome 21) {1561,1597}.

ICD-O code   9811/3

Epidemiology
This disease is most often identified in children with ALL, and is more common in older children who present with low white blood cell counts. It accounts for about 2% of cases of B-ALL. The incidence in adult ALL has not been established, but appears to be lower than in children.

Etiology
Although the etiology of this entity is not fully understood, mechanistic clues have been derived from the observation that

individuals with the rare constitutional Robertsonian translocation rob(15;21)(q10;q10)c have a nearly 3000-fold increased risk of developing this leukaemia, which appears to involve chromothripsis; this mechanism is likely to be contributory in sporadic cases as well {2314}.

Microscopy

There are no unique morphological or cytochemical features that distinguish this entity from other types of ALL.

Immunophenotype

Other than the observation that these cases occur exclusively in B-ALL, no detailed immunophenotypic information is known.

Genetic profile

This leukaemia is recognized by FISH with the probes used to identify *ETV6-RUNX1* translocation. However, the pathogenesis of the disease does not involve *RUNX1*, although it is part of the critical region consistently amplified. In about 20% of cases, this is the only cytogenetic abnormality; in the remainder, many other chromosomal abnormalities are seen, the most common of which include gains of the X chromosome and abnormalities of chromosome 7. This entity is associated with deletions of *RB1* and *ETV6*, and with rearrangements of *CRLF2* at a frequency greater than is seen in other ALLs, but the role of these additional alterations in this leukaemia is uncertain. Given the unique nature of the iAMP21 alteration, cases with genetic lesions that might suggest another category of classification, such as *CRLF2* translocations, should still be included as B-ALL/LBL with iAMP21.

Prognosis and predictive factors

ALL with iAMP21 has a relatively poor prognosis among children with cases that would otherwise be classified and treated as standard-risk ALL, although it appears that treatment of these children with more intensive therapy overcomes this adverse risk {1561}. Children with high-risk ALL with iAMP21 probably do not require any special therapy.

T-lymphoblastic leukaemia / lymphoma

Borowitz M.J.
Chan J.K.C.
Béné M.-C.
Arber D.A.

Definition

T-lymphoblastic leukaemia/lymphoma (T-ALL/LBL) is a neoplasm of lymphoblasts committed to the T-cell lineage, typically composed of small to medium-sized blast cells with scant cytoplasm, moderately condensed to dispersed chromatin, and inconspicuous nucleoli, involving bone marrow and blood (T-ALL) or presenting with primary involvement of the thymus or of nodal or extranodal sites (T-LBL). By convention, the term lymphoma is used when the process is confined to a mass lesion with no or minimal evidence of peripheral blood and bone marrow involvement. With extensive bone marrow and peripheral blood involvement, the appropriate term is T-ALL. If a patient presents with a mass lesion and lymphoblasts in the bone marrow, the distinction between leukaemia and lymphoma is arbitrary. In many treatment protocols, a value of > 25% bone marrow blasts is used to define leukaemia. Unlike with myeloid leukaemias, there is no agreed-upon lower limit for the proportion of blasts required to establish a diagnosis of ALL. In general, the diagnosis should be avoided when there are < 20% blasts.

ICD-O code   9837/3

Synonyms

Precursor T-lymphoblastic leukaemia/lymphoma; T acute lymphoblastic leukaemia

Epidemiology

T-ALL accounts for about 15% of childhood ALL cases; it is more common in adolescents than in younger children, and more common in males than in females. T-ALL accounts for approximately 25% of cases of adult ALL. T-LBL accounts for approximately 85–90% of all LBLs; like its leukaemic counterpart, it is most frequent in adolescent males, but can occur in any age group.

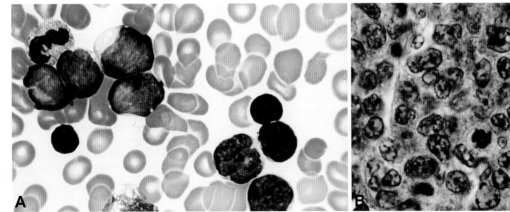

Fig. 12.11 T-lymphoblastic leukaemia. **A** Blood smear. The lymphoblasts vary in size from large cells to small cells with a very high N:C ratio. **B** Bone marrow biopsy section showing mitotic activity in the lymphoblasts.

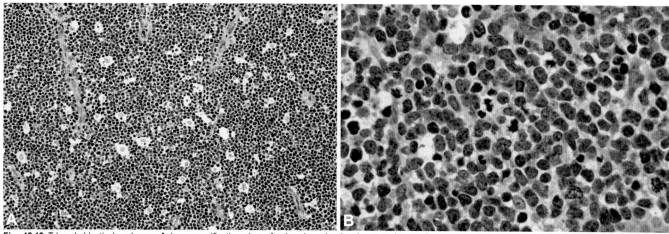

Fig. 12.12 T-lymphoblastic lymphoma. **A** Low-magnification view of a lymph node showing complete replacement by lymphoblastic lymphoma. Numerous tingible-body macrophages are scattered throughout the node. **B** High-magnification view of the same specimen, showing lymphoblasts with round to oval to irregularly shaped nuclei with dispersed chromatin and distinct but not unusually prominent nucleoli. Several mitotic figures are present.

Etiology

One study reported a set of T-ALL cases in monozygotic twins that shared the same TR gene rearrangement {1235}, suggesting an in utero origin of the earliest genetic lesions.

Localization

The bone marrow is involved in all cases of T-ALL. Unlike in B-ALL, aleukaemic presentations in the setting of bone marrow replacement are uncommon. T-LBL frequently shows mediastinal (thymic) involvement, although it may involve any lymph node or extranodal site. The skin, tonsils, liver, spleen, CNS, and testes may be involved, although presentation at these sites without nodal or mediastinal involvement is uncommon.

Clinical features

T-ALL typically presents with a high leukocyte count, and often with a large mediastinal mass or other tissue mass. Lymphadenopathy and hepatosplenomegaly are common. For a given leukocyte count and tumour burden, T-ALL often shows relative sparing of normal bone marrow haematopoiesis compared to B-ALL.

T-LBL frequently presents with a mass in the anterior mediastinum, often exhibiting rapid growth and sometimes presenting as a respiratory emergency. Pleural effusions are common.

Microscopy

The lymphoblasts in T-ALL/LBL are morphologically indistinguishable from those of B-ALL/LBL. In smears, the cells are of medium size with a high N:C ratio; there may be a considerable size range, from small lymphoblasts with very condensed nuclear chromatin and no evident nucleoli to larger blasts with finely dispersed chromatin and relatively prominent nucleoli. Nuclei range from round to irregular to convoluted. Cytoplasmic vacuoles may be present. Occasionally, blasts of T-ALL may resemble more mature lymphocytes; in such cases, immunophenotypic studies may be required to distinguish this disease from a mature (peripheral) T-cell leukaemia.

In bone marrow sections, the lymphoblasts have a high N:C ratio, a thin nuclear membrane, finely stippled chromatin, and inconspicuous nucleoli. The number of mitotic figures is reported to be higher in T-ALL than in B-ALL. In T-LBL, the lymph node generally shows complete effacement of architecture and involvement of the capsule. Partial involvement in a paracortical location with sparing of germinal centres may occur. Sometimes, a multinodular pattern is produced due to stretching of the fibrous framework, mimicking follicular lymphoma. A starry-sky effect may be present, sometimes mimicking Burkitt lymphoma, although the nucleoli and cytoplasm are typically less prominent in T-LBL. The blasts can have round or convoluted nuclei. Mitotic figures are often numerous. In the thymus, there is extensive replacement of the thymic parenchyma and permeative infiltration of the surrounding fibroadipose tissue.

Cases with histological findings of T-LBL with a significant infiltrate of eosinophils among the lymphoma cells may be associated with eosinophilia, myeloid neoplasia, and an 8p11.2 cytogenetic abnormality involving the *FGFR1* gene (see *Myeloid/lymphoid neoplasms with FGFR1 rearrangement*, p. 77) {15,1760}.

Cytochemistry

T-lymphoblasts frequently show focal acid phosphatase activity in smear and imprint preparations, although this is not specific.

Immunophenotype

The lymphoblasts in T-ALL/LBL are usually TdT-positive and variably express CD1a, CD2, CD3, CD4, CD5, CD7, and CD8. Of these markers, CD7 and CD3 (cytoplasmic) are most often positive, but only CD3 is considered lineage specific. CD4 and CD8 are frequently coexpressed on the blasts, and CD10 may be positive; however, these immunophenotypes are not specific for T-ALL, because CD4 and CD8 double positivity can also be seen in T-cell prolymphocytic leukaemia and CD10 positivity in peripheral T-cell lymphomas (most commonly angioimmunoblastic T-cell lymphoma). In addition to TdT and CD34, CD1a and CD99 may help to indicate the precursor nature of T-lymphoblasts {3373}. In 29–48% of cases, there is nuclear staining for TAL1, but this does not necessarily correlate with presence of *TAL1* gene alteration {695,931}.

CD79a positivity has been observed in approximately 10% of cases {3188}. One or both of the myeloid-associated antigens CD13 and CD33 are expressed in 19–32% of cases {1998,4088}. KIT (CD117) is positive in occasional cases; such cases have been associated with activating mutations of *FLT3* {3027}. The

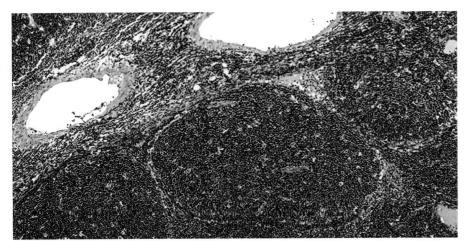

Fig. 12.13 T-lymphoblastic lymphoma. Low-magnification view showing a multinodular or so-called pseudofollicular pattern that can sometimes mimic follicular lymphoma.

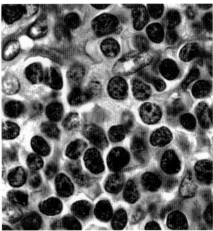

Fig. 12.14 T-lymphoblastic leukaemia. In this example, the lymphoblasts lack nuclear convolutions. The chromatin is finely stippled.

presence of myeloid markers does not exclude the diagnosis of T-ALL/LBL, nor does it indicate T/myeloid mixed-phenotype acute leukaemia.

Many markers characteristic of immature T cells, such as CD7, CD2, and even CD5 and cCD3-epsilon, may also be seen in NK-cell precursors. Therefore, it can be very difficult to distinguish the rare true NK-cell ALL/LBL from T-ALL that expresses only immature markers. CD56 expression, although characteristic of NK cells, does not exclude T-cell leukaemia. T-ALL/LBL has previously been stratified into four stages of intrathymic differentiation according to the antigens expressed {332}: (1) pro-T/T-I, (2) pre-T/T-II, (3) cortical T/T-III, and (4) medullary T/T-IV. Many cases previously classified as pro-T or pre-T would now meet the criteria for early T-cell precursor ALL (see next section). Like normal thymocytes, T-ALL of the cortical T stage often has a double-positive (CD4+, CD8+) immunophenotype together with CD1a positivity, whereas the medullary T stage expresses either CD4 or CD8. Some studies have shown a correlation between the stages of T-cell differentiation and survival. T-ALL tends to have a more immature immunophenotype than does T-LBL, but the groups overlap {4287}.

Postulated normal counterpart

A T-cell progenitor (T-ALL) or a thymic lymphocyte (T-LBL)

Genetic profile

Antigen receptor genes
T-ALL/LBL almost always shows clonal rearrangements of the T-cell receptor (TR) genes, and there is simultaneous presence of IGH gene rearrangements in approximately 20% of cases {3187,3860}.

Cytogenetic abnormalities and oncogenes
An abnormal karyotype is found in 50–70% of cases of T-ALL/LBL {1426, 1534}. The most common recurrent cytogenetic abnormality involves the alpha and delta TR loci at 14q11.2, the beta locus at 7q34, and the gamma locus at 7p14.1, with a variety of partner genes {1426,1534}. In most cases, these translocations lead to a dysregulation of transcription of the partner gene by juxtaposition with the regulatory region of one of the TR loci. The most commonly involved genes include the transcription factors *TLX1* (also called *HOX11*) at 10q24.3, which is involved in 7% of childhood and 30% of adult cases, and *TLX3* (also called *HOX11L2*) at 5q35.1, which is involved in 20% of childhood and 10–15% of adult cases {1426}. Other transcription factors that may be involved in translocations include *MYC* at 8q24.2, *TAL1* at 1p33, *LMO1* (also called *RBTN1*) at 11p15.4, *LMO2* (also called *RBTN2*) at 11p13, and *LYL1* at 19p13.1 {897,1426}. The cytoplasmic tyrosine kinase *LCK* at 1p35.2 can also be involved in a translocation. In many cases, translocations are not detected by karyotyping but only by molecular genetic studies. For example, the *TAL1* locus is altered by translocation in about 20–30% of cases of T-ALL, but a t(1;14)(p33;q11.2) translocation can be detected in only about 3% of cases. Much more often, *TAL1* is fused to *STIL* (also called *SIL*) as a result of

a cryptic interstitial deletion at chromosome 1p33 {467,1596,1837}. Aberrant *TAL1* expression interferes with differentiation and proliferation by inhibiting the transcriptional activity of *TCF3* (also called *E47*) and *TCF12* (also called *HEB*) {2919}. Other important translocations in T-ALL include t(10;11)(p12.3;q14.2), which results in *PICALM-MLLT10* (also called *CALM-AF10*) and is found in 10% of cases, and translocations involving *KMT2A* (also called *MLL*), which occur in 8% of cases, most often with the partner *MLLT1* (also called *ENL*) at 19p13.1 {1426}; both result in activation of HOXA genes {2614}. It has been proposed that T-ALL be divided into four distinct, non-overlapping genetic subgroups based on specific translocations that lead to aberrant expression of (1) TAL or LMO genes, (2) *TLX1*, (3) *TLX3*, and (4) HOXA genes, resulting in arrest of T-cell maturation at distinct stages of thymocyte development {2614,4143}. The *TLX1* group appears to have a relatively favourable prognosis {1189}. Another group, characterized by overexpression of *LYL1*, may correspond more closely to early T-cell precursor ALL {2614}.

Deletions also occur in T-ALL. The most important is del(9p), resulting in loss of the tumour suppressor gene *CDKN2A* (an inhibitor of the cyclin-dependent kinase *CDK4*), which occurs at a frequency of about 30% by cytogenetics, and a greater frequency by molecular testing. This leads to loss of G1 control of the cell cycle.

About 50% of cases have activating mutations involving the extracellular heterodimerization domain and/or the C-terminal

PEST domain of *NOTCH1*, which encodes a protein critical for early T-cell development {4294}. The direct downstream target of *NOTCH1* appears to be *MYC*, which contributes to the growth of the neoplastic cells {4295}. According to one study, *NOTCH1* mutation is associated with shorter survival in adults but not in paediatric patients {4492}. In about 30% of cases, there are mutations in *FBXW7*, a negative regulator of *NOTCH1*. These missense mutations result in an increased half-life of the NOTCH1 protein {2478}.

Prognosis and predictive factors

T-ALL in childhood is generally considered a higher-risk disease than B-ALL, although this is in part due to the frequent presence of high-risk clinical features (i.e. older age and higher white blood cell count). However, patients with T-ALL lacking high-risk features do not fare as well as those with standard-risk B-ALL unless intensive therapy is given. Compared to B-ALL, T-ALL is associated with a higher risk of induction failure, early relapse, and isolated CNS relapse {1393}. Unlike in B-ALL, white blood cell count does not appear to be a prognostic factor. Minimal residual disease following therapy is a strong adverse prognostic factor {4319}, although there is evidence that patients who are positive for minimal residual disease at the end of induction therapy still do very well if the minimal residual disease is cleared by day 78 {3584}. In adult protocols, T-ALL is treated similarly to other types of ALL. The prognosis of T-ALL may be better than that of B-ALL in adults, although this may reflect the lower incidence of adverse cytogenetic abnormalities. The prognosis of T-LBL, like that of other lymphomas, depends on patient age, disease stage, and lactate dehydrogenase levels {2727}.

Several cases of an entity referred to as indolent T-lymphoblastic proliferation have been described. These typically involve the upper aerodigestive tract and are characterized by multiple local recurrences without systemic dissemination {2941}. These cases are morphologically and immunophenotypically similar to T-LBL, but are cytologically less atypical, show a developmentally normal (rather than aberrant) thymic phenotype, and lack clonal rearrangements of the TR genes {2941}.

Early T-cell precursor lymphoblastic leukaemia

Definition

Early T-cell precursor (ETP) lymphoblastic leukaemia (ETP-ALL) is a neoplasm composed of cells committed to the T-cell lineage but with a unique immunophenotype indicating only limited early T-cell differentiation.

ICD-O code   9837/3

Epidemiology

This is an uncommon neoplasm found in both children and adults, accounting for approximately 10–13% of cases of T-ALL in childhood, and for 5–10% of cases of adult ALL.

Microscopy

Blasts from patients with ETP-ALL are similar to those from patients with other ALLs: small to medium-sized with scant cytoplasm and inconspicuous nucleoli.

Immunophenotype

ETP-ALL expresses CD7 but by definition lacks CD8 and CD1a and is positive for one or more of the myeloid / stem cell markers CD34, KIT (CD117), HLA-DR, CD13, CD33, CD11b, and CD65. Blasts also express cytoplasmic, or in rare cases surface CD3, and may express CD2 and/or CD4. CD5 is often negative; when positive, it is present on < 75% of the blast population {828}. It has been suggested that leukaemias that express brighter or more uniform CD5 but otherwise meet the criteria for ETP-ALL be called near–ETP-ALL {4362}. By definition, MPO is negative, because a leukaemia with an otherwise ETP immunophenotype that also expresses MPO would most likely meet the criteria for T/myeloid mixed-phenotype acute leukaemia. A unique case of an MPO-negative leukaemia with an ETP phenotype with blasts containing Auer rods has been described {1275}. This finding, coupled with the frequent expression of myeloid markers in ETP-ALL, as well as the genetic findings outlined below, underscores the promiscuity between immature precursor T cells and the myeloid lineage, supporting the notion of lymphocyte-primed multipotent progenitors {3342}.

Cell of origin

ETP-ALL is postulated to derive from a subset of cells that have immigrated to the thymus from the bone marrow but are not yet irreversibly committed to the T-cell lineage and retain the potential for myeloid/dendritic-cell differentiation.

Genetic profile

Gene expression profiling studies of ETP-ALL have identified an expression profile similar to that of normal early thymocyte precursors and different from that of cases of T-ALL corresponding to later maturational stages. The overexpressed genes included many that are more typically associated with myeloid or stem cell profiles, such as *CD44*, *CD34*, *KIT*, *GATA2*, and *CEBPA* {828, 4475}. In addition, previously described cases of the immature T-ALL characterized by *LYL1* overexpression {1189} likely constitute ETP-ALL. The mutation profile is also more similar to that of myeloid leukaemias than to those of other T-cell leukaemias {2855,2856,4142,4475}, with mutations reported at high frequencies in *FLT3*, the RAS family of genes, *DNMT3A*, *IDH1*, and *IDH2*; more-typical ALL lesions, such as *NOTCH1* activating mutations and mutations in *CDKN1/2* genes, are reported at low frequencies {4142}.

Prognosis and predictive factors

Initial descriptions of this entity suggested that the outcome of the small numbers of children with ETP-ALL was very poor compared with that of other patients with T-ALL {828}, and other small series showed similar results {1765,2420}. However, more recent, larger series with more effective therapy showed either a small but statistically non-significant difference in outcome {3106} or (in the largest series to date) no effect whatsoever {4362}, despite the fact that rates of minimal residual disease in ETP-ALL at the end of induction therapy are higher than among other patients with T-ALL. There are fewer data in adults, but one small study suggested no prognostic effect of ETP-ALL {1497}. Therefore, although the kinetics of response to therapy appears to be very different in ETP-ALL compared with other T-ALL, the ultimate outcome with appropriate therapy appears to be the same.

NK-lymphoblastic leukaemia / lymphoma

Borowitz M.J.
Béné M.-C.
Harris N.L.
Porwit A.
Matutes E.
Arber D.A.

Definition

NK-lymphoblastic leukaemia / lymphoma has been very difficult to define, and there is considerable confusion in the literature. Contributing to this confusion is the fact that many cases reported as NK-leukaemia due to expression of CD56 (NCAM) are now recognized to in fact be blastic plasmacytoid dendritic cell neoplasms {3151,3152}. Similarly, the entity known as myeloid/NK acute leukaemia {3599,3841}, which has been suggested to be of precursor NK-cell origin {3000}, has a primitive immunophenotype indistinguishable from that of acute myeloid leukaemia with minimal differentiation. Until further evidence emerges, these should be considered as cases of acute myeloid leukaemia.

Early in their development, NK-cell progenitors express no specific markers {1255}, or express markers that overlap with those seen in T-ALL, including CD7, CD2, and even CD5 and cCD3-epsilon {3757}; therefore, distinguishing between T-ALL and NK-cell tumours can be difficult. More-mature but more-specific markers such as CD16 are rarely expressed in any acute leukaemia; some markers that might be considered relatively specific but that are still expressed on NK-cell progenitors (e.g. CD94 and CD161 {1255}) are not commonly tested. Some well-characterized cases of NK precursor tumours with lymphomatous presentations that expressed NK-specific CD94 1A transcripts have been described {2338}. It is hoped that wider availability of more specific NK-cell markers, including panels of antibodies against killer-cell immunoglobulin-like receptors, will help clarify this disease, but until then, NK-ALL/LBL is best considered a provisional entity. The diagnosis of precursor NK-ALL/LBL may be considered in a case that expresses CD56 along with immature T-associated markers such as CD7 and CD2, and even including cCD3, provided that the case lacks B-cell and myeloid markers, TR and IG genes are in the germline configuration {1975,2070,3000}, and blastic plasmacytoid dendritic cell neoplasm has been excluded.

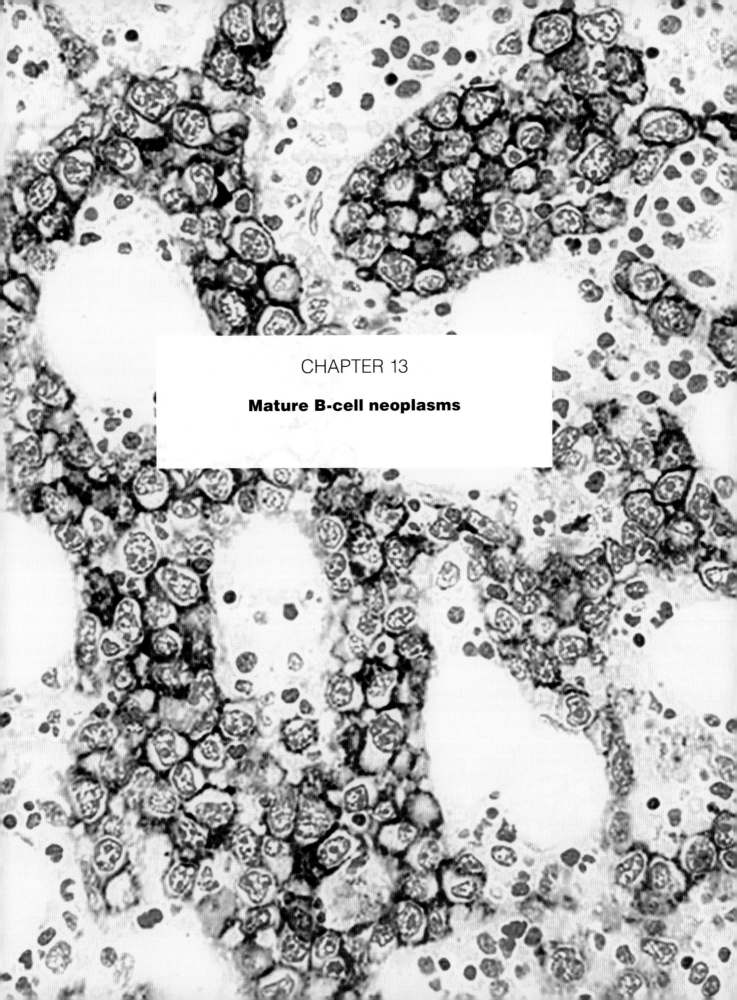

CHAPTER 13

Mature B-cell neoplasms

Chronic lymphocytic leukaemia/ small lymphocytic lymphoma

Campo E.
Ghia P.
Montserrat E.
Harris N.L.

Müller–Hermelink
H.K.
Stein H.
Swerdlow S.H.

Definition

Chronic lymphocytic leukaemia/small lymphocytic lymphoma (CLL/SLL) is a neoplasm composed of monomorphic small mature B cells that coexpress CD5 and CD23. There must be a monoclonal B-cell count $\geq 5 \times 10^9$/L, with the characteristic morphology and phenotype of CLL in the peripheral blood. Individuals with a clonal CLL-like cell count $<5 \times 10^9$/L and without lymphadenopathy, organomegaly, or other extramedullary disease are considered to have monoclonal B-cell lymphocytosis. Although CLL and SLL are the same disease, the term SLL is used for cases with a circulating CLL cell count $<5 \times 10^9$/L and documented nodal, splenic, or other extramedullary involvement {1523}.

ICD-O code   9823/3

Synonyms

Chronic lymphocytic leukaemia, B-cell type; chronic lymphoid leukaemia; chronic lymphatic leukaemia

Epidemiology

CLL is the most common leukaemia of adults in western countries. The annual incidence rate is about 5 cases per 100 000 population, and dramatically increases with age, to as many as >20 cases per 100 000 individuals aged >70 years. The median patient age at diagnosis of CLL is approximately 70 years, but CLL can also present in younger adults {3060}. There is a male preponderance, with a male-to-female ratio of 1.5–2:1. CLL/SLL accounts for 7% of non-Hodgkin lymphomas {2759, 3515}. The disease is rare in Asian countries, with the low incidence maintained in emigrant populations {2451}. This finding, together with the reported familial cases, indicates a genetic basis and predisposition for the disease.

Etiology

B-cell receptors of CLL cells demonstrate highly selected IGHV gene usage or even very similar antigen-binding sites, coded by both heavy and light chain genes (so-called stereotypes), and thus differ from the B-cell receptors of much broader diversity found in normal B lymphocytes. These findings support the concept of a limited set of (auto-)antigenic elements promoting division of precursor cells and clonal evolution {28}.

Localization

CLL/SLL involves the blood, bone marrow, and secondary lymphoid tissues such as the spleen, lymph nodes, and Waldeyer ring. Extranodal involvement (e.g. of the skin, gastrointestinal tract, or CNS) occurs in a small subset of cases {3315}. SLL is diagnosed in 10–20% of cases, and as many as 20% evolve into frank CLL {3516}.

Clinical features

Most cases of CLL in western countries are diagnosed on the basis of routine blood analysis in asymptomatic subjects. Less often, lymphadenopathy, splenomegaly, anaemia, or thrombocytopenia can lead to the diagnosis. In a few cases, the diagnosis is reached after work-up for other manifestations of CLL/SLL, such as an autoimmune cytopenia (i.e. autoimmune haemolytic anaemia, immune thrombocytopenia, or erythroblastopenia) {1652} or an infection, most frequently pulmonary. A small paraprotein, usually of IgM type, can be observed in approximately 10% of the patients {87}. The frequency of hypogammaglobulinaemia is about 30% at diagnosis and increases over time, to as much as 60% among patients with advanced disease {3059}. Extramedullary involvement (e.g. of the skin, gastrointestinal tract, kidneys, or CNS) occurs in a small proportion of patients {3315}. Patients with CLL can experience severe allergic reactions to insect bites {235}.

Microscopy

Lymph nodes and spleen

Enlarged lymph nodes show diffuse architectural effacement by a proliferation of small lymphocytes with variably prominent scattered paler proliferation centres (so-called pseudofollicles) {2267}. In some cases, there is a vaguely nodular appearance. Only partial nodal involvement with an interfollicular or perifollicular infiltration pattern may be seen {224, 3894}. The predominant cell in the diffuse areas is a small lymphocyte with scant cytoplasm, usually a round nucleus with clumped chromatin, and occasionally a

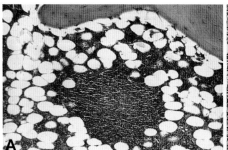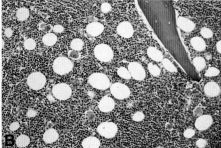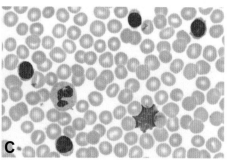

Fig. 13.01 Chronic lymphocytic leukaemia / small lymphocytic lymphoma (CLL/SLL). **A** Bone marrow trephine section illustrating a nodular pattern of infiltration. **B** Bone marrow trephine section illustrating an interstitial pattern of lymphocytic infiltration. **C** Peripheral blood. The CLL lymphocytes are small and round, with distinct clumped chromatin. Smudge cells are commonly seen.

small nucleolus. Mitotic activity is usually very low. In some cases, the small lymphoid cells show moderate nuclear irregularity, which can lead to a differential diagnosis of mantle cell lymphoma {411}. Some cases show plasmacytoid differentiation. The proliferation centres are composed of a continuum of small lymphocytes, prolymphocytes, and paraimmunoblasts. Prolymphocytes are small to medium-sized cells with relatively clumped chromatin and small nucleoli; paraimmunoblasts are larger cells with round to oval nuclei, dispersed chromatin, central eosinophilic nucleoli, and slightly basophilic cytoplasm {411,2267}. In some cases, the proliferation centres are very large (broader than a 20× field) and confluent {760,1373}. Such cases are usually associated with increased proliferation, deletion in 17p13.1, trisomy 12, and a more aggressive course compared to cases with smaller proliferation centres {760,1134,1373}. In the spleen, white pulp involvement is usually prominent, but the red pulp is also involved; proliferation centres may be seen but are less conspicuous than in lymph nodes.

Bone marrow and blood
CLL cells are small lymphocytes with clumped chromatin and scant cytoplasm. Smudge or basket cells are typically seen in peripheral blood smears. In most cases, besides typical CLL cells, other lymphoid cells (e.g. prolymphocytes, cells with irregular nuclear contours, and larger cells with more dispersed chromatin and more abundant cytoplasm) are also observed, but they usually constitute < 15% of the lymphoid cells. Cases with a higher proportion of these cells but < 55% prolymphocytes have been called atypical CLL. In such cases, trisomy 12 and strong positivity for surface immunoglobulin, CD20, and FMC7 are frequently found {341}. The finding of >55% prolymphocytes defines B-cell prolymphocytic leukaemia {341,1523}. Bone marrow biopsy may show interstitial, nodular, mixed (nodular and interstitial), or diffuse involvement; diffuse involvement is usually associated with more advanced disease {2720}. Paratrabecular aggregates are not typical. Proliferation centres can be observed, although they are not as prominent as in lymph nodes, and follicular dendritic cells may be present {716}. Most cases have >30% CLL cells in the bone marrow aspirate {1523}.

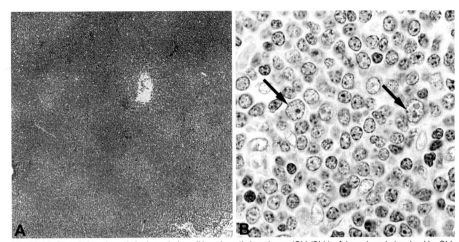

Fig. 13.02 Chronic lymphocytic leukaemia / small lymphocytic lymphoma (CLL/SLL). **A** Lymph node involved by CLL showing regularly spaced proliferation centres in a dark background (Giemsa stain). **B** High-magnification showing a mixture of small lymphocytes with scant cytoplasm and clumped chromatin, slightly larger prolymphocytes with more dispersed chromatin and small nucleoli, and individual paraimmunoblasts (arrows), which are larger cells with round to oval nuclei, dispersed chromatin, and a central nucleolus.

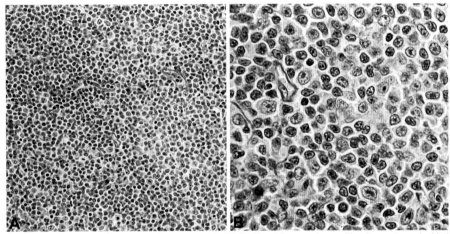

Fig. 13.03 CLL/SLL in lymph node. **A** Periodic acid–Schiff (PAS) staining reveals a proliferation centre embedded in a darker background of small lymphocytes. **B** High-magnification view of lymph node shows clustering of larger lymphoid cells (prolymphocytes and paraimmunoblasts) in the proliferation centre.

Immunophenotype

Circulating leukaemic B cells express CD19 and dim surface IgM/IgD, CD20, CD22, and CD79b. They are also positive for CD5 and CD43 and strongly positive for CD23 and CD200 {1027}. CD10 is negative and FMC7 is usually negative or only weakly expressed. The immunophenotype of CLL cells has been integrated into a scoring system that helps in the differential diagnosis of CLL and other B-cell leukaemias {2582,2722}. Some cases have an atypical immunophenotype (e.g. CD5– or CD23–, FMC7+, strong surface immunoglobulin, or CD79b+) {838, 2580}. However, in these cases it is imperative that the possibility of some other type of B-cell neoplasm, such as splenic marginal zone lymphoma in CD5– cases, be excluded.

In tissue sections, cytoplasmic immunoglobulin may be detectable. CD20 and CD23 expression is usually stronger in cells of the proliferation centres than in the diffuse areas {2202}. Follicular dendritic cell meshworks are present in some cases, and may be associated with the proliferation centres. LEF1 is useful to identify CLL/SLL infiltration in tissues, because it is aberrantly expressed in almost all CLL/SLL, whereas normal mature B lymphocytes and virtually all other small B-cell lymphomas are negative {3893}. Cyclin D1 is not expressed, but some positive cells can be seen in proliferation centres in about 30% of cases. These cells are SOX11-negative and do not carry chromosomal translocations affecting the *CCND1* gene {1419}. MYC and NOTCH1 proteins may also be expressed

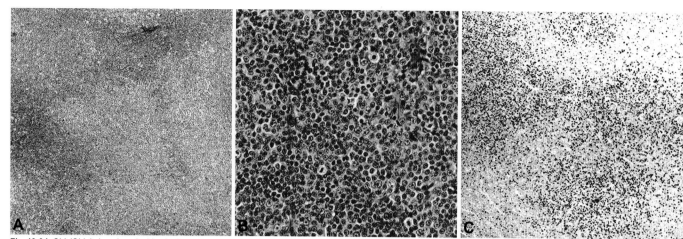

Fig. 13.04 CLL/SLL in lymph node, histologically aggressive. **A** The pale areas, corresponding to proliferation centres, are expanded and confluent. **B** Note the larger cells in the proliferation centre and the mitotic figures. **C** Ki-67 staining highlights the expansion and high proliferation rate of the cells in the proliferation centres.

in proliferation centres independently of gene alterations {2047,2123}.

Postulated normal counterpart

An antigen-experienced mature CD5+ B cell with mutated or unmutated IGHV genes {721}

Genetic profile

Antigen receptor genes

IGHV gene usage in CLL is highly skewed; IGHV genes are mutated (i.e. < 98% identity with the germline) in 50–70% of cases and unmutated (i.e. ≥98% identity) in 30–50% {863,1528}. Patients

can have very similar, if not identical, immunoglobulin sequences, a phenomenon that is present in 30% of all CLL cases and termed 'BCR stereotypy' {28}. BCR signalling is more active in CLL with unmutated IGHV genes {4483}, whereas other cases, in particular those with mutated IGHV genes, have a response resembling anergy. CLL B-cell receptors have been shown to recognize both foreign and self antigens, including the possibility of the monoclonal immunoglobulin recognizing itself on the same or an adjacent cell (so-called autonomous signalling) {1072}.

Cytogenetic abnormalities and oncogenes

CLL has no specific genetic markers. About 80–90% of the cases have cytogenetic abnormalities detected by FISH or copy-number arrays {1073,2469,3244}. The most common alterations are deletions in 13q14.3 (miR-16-1 and miR-15a; present in ~50% of cases) and trisomy 12 or partial trisomy 12q13 (present in ~20%); less commonly, there is deletion in 11q22-23 (ATM and BIRC3), 17p13.1 (TP53), or 6q21 {1073,1510,4469}. The distribution of these abnormalities varies depending on the IGHV mutation status (see Table 13.01). High-resolution genomic arrays have helped to refine and expand the known DNA copy-number alterations, identifying gains in 2p (present in 7% of cases) and 8q24.2 (MYC; in 3%), as well as losses of 14q (in 4%), among others {1079,2469,3244}. Chromosomal translocations in CLL are uncommon, but t(14;18)(q32;q21), resulting in IGH/BCL2, can be found, most likely as a secondary change, in 2% of cases, usually with mutated IGHV. Translocations involving the 13q14 region, present in 2% of cases, are associated with miR-16-1 and miR-15a deletions {3244,3247}. The t(14;19)(q32;q13) translocation, resulting in IGH/BCL3, is present in occasional cases of CLL with unmutated IGHV genes {1730}. Complex rearrangements within single chromosomes (chromothripsis) and among chromosomes have been identified in 2% of cases, mainly with unmutated IGHV genes and frequently in association with TP53 mutations {1079, 3244}. The most commonly mutated genes, affected in 3–15% of cases, are NOTCH1,

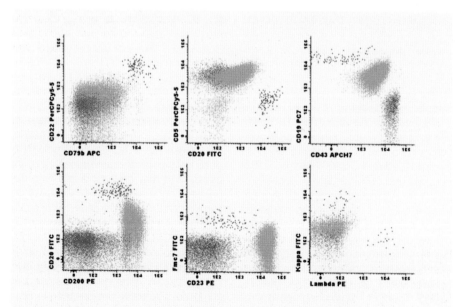

Fig. 13.05 Chronic lymphocytic leukaemia. Immunophenotype of CLL (orange), normal B cells (blue), and T cells (green) by flow cytometry. CLL cells have weak expression of CD22, CD79b (top-left plot), and CD20 (top-middle plot); coexpression of CD5 (top-middle plot) and CD43 (top-right plot); strong expression of CD200 (bottom-left plot) and CD23 (bottom-middle plot); negative FMC7 (bottom-middle plot); and restricted expression of dim kappa light chain (bottom-right plot).

SF3B1, TP53, ATM, BIRC3, POT1, and MYD88. Many other genes are mutated at lower frequencies. The mutation profile varies with the evolution of the disease; aberrations of some genes, in particular TP53, BIRC3, NOTCH1, and SF3B1 are more frequently present at relapse {2207, 2208,3244,4242}.

Whole-genome DNA methylation studies have identified three epigenetic subgroups of CLL with methylation signatures closely related to different stages of B-cell differentiation: one resembling naïve B cells, one resembling memory B cells, and one with a signature intermediate between those of naïve and memory B cells {2130}. These three epigenetic CLL subgroups (naïve-like, memory-like, and intermediate) have different biological characteristics and only partially overlap with IGHV mutation status {2921,3259}. Naïve-like CLLs have mainly unmutated IGHV genes, whereas most epigenetically intermediate and memory-like CLLs have mutated IGHV genes. However, the clinical behaviour of the intermediate subgroup is more aggressive than that of memory-like CLL {3259}. Although these epigenetic subgroups have been identified using genome-wide methylation arrays, they can also be reproducibly identified in clinical practice using pyrosequencing of only five epigenetic biomarkers {3259}.

Genetic susceptibility

CLL is a multifactorial disease with considerable heritability. A familial predisposition can be documented in 5–10% of patients with CLL {1396,3697}. The overall risk of developing CLL is 2–7 times higher in first-degree relatives of CLL patients. These patients also have an increased risk for other lymphoid neoplasms {603}. Family members of patients with CLL also show an increased incidence of CLL-like monoclonal B-cell lymphocytosis. Genetic studies have identified as many as 30 genomic loci related to inherited susceptibility to CLL {355,3747}.

Prognosis and predictive factors

The Rai and Binet clinical staging systems are used to define disease extent and prognosis {382,3283}. Patients with mutated IGHV genes have a better prognosis than do those with unmutated genes {4469}. Expression of ZAP70, CD38, or CD49d is associated with an adverse prognosis {833}. The three epi-

Table 13.01 Relation of IGHV mutation status and genomic aberrations in 300 cases of chronic lymphocytic leukaemia. From: Kröber A, et al. {2120A}

Aberration(s)	Frequency	
	Mutated IGHV n = 132 (44% of cases)	**Unmutated IGHV** n = 168 (56% of cases)
Clonal aberrations	80%	84%
13q deletion*	65%	48%
Isolated 13q deletion*	50%	26%
Trisomy 12	15%	19%
11q deletion*	4%	27%
17p deletion*	3%	10%
17p or 11q deletion*	7%	35%

*Significant difference between cases with and without IGHV mutation.

genetic subtypes are also of prognostic significance; naïve-like cases have the worst prognosis and memory-like cases the best {2921,3259}. Deletion in 11q and in particular deletion in 17p confers a worse clinical outcome, whereas isolated deletion in 13q14 is associated with a more favourable clinical course {833}. CLL with a high proportion of cells with isolated 13q deletion, however, do not do as well {1722A,3246A,4132A}. TP53 abnormalities (i.e. deletion in 17p13.1 and TP53 mutations) are predictive of lack of response to fludarabine-containing regimes; therefore, these aberrations should be checked for in all patients before starting any line of therapy. Prognostic and predictive factors need to be more firmly established for newer therapeutic strategies such as B-cell receptor or BCL2 inhibitors. Complex karyotype also correlates with poor outcome {940, 3012}. The presence of a stereotyped B-cell receptor utilizing the IGHV3-21 gene (so-called subset #2) is an adverse pro-

gnostic marker independent of IGHV mutations {240}. Additional adverse predictive factors include a rapid lymphocyte doubling time in the blood (< 12 months) and serum markers of rapid cell turnover, including elevated thymidine kinase and beta-2 microglobulin {383}. Mutations in TP53, ATM, NOTCH1, SF3B1, and BIRC3, among others, are associated with a poor outcome {2208,3244}. The integration of these results with other prognostic parameters requires further study {241}.

Progression and transformation of chronic lymphocytic leukaemia into high-grade lymphoma

Clinical progression of CLL/SLL is often associated with an increase in size and proliferative activity of the CLL cells. Proliferation centres in lymph nodes may expand with a higher proliferation rate and become confluent {760,1134,1373}. Histologically aggressive CLLs are recognized by proliferation centres that are

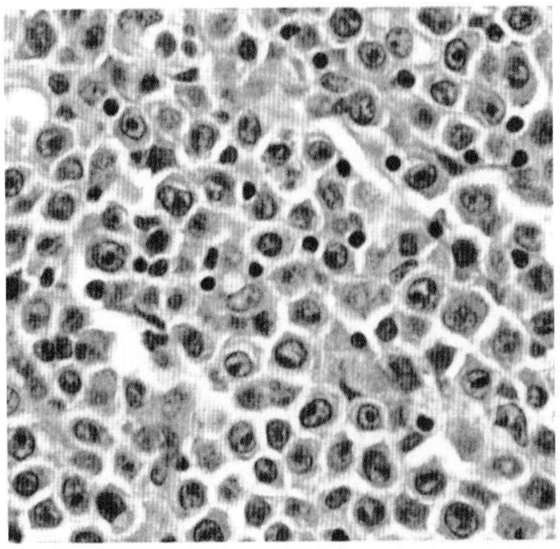

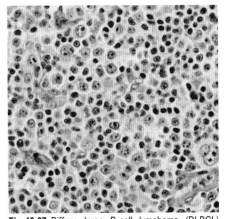

Fig. 13.06 Diffuse large B-cell lymphoma (DLBCL) transformed from chronic lymphocytic leukaemia. The area with DLBCL is composed of a monotonous population of large cells with immunoblastic features.

Fig. 13.07 Diffuse large B-cell lymphoma (DLBCL) transformed from chronic lymphocytic leukaemia. The transformed DLBCL cells are intermingled with residual small lymphocytes.

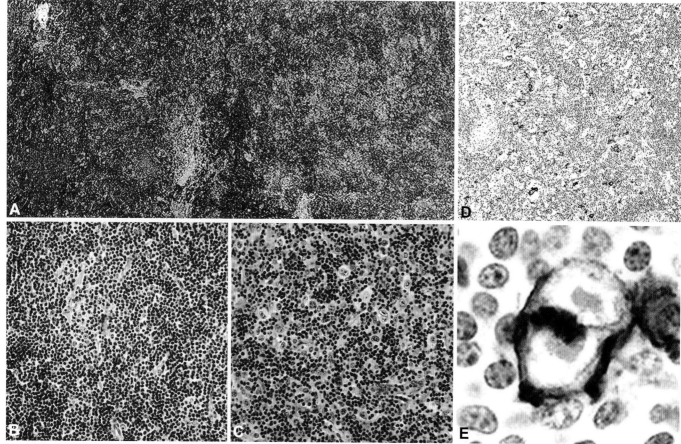

Fig. 13.08 Classic Hodgkin lymphoma–type Richter transformation of chronic lymphocytic leukaemia/small lymphocytic lymphoma (CLL/SLL). **A** The CLL/SLL, with paler proliferation centres, is seen on the left and classic Hodgkin lymphoma on the right. **B** Area of CLL/SLL, with paler proliferation centres, that includes some paraimmunoblasts. **C** Areas with CHL contain many Reed–Sternberg cells and variants, as well as eosinophils, some histiocytes, and small lymphocytes. **D** The Reed–Sternberg cells and variants are CD15-positive. **E** CD15+ Reed–Sternberg cell.

broader than a 20× field or becoming confluent. Although data are limited, cases may also belong in this category when the Ki-67 proliferation index is >40% or there are >2.4 mitoses in the proliferation centres {760,1373}. These cases are reported to have an outcome intermediate between those of typical CLL and classic Richter syndrome (diffuse large B-cell lymphoma; DLBCL) {760,1373}. An increasing proportion of prolymphocytes in the blood may also be seen (prolymphocytoid transformation). However, progression of CLL into B-cell prolymphocytic leukaemia does not occur, by definition. Approximately 2–8% of patients with CLL develop DLBCL, and < 1% develop classic Hodgkin lymphoma {453,2492,4006}. Most cases of DLBCL-type Richter syndrome are clonally related to the previous CLL, i.e. they express the same immunoglobulin gene rearrangement, and are IGHV-unmutated, whereas clonally unrelated cases usually occur in IGHV-mutated CLL {2492,

4006}. The former are associated with a median survival time of < 1 year, whereas the prognosis of the latter is identical to that of a de novo DLBCL {3058}. DLBCL transformation is associated with *TP53* and *NOTCH1* mutations, *CDKN2A* deletions, and *MYC* translocations {712, 1125,3245}. The vast majority of Hodgkin lymphoma cases occur in mutated CLL, are EBV-positive, and are unrelated to the CLL clone {2492}. The diagnosis of Hodgkin lymphoma in the setting of CLL requires classic Reed–Sternberg cells in an appropriate background. The presence of scattered EBV-positive or sometimes EBV-negative Reed–Sternberg cells in the background of CLL does not fulfil the criteria for the diagnosis of Hodgkin lymphoma. EBV-associated lymphoproliferative disorders, including Hodgkin lymphoma–type proliferations, may occur in patients with CLL following immunosuppressive therapy {16,3993}.

Monoclonal B-cell lymphocytosis

Definition
Monoclonal B-cell lymphocytosis (MBL) is defined by a monoclonal B-cell count <5×10⁹/L in the peripheral blood in subjects who have no associated lymphadenopathy, organomegaly, other extramedullary involvement, or any other feature of a B-cell lymphoproliferative disorder {2516}. MBL is classified into three categories on the basis of phenotype: (1) chronic lymphocytic leukaemia (CLL)-type, (2) atypical CLL-type, and (3) non–CLL-type. Caution is advised, because many small B-cell lymphomas/leukaemias have low-level peripheral blood involvement.

MBL with a CLL-type phenotype is the most common, accounting for as many as 75% of all cases. It is characterized by coexpression of CD19, CD5, CD23, and CD20 (dim). The B cells show light chain class restriction or ≥25% lack surface immunoglobulin. More than one clone may coexist. The reported frequency of CLL-type MBL in the general population depends on the sensitivity of the method used for detection, ranging from 3.5% to 12% among healthy individuals {1167, 2876,3320}. The frequency increases with age; it is negligible among individuals aged < 40 years and 50–75% among 90-year-old individuals {1353,2876, 3320}. It has been reported that virtually all CLLs are preceded by MBL, although not all MBL progresses to CLL {1167}. Some patients have counts that oscillate between MBL and CLL for some time. CLL-type MBL must be further classified on the basis of the size of the monoclonal population, as low-count ($<0.5 \times 10^9$/L) or high-count ($\geq 0.5 \times 10^9$/L) MBL. Low-count MBL has some biological differences from high-count MBL and CLL, and does not seem to progress, whereas high-count MBL has biological features identical to those of low-stage (Rai stage 0) CLL, and progresses to frank leukaemia requiring therapy at an annual rate of 1–2% {1167,3319,3666}. The higher the MBL count, the more likely there will be progression. The adverse prognostic indicators identified in patients with CLL are also associated with progression from MBL to CLL and shorter time to treatment {1949,1992}. MBL cases usually have mutated IGHV genes (present in 75–90% of cases) and may carry the same chromosomal abnormalities and somatic mutations as CLL, including *NOTCH1*, *SF3B1*, *ATM*, and *TP53* aberrations, although at lower frequencies {1992,3244}. Nodal infiltration by CLL-type cells without apparent proliferation centres in individuals without lymphadenopathy > 1.5 cm on CT who

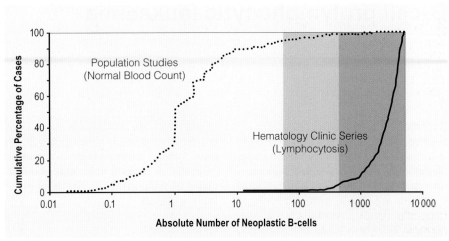

Fig. 13.09 Low-count and high-count chronic lymphocytic leukaemia (CLL)-type monoclonal B-cell lymphocytosis (MBL). The cumulative percentage of cases according to the absolute number of clonal B cells in studies of individuals from the general population with a normal blood count (dotted line) and in series of individuals referred for clinical haematology investigations, usually with current or prior lymphocytosis (solid line). There is a marked difference in the clonal B-cell count in CLL-type MBL in cases from population studies versus clinical haematology series. In population studies, the median clonal B-cell count is 1/μL, with 95% of cases having < 56/μL (white background). In clinical haematology series, the median is 2939/μL, with 95% of cases having > 447/μL (dark-grey background). Very few cases from either series have a clonal B-cell count within the same range as polyclonal B-cell levels in individuals with no detectable abnormal B cells (light-grey background). From Rawstron AC et al. {3321}.

otherwise have MBL may constitute a nodal equivalent of MBL rather than small lymphocytic lymphoma {1369}.

MBL with an atypical CLL phenotype expresses CD19, CD5, CD20 (bright), and moderate to bright surface immunoglobulin. CD23 may be negative. It is critical to exclude the possibility of mantle cell lymphoma or other B-cell lymphoma in these cases.

MBL with a non-CLL phenotype is characterized by CD5– (or CD5 (dim) in 20% of cases), CD19+, CD20+ B cells with moderate to bright surface immunoglobulin expression {1353,3631}. Some of these clonal expansions may be transient and self-limited. Additional phenotypic and cytogenetic studies are mandatory

to rule out a specific lymphoid neoplasm {1949}. Some cases have aberrant karyotypes involving chromosome 7q, and as many as 17% may eventually develop splenomegaly, suggesting a relationship to splenic marginal zone lymphoma {4390}. Some very similar cases with a low rate of progression may have a monotypic B-cell count $>5 \times 10^9$/L, therefore not fulfilling the criteria for MBL {4390}. Some cases of diffuse large B-cell lymphoma with simultaneous MBL with a CLL or non-CLL phenotype are clonally related {2468}.

ICD-O codes
MBL, CLL-type	9823/1
MBL, non-CLL-type	9591/1

B-cell prolymphocytic leukaemia

Campo E.
Matutes E.
Montserrat E.

Harris N.L.
Stein H.
Müller–Hermelink H.K.

Definition
B-cell prolymphocytic leukaemia (B-PLL) is a neoplasm of B-cell prolymphocytes affecting the peripheral blood, bone marrow, and spleen. Prolymphocytes must constitute >55% of lymphoid cells in peripheral blood. Cases of chronic lymphocytic leukaemia (CLL) with increased prolymphocytes and lymphoid proliferations with relatively similar morphology but with a t(11;14)(q13;q32) (IGH/CCND1) translocation or SOX11 expression are excluded; they instead constitute mantle cell lymphoma with leukaemic expression.

ICD-O code   9833/3

Synonym
Prolymphocytic leukaemia, B-cell type

Epidemiology
B-PLL is an extremely rare disease, accounting for approximately 1% of lymphocytic leukaemias. Most patients are aged >60 years, with a median age of 65–69 years. The frequencies in males and females are similar {2621}.

Localization
The leukaemic cells are found in the peripheral blood, bone marrow, and spleen.

Clinical features
Most patients present with B symptoms, massive splenomegaly with absent or minimal peripheral lymphadenopathy, and a rapidly increasing lymphocyte count, usually >100 × 10⁹/L. Anaemia and thrombocytopenia are seen in 50% of cases {2117}.

Microscopy
Peripheral blood and bone marrow
The majority (>55% and usually >90%) of the circulating cells are prolymphocytes. These are medium-sized lymphoid cells (twice the size of a normal lymphocyte) with a round nucleus, moderately condensed nuclear chromatin, a prominent central nucleolus, and a relatively small amount of faintly basophilic cytoplasm {1284,2621}. Although the nucleus is typically round, in some cases it can be indented. The bone marrow shows an interstitial or nodular intertrabecular infiltration of lymphoid cells similar to those found in blood.

Other tissues
The morphology of B-PLL in tissues is not well characterized, because initial descriptions of the disease included cases with the t(11;14)(q13;q32) (IGH/CCND1) translocation characteristic of mantle cell lymphoma {3449,3563}. The spleen shows expanded white pulp nodules and red pulp infiltration by intermediate to large cells with abundant cytoplasm and irregular or round nuclei with a central eosinophilic nucleolus {3449}. Lymph nodes display diffuse or vaguely nodular infiltration by similar-looking cells. Proliferation centres (pseudofollicles) are not seen.

Distinguishing B-PLL from pleomorphic mantle cell lymphoma, splenic marginal zone lymphoma, and CLL with an increased number of prolymphocytes can be difficult on morphological grounds. The diagnosis of B-PLL cannot be made without excluding other conditions, because there are no specific markers for B-PLL. The diagnosis of mantle cell lymphoma, for example, is based on immunophenotyping and genetic studies to detect cyclin D1 overexpression and t(11;14)(q13;q32). Evaluation of SOX11 expression may be useful to exclude leukaemic cyclin D1–negative mantle cell lymphoma {3492}. In pure leukaemic cases, the evaluation of SOX11 and cyclin D1 expression may require mRNA analysis by quantitative PCR {3439}.

Immunophenotype
B-PLL cells strongly express surface IgM/IgD, as well as B-cell antigens (CD19, CD20, CD22, CD79a, CD79b, and FMC7). CD5 and CD23 are only positive in 20–30% and 10–20% of cases, respectively, and CD200 is weakly positive or negative {927,2117,3449}. ZAP70 and CD38 are expressed in approximately 50% of cases. ZAP70 expression does not correlate with IGHV mutation status {927}.

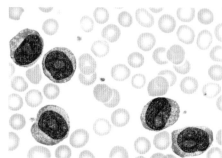

Fig. 13.10 B-cell prolymphocytic leukaemia. Peripheral blood smear. The cells are medium-sized, with moderately condensed chromatin and prominent vesicular nucleoli. The nuclear outline is regular and the cytoplasm faintly basophilic.

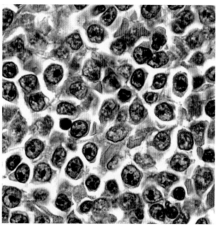

Fig. 13.11 B-cell prolymphocytic leukaemia. Spleen, showing an infiltrate of prolymphocytes.

Postulated normal counterpart
A mature B cell of unknown type

Genetic profile
Antigen receptor genes
IG genes are clonally rearranged, with an unmutated IGH gene in about half of the cases. B-PLL has been reported to use members of the IGHV3 and IGHV4 gene families in 68% and 32% of cases, respectively {927}.

Cytogenetic abnormalities and oncogenes

Initial studies demonstrated t(11;14) (q13;q32) (IGH/*CCND1*) in as many as 20% of B-PLLs {459}. However, these cases are now considered to be leukaemic variants of mantle cell lymphoma {3449,3563,4358}. Complex karyotypes are common {3563}. Deletion in 17p13 is detected in 50% of the cases {927} and is associated with *TP53* mutations {2270}. This probably underlies the progressive course and relative treatment resistance of B-PLL. FISH analysis detects deletions at 13q14 in 27% of the cases {927}. Trisomy 12 is uncommon {927}. Aberrations of *MYC*, including gains, amplifications, and translocations with the IGH, IGK, or IGL loci, have been reported {1224}. This is consistent with the documented increased expression of MYC mRNA and protein {929,1224}. B-PLL has a transcriptional profile different from those of CLL and CLL with increased prolymphocytes, but has features that overlap those of some other lymphomas, such as mantle cell lymphoma {929,4127}. However, the number of investigated cases is limited, and the relationship of B-PLL without *CCND1* rearrangement to mantle cell lymphoma is still uncertain {4127}.

Prognosis and predictive factors

B-PLL responds poorly to therapies for CLL, with a median survival of 30–50 months {927,3449}. There is no correlation between survival and ZAP70 expression, CD38 positivity, deletion in 17p, or IGHV mutation status {927}. Splenectomy may improve symptoms. Responses have been recorded with the CHOP chemotherapy regimen, fludarabine, and cladribine. A combination of chemotherapy and rituximab may be a reasonable treatment approach {2117}. In selected cases, allogeneic bone marrow transplantation should be considered.

Splenic marginal zone lymphoma

Piris M.A.
Isaacson P.G.
Swerdlow S.H.
Thieblemont C.

Pittaluga S.
Rossi D.
Harris N.L.

Definition

Splenic marginal zone lymphoma (SMZL) is a B-cell neoplasm composed of small lymphocytes that surround and replace the splenic white pulp germinal centres, efface the follicle mantle, and merge with a peripheral (marginal) zone of larger cells, including scattered transformed blasts; both small and larger cells infiltrate the red pulp. Splenic hilar lymph nodes and bone marrow are often involved; lymphoma cells are frequently found in the peripheral blood as villous lymphocytes.

ICD-O code   9689/3

Synonyms

Splenic B-cell marginal zone lymphoma; splenic lymphoma with villous lymphocytes; splenic lymphoma with circulating villous lymphocytes (no longer used)

Epidemiology

SMZL is a rare disorder, accounting for <2% of lymphoid neoplasms {148}, but it may account for most cases of otherwise unclassifiable chronic lymphocytic leukaemias that are CD5-negative. Most patients are aged >50 years, with a median age of 67–68 years. The incidence rates among males and females are equal {347, 1999,4388}.

Localization

The tumour involves the spleen and splenic hilar lymph nodes, the bone marrow, and often the peripheral blood. The liver may also be involved. Peripheral lymph nodes are not typically involved {347,2691}.

Clinical features

Patients present with splenomegaly, sometimes accompanied by autoimmune thrombocytopenia or anaemia and a variable presence of peripheral blood villous lymphocytes. The bone marrow is regularly involved, but peripheral lymphadenopathy and extranodal infiltration are extremely uncommon. About one third of patients have a small para-

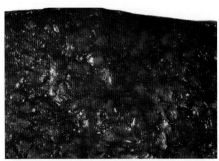

Fig. 13.12 Splenic marginal zone lymphoma. Gross photograph of spleen showing marked expansion of the white pulp and infiltration of the red pulp.

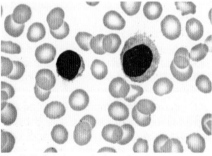

Fig. 13.13 Splenic marginal zone lymphoma. Peripheral blood containing tumour cells with polar villi (villous lymphocytes).

protein, but marked hyperviscosity and hypergammaglobulinaemia are uncommon {347,2691}. An association with hepatitis C virus has been described in southern Europe {135,1620}.

Macroscopy

Gross examination of the spleen reveals marked expansion of the white pulp and infiltration of the red pulp.

Microscopy

In the splenic white pulp, a central zone of small round lymphocytes surrounds or, more commonly, replaces reactive germinal centres, with effacement of the normal follicle mantle {1783,2691}. This zone

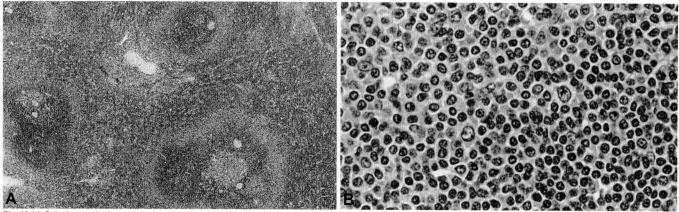

Fig. 13.14 Splenic marginal zone lymphoma, spleen. **A** Infiltration of white and red pulp. The white pulp nodules show a central dark zone of small lymphocytes (sometimes surrounding a residual germinal centre) giving way to a paler marginal zone. **B** High-magnification view of white pulp nodule showing the small lymphocytes merging with a marginal zone consisting of larger cells with pale cytoplasm and occasional transformed blasts.

merges with a peripheral zone of small to medium-sized cells with more dispersed chromatin and abundant pale cytoplasm, which resemble marginal zone cells, and interspersed transformed blasts. The red pulp is always infiltrated, with small nodules of the larger cells and sheets of the small lymphocytes, which often invade sinuses. Epithelioid histiocytes may be present in the lymphoid aggregates. Some cases have a markedly predominant population of the larger marginal zone–like cells {1532,1793}. Plasmacytic differentiation may occur, and in rare cases, clusters of plasma cells are present in the centres of the white pulp nodules. In splenic hilar lymph nodes, the sinuses are dilated and lymphoma surrounds and replaces germinal centres, but the two cell types, small lymphocytes and marginal zone cells, are often more intimately admixed, without the formation of a distinct so-called marginal zone. In the bone marrow, there is a nodular interstitial infiltrate cytologically similar to that in the lymph nodes. Occasionally, neoplastic cells surround reactive follicles. Intrasinusoidal lymphoma cells, which are more apparent after CD20 immunostaining,

are a helpful feature, although they are sometimes observed in other lymphomas {1242}. When lymphoma cells are present in the peripheral blood, they are usually characterized by short polar villi. Some may appear plasmacytoid {2622}.

Differential diagnosis
The differential diagnosis includes other small B-cell lymphomas/leukaemias, including chronic lymphocytic leukaemia (CLL), hairy cell leukaemia (HCL), mantle cell lymphoma, follicular lymphoma, and lymphoplasmacytic lymphoma. It is also important to recognize that many small B-cell lymphomas (other than HCL, which diffusely involves the red pulp) can have slightly larger cells with pale cytoplasm when they involve the splenic marginal zone, mimicking SMZL {3197}. The nodular pattern on bone marrow biopsy excludes HCL, but the morphological features on bone marrow examination may not be sufficient to distinguish between the other small B-cell neoplasms. Immunophenotypic and molecular/cytogenetic findings may also be very helpful, but the diagnosis can be rendered most confidently from a splenectomy specimen;

however, such a specimen is often not available.

Immunophenotype
Tumour cells express surface IgM and usually IgD. They are positive for CD20 and CD79a and negative for CD5, CD10, CD23, CD43, and annexin A1 {1783, 2579}. CD103 is usually negative, and cyclin D1 is absent {3540}. Ki-67 staining shows a distinctive targetoid pattern due to an increased growth fraction in both the germinal centre, if present, and the marginal zone. The absence of cyclin D1 and LEF1 is useful in excluding mantle cell lymphoma and CLL, respectively. The absence of annexin A1 excludes HCL, and lack of CD10 and BCL6 helps to exclude follicular lymphoma {3540}. A group of CD5+ SMZL cases has been described, distinguished by a higher lymphocytosis and diffuse bone marrow infiltration {285}.

Postulated normal counterpart
A marginal-zone B cell that may or may not demonstrate evidence of antigen exposure

Genetic profile
Antigen receptor genes
IG heavy and light chain genes have clonal rearrangements, and approximately half of the cases have somatic hypermutation. Bias in IGHV1-2*04 usage has been found in 30% of SMZL cases, suggesting that this tumour derives from a highly selected B-cell population {62, 378}. Stereotyped HCDR3 sequences, specific for SMZL, support a potential role of antigen selection in the pathogenesis of these lymphomas {4493}.

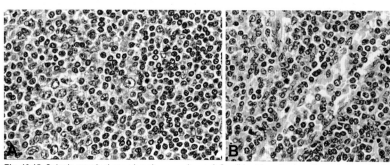

Fig. 13.15 Splenic marginal zone lymphoma, spleen. **A** Small lymphocytes invading splenic red pulp, with a poorly defined nodule of larger cells. **B** Small lymphocytes invading red pulp sinuses.

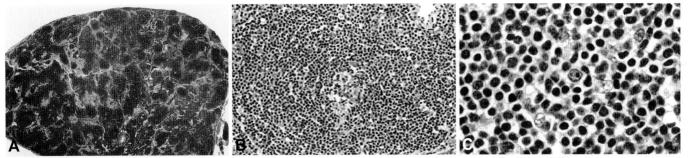

Fig. 13.16 Splenic marginal zone lymphoma, splenic hilar lymph node. **A** There is a nodular proliferation with preservation of the sinuses. **B** This nodule has a central small residual germinal centre. **C** High magnification shows a mixture of small lymphocytes and larger cells.

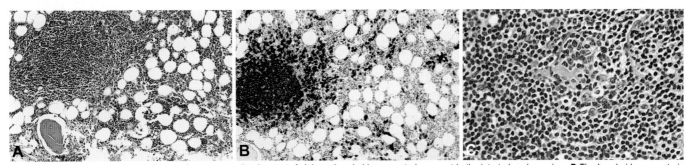

Fig. 13.17 Splenic marginal zone lymphoma, bone marrow involvement. **A** A large lymphoid aggregate is present in the intertrabecular region. **B** The lymphoid aggregate is CD20-positive, and CD20+ B cells infiltrate the sinusoids of the marrow. **C** Lymphoid aggregate with a small residual germinal centre.

Cytogenetic abnormalities and oncogenes

SMZL lacks recurrent chromosomal translocations, including translocations that are typical of other lymphoma types, such as the t(14;18)(q32;q21) translocation affecting *BCL2* in follicular lymphoma; the t(11;14)(q13;q32) translocation affecting *CCND1* in mantle cell lymphoma; and the t(11;18)(q21;q21), t(14;18)(q32;q21), and t(1;14)(p22;q32) translocations resulting in *BIRC3-MALT1*, IGH/*MALT1*, and IGH/*BCL10* juxtaposition, respectively, in extranodal marginal zone lymphoma of mucosa-associated lymphoid tissue (MALT lymphoma). The absence of these abnormalities helps distinguish SMZL from some of the lymphomas that can mimic it. A small number of SMZLs carry a recurrent t(2;7) (p12;q21) translocation, which activates the *CDK6* gene through juxtaposition with the IGK locus {810}. Approximately 30% of SMZLs show a heterozygous deletion in 7q, which is rarely found in other lymphoma subtypes {3362,3497}. The gene(s) targeted by the 7q deletion remain unknown, despite the combined investigation of genomic and transcriptomic profiles and mutation analysis of a number of candidate genes {1254,3376, 4268}. Gain of 3q is present in a considerable subset of cases.

NOTCH2 is one of the most frequently mutated genes in SMZL, mutated in approximately 10–25% of cases {771,2006, 2532,3070,3203,3419}. Although diagnostically useful, *NOTCH2* mutations are also seen in infrequent other small B-cell lymphomas {305,1945,2006, 3419}. *KLF2* is somatically mutated in approximately 10–40% of SMZLs {771, 3070,3203}, but these mutations are also found in some other small B-cell neoplasms {3203}. Mutations in both of these genes have been associated with SMZLs that have deletion in 7q. *MYD88* mutations are rare in SMZL, and may therefore be a useful biomarker for the differentiation of SMZL from lymphoplasmacytic lymphoma in pathologically challenging cases with evidence of plasmacytic differentiation {2534,3070}. The fact that the most frequently mutated genes in SMZL (i.e. *NOTCH2* and *KLF2*) are physiologically involved in proliferation and commitment of mature B cells to the marginal zone, points to homing to the spleen compartment and marginal zone differentiation as the major programmes deregulated in this lymphoma. Congruently, SMZL has an expression signature characterized by the upregulation of genes belonging to the marginal zone differentiation programme {3455, 4064}.

Prognosis and predictive factors

The clinical course is indolent, with a 10 year survival probability from 67% to 95% {135,347,2266,2781,3956,3957,3768A}. Response to chemotherapy of the type that is typically effective in other small B-cell neoplasms is often poor, but patients generally have haematological responses to splenectomy and/or rituximab, with long-term survival {2266,3139A,3768A}. Transformation to large B-cell lymphoma occurs in 10–15% of cases {4388}, and is usually associated with a shorter time to progression {2266,2781}. Hepatitis C virus–positive cases have been reported to respond to antiviral treatment using interferon gamma, with or without ribavirin {1620,3955}. Adverse clinical prognostic factors include a large tumour mass and poor general health status {627}. A clinical scoring system has been proposed that incorporates haemoglobin concentration, platelet count, lactate dehydrogenase level, and presence of extrahilar lymphadenopathy {2696}. Although data are limited, *NOTCH2*, *KLF2*, and in particular *TP53* mutations have been reported to be adverse prognostic indicators {3070}.

Hairy cell leukaemia

Foucar K.
Falini B.
Stein H.

Definition

Hairy cell leukaemia (HCL) is a cytologically and immunophenotypically distinct, indolent neoplasm of small mature lymphoid cells with oval nuclei and abundant cytoplasm with so-called hairy projections involving peripheral blood and diffusely infiltrating the bone marrow and splenic red pulp.

ICD-O code   9940/3

Synonym

Leukaemic reticuloendotheliosis (obsolete)

Epidemiology

HCL is a rare disease, accounting for 2% of lymphoid leukaemias. The annual incidence rate in the USA is 0.32 cases per 100 000 population {1025}. Patients are predominantly middle-aged to elderly adults, with a median age of 58 years; HCL has been diagnosed rarely in patients in their 20s, but it is exceptionally uncommon in children. The male-to-female ratio is 4:1, and the incidence is substantially higher in White versus Black populations {1025}.

Etiology

The presence of the *BRAF* V600E mutation in virtually 100% of cases of HCL is strong evidence of a disease-defining genetic event {3998}. This leads to constitutive activation of MAPK {3997}.

Localization

Tumour cells are found predominantly in the bone marrow and spleen. Typically, a small number of circulating cells are noted. Tumour infiltrates may occur in the liver and lymph nodes, and occasionally also in the skin. Rare patients demonstrate prominent abdominal lymphadenopathy {3638}.

Clinical features

The most common presenting symptoms include weakness and fatigue, left upper quadrant pain, fever, and bleeding. Most patients present with splenomegaly and

Table 13.02 Pathogenesis of hairy cell leukaemia (HCL) {287,586,3160,3994,3998}

Property	Proposed pathogenetic mechanism(s)
Clonal B cell	Derived from a *BRAF* V600E–mutant mature memory B cell *BRAF* V600E mutation in virtually all cases
Hairy cell morphology	Shaped by *BRAF* V600E mutation and influenced by overexpression and constitutive activation of members of the RHO family of small GTPases and upregulation of the growth arrest–specific molecule GAS7
Reticulin fibrosis	HCL cells synthesize and bind to fibronectin in bone marrow microenvironment Production rate of fibronectin is under control of autocrine bFGF secreted by hairy cells TGF-beta 1 also plays a role in reticulin fibrosis
Homing to bone marrow, splenic red pulp, and hepatic sinusoids	Hairy cells home to blood-related compartments via constitutively activated integrin receptors and overexpression of matrix metalloproteinase inhibitors Downregulation of chemokine receptors such as CCR7 and CXCR5 explains absence of lymph node involvement
Phagocytosis	Overexpression of annexin A1 and actin possible mediators
Pseudosinus formation in spleen	Interaction of hairy cells with endothelial cells resulting in replacement of endothelial cells by HCL cells
CD25 and tartrate-resistant acid phosphatase expression	Induced by *BRAF* V600E
Prolonged cell survival	Mediated by *BRAF* V600E; also influenced by constitutive production of tumour necrosis factor and IL6, and overexpression of the apoptosis inhibitor BCL2
Inhibition of normal haematopoiesis (hypocellular HCL)	Constitutive production of TGF-beta by hairy cells

pancytopenia, with few circulating neoplastic cells. Monocytopenia is characteristic. Other common distinctive manifestations include hepatomegaly and recurrent opportunistic infections; less common unique findings include vasculitis, bleeding disorders, neurological disorders, skeletal involvement, and other immune dysfunction {364}.

Macroscopy

Diffuse expansion of the red pulp with variably sized blood lakes in markedly enlarged spleen

Microscopy

Peripheral blood and bone marrow
Hairy cells are small to medium-sized lymphoid cells with an oval or indented (kidney-shaped) nucleus with homogeneous, spongy, ground-glass chromatin that is slightly less clumped than that of a normal lymphocyte. Nucleoli are typically absent or inconspicuous. The cytoplasm is abundant and pale blue, with circumferen-

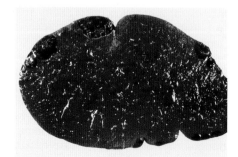

Fig. 13.18 Hairy cell leukaemia (HCL). The spleen is markedly enlarged, with diffuse expansion of the red pulp. White pulp is not discernible. Numerous blood lakes of varying size are visible.

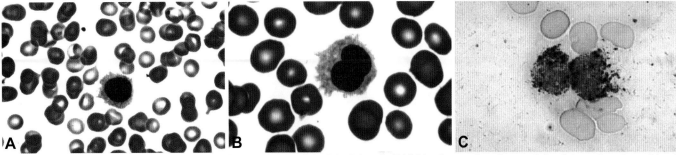

Fig. 13.19 Hairy cell leukaemia. **A,B** Note the typical morphological features of circulating hairy cells highlighting the range in nuclear morphology between these two peripheral blood smear photomicrographs. **C** There is strong tartrate-resistant acid phosphatase positivity, characteristic of hairy cell leukaemia.

tial so-called hairy projections on smears {364,3638}. Occasionally, the cytoplasm contains discrete vacuoles or rod-shaped inclusions that represent the ribosome lamellar complexes that have been identified by electron microscopy {3638}.

The diagnosis is best made on bone marrow biopsy. The extent of bone marrow effacement in HCL varies. The primary pattern is interstitial or patchy with some preservation of fat and haematopoietic elements. The infiltrate is characterized by widely spaced lymphoid cells with oval or indented nuclei, in contrast to the closely packed nuclei of most other indolent lymphoid neoplasms involving the bone marrow. The abundant cytoplasm and prominent cell borders may produce a so-called fried-egg appearance. Mitotic figures are virtually absent. When infiltration is minimal, the subtle clusters of hairy cells can be overlooked. In patients with advanced disease, a diffuse solid infiltrate may be evident. The obvious discrete aggregates that typify bone marrow infiltrates of many other chronic lymphoproliferative neoplasms are not a feature of HCL. An increase in reticulin fibres is associated with all hairy cell infiltrates in bone marrow and other sites, and often results in a so-called dry tap (i.e. failure to obtain aspirate on attempted bone marrow aspiration). In some cases, the bone marrow is hypocellular, with a loss of haematopoietic elements, in particular of the granulocytic lineage, which can lead to an incorrect diagnosis of aplastic anaemia. In such cases, immunostaining for a B-cell antigen such as CD20 is essential for the identification of an abnormal B-cell infiltrate, prompting the use of immunohistochemical stains more specific for HCL. In some cases, the morphological appearance of HCL overlaps with that of splenic marginal zone lymphoma or splenic B-cell lymphoma/leukaemia, unclassifiable, requiring correlation with the immunophenotypic studies.

Spleen and other tissues

In the spleen, HCL infiltrates are found in the red pulp. The white pulp is typically atrophic. The cells characteristically fill the red pulp cords. Red blood cell lakes, collections of pooled erythrocytes surrounded by elongated hairy cells, are the presumed consequence of disruption of normal blood flow in the red pulp {364, 3638}. The liver may show infiltrates of hairy cells, predominantly in the sinusoids. Lymph node infiltration may occur, especially with advanced disease, and is variably interfollicular/paracortical, with sparing of follicles and intact sinuses.

Cytochemistry

The only cytochemical stain used in the diagnosis is tartrate-resistant acid phosphatase, but the use of this technically challenging stain has been largely sup-

planted by immunophenotypic/immuno-histochemical techniques. When appropriate air-dried unfixed slide preparations are available, virtually all cases of HCL are found to contain at least some cells with strong, granular cytoplasmic tartrate-resistant acid phosphatase positivity; weak staining is of no diagnostic utility.

Immunophenotype

The classic immunophenotypic profile of HCL consists of bright monotypic surface immunoglobulin; bright coexpression of CD20, CD22, and CD11c; and expression of CD103, CD25, CD123, TBX21 (also called TBET), annexin A1, FMC7, CD200, and cyclin D1 {1153,1302,1896, 3643}. Most cases of HCL lack both CD5 and CD10, but CD10 expression is reported in about 10–20% of cases and CD5 expression in about 0–2% {685,

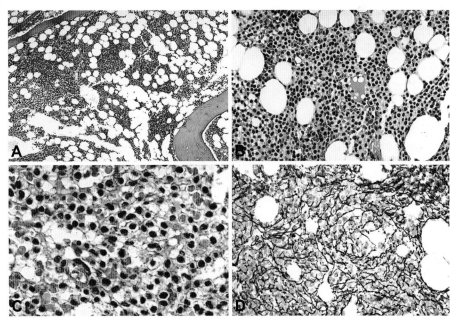

Fig. 13.20 Hairy cell leukaemia (HCL), bone marrow biopsy. **A** Low-magnification view showing a subtle diffuse interstitial infiltrate of hairy cells. **B** Extensive diffuse interstitial infiltration by hairy cell leukaemia. Note the widely spaced oval nuclei and paucity of mitotic activity. **C** The so-called fried-egg appearance of hairy cells is evident on high magnification. **D** Note the diffuse increase in reticulin fibres.

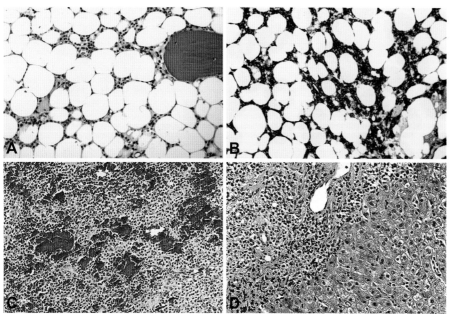

Fig. 13.21 Hairy cell leukaemia (HCL). **A** Hypocellular HCL with interstitial infiltrates in bone marrow biopsy. **B** CD20 immunohistochemical staining highlights the subtle leukaemic infiltrate in this case. **C** Spleen shows red pulp infiltration with numerous red blood cell lakes. **D** There is both portal and sinusoidal infiltration in the liver.

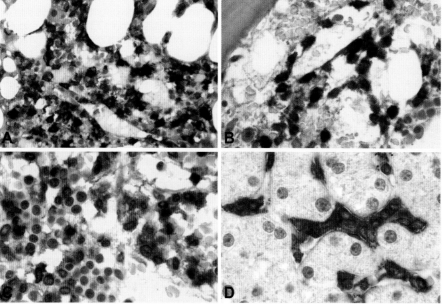

Fig. 13.22 Hairy cell leukaemia (HCL), immunohistochemical features (A, B, C bone marrow biopsy, D liver). **A** CD72 (DBA.44) positivity of hairy cells, accentuating hairy projections. **B** CD123 positivity of hairy cells. **C** The hairy cells express annexin A1, whereas erythroid precursors are negative. **D** There is sinusoidal infiltration by annexin A1–positive leukaemic hairy cells in this liver.

1024,1844,3632}. Other immunophenotypic variants are also recognized {685}. Annexin A1 is the most specific marker; it is not expressed in any B-cell lymphoma other than HCL {1153}. Expression of annexin A1 can be used to distinguish HCL from splenic marginal zone lymphoma and HCL variant, which are both annexin A1–negative. Immunostaining for annexin A1 must always be compared with

staining for a B-cell antigen (e.g. CD20), because annexin A1 is also expressed by myeloid cells and a proportion of T cells. For this reason, annexin A1 is not a suitable marker for monitoring minimal residual disease. A more suitable approach for assessment for residual disease after therapy is multicolour flow cytometry targeting the distinctive HCL profile or immunostaining for TBX21 {1896,2730,

3185,3643}. Immunohistochemical staining for V600E-mutant BRAF protein can also be helpful and may be useful for recognizing residual disease {4076}.

Postulated normal counterpart

Although the *BRAF* V600E mutation has been detected in the haematopoietic stem cell compartment of patients with HCL, the postulated normal counterpart is a late, activated memory B cell, as suggested by gene expression profiling studies {287,755}.

Genetic profile

Antigen receptor genes

Although exceptions have been reported, the majority (>85%) of cases of HCL demonstrate IGHV genes with somatic hypermutation indicative of a post–germinal centre stage of maturation {152, 586,3994}. A unique feature of HCL is the common coexpression of multiple clonally related immunoglobulin isotypes, suggesting arrest at some point during isotype switching {3994}.

Cytogenetic abnormalities and oncogenes

No cytogenetic abnormality is specific for HCL; numerical abnormalities of chromosomes 5 and 7 have been rarely described, but translocations are distinctly uncommon {586}. The high frequency of *BRAF* V600E mutation, confirmed by multiple investigators, suggests a key role in the pathogenesis of HCL {3160}. Sensitive methods for the detection of this HCL-defining mutation have been published {138,3997,3998}. It remains to be established whether cases that lack *BRAF* V600E mutation, use the IGHV4-34 family, and have *MAP2K1* mutations are more closely related to classic HCL or HCL variant {4267,4382}.

Prognosis and predictive factors

HCL is uniquely sensitive to either interferon alfa or nucleosides (purine analogues) such as pentostatin and cladribine. Patients receiving purine analogues often achieve complete and durable remission {1458}. However, as many as 50% of patients with HCL relapse. In refractory or relapsed cases, salvage therapeutic options include chemotherapy combined with rituximab, anti-CD22 immunotoxin therapy, and, more recently, BRAF inhibitors {3160,3995}.

Splenic B-cell lymphoma/leukaemia, unclassifiable

Piris M.A.
Foucar K.
Mollejo M.
Matutes E.
Campo E.
Falini B.
Swerdlow S.H.

Definition

There are a number of variably well-defined entities that constitute small B-cell clonal lymphoproliferations involving the spleen but that do not fit into any of the other categories of B-cell lymphoid neoplasms in the WHO classification. The best-defined of these relatively rare provisional entities are splenic diffuse red pulp small B-cell lymphoma and hairy cell leukaemia variant.

The relationship of splenic diffuse red pulp small B-cell lymphoma to hairy cell leukaemia variant and other primary splenic B-cell lymphomas remains uncertain; the precise diagnostic criteria and most-appropriate terminology for these provisional entities have not yet been fully established.

Other splenic small B-cell lymphomas that do not fulfil the criteria for either of these provisional entities should be diagnosed as splenic B-cell lymphoma/leukaemia, unclassifiable, until more is known {3848}.

ICD-O code 9591/3

Synonyms

Splenic marginal zone lymphoma, diffuse variant; splenic red pulp lymphoma with numerous basophilic villous lymphocytes; splenic lymphoma with villous lymphocytes; prolymphocytic variant of hairy cell leukaemia

Splenic diffuse red pulp small B-cell lymphoma

Definition

Splenic diffuse red pulp small B-cell lymphoma (SDRPL) is an uncommon lymphoma with a diffuse pattern of involvement of the splenic red pulp by small monomorphous B lymphocytes. The neoplasm also involves bone marrow sinusoids and peripheral blood, commonly with a villous cytology {1921,4043,4044}. This is a provisional entity that requires additional molecular studies for defining its main features and diagnostic markers. This

diagnosis should be restricted to characteristic cases fulfilling the major features described here, and should not be applied to any lymphoma growing diffusely in the spleen. Chronic lymphocytic leukaemia, hairy cell leukaemia, lymphoplasmacytic lymphoma, and B-cell prolymphocytic leukaemia should be excluded through appropriate studies. A diagnosis of SDRPL may be suggested for cases showing purely intrasinusoidal bone marrow involvement and villous lymphocytes in the peripheral blood, but the differential with splenic marginal zone lymphoma (SMZL) may require examination of the spleen {3216}. In case of doubt, the use of the term splenic B-cell lymphoma/leukaemia, unclassifiable, is warranted.

There is some degree of overlap with cases that fulfil the criteria for hairy cell leukaemia variant; however, additional studies are required to further evaluate the extent of overlap between these entities, particularly given that not all studies report the same phenotypic, cytogenetic, or molecular findings {2584,3481}. Although the rare large B-cell lymphomas that involve the splenic and bone marrow sinusoids may be related to SDRPL, they should not be included in this category, which is restricted to indolent lymphomas composed of small lymphocytes {2688, 2743}.

ICD-O code 9591/3

Epidemiology

SDRPL is a rare disorder, accounting for < 1% of non-Hodgkin lymphomas. It accounts for about 10% of the B-cell lymphomas diagnosed in splenectomy specimens. Most patients are aged > 40 years, and there is no sex predilection.

Localization

All cases are diagnosed at clinical stage IV, with spleen, bone marrow, and peripheral blood involvement. Peripheral lymph node involvement is only rarely reported.

Clinical features

SDRPL is a leukaemic neoplasm, usually with a relatively low lymphocytosis. Almost all patients have splenomegaly (frequently massive). Although not consistent among all studies, thrombocytopenia and leukopenia are frequently present, whereas anaemia has been reported more rarely. B symptoms are infrequent. The presence of a paraprotein has not been reported.

Microscopy

Peripheral blood

Villous lymphocytes similar to those

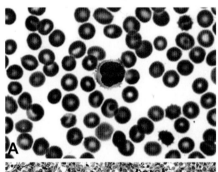
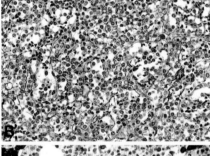
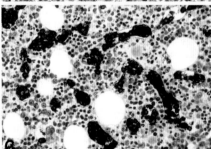

Fig. 13.23 Splenic diffuse red pulp small B-cell lymphoma. **A** Peripheral blood cytology with villous cell. **B** Reticulin staining in spleen outlines the infiltration of red pulp cords and sinusoids. **C** Bone marrow intrasinusoidal infiltration highlighted by CD20 staining.

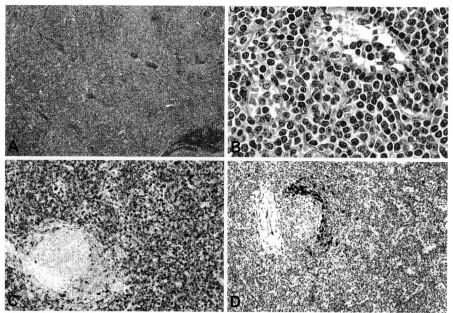

Fig. 13.24 Splenic diffuse red pulp small B-cell lymphoma, spleen. **A** Diffuse infiltration of the red pulp. **B** High-magnification view showing the infiltration of both red pulp cord and sinusoids. **C** CD72 (DBA.44) staining of the tumoural cells. **D** IgD staining is usually negative, outlining residual IgD+ mantle zone cells.

reported in SMZL are present. Clonal B-cell expansions with an immunophenotype consistent with marginal zone lymphoma presenting with isolated lymphocytosis may constitute an early stage of splenic B-cell lymphoma/leukaemia, unclassifiable, or of SMZL, although most of these cases remain stable over time {4390}. Some of these cases fulfil the criteria for non-chronic lymphocytic leukaemia–type monoclonal B-cell lymphocytosis.

Bone marrow
Intrasinusoidal infiltration is the rule, occasionally as a sole finding. This can be accompanied by interstitial and nodular infiltration. Lymphoid follicles, as seen in SMZL, have not been reported.

Spleen
There is a diffuse pattern of involvement of the red pulp, with both cord and sinusoid infiltration. Characteristic blood lakes lined by tumoural cells may be seen. Unlike in SMZL, white pulp involvement is absent, although there may be residual lymphoid nodules composed of T cells or, much less often, residual white pulp nodules {2530}. The neoplastic infiltrate is composed of a monomorphic population of small to medium-sized lymphocytes, with round and regular nuclei, compact chromatin, and occasional distinct small nucleoli, with scattered nucleolated blast cells. The tumoural cells have pale cytoplasm and plasmacytoid features but lack phenotypic features of plasmacytic differentiation such as cytoplasmic immunoglobulin and CD38 expression. Some cases show focal plasmacytic differentiation. Rare cases have clusters of large cells {2530}.

Cytochemistry
Tartrate-resistant acid phosphatase staining is negative.

Immunophenotype
SDRPL is characteristically positive for CD20, CD72 (DBA.44), and IgG and negative for IgD, annexin A1, CD25, CD5, CD103, CD123, CD11c, CD10, and CD23 {2581,2689,3499}. IgD+ cases can be seen with similar features. There have also been reports of cases that are positive for IgM (with or without IgG), CD103, and CD11c, with infrequent CD5 and CD123 expression {4043}.

Postulated normal counterpart
A mature B cell of unknown type

Genetic profile
Somatic hypermutation in IGHV genes is present in most cases, but about 20–30% of cases are unmutated {2530,4043}. Overrepresentation of IGHV3-23 and IGHV4-34, as is seen in hairy cell leukaemia, has been reported {4043}. The reported proportion of cases that use the IGHV1-2 gene, which is overrepresented in SMZL, has varied; in one series, its use was reported in 3 of 13 cases; the same number of cases used IGHV4-34 {2530,4043}.
Complex cytogenetic alterations, including t(9;14)(p13.2;q32.3) involving *PAX5* and IGH genes, have been found in some cases, but the neoplasms lack *CCND1* rearrangements, and usually do not demonstrate deletions in 7q or trisomies of chromosomes 3 or 18 {262, 2530,4043}. Copy-number arrays have identified abnormalities in almost 70% of cases {2530}. *TP53* mutations have been reported in a small number of cases, and some cases show increased p53 expression {2530,2689}. Sequencing studies have shown that SDRPL has a distinct pattern of somatic mutations amongst B-cell malignancies {4047A}, with an increased expression of cyclin D3 and recurrent mutations in the *CCND3* PEST domain in a high proportion of SDRPL cases {848A}. Infrequent mutations in *NOTCH1*, *MAP2K1*, *BRAF*, and *SF3B1* have also been reported {2530}.

Prognosis and predictive factors
This is an indolent but incurable disease, with good responses after splenectomy in most patients; however, some patients do develop progressive disease and have an adverse outcome. The small number of patients with mutations in *NOTCH1*, *MAP2K1*, and *TP53* have been reported to have shorter progression-free survival {2530}.

Hairy cell leukaemia variant

Definition
The designation of hairy cell leukaemia variant (HCL-v) encompasses cases of B-cell chronic lymphoproliferative disorders that resemble classic HCL but exhibit variant cytological and haematological features such as leukocytosis, presence of monocytes, cells with prominent nucleoli, cells with blastic or convoluted nuclei, and/or absence of circumferential shaggy contours. They also have a variant immunophenotype (including absence of CD25, CD123, annexin A1, and tartrate-resistant acid phosphatase), have wildtype *BRAF*, and are resistant to conventional HCL therapy (i.e. show lack of response to cladribine). These cases are not considered to be biologically related to HCL.

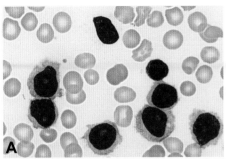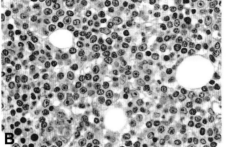

Fig. 13.25 Hairy cell leukaemia variant. **A** Blood smear. The cells have abundant, moderately basophilic cytoplasm with villous projections, but unlike the cells of typical hairy cell leukaemia, they have visible nucleoli, resembling prolymphocytes. **B** The bone marrow biopsy shows a diffuse, interstitial pattern of infiltration similar to that of typical hairy cell leukaemia.

ICD-O code   9591/3

Synonym
Prolymphocytic variant of hairy cell leukaemia

Epidemiology
HCL-v is about one tenth as common as HCL, with an annual incidence of approximately 0.03 cases per 100 000 population {3367}. Middle-aged to elderly patients are affected, and there is a slight male predominance {1647,2584}. Cases of HCL-v have been described in Asian populations where HCL-v may be more common than HCL {2584}.

Localization
The spleen, bone marrow, and peripheral blood are involved, but lymphadenopathy is relatively uncommon {2584}. Hepatomegaly is seen in less than one third of patients. Involvement of other solid tissues is rare.

Clinical features
Patients with HCL-v typically manifest signs and symptoms related to either splenomegaly or cytopenias. Leukocytosis is a consistent feature, with an average white blood cell count of about 30×10^9/L. Thrombocytopenia is present in about half of the patients and anaemia in one quarter {1647}. The absolute monocyte count is typically within normal range.

Microscopy
Circulating HCL-v cells are readily apparent on the peripheral blood smear; the cells commonly exhibit hybrid features of prolymphocytic leukaemia and classic HCL, although several other morpho-

logical subtypes (e.g. blastic and convoluted) have also been described {3367}. Nuclear features range from condensed chromatin with the prominent central nucleolus of a prolymphocytic cell to dispersed chromatin with highly irregular nuclear contours. Cytoplasmic features are similarly variable, although some degree of hairy projections is typically noted. Transformation to large cells with convoluted nuclei has been described, and cases of so-called convoluted HCL may be explained by this phenomenon {2584,4461}. Unlike in classic HCL, the bone marrow is aspirable, without significant reticulin fibrosis {1920}. The infiltrates of HCL-v may be subtle and very inconspicuous, often requiring immunohistochemical staining to highlight the pattern and extent of infiltration {624}. A distinct predilection for sinusoidal infiltration has been described {624}.

Like in HCL and splenic diffuse red pulp small B-cell lymphoma, the red pulp of the spleen is diffusely involved and expanded in HCL-v, with regressed or absent white pulp follicles {1920}. The leukaemic cells fill dilated sinusoids, and red blood cell lakes may be noted {2584}. Liver involvement is characterized by both portal tract and sinusoidal infiltrates.

Cytochemistry
Unlike in classic HCL, cytochemical staining for tartrate-resistant acid phosphatase is weak to negative in HCL-v {1920,2584}.

Immunophenotype
Cases of HCL-v share many phenotypic features with HCL, although HCL-v cells characteristically lack several key HCL

antigens, usually including CD25, annexin A1, tartrate-resistant acid phosphatase, CD200, and CD123 {52,1024, 1153,3367}. Positive markers in HCL-v include CD72 (DBA.44), pan–B-cell antigens, CD11c, bright monotypic surface immunoglobulin (most frequently IgG), CD103, and FMC7 {2574}.

Postulated normal counterpart
An activated B cell at a late stage of maturation

Genetic profile
Studies are limited, but about one third of cases of HCL-v demonstrate no somatic mutations of IGHV; these unmutated cases have a high frequency of *TP53* mutation {1647}. There is preferential usage of the IGHV4-34 gene family, although this is not a feature exclusive to HCL-v {1648}. High-resolution genomic profiling has shown a large number of DNA copy-number alterations, the most frequent being gains on chromosome 5 and losses on 7q and 17p {1649}. *BRAF* V600E mutations have not been documented in HCL-v {3278,3997,3998,4382}. Recurrent *MAP2K1* mutations have been found in HCL-v and in cases described as classic HCL with IGHV4-34 gene family usage {4267}.

Prognosis and predictive factors
The 5-year survival rate is reported to be 57% {1647}. Most patients with HCL-v require therapy, which can range from splenectomy to combination chemotherapy with rituximab {1647}. Agents that are effective in classic HCL (i.e. cladribine and pentostatin) are not effective in HCL-v {1024,3367}. However, patients seem to achieve a long-lasting response to the combination of cladribine and rituximab {2106}. Significant adverse prognostic factors include older patient age, greater severity of anaemia, and *TP53* mutations {1647}.

Lymphoplasmacytic lymphoma

Swerdlow S.H.
Cook J.R.
Sohani A.R.
Pileri S.A.

Harris N.L.
Jaffe E.S.
Stein H.

Definition

Lymphoplasmacytic lymphoma (LPL) is a neoplasm of small B lymphocytes, plasmacytoid lymphocytes, and plasma cells, usually involving bone marrow and sometimes lymph nodes and spleen, which does not fulfil the criteria for any of the other small B-cell lymphoid neoplasms that can also have plasmacytic differentiation. Because the distinction between LPL and some of the other small B-cell lymphoid neoplasms, especially some marginal zone lymphomas (MZLs), is not always clear-cut, some cases may need to be diagnosed as a small B-cell lymphoid neoplasm with plasmacytic differentiation and a differential diagnosis provided. The great majority (>90%) of LPLs have *MYD88* L265P mutation, which can make the diagnosis either more or less likely; however, this abnormality is neither specific nor required. Although LPL is often associated with a paraprotein, usually of IgM type, this is not required for the diagnosis. Waldenström macroglobulinaemia (WM) is found in a substantial subset of patients with LPL, but is not synonymous with it; it is defined as LPL with bone marrow involvement and an IgM monoclonal gammopathy of any concentration {3017}. Cases of gamma heavy chain disease are no longer considered a variant of LPL {1526}.

ICD-O codes

Lymphoplasmacytic lymphoma   9671/3
Waldenström macroglobulinaemia
                              9761/3

Synonym

Malignant lymphoma, lymphoplasmacytoid

Epidemiology

LPL occurs in adults, with a median age in the seventh decade of life, and shows a slight male predominance {991,4195}.

Etiology

Hepatitis C virus is associated with type II cryoglobulinaemia and with LPL in some series, perhaps related to geographical differences {908,2263,2616,2875,3037, 3263,3514,3913}. Some of the hepatitis C virus–associated lymphoplasmacytic proliferations, even if monotypic, are non-progressive and may be similar to monoclonal B-cell lymphocytosis {2690,2717}. Treatment of these patients with antiviral agents may lead to regression of the lymphoplasmacytic proliferations {2589,3913}. So-called immune-stimulating conditions, such as autoimmune disorders, are associated with an increased risk {2483}.

Localization

Most cases involve the bone marrow, and some cases involve the lymph nodes and other extranodal sites. About 15–30% of patients with WM also have splenomegaly, hepatomegaly, and/or adenopathy, with a higher proportion with disease progression {991,4051}. The peripheral blood may also be involved. Rare involvement of the CNS, associated with WM, is known as Bing–Neel syndrome {3225}. LPL can occur at sites typically involved by extranodal MZL of mucosa-associated lymphoid tissue (MALT lymphoma), such as the ocular adnexa {2347,3851}.

Clinical features

Most patients present with weakness and fatigue, usually related to anaemia. Most patients have an IgM serum paraprotein, and would therefore also fulfil the criteria for WM. Some, however, have a different paraprotein or no paraprotein at all. A minority have both IgM and IgG or other paraproteins. Hyperviscosity occurs in as many as 30% of cases. The paraprotein may also have autoantibody or cryoglobulin activity, resulting in autoimmune phenomena or cryoglobulinaemia (seen in as many as ~20% of patients with WM). Cold agglutinins may also be present; however, primary cold agglutinin disease may be distinct from LPL {3301}. Neuropathies occur in a minority of patients and may result from reactivity of the IgM paraprotein with myelin sheath antigens,

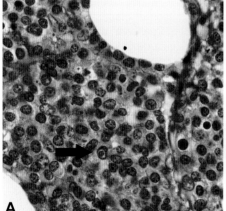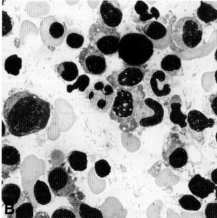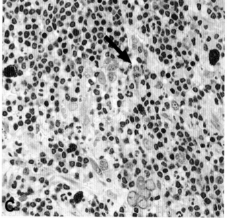

Fig. 13.26 Lymphoplasmacytic lymphoma. **A** Bone marrow biopsy shows a lymphoplasmacytic infiltrate with a Dutcher body (arrow), which gives a positive periodic acid–Schiff (PAS) reaction. **B** The lymphoplasmacytic infiltrate is also seen in the aspirate smear. **C** Giemsa staining highlights the characteristic increased mast cells and haemosiderin (arrow).

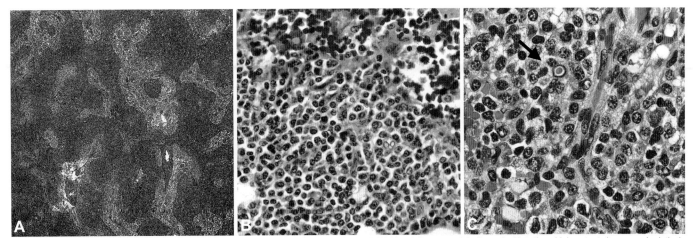

Fig. 13.27 Lymphoplasmacytic lymphoma (LPL). Lymph node. **A** Classic LPL in a patient with Waldenström macroglobulinaemia. Note the widely patent sinuses and relatively monotonous lymphoplasmacytic infiltrate in the intersinus regions. **B** Typical relatively monotonous appearance of lymphocytes, plasmacytoid lymphocytes, and plasma cells adjacent to an open sinus. **C** A Dutcher body (arrow) is seen with H&E staining in this relatively plasma cell–rich case.

cryoglobulinaemia, or paraprotein deposition. Deposits of IgM may occur in the skin or the gastrointestinal tract, where they may cause diarrhoea. Coagulopathies may be caused by IgM binding to clotting factors, platelets, and fibrin. IgM paraproteins are not diagnostic of either LPL or WM, because they can also occur in patients with other lymphoid neoplasms or without an overt neoplasm. A minority of patients initially present with an IgM-related disorder such as cryoglobulinaemia or IgM monoclonal gammopathy of undetermined significance (see below) and only later develop an overt LPL {621,2173,2752}.

Microscopy

Bone marrow and peripheral blood

Bone marrow involvement is characterized by a nodular, diffuse, and/or interstitial infiltrate, sometimes even with paratrabecular aggregates. The infiltrate is usually composed predominantly of small lymphocytes admixed with variable numbers of plasma cells, plasmacytoid lymphocytes, and often increased mast cells {2347,3016,3017}. The plasma cells may also form distinct clusters separate from the lymphoid component {2347, 2736}. Residual disease after treatment may demonstrate virtually all plasma cells {2347,4157}. A similar spectrum of cells as are present in the bone marrow may be present in the peripheral blood, but the white blood cell count is typically lower than in chronic lymphocytic leukaemia.

Lymph nodes and other tissues

In the most classic cases, which are usually associated with WM, the lymph nodes show retention of normal architectural features with dilated sinuses with periodic acid-Schiff (PAS) positive material and sometimes small portions of re-sidual germinal centres. There is a relatively monotonous proliferation of small lymphocytes, plasma cells, and plasmacytoid lymphocytes, with relatively few transformed cells. Dutcher bodies (PAS-positive intranuclear pseudoinclusions), increased mast cells, and haemosiderin are also typical features. Other cases show greater architectural destruction and may have a vaguely follicular growth pattern, more prominent residual germinal centres (even with follicular colonization), epithelioid histiocyte clusters, sometimes a much greater proportion of plasma cells, and sometimes a paucity of frank plasma cells {3521,3851}. The presence of prominent large transformed cells should raise the possibility of either disease progression or a diagnosis other than LPL. Proliferation centres like those seen in chronic lymphocytic leukaemia / small lymphocytic lymphoma must be absent, and the presence of paler

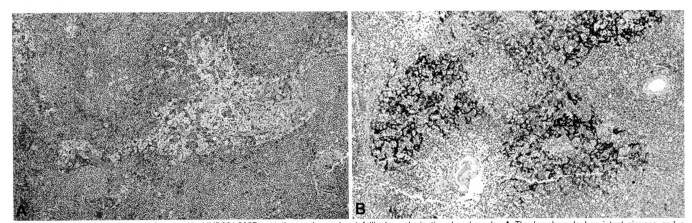

Fig. 13.28 Lymphoplasmacytic lymphoma with *MYD88* L265P mutation and prominent follicular colonization, lymph node. **A** The lymph node has intact sinuses and a monotonous lymphoplasmacytic proliferation with a somewhat follicular growth pattern. **B** CD21 immunohistochemical staining highlights the prominent infiltration of distorted follicular structures by the lymphoma.

appearing marginal zone–type differentiation should suggest a diagnosis of one of the MZLs. There may be associated amyloid, other immunoglobulin deposition, or crystal-storing histiocytes. The growth pattern in spleen is not well established, but there should be a lymphoplasmacytic infiltrate with diffuse and/or nodular red pulp involvement and sometimes white pulp nodules {1527,2343}.

Immunophenotype

Most cells express surface immunoglobulin, and the light chain–restricted plasmacytic cells express cytoplasmic immunoglobulin (usually IgM, sometimes IgG, and rarely IgA). LPLs are typically IgD-negative; express B-cell–associated antigens (CD19, CD20, CD22, and CD79a); and are most typically negative for CD5, CD10, CD103, and CD23, with frequent CD25 and CD38 expression. However, a minority of cases are positive for CD5 or CD10 (but BCL6-negative), and CD23 expression is not at all uncommon in some studies {2347,2736,3851}. The precise phenotype may also change over time {2347}. The plasma cells are CD138-positive; unlike in plasma cell myeloma, they are usually also positive for CD19 and often for CD45 {2736,3401}. The CD138+ plasma cells in LPL, although usually positive for IRF4/MUM1, are more likely to be IRF4/MUM1-negative and PAX5-positive compared with normal plasma cells or those in MZL {1502,2736, 3372}. These differences are not easily assessed in daily practice. In addition to the neoplastic plasma cells, polytypic plasma cells may also be present.

Postulated normal counterpart

A post-follicular B cell that differentiates into plasma cells

Genetic profile

Antigen receptor genes

IG genes are rearranged, usually with variable regions that show somatic hypermutation but lack ongoing mutations {4226}. There may be biased IGHV gene usage {1801,2114}. Clonal cytotoxic T-cell populations may be present, at least in the peripheral blood {2299}.

Cytogenetic abnormalities and oncogenes

No specific chromosomal abnormalities are recognized in LPL; however, >90% of cases have MYD88 L265P mutation,

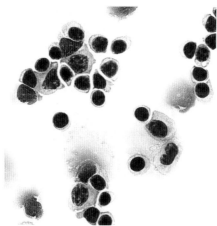

Fig. 13.29 Lymphoplasmacytic lymphoma with MYD88 L265P mutation involving cerebrospinal fluid (Bing–Neel syndrome). Cytology preparation of the cerebrospinal fluid shows a population of small lymphocytes, as well as small and larger plasmacytoid forms (Diff-Quik stain). The patient had an IgM monoclonal gammopathy with bone marrow involvement (Waldenström macroglobulinaemia).

and approximately 30% have truncating CXCR4 mutations (most frequently CXCR4 S338X or frameshift mutations) similar to those seen in the syndrome of warts, hypogammaglobulinaemia, immunodeficiency, and myelokathexis (WHIM syndrome) {1527,1735,3379,3567,3851, 4052,4057}. ARID1A mutations have been identified in 17% of patients, and less commonly, other somatic mutations, such as mutations of TP53, CD79B, KMT2D (previously designated MLL2), and MYBBP1A {1735}.

Documenting MYD88 L265P mutation may be helpful in cases in which LPL is in the differential diagnosis but there is some diagnostic uncertainty; however, some cases lack at least a demonstrable

mutation, and there is a small proportion of other small B-cell lymphomas in which it is present {3851}. MYD88 L265P mutation is also seen in some non-germinal centre subtype DLBCL, NOS, primary cutaneous DLBCL, leg type, and primary CNS and testicular DLBCL cases. Similarly, CXCR4 mutations are also present in a very small proportion of other small B-cell lymphomas. These mutations are important in the pathogenesis of LPL, at least in part by leading to NF-kappaB signalling, and for developing improved therapeutic strategies {548,549,3379}. The previously reported t(9;14)(p13.2;q32.33) translocation leading to IGH/PAX5 juxtaposition is rarely, if ever, found in LPL {792,1328,2489}. Deletion in 6q is reported in somewhat more than half of bone marrow–based cases, but it is not a specific finding and may be less frequent in tissue-based LPL {793,2489,2925,3582}. Small copy-number abnormalities leading to varied B-cell regulatory gene losses are also commonly found {1735}. Trisomies 3 and 18 are infrequent. Trisomy 4, present in about 20% of WM, is another finding that can be used to support the diagnosis {444,3941}. LPLs do not demonstrate the translocations associated with other B-cell lymphomas (e.g. those involving CCND1, MALT1, or BCL10), with the possible rare exception of BCL2 gene rearrangements. One study found that WM had a homogeneous gene expression profile, independent of 6q deletion, which is more similar to chronic lymphocytic leukaemia and normal B cells than to myeloma {727}. The study also suggested the importance of upregulated IL6 and its downstream MAPK signalling pathway.

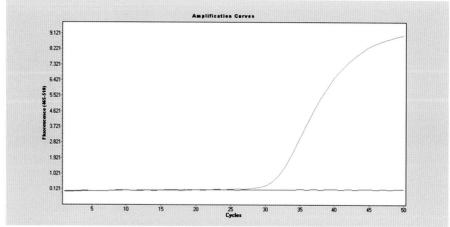

Fig. 13.30 Lymphoplasmacytic lymphoma (LPL). Real-time PCR with MYD88 L265P–specific primers shows positive amplification in a case of LPL (blue) and no amplification in a negative control cell line (red).

Genetic susceptibility

A familial predisposition may exist in as many as 20% of patients with WM {80, 4053,4054}. These patients are diagnosed at a younger age and with greater bone marrow involvement. There may also be prognostic and therapeutic implications {4054}.

Prognosis and predictive factors

The clinical course is typically indolent, with median survival times of 5–10 years, and with improved survival in more recent years {579,991,4195}. Advanced patient age, peripheral blood cytopenias (especially anaemia), poor performance status, and high beta-2 microglobulin levels have been reported to be associated with a worse prognosis {991,4195}. An international prognostic scoring system for WM has been proposed that also includes a high (> 7.0 g/dL) serum paraprotein level but not performance status {2726}. Cases with increased numbers of transformed cells/immunoblasts may also be associated with an adverse prognosis; however, a validated grading system does not exist {103,346}. Cases with del(6q) have been associated with adverse prognostic features {2925}. Cases lacking MYD88 L265P mutation are reported to have an adverse prognosis and a lower response to ibrutinib; however, the diagnosis in these cases may be less certain, and data are limited {4052,4055}. Although there are no documented survival differences, CXCR4-mutated LPL (in particular cases with nonsense mutations), has been associated with more-symptomatic/active disease, other clinical and laboratory findings, and greater resistance to ibrutinib and possibly other therapeutic agents {4051,4052,4055, 4056}. Transformation to diffuse large B-cell lymphoma occurs in a small proportion of cases and is associated with poor survival {2346}.

IgM monoclonal gammopathy of undetermined significance

Cook J.R.
Swerdlow S.H.
Sohani A.R.
Pileri S.A.
Harris N.L.
Jaffe E.S.
Stein H.

Definition

IgM monoclonal gammopathy of undetermined significance (MGUS) is defined by a serum IgM paraprotein concentration <30 g/L; bone marrow lymphoplasmacytic infiltration of < 10%; and no evidence of anaemia, constitutional symptoms, hyperviscosity, lymphadenopathy, hepatosplenomegaly, or other end-organ damage that can be attributed to the underlying lymphoproliferative disorder {3290}. IgM MGUS is a precursor condition that may progress to overt lymphoma or primary amyloidosis.

ICD-O code   9761/1

Epidemiology

MGUS of any isotype is reported in approximately 3% of individuals aged ≥50 years; of these cases, approximately 15% are of IgM type, yielding a prevalence of approximately 0.5% {1004,1085, 2175}. The proportion of MGUS due to IgM is higher among White populations than among Black or Asian populations {2215}. The median patient age at diagnosis is 74 years, and there is a male predominance, with a male-to-female ratio of 1.4:1 {2177}.

Localization

There may be bone marrow infiltration by an IgM+ clonal lymphoplasmacytic population, but it must be < 10%. Cases with any degree of bone marrow infiltration are considered by some pathologists to constitute asymptomatic Waldenström macroglobulinaemia (WM), lymphoplasmacytic lymphoma (LPL).

Clinical features

Patients with IgM MGUS lack the signs and symptoms of an overt lymphoproliferative disorder or plasma cell neoplasm, and the paraprotein is typically discovered incidentally on serum protein electrophoresis. Reduced polyclonal

Table 13.03 Diagnostic criteria for IgM monoclonal gammopathy of undetermined significance; adapted from the International Myeloma Working Group (IMWG) updated criteria for the diagnosis of multiple myeloma From: Rajkumar SV, et al. {3290}.

- Serum IgM monoclonal protein concentration < 30 g/L
- Bone marrow lymphoplasmacytic infiltration of < 10%
- No evidence of anaemia, constitutional symptoms, hyperviscosity, lymphadenopathy, hepatosplenomegaly, or other end-organ damage that can be attributed to the underlying lymphoproliferative disorder

immunoglobulins are reported in 35% of cases, and Bence Jones proteinuria has been reported in approximately 20% {2162,2751}. The term IgM-related disorder has been proposed for cases in patients who have no evidence of an overt lymphoma or plasma cell neoplasm but have symptoms related to the IgM paraprotein, such as anti-myelin-associated glycoprotein–mediated peripheral neuropathy, cold agglutinin disease, or cryoglobulinaemia {3017}.

Microscopy

By definition, IgM MGUS lacks findings diagnostic of LPL, another lymphoproliferative disorder, or plasma cell neoplasm. Distinguishing IgM MGUS from LPL and other lymphomas requires examination of a bone marrow biopsy {3017}. The marrow contains clonal lymphoplasmacytic cells; however, they must not represent an infiltrate of ≥10%. In addition, sometimes the clonal cells are not easily identified in the background of normal polytypic plasma cells.

Immunophenotype

On sensitive multiparameter flow cytometry, clonal B cells are reported in as many as 75% of IgM MGUS bone marrows, although complex gating strategies

may be required to identify the clonal population within the background of benign polytypic B cells {2924,3032,3034}. When present, the clonal B-cell population shows a non-specific phenotype similar to that of LPL (CD19+, CD20+, CD5−, CD10−, and CD103−). The plasma cells in IgM MGUS lack expression of CD56 {3034}.

Postulated normal counterpart

B cells with somatic hypermutation of the IGHV genes but without class switching {2177}

Genetic profile

The gene expression profile of IgM MGUS is similar to that of LPL {3032}. Approximately half of IgM MGUS cases are positive for the *MYD88* L265P mutation {1861,2214,4155,4393}, and 20% have been reported to have *CXCR4* S338X mutations {3379}, but further genetic data are limited. Deletions of chromosome 6q have been reported, but are non-specific and appear to be less frequent than in LPL and WM {3032,3582}.

Prognosis and predictive factors

IgM MGUS progresses to LPL/WM, other B-cell neoplasms, or primary amyloidosis at a rate of 1.5% per year. Progression to plasma cell myeloma occurs rarely, if at all. The rate of progression in patients with symptomatic IgM-related disorders appears similar to that in patients without monoclonal protein–related symptoms {2751}. Patients remain at risk for progression even after having stable disease for 20 years {2177}. A detectable *MYD88* L265P mutation and higher levels of serum monoclonal protein are independent risk factors for progression {239,4116,4155,4156}. In one study, the risk of progression doubled for every increase of 7 g/L in serum monoclonal protein {239}.

Heavy chain diseases

Cook J.R.
Harris N.L.
Isaacson P.G.
Jaffe E.S.

Definition

The heavy chain diseases (HCDs) are three rare B-cell neoplasms characterized by the production of monoclonal immunoglobulin heavy chains (IgG in gamma HCD, IgA in alpha HCD, and IgM in mu HCD) and typically no light chains {370,4230}. The heavy chain is usually truncated, preventing normal assembly with light chains. Variably sized proteins are produced, which may not yield a characteristic monoclonal peak by routine serum protein electrophoresis, and require immunoelectrophoresis or immunofixation to detect.

In some cases, HCD can show morphological features consistent with another well-defined histological entity. Some cases of gamma HCD resemble typical examples of splenic marginal zone lymphoma or extranodal marginal zone lymphoma of mucosa-associated lymphoid tissue (MALT lymphoma) {371}, whereas mu HCD typically resembles chronic lymphocytic leukaemia, and alpha HCD is considered a variant of MALT lymphoma {370,4230}. However, each of these HCDs is sufficiently distinct to be considered a separate entity. Establishing the diagnosis of an HCD requires demonstration of free heavy chains by protein electrophoresis/immunofixation.

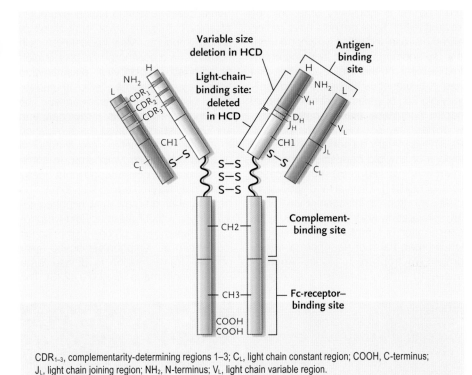

CDR$_{1-3}$, complementarity-determining regions 1–3; C$_L$, light chain constant region; COOH, C-terminus; J$_L$, light chain joining region; NH$_2$, N-terminus; V$_L$, light chain variable region.

Fig. 13.31 Structure of the immunoglobulin molecule in heavy chain disease. An immunoglobulin molecule is composed of two heavy chains (H) and two light chains (L), which are joined by disulfide bonds (S–S). The normal heavy chain constant region has three constant domains: CH1 is responsible for binding to the light chain, CH2 for binding to complement, and CH3 for binding to Fc receptors. In the absence of an associated light chain, the CH1 domain binds to HSP78 and undergoes proteasomal degradation; thus, normal free heavy chains are not secreted. In heavy chain diseases, non-contiguous deletions in the CH1 domain prevent both binding of the heavy chain to the light chain and degradation in the proteasome, and free heavy chains are secreted. Variably sized deletions also occur in the heavy chain diversity region (D$_H$), the heavy chain joining region (J$_H$), and the heavy chain variable region (V$_H$). Reprinted with permission from Munshi NC et al. {2785}.

Mu heavy chain disease

Definition

Mu heavy chain disease (HCD) is a B-cell neoplasm resembling chronic lymphocytic leukaemia (CLL), in which a defective mu heavy chain lacking a variable region is produced. The bone marrow contains an infiltrate of characteristic vacuolated plasma cells, admixed with small, round lymphocytes.

ICD-O code   9762/3

Epidemiology

This is an extremely rare disease of adults, with only 30–40 cases reported, a median patient age of 60 years, and an approximately equal frequency in males and females {370,4230}.

Localization

The spleen, liver, bone marrow, and peripheral blood may be involved; peripheral lymphadenopathy is usually absent.

Clinical features

Most patients present with a slowly progressive disease resembling CLL. Mu HCD differs from most cases of CLL in the high frequency of hepatosplenomegaly and the absence of peripheral lymphadenopathy. Routine serum protein electrophoresis is frequently normal. Immunoelectrophoresis reveals reactivity to anti-mu in polymers of diverse sizes. Although mu chain is not found in the urine, Bence Jones light chains (particularly kappa chains) are common (found in the urine in 50% of cases). Light chains, although still produced in mu HCD, are not assembled into a complete immunoglobulin protein, due to IGH gene aberrancies leading to truncated forms {242, 4229,4230}.

Microscopy

The bone marrow contains vacuolated plasma cells, which are typically admixed with small, round lymphocytes similar to CLL cells.

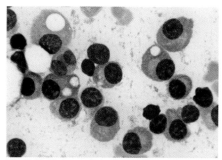
Fig. 13.32 Mu heavy chain disease. Bone marrow aspirate shows predominantly plasma cells with prominent cytoplasmic vacuolation.

Immunophenotype
The cells contain monoclonal cytoplasmic mu heavy chain (with or without monotypic light chain), express B-cell antigens, and are usually negative for CD5 and CD10.

Postulated normal counterpart
A post–germinal centre B cell that can differentiate into a plasma cell, with an abnormal IGHM gene

Genetic profile
Immunoglobulin genes are clonally rearranged and contain high levels of somatic hypermutation {370,4230}. Deletions in the IGHM gene are present that result in expression of a defective heavy chain protein that cannot bind light chain to form a complete immunoglobulin molecule. These deletions involve IGHV and variable proportions of the CH1 domain, and there may be insertions of large amounts of DNA of unknown origin {1244, 4230}.

Prognosis and predictive factors
The clinical course is slowly progressive in most cases {242,1244,4229,4230}.

Gamma heavy chain disease

Definition
Gamma heavy chain disease (HCD) is a small B-cell neoplasm with plasmacytic differentiation that produces a truncated immunoglobulin gamma heavy chain that lacks light chain–binding sites and therefore cannot form a complete immunoglobulin molecule.

ICD-O code   9762/3

Synonym
Franklin disease

Epidemiology
This is a rare disease of adults, with a median patient age of 60 years; approximately 150 cases have been described. There is no particular geographical distribution, and recent series report a female predominance {371,4231}.

Localization
The tumour may involve the lymph nodes, Waldeyer ring, gastrointestinal tract and other extranodal sites, bone marrow, liver, spleen, and peripheral blood.

Clinical features
Most patients have systemic symptoms such as anorexia, weakness, fever, weight loss, and recurrent bacterial infections. Autoimmune manifestations are reported in 25–70% of cases, most frequently rheumatoid arthritis and systemic lupus erythematosus, but also autoimmune haemolytic anaemia, thrombocytopenia, or both; vasculitis; Sjögren syndrome; myasthenia gravis; and thyroiditis {371, 1739,4231}. Autoimmune disease may precede the diagnosis of lymphoma by several years. Most patients have generalized disease, including lymphadenopathy, splenomegaly, and hepatomegaly. Involvement of the Waldeyer ring, skin and subcutaneous tissues, thyroid, salivary glands, or gastrointestinal tract may occur. Circulating plasma cells or lymphocytes may occasionally be present. Patients generally do not have lytic bone lesions or amyloid deposition. The bone marrow is involved in 30–60% of cases {371,1739,4231}. Clinical and laboratory distinction from an infection or inflammatory process may be difficult given the constellation of symptoms and the sometimes broad band or near-normal serum protein electrophoresis results. Approximately 10–20% of patients have no overt

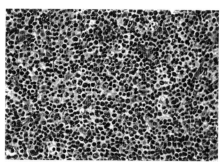
Fig. 13.34 Gamma heavy chain disease. This case displays a diffuse proliferation of small lymphocytes, plasmacytoid cells, plasma cells, and scattered large transformed cells.

lymphadenopathy or other mass lesions; most of these patients have autoimmune disorders.

The diagnosis is made by demonstration of IgG without light chains by immunofixation in the peripheral blood, the urine, or both.

Microscopy
The morphological findings in gamma HCD are heterogeneous {371,2785,4231}. Some cases resemble typical examples of splenic marginal zone lymphoma or MALT lymphoma. Most frequently, lymph nodes show a polymorphous proliferation of admixed lymphocytes, plasmacytoid lymphocytes, plasma cells, immunoblasts, histiocytes, and eosinophils. The presence of eosinophils, histiocytes, and immunoblasts may cause a resemblance to angioimmunoblastic T-cell lymphoma or classic Hodgkin lymphoma. In some cases, plasma cells predominate; these cases may resemble plasmacytoma. The peripheral blood may show lymphocytosis with or without plasmacytoid lymphocytes, resembling chronic lymphocytic leukaemia or lymphoplasmacytic lymphoma. Transformation to diffuse large B-cell lymphoma is rare {370,4230}. The

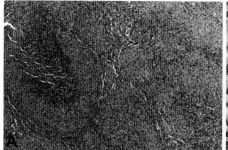 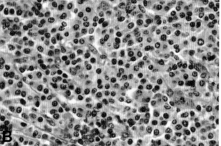
Fig. 13.33 Gamma heavy chain disease. This case presented with splenomegaly. The white pulp contains a nodular proliferation (A) of small lymphocytes with abundant pale cytoplasm (B), morphologically suggestive of a splenic marginal zone lymphoma. The diagnosis of gamma heavy chain disease was established by serum immunofixation studies and the finding of gamma heavy chain–expressing plasma cells that lacked kappa and lambda staining.

bone marrow may show lymphoplasma-cytic aggregates or only a subtle increase in plasma cells with monotypic gamma heavy chains without light chains.

Immunophenotype

The cells express CD79a and cytoplasmic gamma chain and are negative for CD5 and CD10. CD20 is found on the lymphocytic component and CD138 on the plasma cell component. Kappa and lambda light chains are typically not expressed, but a minority of cases show staining for monotypic light chains by immunohisto-chemistry or in situ hybridization, despite the absence of light chains on immuno-fixation studies {370,371,4230}.

Postulated normal counterpart

A post–germinal centre B cell that can differentiate into a plasma cell, with a defective IGHG gene

Genetic profile

IG genes are clonally rearranged and contain high levels of somatic hypermu-tation. Deletions in the IGHG gene are present that result in expression of an abnormally truncated heavy chain pro-tein that cannot bind light chain to form a complete immunoglobulin molecule. These deletions involve IGHV and vari-able proportions of the CH1 domain, and there may be insertions of large amounts of DNA of unknown origin {57,370,1132, 1243,1249,4230}.

Abnormal karyotypes have been found in about half of the reported cases, but no specific or recurrent genetic abnor-mality has been reported {371,4231}. The MYD88 L265P mutation that is character-

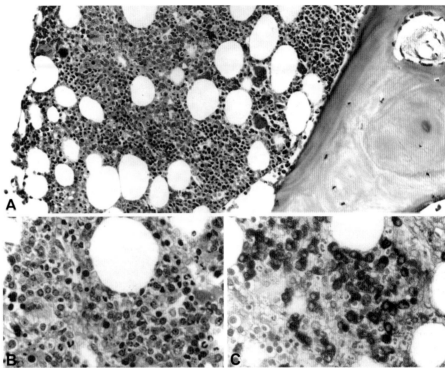

Fig. 13.35 Gamma heavy chain disease. Bone marrow biopsy. A Small aggregates composed of plasma cells and lymphoid cells are present, constituting approximately 5% of the overall marrow cellularity. B Some plasma cells appear mature; others are atypical, with open chromatin. C Immunohistochemical staining shows cIgG. Images from Munshi NC et al. {2785}.

istic of lymphoplasmacytic lymphoma is absent in gamma HCD {1526}.

Prognosis and predictive factors

The clinical course is highly variable, ranging from indolent to rapidly progres-sive. One study of 23 cases reported a median survival time of 7.4 years, with more than half of the deaths unrelated to the lymphoproliferative disorder {4231}. There is no standardized therapy. Most patients with low-grade–appearing lym-

phoplasmacytic infiltrates appear to re-spond to non–anthracycline-containing chemotherapy, and responses to rituxi-mab and other single agents have also been reported {370,4230}.

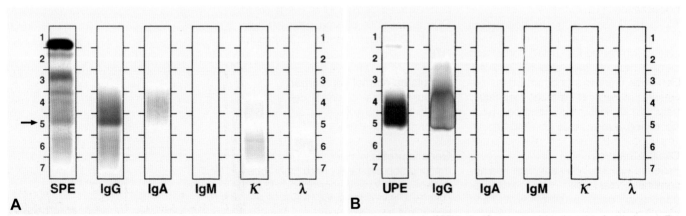

Fig. 13.36 Gamma heavy chain disease. A A distinct band was identified by serum protein electrophoresis (SPE) in the IG region anodal to the point of origin (arrow). The M protein (also called M component) typed as IgG (denoted by the band seen in the IgG lane), but without a corresponding light chain (only faint polyclonal patterns were seen in the kappa and lambda lanes). B Urine protein electrophoresis (UPE) revealed similar results, with a broad monoclonal band corresponding to IgG without a corresponding light chain. Reprinted from Munshi NC et al. {2785}.

Alpha heavy chain disease

Definition
Alpha heavy chain disease (HCD), also known as immunoproliferative small intestinal disease, is a variant of extranodal marginal zone lymphoma of mucosa-associated lymphoid tissue (MALT lymphoma) in which defective immunoglobulin alpha heavy chains are secreted {48, 4230}.

ICD-O code   9762/3

Synonyms
Mediterranean lymphoma; immunoproliferative small intestinal disease

Epidemiology
Alpha HCD is the most common of the HCDs. Unlike the other HCDs, alpha HCD involves a young age group, with a peak incidence rate in the second and third decades; it is rare in young children and older adults, and there is an equal incidence in males and females. It is most common in areas bordering the Mediterranean Sea, including northern Africa, Israel and Saudi Arabia. It is associated with factors linked to low socioeconomic status, including poor hygiene, malnutrition, and frequent intestinal infections {48,3298,3617,4230}.

Etiology
Chronic intestinal infection, in some cases with *Campylobacter jejuni*, is believed to result in chronic inflammation, a setting in which neoplastic transformation of a clone of abnormal B cells develops {2248,3072}.

Localization
Alpha HCD involves the gastrointestinal tract (mainly the small intestine) and mesenteric lymph nodes. The gastric and colonic mucosa may also be involved. The bone marrow and other organs are usually not involved, although respiratory tract and thyroid involvement has been described in rare cases {3617,4040}.

Clinical features
Patients typically present with malabsorption, diarrhoea, hypocalcaemia, abdominal pain, wasting, fever, and steatorrhoea. Typically, serum protein electrophoresis is normal, and identification of the abnormal alpha heavy chain requires immunofixation, immunoelectro-

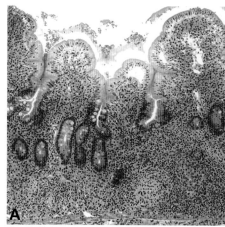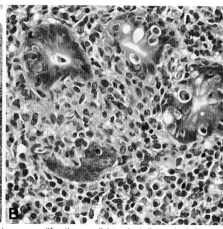

Fig. 13.37 Alpha heavy chain disease (also known as immunoproliferative small intestinal disease). **A** Partially colonized reactive follicle centre is present just above the muscularis mucosae at the right. Clusters of pale-staining marginal zone cells are present adjacent to the follicle and elsewhere in the biopsy. The lamina propria and small intestinal villi are expanded by plasma cells. **B** A lymphoepithelial lesion in a case of alpha heavy chain disease showing destruction of intestinal crypts by marginal zone cells, with surrounding plasma cells.

phoresis, or immunoselection techniques {370,4230}.

Microscopy
The lamina propria of the bowel is heavily infiltrated with plasma cells and admixed small lymphocytes; marginal zone B cells may be present, with formation of lymphoepithelial lesions. The lymphoplasmacytic infiltrate separates the crypts, and villous atrophy may be present {1781, 3239,3298}. Sheets of large plasmacytoid cells and immunoblasts that form solid, destructive aggregates with ulceration characterize progression to diffuse large B-cell lymphoma {370,4230}.

Immunophenotype
The plasma cells and marginal zone cells express monoclonal cytoplasmic alpha chain without light chains. Marginal zone cells express CD20 and are negative for CD5 and CD10; plasma cells are typically CD20-negative and CD138-positive {1781}.

Postulated normal counterpart
A post–germinal centre B cell that can differentiate into a plasma cell, with an abnormal IGHA gene

Genetic profile
Immunoglobulin heavy and light chain genes are clonally rearranged {3710}. Deletions in the IGHA gene are present that result in expression of a defective heavy chain protein that cannot bind light chain to form a complete immunoglobulin molecule. These deletions involve IGHV

and the CH1 domain, and there may be insertions of DNA of unknown origin {48, 4230}. Cytogenetic abnormalities have been reported in rare single cases. The t(11;18)(q21;q21) (*BIRC3-MALT1*) translocation associated with gastric and pulmonary MALT lymphomas has not been described {4421}.

Prognosis and predictive factors
In the early phase, alpha HCD may completely remit with antibiotic therapy. In patients with more advanced disease, multiagent chemotherapy is typically required. Treatment with anthracycline-containing regimens has been reported to result in remission and long-term survival in 67% of patients {48,3295,4230}.

Plasma cell neoplasms

McKenna R.W.
Kyle R.A.
Kuehl W.M.
Harris N.L.
Coupland R.W.
Fend F.

Plasma cell neoplasms result from expansion of a clone of immunoglobulin-secreting, heavy chain class-switched, terminally differentiated B cells that typically secrete a single homogeneous monoclonal immunoglobulin called an M protein; the presence of such a protein is called monoclonal gammopathy. The plasma cell neoplasms discussed in this section include plasma cell myeloma, plasmacytoma, disorders defined by tissue immunoglobulin deposition (primary amyloidosis and light and heavy chain deposition diseases), and clonal plasma cell proliferations with an associated paraneoplastic syndrome (POEMS syndrome and TEMPI syndrome) (see Table 13.04). Non-IgM monoclonal gammopathy of undetermined significance, a precursor lesion with the potential to evolve to a malignant plasma cell neoplasm, is also included. Other immunoglobulin-secreting disorders that consist of both clonal lymphocytes and plasma cells, including lymphoplasmacytic lymphoma, the heavy chain diseases, and IgM monoclonal gammopathy of undetermined significance, are discussed in other sections.

Non-IgM monoclonal gammopathy of undetermined significance

Definition

There are two major types of monoclonal gammopathy of undetermined significance (MGUS): plasma cell and lymphoid/lymphoplasmacytic, which have different genetic bases and different outcomes in terms of malignant progression. Plasma cell MGUS and lymphoid/lymphoplasmacytic MGUS can usually be distinguished by morphology, but this analysis is not always precise. Instead, MGUS is classified as IgM MGUS, which is mostly lymphoid/lymphoplasmacytic, or non-IgM MGUS, which is mostly plasma cell, although about 1% of plasma cell MGUS cases actually produce an IgM M protein. Features of IgM MGUS

Table 13.04 Plasma cell neoplasms

Non-IgM (plasma cell) monoclonal gammopathy of undetermined significance (precursor lesion)
Plasma cell myeloma
Clinical variants:
Smouldering (asymptomatic) plasma cell myeloma
Non-secretory myeloma
Plasma cell Leukemia
Plasmacytoma
Solitary plasmacytoma of bone
Extraosseous (extramedullary) plasmacytoma
Monoclonal immunoglobulin deposition diseases
Primary amyloidosis
Systemic light and heavy chain deposition diseases
Plasma cell neoplasms with associated paraneoplastic syndrome
POEMS syndrome
TEMPI syndrome (provisional)

are detailed in the section on lymphoplasmacytic lymphoma and will not be discussed further in this section.

Non-IgM (plasma cell) MGUS is defined as the presence in the serum of an IgG, IgA, or (rarely) IgD M protein at a concentration <30 g/L; clonal bone marrow plasma cells <10%; and absence of end-organ damage such as hypercalcaemia, renal insufficiency, anaemia, and bone lesions (CRAB) and amyloidosis attributable to the plasma cell proliferative disorder (Table 13.05) {3290}. The risk of progression to plasma cell myeloma, light-chain amyloidosis, or a related disorder is 1% per year. Light-chain MGUS consists only of monoclonal light chains. It is defined by an abnormal free light chain ratio and an increase of involved light chain with complete loss of heavy chain expression. The urinary light chain excretion must be <0.5 g/24 hour. The plasma cell content is <10%, and there is no end-organ damage attributable to the plasma cell disorder {1004,2167}. The rate of progression of light-chain MGUS is approximately 0.3% per year (Table 13.06). Although the M protein reflects the presence of an expanded clone of immunoglobulin-secreting plasma cells, non-IgM MGUS is considered a premalignant neoplasm, which in most cases does not progress to overt malignancy.

ICD-O code   9765/1

Synonym

Monoclonal gammopathy, NOS

Epidemiology

MGUS is uncommon in patients aged <40 years but is found in approximately 3–4% of individuals aged >50 years and in >5% of individuals aged >70 years; 80–85% of cases are non-IgM MGUS {2175, 2176}. Approximately 60% of patients with non-IgM MGUS are men, and it is nearly twice as frequent in Black populations as in White populations {2171, 2210,2211,3685}.

Etiology

No cause of MGUS has been identified, but there is an increased prevalence in families with members with a lymphoid or plasma cell proliferative disorder {1441, 2212}. Transient oligoclonal and monoclonal gammopathies may occur in solid organ and bone marrow / stem cell transplant recipients {2171,2679,3330}.

Localization

The clonal plasma cells producing non-IgM MGUS are in the bone marrow.

Clinical features

Patients exhibit no symptoms or physical findings related to non-IgM MGUS, and the typical laboratory and radiographical abnormalities associated with plasma cell myeloma are lacking. The M protein is often identified in the course

Table 13.05 Diagnostic criteria for non-IgM monoclonal gammopathy of undetermined significance (MGUS) and light-chain MGUS. Adapted from the International Myeloma Working Group (IMWG) updated criteria for the diagnosis of multiple myeloma. From: Rajkumar SV et al. {3290}.

Non-IgM MGUS:	Serum M protein (non-IgM) concentration < 30 g/L Clonal bone marrow plasma cells < 10% Absence of end-organ damage; e.g. hypercalcaemia, renal insufficiency, anaemia, and bone lesions (CRAB) and amyloidosis attributable to the plasma cell proliferative disorder
Light-chain MGUS:	Abnormal free light chain ratio (< 0.26 or > 1.65) Increased level of the involved free light chain No abnormal immunoglobulin heavy chain expression on immunofixation electrophoresis Urinary M protein < 500 mg/24 hours Clonal plasma cells < 10% Absence of end-organ damage (CRAB) and amyloidosis

Table 13.06 Diagnostic criteria for monoclonal plasma cell proliferative disorders with complete loss of immunoglobulin heavy chain (HC) expression, i.e. with light chain (LC) expression only. Adapted from Kyle RA et al. {2167}

Feature	Plasma cell disorder		
	LC-MGUS	**LC-SPCM**	**LC-PCM**
M protein concentration	Abnormal FLC ratio and increase of involved LC with absence of abnormal HC expression in serum; urinary LC M protein < 0.5 g/24 hours	Urinary LC M protein ≥ 0.5 g/24 hours	Presence of LC-only M protein (usually in urine but can sometimes be seen in serum)
Percentage of plasma cells in bone marrow[a]	< 10%	≥ 10%	≥ 10% or biopsy-proven plasmacytoma
End-organ damage attributable to the plasma cell disorder	Absent	Absent	Present
Annual rate of progression	0.3%	First 5 years: 5% Next 5 years: 3% Following 5 years: 2%	n/a

FLC, free light chain; LC-MGUS, light-chain monoclonal gammopathy of undetermined significance; LC-PCM, light-chain plasma cell myeloma; LC-SPCM, light-chain smouldering plasma cell myeloma; n/a, not applicable.

[a] For the diagnosis of LC-MGUS, both M protein and bone marrow plasma cell percentage criteria must be fulfilled; in contrast, the diagnosis of LC-SPCM requires only that at least one of these two criteria is fulfilled.

of evaluation for another disorder, but there is no specific association with any particular disease {2171}. The M proteins are usually discovered unexpectedly on serum protein electrophoresis. Approximately 60% are IgG, 15% IgA, 1% IgD, 1% IgE, and 3% biclonal {2171}. About 20% of non-IgM MGUS consists only of an immunoglobulin light chain, which can be detected with the serum free light chain assay {1004,1969,2476,3290}. Reduction of uninvolved immunoglobulin is found in 30–40% of patients with non-IgM MGUS, and monoclonal light chain in urine in nearly one third {2171,2176, 3330}.

Microscopy
Marrow aspirates contain a median of 3% plasma cells, and trephine biopsies show no or only a minimal increase in plasma cells, which are interstitial and evenly scattered throughout the bone marrow or occasionally in small clusters {1762,3330}. They are usually mature-appearing, but mild changes, including cytoplasmic inclusions and nucleoli, are occasionally observed.

Immunophenotype
Immunohistochemical staining for CD138 facilitates enumeration of plasma cells on bone marrow biopsy sections. The detection of plasma cells that express monotypic cytoplasmic light chain of the same isotype as the M protein is often problematic, because the clone may be small and may occur in a background of normal polytypic plasma cells. In some non-IgM MGUSs, the kappa/

lambda ratio is within the normal reference range; in others, it is skewed (but less so than in myeloma) {2450,3147}. Flow cytometry frequently shows two populations of plasma cells: a polyclonal population with a normal immunophenotype (CD38bright, CD19+, CD56−) and a monoclonal population with an aberrant phenotype (most often either CD19−/CD56+ or CD19−/CD56−) {2974,3138}. The monoclonal population may exhibit weaker expression of CD38 than normal, along with other aberrant antigen expression {2926,2974,3138}. Residual normal polyclonal bone marrow plasma cells are a consistent finding by flow cytometry in non-IgM MGUS, whereas they are absent or present in only very low numbers in myeloma {2926,2974}.

Cell of origin
Non-IgM (plasma cell) MGUS is produced by post–germinal centre plasma cells with IG genes that have somatic hypermutation of the variable regions and are class-switched.

Genetic profile
Abnormal karyotypes are rarely found in non-IgM MGUS, but FISH identifies numerical and/or structural abnormalities in most cases {202, 728,1230,1231}. The abnormalities are the same as those found in myeloma, although the prevalence may differ. Translocations involving the IGH locus (14q32) are found in nearly half of non-IgM MGUSs, with various studies showing t(11;14)(q13;q32) (IGH/CCND1) in 15–25%, t(4;14)(p16.3;q32) (IGH/NSD2, also called IGH/MMSET) in 2–9%, and t(14;16)(q32;q23) (IGH/MAF) in 1–5% {202,1230}. Hyperdiploidy is observed in about 40% of non-IgM MGUSs, with chromosomal trisomies similar to those in myeloma {728}. Deletions of 13q are present in about 35–40% of non-IgM MGUSs, versus about 50% of myelomas {1230,1231,1970,2179}. Activating NRAS mutations are much less frequent in MGUS (present in ~7%) compared with myeloma (~15–20%), whereas activating KRAS mutations have not been detected in MGUS but are present in about 15–20% of myelomas {2128,3312}. No obvious clinical correlations are associated with chromosome abnormalities, but this may reflect a lack of sufficient data {1230}. Although genetic alterations and gene expression patterns can probably distinguish advanced myeloma from

MGUS, there are no unequivocal intrinsic differences that distinguish the two.

Prognosis and predictive factors

In most cases, the clinical course of MGUS is stable, with no increase in M protein or other evidence of progression, but in a substantial minority, there is evolution to an active plasma cell myeloma, solitary plasmacytoma, or amyloidosis {1762, 2171}. The risk of progression is about 1% per year (0.3% for light-chain MGUS) and indefinite, persisting even after 30 years {2171,2176}. The size and type of M protein and serum free light chain ratio are significant prognostic indicators {1762, 2172,2176,3080,4078}. The risk of progression for patients with an M protein concentration of 25 g/L is > 4 times that of patients with a concentration < 5 g/L. Patients with IgA MGUS are at greater risk of progression (~1.5% per year) to a malignant disorder than are patients with IgG or light-chain MGUS {2171}. Patients with IgG or IgA MGUS with an abnormal serum free light chain ratio at diagnosis are at higher risk of progression than are patients with a normal ratio {2171,3292}. Individuals with marked predominance of aberrant plasma cells (> 90%) on flow cytometry have a significantly higher risk of progression to myeloma {2974,3138}. DNA aneuploidy and subnormal levels of polyclonal immunoglobulin appear to be additional clinical risk factors {3138}. An evolving clinical phenotype also predicts an increased probability of progression to myeloma {3137}. Several risk stratification models identify subgroups of cases of non-IgM MGUS that progress to myeloma at rates ranging from approximately 0.3% to 12% per year {2167,3137,3138, 3292,4496}.

Plasma cell myeloma

Definition

Plasma cell myeloma (PCM) is a bone marrow–based, multifocal neoplastic proliferation of plasma cells, usually associated with an M protein in serum and/or urine and evidence of organ damage related to the plasma cell neoplasm. Bone marrow is the site of origin of nearly all PCMs, and in most cases there is disseminated bone marrow involvement. Other organs may be secondarily involved. The disease spans a clinical spectrum from asymptomatic to highly aggressive. Diagnosis is

Table 13.07 Diagnostic criteria for plasma cell myeloma (PCM) and smouldering (asymptomatic) PCM. Adapted from the International Myeloma Working Group (IMWG) updated criteria for the diagnosis of multiple myeloma {3290}

PCM
Clonal bone marrow plasma cell percentage ≥ 10% or biopsy-proven plasmacytoma and ≥ 1 of the following myeloma-defining events:

  End-organ damage attributable to the plasma cell proliferative disorder:
    - Hypercalcaemia: serum calcium > 0.25 mmol/L (> 1 mg/dL) higher than the upper limit of normal or > 2.75 mmol/L (> 11 mg/dL)
    - Renal insufficiency:
      creatinine clearance < 40 mL/minute or serum creatinine > 177 µmol/L (> 2 mg/dL)
    - Anaemia: a haemoglobin value of > 20 g/L below the lower limit of normal or a haemoglobin value < 100 g/L
    - Bone lesions: ≥ 1 osteolytic lesion on skeletal radiography, CT, or PET/CT

  ≥ 1 of the following biomarkers of malignancy:
    - Clonal bone marrow plasma cell percentage ≥ 60%
    - An involved-to-uninvolved serum free light chain ratio ≥ 100
    - > 1 focal lesion on MRI

Smouldering (asymptomatic) PCM
Both criteria must be met:

    - Serum M protein (IgG and/or IgA) ≥ 30 g/L and/or urinary M protein ≥ 500 mg/24 hours and/or clonal bone marrow plasma cell percentage of 10–60%
    - Absence of myeloma-defining events or amyloidosis

based on a combination of clinical, morphological, immunological, and radiological features. The diagnostic criteria for PCM are listed in Table 13.07.

ICD-O code   9732/3

Synonyms

Multiple myeloma; medullary plasmacytoma; myelomatosis; Kahler disease (no longer used); myeloma, NOS

Epidemiology

PCM accounts for about 1% of malignant tumours, 10–15% of haematopoietic neoplasms, and 20% of deaths from haematological malignancies {1851, 2164,3357}. In the USA in 2015, an estimated 26 000 cases were diagnosed and > 11 000 patients died of PCM {3673}. PCM is more common in men than in women, with a male-to-female ratio of 1.1:1. It is nearly twice as frequent in Black populations as in White populations {2164,3357,3673}. PCM is almost never found in children and very infrequently in adults aged < 30 years {840, 390}; the incidence increases progressively with patient age thereafter, with about 90% of cases occurring in patients aged > 50 years (median patient age at diagnosis: ~70 years).

Etiology

Chronic antigenic stimulation from infection or other chronic disease and exposure to specific toxic substances or radiation has been associated with an increased incidence of PCM {2292,2353}. An antigenic stimulus giving rise to multiple benign clones could be followed by a mutagenic event initiating malignant transformation {1522}. Most patients have

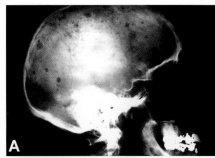

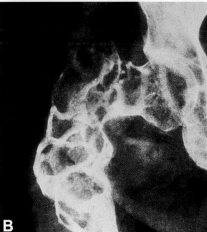

Fig. 13.38 Plasma cell myeloma. Radiographs of skull (**A**) and femoral head (**B**) demonstrate multiple lytic bone lesions.

no identifiable toxic exposure or known chronic antigenic stimulation {2353}. Almost all PCMs arise in patients with a precursor monoclonal gammopathy of undetermined significance (MGUS) {2213,4284}.

Localization

Generalized or multifocal bone marrow involvement is typically present. Lytic bone lesions and focal tumoural masses of plasma cells also occur, most commonly in sites of active haematopoiesis. Extramedullary involvement is usually a manifestation of advanced disease.

Clinical features

In most patients, there is clinical evidence of PCM-related end-organ damage in the form of one or more of the following: hypercalcaemia, renal insufficiency, anaemia, and bone lesions (CRAB). Renal failure occurs due to tubular damage resulting from monoclonal light chain proteinuria, and anaemia results from bone marrow replacement and renal damage. Bone pain and hypercalcaemia result from PCM-induced lytic lesions and osteoporosis {2164}. Other presenting findings may include infections (partly a consequence of depressed normal immunoglobulin [Ig] production), bleeding, and occasionally neurological manifestations due to spinal cord compression or peripheral neuropathy {1762,2164, 3348}. Physical findings are often absent or non-specific. Pallor is most common. Mass disease or organomegaly due to extramedullary plasmacytomas or amyloidosis is found in approximately 10% of patients. Skin lesions resulting from plasma cell infiltrates and purpura are observed rarely {2164}.

An M protein is found in the serum or urine in about 97% of cases: IgG in 50% of these cases; IgA in 20%; light chain in 20%; and IgD, IgE, IgM, or biclonal in < 10%. About 3% of cases are non-secretory {1762,2164}. The serum M protein is usually > 30 g/L of IgG and > 20 g/L of IgA. In 90% of patients, there is a decrease in polyclonal Ig (< 50% of normal). Other laboratory findings include hypercalcaemia (found in up to 10% of cases), elevated creatinine (in 20–30%), hyperuricaemia (in > 50%), and hypoalbuminaemia (in ~15%) {1456,2164}.

Imaging

Bone lesions are found on radiographical skeletal survey in about 70% of cases of PCM, and even more frequently by MRI and PET/CT {988,2164,3348,4455}. Lytic lesions are most common (accounting for ~70% of the bone lesions found), but abnormalities also include osteoporosis (accounting for 10–15% of bone lesions), pathological fractures, and vertebral compression fractures. The most frequent sites of lesions, in decreasing order, are the vertebrae, ribs, skull, shoulders, pelvis, and long bones {4455}.

Macroscopy

The bone defects apparent on gross examination are filled with soft, gelatinous, fish-flesh haemorrhagic tissue.

Microscopy

Bone marrow biopsy

Monoclonal plasma cells may be scattered interstitially, in small clusters, in focal nodules, or in diffuse sheets {281, 480,3330}. There is often bone marrow sparing and preservation of normal haematopoiesis, with interstitial and focal patterns of involvement. With diffuse involvement, expansive areas of the bone marrow are replaced and haematopoiesis may be markedly decreased. There is typically progression from interstitial and focal disease in early PCM to diffuse involvement in advanced stages of disease {281}. Generally, when 30% of the bone marrow volume is composed of plasma cells, a diagnosis of myeloma is likely, although rare cases of reactive plasmacytosis can reach that level. A tumoural

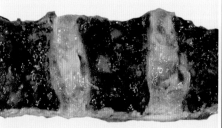
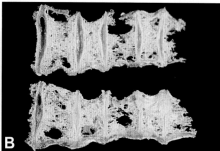

Fig. 13.39 Plasma cell myeloma. **A** Gross photograph of the vertebral column, showing multiple lytic lesions filled with grey, fleshy tumour. **B** Vertebral column after maceration, showing multiple lytic lesions.

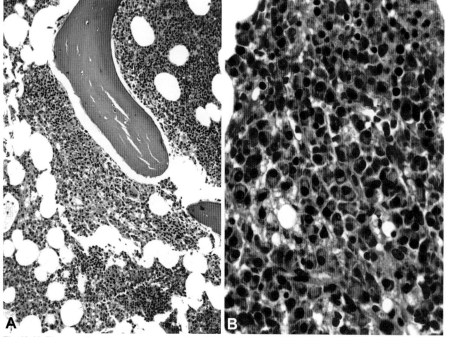

Fig. 13.40 Plasma cell myeloma. Low-magnification (**A**) and high-magnification (**B**) views of a bone marrow biopsy. There is extensive marrow replacement with neoplastic plasma cells. The pattern of involvement is mixed, interstitial, and focal. The plasma cells exhibit mature features, with abundant cytoplasm and eccentric nuclei with coarse chromatin; most lack visible nucleoli.

mass of plasma cells displacing normal bone marrow elements strongly favours a diagnosis of PCM, even if the volume of bone marrow replaced is <30%. Prominent osteoclastic activity is observed in some cases.

Immunohistochemistry is useful in quantifying plasma cells on biopsies, in confirming a monoclonal proliferation, and in distinguishing PCM from other neoplasms. CD138 staining is useful for quantifying plasma cells, and clonality can usually be established with staining for Ig kappa and lambda light chains {1762,3147}. Staining for commonly expressed aberrant antigens such as CD56 and KIT (CD117) may be used to detect populations of neoplastic plasma cells. The small-cell or lymphoplasmacytic variant of PCM may be confused with small B-cell lymphoma or mantle cell lymphoma, especially given that these cases frequently show strong CD20 expression and/or strong cyclin D1 expression, due to the common presence of a t(11;14)(q13;q32) (IGH/*CCND1*) translocation {3242,3744}.

Bone marrow aspiration

The proportion of plasma cells on aspirate smears varies from barely increased to >90% {2164}. Myeloma plasma cells vary from mature forms indistinguishable from normal cells to immature, plasmablastic, and pleomorphic cells {281,480,1454}. Mature plasma cells are usually oval, with a round eccentric nucleus and so-called spoke-wheel or clock-face chromatin without nucleoli. There is generally abundant basophilic cytoplasm and a perinuclear hof. The small-cell variant shows a lymphoplasmacytic appearance, with a narrow rim of basophilic cytoplasm and the occasional perinuclear hof. In contrast, immature forms have more-dispersed nuclear chromatin, a higher N:C ratio, and (often) prominent nucleoli. In almost 10% of cases, there is plasmablastic morphology {1454}. Multinucleated, multilobed, pleomorphic plasma cells are prominent in some cases {281,480}. Because nuclear immaturity and pleomorphism rarely occur in reactive plasma cells, they are reliable indicators of neoplastic plasma cells. The cytoplasm of myeloma cells has abundant endoplasmic reticulum, which may contain condensed or crystallized cytoplasmic Ig producing a variety of morphological findings, including multiple pale bluish-white, grape-like accumulations (Mott cells and morula cells); cherry-

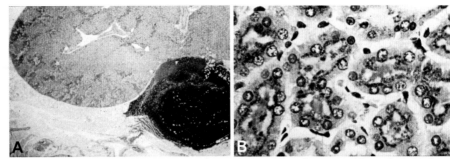

Fig. 13.41 Plasma cell myeloma. **A** Perirenal involvement (extramedullary plasmacytoma) in a patient with plasma cell myeloma. Immunohistochemical assay reveals lambda light chain–bearing perirenal plasmacytoma. **B** Section of kidney showing renal tubular lambda deposition, with casts reflecting renal tubular Bence Jones protein reabsorption (immunoperoxidase and anti–lambda light chain).

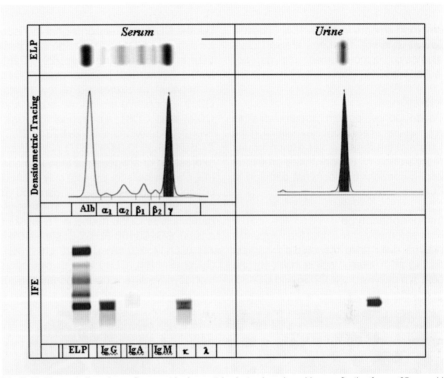

Fig. 13.42 Plasma cell myeloma. Serum and urine protein electrophoresis and immunofixation from a 65-year-old woman with plasma cell myeloma who presented with back, neck, and pelvic pain and generalized weakness. There was no hypercalcaemia, renal failure, or anaemia. However, a skeletal survey revealed multiple lytic lesions in the skull, ribs, pelvis, clavicles, scapula, and spine. A bone marrow biopsy showed 13% plasma cells. Protein electrophoresis (ELP) revealed a serum IgG kappa M protein value of 31 g/L and a urine M protein value of 347.4 mg/24 hours. The M protein was identified by immunofixation electrophoresis (IFE) as IgG kappa. Courtesy of Drs Frank H. Wians, Jr. and Dennis C. Wooten

red refractive round bodies (Russell bodies); vermilion-staining glycogen-rich IgA (flame cells); overstuffed fibrils (pseudo-Gaucher cells and thesaurocytes); and crystalline rods {480}. These changes are not pathognomonic of PCM; they can also be found in reactive plasma cells.

In about 5% of cases of PCM, there are <10% plasma cells in the bone marrow aspirate smears {1762}. This may be due to a suboptimal bone marrow aspirate or the frequent focal distribution of PCM in the bone marrow. In such instances,

larger numbers of plasma cells and focal clusters are sometimes observed in the trephine biopsy sections. Biopsies directed at radiographical lesions may be necessary to establish the diagnosis in some patients.

Peripheral blood

Rouleaux formation is the most striking feature on blood smears and is related to the quantity and type of M protein. A leukoerythroblastic reaction is observed in some cases. Plasma cells are found

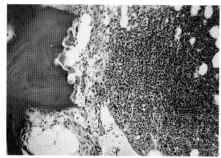

Fig. 13.43 Plasma cell myeloma. Bone marrow biopsy. A discrete plasma cell mass displaces normal marrow fat cells and haematopoietic elements. Note the prominent osteoclastic activity in the trabecular bone near the myeloma mass.

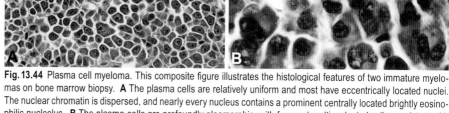

Fig. 13.44 Plasma cell myeloma. This composite figure illustrates the histological features of two immature myelomas on bone marrow biopsy. **A** The plasma cells are relatively uniform and most have eccentrically located nuclei. The nuclear chromatin is dispersed, and nearly every nucleus contains a prominent centrally located brightly eosinophilic nucleolus. **B** The plasma cells are profoundly pleomorphic, with frequent multinucleated cells consistent with the term "anaplastic plasma cell myeloma".

on blood smears in about 15% of cases, usually in small numbers. Marked plasmacytosis accompanies plasma cell leukaemia.

Kidney

Bence Jones protein accumulates as aggregates of eosinophilic material in the lumina of the renal tubules. Renal tubular reabsorption of Bence Jones protein is largely responsible for renal damage in PCM.

Immunophenotype

Flow cytometry shows that the neoplastic plasma cells have monotypic cytoplasmic Ig and usually lack surface Ig; the cells typically express CD38 and CD138, but the CD38 expression signal tends to be dimmer and the CD138 signal brighter than in normal plasma cells {291,2926}. Unlike in normal plasma cells, CD45 is negative or expressed at low levels; CD19 is negative in 95% of cases, and CD27 and CD81 are frequently negative or underexpressed {291,2348,2557, 2725,2926,3033,3474,3937}. Aberrant expression of antigens not found on normal plasma cells (or present only in small subsets of normal cells) is identified in nearly 90% of cases {2348}. These antigens include CD56 (found in 75–80% of cases), CD200 (60–75%), CD28 (~40%), KIT (CD117; 20–35%), CD20 (10–20%), CD52 (8–14%), CD10 and myeloid and monocytic antigens (found occasionally), and stem cell–associated antigens (found rarely) {73,291,292,2348,2973, 3123,3227,3286,3375,3474}. Increased expression of MYC may be detected on immunohistochemistry, and cyclin D1 is expressed in cases with t(11;14)(q13;q32) (IGH/CCND1) and some cases with hyperdiploidy {795,3744,4384}.

There is conflicting evidence regarding the value of immunophenotype as an indicator of prognosis in PCM {2724,3124}. Expression of CD19, CD28, and CD200; lack of expression of CD45 or KIT (CD117); and underexpression of CD27 have all been associated with more-aggressive disease; however, none of these markers has been proven by multivariate analysis to have independent prognostic significance {52,2557,2725,2973}.

Postulated normal counterpart

The postulated normal counterparts are post–germinal centre long-lived plasma cells in which the IG genes have undergone class switch and somatic hypermutation.

Genetic profile

Antigen receptor genes

IG heavy and light chain genes are clonally rearranged. There is a high load of IGHV gene somatic hypermutation without ongoing mutations, consistent with derivation from a post–germinal centre, antigen-driven B cell {237}.

Cytogenetic abnormalities and oncogenes

Abnormalities are detected by karyotype cytogenetics in about one third of PCMs, and by FISH in >90% {200,728,1231, 2180,2188,3541}. Abnormalities are both numerical and structural and include

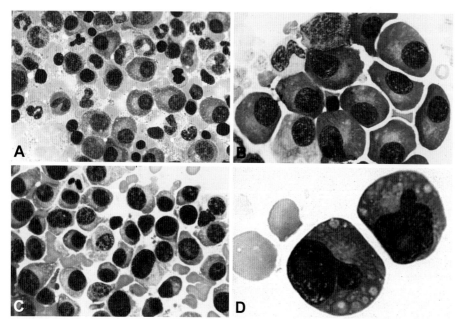

Fig. 13.45 Plasma cell myeloma. Cytological features in marrow aspirations showing variation from mature (**A,B**) to immature (**C,D**) plasma cells. The more mature cells have clumped nuclear chromatin, abundant cytoplasm, a low N:C ratio, and only rare nucleoli. In contrast, the less mature cells have more-prominent nucleoli, loose reticular chromatin, and a higher N:C ratio.

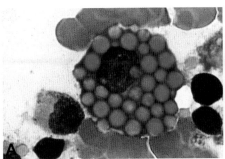 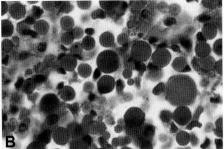

Fig. 13.46 Plasma cell myeloma. Morphological variants based on cytoplasmic features. **A** So-called Mott cell with abundant grape-like cytoplasmic inclusions of immunoglobulin. **B** Numerous Russell bodies.

trisomies and whole or partial chromosome deletions and translocations; complex cytogenetic abnormalities are common. A molecular cytogenetic classification of PCM proposed by the International Myeloma Working Group (IMWG) is shown in Table 13.08 {1232}. The genetic categories are major indicators of prognosis and form the basis for risk stratification of PCM (see *Prognosis and predictive factors*). The IMWG consensus recommendations on genetic testing are listed in Table 13.09 {1232}.

The most frequent chromosome translocations involve IGH on chromosome 14q32 and are present in 55–70% of PCMs {202,1231}. Seven recurrent oncogenes are involved in 14q32 translocations: *CCND1* on 11q13 (involved in 16% of cases), *MAF* on 16q23 (in 5%), *FGFR3/NSD2* (also called *FGFR3/MMSET*) on 4p16.3 (in 15%), *CCND3* on 6p21 (in 2%), *MAFB* on 20q11 (in 2%), *MAFA* on 8q24 (in < 1%), and *CCND2* on 12p13 (in < 1%) (see Table 13.08 and Table 13.10) {200,1232,2128}. Together these seven translocations are found in about 40% of cases of PCM, most of which are non-hyperdiploid (i.e. with < 48 or > 75 chromosomes). The remaining PCMs are mostly hyperdiploid (usually with gains in three or more of the odd-numbered chromosomes 3, 5, 7, 9, 11, 15, 19, and 21) and only infrequently have one of the seven recurrent IGH translocations listed above {728,729,1231}.

IGH translocations and hyperdiploidy appear to be early events in the genesis of plasma cell neoplasms, unified by associated upregulation of one of the cyclin D genes (*CCND1*, *CCND2*, or *CCND3*) {351,2128}. Gene expression profiling can determine the expression levels of *CCND1*, *CCND2*, and *CCND3* RNA and identify tumours that overexpress oncogenes dysregulated by the seven recurrent IGH translocations. On the basis of

patterns of translocations and cyclin D expression (TC groups), non-IgM MGUS and PCM can be classified into groups that are based mostly on early pathogenic events (Table 13.10). Some or all of these groups may represent distinct disease entities that require different therapeutic strategies {2128,3798}. Two other molecular classifications based on unsupervised clustering of tumours by gene expression profiles are similar to the TC groups {473,4474}. However, they are not generally applicable for non-IgM MGUS, because some of the groups are based on progression events not found in MGUS (e.g. proliferation) {2128}.

Monosomy or partial deletion of chromosome 13 (13q14) is found by FISH in nearly half of PCMs. It is sometimes an early event (present in about 35% of non-IgM MGUSs) but can also be a progression event, particularly in PCM with t(11;14) {711,1231}. *MYC* (and rarely *MYCN*) locus rearrangements are present in nearly half of PCM tumours. These reposition *MYC* near a promiscuous array of plasma cell–specific super-enhancers (including IGH, IGK, and IGL super-enhancers). The *MYC* rearrangements may sometimes contribute to the progression from non-IgM MGUS to PCM, but can also occur at later stages of PCM progression {26}. Mutually exclusive activating mutations of *KRAS*, *NRAS*, or *BRAF* are present in about 40% of PCMs and are candidates for mediating the transition of non-IgM MGUS to myeloma in some patients {2383,3312,4496}.

Other recurrent genetic changes associated with disease progression include secondary IGH or IGL translocations; deletion and/or mutation of *TP53* (17p13.1); gains of chromosome 1q and loss of 1p; mutations of genes that result in activation of the NF-kappaB pathway; mutations of *FGFR3* in tumours with t(4;14); and inactivation of *CDKN2C*, *RB1*, *FAM46C*, and

Table 13.08 The International Myeloma Working Group (IMWG) molecular cytogenetic classification of plasma cell myeloma. Adapted from Fonseca R, et al. {1232}

Genetic category	Proportion of cases	
Hyperdiploid	45%	
Non-hyperdiploid	40%	
Cyclin D translocation	18%	
t(11;14)(q13;q32)		16%
t(6;14)(p25;q32)		2%
t(12;14)(p13;q32)		< 1%
NSD2 (also called *MMSET*) translocation	15%	
t(4;14)(p16;q32)		15%
MAF translocation	8%	
t(14;16)(q32;q23)		5%
t(14;20)(q32;q11)		2%
t(8;14)(q24;q32)		1%
Unclassified (other)	15%	

Table 13.09 The International Myeloma Working Group (IMWG) consensus recommendations on genetic testing. Adapted from Fonseca R, et al. {1232}

FISH (on cell-sorted samples or cytoplasmic immunoglobulin FISH)

Minimal panel:
  t(4;14)(p16;q32),
  t(14;16)(q32;q23),
  del(17p13.1)

More comprehensive panel:
  t(11;14)(q13;q32),
  del 13,
  ploidy category,
  chromosome 1 abnormalities

Clinical trials should incorporate gene expression profiling

DIS3 {109,1232,2128,2383}. Epigenetic changes manifested by DNA methylation are also associated with tumour progression.

Myeloma tumour cells from individual patients often have heterogeneous somatic genetic abnormalities reflecting the presence of multiple subclones. Tumour subclones can have activating mutations of *NRAS*, *KRAS*, or *BRAF*; although each subclone can have only one of these mutations. This has important therapeutic implications, because a specific therapeutic regimen may target one or more specific subclones but have little or no effect on other subclones {1979, 2383}. Although genetic events appear to play the key role in initiation and progression

Table 13.10 Molecular classifications of plasma cell myeloma[a]; modified from Kuehl WM and Bergsagel PL {2128}

Group	TC[b]	Gene[c]	Ploidy	%[d]	UAMS	HOVON-GMMG
Cyclin D TLC	11q13	CCND1	N	15	CD1, CD2	CD1, CD2
	6p21	CCND3	N	2	CD1, CD2	CD1, CD2
	12p13	CCND2	N	< 1	CD1, CD2	CD1, CD2
NSD2[e] TLC	4p16	NSD2, FGFR3 (CCND2)	N > H	15	MS	MS
MAF TLC	16q23	MAF (CCND2)	N	5	MF	MF
	20q12	MAFB (CCND2)	N	2	MF	MF
	8q24	MAFA (CCND2)	N	< 1	MF	MF
No primary TLC	D1	CCND1	H	33	HY	Y, CD1, NFKB, CTA, PRL3
	D1 + D2	CCND1, CCND2	H	7	PR	PR, CTA
	D2	CCND2	H, NH	18	PR, LB	LB, CTA, PRL3
	None[f]	No cyclin D genes	N	2	PR	PR, CTA

H, mostly hyperdiploid; HOVON-GMMG, Dutch-Belgian Cooperative Trial Group for Hematology-Oncology and German Multiple Myeloma Group classification; N, mostly non-hyperdiploid; PR, proliferation; TC, translocations and cyclin D classification; TLC, IGH translocation; UAMS, University of Arkansas for Medical Science classification.

[a] The TC classification is generally valid for monoclonal gammopathy of undetermined significance (MGUS) and multiple myeloma. The UAMS and HOVON-GMMG classifications include plasma cell myeloma progression events and are probably not generally valid for MGUS.
[b] 11q13 and 6p21 are combined into one TC group; 12p13 is rarely identified and thus usually in the D2 group.
[c] TLC target and/or cyclin D upregulated
[d] The percentage of patients with plasma cell myeloma in each group. [e]NSD2 is also known as MMSET.
[f]None refers to a group of patients with no cyclin D expression.

Table 13.11 International Staging System (ISS) for plasma cell myeloma. From Greipp PR, et al. {1456}

Stage	Criteria	Median survival (months)
I	Serum beta-2 microglobulin < 3.5 g/dL Serum albumin ≥ 3.5 g/dL	62
II	Not stage I or III[a]	44
III	Serum beta-2 microglobulin ≥ 5.5 mg/L	29

[a] There are two categories for stage II:
(1) serum beta-2 microglobulin < 3.5 mg/L but serum albumin < 3.5 g/dL and
(2) serum beta-2 microglobulin of 3.5 to < 5.5 mg/L, irrespective of the serum albumin level.

Table 13.12 Mayo Stratification of Myeloma and Risk-Adapted Therapy. Adapted from Chesi M and Bergsagel PL {690}

Standard risk (60%)	Intermediate risk (20%)	High risk (20%)
t(11;14)	t(4;14)	Del 17p
t(6;14)	Del 13	t(14;16)
Hyperdiploid	Hypodiploid	t(14;20)
All others		GEP high-risk signature
OS: 8–10 years	OS: 4–5 years	OS: 3 years

GEP, gene expression profiling; OS, overall survival.

of PCM, the bone marrow microenvironment is also important in pathogenesis and progression {97}. Extracellular matrix proteins, secreted cytokines and growth factors (including IL6), and/or the functional consequences of direct interaction of the bone marrow stromal cells with neoplastic plasma cells are major constituents that influence the pathophysiology of PCM {2677}.

Genetic susceptibility

The risk of PCM in individuals with a first-degree relative with PCM or MGUS is 3.7 times that in the general population {468,1441}.

Prognosis and predictive factors

For most patients, PCM is an incurable progressive disease, but newer therapeutic approaches have significantly improved quality of life and survival {2723}. Survival ranges from < 6 months to > 10 years (median: ~5.5 years) {666}. Patients aged > 70 years and those with significant comorbidities and poor performance status have a less favourable prognosis. The International Staging System (ISS) for PCM, based on pretreatment serum beta-2 microglobulin and albumin levels, provides a strong predictor of survival (Table 13.11) {1456}. Treatment response as measured by minimal residual disease detection by flow cytometry is a significant predictor of both progression-free and overall survival, especially following autologous stem cell transplantation {3035,3036}.

Genetics is a powerful predictor of prognosis and has been combined with the ISS (R-ISS) to provide improved risk stratification {3041}. Genetic risk stratification based primarily on FISH analysis stratifies cases into standard-risk, intermediate-risk, and high-risk categories {690,1232,2661}. The most important genetic indicators of high-risk myeloma are deletion of 17p/TP53 sequences and the MAF translocations t(14;16) and t(14;20) (Table 13.12). Several high-risk molecular signatures, based on gene expression profiling using various panels of genes, serve as prognostic indicators for PCM. Increased expression of genes associated with proliferation is an important component of these prognostic signatures. The UAMS-70 and related UAMS-17 prognostic scores {3639} and the EMC-92-gene signature {2129} appear to be the most robust prognostic gene signature models when applied to cohorts of PCMs from various institutions. Other reported indicators of less favourable risk include reduced polyclonal (uninvolved) serum Igs, elevated lactate dehydrogenase, high C-reactive protein, increased plasma cell proliferative activity, a high degree of bone marrow replacement, plasmablastic morphology, and elevated serum soluble receptor for IL6 {281,289, 290,1454,1455,2164,3291}.

Plasma cell myeloma variants

Smouldering (asymptomatic) plasma cell myeloma

Patients with smouldering plasma cell myeloma (SPCM) have 10–60% clonal plasma cells in their bone marrow and/or an M protein at myeloma levels but absence of myeloma-defining events (i.e. hypercalcaemia, renal insufficiency, anaemia, and bone lesions; CRAB) and amyloidosis (see Table 13.06, p. 242, and Table 13.07, p. 243) {2165,2174,3290}. Approximately 8–14% of patients with plasma cell myeloma (PCM) are initially diagnosed with SPCM {2119,2174}. The disorder is similar to monoclonal gammopathy of undetermined significance in its lack of clinical manifestations, but is much more likely to progress to symptomatic PCM {992,2165,2174,2176}. Most patients have 10–20% bone marrow plasma cells, and the median level of serum M protein is nearly 30 g/L. Normal polyclonal immunoglobulins (Igs) are reduced in >83% of patients, and 53% of patients have monoclonal light chains in the urine {2164,2165}. Light chain SPCM is characterized by 10–60% bone marrow clonal plasma cells and urinary light chain M protein excretion of ≥0.5 mg/24 hours.

Some patients with SPCM have stable disease for long periods, but the cumulative probability of progression to symptomatic PCM or amyloidosis is approximately 10% per year for the first 5 years, 3% per year for the next 5 years, and 1% per year thereafter; the median time to progression is about 5 years {2174}. For light chain SPCM, the rate of progression is 5% per year for the first 5 years, 3% per year for the next 5 years, and then 2% per year for the following 5 years. Risk factors for earlier progression to symptomatic PCM include the presence of both >10% bone marrow plasma cells and >30 g/L M protein, detection of bone lesions by MRI, a high percentage of bone marrow plasma cells with an aberrant immunophenotype, an abnormal serum free light chain ratio, a high-risk gene expression profile, a high plasma cell proliferation rate, and circulating plasma cells {969,1005,1007,2174,2558}. Therapeutic intervention for the highest-risk patients has been shown to delay progression to symptomatic PCM and to improve overall survival {1007,2558,3293}.

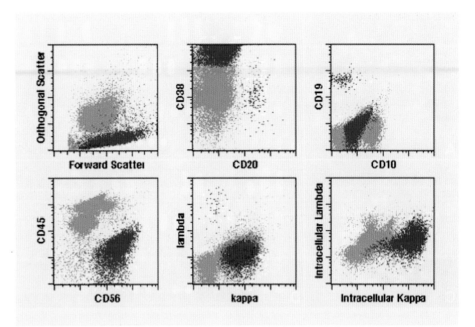

Fig. 13.47 Plasma cell myeloma. Flow cytometry histograms of bone marrow. The neoplastic plasma cells are indicated in red and normal B lymphocytes in blue. The myeloma cells express bright CD38 and are negative for CD20, CD19, and CD10. They express CD56 and partial CD45, are negative for surface light chains, and express cytoplasmic kappa.

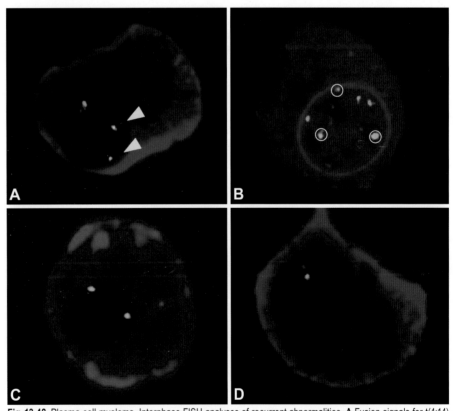

Fig. 13.48 Plasma cell myeloma. Interphase FISH analyses of recurrent abnormalities. **A** Fusion signals for t(4;14) (p16;q32). Probes for IGH are green and probes for *FGFR3/NSD2* (also called *FGFR3/MMSET*) are red. Two fusion signals (indicated by arrowheads) most likely identify der(4) and der(14), but could represent two copies of der(4). **B** Extra copies of three chromosomes in a hyperdiploid tumour. Three copies of chromosome 5 (LSI D5S23/D5S721, green) and chromosome 9 (CEP 9, aqua, circled) and four copies of chromosome 15 (CEP 15, red). **C** Two copies of chromosome 17 (CEP 17, green) and deletion of one copy of *TP53* (red). **D** Loss of one copy of chromosome 13/13q. LSI 13 containing *RB1* (green), D13S19 (red). In all four panels, the cytoplasm is blue due to immunostaining of Ig-kappa or Ig-lambda expressed by the tumour plasma cells, and the probes are from Vysis. Courtesy of Dr R. Fonseca.

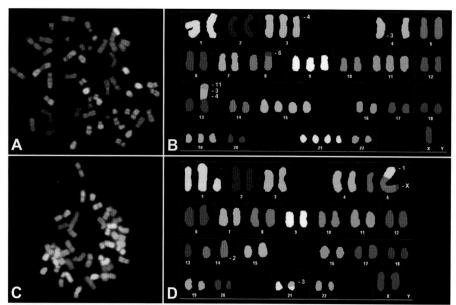

Fig. 13.49 Plasma cell myeloma. Spectral karyotypic analysis of hyperdiploid and non-hyperdiploid cases, showing metaphase spreads in display colours (**A,C**) and classification of chromosomes (**B,D**). **A,B** Hyperdiploid tumour with 53 chromosomes, including 4 rearranged chromosomes involving ≥2 different chromosomes; trisomies of chromosomes 3, 9, 11, and 19; and tetrasomies of chromosomes 15 and 21. From FISH analyses (not shown), there is no IGH or IGL translocation, but *MYC* is inserted on chromosome 6p23. **C,D** Non-hyperdiploid tumour with 46 chromosomes, including at least 3 rearranged chromosomes involving ≥2 different chromosomes, an internally deleted chromosome 14, and loss of one copy of chromosome 13. FISH analyses (not shown) confirm the presence of a t(2;14)(p23;q32) translocation involving *MYCN* (also called *NMYC*) and a karyotypically silent t(4;14)(p16;q32) translocation. Courtesy of Roschke A, Gabrea A, Kuehl MW.

The highest-risk asymptomatic patients are defined as those with extreme bone marrow plasmacytosis (>60%), an extremely abnormal serum free light chain ratio (> 100), or ≥2 bone lesions detected only by modern imaging {1007,3290}. Asymptomatic patients with any one or more of these biomarkers should be considered to have active PCM for the purpose of treatment; such cases should not be classified as SPCM {1007,3293}.

Non-secretory myeloma

Approximately 1% of PCMs are non-secretory. In these, there is absence of an M protein by serum and urine immunofixation electrophoresis {1762,2164}. Cytoplasmic M protein is present in the neoplastic plasma cells in about 85% of cases when evaluated by immunohistochemistry, consistent with production but impaired secretion of Ig {1762}. Elevated serum free light chains and/or an abnormal free light chain ratio is found in as many as two thirds of cases considered to be non-secretory by immunofixation electrophoresis, suggesting that many such cases are at least minimally secretory or oligosecretory {1036,1762}. In about 15% of non-secretory myelomas, no cytoplasmic Ig synthesis is detect-

ed (non-producer myeloma). Acquired mutations of the IG light chain variable genes and alteration in the light chain constant region have been implicated in the pathogenesis of the non-secretory state {813,1053}.

The clinical features of non-secretory myeloma are similar to those of other PCMs, except for a lower incidence of renal insufficiency and hypercalcaemia and less depression of normal Ig {1762,3705}. The immunophenotype, genetics, and prognosis of non-secretory myeloma are similar to those of other PCMs {666}. Survival appears to be better for patients with a normal baseline serum free light chain ratio than those with an abnormal ratio {666}. Non-secretory myeloma must be distinguished from the rare IgD and IgE myelomas, which have low serum M protein and may not be routinely screened for by immunofixation electrophoresis.

Plasma cell leukaemia

Plasma cell leukaemia (PCL) is a PCM in which clonal plasma cells constitute > 20% of total leukocytes in the blood or the absolute count is >2.0 × 10⁹/L {1185, 1762}. The bone marrow is usually extensively and diffusely infiltrated. Neoplastic plasma cells are frequently found

in extramedullary sites such as the liver, spleen, body cavity effusions, and spinal fluid. PCL is an initial presentation (primary PCL) in 2–4% of myelomas. Secondary PCL is a leukaemic transformation occurring in approximately 1% of previously diagnosed PCMs {1400}. 60–70% of all PCLs are primary {201,993,1185,1300}. The median patient age at diagnosis is younger than for other myelomas. Lymphadenopathy, organomegaly, and renal failure are more common, and lytic bone lesions and bone pain less common {1300}. A higher proportion of cases of light chain–only, IgE, and IgD myelomas present as PCL compared with IgG or IgA myelomas {1300,1600}. The immunophenotype of PCL differs from other PCMs by its more frequent expression of CD20 and less frequent expression of CD56, which is negative in about 80% of PCLs {1185,1300,3123,3474}. PCL has a higher incidence of high-risk genetic findings {201,1185,1862,4000}. The t(11;14) translocation, typically associated with a more favourable prognosis in PCM, is also overrepresented in primary PCL {201, 4000}. Patients with PCL have aggressive disease, poor response to therapy, and a relatively short survival {201,993, 1185,1300,1400,2169,2886,4000}.

Plasmacytoma

Definition

Solitary plasmacytomas are single localized tumours consisting of monoclonal plasma cells with no clinical features of plasma cell myeloma (PCM) and no physical or radiographical evidence of additional plasma cell tumours. There are two types of plasmacytoma: solitary plasmacytoma of bone and extraosseous (extramedullary) plasmacytoma.

Solitary plasmacytoma of bone

Definition

Solitary plasmacytoma of bone (SPB) is a localized tumour consisting of monoclonal plasma cells with no clinical features of PCM. Radiographical studies, including MRI and CT, show no other bone lesions {988,2324,3290,3742}. Approximately 30% of patients with a solitary plasmacytoma defined only by radiographical skeletal survey have additional lesions identified on MRI or CT {988,2765}. These patients are consid-

Table 13.13 Diagnostic criteria for solitary plasmacytoma. Adapted from the International Myeloma Working Group (IMWG) updated criteria for the diagnosis of multiple myeloma. From: Rajkumar SV, et al. {3290}

Solitary plasmacytoma
    Biopsy-proven solitary lesion of bone or soft tissue consisting of clonal plasma cells
    Normal random bone marrow biopsy with no evidence of clonal plasma cells
    Normal skeletal survey and MRI or CT (except for the primary solitary lesion)
    Absence of end-organ damage, such as hypercalcaemia, renal insufficiency, anaemia, and bone lesions
    (CRAB) attributable to a plasma cell proliferative disorder

Solitary plasmacytoma with minimal bone marrow involvement
    Same as above plus clonal plasma cells < 10% in random bone marrow biopsy
    (usually identified by flow cytometry)

ered to have PCM {2324,3290,4260}. There are two distinct types of SPB, with different prognoses: those with no clonal bone marrow plasmacytosis except for the solitary lesion and those with minimal (< 10%) clonal bone marrow plasma cells, often identified only by flow cytometry {3290}. The diagnostic criteria for solitary plasmacytoma, adapted from the International Myeloma Working Group (IMWG) updated criteria for the diagnosis of multiple myeloma {3290}, are listed in Table 13.13).

ICD-O code   9731/3

Synonyms
Plasma cell tumour; solitary myeloma; solitary plasmacytoma; osseous plasmacytoma; plasmacytoma of bone

Epidemiology
SPB accounts for 1–2% of plasma cell neoplasms {1762}. It is more common in men (accounting for 65% of cases), and the median patient age at diagnosis is 55 years {992,1762}.

Localization
The most common sites are bones with active bone marrow haematopoiesis, in order of frequency: the vertebrae, ribs, skull, pelvis, femora, humeri, clavicles, and scapulae {992}. Thoracic vertebrae are more commonly involved than are cervical or lumbar vertebrae; long bone involvement below the elbow or knee is rare {934,1762}.

Clinical features
Patients most frequently present with localized bone pain or a pathological fracture. Vertebral lesions may be associated with symptomatic cord compression {934}. Soft tissue extension may produce a palpable mass {1762}.

An M protein is found in the serum or urine in 24–72% of patients; the serum free light chain ratio is abnormal in about half {992,997,1762,3742,4315}. In most cases, polyclonal immunoglobulins are at normal levels {992,3742}. There is no anaemia, hypercalcaemia, or renal failure related to the plasmacytoma {1762}.

Microscopy
Plasmacytomas have features similar to those of PCM and are easily recognizable in tissue sections, except in rare poorly differentiated cases (e.g. plasmablastic or anaplastic cases). Plasma cell clonality can be confirmed by immunohistochemistry.

Immunophenotype
The immunophenotype is similar to that of PCM.

Genetic profile
The genetic findings are similar to those in PCM.

Prognosis and predictive factors
Local control is achieved by radiotherapy in most cases, but as many as two thirds of cases eventually evolve to generalized PCM or additional solitary or multiple plasmacytomas {934,1664,1762,2765, 4315,4335}. Progression occurs within 3 years in about 10% of cases of SPB and no detectable bone marrow involvement and in 60% of those with minimal bone marrow involvement (< 10% bone marrow clonal plasma cells) {1635,3031,3290, 4260}. Approximately one third of patients remain disease free for > 10 years; median overall survival is about 10 years {990,1762}. Older patients and patients with an SPB >5 cm or persistence of an M protein for > 1 year following local radiotherapy have a higher incidence of progression {992,1762,2324,3742,4068,

4315}. Other reported risk factors for progression to myeloma are an abnormal serum free light chain ratio, monoclonal urinary free light chains, low levels of uninvolved immunoglobulin, and osteopenia {992,997,1635,1811,3031,4315}.

Extraosseous plasmacytoma

Definition
Extraosseous (extramedullary) plasmacytomas are localized plasma cell neoplasms that arise in tissues other than bone (Table 13.13). Lymphomas with prominent plasmacytic differentiation, especially extranodal marginal zone lymphoma (MZL) of mucosa-associated lymphoid tissue (MALT lymphoma), must be excluded (Table 13.14).

ICD-O code   9734/3

Epidemiology
Extraosseous (extramedullary) plasmacytomas constitute approximately 1% of plasma cell neoplasms {61}. Two thirds of patients are male, and the median patient age at diagnosis is about 55 years.

Localization
Extraosseous plasmacytomas occur most commonly in the mucous membranes of the upper air passages, but they can also occur in numerous other sites, including the gastrointestinal tract, lymph nodes, bladder, breasts, thyroid, testes, parotid glands, skin, and CNS {61, 1279}. Plasmacytomas of the upper respiratory track spread to cervical lymph nodes in about 15% of cases {2631}. An indolent variant of IgA-expressing, predominantly nodal plasmacytoma has been described in younger adults, with frequent signs of immune dysfunction {3634}.

Clinical features
Symptoms are generally related to the tumour mass. With masses in the upper airway, symptoms may include rhinorrhoea, epistaxis, and nasal obstruction. Radiographical and morphological assessments show no evidence of bone marrow involvement. Approximately 20% of patients have a small M protein, most commonly IgA {1279,1762,3742}. In extraosseous plasmacytoma there are no clinical features of plasma cell myeloma.

Table 13.14 Differential diagnosis of neoplasms with plasmacytic (PC) or plasmablastic (PB) differentiation in extraosseous locations

	Extraosseous infiltrates of plasma cell myeloma (PCM)	Plasmablastic lymphoma	Primary extraosseous plasmacytoma
Clinical features and predisposing factors	Usually in advanced PCM, sometimes pure extraosseous relapse after treatment	HIV infection and iatrogenic immunosuppression, elderly immunocompetent patients	No known predisposing factors, broad patient age range, rare cases in post-transplantation setting {3352}
Location	Any site, with or without leukaemic peripheral blood involvement	Predominantly extranodal, oral cavity, gastrointestinal tract, skin, and lymph nodes; 50% in immunocompetent patients	80% in head and neck region, mostly extranodal
Osteolytic lesions	Common, disseminated	Rare	Rare local infiltration (skull)
M protein	>95%	Rare	20%, low level
Bone marrow involvement	Yes	Rare	No manifest involvement (by definition), 15% during disease evolution
Disease stage	Usually in advanced-stage PCM	>90% either stage I or IV	Mostly stage IE–IIE
Morphology	PB/PC	Immunoblastic/PB, occasionally PC component	Usually mature PC
Immunophenotype	PC markers and cytoplasmic immunoglobulin light chains positive CD56+ in 70–80% (PC leukaemia usually CD56–)	PC markers positive Immunoglobulin light chains positive in 50% B-cell markers negative CD56+ in 10–30%	PC markers and cytoplasmic immunoglobulin light chains positive CD56 less common, weak Cyclin D1 negative
Molecular alterations	PCM cytogenetics, with 50–70% IG translocations MYC rearrangement frequent with PB morphology	PCM-type translocations absent 50% MYC rearrangement	t(11;14) translocation and MYC rearrangement absent
EBV infection	Absent	50–75%, depending on patient background	Rare, 50–70% in extramedullary plasmacytoma–like post-transplant lymphoproliferative disorder
Outcome	Poor	Poor	Good, progression to PCM in 15%

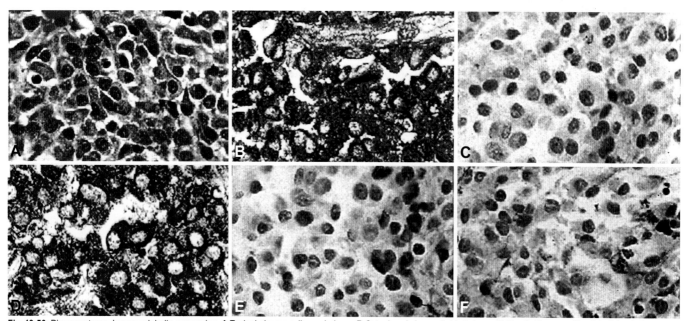

Fig. 13.50 Plasmacytoma. Immunoglobulin expression. **A** Typical plasma cell morphology. **B** Cytoplasmic kappa light chain positivity. **C** Absence of lambda light chain expression. **D** Expression of cytoplasmic gamma heavy chain. **E,F** Absence of mu and alpha heavy chains.

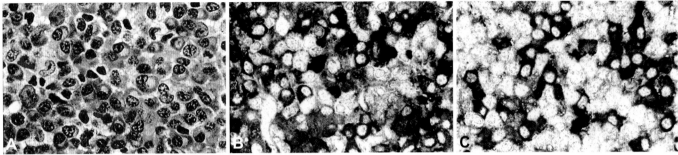

Fig. 13.51 A The so-called mass effect of plasma cells simulates a neoplasm. **B,C** Immunoperoxidase staining reveals polytypic cytoplasmic immunoglobulin, with some plasma cells expressing kappa light chains (B) and some expressing lambda light chains (C).

Microscopy

The morphological features are similar to those of SPB. However, in extraosseous sites, the distinction between lymphomas that exhibit extreme plasma cell differentiation and plasmacytoma can be difficult {990}. MZL of the mucosa-associated lymphoid tissue type, lymphoplasmacytic lymphoma, and (possibly) plasmablastic lymphoma may be misdiagnosed as plasmacytoma {990,1742}. Distinction from an MZL with marked plasma cell differentiation is especially problematic, particularly in the skin, upper airway, and gastrointestinal tract, and may not be possible by morphological assessment. A search for areas of a biopsy with lymphocyte proliferation typical of MZL is fruitful in some cases. In others, a clonally related lymphocyte population may be identified by flow cytometry {1742,3609}. Distinguishing plasmacytoma from extraosseous

infiltrates of PCM is impossible by morphology, although extraosseous PCM more frequently shows cellular atypia or blastic features {2107}. The differential diagnosis of extraosseous tumours with plasmacytic or plasmablastic features is detailed in Table 13.14. Rarely, extraosseous plasmacytoma is accompanied by a local, occasionally tumour-forming amyloid deposit.

Immunophenotype

The immunophenotype appears to be similar to that of PCM, although certain differences may be helpful for diagnosis. Extraosseous plasmacytoma usually lacks cyclin D1 expression and shows less-frequent and weaker positivity for CD56 {2107}. Immunohistochemistry or in situ hybridization for immunoglobulin light chains can be useful in distinguishing a monotypic plasmacytoma from polytypic reactive plasma cell infiltrates. Expression of CD20 by lymphocytes within the lesion or by the plasmacytoid cells, or expression of mu rather than alpha or gamma heavy chain, favours a diagnosis of lymphoma over plasmacytoma. On flow cytometry, the clonal plasma cells of lymphomas are more likely than those of PCM or plasmacytoma to express CD19 (positive in 95% vs 10%) and CD45 (in 91% vs 41%) and to lack CD56 (positive in 33% vs 71%) {3609}. In some cases, extraosseous plasmacytoma and lymphoma with extreme plasma cell differentiation cannot be immunophenotypically distinguished with certainty.

Genetic profile

The genetic features have not been extensively studied, but appear to be similar to those of PCM, with the exception of a lack of t(11;14)(q13;q32) (IGH/*CCND1*) translocations and aberrations of *MYC* {379,384,410}.

Prognosis and predictive factors

In most cases, the lesions are eradicated with local radiation therapy. Regional recurrences develop in as many as 25% of patients, and occasionally there is metastasis to distant extraosseous sites. Progression to PCM is infrequent, occurring in about 15% of cases {61,662,4335}. Cases with minimal bone marrow involvement have a higher rate of progression to PCM {410,3290}. About 70% of patients remain disease free at 10 years {989}.

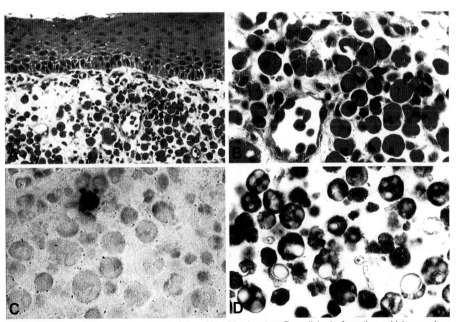

Fig. 13.52 Extramedullary plasmacytoma of the skin with abundant Russell body formation, which can show non-specific staining by immunohistochemistry (**A,B**). Monoclonality is demonstrated by non-radioactive in situ hybridization showing absence of kappa (**C**) and presence of lambda (**D**) mRNA transcripts.

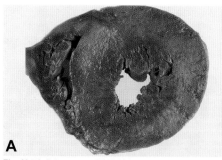
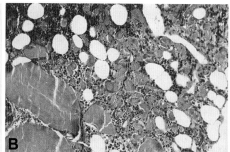
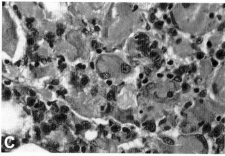

Fig. 13.53 Primary amyloidosis in a patient with plasma cell myeloma. **A** Gross photograph of a section of heart shows the diffuse enlargement characteristic of amyloid deposition, especially in the left ventricle. **B,C** Bone marrow biopsy of primary amyloidosis showing characteristic pale, waxy amorphous deposits (B) and associated histiocytes, often multinucleated, and neoplastic plasma cells (C).

Monoclonal immunoglobulin deposition diseases

Definition

The monoclonal immunoglobulin (Ig) deposition diseases are closely related disorders characterized by visceral and soft tissue deposition of aberrant Ig, resulting in compromised organ function {190,509, 913,1627,1906,2163,3234,3300,3626}. The underlying disorder is typically a plasma cell neoplasm, or rarely a lymphoplasmacytic neoplasm; however, the Ig molecule usually accumulates in tissue before the development of a large tumour burden {1346,1347}. Therefore, patients typically do not have overt myeloma or lymphoma at the time of the diagnosis. There are two major categories of monoclonal Ig deposition diseases: primary amyloidosis and light chain and heavy chain deposition diseases. These disorders appear to be chemically different manifestations of similar pathological processes, resulting in clinically similar conditions.

Primary amyloidosis

Definition

Primary amyloidosis is caused by a plasma cell or (rarely) a lymphoplasmacytic neoplasm in which the monoclonal plasma cells secrete intact or fragments of abnormal immunoglobulin light chains that deposit in various tissues and form a beta-pleated sheet structure (amyloid light chain). The abnormal light chains include the N-terminal (variable) region and part of the constant region of the light chain {509}. Most light chain variable (V) region subgroups are potentially amyloidogenic, but V lambda VI is always associated with amyloidosis {509}. The amyloid tissue deposits accumulate and lead to organ dysfunction {1487}. In most cases, the diagnostic criteria for plasma

cell myeloma (PCM) are lacking, but there is a moderate increase in monoclonal plasma cells in the bone marrow.

ICD-O code   9769/1

Synonyms

Immunoglobulin deposition disease; systemic light chain disease

Epidemiology

The reported annual incidence of primary amyloidosis is approximately 1 case per 100 000 population, and appears to have been stable {2163,2168}. The median patient age at diagnosis is 64 years, and >95% of patients are aged >40 years; 65–70% are male {2163,2166,2168}. Approximately 20% of patients with primary amyloidosis have PCM {1762,2163,2164, 2168,3626}.

Localization

Amyloid light chain accumulates in many tissues and organs, including the subcutaneous fat, kidneys, heart, liver, gastrointestinal tract, peripheral nerves, and bone marrow. The diagnostic biopsy site is typically the abdominal subcutaneous fat pad or bone marrow {2163,3626}. In most cases, the monoclonal plasma cell proliferation is in the bone marrow.

Clinical findings are usually related to deposition of amyloid in organs and tissues. Early signs of disease include peripheral neuropathy (present in 17% of cases), carpal tunnel syndrome (in 21%), and bone pain (in 5%). Symptoms referable to congestive heart failure (present in 17% of cases), nephrotic syndrome (in 28%), or malabsorption (in 5%) are relatively common {2163}. Physical findings include hepatomegaly in 25–30% of patients, macroglossia in about 10%, and purpura (most commonly periorbital or facial) in about 15% {2163}. Haemorrhagic manifestations can result from factor X binding to amyloid, fibrinolysis, disseminated intravascular coagulation, and loss of vascular integrity due to amyloid deposition. Oedema is often present in patients with congestive heart failure or nephrotic syndrome {2163}. Splenomegaly and lymphadenopathy are uncommon. Radiographical lesions of bone are restricted to patients with myeloma and amyloidosis.

Clinical features

An M protein is detected in the serum or urine by the combination of immunofixation and serum free light chain ratio in 99% of patients {1487,1968,2163}. The median concentration of the serum M protein is

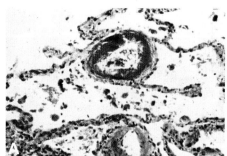
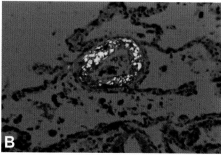

Fig. 13.54 Primary amyloidosis. Pulmonary blood vessel with amyloid deposition, showing Congo red staining (**A**) and apple-green birefringence in polarized light (**B**).

1.4 g/dL. IgG is most frequent, followed by light chain only, IgA, IgM, and IgD; the light chain is lambda in 70% of cases {1345,2163,4272}. About 20% of patients present with hypogammaglobulinaemia {2163}. Proteinuria is present in >80% of patients and nephrotic syndrome or renal failure in approximately 30%, with serum creatinine >2.0 mg/dL in 20–25% of cases {2163}. Hypercalcaemia is occasionally found, most often in patients with myeloma.

Macroscopy
On gross inspection, amyloid has a dense so-called porcelain-like or waxy appearance.

Microscopy
Bone marrow specimens vary from revealing no pathological findings to showing extensive replacement with amyloid, overt PCM, or (rarely) involvement with lymphoplasmacytic lymphoma. The most common finding is a mild increase in plasma cells, which may appear normal or may exhibit any of the changes found in myeloma. Amyloid deposits are found in the bone marrow in about 60% of cases {2163,3159,3843}. Amyloid is also present in many other tissues and organs. On H&E-stained sections, amyloid is a pink, amorphous, waxy-looking substance with a characteristic cracking artefact. Typically, it is found focally in thickened blood vessel walls, on basement membranes, and in the interstitium of tissues such as fat and bone marrow {3843}. Macrophages and foreign-body giant cells may be found around deposits. Rarely, organ parenchyma may be massively replaced by amyloid. Plasma cells may be increased in the adjacent tissues. Congo red stains amyloid pink to red by standard light microscopy, and under polarized light produces a charac-

teristic apple-green birefringence. Congo red fluorescence microscopy may be a more sensitive method for amyloid detection {2503}. Electron microscopic studies can differentiate light-chain amyloidosis from non-amyloid immunoglobulin deposition diseases.

It is essential to characterize the amyloid type even when there is an associated serum or urine M protein. Secondary or familial amyloidosis may be incidentally present in patients with monoclonal gammopathy of undetermined significance or another plasma cell proliferative disorder {788,2182}. Laser microdissection of the amyloid in a biopsy specimen and analysis by mass spectrometry is the most effective method of characterizing amyloid type, with nearly 100% sensitivity and specificity {4221}.

Immunophenotype
The immunophenotypic features of the monotypic plasma cells in primary amyloidosis are similar to those of PCM. Immunohistochemical staining for immunoglobulin kappa and lambda light chains on bone marrow sections usually shows a monoclonal plasma cell staining pattern, but if the clone is small, it may be masked by normal polyclonal plasma cells {4349,4376}.

Genetic profile
The genetic abnormalities reported in primary amyloidosis are similar to those in non-IgM monoclonal gammopathy of undetermined significance and PCM. One exception is the unexplained observation that t(11;14) is present in >40% of individuals with amyloidosis but only 15–20% of those with non-IgM monoclonal gammopathy of undetermined significance or myeloma {484,1231,1594}. Other frequent chromosomal abnormalities include 13q14 deletion and gain of 1q21 {396}.

Prognosis and predictive factors
In recent years, the survival of patients with primary amyloidosis (especially low-stage disease) has greatly improved, but prognosis remains poor for those with high-stage disease {2131,3502}. The major determinant of outcome is extent of cardiac involvement. Other indicators of higher risk are bone marrow monoclonal plasma cells >10%, a high serum free light chain level, and elevated beta-2 microglobulin {2131,2640}. Multiple organ involvement and an elevated serum uric acid level also have negative prognostic significance {1345}. A recently revised staging system for primary amyloidosis uses two cardiac biomarkers and the free light chain level {2131}. Four stages are defined by the elevation of 0, 1, 2, or all 3 of these parameters. Stages 1 and 2 are associated with median overall survivals of 94 and 40 months, and stages 3 and 4 with median overall survivals of only 14 and 6 months, respectively {2131}. The single most frequent cause of death (responsible for ~40% of deaths) is amyloid-related cardiac disease {2166}.

Light chain and heavy chain deposition diseases

Definition
Monoclonal light chain and heavy chain deposition diseases are plasma cell or (rarely) lymphoplasmacytic neoplasms that secrete an abnormal light or (less often) heavy chain, or both, which deposit in tissues, causing organ dysfunction, but do not form amyloid beta-pleated sheets, bind Congo red stain, or contain an amyloid P component. These disorders comprise light chain deposition disease (LCDD), heavy chain deposition disease (HCDD), and light and heavy chain deposition disease (LHCDD) {190,509,510, 1283,1627,1906,2537,3230,3234,3300}.

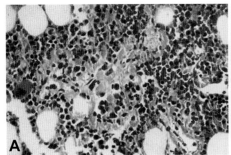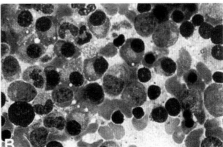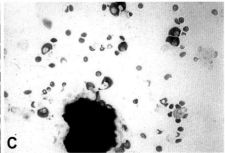

Fig. 13.55 Light chain deposition disease. **A** Bone marrow biopsy showing patches of pale amorphous material. **B** Bone marrow aspirate showing numerous plasma cells. **C** Joint fluid aspirate showing clumps of amorphous material and plasma cells, both staining for kappa light chain by immunoperoxidase.

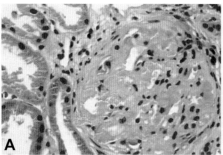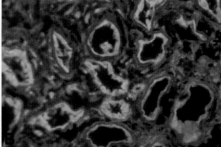

Fig. 13.56 Light chain deposition disease in kidney showing (**A**) pale amorphous patches within glomeruli (nodular glomerulosclerosis and (**B**) immunofluorescence stain showing renal tubular and extratubular deposition of kappa light chain in a smooth linear pattern.

ICD-O code   9769/1

Synonym
Randall disease

Epidemiology
These are rare diseases occurring at a median patient age of 58 years (range: 33–79 years); 60–65% of patients are men {509,1906,3230,3234,3542}. There is no evidence of an ethnicity effect. LCDD is the most common, and frequently occurs in association with plasma cell myeloma (PCM; in 40–65% of cases) or in patients with M protein and marrow plasma cells at monoclonal gammopathy of undetermined significance levels. Some cases are idiopathic or occur with a lymphoproliferative disorder {510,3230}.

Localization
The plasma cell proliferative disorder is in the bone marrow. Deposition of aberrant immunoglobulin (Ig) may involve many organs, most commonly the kidneys {3230}. The liver, heart, peripheral nerves, blood vessels, and occasionally joints may also be involved {366,2641,3230}. Diffuse or nodular pulmonary involvement has also been reported {366,3420}. There is prominent deposition of the aberrant Ig on basement membranes, elastic fibres, and collagen fibres.

Clinical features
Patients have symptoms of organ dysfunction as a result of diffuse, systemic Ig deposits. As many as 96% of patients with LCDD present with renal manifestations {3230}. Nephrotic syndrome and renal failure are the most common features {968,3230,3542}. Symptomatic extrarenal deposition, which is uncommon in LCDD, involves the heart (in 21% of cases), liver (in 19%), and peripheral nervous system (in 8%) {366,2641,3230}. HCDD of the IgG3 or IgG1 isotype results in hypocomplementaemia, because the IgG3 and IgG1 subclasses most readily fix complement {1627,1906,2340}. There is a detectable M protein in about 85% of cases. Kappa deposition is found in at least two thirds of cases of LCDD. Gamma deposits are most common in HCDD, but alpha deposition has also been reported {2340}.

Microscopy
In most cases, bone marrow is involved with a plasma cell proliferative disorder, most frequently PCM {3230}. Rarely, lymphoplasmacytic lymphoma, marginal zone lymphoma, or chronic lymphocytic leukaemia is the associated neoplasm {4299}. Deposition of the light or heavy chains is most frequently found in renal biopsies but can be observed in bone marrow and other tissues in some cases.

The aberrant Ig deposits consist of amorphous eosinophilic material that is non-amyloid and non-fibrillary, and does not stain with Congo red. In LCDD, renal biopsies typically show nodular sclerosing glomerulonephritis. The deposits consist of refractile eosinophilic material in the glomerular and tubular basement membranes. Immunofluorescence microscopy most often identifies kappa chains. A hallmark of LCDD is prominent, smooth, ribbon-like linear peritubular deposits of monotypic Ig along the outer edge of the tubular basement membrane. By electron microscopy, these deposits are typically non-fibrillary, powdery, and electron-dense, with an absence of the beta-pleated sheet structure by X-ray diffraction {2340,2537,3230}. In some cases, plasma cells are found in the vicinity of Ig deposits in visceral organs, but most commonly, few if any are present {366,510}.

Immunophenotype
LCDD has a high prevalence of kappa light chains (80%), with overrepresentation of the V kappa IV variable region {510,3230}. Immunohistochemistry on bone marrow sections may reveal an aberrant kappa/lambda ratio {4349}.

Genetic profile and pathophysiology
The genetic profile of cases associated with PCM is similar to that of other PCMs. The M protein in non-amyloid Ig deposition diseases has undergone structural change due to deletion and mutation events {509,510,1906,3234}. In LCDD, the primary defect involves multiple mutations of the IG light chain variable region, with kappa light chain of V kappa IV type notably overrepresented {509,510,3234}. In HCDD, the critical event is deletion of the CH1 constant domain, which causes failure to associate with heavy chain–binding protein, resulting in premature secretion {190,1627,1906,2340,3234}. In HCDD, the variable regions also contain amino acid substitutions that cause an increased propensity for tissue deposition and for binding blood elements {190,509, 1906}.

Prognosis and predictive factors
Older patient age, associated PCM, and extrarenal light chain deposition are predictors of higher risk and unfavourable survival {2641,3230}. The median overall survival of patients with LCDD varies from 4 years to 14 years in one recent series {3230,3542}.

Plasma cell neoplasms with associated paraneoplastic syndrome

POEMS syndrome

Definition
POEMS syndrome is a paraneoplastic syndrome associated with a plasma cell neoplasm, usually characterized by fibrosis and osteosclerotic changes in bone trabeculae, and often with lymph node changes resembling the plasma cell variant of Castleman disease. The POEMS acronym stands for polyneuropathy, organomegaly, endocrinopathy, mono-

clonal gammopathy, and skin changes {1983}, but these components are not all required for diagnosis; in many cases, not all are present. The diagnostic criteria for POEMS syndrome are shown in Table 13.15 {1001}.

Synonyms
Osteosclerotic myeloma; Crow–Fukase syndrome

Epidemiology
POEMS syndrome is a rare disease, estimated to account for < 1% of plasma cell neoplasms. Many cases have been reported from Asia. Men are affected more often than women, with a male-to-female ratio of 1.4:1, and the median patient age is about 50 years {1006}.

Etiology
The etiology and pathogenesis of POEMS syndrome are not well understood, but markedly elevated levels of VEGF are present and appear to be an important pathogenic factor and to be responsible for some of the symptoms {1070,3737, 4266}. The pathophysiological connection between POEMS syndrome, osteosclerotic myeloma, and Castleman disease is not clearly defined. A few reported patients, typically with cases associated with Castleman disease, have been infected with HHV8 {318,1002,2671}.

Clinical features
The mandatory criteria for diagnosis of POEMS syndrome are a chronic progressive polyneuropathy and a monoclonal plasma cell proliferative disorder. There is usually an associated M protein of either IgG or IgA type, with lambda light chain restriction in almost all cases. The quantity of M protein is typically below myeloma levels (median: 1.1 g/dL) {1006}. In addition, patients must have one or more major and one or more minor criteria (Table 13.15) {1001,1003,2300}. Two thirds of patients with lymphadenopathy have changes consistent with the plasma cell variant of Castleman disease {1006}. Osteosclerotic bone lesions are present in >95% of cases {1003,1006}. These vary from single sclerotic lesions (seen in about half of patients) to >3 lesions (in one third of patients) {1006}. Plasma and serum VEGF is markedly elevated in nearly all cases, and the levels correlate with disease activity {1003,2300}. Organomegaly, primarily hepatomegaly or

Table 13.15 Diagnostic criteria for POEMS syndrome; adapted from Dispenzieri A {1001}

Mandatory criteria
Polyneuropathy (typically demyelinating)
Monoclonal plasma cell proliferative disorder
Major criteria (≥ 1 required)
Castleman disease
Osteosclerotic bone lesions
VEGF elevation
Minor criteria (≥ 1 required)
Organomegaly
Endocrinopathy
Skin changes
Papilloedema
Thrombocytosis
Extravascular volume overload

splenomegaly, is present in at least half of patients, and an endocrinopathy, most frequently hypogonadism or thyroid abnormality is found in more than two thirds of patients. Skin changes occur in more than two thirds of cases, most commonly hyperpigmentation and hypertrichosis {1003,1006,2300}. Other relatively common clinical findings include papilloedema, thrombocytosis, oedema and serous cavity effusions, weight loss, fatigue, fingernail clubbing, bone pain, and arthralgias. Hypercalcaemia, renal insufficiency, and pathological fractures are rare.

Microscopy
The characteristic lesion in bone marrow is a single or multiple osteosclerotic plasmacytoma. The lesion is composed of focally thickened trabecular bone with associated paratrabecular fibrosis containing entrapped plasma cells. The plasma cells may appear elongated due to distortion by small bands of connective tissue. In the bone marrow away from the osteosclerotic lesion, plasma cells are usually <5%, but can be >50% in patients with disseminated disease {867, 3738}. The plasma cells are distributed interstitially or in small or large clusters, depending on their abundance. Lymphoid aggregates rimmed by monotypic or polytypic plasma cells are found in half of patients. Megakaryocyte hyperplasia in clusters and often with atypical morphological features similar to those seen in myeloproliferative neoplasms is frequently observed {867}. Lymph node biopsies commonly reveal features of the plasma cell variant of Castleman disease {1006}.

Immunophenotype
In most patients with POEMS syndrome, a bone marrow monoclonal plasma cell population is detectable by flow cytometry or immunohistochemistry, frequently in a background of polyclonal plasma cells. The neoplastic plasma cells are of IgG or IgA type, and are lambda-restricted in almost all cases. The common phenotypic aberrancies found in other plasma cell neoplasms are also seen in POEMS syndrome {867,1006,3738}.

Genetic profile
The few published studies on the genetics of POEMS syndrome report abnormalities similar to those in plasma cell myeloma but with different prevalence rates {483,1924}. No significant correlations between genetic abnormalities and clinical features have been established {1924}.

Prognosis and predictive factors
In most cases, POEMS syndrome is a chronic and progressive disease but with a median overall survival as long as 165 months and a 5-year survival rate of 60–94% {856,1006,1983,2300}. Patients with localized plasma cell tumours treated with radiation therapy fare best, with improvement of the paraneoplastic symptoms and in some instances apparent cure {1003}. Several clinical factors are associated with shorter survival, including extravascular fluid overload, fingernail clubbing, respiratory symptoms, and pulmonary hypertension {1003,2300}. There are no known genetic findings that are predictors of prognosis {1003,1006}.

TEMPI syndrome

Definition
TEMPI syndrome is a paraneoplastic syndrome associated with a plasma cell neoplasm. The acronym stands for telangiectasias, elevated erythropoietin and erythrocytosis, monoclonal gammopathy, perinephric fluid collection, and intrapulmonary shunting. TEMPI syndrome is similar to POEMS syndrome in that its manifestations appear to result from the monoclonal plasma cell proliferation and associated M protein. However, the clinical and laboratory findings are mostly distinct from those of POEMS syndrome. Because TEMPI syndrome is a rare and only recently described disease, it is

included in the WHO classification as a provisional category of plasma cell neoplasm {17,2153,2684,3402,3585,3858}.

Epidemiology

TEMPI syndrome is a rare disease, with only 11 cases reported in the medical literature as of mid-2015 {3402}. The lack of familiarity with this disease until very recently and its propensity to mimic other disorders suggest that TEMPI syndrome may be underrecognized. The reported patient age range is 35–58 years, and it occurs in both men and women.

Etiology

There is no published information on the etiology of TEMPI syndrome. The successful results of treatment aimed at ablation of the monoclonal plasma cells suggest that the monoclonal plasma cells and their M protein product play a major role in the pathophysiology of the disease and its paraneoplastic manifestations {2153,3585}.

Localization

The clonal plasma cells producing TEMPI syndrome are in the bone marrow.

Clinical features

TEMPI syndrome has an insidious onset with slowly progressive symptoms, which may cause delay in diagnosis. Erythrocytosis seems to be a uniform feature, associated with a steadily progressive increase in erythropoietin to very high levels exceeding those produced by most other causes of erythrocytosis. Telangiectasia is reported in most cases, prominent on the face, trunk, arms, and hands. These findings appear to precede development of intrapulmonary shunting and hypoxia. The perinephric fluid, which collects between the kidney and its capsule, is clear, serous, and of low protein content. Spontaneous intracranial haemorrhage and venous thrombosis have been reported in some patients {3858}. M protein has been present in all reported cases. IgG kappa predominates; both IgG and IgA lambda have been reported in single cases {2153,2684,3402,3858}. In at least one patient, the serum free light chain ratio was skewed {2153}. Unlike in POEMS syndrome, VEGF levels are reportedly normal {3402}.

Microscopy

There are no reported blood or bone marrow morphological findings that are specific for TEMPI syndrome, but erythrocytosis and a hypercellular marrow due to erythroid hyperplasia are recurrent findings {3402}. Mild erythroid and megakaryocytic atypia has been described in one patient, and reactive lymphoid aggregates were present in another {3402}. Most patients have a percentage of bone marrow clonal plasma cells in the range of monoclonal gammopathy of undetermined significance (< 10%). Two patients have been reported to have had > 10% plasma cells (one diagnosed with smouldering plasma cell myeloma), but no case reported to date has fulfilled the criteria for the diagnosis of symptomatic plasma cell myeloma. Slight plasma cell atypia is generally present, with prominent cytoplasmic vacuolization reported in one case {2153,3402}.

Immunophenotype

The monoclonal plasma cell proliferation is most commonly IgG kappa, but both IgG and IgA lambda have also been reported. There are no detailed descriptions of the immunophenotype of the monoclonal plasma cells.

Prognosis and predictive factors

There is insufficient experience with TEMPI syndrome to predict its overall prognosis or risk factors, but it seems to be an indolent plasma cell neoplasm of low tumour burden, with symptomatology related to the constellation of paraneoplastic manifestations. Recognition of the disease and initiation of treatment before advanced symptoms develop seems key to successful management.

Complete or partial resolution of symptoms has been achieved through treatment with the proteasome inhibitor bortezomib {2153,3585}. A significant decrease in erythropoietin level following treatment is one indicator of good therapeutic response {3402}. In at least one case, a bortezomib regimen was followed by autologous stem cell transplantation, with complete remission and resolution of symptoms {3402}.

Extranodal marginal zone lymphoma of mucosa-associated lymphoid tissue (MALT lymphoma)

Cook J.R.
Isaacson P.G.
Chott A.
Nakamura S.
Müller-Hermelink H.K.
Harris N.L.
Swerdlow S.H.

Definition

Extranodal marginal zone lymphoma of mucosa-associated lymphoid tissue (MALT lymphoma) is an extranodal lymphoma composed of morphologically heterogeneous small B cells including marginal zone (centrocyte-like) cells, cells resembling monocytoid cells, small lymphocytes, and scattered immunoblasts and centroblast-like cells. There is plasmacytic differentiation in some cases. The neoplastic cells reside in the marginal zones of reactive B-cell follicles and extend into the interfollicular region as well as into the follicles (follicular colonization). In epithelial tissues, the neoplastic cells typically infiltrate the epithelium, forming lymphoepithelial lesions {1044,1782}. Thus, MALT lymphomas variably recapitulate Peyer's patch–type lymphoid tissue, the prototypical normal mucosa-associated lymphoid tissue (MALT). MALT lymphomas arising at any anatomical site share many characteristics, but there are also site-specific differences with respect to etiology, morphological features, molecular cytogenetic abnormalities, and clinical course {502, 1044,2140}.

ICD-O code   9699/3

Epidemiology

MALT lymphoma accounts for 7–8% of all B-cell lymphomas {1} and for as many as 50% of primary gastric lymphomas {1016,3275}. Most cases occur in adults, with a median patient age in the seventh decade of life. Men and women are about equally affected, although there are site-specific sex differences, with a female predominance reported for cases in the thyroid and salivary glands {1, 1999}. There is geographical variability, with a higher incidence of gastric MALT lymphoma reported in north-eastern Italy {1016}, and a special subtype called alpha heavy chain disease (also known as immunoproliferative small intestinal disease) occurs in the Middle East {48,4230}, the Cape region of South Africa {3239}, and a variety of other tropical and subtropical locations (see *Alpha heavy chain disease*, p. 240).

Etiology

In many MALT lymphoma cases, there is a history of a chronic inflammatory disorder that results in accumulation of extranodal lymphoid tissue (called acquired MALT). The chronic inflammation may be the result of infection, autoimmunity, or unknown other stimuli.

The link between infection and MALT lymphoma is most clearly established for *Helicobacter pylori* and gastric MALT

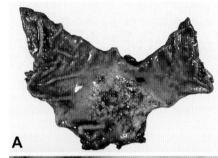
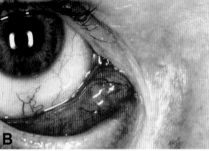

Fig. 13.57 MALT lymphoma. **A** Resection specimen of a gastric MALT lymphoma. **B** MALT lymphoma of the conjunctiva.

lymphoma {1199,3954}. The continued proliferation of gastric MALT lymphoma cells from patients infected with *H. pylori* depends on the presence of T cells specifically activated by *H. pylori* antigens and/or direct oncogenic effects of *H. pylori* proteins on B cells {1741,2137}. The importance of this stimulation in vivo has been clearly demonstrated by the

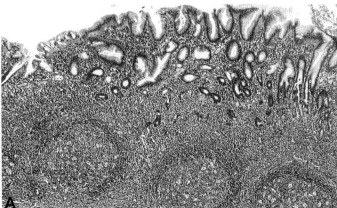
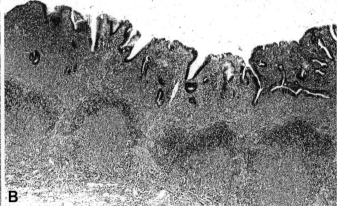

Fig. 13.58 Gastric MALT lymphoma. **A** The tumour cells surround reactive follicles and infiltrate the mucosa. The follicles have a typical starry-sky appearance. **B** The marginal zone cells infiltrate the lamina propria in a diffuse pattern and have colonized the germinal centres of reactive B-cell follicles. The colonized follicles do not show a starry-sky pattern.

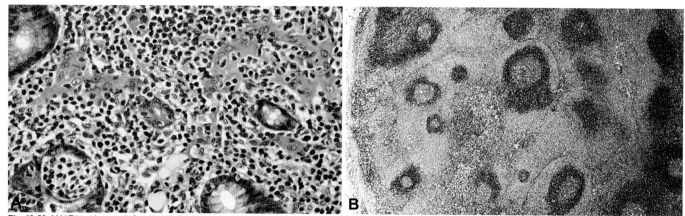

Fig. 13.59 MALT lymphoma. **A** Gastric MALT lymphoma with prominent lymphoepithelial lesions. **B** Gastric lymph node involved by MALT lymphoma. The tumour cells infiltrate the marginal zones and spread into the interfollicular areas.

induction of remissions in gastric MALT lymphomas with antibiotic therapy to eradicate *H. pylori* {4366}. In the first study in which the association of gastric MALT lymphoma with *H. pylori* infection was examined, the organism was present in >90% of cases {4367}. More recent studies, in the era of antibiotic eradication therapy for *H. pylori* gastritis, suggest that the overall incidence of gastric MALT lymphoma is decreasing, and that a much smaller proportion of cases (32%) are now associated with *H. pylori* at diagnosis {2414, 3621}.

A role for antigenic stimulation by *Chlamydia psittaci* and *Borrelia burgdorferi* has been proposed for some cases of ocular adnexal MALT lymphoma and cutaneous MALT lymphoma, respectively {611,1199,1201}. There is great variation in the strength of these associations, which might relate in part to geographical diversity {658,2296,3454}. A similar role has been proposed for *Campylobacter* infection in patients with alpha heavy chain disease.

In other cases, acquired MALT secondary to autoimmune disease may serve as the substrate for lymphoma development {1779}. Autoimmune-based chronic inflammation in the form of Sjögren syndrome and Hashimoto thyroiditis is known to precede salivary gland and thyroid MALT lymphomas, respectively. Patients with primary Sjögren syndrome have an estimated risk of lymphoma 14–19 times that of the general population {2319, 4497}; most lymphomas in patients with Sjögren syndrome are MALT lymphomas. In patients with Hashimoto thyroiditis, the risk of developing lymphoma is 3 times that in the general population, and the risk of thyroid lymphoma 70 times that in the general population, for an overall lymphoma risk of 0.5–1.5% {117,1671, 1959}. Approximately 90% of thyroid lymphomas have evidence of lymphocytic thyroiditis {957,4265}.

Localization

The stomach is the most common site of MALT lymphoma, affected in 35% of all cases. Other common sites include the eyes and ocular adnexa (affected in 13% of cases), skin (9%), lungs (9%), salivary glands (8%), breasts (3%), and thyroid (2%) {1999}.

Clinical features

Most patients present with stage I or II disease, but 23–40% have involvement of multiple extranodal sites {1905, 2140}. Staging in patients with multiple extranodal lesions may be challenging, because at least some cases constitute multiple clonally unrelated proliferations rather than truly disseminated disease {2081}. Making this distinction may not be possible in routine practice. A minority of patients (2–20%) have bone marrow involvement {148,3276,3953}. The frequency of bone marrow involvement and involvement of multiple extranodal sites is higher in non-gastric MALT lymphoma than in gastric cases. Generalized nodal involvement is rare (reported in < 10% of cases) {1905,2140,3952}. Plasmacytic

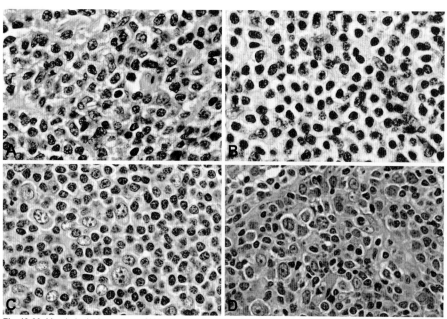

Fig. 13.60 Morphological spectrum of MALT lymphoma cells. **A** Neoplastic marginal zone B cells with nuclei resembling those of centrocytes, but with more-abundant cytoplasm. **B** The cells of this MALT lymphoma have abundant pale-staining cytoplasm, resulting in a monocytoid appearance. **C** Lymphoma cells resembling small lymphocytes. There are scattered transformed cells. **D** Increased number of large cells.

differentiation is a feature of many of the cases, and a serum paraprotein can be detected in one third of patients with MALT lymphoma {4381}.

Microscopy

The characteristic marginal zone B cells have small to medium-sized, slightly irregular nuclei with moderately dispersed chromatin and inconspicuous nucleoli, resembling those of centrocytes, and relatively abundant, pale cytoplasm. The accumulation of even more pale-staining cytoplasm may lead to a monocytoid appearance, which is especially common in salivary gland MALT lymphomas. Alternatively, the marginal zone cells may more closely resemble small lymphocytes. Plasmacytic differentiation is present in approximately one third of gastric MALT lymphomas, is frequently found in cutaneous MALT lymphomas, and is a constant and often striking feature in thyroid MALT lymphomas. In some MALT lymphomas, there is a marked predominance of plasma cells, resulting in resemblance to an extramedullary plasmacytoma. Cutaneous plasmacytomas are diagnosed as MALT lymphoma. Amyloid deposition is seen in some cases. Large cells resembling centroblasts or immunoblasts are usually present, but are in the minority.

The lymphoma cells infiltrate around reactive B-cell follicles external to a preserved mantle in a marginal zone distribution, and spread out to form larger confluent areas that eventually replace some or most of the follicles, often leaving small remnants of germinal centres, which can be highlighted by negativity for BCL2 {1784,1785}. The lymphoma cells sometimes specifically colonize reactive germinal centres; in extreme ex-

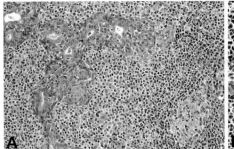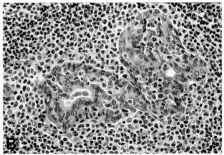

Fig. 13.61 MALT lymphoma of salivary gland. **A** Reactive B-cell follicle is surrounded by neoplastic marginal zone cells that invade salivary duct remnants. **B** Lymphoid cells with pale cytoplasm are present in and around the lymphoepithelial lesions.

amples, this can lead to a close resemblance to follicular lymphoma. Lymphoepithelial lesions, defined as aggregates of ≥3 marginal zone cells with distortion or destruction of the epithelium, may be seen in glandular tissues, often together with eosinophilic degeneration (oxyphilic change) of epithelial cells.

In lymph nodes, MALT lymphoma invades the marginal zone, with subsequent interfollicular expansion. Discrete aggregates of monocytoid-like B cells may be present in a parafollicular and perisinusoidal distribution. Cytological heterogeneity is still present, and both plasmacytic differentiation and follicular colonization may be seen.

MALT lymphoma, by definition, is a lymphoma composed predominantly of small cells. Transformed centroblast-like or immunoblast-like cells may be present in variable numbers, but when solid or sheet-like proliferations of transformed cells are present, the tumour should be diagnosed as diffuse large B-cell lymphoma (DLBCL) and the presence of accompanying MALT lymphoma noted. The term 'high-grade MALT lymphoma' should not be used, and the term 'MALT lymphoma'

should not be applied to a DLBCL even if it has arisen in a MALT site or is associated with lymphoepithelial lesions.

Immunophenotype

The neoplastic cells of MALT lymphoma are CD20+, CD79a+, CD5–, CD10–, CD23–, CD43+/–, and CD11c+/– (weak). Infrequent cases are CD5+, and very rare cases are CD10+ but BCL6– {2140,3954}. Staining for CD21, CD23, and CD35 typically reveals expanded meshworks of follicular dendritic cells, corresponding to colonized follicles. The demonstration of light chain restriction is helpful in the differential diagnosis with reactive hyperplasia. Recent reports have highlighted IRTA1 as a possible specific marker for marginal zone lymphomas, including MALT lymphoma, although IRTA1 antibodies are not yet widely available {1137, 1154}. MNDA staining may facilitate the differential diagnosis of MALT lymphoma versus follicular lymphoma, because this nuclear antigen is expressed in 61–75% of MALT lymphomas but < 10% of follicular lymphomas {1922,2645}.

The tumour cells of MALT lymphoma typically express IgM heavy chains, and less

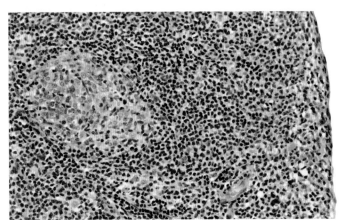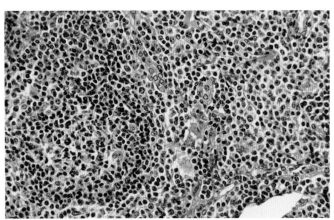

Fig. 13.62 Conjunctival MALT lymphoma. Neoplastic marginal zone cells infiltrate around a reactive follicle and infiltrate overlying epithelium.

Fig. 13.63 Pulmonary MALT lymphoma showing a reactive B-cell follicle surrounded by neoplastic marginal zone cells that infiltrate bronchiolar epithelium (lower right).

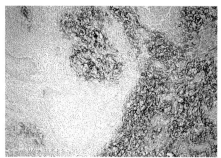

Fig. 13.64 MALT lymphoma. Immunohistochemistry for CD21 highlights expanded and distorted follicular dendritic cell meshworks in this salivary gland MALT lymphoma with follicular colonization.

often IgA or IgG. A notable exception is cutaneous marginal zone lymphoma, of which two subsets have been described: a more common class-switched subset (accounting for 75–85% of cases) with IgG (including many IgG4+ cases) or IgA expression and usually a T-cell–predominant background, and a less common (15–25% of cases) IgM+ subset that tends to be B-cell–predominant {455, 1080,4137}.

Postulated normal counterpart

A post–germinal centre marginal-zone B cell

Genetic profile

IG heavy and light chain genes are rearranged and show somatic hypermutation of variable regions {1043,3254}. There is biased usage of certain IGHV gene families at different anatomical sites, suggesting antigen-induced clonal expansion during the process of lymphomagenesis {1905,3954}.
Chromosomal translocations associated with MALT lymphomas include t(11;18)

(q21;q21), t(1;14)(p22;q32), t(14;18) (q32;q21), and t(3;14)(p14.1;q32), resulting in the production of a chimeric protein (BIRC3-MALT1) and in transcriptional deregulation of *BCL10*, *MALT1*, and *FOXP1*, respectively {1044,3813}. Trisomy of chromosome 3 or 18 (or less commonly of other chromosomes) is a non-specific but also not infrequent finding in MALT lymphomas. The frequencies at which the translocations or trisomies occur vary markedly with the primary site of disease. The t(11;18)(q21;q21) translocation is mainly detected in pulmonary and gastric tumours; t(14;18)(q32;q21) in ocular adnexa, orbit, and salivary gland lesions; and t(3;14)(p14.1;q32) in MALT lymphomas arising in the thyroid, ocular adnexa, orbit, and skin (Table 13.16). Similarly, geographical variability in incidence and anatomical site specificity of the translocations has been noted, suggesting different environmental influences, such as infectious and other etiological factors {3340,3813}.
Abnormalities of *TNFAIP3* on chromosome 6q23, which may include deletions, mutations, and promoter methylation, occur in 15–30% of cases, most frequently cases lacking specific translocations {657,1045,2898}. However, *TNFAIP3* abnormalities are not specific for MALT lymphoma, and can be found in many types of non-Hodgkin lymphoma {1681}. *MYD88* L265P mutation has been reported in 6–9% of MALT lymphomas {1267, 2315,2860}.

Prognosis and predictive factors

MALT lymphomas have an indolent natural course and are slow to disseminate. Recurrences, which can occur after many

years, may involve other extranodal sites and occur more often in patients with extragastric MALT lymphomas than in patients with primary gastric disease {3276}. Cutaneous marginal zone lymphomas have a particularly indolent course, with 5-year survival rates approaching 100% {4320}. MALT lymphomas are sensitive to radiation therapy, and local treatment may be followed by prolonged disease-free intervals. Involvement of multiple extranodal sites and even bone marrow involvement do not appear to confer a worse prognosis {3953,3954}.
Protracted remissions may be induced in *H. pylori*–associated gastric MALT lymphoma by antibiotic therapy for *H. pylori* {2853,4366}. The presence or absence of *H. pylori* should be investigated in both gastric MALT lymphoma and gastric DLBCL, because some primary gastric DLBCLs may also respond to antibiotic eradication therapy alone {676,1200}. Cases with t(11;18)(q21;q21) appear to be resistant to *H. pylori* eradication therapy {2366}. Antibiotics have also been used to successfully treat selected other MALT lymphomas. Transformation to DLBCL may occur but is uncommon (reported in < 10% of cases) {3953,3954}.

Table 13.16 Anatomical site distribution and frequency of chromosomal translocations and trisomies 3 and 18 in MALT lymphomas. Data summarized according to Streubel B et al. {3812} and Remstein ED et al. {3340}

| Site of disease | Frequency (%) | | | | | |
	t(11;18)(q21;q21)	t(14;18)(q32;q21)	t(3;14)(p14.1;q32)	t(1;14)(p22;q32)	+3	+18
Stomach	6–26	1–5	0	0	11	6
Intestine	12–56	0	0	0–13	75	25
Ocular adnexa / orbit	0–10	0–25	0–20	0	38	13
Salivary gland	0–5	0–16	0	0–2	55	19
Lung	31–53	6–10	0	2–7	20	7
Skin	0–8	0–14	0–10	0	20	4
Thyroid	0–17	0	0–50	0	17	0

Nodal marginal zone lymphoma

Campo E.
Pileri S.A.
Jaffe E.S.

Nathwani B.N.
Stein H.
Müller-Hermelink H.K.

Definition
Nodal marginal zone lymphoma (NMZL) is a primary nodal B-cell neoplasm that morphologically resembles lymph nodes involved by marginal zone lymphoma (MZL) of the extranodal or splenic types, but without evidence of extranodal or splenic disease.

ICD-O code
9699/3

Synonyms
Monocytoid B-cell lymphoma; parafollicular B-cell lymphoma (obsolete)

Epidemiology
NMZL accounts for only 1.5–1.8% of all lymphoid neoplasms, and has an annual incidence of 0.8 cases per 100 000 adults {106,347,2834}. Most cases occur in adults, with a median age of ~60 years, and the proportion of males and females affected is similar {106,4123}. This lymphoma can also occur in children, and is then separately designated as paediatric NMZL {3866}. A significantly increased incidence has been observed among females with autoimmune disorders {442}. A relationship to hepatitis C virus infection has been detected in some studies {137,4503}, but not in others {442,4046}.

Localization
NMZL involves peripheral lymph nodes, but can also involve the bone marrow and occasionally the peripheral blood {106,347,2834,4123}.

Clinical features
Most patients present with asymptomatic, localized, or generalized peripheral lymphadenopathy {137,347}. The head and neck lymph nodes are more frequently involved {4123}. B symptoms are present in 10–20% of patients. Bone marrow infiltration is seen in one third of patients {4123}. The presence of a primary extranodal MZL should be ruled out, because approximately one third of cases presenting as NMZL in fact constitute nodal dissemination of a MALT lymphoma, which is particularly common in patients with Hashimoto thyroiditis or Sjögren syndrome {542}.

Microscopy
Lymph nodes demonstrate a small-cell lymphoid proliferation that surrounds reactive follicles and expands into the interfollicular areas. Follicular colonization may be present. In cases with a diffuse pattern, follicle remnants may be detected with immunohistochemical stains for follicular dendritic cells and germinal centre markers. The neoplastic cells are composed of variable numbers of marginal zone (centrocyte-like and monocytoid) B cells, plasma cells in some cases, and scattered transformed B cells {533, 2834,2884,4046}. Cases with a predominant monocytoid B-cell population are uncommon. Plasma cell differentiation may be prominent, and the differential diagnosis with lymphoplasmacytic lymphoma or even nodal plasmacytoma may be difficult. The presence of remnants of follicular dendritic cell meshworks suggestive of colonized follicles favours the diagnosis of NMZL. Prominent eosinophilia may be present. Some cases have more-numerous large transformed cells (sometimes > 20%). However, these cells are usually mixed with small cells and may be more common in the colonized germinal centres {2834,4046}. Some cases mimic splenic MZL, with the neoplastic cells being small to medium-sized lymphocytes with pale cytoplasm and occasional transformed cells growing inside an attenuated mantle zone and often around a residual germinal centre {542}. Composite NMZL and Hodgkin lymphoma have been reported {4473}.

Bone marrow involvement is usually interstitial or nodular, with an intertrabecular or paratrabecular distribution. An intrasinusoidal infiltration may be seen but is less common {437,1757}.

Immunophenotype
Most NMZLs express pan–B-cell markers, with CD43 coexpression in 20–75% of cases {3486}. CD23 is usually negative, but may be expressed in as many as 29% of cases {4123}. CD5 expression

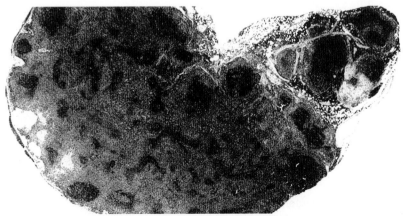
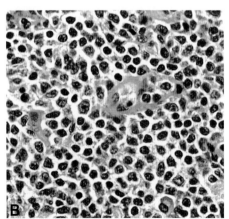

Fig. 13.65 Nodal marginal zone lymphoma. **A** Reactive follicles are separated by an interfollicular infiltrate of paler-staining cells. **B** The neoplastic cells have irregularly shaped nuclei and moderately abundant pale cytoplasm. Occasional plasma cells and transformed blasts are present.

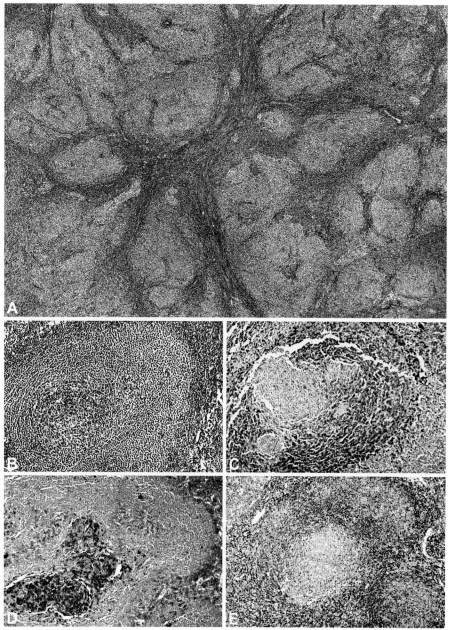

Fig. 13.66 Splenic-type nodal marginal zone lymphoma. **A** At low magnification, note the follicular growth pattern, with pale cells that focally surround portions of reactive germinal centres. **B** The tumour is composed of a proliferation of small cells growing between a reactive germinal centre and an attenuated mantle zone. **C** IgD stain shows the weak positivity of the tumour cells that surround the negative germinal centre, whereas the residual mantle cells are strongly positive. **D** CD10 stain. The tumour cells are negative, whereas the residual germinal centre is positive. **E** BCL2 stain. The tumour cells are positive, whereas the reactive germinal centre is negative.

may be seen in as many as 17% of tumours, which tend to have more disseminated disease, although with no impact on prognosis {1845,4123}. Cyclin D1 is negative {4123}. Germinal centre markers (CD10, BCL6, HGAL, and LMO2) are rarely reported. The coexpression of more than one of these germinal centre markers in interfollicular areas is very unusual and favours the diagnosis of follicular lymphoma {1071}. BCL2 is positive in most cases {4123}. MNDA and IRTA1 are expressed in 75% of cases, and are usually negative in follicular lymphoma {394,1922,4123}. IgD is usually negative. Tumours mimicking splenic MZL have a similar phenotype but are usually IgD-positive {542}.

Postulated normal counterpart

A post–germinal centre marginal-zone B cell

Genetic profile

The IG genes are clonally rearranged, with a predominance of mutated IGHV3 and IGHV4 family members, in particular IGHV4-34 {533,4045}. Cases associated with hepatitis C virus preferentially use IGHV1-69 {2499,4123}.

NMZL shares gains of chromosomes 3 and 18 and loss of 6q23-24 with extranodal MZL of mucosa-associated lymphoid tissue (MALT lymphoma) and splenic MZL. However, deletions in 7q31 and the recurrent translocations associated with extranodal MZL are not detected {443,983,3362,4046}.

Gene expression profiling analysis has demonstrated an increased expression of NF-kappaB–related genes {154}. *MYD88* L265P mutation is usually absent but has been detected in occasional cases not specifically associated with plasmacytic differentiation {1527,2534,3851}.

Prognosis and predictive factors

The 5-year overall survival rate is about 60–70% {137}. Advanced patient age, B symptoms, and advanced disease stage are associated with a worse prognosis {106}. However, on a multivariate analysis, only the Follicular Lymphoma International Prognostic Index (FLIPI) applied to these patients predicted overall survival {137}. The proportion of scattered or clustered large cells does not appear to be of prognostic significance {4046}. However, transformation to diffuse large B-cell lymphoma may occur. This diagnosis requires the presence of sheets of large cells {2687}.

Paediatric nodal marginal zone lymphoma

Definition

Paediatric nodal marginal zone lymphoma (NMZL) has distinctive clinical and morphological characteristics {3866}. It presents predominantly in males (with a male-to-female ratio of 20:1) with asymptomatic and localized disease (stage I in 90% of cases), mainly in the head and neck lymph nodes. Histologically, it is similar to adult NMZL, except that there are often large follicles with extension of mantle zone B cells into the germinal centres, resembling progressively transformed germinal centres. The immunophenotype is similar to that of adult NMZL, with expansion of the interfollicu-

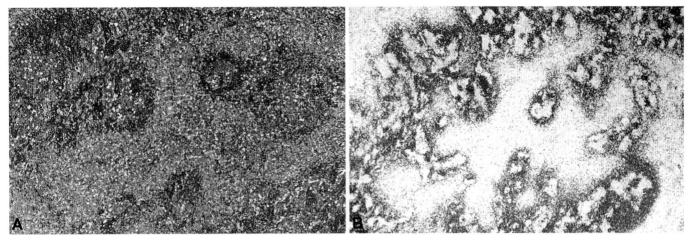

Fig. 13.67 Paediatric nodal marginal zone lymphoma. **A** These lymphomas commonly exhibit progressive transformation of germinal centres. The atypical cells are found primarily in the interfollicular areas and may disrupt the follicles. **B** IgD stain highlights the disrupted and expanded mantle zone; the tumour cells are IgD-negative.

lar areas by CD20+ B cells that commonly coexpress CD43 {3866}. Light chain restriction can often be demonstrated by immunohistochemistry or flow cytometry {3366}. IgD staining may help to delineate an irregular and expanded mantle zone. BCL2 is positive in half of the cases. CD10 is usually negative {3272}. Staining for CD279/PD1 shows numerous positive cells in the reactive germinal centres, a feature that may help in the differential diagnosis with paediatric-type follicular lymphoma, in which these cells are less numerous and pushed to the periphery of the germinal centre {2369,3272}.

Clonal rearrangements of the IGHV region are detected in almost all cases {3366}. Trisomy 18 may be present in approximately one fifth of cases, and occasionally trisomy 3 {3366}. The prognosis of paediatric NMZL is excellent, with a very low relapse rate and long survival following conservative treatment {3272, 3866}.

The differential diagnosis with atypical marginal zone hyperplasia with monotypic immunoglobulin expression may be difficult, because the large cells in this condition also express CD43 {183}; although this type of hyperplasia has been

reported in extranodal sites, some caution is advised because a similar process might also occur in the lymph nodes. Particularly for these reasons, genetic studies in paediatric marginal zone lymphomas are strongly recommended {3866}. A marginal zone hyperplasia mimicking NMZL in head and neck lymph nodes of children has been associated with *Haemophilus influenzae*. The marginal zone cells in these cases are IgD-positive {2046}.

ICD-O code   9699/3

Follicular lymphoma

Jaffe E.S.
Harris N.L.
Swerdlow S.H.
Ott G.
Nathwani B.N.

de Jong D.
Yoshino T.
Spagnolo D.
Gascoyne R.D.

Definition

Follicular lymphoma (FL) is a neoplasm composed of follicle centre (germinal centre) B cells (typically both centrocytes and centroblasts/large transformed cells), which usually has at least a partially follicular pattern. Lymphomas composed of centrocytes and centroblasts with an entirely diffuse pattern in the sampled tissue may be included in this category, but are relatively rare at presentation. Progression in cytological grade is common during the natural history of the disease. A diffuse lymphoma composed of centroblasts is considered evidence of progression to diffuse large B-cell lymphoma (DLBCL). Four variants of FL are recognized: (1) in situ follicular neoplasia, formerly called FL in situ; (2) duodenal-type FL; (3) testicular FL; and (4) the diffuse variant of FL.

Primary cutaneous follicle centre lymphomas are separately classified {2242, 3848}. FL is nearly exclusively a disease of adults, and very rarely occurs in patients aged < 18 years. Paediatric-type FL, which is a nodal lymphoma that occurs in children and young adults, is considered a separate entity.

ICD-O codes

Follicular lymphoma	9690/3
Grade 1	9695/3
Grade 2	9691/3
Grade 3A	9698/3
Grade 3B	9698/3

Epidemiology

FL accounts for about 20% of all lymphomas. The highest incidence rates are reported in the USA and western Europe. In eastern Europe, Asia, and developing countries, the incidence is much lower {95}. It affects predominantly adults, with a median age in the sixth decade of life and a male-to-female ratio of 1:1.7 {1}. FL is 2–3 times as common in White populations as in Black populations {1477}. Unlike paediatric-type FL, usual FL rarely occurs in individuals aged < 18 years. Agricultural exposure to pesticides and herbicides has been associated with an increased risk {33,1257,3678}.

Etiology

Individuals with a high environmental exposure to pesticides and herbicides have increased numbers of cells carrying t(14;18)(q32;q21) (IGH/BCL2) in the peripheral blood {33}. This may help explain the reported increased risk of FL among such individuals.

Localization

FL predominantly involves the lymph nodes, but also involves the spleen, bone marrow, peripheral blood, and less commonly Waldeyer ring. Any nodal group can be involved, but most patients present with peripheral lymphadenopathy. Pure extranodal presentations are uncommon. The most commonly affected extranodal sites include the gastrointestinal tract (often in association with mesenteric lymph node involvement), soft tissue, breast, and ocular adnexa. FL arising in the small intestine, in particular the duodenum, has distinctive features (duodenal-type FL).

FLs can occur in almost any extranodal site {1203}. In some cases, the morphology, phenotype, and genetics are similar to those of nodal FL. However, many FLs in extranodal sites tend to be of higher grade (grade 3), and may lack BCL2 protein and the BCL2 translocation {3021, 4148}.

Clinical features

Most patients have widespread disease at diagnosis, including peripheral and central (abdominal and thoracic) lymphadenopathy and splenomegaly. The bone marrow is involved in 40–70% of cases. Only 15–25% of cases are stage I or II at the time of diagnosis {1632}. Despite widespread disease, patients are usually otherwise asymptomatic. B symptoms such as fever and weight loss are uncommon. Waxing and waning of the disease without therapy is common. The disease follows a chronic relapsing clinical course.

Imaging

Conventional imaging tools such as CT and MRI are useful in assessing the de-

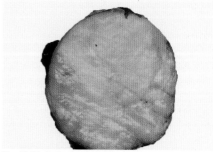

Fig. 13.68 Follicular lymphoma, lymph node. Vague nodules bulge from the cut surface.

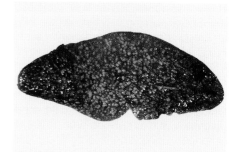

Fig. 13.69 Follicular lymphoma, spleen. The white pulp is expanded, with multiple pale nodules throughout the spleen. The red pulp is unremarkable.

gree of lymphadenopathy and extent of disease. FDG-PET is less useful in assessing disease than in more aggressive lymphomas. However, the detection of PET-avid disease may be useful in identifying patients with higher risk for progression {112}.

Staging

The stage of the disease is now determined using the Lugano classification, a modification of the Ann Arbor staging system {691}. Assessment of bone marrow involvement should be accomplished with bone marrow biopsy. Bone marrow aspiration has a lower yield, due to the difficulty is aspirating cells from the paratrabecular lymphoid aggregates. The designation of a case as A or B (asymptomatic or symptomatic) is no longer required for non-Hodgkin lymphoma subtypes, according to the Lugano system.

Macroscopy

The cut surface of lymph nodes involved

by FL displays a vaguely nodular pattern that can be seen macroscopically. The neoplastic follicles often have a bulging appearance. However, reactive follicular hyperplasia can display the same pattern. Spleens involved by FL show uniform expansion of the white pulp, usually with no evidence of involvement of the red pulp.

Microscopy

Pattern

Most cases of FL have a predominantly follicular pattern, with closely packed follicles that efface the nodal architecture. Neoplastic follicles are often poorly defined and usually have attenuated or absent mantle zones. Unlike in reactive germinal centres, where the proportion of centroblasts and centrocytes varies in different zones (polarization), in FL the two types of cells are randomly distributed. Similarly, tingible body macrophages, characteristic of reactive germinal centres, are usually absent in FL. In some cases, follicles may be irregular and serpiginous, but this growth pattern does not constitute progression to a diffuse growth pattern. Staining for follicular dendritic cell (FDC) markers (CD21 and/ or CD23) can be helpful in highlighting the follicular pattern. Interfollicular infiltration by neoplastic cells is common and does not constitute a diffuse pattern. The interfollicular neoplastic cells are often centrocytes that are smaller than those in the germinal centres, with a less irregular nuclear contour, and they may show immunophenotypic differences from the cells in the germinal centres {1015}. Infrequent cases have a so-called floral growth pattern that resembles progressively transformed germinal centres {4004}.

Spread beyond the lymph node capsule is often associated with sclerosis, particularly in mesenteric and retroperitoneal locations. With limited sampling in small biopsies, it may be difficult to appreciate a follicular pattern. A diffuse area is defined as an area of the tissue completely lacking follicles as evidenced by the absence of CD21+/CD23+ FDCs. The distinction between an extensive interfollicular component and a diffuse component is sometimes arbitrary. Diffuse areas composed predominantly of centrocytes are not thought to be clinically significant. Nevertheless, it is recommended that the relative proportions

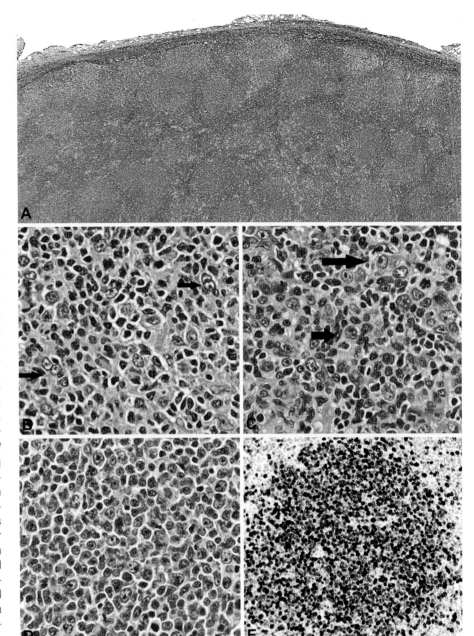

Fig. 13.70 Follicular lymphoma. **A** The neoplastic follicles are closely packed, focally show an almost back-to-back pattern, and lack mantle zones. **B,C** Follicular lymphoma, grade 1–2. **B** Most of the cells in the field are centrocytes. Follicular dendritic cells with so-called kissing nuclei are noted (arrows). **C** There are < 15 centroblasts per high-power field. Two centroblasts are noted with arrows. **D,E** Follicular lymphoma, grade 3A. **D** Both centrocytes and centroblasts are present, but there are > 15 centroblasts per high-power field. Both small and large centroblasts are present. **E** MIB1 antibody staining for Ki-67 highlights both small and large centroblasts and indicates a high proliferation rate.

of follicular and diffuse areas be noted in the pathology report as follicular (> 75% follicular), follicular and diffuse (25–75% follicular), or focally follicular / predominantly diffuse (< 25% follicular) {1556}. However, the presence of diffuse areas composed entirely or predominantly of large centroblasts (that would fulfil the criteria for grade 3 FL) in FL of any grade is equivalent to DLBCL, and a separate

diagnosis of DLBCL should be made {1556} (see *Grading*).

Some cases have the morphology and immunophenotype of FL but with no evidence of a follicular growth pattern. This phenomenon is usually seen in small biopsy specimens, and likely constitutes a diffuse area in an FL that was not adequately sampled. A repeat biopsy in the same or another site may reveal a follicu-

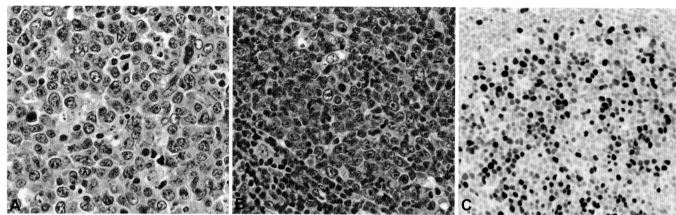

Fig. 13.71 Follicular lymphoma, grade 3B. **A** The follicle is composed of a uniform population of centroblasts, with no evident centrocytes. **B** This case was negative for CD10 but positive for IRF4/MUM1. Such cases are often negative for the *BCL2* translocation {1944}. The border of the neoplastic follicle is shown at lower left. **C** The neoplastic cells show nuclear staining for IRF4/MUM1, but are negative for CD10.

lar pattern. This situation should be distinguished from the diffuse variant of FL usually lacking the *BCL2* rearrangement described below.

Cytology

FL is typically composed of the two types of B cells normally found in germinal centres. Small to medium-sized cells with angulated, elongated, twisted, or cleaved nuclei; inconspicuous nucleoli; and scant pale cytoplasm are called centrocytes. Large centrocytes with dispersed chromatin and inconspicuous nucleoli may also be present. Large cells with usually round or oval nuclei, vesicular chromatin, 1–3 peripheral nucleoli, and a rim of cyto-

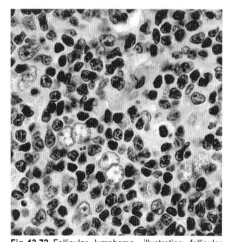

Fig. 13.72 Follicular lymphoma, illustrating follicular dendritic cells (FDCs). Two binucleate FDCs are present in the centre of the field. The nuclei are round (but with flattening of adjacent nuclear membranes) and have bland, dispersed chromatin with one small, centrally located nucleolus. The cytoplasm is not seen in H&E-stained or Giemsa-stained sections. Centroblasts, unlike FDCs, have vesicular chromatin and multiple distinct nucleoli that are usually located adjacent to the nuclear membranes.

plasm are called centroblasts. Typically, they are ≥3 times the size of lymphocytes, but they may be smaller in some cases. Centrocytes predominate in most cases; centroblasts are always present, but are usually in the minority. The number of centroblasts varies from case to case and is the basis of grading. In some cases, neoplastic centroblasts have irregular or multilobed nuclei. Rare cases of FL are composed of blastoid-appearing cells with dispersed chromatin resembling lymphoblasts {4250}. This variant appears to have an aggressive clinical course, equivalent to grade 3. Unlike in reactive germinal centres, polarization is usually absent, and starry-sky histiocytes are absent or few in number.

In about 10% of FLs, there are discrete foci of marginal zone or monocytoid-appearing B cells, typically at the periphery of the neoplastic follicles {1407, 2833,4029}. These cells are part of the neoplastic clone {3374}. Plasmacytic differentiation can be seen uncommonly. In cases with plasmacytic differentiation, the plasmacytoid cells have an interfollicular distribution and carry the *BCL2* translocation, indicating they are part of the neoplastic clone {1418}. Other cases resembling FL have intrafollicular plasmacytoid cells and lack the translocation. Such t(14;18)-negative cases might constitute an unusual variant of marginal zone lymphoma with follicular colonization.

Bone marrow and blood

In bone marrow, FL characteristically localizes to the paratrabecular region and may spread into the interstitial areas. A follicular growth pattern with a meshwork

of FDCs can be rarely seen. The morphology of the tumour cells most commonly resembles that of the neoplastic interfollicular cells in lymph nodes. The same cells may be seen in the peripheral blood.

Diffuse follicular lymphoma variant

A novel diffuse FL variant is characterized by a predominantly diffuse growth pattern and consistent absence of the t(14;18)(q32;q21) (IGH/*BCL2*) chromosomal translocation {1962,3670A}. In all cases, small follicles or so-called microfollicles are seen, with weak to absent BCL2 staining. This particular FL variant mainly occurs in the inguinal region, forming larger tumours, but with little tendency to disseminate. The neoplastic cells are usually CD10-positive, and in almost all cases express the CD23 antigen as well. These cases cluster with typical FL by gene expression profiling. A recurrent genetic aberration, deletion in 1p36, is seen in most cases. These alterations are not specific to this variant; the region at 1p36, which contains *TNFRSF14*, is also commonly affected in t(14;18)–positive FL.

Testicular follicular lymphoma

Testicular FLs {1219} are a distinctive variant of FL. They are reported with higher frequency in children, but are also seen rarely in adults {214}. They differ biologically from nodal FL in that they lack evidence of the *BCL2* translocation. Cytologically they are of high cytological grade, usually grade 3A, but have a good prognosis, even without additional therapy beyond surgical excision {1608, 2369,2386}.

Immunophenotype

The tumour cells are usually positive for surface immunoglobulin (IgM with or without IgD, IgG, or rarely IgA). They express B-cell–associated antigens (CD19, CD20, CD22, and CD79a) and are usually positive for BCL2, BCL6, and CD10 and negative for CD5 and CD43. Some cases, that are most commonly grade 3B, lack CD10 but retain BCL6 expression {424,584,1944,2190,3008,3199}. CD10 expression is often stronger in the follicles than in interfollicular neoplastic cells, and may be absent in the interfollicular component as well as in areas of marginal zone differentiation, peripheral blood, and bone marrow {1015,1558}. BCL6 is frequently downregulated in the interfollicular areas and is more variably expressed than in normal germinal centres. Other germinal centre markers, such as LMO2, GCET1, and HGAL (also called GCET2), are positive, but are generally not required for routine diagnosis {2634, 2840,3043}. However, they may be useful in the differential diagnosis of FL and marginal zone lymphoma with follicular colonization. CD5 is expressed in rare cases of FL, possibly more frequently in those with a floral growth pattern {2313, 4004}. Meshworks of FDCs are present in follicular areas {4505} but are usually sparser and more irregularly distributed than in normal follicles. They may variably express CD21 and CD23, so antibodies to both antigens may be needed to detect FDC meshworks.

BCL2 overexpression is the hallmark of FL, and BCL2 protein is expressed by a variable proportion of the neoplastic cells in 85–90% of cases of grade 1–2 FL, but in <50% of grade 3 FLs {2189}. In some cases, the apparent absence of

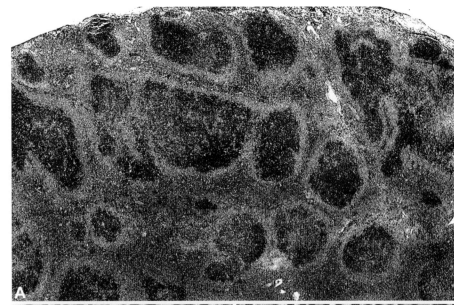

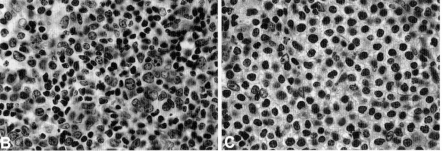

Fig. 13.73 Follicular lymphoma, grade 1–2, with marginal zone differentiation. **A** At the periphery of the follicles, there is a pale rim corresponding to marginal zone differentiation. **B** The centres of the follicles contain the typical mixture of centrocytes and centroblasts. **C** The cells at the periphery of the follicles are medium-sized cells with slightly irregular nuclei and abundant lightly eosinophilic to pale-staining cytoplasm, consistent with marginal zone or monocytoid B cells.

BCL2 protein is due to mutations in the *BCL2* gene that eliminate the epitopes recognized by the most commonly used antibody; however, BCL2 can be detected in those cases using antibodies to other BCL2 epitopes {1990,2540, 3583}. BCL2 protein can be useful in distinguishing neoplastic from reactive follicles, although absence of BCL2 protein does not exclude the diagnosis of a FL. BCL2 protein is not useful in distinguishing FL from other types of low-grade B-cell lymphomas, most of which also express BCL2. The interpretation of BCL2

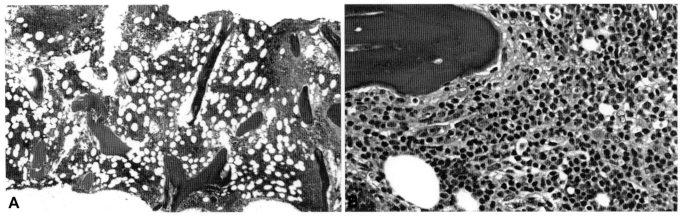

Fig. 13.74 Bone marrow involvement by follicular lymphoma. **A** At low magnification, paratrabecular lymphoid aggregates are visible. **B** The cells are small centrocytes.

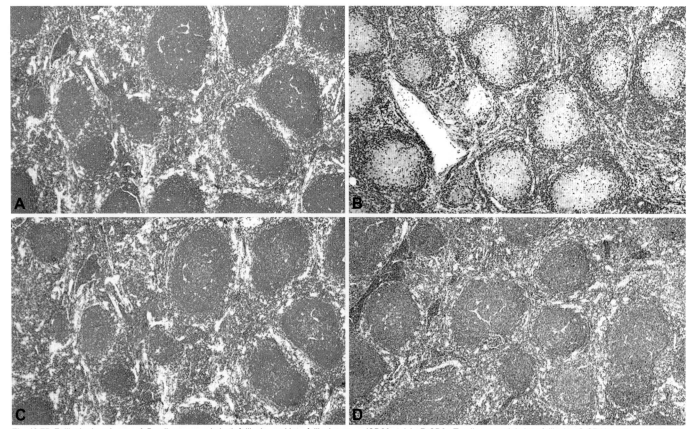

Fig. 13.75 Follicular lymphoma. **A** B cells are seen in both follicular and interfollicular areas (CD20 stain). **B** CD3+ T cells are mainly interfollicular. **C** CD10+ cells are within the follicles and also infiltrate the interfollicular region. In some cases, CD10 is downregulated in the interfollicular zone. **D** Follicles are strongly positive for BCL2.

immunostaining in germinal centre cells requires caution, because T cells, primary follicles, and mantle zones normally express this protein.

In addition to FDCs, neoplastic follicles contain numerous other non-neoplastic cells normally found in germinal centres, including follicular T cells (CD3+, CD4+, CD57+, PD1/CD279+, CXCL13+) and varying numbers of histiocytes. Consistent with the germinal centre phenotype of the neoplastic cells, most cases are negative for IRF4/MUM1. However, a subset of FLs negative for CD10 are positive for IRF4/MUM1 {1944}. Such tumours typically lack the *BCL2* translocation but show amplification of *BCL6* {1950}. They tend to occur in elderly patients and cytologically are of higher grade (3A or 3B). These cases must be distinguished from large B-cell lymphoma with *IRF4* rearrangement, which often has at least a partially follicular growth pattern {2369, 3491}.

The Ki-67 proliferation index in FL generally correlates with histological grade; most grade 1–2 cases have a proliferation index < 20%, whereas most grade 3 cases have a proliferation index > 20%, although there is considerable variation among studies, probably due to technical differences in immunostaining {2088, 2520,3008,4250}. A subgroup of morphologically low-grade FLs with a high proliferation index has been described {2088,4250}; these cases behaved more aggressively than did those with a low proliferation index, and similarly to grade 3 FL {4250}. Therefore, Ki-67 staining should be considered as an adjunct to histological grading, and its use is clinically justified, although not formally required at this time.

Postulated normal counterpart

The postulated normal counterpart is a germinal centre B cell. In cases with t(14;18)(q32;q21), the IGH/*BCL2* translocation occurs in bone marrow pre–B cells; fully malignant transformation of these t(14;18)-positive primed cells occurs during (re)entry into the germinal centres in secondary lymphoid organs {3425,3426}.

Grading

FL is graded by counting or estimating the absolute number of centroblasts (large or small) in 10 neoplastic follicles, expressed per high-power (40× magnification, 0.159 mm^2) microscopic field (HPF) {1820,2485,2835}. At least 10 HPFs within different follicles must be evaluated; these should be representative follicles, not those with the most numerous large cells.

Grade 1–2 cases have a marked predominance of centrocytes, with few centroblasts (grade 1: 0–5 centroblasts per HPF; grade 2: 6–15 centroblasts per HPF). As recommended in the 2008 WHO classification, the combined designation of grade 1–2 is preferred, due to the lack of clinically significant differences between grades 1 and 2, the considerable interobserver variation in grading, and variations in grade within a given biopsy.

Grade 3 cases have > 15 centroblasts per HPF. Grade 3 is further subdivided on the basis of the presence or absence of centrocytes. In grade 3A, centrocytes are still present, whereas grade 3B follicles are composed entirely of large blastic cells (centroblasts or immunoblasts). Recent data indicate that grade 3B FL differs from other forms of FL both biologically and clinically, as discussed below. If distinct areas of grade 3 FL are present in a biopsy of an otherwise grade 1–2 FL, a separate diagnosis of grade 3 FL should also be made and the approximate percentages of each grade reported. Because both pattern and cytology vary among follicles, lymph nodes must be adequately sampled. Accurate grading cannot be performed on fine-needle aspirations and may be difficult on core needle biopsies. Therefore, an excisional biopsy is recommended for primary diagnosis. The presence of a diffuse component with grade 3 cytology always warrants an additional diagnosis of DLBCL.

The vast majority of FLs (80–90% in most unselected series) are of grade 1–2 {4228}. Only a few studies have compared the frequency of grade 3A versus 3B cases. However, pure grade 3B FL is rare, with most cases containing at least focal diffuse areas composed mainly of centroblasts, constituting DLBCL {1963,3008}.

Grade 3B FL is biologically more closely related to DLBCL than to other FLs {1684}. Translocations involving *BCL2* are relatively rare in such cases {3493}. In addition, biopsies frequently contain diffuse areas composed mainly of centroblasts, constituting DLBCL. The natural history appears to differ from that of other forms of FL. There may be higher short-term mortality, but patients in remission after anthracycline-based therapy at 5 years, are likely cured of disease {4228}. Thus, the clinical course resembles that of DLBCL. However, some studies have not found significant differences between grade 3A and 3B FL {3668}. These data underscore the often subjective nature of grading in FL, with considerable interobserver variation.

Genetic profile

Antigen receptor genes

IG heavy and light chain genes are rearranged; IGV genes show extensive and ongoing somatic hypermutation {765, 3010}. As a result of mutations in the complementarity-determining regions, a high false-negative rate on IGH PCR was observed with older primer sets. Multiplex PCR reactions using BIOMED-2 expanded primer sets detect closer to 90% of IGH VDJ gene rearrangements, and clonality detection approximates 100% when primers detecting IGH DJ and light chain gene rearrangements are included {1117}. FL undergoes genetic evolution over time, which can be linear, but in most cases follows a pattern of divergent evolution rather than direct evolution. FL is associated with the development of multiple subclones {1434}. This observation has relevance for histological

Table 13.17 Follicular lymphoma grading, based on the absolute number of centroblasts per high-power (40 × objective, 0.159 mm^2) microscopic field (HPF)[a]

Grading	Definition
Grade 1–2 (low grade)	0–15 centroblasts per HPF
1	0–5 centroblasts per HPF
2	6–15 centroblasts per HPF
Grade 3	> 15 centroblasts per HPF
3A	Centrocytes present
3B	Solid sheets of centroblasts
Reporting of pattern	**Proportion follicular**
Follicular	> 75%
Follicular and diffuse	25–75%[b]
Focally follicular / predominantly diffuse	< 25%[b]
Diffuse	0%[c]

Diffuse areas containing > 15 centroblasts per HPF are reported as diffuse large B-cell lymphoma with follicular lymphoma (grade 1–2, grade 3A, or grade 3B)[b].

[a] To determine the number of centroblasts per 0.159 mm^2 HPF: if using an 18 mm field of view ocular, count the centroblasts in 10 fields and divide by 10; if using a 20 mm field of view ocular, count in 8 fields and divide by 10 or count in 10 fields and divide by 12; if using a 22 mm field of view ocular, count in 7 fields and divide by 10 or count in 10 fields and divide by 15.
[b] Mention the approximate percentage of each component in the report.
[c] If the biopsy specimen is small, a note should be added that the absence of follicles may reflect sampling error.

Table 13.18 Frequency of genetic alterations in follicular lymphoma at diagnosis

Gene	Frequency of alterations (%)[a]	Predominant type of alteration
BCL2	85–90	Translocation, mutation
KMT2D (MLL2)	85	Mutation
TNFRSF14	45–65	Deletion, mutation
EZH2	60	Mutation (Y641)
EPHA7	70	Mutation
CREBBP	33	Deletion, mutation
BCL6	45	Translocation, mutation
MEF2B	15	Mutation
EP300	10	Deletion, mutation
TNFAIP3 (also called A20)	20	Deletion, mutation
FAS	5	Mutation
TP53	< 5	Deletion, mutation
MYC	< 5	Translocation, gain

[a] Approximate frequency of alterations; some alterations may be subclonal.

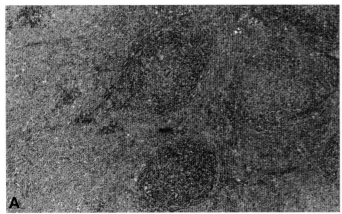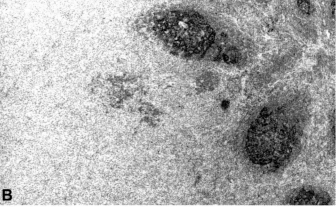

Fig. 13.76 Follicular lymphoma associated with diffuse large B-cell lymphoma (DLBCL). **A** Neoplastic follicles are present on the right, with a diffuse area on the left. The diffuse area consists predominantly of large cells, so a separate diagnosis of DLBCL is made. **B** Staining for CD21 shows follicular dendritic cell meshworks in the follicles, but not in the areas of DLBCL.

progression in FL, in which transformation develops in an earlier common progenitor rather than one of the later subclones {1432}.

Cytogenetic abnormalities and oncogenes

FL is genetically characterized by the t(14;18)(q32;q21) translocation between the IGH and *BCL2* genes. Alternative *BCL2* translocations to IG light chain genes have been reported. The t(14;18) translocation is present in as many as 90% of grade 1–2 FLs {1700,3434}. Due to the variation in breakpoint regions, FISH is more sensitive than PCR-based approaches for detecting the translocation {4094}. Caution is advised because classic cytogenetics cannot be used to distinguish IGH/*BCL2* from IGH/*MALT1* translocations. FLs negative for *BCL2* rearrangement are more likely to have a late germinal centre gene expression profile {2259}, but the absence of the translocation has no apparent impact on prognosis {2258}. However, *BCL2* rearrangements are much less frequent in grade 3B FL {3008}. Similarly, testicular FL, seen mainly in young boys, is negative for the *BCL2* rearrangement. Abnormalities of 3q27.3 and/or *BCL6* rearrangement are found in 5–15% of FLs, and have also been reported in testicular FL {1219}.

In addition to t(14;18), other genetic alterations are found in 90% of FLs: most commonly, loss of 1p, 6q, 10q, and 17p and gains of chromosomes 1, 6p, 7, 8, 12q, X, and 18q {1750,2931,4005}. One of the most commonly affected regions is 1p36, which contains *TNFRSF14* {1434}. Copy-number alterations, acquired copy-

neutral LOH, and mutations in *TNFRSF14* are among the most common findings in all forms of FL, including the diffuse variant of FL and paediatric-type FL {2228}. *TNFRSF14* mutations were initially suggested to be associated with an adverse prognosis {702}, but other studies have not confirmed this association {2228}. The number of additional alterations increases with histological grade and transformation {3508}. Rare cases of FL carry t(8;14)(q24;q32) or variants together with t(14;18) {185,4214}, and progression to a high-grade so-called double-hit lymphoma may occur, with translocations affecting both *BCL2* and *MYC* {3082}.

Gain-of-function mutations in the H3K27 methyltransferase *EZH2* are relatively common in FL, and appear to be an early event in the evolution of the disease {513}. Additionally, driver mutations in the chromatin regulator genes *CREBBP* and

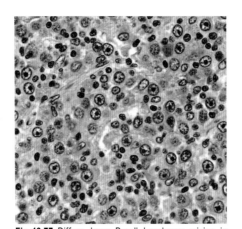

Fig. 13.77 Diffuse large B-cell lymphoma arising in follicular lymphoma. The infiltrate is dominated by large blastic cells with prominent central nucleoli resembling immunoblasts. This case was associated with secondary *TP53* mutation and overexpression of p53.

KMT2D (*MLL2*) play a key role {1435, 2966}. *EZH2*, *KMT2D*, and *CREBBP* have all been proposed as possible therapeutic targets. More recently, activating somatic mutations in *RRAGC* have been found in approximately 17% of cases {2967}.

Gene expression studies have shown the importance of the microenvironment in the pathogenesis, evolution, and prognosis of FL {878,1382}. Transformation to DLBCL may occur via various genetic pathways, including inactivation of *TP53* and *CDKN2A* and activation of *MYC* {884,1089,2395,3195,3508}.

Genetic susceptibility

Genome-wide association studies have identified five susceptibility loci for FL outside the HLA region {3690}. Consistent with these data, FL has an increased incidence in patients with a history of lymphoma in first-degree family members {2354}.

Prognosis and predictive factors

The prognosis of FL is closely related to the extent of the disease at diagnosis. The FLIPI, a modification of the International Prognostic Index (IPI), is useful in predicting outcome {1,2,3720}. The FLIPI uses five independent predictors of inferior survival: age >60 years, haemoglobin concentration <12 g/dL, elevated serum lactate dehydrogenase, Ann Arbor stage III/IV (disseminated disease in the Lugano system), and >4 involved nodal areas. The presence of 0–1, 2, 3–5 of these adverse factors, respectively, defines low-risk, intermediate-risk, and high-risk disease. Genetic profiling may provide additional information {3094}.

Most published studies show a more aggressive clinical course for FLs classified as grade 3, but the use of regimens containing doxorubicin and/or rituximab may obviate these differences, and requires further study {1252,4228,4293}. With current therapies, the median survival for patients with FL of grades 1–3A is > 12 years {4228}. There are continued relapses over time, with no plateau in the survival curves.

Transformation or so-called progression usually to DLBCL occurs in 25–35% of patients with FL. Rare patients with initial DLBCL develop a late relapse as FL {2249}. This sequence is analogous to chronic myeloid leukaemia presenting in blast-phase crisis. The clinical outcome for patients with histological progression is better than in past years {4227}. FL may also progress to a lymphoma resembling Burkitt lymphoma or with features intermediate between those of DLBCL and Burkitt lymphoma {77,1280,1689,3279}. Transformation typically involves additional genetic abnormalities, in particular MYC translocations; the combination of a BCL2 and a MYC rearrangement is associated with a particularly aggressive course {1212,2252,4394,4420}; cases with this combination should be diagnosed as high-grade B-cell lymphoma with MYC and BCL2 rearrangements, transformed from FL, so-called double-hit lymphoma.

Rarely, patients develop B-lymphoblastic leukaemia/lymphoma, which in the cases studied is clonally related to the original B-cell tumour {896,1311,2061, 2121}. This form of transformation also involves the acquisition of a MYC rearrangement in addition to the underlying BCL2 rearrangement. However, the term 'high-grade B-cell lymphoma with MYC and BCL2 rearrangements' should not be used in the setting of lymphoblastic transformation.

FL can relapse as classic Hodgkin lymphoma. The association of FL and other B-cell lymphomas with classic Hodgkin lymphoma provided early evidence for the B-cell origin of the Hodgkin/Reed–Sternberg cell {1825}. Genetic studies identified the BCL2 translocation in cases of classic Hodgkin lymphoma associated with FL {2244} and established a common clonal identity for the two morphologically different neoplasms {486}.

Rarely, the occurrence of histiocytic or dendritic cell sarcoma has been described in patients with FL, in which the sarcomas also had the IGH and BCL2 rearrangements. However, the histiocytic cells show loss of PAX5 activity and loss of all B-cell markers {1172}. Genetic studies show that the histiocytic sarcoma and the FL both arise from a common precursor, rather than constituting dedifferentiation of the mature FL B cell {479}. However, this precursor is beyond the haematopoietic stem cell level, and has already undergone IG rearrangement.

In situ follicular neoplasia

Definition
In situ follicular neoplasia (ISFN), formerly referred to as follicular lymphoma in situ {789}, is defined as partial or total colonization of germinal centres by clonal B cells carrying the *BCL2* translocation characteristic of FL in an otherwise reactive lymph node. It can also be seen in reactive follicles in lymphoid tissue in other sites, including the spleen. ISFN is biologically similar to the presence of cells carrying the *BCL2* rearrangement found in the peripheral blood of otherwise healthy individuals by PCR amplification for *BCL2* rearrangement {2479}, referred to as FL-like B cells. Both FL-like B cells and ISFN have been described in the same patient {703}. ISFN may be seen uncommonly in patients with overt FL at another site or subsequently. In the few such cases studied, there have been differences in the genetic profiles of the two lesions, suggesting that in at least some cases the ISFN lesion does not simply constitute secondary spread of FL from

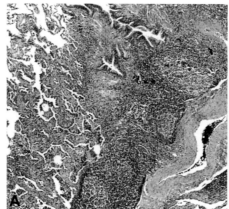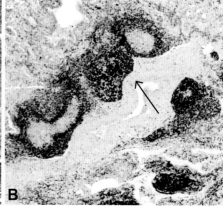

Fig. 13.78 In situ follicular neoplasia in the lung. **A** Lung resection was performed for adenocarcinoma. A focal peribronchial lymphoid infiltrate was noted. **B** One of the follicles shows centrocytes strongly positive for BCL2 within the germinal centre (arrow).

another site {3568}. ISFN should be distinguished from lymph nodes showing only partial involvement by FL. Although patients with partial involvement tend to have lower-stage disease, partial involvement is considered a form of FL for clinical purposes {21}.

ICD-O code 9695/1

Synonyms
Intrafollicular neoplasia; follicular lymphoma in situ

Epidemiology
ISFN can be detected in approximately 2% of randomly selected reactive lymph node biopsies {353,1610}. Epidemiological studies have shown that FL-like B cells are more commonly found in patients with increased environmental risk, such as prolonged exposure to herbicides and pesticides {33}. FL-like B cells can be detected in as many as 70% of adults aged >50 years. The incidence of this finding increases with age, and is uncommon in individuals aged <18 years, in whom FL is rare {1076,3424}. Some cases of ISFN are discovered incidentally in lymph nodes involved by other forms of lymphoma, most often other B-cell lymphomas {353,1848,2698,3184}. ISFN has also been observed in lymph nodes from nodal dissections performed in connection with surgery for other cancers {353, 2747}. In patients with subsequent FL, the in situ lesion preceded the lymphoma diagnosis by 23 months to 10 years.

Microscopy
ISFN is generally not apparent in routine H&E-stained sections {789}. Lymph nodes contain reactive follicles with well-formed germinal centres. The affected follicles are similar in size and shape to adjacent uninvolved follicles, although on close inspection closely packed centrocytes may be appreciated. The lesion can also be seen in reactive follicles in extranodal sites, i.e. any location where reactive follicles are identified. ISFN is distinct from partial involvement by FL,

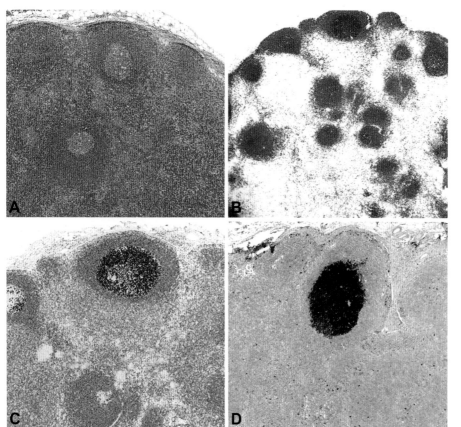

Fig. 13.79 In situ follicular neoplasia. **A** The lymph node is unremarkable, with preserved nodal architecture. **B** CD20 staining shows a normal distribution of follicles. **C** BCL2 staining highlights strongly positive centrocytes within the affected germinal centre. **D** The atypical cells show strong staining for CD10.

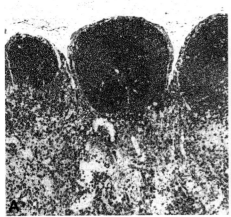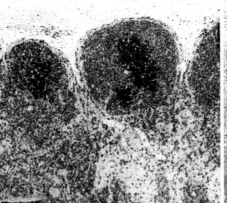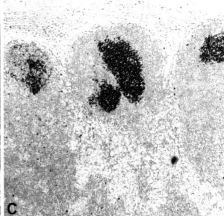

Fig. 13.80 In situ follicular neoplasia. **A** The lymph node architecture is preserved, with CD20-positive cells present in follicles. **B** Several germinal centres contain strongly BCL2-positive cells. **C** The BCL2-positive follicles are strongly CD10-positive.

in which only selected follicles within a lymph node may be involved {1848}. Partial involvement can usually be suspected based on H&E-stained sections, whereas ISFN can only be observed with subsequent immunohistochemical stains. Partial involvement is associated with lower-stage disease {21}, but progression can occur.

ISFN may be detected in lymph nodes involved by other forms of lymphoma, most often other lymphomas of B-cell lineage, which include chronic lymphocytic leukaemia, mantle cell lymphoma, marginal zone lymphoma, diffuse large B-cell lymphoma, and classic Hodgkin lymphoma {1848,2698,3184}. ISFN has also been reported to coexist in the same anatomical site with in situ mantle cell neoplasia {3428}. Activation-induced cytidine deaminase is involved in initiating chromosomal breaks that lead to both the t(14;18) and the t(11;14) translocations, which is suggestive of

common molecular mechanisms {1457}.

Immunophenotype
ISFN can only be detected by immunohistochemistry for BCL2, and is generally not suspected on H&E staining. The BCL2-positive cells are exclusively centrocytes, and BCL2 is very strongly expressed, with a higher intensity than in adjacent T cells or mantle zone cells. The BCL2-positive centrocytes also show increased expression of CD10. Flow cytometry may demonstrate CD10-positive, BCL2-positive, light chain restricted B cells, often in the presence of more numerous other CD10-positive or CD10-negative B cells {3184}.

Genetic profile
ISFN cells are positive for t(14;18), but are found to have very few other genetic aberrations when examined by array comparative genomic hybridization {2480,3568}, suggesting that this is a

very early step in lymphomagenesis. In addition to the *BCL2* translocation, mutations in *EZH2* (Y641) were also reported {3568}. Deletions at 1p36 encompassing the *TNFRSF14* gene have also been seen {2480}. This aberration is common to many B-cell lymphomas. Lymph nodes showing partial involvement by FL have also been found to have a relatively low level of genomic alterations {2480, 3568}. In cases in which ISFN and overt FL are seen in the same patient, there are additional genetic alterations in the FL that are not present in the ISFN {414, 3568}. Some of these secondary events lead to mutations in *BCL2*, resulting in negative staining of the FL with the commonly used clone 124 antibody to BCL2 {414,1848}.

Prognosis and predictive factors
For patients with incidentally diagnosed ISFN and no other evidence of FL on clinical evaluation, the risk of subsequent FL is very low (≤ 5%) {353,1848}. Most studies have not found that the number of follicles involved within a single lymph node showing ISFN predicts the subsequent risk of lymphoma {1848, 3184}. High levels of FL-like B cells in the peripheral blood are associated with an increased risk of subsequent FL {3425}, but levels so low that the cells can only be identified with multiple rounds of PCR amplification carry no increased risk. For patients with other sites of lymphadenopathy at presentation with ISFN, additional biopsy is recommended, because other forms of lymphoma (usually B-cell lymphomas) may exist with ISFN {353,1288, 1848,3184}.

Table 13.19 Histological features distinguishing *in situ* follicular neoplasia (ISFN) from partial involvement by follicular lymphoma (FL). Modified from Jegalian AG et al. {1848}

In situ follicular neoplasia	Partial involvement by FL
Nodal architecture intact	Altered architecture evident on H&E staining
Follicle size normal	Follicle size often expanded
Involved follicles widely scattered	Involved follicles grouped together
Mantle cuff intact, with sharp border to germinal centre	Mantle cuff often attenuated or with blurred border to germinal centre
BCL2 and CD10 immunostaining very strongly positive	BCL2 and CD10 immunostaining more variable in intensity
Composed almost exclusively of centrocytes	Composed of centrocytes and few centroblasts
Atypical cells confined to the germinal centre	Atypical cells (CD10+, BCL2+) may be found outside the germinal centre

Duodenal-type follicular lymphoma

Definition
Most cases of primary follicular lymphoma (FL) in the gastrointestinal tract occur in the small intestine, usually with involvement of the duodenum {2675,3530,3648, 4439}. Duodenal-type FL is a specific variant of FL defined by distinctive clinical and biological features. The lesions are predominantly found in the second portion of the duodenum, presenting as multiple small polyps, often as an incidental finding on endoscopy performed for other reasons {3564}. The immunophenotype is similar to that of nodal FLs. Most patients have localized disease (stage IE or IIE), and survival appears to be excellent even without treatment. Surveillance of the small bowel in patients with duodenal-type FL reveals involvement of the more distal small intestine in approximately 80–85% of cases {3564,3876}.

Cases not exhibiting the typical features of duodenal-type FL should be evaluated for evidence of FL at other sites. Classic FL can involve the intestine, usually in association with involvement of mesenteric lymph nodes. Such cases lack the indolent clinical features of the duodenal-type variant {2676}. They usually show more-extensive involvement of the intestinal wall, with infiltration into the muscularis propria. They show variation in cytological grade (similar to that seen in nodal FL) and are distinct from duodenal-type FL {3648}.

ICD-O code
9695/3

Synonym
Primary intestinal follicular lymphoma

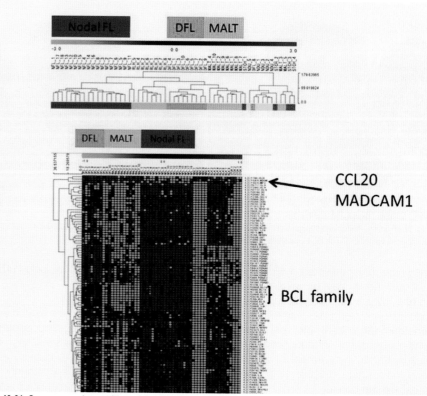

Fig. 13.81 Gene expression profiling of duodenal-type follicular lymphoma (DFL), extranodal marginal zone lymphoma of mucosa-associated lymphoid tissue (MALT lymphoma), and nodal follicular lymphoma (nodal FL). The gene expression pattern of DFL is closer to that of *Helicobacter*-associated gastric MALT lymphoma than to that of nodal FL. DFL and MALT lymphoma both show high expression of *CCL20* and *MADCAM1*, which are expressed at low levels in nodal FL. In contrast, for the BCL gene family, DFL and nodal FL show similar patterns, which are distinct from that of MALT lymphoma. These data were compared with data from 17 normal control samples: 5 normal duodenal mucosa (yellow), 8 nodal reactive lymphoid hyperplasia (green), and 4 normal gastric mucosa (vermilion) samples. {3879}.

Epidemiology
Most patients are middle-aged, with an equal male-to-female ratio in most large series {2732,3564}. Several large series have been reported from Japan, but it is not clear that this reflects an increased incidence; it could instead be a result of increased surveillance by endoscopy in this population {1802,2732}.

Microscopy
Duodenal-type FL demonstrates neoplastic follicles in the mucosa/submucosa. The atypical follicles are composed almost uniformly of centrocytes (with only infrequent centroblasts), constituting grade 1–2 disease in the grading system for nodal FL. The neoplastic cells also infiltrate the lamina propria outside of the follicles, a feature best illustrated with immunohistochemical staining.

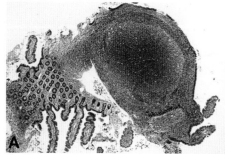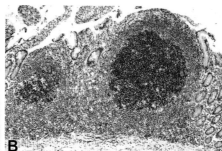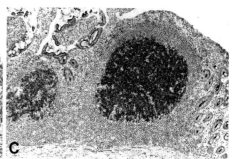

Fig. 13.82 Duodenal-type follicular lymphoma. Large nodules of lymphoid cells are present in the mucosa (**A**). The follicles are uniformly positive for BCL2 (**B**) and positive for CD10 (**C**).

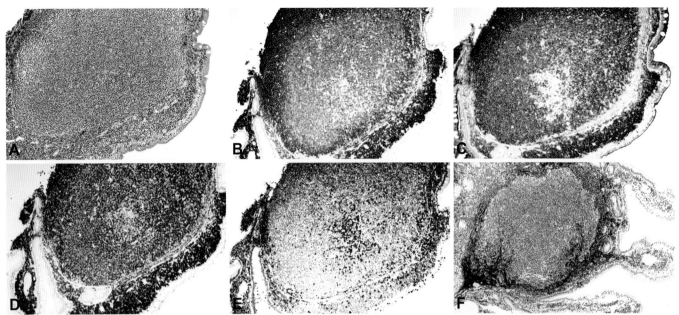

Fig. 13.83 Duodenal-type follicular lymphoma. **A** This duodenal polyp was an incidental finding in a patient undergoing screening endoscopy. Another similar polypoid lesion was observed. **B** CD20 stain. Note the extension of the infiltrate into the lamina propria. **C** The cells are strongly positive for CD10. **D** The cells are intensely BCL2-positive. **E** CD3 stain. Few T cells are present surrounding the abnormal follicle. **F** CD21 stain shows that the follicular dendritic cells are few in number and mainly located in the periphery of the lymphoid infiltrate.

Immunophenotype

The immunophenotype of duodenal-type FL is similar to that of nodal FL. The cells are positive for CD20, BCL2, and CD10, with variable expression of BCL6 {3564}. The proliferation rate is generally low. The cells are negative for activation-induced cytidine deaminase {3878}, which plays a key role in class switching and in somatic hypermutation in normal and neoplastic B cells. Follicular dendritic cells (as identified by CD21) are usually restricted to the periphery of the follicle {3878}. The cells express the intestinal homing receptor alpha4beta7 {328}. Consistent with the intestinal origin of the neoplastic cells, they usually express IgA heavy chain.

Postulated normal counterpart

A B cell that expresses germinal centre markers and has features of a memory B cell {3878}

Genetic profile

The cells carry the t(14;18)(q32;q21) (IGH/*BCL2*) translocation. They are thought to be memory B cells and show evidence of somatic hypermutation of the IGH gene {3877}. Restricted IGHV usage suggests similarities to MALT lymphomas {3879}. Gene expression studies have also suggested an overlap with MALT lymphoma, showing overexpression of *CCL20* and *MADCAM1*, genes that were not found to be upregulated in nodal FL {3879}. A study using array comparative genomic hybridization showed that although duodenal-type FL is positive for the IGH/*BCL2* translocation, it has a lower frequency of other genetic aberrations than does nodal FL, consistent with its indolent clinical course and low incidence of progression {2480}. However, in common with nodal FL, recurrent deletion of chromosome 1p was observed, encompassing the *TNFRSF14* gene, as well as

mutations in *TNFRSF14* exons {2480}. The same study identified a limited set of amplified oncogenes (*BCL2*, *BCL6*, *FGFR1*, *EIF4A2*, and *TFRC*) and deleted tumour suppressor genes (*PTEN*, *FAS*, and *TP73*) in some cases of duodenal-type FL {2480}. These aberrations are also found in nodal FL.

Prognosis and predictive factors

Long-term survival is excellent, even with local recurrences in the intestine {2732,3564}. There is a low (< 10%) risk of progression to nodal disease. Various therapies have been used, including local radiation therapy, chemotherapy, and rituximab. Given the indolent clinical course, a watch-and-wait approach is reasonable for most patients {1288,3564, 3903}.

Paediatric-type follicular lymphoma

Jaffe E.S.
Harris N.L.
Siebert R.

Definition

Paediatric-type follicular lymphoma (PTFL) is an uncommon nodal follicular lymphoma (FL) that occurs primarily in children and young adults, but also occurs sporadically in older individuals {2369,2400}. This term should not be used for cases with areas of diffuse large B-cell lymphoma (DLBCL) or other lymphomas of follicle centre derivation that occur in the paediatric age group. In particular, this category does not include testicular FLs {1219,2386} or large B-cell lymphomas with *IRF4* rearrangement, which often have a follicular or partially follicular growth pattern {2369,3491}. PTFL most often involves lymph nodes of the head and neck, and usually presents with stage I disease. The median age at onset is 15–18 years, with only rare cases presenting in patients aged >40 years. The male-to-female ratio is ≥10:1. Cytologically, the lesions appear to be of high grade, most often with a high proliferation rate, but the prognosis is excellent, and many patients achieve continuous complete remission following only complete surgical excision of the affected lymph node. The usual translocations found in other B-cell lymphomas of germinal centre origin (i.e. of *BCL2* and *BCL6*) are absent.

ICD-O code   9690/3

Epidemiology

There are no known risk factors and no known associations with immunodeficiency or autoimmune disease. Most patients are aged 5–25 years. There is a marked male predominance, with a male-to-female ratio of ≥10:1.

Localization

Most patients present with enlarged lymph nodes in the head and neck region (i.e. the cervical, submental, submandibular, postauricular, and periparotid nodes) {2369,2400}. The inguinal and femoral lymph nodes are less often the presenting site. Virtually all patients present with isolated peripheral lymphadenopathy, without involvement of the para-aortic or mesenteric lymph nodes.

Clinical features

Most patients present with isolated, asymptomatic lymph node enlargement. Occasional cases of FL in children have been reported with more extensive disease or focal progression to DLBCL {2393,2524}. However, these reports did not use the current WHO definition of PTFL, and at least some of the reported cases had significant genetic or immunophenotypic differences from PTFL as it is currently defined {1817}. In clinical practice, cases with areas of DLBCL or disseminated disease are excluded from this category.

Imaging

Imaging studies confirm the localized nature of the disease, with absence of radiological evidence of mediastinal or intra-abdominal lymph node involvement.

Staging

The vast majority of patients present with a single site of lymph node enlargement. Bone marrow involvement has not been reported. B symptoms such as fever and weight loss are absent.

Microscopy

Lymph node architecture is totally or subtotally effaced by large expansile follicles, often with a serpiginous growth pattern. Partial involvement can be seen, with a rim of normal node at the edge of the biopsy. On low-power magnification, the follicles show a starry-sky pattern and thin or absent mantle zones. In some cases, evidence of marginal zone differentiation may be seen peripheral to the neoplastic follicles. The cellular composition is typically monotonous; the atypical cells are intermediate in size, often have a blastoid appearance, and lack prominent nucleoli {2369}. Mitotic figures are readily apparent. Some cases contain more typical centroblasts. Areas of DLBCL preclude the diagnosis of PTFL. Historically, most cases have been reported as grade 3A or 3B {2393,2997}, but grading is not typically used, unlike for usual FL.

Immunophenotype

The cells have a mature B-cell phenotype and are positive for CD20, CD79a, and PAX5. CD10 is usually strongly expressed, and BCL6 is positive. Most cases are negative for BCL2 expression, but weak staining is seen in a minority of cases. Ki-67 staining usually reveals a

Table 13.20 Primary diagnostic criteria for paediatric-type follicular lymphoma (PTFL)

Morphology	At least partial effacement of nodal architecture (required)
	Pure follicular proliferation (required)[a]
	Expansile follicles[b]
	Intermediate-sized so-called blastoid cells (not centrocytes)[b]
Immunohistochemistry (required)	BCL6 positivity
	BCL2 negativity or weak positivity
	High proliferative fraction (>30%)
Genomics (required)	No *BCL2*, *BCL6*, *IRF4*, or aberrant IG rearrangement
	No *BCL2* amplification
Clinical features	Nodal disease (required)
	Stage I–II disease (required)
	Patient age <40 years[b]
	Marked male predominance

[a] The presence of any component of diffuse large B-cell lymphoma or advanced-stage disease excludes PTFL
[b] These are common features of PTFL, but not required for diagnosis.

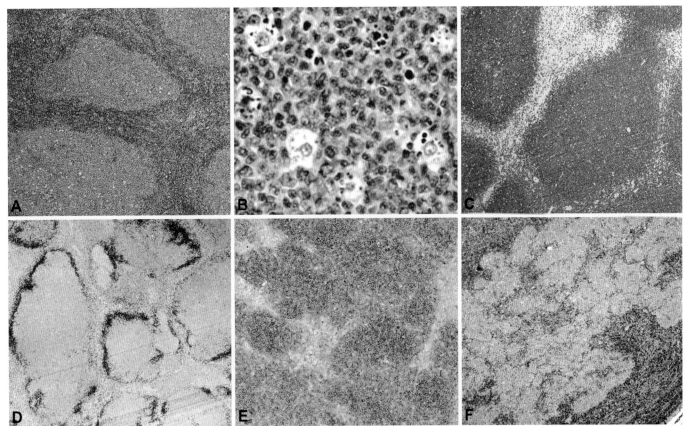

Fig. 13.84 Paediatric-type follicular lymphoma. **A** The follicles are large and lack mantle zones. No polarization is evident, and the cellular composition is monotonous. **B** High-magnification view shows that the follicles are composed of monotonous, medium-sized lymphoid cells. Abundant starry-sky histiocytes are present. **C** CD20 stain. The follicles are closely packed. **D** IgD stain. The mantle zones are attenuated. **E** Serpiginous follicles are strongly CD10-positive. **F** BCL2 protein is negative in the neoplastic follicles.

moderate to high proliferation rate (> 30% of follicular cells), usually without evidence of polarization in the follicles. The follicular dendritic cell markers (CD21 and CD23) outline meshworks within the follicles. IgD is negative and shows either absent or attenuated mantle cuffs. IRF4/MUM1 is negative; strong positivity should raise the possibility of large B-cell lymphoma with *IRF4* rearrangement.

Plasma cells are sparse; an abundance of plasma cells raises the possibility of reactive hyperplasia. Flow cytometry identifies a monotypic population of B cells positive for CD10 and negative for CD5. However, rare cases of florid follicular hyperplasia, most commonly in young boys, can have clonal populations of CD10+ B cells detected by flow cytometry that are usually small, with monoclonality in IG rearrangement studies {2145}. Architectural effacement is a key feature that distinguishes PTFL from reactive follicular hyperplasia with clonal B cells.

Postulated normal counterpart

A germinal centre B cell

Grading

Although most cases would meet the criteria for grade 3 FL, grading is not used if the criteria for the diagnosis of PTFL are met.

Genetic profile

PCR techniques for the detection of IG gene rearrangements are positive, which is helpful in ruling out many, but not all, cases of florid follicular hyperplasia {2145}. Aberrations affecting the *BCL2*, *BCL6*, or *IRF4* loci are absent. PT-FLs generally lack mutations in *KMT2D* (*MLL2*), *CREBBP*, and *EZH2*, genes frequently mutated in usual FL {1435,2966}, including cases negative for *BCL2* rearrangements {2400A,3567A}. The most common genetic aberrations are deletion at 1p36 and deletions or mutations affecting *TNFRSF14* {2400A,2524,

3567A}. *MAP2K1* mutations are identified in approximately 40–50% of cases {2400A,3567B}.

Prognosis and predictive factors

The prognosis is excellent. Most data indicate that patients with localized disease amenable to surgical excision do not require radiation or chemotherapy {176,2400}. In one study, there was no difference in clinical outcome between patients with and without genetic aberrations {2524}; however, most of the patients received multiagent chemotherapy. Areas of DLBCL exclude the diagnosis of PTFL as it is currently defined {2997}. The diagnosis should be made with caution in patients aged > 25 years, because the differential diagnosis with usual FL of grade 3A or 3B can be challenging. Correlation with clinical features is essential in older patients.

Large B-cell lymphoma with *IRF4* rearrangement

Pittaluga S.
Harris N.L.
Siebert R.
Salaverria I.

Definition

Large B-cell lymphoma (LBCL) with *IRF4* rearrangement is an uncommon subtype of LBCL that can be entirely diffuse, follicular and diffuse, or entirely follicular. It is characterized by strong expression of IRF4/MUM1, usually with *IRF4* rearrangement. It occurs primarily in children and young adults, with predominantly Waldeyer ring or head and neck lymph node involvement {2369,3491}. Despite its common occurrence in the paediatric age group, it is distinct from paediatric-type follicular lymphomas, even when purely follicular {2369,2400}.

ICD-O code   9698/3

Epidemiology

LBCL with *IRF4* rearrangement is rare, accounting for just 0.05% of diffuse LBCLs. The patient age range at presentation is 4–79 years, with a median age of 12 years and an equal sex distribution. This entity is significantly more frequent in children (individuals aged < 18 years) than in adults ($P < 0.001$) {3491}.

Localization

Most patients present with enlarged lymph nodes of the head and neck region. The Waldeyer ring is also a frequent site of disease. Another reported site of involvement is the gastrointestinal tract {898,2369,3491}.

Clinical features

Most patients present with isolated lymph node or tonsillar enlargement (stage I–II) {3491}.

Microscopy

The neoplastic cells are medium-sized to large, with chromatin which is more open than typically seen in centrocytes and small, basophilic nucleoli. Mitotic figures are infrequent, and a starry-sky pattern is absent. When a follicular pattern is present, the neoplastic follicles are large, with a back-to-back growth pattern and absent or attenuated mantle zones. Many cases have an entirely diffuse growth

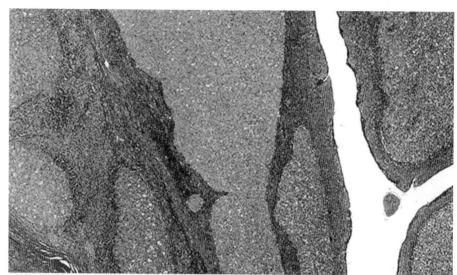

Fig. 13.85 Large B-cell lymphoma with *IRF4* rearrangement. Low-magnification view of tonsil shows large abnormal follicles. Residual reactive germinal centres are visible at lower left.

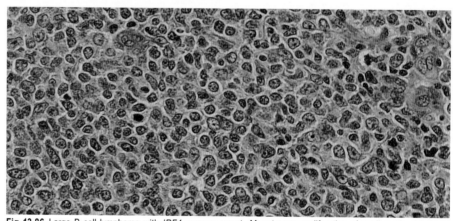

Fig. 13.86 Large B-cell lymphoma with *IRF4* rearrangement. Monotonous proliferation of medium-sized to large cells which appear distinct from both typical centrocytes and centroblasts and that lacks a starry-sky pattern.

pattern. Unlike in paediatric-type follicular lymphoma, the follicles generally lack a serpiginous configuration and starry-sky pattern.

Immunophenotype

The atypical cells have a mature B-cell phenotype and are positive for CD20, CD79a, and PAX5. IRF4/MUM1 is typically strongly expressed, and BCL6 is positive, whereas PRDM1 (also known as BLIMP1) is usually negative. CD10 and BCL2 expression is observed in 66% of cases {3491}. The proliferation

rate is usually high, with no evidence of polarization in the neoplastic follicles. In the appropriate clinical context, cases with coexpression of CD10, BCL6, and IRF4/MUM1 should be screened for *IRF4* rearrangements.

Postulated normal counterpart

Germinal centre B cell with *IRF4* rearrangement resulting in IRF4/MUM1 expression

Genetic profile

Immunoglobulin genes are clonally re-

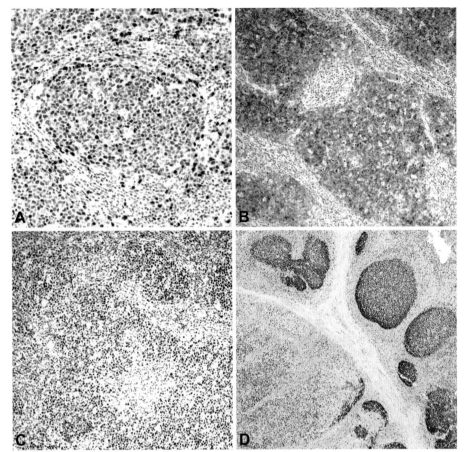

Fig. 13.87 Large B-cell lymphoma with *IRF4* rearrangement. **A** There is uniform expression of IRF4/MUM1, **(B)** CD10 and **(C)** BCL6. **D** MIB-1/Ki-67 stain shows numerous positive cells in the reactive germinal centres (upper right) and somewhat fewer positive cells in the neoplastic follicles (lower left).

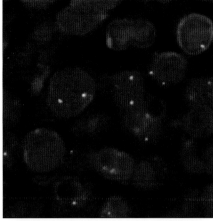

Fig. 13.88 Large B-cell lymphoma with *IRF4* rearrangement. FISH for *IRF4* rearrangement using a break-apart probe demonstrates many cells with one fused normal signal plus one green and one red split signal indicative of the rearrangement (*IRF4* proximal in green, *IRF4* distal in red).

arranged. A cytogenetically cryptic re-arrangement of *IRF4* with an IGH locus is detected in most cases, whereas light chains are rarely involved in the transloca-tion {3491}. In rare cases with similar clinical and pathological features, the *IRF4* translocation may not be demon-strated with current techniques. However, an IGH rearrangement may be detected in these cases. *BCL6* locus breakpoints may be seen in some cases, but virtually all cases lack *MYC* and *BCL2* rearrange-ments {3272,3491}. These cases display a complex pattern of genetic changes, including loss of *TP53* in a subset of patients, independent of age, but these changes are most likely not predictors of clinical behaviour {3489}. Although most cases are found to have a germinal cen-tre B-cell origin (either by gene expres-sion profiling or by immunohistochem-istry), the cases have a unique gene expression signature that is distinct from those of both germinal centre B cells and activated B cells {3491}.

Prognosis and predictive factors
Patients have favourable outcome after treatment (combination immunochemo-therapy with or without radiation) {3491}. This clinical picture is in contrast with that of paediatric-type follicular lymphoma, which tends to have a good prognosis with local management.

Primary cutaneous follicle centre lymphoma

Willemze R.
Swerdlow S.H.
Harris N.L.
Vergier B.

Definition

Primary cutaneous follicle centre lymphoma (PCFCL) is a tumour of neoplastic follicle centre cells, including centrocytes and variable numbers of centroblasts, with a follicular, follicular and diffuse, or diffuse growth pattern. It generally presents on the head or trunk {4320}. Lymphomas with a diffuse growth pattern and a monotonous proliferation of centroblasts and immunoblasts are classified, irrespective of site, as primary cutaneous diffuse large B-cell lymphoma, leg type {4320}.

ICD-O code   9597/3

Synonyms

Reticulohistiocytoma of the dorsum; Crosti lymphoma

Epidemiology

PCFCL accounts for approximately 50% of primary cutaneous B-cell lymphomas. It mainly affects middle-aged adults, with a male-to-female ratio of approximately 1.5:1 {1530,3623,4499}.

Localization

PCFCL characteristically presents with solitary or localized skin lesions on the scalp, forehead, or trunk. Approximately 5% of cases present with skin lesions on the legs, and 15% with multifocal skin lesions {2062,3623,4499}.

Clinical features

The clinical presentation consists of firm erythematous to violaceous plaques, nodules, or tumours of variable size. Particularly on the trunk, tumours may be surrounded by erythematous papules and slightly infiltrated, sometimes figurate plaques, which may precede the development of tumorous lesions by months or years {358,3517,4322}. PCFCL with this typical presentation on the back was formerly referred to as reticulohistiocytoma of the dorsum or Crosti lym-

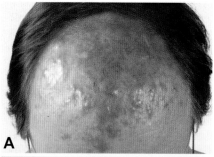

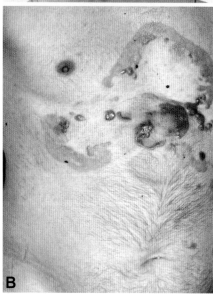

Fig. 13.89 Primary cutaneous follicle centre lymphoma. **A** Characteristic clinical presentation on the scalp. **B** Characteristic clinical presentation with localized skin lesions on the chest.

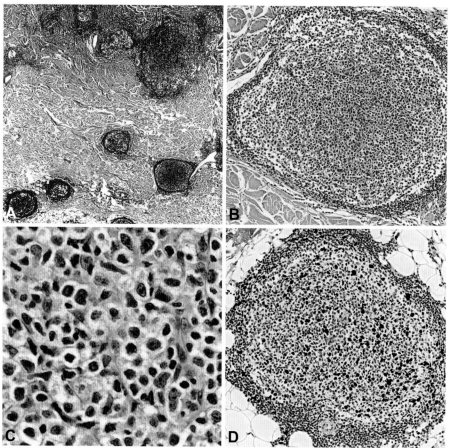

Fig. 13.90 Primary cutaneous follicle centre lymphoma with a follicular growth pattern. **A** Note the distinct follicular structures. **B** Detail of neoplastic follicle showing a monotonous proliferation of follicle centre cells with no polarization, attenuated mantle zone and absence of tingible body macrophages. **C** Monotonous neoplastic follicle centre cells are seen at higher magnification. **D** Unlike in reactive germinal centres, the Ki-67 stain shows only scattered positive cells in the neoplastic follicle.

phoma {358}. The skin surface is smooth and ulceration is rarely observed. Presentation with multifocal skin lesions is observed in a minority of patients, but is not associated with a more unfavourable prognosis {1421,3623}. If left untreated, the skin lesions gradually increase in size over the course of several years, but dissemination to extracutaneous sites is uncommon (occurring in ~10% of cases) {3623,4499}. Recurrences tend to be proximate to the initial site of cutaneous presentation.

Microscopy

PCFCL shows perivascular and periadnexal to diffuse infiltrates, with almost invariable sparing of the epidermis. The infiltrates show a spectrum of growth patterns, with a morphological continuum from follicular to follicular and diffuse to diffuse {3517,4320,4322}. Cases with a follicular growth pattern show nodular infiltrates throughout the entire dermis, often extending into the subcutis. Unlike in cutaneous follicular hyperplasias, the follicles in PCFCL may be poorly defined, show a monotonous proliferation of BCL6+ follicle centre cells enmeshed in a meshwork of CD21+/CD35+ follicular dendritic cells, lack tingible body macrophages, generally have an attenuated or absent mantle zone, and show a low proliferation rate {606,1408}. Reactive T cells may be numerous, and a prominent stromal component is usually present.

Cases with a diffuse growth pattern usually show a monotonous population of large centrocytes, some of which may have a multilobated appearance, and variable numbers of admixed centroblasts {358,1421,3517,4322}. In rare cases, the large centrocytes may be spindle-shaped {607,1406}. In some cases, foci of CD21+/CD35+ follicular dendritic cells may still be present; in other cases, they may be totally absent {1494}. The proliferative fraction in these diffuse PCFCLs is generally high.

Immunophenotype

The neoplastic cells express CD20 and CD79a, but are usually immunoglobulin-negative by immunohistochemistry. Flow cytometric studies are reported to demonstrate restricted light chain expression in almost 3/4 of cases {3549A}. PCFCLs consistently express BCL6. CD10 may be positive in cases with a follicular growth pattern, but is generally negative in cases

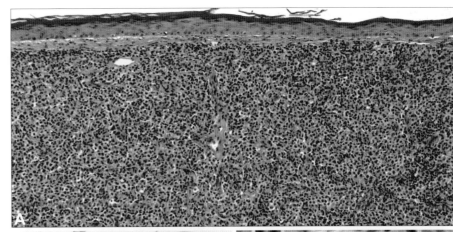

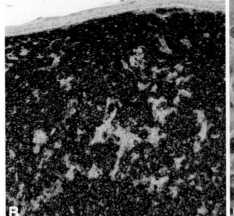
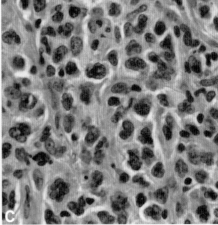

Fig. 13.91 Primary cutaneous follicle centre lymphoma with a diffuse growth pattern. **A** Diffuse non-epidermotropic infiltrate. **B** The tumour cells express CD20. **C** Higher magnification shows that the cellular infiltrate contains many multilobated cells.

with a diffuse growth pattern {903,1409, 1654,2016,2062,2674,3623}. Most cases either do not express BCL2 or only show faint BCL2 staining (weaker than in admixed T cells) in a minority of neoplastic B cells {606,610,715,1318,1654,2062, 3623}. However, several studies have reported BCL2 expression in a substantial proportion of PCFCLs with at least a partially follicular growth pattern {37,1409, 2016,2674,3164}. Strong expression of both BCL2 and CD10 by the neoplastic B cells should always raise suspicion of a nodal follicular lymphoma involving the skin secondarily. Staining for IRF4/MUM1 and FOXP1 is negative in most cases; staining for CD5 and CD43 is always negative {2062,3623}.

Postulated normal counterpart

A mature germinal centre B cell

Genetic profile

Antigen receptor genes

Clonally rearranged IG genes with so-

matic hypermutation are present, but may not be detectable by PCR {6,1325}.

Cytogenetic abnormalities and oncogenes

In many studies, PCFCLs, including cases with a follicular growth pattern, do not show (or rarely show) *BCL2* rearrangements {10,610,715,1318,1408, 1409,1494,1524,1525,3164,4183}. However, other studies using PCR and/or FISH report *BCL2* rearrangements in about 10–40% of PCFCLs with a follicular growth pattern, as well as in some totally diffuse cases {37,2016,2674,3859}. PCFCLs have the same gene expression profile as germinal centre B-cell–subtype diffuse large B-cell lymphomas, and often show amplification of *REL* {6, 986,1653}. Deletion of chromosome 14q32.33 has been reported {986}. Unlike in primary cutaneous diffuse large B-cell lymphoma, leg type, inactivation of *CDKN2A* and *CDKN2B* gene loci on chromosome 9p21.3 by deletion or promotor hypermethylation is only rarely found in PCFCL {986}.

Prognosis and predictive factors

Irrespective of the growth pattern (follicular or diffuse), the number of centroblasts, the presence of t(14;18) and/or BCL2 expression, or the presence of either localized or multifocal skin disease, PCFCLs have an excellent prognosis, with a 5-year survival rate of > 95% {1408,1421,2674,3517,3623,4499}. PCFCLs presenting on the leg are reported to have a less favourable prognosis {2062, 3623}. In patients with localized or few scattered lesions, local radiotherapy is the preferred treatment {1530,3624}. Cutaneous relapses, observed in about 30% of cases, do not indicate progressive disease. Systemic therapy is only required for patients with very extensive cutaneous disease, extremely thick skin tumours, or extracutaneous disease.

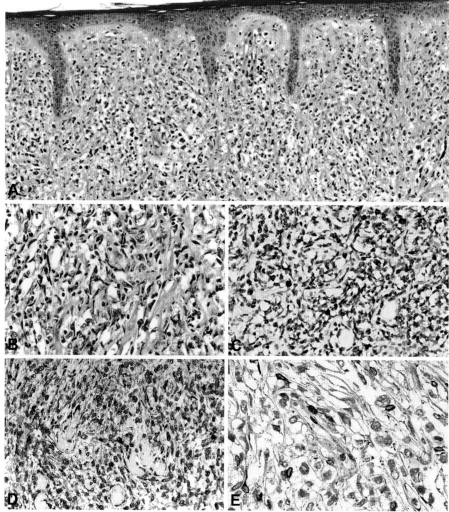

Fig. 13.92 Primary cutaneous follicle centre lymphoma, spindle-shaped morphology. **A** Diffuse proliferation of centrocytes with a spindled morphology. **B** Detail of spindle-shaped cells. **C** Ki-67 stain shows high proliferation rate. **D** The cells are strongly positive for CD79a but (**E**) negative for BCL2.

Mantle cell lymphoma

Swerdlow S.H.
Campo E.
Seto M.
Müller-Hermelink H.K.

Definition

Mantle cell lymphoma is a mature B-cell neoplasm usually composed of monomorphic small to medium-sized lymphoid cells with irregular nuclear contours; in >95% of cases, there is a *CCND1* translocation {245,543,2219,2269,3849, 4018}. Neoplastic transformed cells (centroblasts), paraimmunoblasts, and proliferation centres are absent. Mantle cell lymphoma has traditionally been considered a very aggressive and incurable lymphoma, but more indolent variants, including leukaemic non-nodal mantle cell lymphoma and in situ mantle cell neoplasia, are now also well recognized.

ICD-O codes

Mantle cell lymphoma   9673/3
In situ mantle cell neoplasia   9673/1

Synonyms

Mantle zone lymphoma (obsolete); malignant lymphoma, lymphocytic, intermediate differentiation, diffuse (obsolete); malignant lymphoma, centrocytic (obsolete); malignant lymphomatous polyposis; in situ mantle cell lymphoma (for in situ mantle cell neoplasia)

Epidemiology

Mantle cell lymphoma accounts for approximately 3–10% of non-Hodgkin lymphomas {1}. It occurs in middle-aged to older individuals, with a median age of about 60 years. There is a variably marked male predominance, with a male-to-female ratio of ≥2:1 {139,423,543, 2219,3849,3854}.

Localization

Lymph nodes are the most commonly involved site. The spleen and bone marrow, with or without peripheral blood involvement, are also important sites of disease {139,423,2896,3849}. Other extranodal sites are also frequently involved, including the gastrointestinal tract (where infiltration may be subclinical), Waldeyer ring, lungs, and pleura {1324,3487}. An uncommon but distinctive presentation is

Table 13.21 Morphological variants of mantle cell lymphoma

Aggressive variants	**Blastoid:** Cells resemble lymphoblasts with dispersed chromatin and a high mitotic rate (usually ≥20–30 mitoses per 10 high-power fields). **Pleomorphic:** Cells are pleomorphic, but many are large with oval to irregular nuclear contours, generally pale cytoplasm, and often prominent nucleoli in at least some of the cells.
Other variants	**Small-cell:** Cells are small round lymphocytes with more clumped chromatin, either admixed or predominant, mimicking a small lymphocytic lymphoma. **Marginal zone–like:** There are prominent foci of cells with abundant pale cytoplasm resembling marginal zone or monocytoid B cells, mimicking a marginal zone lymphoma; sometimes these paler foci also resemble proliferation centres of chronic lymphocytic leukaemia / small lymphocytic lymphoma.

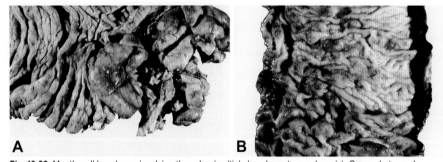

Fig. 13.93 Mantle cell lymphoma involving the colon (multiple lymphomatous polyposis). Gross photographs. **A** Overview showing one large and multiple small polypoid mucosal lesions. **B** Closer view showing tiny polypoid mucosal lesions.

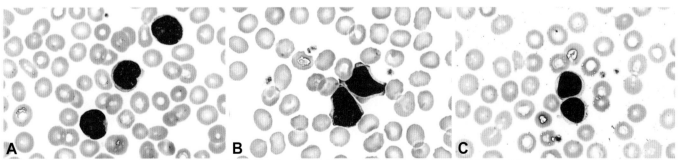

Fig. 13.94 Mantle cell lymphoma, peripheral blood, cytological variation. **A** This typical mantle cell lymphoma demonstrates relatively small lymphoid cells with clumped chromatin and prominent nuclear clefts. **B** In contrast, the cells in this blastoid mantle cell lymphoma are larger and have prominent nucleoli. **C** This mantle cell lymphoma could easily be confused morphologically with chronic lymphocytic leukaemia.

with multiple intestinal polyps (so-called multiple lymphomatous polyposis), although these findings are not specific for mantle cell lymphoma {2134,2910,3459}. CNS involvement may occur, most commonly at the time of relapse {667}.

Clinical features

Most patients present with stage III or, usually, stage IV disease with lymphadenopathy, hepatosplenomegaly, and bone marrow involvement {423,543,2896, 3854}. Extranodal involvement, usually in the presence of extensive lymphadenopathy, is common. Peripheral blood involvement is also common, and can be identified by flow cytometry in almost all patients {1192}. Some patients have a marked lymphocytosis, which can closely mimic prolymphocytic leukaemia {139, 423,2896}, an acute leukaemia {4204}, or chronic lymphocytic leukaemia. Some patients present with leukaemic non-nodal disease, sometimes with splenomegaly. These cases constitute a different variant of the disease (see below).

Macroscopy

Most cases of multiple lymphomatous polyposis constitute mantle cell lymphoma.

Microscopy

Classic mantle cell lymphoma is a monomorphic lymphoid proliferation with a vaguely nodular, diffuse, mantle zone, or rarely follicular growth pattern {245,2219, 2269,3849,4018}. Mantle cell lymphoma with a mantle zone growth pattern should be distinguished from in situ mantle cell neoplasia (see discussion below). Most cases are composed of small to medium-sized lymphoid cells with slightly to markedly irregular nuclear contours, most closely resembling centrocytes. The nuclei have at least somewhat dispersed chromatin but inconspicuous nucleoli. Neoplastic transformed cells resembling centroblasts, immunoblasts, or paraimmunoblasts and proliferation centres are absent; however, foci mimicking proliferation centres may be present {3855A}, and a spectrum of morphological variants is recognized, which can also cause diagnostic confusion (Table 13.21, p.285). The blastoid and pleomorphic variants are considered to be of important clinical significance. The small-cell variant is overrepresented among cases of leukaemic, non-nodal mantle cell lymphoma

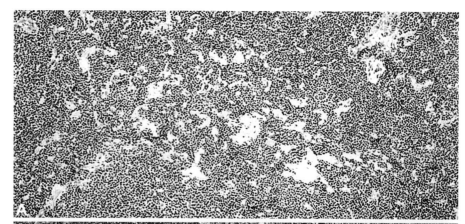

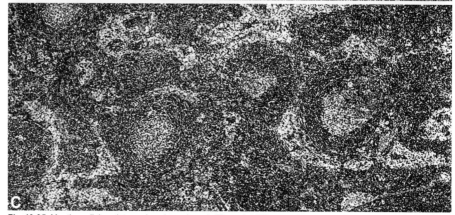

Fig. 13.95 Mantle cell lymphoma, lymph nodes. **A** There is diffuse architectural effacement and typical pale hyalinized vessels. **B** In addition to diffuse areas, note the prominent vague neoplastic nodules. **C** A mantle zone growth pattern is seen in this lymph node with an intact architecture.

{1187}, and the marginal zone–like variant is of greatest interest because of its potential confusion with marginal zone lymphomas. Mantle cell lymphoma in the peripheral blood or in bone marrow aspirates shows the same cytological spectrum that is seen in tissue sections; however, nucleoli are sometimes more prominent, even in cases of classic type. Although mantle cell lymphoma is not graded, evaluation of the proliferative fraction (either by counting mitotic figures or estimating the proportion of Ki-67–

positive nuclei) is critical because of its prognostic impact.

Hyalinized small vessels are commonly seen. Many cases have scattered single epithelioid histiocytes, which in occasional blastoid or pleomorphic cases can create a so-called starry-sky appearance. Non-neoplastic plasma cells may be present, but true plasmacytic differentiation, which can be very marked, is seen only rarely {2645,3347,3851,4444,4445}. Splenic involvement, characterized by white pulp and variable red pulp infiltra-

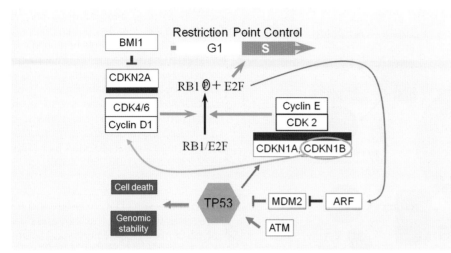

Fig. 13.96 Mantle cell lymphoma (MCL). Cell-cycle and DNA damage repair pathways altered in MCL. The cyclin D1 / CDK4/6 complex promotes phosphorylation of RB (also called RB1). This leads to release of the E2F transcription factors, which then lead to progression of the cell cycle into the S phase. The cyclin D1 / CDK4/6 complex is inhibited by p16 (also called CDKN2A). BMI1 is a transcriptional repressor of the *CDKN2A/ARF* locus. Abnormalities in MCL that lead to progression of cells from G1 to S phase include increased cyclin D1 in almost all cases, as well as loss of p16, *RB1* deletions, increased CDK4, and increased BMI1 in a minority of cases, especially those that are more aggressive. Deregulated E2F also induces ARF transcription. ARF leads to stabilization of p53 by inhibiting the activity of MDM2, which leads to the degradation of p53. The tumour suppressor p53 leads to increased expression of p21 (also called CDKN1A) and to cell-cycle arrest or apoptosis. *ATM* is required for activation of p53 after DNA damage. Many MCLs have *ATM* abnormalities, and some patients have germline mutations of this gene. Some MCLs have loss or transcriptional repression of the *CDKN2A/ARF* locus (lacking p16/ARF), loss or mutation of *TP53*, or high levels of MDM2. Finally, cyclin E / CDK2 complexes also lead to cell-cycle progression, and are inhibited by p21 and p27 (also called CDKN1B). In MCL, increased levels of cyclin D1 lead to sequestration of these cell-cycle inhibitors, and they may also increase p27 degradation {1843}.

tion, can mimic a splenic marginal zone lymphoma, with smaller cells with little cytoplasm centrally in the white pulp nodules and a peripheral zone where the neoplastic cells more closely resemble marginal zone cells, being somewhat larger and with more abundant cytoplasm.

Histological transformation to a typical diffuse large B-cell lymphoma does not occur; however, loss of a mantle zone growth pattern, increase in nuclear size, pleomorphism and chromatin dispersal, and increase in mitotic activity and Ki-67 proliferation index can be seen in some cases at relapse {139,2219,2896,3849, 4208}. Some such cases fulfil the criteria for a blastoid or pleomorphic mantle cell lymphoma (see below). Cases that are blastoid at diagnosis may relapse with classic morphology {4208}.

Immunophenotype

The cells express relatively intense surface IgM/IgD, more frequently with lambda than kappa restriction {543,3849, 4018}. They are uniformly BCL2-positive {3853}; usually positive for CD5, FMC7, and CD43; sometimes positive for IRF4/ MUM1; and negative for CD10 and BCL6.

CD23 is negative or weakly positive. Nuclear cyclin D1 is expressed by >95% of mantle cell lymphomas, including the minority of cases that are CD5-negative {700,3855,4026}. SOX11 is positive with the most sensitive monoclonal antibody in >90% of mantle cell lymphomas, including cyclin D1–negative and blastoid cases {2769,2816,3721}. Caution is advised, because the specificity and sensitivity of SOX11 antibodies vary widely. Aberrant phenotypes have been described (sometimes in association with blastoid or pleomorphic variants), including absence of CD5 and expression of CD10 and BCL6 {41,535,1294, 2737,4425}. Rare cases express other antigens more typically associated with chronic lymphocytic leukaemia, such as LEF1 or CD200, with LEF1 more likely to be seen in blastoid or pleomorphic mantle cell lymphoma and CD200 in the leukaemic non-nodal variant {636,1115, 1157,2633,3505}. Immunohistochemical staining often reveals loose meshworks of follicular dendritic cells.

Postulated normal counterpart

The postulated normal counterpart is a peripheral B cell of the inner mantle zone;

this postulate is based in part on the growth pattern, with early involvement in lymphoid organs. The possibility that mantle cell lymphoma may derive from more than one B-cell compartment has also been suggested {2075}. Most cases are of pre–germinal centre origin, but some are of post–germinal centre origin.

Genetic profile

Antigen receptor genes

IG genes are clonally rearranged. IGV genes are unmutated or minimally mutated in most cases, but in 15–40% of cases, IG genes show somatic hypermutation, although the load of mutations is usually lower than in mutated chronic lymphocytic leukaemia {534,2008,2992, 3950}. A biased use of the IGHV genes has been reported, suggesting that mantle cell lymphoma may originate from specific subsets of B cells {534,2008, 2992,3950}. Together with other observations, this finding suggests that at least a substantial proportion of mantle cell lymphomas show evidence of antigenic drive {1509,4391}.

Cytogenetic abnormalities and oncogenes

The t(11;14)(q13;q32) translocation between an IGH gene and *CCND1* (encoding cyclin D1) is present in >95% of cases and is considered to be the primary genetic event {2301,3408,4095,4146,4323, 4324}. Variant *CCND1* translocations with the IG light chains have also been reported but are very uncommon. The translocation results in deregulated overexpression of CCND1 mRNA and protein {422, 889,3627}. Some mantle cell lymphomas express aberrant transcripts, resulting in an increased half-life of cyclin D1. Tumours with these truncated transcripts have very high levels of cyclin D1 expression {422,889,3627}, high proliferation rates, and more-aggressive clinical behaviour {3413}. Deregulated expression of cyclin D1 is assumed to overcome the cell cycle suppressive effect of RB and p27 in addition to other effects, leading to the development of mantle cell lymphoma {1841,3264}. Nevertheless, it is not sufficient by itself to lead to mantle cell lymphoma, as demonstrated both with animal models and by observations related to *CCND1*-rearranged clonal populations in the peripheral blood of healthy individuals {2247}. In addition to the molecular cytogenetic abnormalities described below,

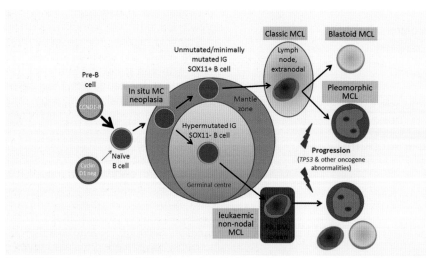

Fig.13.97 Mantle cell lymphoma (MCL). Proposed model of molecular pathogenesis in the development and progression of major subtypes of MCL. Precursor B cells, usually with but sometimes without a *CCND1* rearrangement (*CCND1-R*), mature to abnormal naïve B cells, which may initially colonize the inner portion of the mantle zones, constituting in situ mantle cell (MC) neoplasia. These cells already have additional molecular genetic abnormalities, such as inactivating *ATM* mutations. They may progress to classic MCL, which is most frequently SOX11-positive; has no evidence of transit through the germinal centre; and is genetically unstable, acquiring additional abnormalities related to cell-cycle dysregulation, the DNA damage response pathway, cell survival, and other pathways. Ultimately, progression to blastoid or pleomorphic MCL may occur. A smaller proportion of neoplastic MCs, usually SOX11 negative, may undergo somatic hypermutation, presumably in germinal centres, developing tumours that are more genetically stable for long periods of time and that preferentially involve the peripheral blood (PB), bone marrow (BM), and sometimes the spleen. However, even these MCLs can acquire additional molecular and cytogenetic abnormalities, in particular *TP53* abnormalities, leading to clinical and sometimes morphological progression. Modified from Jares P et al. {1843}.

the abnormal SOX11 expression found in many mantle cell lymphomas is thought to be important in the pathogenesis of mantle cell lymphoma {1188,3039,4169}.

Mantle cell lymphoma carries a high number of non-random secondary chromosomal aberrations, including gains of 3q26 (in 31–50% of cases), 7p21 (in 16–34%), and 8q24.2 (*MYC*, in 16–36%), as well as losses of 1p13-31 (in 29–52% of cases), 6q23-27 (*TNFAIP3*, in 23–38%), 9p21 (*CDKN2A* which codes for p16INK4a and p14ARF, in 18–31%), 11q22-23 (*ATM*, in 21–59%), 13q11-13 (in 22–55%), 13q14-34 (in 43–51%), and 17p13.1 (*TP53*, in 21–45%) {302,3444,3627}. SNP studies also demonstrate copy-neutral LOH in as many as approximately 60% of cases, often involving the same regions where copy losses are found, such as in the region of *TP53* {303,3440}. High-level amplifications, such as of 18q21 (the site of the *BCL2* locus) or of the translocated *CCND1* region, are also found in a minority of cases {303}. Trisomy 12 has been reported in 25% of cases, but usually in the context of other alterations {847}. In addition to chromosomal imbalances, mantle cell lymphoma may also demonstrate tetraploid clones, which are more common in the pleomorphic variant (present

in 80% of these cases) and the blastoid variant (in 36%) than in cases with typical morphology (present in 8%) {3007}. The t(8;14)(q24;q32) translocation and variant *MYC* translocations are rarely present, and are associated with an aggressive clinical course {4098}. *BCL6* (3q27.3) translocations also occur uncommonly and are reportedly associated with BCL6 expression {535}. Some cytogenetic abnormalities may also have associations with various clinical parameters, including a leukaemic presentation {1192,3071}.

Oncogenic alterations have been found in genes targeting cell-cycle regulatory elements, the DNA damage response pathway, cell survival, and other pathways {305,1186,2115,2615,3280,4477}. Inactivating mutations of *ATM* at 11q22-23 have been detected in 40–75% of mantle cell lymphomas, as well as in the germline of some patients with mantle cell lymphoma {305,532,3550}. *CCND1* is reported to be mutated in 35% of cases (usually IGHV-mutated cases), *KMT2D* (*MLL2*) in 14%, *NOTCH1* in 5–12%, and many other genes in ≤ 10% of cases; some mutations, such as those of *NOTCH1/2*, are of prognostic and potential therapeutic importance {305,2115,2615,4477}. Mutations in some genes (*ATM*, *KMT2D*, and

NOTCH1/2) have been reported only in SOX11-positive mantle cell lymphomas. Highly proliferative variants of mantle cell lymphoma have frequent *TP53* mutations, homozygous deletions of *CDKN2A* and the cyclin-dependent kinase inhibitor *CDKN2C*, amplifications and overexpression of the *BMI1* polycomb and *CDK4* genes, and occasional microdeletions of the *RB1* gene {302,304,543,1453, 1622,2399,3194,3196,4325,4326}.

Cyclin D1–negative mantle cell lymphoma

Rare cases with the morphology and phenotype of mantle cell lymphoma are negative for cyclin D1 and t(11;14)(q13;q32) (IGH/*CCND1*) but have gene expression and global genomic profiles as well as other features, including clinical presentation and evolution, indistinguishable from those of cyclin D1–positive mantle cell lymphoma {1262,3413,3492,3494}. Cyclin D2 or cyclin D3 is highly expressed. Approximately half of these cases have *CCND2* translocations, usually with an IG partner (often either IGK or IGL), and are associated with high cyclin D2 expression levels {3492}. Immunostaining for cyclin D2 or D3 is not useful in recognizing these cases, because such staining is also positive in other B-cell lymphomas; however, SOX11 staining is very useful {3492}. Diminished p27 staining (less intense than in the T-cell population) may also be helpful {3264}. In the absence of SOX11 staining, this diagnosis must be made with extreme caution, if at all, given the many lymphomas that can mimic mantle cell lymphoma. Very rare cases in which cyclin D1 expression cannot be demonstrated despite the presence of the *CCND1* rearrangement do occur {3505}. Conversely, rare cases express cyclin D1 but lack a demonstrable *CCND1* rearrangement {3851}.

Genetic susceptibility

Familial aggregation of mantle cell lymphoma and of mantle cell lymphoma with other B-cell neoplasms has been reported {4032}.

Prognosis and predictive factors

Mantle cell lymphoma is associated with a median survival of 3–5 years, with the vast majority of patients not being cured even with the newer therapeutic modalities being used today {46,543,544, 651A,1037,1115,1187,2992,3854,4218}.

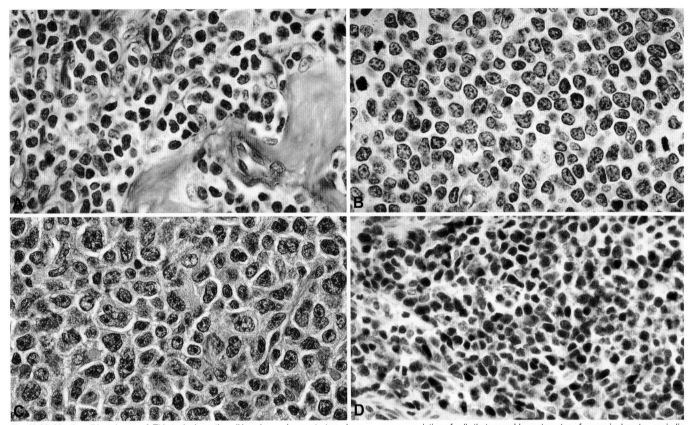

Fig. 13.98 Mantle cell lymphoma. **A** This typical mantle cell lymphoma demonstrates a homogeneous population of cells that resemble centrocytes of a germinal centre, periodic acid–Schiff (PAS) stain. **B** The cells in the blastoid variant resemble lymphoblasts and have a high mitotic rate. **C** Note the large and pleomorphic cells, including cells with prominent nucleoli, in the pleomorphic variant. **D** Cyclin D1 immunostaining shows nuclear positivity.

In recent years, overall survival appears to have improved among at least some subsets of patients. A subset of asymptomatic patients with indolent disease who can be followed, at least initially, without any therapy has also been increasingly recognized and includes many of the patients with one of the clinicopathological mantle cell lymphoma variants described below {571,1037,1118,1187,2522,2992}. Assessment of proliferation rate is critical; high mitotic rate (> 10–37.5 mitoses per 15 high-power fields or > 50 mitoses/mm²) {139,423,3849,4001} and high Ki-67 proliferation index (variably defined,

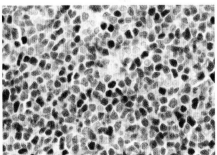

Fig. 13.99 Mantle cell lymphoma. SOX11 immunostaining shows nuclear positivity.

but with > 30% as a currently accepted cut-off point) are associated with an adverse prognosis {962,1038,1416,1964, 4001}. Cases with < 10% Ki-67–positive cells have a more indolent course. Ki-67 expression has also been incorporated into the biological, prognostically important Mantle Cell Lymphoma International Prognostic Index (MIPI) score, which also includes patient age, Eastern Cooperative Oncology Group (ECOG) performance score, lactate dehydrogenase level, and white blood cell count {1319,1704}. In a major gene expression profiling study, the most significant prognostic indicator in mantle cell lymphoma was also the proliferation signature score, which further highlights the clinical importance of proliferation rate in this entity {3413}. The following features have been reported in at least some studies to be adverse prognostic factors (although they are not necessarily all independent of the proliferative fraction): blastoid or pleomorphic morphology, karyotypic complexity, *TP53* mutation/overexpression/loss, *CDKN2A* deletion, and a variety of individual clinical parameters including overt peripheral

blood involvement (at least in patients with adenopathy) {302,423,543,847,939, 1453,2399,2892,3200,3494,3522,3849}. Lack of SOX11 expression has been associated with more-indolent mantle cell lymphoma in some studies; however, other studies have found these cases to be more aggressive, perhaps related to acquisition of *TP53* abnormalities, which are present in a substantial subset of the cases {1187,2841,2892,2908}. The small-cell variant also appears to have a more indolent course; the impact of a mantle zone or nodular pattern is less certain, but at least some nodular cases are probably associated with a more indolent course {423,571,2219,2449,2896,3413,3849, 4001}. The literature is not uniform with regard to the impact of individual chromosomal gains or deletions, limiting their utility. The prognostic value of 9p (*CDKN2A*) and 17p (*TP53*) deletions has been confirmed in clinical trials with new therapies, and seems to be independent of proliferation {939}. Other chromosomal alterations have been associated with a poor prognosis independent of the proliferative fraction, but these associations need to

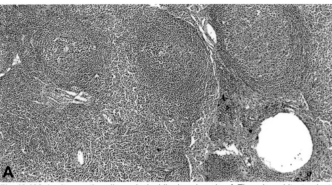
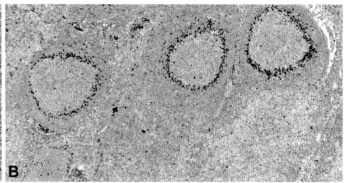

Fig. 13.100 In situ mantle cell neoplasia, hilar lymph node. **A** There is architectural retention, with intact sinuses and scattered follicles with germinal centres and mantle zones (anthracotic pigment is present). **B** The follicles show cyclin D1–positive lymphocytes, mostly in the inner mantle zones.

be confirmed in patients treated with current therapeutic approaches {3494,3522}.

Leukaemic non-nodal mantle cell lymphoma

Leukaemic non-nodal mantle cell lymphoma is defined as mantle cell lymphoma in which the patient presents with peripheral blood, bone marrow, and sometimes splenic involvement but without significant adenopathy (typically defined as peripheral lymph nodes < 1–2 cm and without adenopathy on CT, if performed) {1115,1187,2992}. Like in chronic lymphocytic leukaemia, it appears that these circulating cells may reversibly infiltrate extranodal inflammatory sites (e.g. with *Helicobacter pylori*–associated gastritis) and may remain localized to the mantle zone, overlapping with in situ mantle cell neoplasia. The neoplastic cells in leukaemic non-nodal mantle cell lymphoma are more likely to be small, resembling chronic lymphocytic leukaemia–type cells, SOX11-negative, and to have somatic IG hypermutation {928,1115,1187,2992}. CD5 expression may be less common than in other mantle cell lymphomas. Leukaemic non-nodal mantle cell lymphomas are more likely than classic mantle cell lymphomas to have < 30–40% CD38 positivity, and at least a subset is more likely to have ≥ 2% CD200 positivity, a phenotype that may overlap with that of chronic lymphocytic leukaemia {1115,2992}. Cytogenetic studies show few abnormalities other than the *CCND1* translocation, whereas classic mantle cell lymphoma typically has greater genomic instability and a more complex karyotype {1187,3439}. Although not considered a prognostic indicator, mutated IG genes have been identified in patients with longer-term

survival. Expression profiling and experimental studies suggest that these cases have a lack of tumour invasion properties and angiogenic potential, perhaps accounting for the absence of significant adenopathy {928,3039}. Patients with this variant have been reported to have a better prognosis than those with classic mantle cell lymphoma (median survival: 79 months) and are overrepresented in studies of patients with mantle cell lymphomas that have followed an indolent course, often not requiring therapy for long periods {1115,1187,2992}. However, some cases of this subtype may progress to an aggressive disease, with or without the development of lymphadenopathy, sometimes with rapidly progressive splenomegaly and sometimes with transformation to a blastoid or pleomorphic variant. Acquisition of *TP53* mutations or other oncogenic alterations may be associated with this aggressive evolution {3439}. Although monoclonal B-cell lymphocytosis of mantle cell lymphoma type is not recognized, there is a small proportion of healthy individuals (at least 7%) with circulating cells that have IGH/*CCND1* translocations detected with highly sensitive techniques, which can persist for years and may increase in number over time {2247}. A report of simultaneous development of mantle cell lymphoma in a recipient and donor 12 years after allogeneic bone marrow transplantation is also consistent with a very long latent period for mantle cell lymphoma after an initial event {750}.

In situ mantle cell neoplasia

In situ mantle cell neoplasia, formerly referred to as in situ mantle cell lymphoma or mantle cell lymphoma–like B cells of uncertain/undetermined significance, is

defined as the presence of cyclin D1–positive lymphoid cells with *CCND1* rearrangements restricted to the mantle zones of otherwise hyperplastic-appearing lymphoid tissue {571,2885}. Peripheral blood involvement or involvement at more than one site does not exclude the diagnosis, with some cases probably constituting the leukaemic non-nodal type of mantle cell lymphoma but with involvement of the mantle zone (i.e. in situ) in lymph nodes enlarged for some other reason. Extranodal involvement may also be present. The cyclin D1–positive cells are typically in the inner mantle zone, but may rarely be scattered throughout the mantle zone, in the outer mantle zone, or very rarely intrafollicular. When the mantle zones are expanded and completely replaced by cyclin D1–positive lymphoid cells, the diagnosis of overt mantle cell lymphoma with a mantle zone growth pattern is more appropriate. Compared with classic mantle cell lymphoma, these cases are more likely to be CD5-negative, and they include both SOX11-positive and a moderate number of SOX11-negative cases. These cases are very rare (none were found in two series of at least 100 hyperplastic lymph nodes) and are usually identified as an incidental finding, sometimes associated with other malignant lymphomas, when cyclin D1 immunohistochemical staining is performed {571,22A}. In situ mantle cell neoplasia often has an indolent course with long-term survival, frequently with stable disease even without therapy. However, caution is advised, because rare cases may progress to overt mantle cell lymphoma and occasional patients have been reported who have not done well {571,1949,3351}. The proportion of overt mantle cell lymphoma preceded by in situ mantle cell neoplasia is controversial.

Diffuse large B-cell lymphoma, NOS

Gascoyne R.D.
Campo E.
Jaffe E.S.
Chan W.C.

Chan J.K.C.
Rosenwald A.
Stein H.
Swerdlow S.H.

Definition

Diffuse large B-cell lymphoma (DLBCL) is a neoplasm of medium or large B lymphoid cells whose nuclei are the same size as, or larger than, those of normal macrophages, or more than twice the size of those of normal lymphocytes, with a diffuse growth pattern.

Morphological, biological, and clinical studies have subdivided DLBCLs into morphological variants, molecular subtypes, and distinct disease entities (Table 13.22). However, there remain many cases that may be biologically heterogeneous, but for which there are no clear and accepted criteria for subdivision. These cases are classified as DLBCL, NOS, which encompasses all cases that do not belong to a specific diagnostic category listed in Table 13.22. DLBCL, NOS can be subdivided into germinal centre B-cell (GCB) subtype and activated B-cell (ABC) subtype. Focal involvement of follicular structures in DLBCL, which can be highlighted by immunohistochemical staining for follicular dendritic cells, does not require the additional diagnosis of a grade 3B follicular lymphoma.

ICD-O codes

Diffuse large B-cell lymphoma, NOS
　　　　　　　　　　　　　　9680/3
Germinal centre B-cell subtype　9680/3
Activated B-cell subtype　　　　9680/3

Epidemiology

DLBCL, NOS, constitutes 25–35% of adult non-Hodgkin lymphomas in developed countries, and a higher percentage in developing countries. It is more common in elderly individuals. The median patient age is in the seventh decade of life, but it can also occur in children and young adults. It is slightly more common in males than in females {1,95}.

Etiology

The etiology of DLBCL, NOS, remains unknown. These tumours usually arise de novo (referred to as primary) but can also represent transformation of a less

Table 13.22 Large B-cell lymphomas; italics indicate that an entity is provisional

Diffuse large B-cell lymphoma, NOS
　Morphological variants
　　　　　　　　Centroblastic
　　　　　　　　Immunoblastic
　　　　　　　　Anaplastic
　　　　　　　　Other rare variants
　Molecular subtypes
　　　　　　　　Germinal centre B-cell subtype
　　　　　　　　Activated B-cell subtype

Other lymphomas of large B cells
　T-cell/histiocyte-rich large B-cell lymphoma
　Primary diffuse large B-cell lymphoma of the CNS
　Primary cutaneous diffuse large B-cell lymphoma, leg type
　EBV-positive diffuse large B-cell lymphoma, NOS
　Diffuse large B-cell lymphoma associated with chronic inflammation
　Lymphomatoid granulomatosis
　Large B-cell lymphoma with *IRF4* rearrangement
　Primary mediastinal (thymic) large B-cell lymphoma
　Intravascular large B-cell lymphoma
　ALK-positive large B-cell lymphoma
　Plasmablastic lymphoma
　HHV8-positive diffuse large B-cell lymphoma
　Primary effusion lymphoma

High-grade B-cell lymphoma
　High-grade B-cell lymphoma with *MYC* and *BCL2* and/or *BCL6* rearrangements
　High-grade B-cell lymphoma, NOS

B-cell lymphoma, unclassifiable
　B-cell lymphoma, unclassifiable, with features intermediate between diffuse large B-cell lymphoma and classic Hodgkin lymphoma

aggressive lymphoma (referred to as secondary), such as chronic lymphocytic leukaemia/small lymphocytic lymphoma, follicular lymphoma, marginal zone lymphoma, or nodular lymphocyte predominant Hodgkin lymphoma. Underlying immunodeficiency is a significant risk factor. DLBCLs, NOS, occurring in the setting of immunodeficiency are more often EBV-positive than sporadic cases. In DLBCL cases without an overt immunodeficiency, the EBV infection rate varies from 3% in western populations to approximately 10% in Asian and Latin American populations, and the lymphoma is typically of the ABC subtype {325, 1017,1367,1655,2701,2956,3696}. Importantly, EBV positivity in most tumour cells should lead to a diagnosis of either EBV-positive DLBCL, NOS, or another specific type of EBV-positive lymphoma (e.g.

DLBCL associated with chronic inflammation or lymphomatoid granulomatosis).

Localization

Patients may present with nodal or extranodal disease; as many as 40% of cases are confined to extranodal sites at least initially {1,95}. The most common

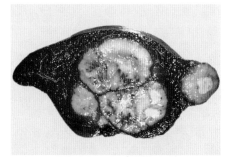

Fig. 13.101 Diffuse large B-cell lymphoma, NOS. Involved spleen contains large tumour nodules.

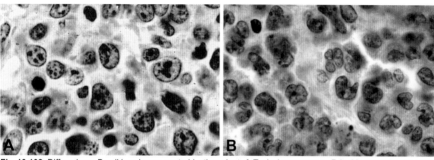

Fig. 13.102 Diffuse large B-cell lymphoma, centroblastic variant. **A** Typical appearance. **B** In this example, the tumour cells have a polymorphic and multilobated appearance.

extranodal site is the gastrointestinal tract (stomach and ileocaecal region), but virtually any extranodal location can be primarily involved. Other common sites of extranodal presentation include the bone, testes, spleen, Waldeyer ring, salivary glands, thyroid, liver, kidneys, and adrenal glands. Primary CNS lymphoma and primary testicular lymphoma are both lymphomas of immune-privileged sites and therefore share some overlapping biology. DLBCLs involving the kidneys and adrenal glands are associated with an increased risk of spread to the CNS. Cutaneous lymphomas composed mostly of large B lymphocytes (i.e. primary cutaneous follicle centre lymphoma and primary cutaneous DLBCL, leg type) are considered distinct entities and discussed separately in this volume.

Bone marrow involvement in DLBCL can be discordant (low-grade B-cell lymphoma in the marrow, seen in 10–25% of cases) or concordant (large cell lymphoma in the marrow, seen in a similar proportion of cases) {128,474,538,3061, 3612}. The detection rate for minimal involvement may be increased with the use of ancillary techniques such as flow cytometry, immunohistochemistry, and

molecular genetics {3883,3884}. Recent studies have suggested that FDG-PET is a sensitive technique for detecting concordant bone marrow involvement, but is not reliable for discordant disease {24, 273,2000}. The most recent consensus criteria for lymphoma staging indicate that a routine staging bone marrow biopsy is no longer required if FDG-PET is negative {691}. Morphologic involvement of the peripheral blood by DLBCL is rare.

Clinical features

Patients usually present with a rapidly enlarging tumour mass at single or multiple nodal or extranodal sites. Almost half of the patients have stage I or II disease, but the inclusion of PET/CT in the initial staging of DLBCL has resulted in stage migration, reducing the percentage of patients with limited-stage disease. Many patients are asymptomatic, but B symptoms may be present. Specific localizing symptoms may be present and are highly dependent on the site of extranodal involvement {1,148}.

Microscopy

Lymph nodes demonstrate partial or more commonly total architectural efface-

ment by a diffuse proliferation of medium or large lymphoid cells. Partial nodal involvement may be interfollicular and/or less commonly sinusoidal. The perinodal tissue is often infiltrated. Broad or fine bands of sclerosis may be present. The morphology of DLBCL, NOS, is diverse and the disease can be divided into common and rare morphological variants. For this reason, ancillary studies are critical before making the diagnosis of DLBCL, NOS. Cases with medium-sized cells are particularly prone to misclassification. Special studies are required to exclude extramedullary leukaemias, Burkitt lymphoma, high-grade B-cell lymphoma with *MYC* and *BCL2* and/or *BCL6* rearrangements, and blastoid mantle cell lymphoma.

Common morphological variants
Three common and several rare morphological variants have been recognized. All variants may be admixed with a high number of T cells and/or histiocytes. These cases should not be categorized as T-cell/histiocyte-rich large B-cell lymphoma as long they do not fulfil all the criteria for that entity.

Centroblastic variant: This is the most common variant. Centroblasts are medium-sized to large lymphoid cells with usually oval to round, vesicular nuclei containing fine chromatin. There are 2–4 nuclear membrane-bound nucleoli. The cytoplasm is usually scant and amphophilic or basophilic. In some cases, the tumour is monomorphic, i.e. it is composed almost entirely (>90%) of centroblasts. Centroblastic cases are more frequently of the GCB subtype {3411}. However, in most cases the tumour is polymorphic with an admixture of

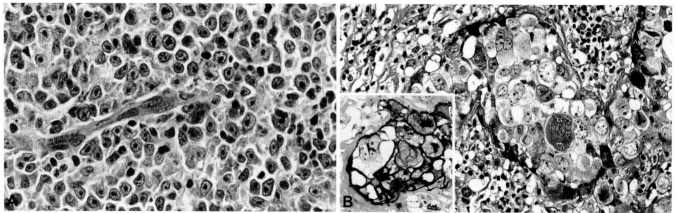

Fig. 13.103 Diffuse large B-cell lymphoma. **A** Immunoblastic variant. The neoplastic cells have a uniform cytological appearance with prominent single central nucleoli. **B** Anaplastic variant. Large lymphoma cells with pleomorphic nuclei infiltrate the sinus. Inset: There is strong membranous and perinuclear labelling of the lymphoma cells for CD20.

centroblasts and immunoblasts (<90%) {1105,3009}. The tumour cells may have multilobated nuclei, which predominate in rare instances, especially in tumours localized to the bone and other extranodal sites.

Immunoblastic variant: In this variant, >90% of the cells are immunoblasts, with a single centrally located nucleolus and an appreciable amount of basophilic cytoplasm. Immunoblasts with plasmacytoid differentiation may also be present. Clinical and/or immunophenotypic findings may be essential in for differentiating this variant from extramedullary involvement by a plasmablastic lymphoma or an immature plasma cell myeloma. The distinction of the immunoblastic variant from the common centroblastic variant has generally shown poor intraobserver and interobserver reproducibility {1105,3009}.

Anaplastic variant: This variant is characterized by large to very large cells with bizarre pleomorphic nuclei that may resemble, at least in part, Hodgkin/Reed–Sternberg cells, and may resemble the neoplastic cells of anaplastic large cell lymphoma. The cells may show a sinusoidal and/or a cohesive growth pattern and may mimic undifferentiated carcinoma {1548}. The anaplastic variant is biologically and clinically unrelated to anaplastic large cell lymphoma, which is often of cytotoxic T-cell derivation, and unrelated to ALK-positive large B-cell lymphoma, which lacks expression of CD20 and CD30.

Rare morphological variants

Rare cases of DLBCL, NOS, have a myxoid stroma or a fibrillary matrix. Pseudorosette formation is rarely seen. Occasionally, the neoplastic cells are spindle-shaped or display features of signet ring cells. Cytoplasmic granules, microvillous projections, and intercellular junctions can also be seen ultrastructurally.

Immunophenotype

The neoplastic cells typically express pan–B-cell markers such as CD19, CD20, CD22, CD79a, and PAX5, but may lack one or more of these. Surface and cytoplasmic immunoglobulin (most commonly IgM, followed by IgG and IgA) can be demonstrated in 50–75% of the cases. The presence of cytoplasmic immunoglobulin does not correlate with the expression of plasma cell–associated markers such as CD138. CD138 is rarely

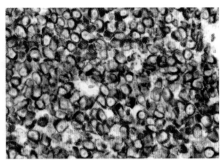

Fig. 13.104 Diffuse large B-cell lymphoma, immunoblastic variant, expressing BCL2.

coexpressed in CD20-positive cells. CD30 may be expressed in 10–20% of cases, especially in the anaplastic variant {1717,3696}. The presence of EBV in most of the cells should lead to a diagnosis of EBV-positive DLBCL, NOS; most of these cases are CD30-positive.

The neoplastic cells express CD5 in 5–10% of the cases {4399,4406}. CD5+ DLBCLs usually constitute de novo DLBCL, only rarely arising from chronic lymphocytic leukaemia / small lymphocytic lymphoma. CD5+ DLBCL can be distinguished from the blastoid or pleomorphic variant of mantle cell lymphoma by the absence of cyclin D1 and/or SOX11 expression {4467}. Rare cases express cyclin D1 in the absence of *CCND1* translocation and SOX11 expression. However, it is usually not as strong and uniform as in MCL {1714,2959,4170}.

The expression of MYC and BCL2 varies considerably, in part depending on the threshold used to define positivity {1440, 1686,1718,1866,2048,2049,2446,3141, 3601,4113,4415}. In most studies, BCL2 is considered positive if ≥50% of the tumour cells are positive, and MYC is considered positive if ≥40% of the tumour cell nuclei are positive. Coexpression of these two proteins (so-called double-expressers) is more frequent in the ABC subtype (see below) {1866,3601}.

The reported incidence of CD10, BCL6, IRF4/MUM1, FOXP1, GCET1, and LMO2 expression varies. The Hans algorithm uses three markers to distinguish the GCB from the non-GCB subtype: CD10, BCL6, and IRF4/MUM1 are each considered positive if ≥30% of the tumour cell stain positively {1537}. CD10 is positive in 30–50% of cases, BCL6 in 60–90%, and IRF4/MUM1 in 35–65% {348,786, 902,2790}. Unlike in normal GCBs, in which expression of IRF4/MUM1 and BCL6 is mutually exclusive, coexpression of these markers is found in 50% of

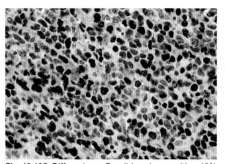

Fig. 13.105 Diffuse large B-cell lymphoma with >40% of the tumour cells expressing nuclear MYC protein.

DLBCLs {1141}. FOXP1 expression has been reported in about 20% of DLBCL cases that lack the germinal centre phenotype and express IRF4/MUM1 and BCL2 in the absence of t(14;18) (q32;q21.3) {271}. GCET1, a germinal centre marker, is expressed in 40–50% of cases and is highly correlated with the GCB type {2703}. LMO2 expression is found in approximately 45% of DLBCL and is highly correlated with the germinal centre markers CD10, BCL6, and HGAL, but not with IRF4/MUM1 or BCL2 {2840}. Expression of BCL2 varies between reports, with a range of 47–84% {902,1305, 1619,1770}. The observed frequency may also vary depending on the BCL2 antibody used {1990}. In the GCB subtype, BCL2 expression is closely linked to the presence of t(14;18)(q32;q21.3), whereas expression is more common in the ABC subtype, but is the result of copy number gains and transcriptional upregulation {2761,3601}.

The Ki-67 proliferation index is high; it is usually much more than 40% and may be >90% in some cases {1468,1589,2069, 2664,4430}. Expression of p53 is seen in 20–60% of cases, but is more common than the presence of mutations, suggesting upregulation of wildtype *TP53* in some cases {701,2279,2312,4400,4445}.

Cell of origin / postulated normal counterpart

The postulated normal counterparts are peripheral mature B cells of either germinal centre origin (GCB subtype) or germinal centre exit / early plasmablastic or post–germinal centre origin (ABC subtype). Cell of origin distinctions underlie fundamentally different biology based on gene expression, chromosomal aberrations, and recurrent mutations; they are also associated with reproducible survival differences in patients treated with the CHOP chemotherapy regimen plus rituximab (R-CHOP). The accurate distinction of the GCB from the ABC subtype is an important predictive factor in DLBCL, NOS.

Cell of origin subtyping
On the basis of gene expression profiling, DLBCL can be divided into two main molecular subgroups: the GCB subtype and the ABC subtype. Approximately 10–15% of cases cannot be included in either of these subtypes and remain unclassified {67,2272,2273,3411,4372}. The relative frequencies of the GCB subtype and the ABC subtype vary based on geographical location, median age of the patient population, and methodology used, but are typically about 60% and 40%, respectively {3601}. The frequency of the GCB subtype is lower in Asian countries {1745,2308,3061,3615,3663,4383}. Low density gene expression analysis platforms can recapitulate these same groups, and many are applicable to formalin-fixed, paraffin-embedded material {2505,3601,3603}. Numerous immunohistochemical algorithms exist, but most are binary classifiers (i.e. two-class predictors) {738,830,1537,2652,2790,2838, 2909,4199}. For example, the Hans algorithm classifies DLBCL into the two subgroups of GCB subtype and non-GCB subtype, and thus does not recognize the unclassified cases. Although routinely available, all immunohistochemical algorithms suffer from a lack of reproducibility and accuracy, but the determination of cell of origin has begun to penetrate clinical practice and is therefore required {830,3325}. Enrolment in current clinical trials requires the determination of cell of origin status, because preliminary data from phase I/II trials suggest that the benefit from the addition of bortezomib, lenalidomide, and ibrutinib to R-CHOP is preferentially seen in the ABC subtype {1057,2562,2902,2903,2932,4334, 4419}. Therefore, the distinction between the GCB subtype and the ABC subtype should be made for all cases of DLBCL, NOS, at diagnosis. If gene expression technologies are not available, then immunohistochemistry technologies are considered an acceptable alternative. The algorithm used should be specified.

Genetic profile
Antigen receptor genes
Clonally rearranged IG heavy and light chain genes are detectable. The IG

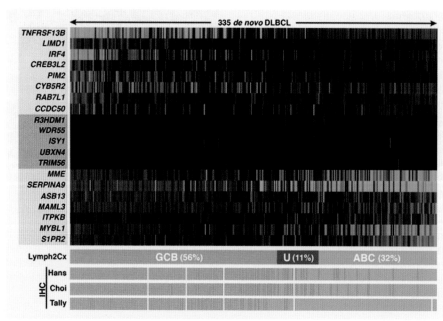

Fig. 13.106 Diffuse large B-cell lymphoma (DLBCL). The Lymph2Cx model is shown in the form of a gene expression heat map. Cases (N = 335) are arrayed from left to right, in ascending order of assay score. The 20 genes that contribute to the model are listed at the left. The top 8 genes are overexpressed in the activated B-cell type (ABC), the middle 5 genes are housekeeping genes, and the bottom 7 genes are overexpressed in the germinal centre B-cell type (GCB). From Scott DW et al. {3601}. Reprinted with permission. © 2015 by American Society of Clinical Oncology. All rights reserved.

genes show ongoing somatic hypermutation in the GCB subtype or evidence of prior somatic hypermutation in the ABC subtype.

Mutation landscape
Several studies have examined the mutation landscape of DLBCL (Table 13.23), implicating many novel mutations in the pathogenesis of this disease {2384, 2745,3085,4476}. For many genes, the frequency of specific mutations varies depending on the cell of origin subtype; others are found in both the GCB subtype and the ABC subtype. For example, mutations in *EZH2* and *GNA13* are seen almost exclusively in the GCB subtype, whereas *CARD11*, *MYD88*, and *CD79B* mutations are characteristic of the ABC subtype {886,2744,2745,2860}. Recurrent copy number changes have also been studied. Gains and deletions of chromosomal material are common and are differentially seen across the cell of origin subtypes (Table 13.23) {2274, 2718}. For example, GCB DLBCLs often harbour gains or amplification of 2p16 and 8q24 and deletions of 1p36 and 10q23; ABC cases show gains of 3q27.3, 11q23-4, and 18q21.3 and deletions of 6q21 and 9p21 {306,1433,1839,2274, 2718,3081,3085,3545,3578,3607}. Copy

number gains and amplifications of the *MYC* locus vary in frequency; they occur in both the GCB subtype and the ABC subtype, but are slightly more common in GCB DLBCL {2404,3601,4432}.
Candidate gene studies of DLBCL arising at specific extranodal sites have, in some cases, shown both overlapping and unique molecular features. Primary breast DLBCL arising in women is uncommon, but studies reveal that most cases are of the ABC subtype and show recurrent *MYD88* L265P and *CD79B* mutations, similar to nodal ABC DLBCL, NOS {3900}. Rearrangements of either *BCL2* or *BCL6* are rare. Primary gastric DLBCLs are mostly of the ABC subtype. Recurrent mutations of *MYD88* and *CD79B* are uncommon. Translocations involving *BCL6* occur in a subset of cases, as do *MYC* rearrangements, but *BCL2* translocations are uncommon {687}. Primary DLBCLs are common testicular tumours in elderly men, and like primary CNS lymphomas, they are considered lymphomas of immune-privileged sites. Testicular DLBCL, NOS, can spread to the CNS and the contralateral testis {954}. Most cases are of the ABC subtype. Molecular studies reveal a high frequency of *MYD88* mutations, accompanied in a subset of cases by *CD79B* mutations {2098}. Occasional

cases show translocations of *MYC* or *BCL6*, but *BCL2* translocations are rare. Recent data reveal copy-number gains of the 9p21 locus, the site of the ligands of PD1 {665}. In addition, rare translocations of the ligands are also seen, characterized by promotor substitution with promiscuous genes actively transcribed in B cells, leading to overexpression of PDL1, PDL2, or both proteins in primary testicular DLBCL {665,4082}. Further evidence of an immune escape phenotype is loss of major histocompatibility complex (MHC) class I and II expression, which is also a common genetic alteration in primary testicular DLBCL resulting from deletion of HLA loci on chromosome 6p21.3 {415,1883,3355,3356}.

Chromosomal translocations

As many as 30% of cases show rearrangement of the 3q27 region involving *BCL6*, which is the most common translocation in DLBCL {40,272,288,1768,2396, 2930,3667}. These rearrangements tend to occur more commonly in the ABC subtype {1768,3601,4422}. Translocation of the *BCL2* gene, i.e. t(14;18)(q32;q21.3), a hallmark of follicular lymphoma, occurs in 20–30% of DLBCL cases, more commonly in the GCB subtype, where it is present in about 40% of cases and is closely associated with BCL2 and CD10 protein expression {270,1719,1769, 1771,3601,4200}. *MYC* rearrangement is observed in 8–14% of cases, evenly distributed between the GCB subtype and the ABC subtype; unlike in Burkitt lymphoma, it is typically associated with a complex karyotype {44,269,802,848, 1440,1686,1718,1866,2074,2100,3537, 4085,4200}. Approximately half of the DLBCL cases that harbour a *MYC* translocation also show a *BCL2* and/or *BCL6* translocation, and therefore belong in the newly created category of high-grade B-cell lymphoma with *MYC* and *BCL2* and/or *BCL6* rearrangements (so-called double-hit lymphoma) {194,802,1865, 1943,2878,3117,3601}. Cases with otherwise typical DLBCL morphology and an isolated *MYC* translocation belong in the category of DLBCL, NOS {802,1865, 4398}. A variable proportion of the *MYC* translocations involve IG loci as partners: IGH, IGK, or IGL. Others partners include non-IG loci such as *PAX5*, *BCL6*, *BCL11A*, *IKZF1 (IKAROS)*, and *BTG1* {193,362,1865,3118}. The ability to detect *MYC* translocations with non-IG partner

Table 13.23 Genetic, molecular, and clinical characteristics of the diffuse large B-cell lymphoma (DLBCL) subtypes and primary mediastinal large B-cell lymphoma (PMBL)

Characteristic	Frequency		
	ABC DLBCL	GCB DLBCL	PMBL
Rearrangements			
BCL2	<5%	40%	0%
BCL6	25–30%	15%	0%
MYC, single hit	5–8%	5–8%	0%
CD274/PDCD1LG2 (also called *PDL1/2*)	Rare	Rare	20%
CIITA	Rare	Rare	38%
TBL1XR1	0%	5%	0%
Copy-number aberrations			
1p36.32 deletion (*TNFRSF14*)	10%	30%	Rare
2p16 gain/amplification (*REL*)	Rare	30%	60–75%
3q27 gain/amplification	45%	15–20%	Rare
6q21 deletion (*PRDM1*)	45%	25%	n/a
9p21 deletion (*CDKN2A*)	40%	20%	Rare
9p24.1 gains/amplification (*CD274/PDCD1LG2*)	Uncommon	Uncommon	60–75%
18q21.3 gain/amplification (*BCL2*)	55%	15%	Rare
Recurrent mutations[a]			
EZH2	Rare	20–25%	n/a
GNA13	Rare	25%	n/a
KMT2D (also called *MLL2*)	35%	40%	n/a
TP53	25%	20%	n/a
MEF2B	5%	15–20%	n/a
SGK1	5–10%	15–20%	n/a
CREBBP	10%	30%	n/a
TNFRSF14	Rare	30%	n/a
SOCS1	Uncommon	10–15%	40%
PTPN1	n/a	n/a	20%
STAT6	Rare	5%	35%
CARD11	10–15%	10–15%	n/a
CD79B	20–25%	Uncommon	n/a
MYD88	35%	Uncommon	n/a
PRDM1	15%	Rare	n/a
B2M	15–20%	20–25%	n/a
CD58	10%	10%	n/a
Pathway perturbations			
NF-kappaB activation	Yes	No	Yes
PI3K/AKT	No	Yes	No
JAK/STAT signalling	Rare	Yes	Yes
Immune escape	Yes	Yes	Yes
Clinical features			
5-year PFS (R-CHOP)	40–50%	70–80%	85–90%

ABC, activated B-cell subtype; **GBC**, germinal centre B-cell subtype; **n/a**, not available; **PFS**, progression-free survival; **R-CHOP, CHOP** chemotherapy regimen plus rituximab.

[a] Some cases with recurrent mutations also harbour copy number alterations of the same locus, in particular alterations associated with loss of function.

genes is heavily dependent on the FISH assay used {802,2784}. Most DLBCL, NOS, cases with a *MYC* translocation are also double expressers (i.e. are positive for both MYC and BCL2 protein) {1440, 1866,3601}. Cases harbouring a *MYC* translocation tend to have a higher Ki-67 proliferation index, although it is highly variable and is not a useful surrogate for selecting cases for FISH testing. Less-common translocations in DLBCL, NOS, include *TBL1XR1* translocations, which are found in the GCB subtype, and re-arrangements of *CD274* (also called *PD-CD1LG1* or *PDL1*) and *PDCD1LG2* (also called *PDL2*), which are more common in primary testicular DLBCL {3602,4082}.

Genetic susceptibility
Recent case control studies have identified genetic loci that may predispose individuals to the development of DLBCL {602,2135,3691,3704}. Some of the findings in European studies have been replicated in eastern Asian populations, suggesting a common risk {286,3888}. The identities of the candidate genes in these loci suggest that immune recognition and immune function may underlie the pathogenesis of DLBCL {602}.

Prognosis and predictive factors
Clinical features
In the R-CHOP era, the 5-year progression-free and overall survival rates are approximately 60% and 65%, respectively {3611}. Disease stage and patient age are significant factors affecting survival. The International Prognostic Index (IPI), which incorporates five clinical variables, remains a valuable prognostic tool, although newer variations have been described that are better able to identify patients with the highest-risk clinical features {3610,4491}. Other clinical prognostic factors associated with inferior outcome include tumour bulk (masses ≥ 10 cm), male sex, vitamin D deficiency, low body mass index, elevated serum free light chains, monoclonal serum IgM proteins, low absolute lymphocyte/monocyte count, and concordant (but not discordant) bone marrow involvement {568, 831,1035,1673,2586,2797,3161,3220, 3612,4314}. Concordant bone marrow involvement also predicts an increased risk of CNS relapse and in some centres dictates CNS prophylaxis.

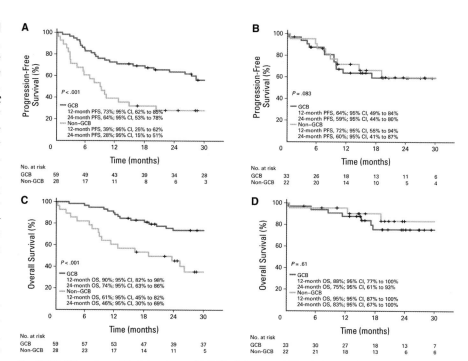

Fig. 13.107 Diffuse large B-cell lymphoma (DLBCL). Outcomes of historical control patients treated with the CHOP chemotherapy regimen plus rituximab (R-CHOP) and study patients treated with lenalidomide added to R-CHOP (R2CHOP), in the germinal centre B-cell (GCB) versus the activated B-cell (ABC; non-GCB) subtypes of DLBCL. **A** Progression-free survival (PFS) of patients treated with R-CHOP. **B** PFS of patients treated with R2CHOP. **C** Overall survival (OS) of patients treated with R-CHOP. **D** OS of patients treated with R2CHOP {2903}. Lenalidomide is effective in patients with ABC lymphomas, mitigating the negative impact of the ABC phenotype on patient outcome.
From: Nowakowski GS, et al. (2015) Lenalidomide combined with R-CHOP overcomes negative prognostic impact of non-germinal center B-cell phenotype in newly diagnosed diffuse large B-cell lymphoma: a phase II study. {2903} Reprinted with permission. © 2015 American Society of Clinical Oncology. All rights reserved.

Morphology
There are many conflicting reports on the prognostic impact of immunoblastic features {1105,3009}. Some studies have found an adverse prognostic impact of immunoblastic morphology, whereas others have not. Reproducibility and variable criteria remain significant obstacles in these studies. The immunoblastic variant is associated with *MYC* translocations, typically involving IG loci. These cases frequently express CD10 {1685}.

Immunophenotype
Many immunohistochemical markers have been reported to have prognostic impact, but most have not been validated and are therefore not accepted as robust or routine biomarkers {212,2397, 2917}. All biomarkers require reassessment using standard of care therapy. De novo CD5+ DLBCL is variably reported to have prognostic importance {754, 2681,2879,4399}. It is often associated with high-risk clinical features, especially in Asian countries, and is usually of ABC subtype {1110,2681,4406}. BCL2

and BCL6 are examples of biomarkers of which the reported prognostic effect was altered by the addition of rituximab to the CHOP chemotherapy regimen {2766,4337}. Many of these immunohistochemistry-based biomarkers reflect biology, but are not predictive. Moreover, the results obtained in these studies are often conflicting, and their interpretation is therefore controversial. The current emphasis is on developing predictive biomarkers in DLBCLs where knowledge of a biomarker impacts an initial or subsequent therapeutic decision. Predictive markers currently include markers for the determination of cell of origin (i.e. GCB subtype vs ABC subtype) being tested now in the context of phase III clinical trials and markers of the presence of relevant oncogene translocations (see below), in particular involving the *MYC* gene {3601}. A recent meta-analysis clearly established the prognostic significance of cell of origin as determined by gene expression profiling, but not based on most immunohistochemical algorithms {3325}. More controversial is the assessment of the double-expression status of MYC and BCL2 proteins, found in approximately 30% of all cases of DLBCL, NOS, and associated with inferior survival in most studies {2686,3523}. Double-expression status also predicts an increased risk of CNS relapse in DLBCL, NOS, and is independent of the CNS International Prognostic Index (CNS-IPI) {3539}. Cases with MYC and BCL2 double-expression that have rearrangements of these genes or of MYC and BCL6 belong in the high grade B-cell lymphoma, with MYC and BCL2 and/or BCL6 rearrangements category. CD30 expression in EBV-negative DLBCL (occurring in ~10–20% of cases), excluding primary mediastinal large B-cell lymphomas, is associated with a favourable outcome in some studies {1542, 1717,3696}. CD30 expression might have therapeutic implications with the existence of anti-CD30 therapy.

Proliferation
The prognostic importance of a high proliferative fraction, as assessed by the Ki-67 proliferation index, is controversial. The findings of studies from both the CHOP and the R-CHOP eras are often conflicting and are typically confounded by the lack of consideration of patient age, other clinical variables, and the cell of origin status {1866,2069,2922,4085}.

Genetics
In some studies, the presence of a BCL2 translocation is associated with inferior outcome in GCB DLBCL in patients treated with R-CHOP {270,1769,4200}. BCL2 copy-number gain predicts inferior survival in the ABC subtype {2404}. Translocation of BCL6 is more frequent in ABC DLBCL, and in some studies it has been associated with improved survival {272, 1768,3667}. MYC translocations occur in about 8–14% of DLBCL, NOS, cases and are associated with inferior survival {269, 802,3537,4085}. Published data are confounded by whether or not FISH is also performed for additional oncogenes,

including BCL2 and BCL6. Most studies have confirmed that MYC and BCL2 double-hit lymphomas are much more common among GCB cases and are associated with inferior survival {194,269, 1865,3601}. The prognostic relevance of MYC and BCL6 translocations is more controversial, because studies are contradictory {2304,3183,4422}; these translocations are more common within the ABC subtype {3183,3601,4422}. These double-hit lymphomas are now excluded from DLBCL, NOS and diagnosed as high-grade B-cell lymphoma with MYC and BCL2 and/or BCL6 rearrangements (p. 335). Cases of DLBCL with MYC translocations only are also associated with decreased survival in some series {551, 778,802,848,4085,4398}. The results for MYC copy-number gains or amplification suggest inferior outcomes, but are inconsistent, in part due to the varying definitions of gain versus amplification {2404, 3770,3947,4109,4432}. TP53 loss and/or mutations are associated with inferior survival {4400,4445}. Deletions of the CDKN2A locus on chromosome 9p21 and trisomy 3 are also associated with diminished survival, in particular with the ABC subtype {1839,2271}. Definitive data regarding the prognostic role of other recurrently mutated genes in DLBCL, with the exception of FOXO1, are lacking {4060}. There are increasing expectations that at least some of the mutations found in DLBCL will become important in the development of future targeted therapies {1763,3405}.

Microenvironment
Gene expression profiling studies indicate a prognostic role for both non-neoplastic cells and extracellular matrix components in the tumour microenvironment in DLBCL {3600}. Stromal-1 (extracellular matrix deposition and histiocytic infiltration) and stromal-2 (tumour blood vessel density/angiogenesis) signatures have been shown to be prognostic in the current R-CHOP treatment era {2273}.

A two-gene expression signature including one gene representing the microenvironment (TNFRSF9) has also been shown to predict prognosis {68}. Mutation landscape studies in DLBCL highlight a number of recurrently mutated genes targeting the cross-talk between malignant B cells and non-neoplastic cells, including mutations and aberrant protein expression of beta-2 microglobulin and CD58 {635,2745}. Congruent data have also shown that loss of MHC class II is associated with decreased tumour-infiltrating CD8+ T cells and inferior outcome {3360,3361}. Immune escape mechanisms are also important oncogenic drivers in DLBCL. Overexpression of PDL1 in DLBCL, NOS, has been shown to be associated with inferior survival {2036}. The prognostic role of other immune cells and the assessment of these cells in the peripheral blood remain less well studied.

MicroRNA
Several studies have linked specific microRNA expression patterns with outcome in DLBCL {56,1772}. More recently, somatic mutations involving microRNAs have been shown to be prognostic in DLBCL and to be independent of both cell of origin and the IPI {2328}.

Host genetics
Analysis of host genetics has recently been shown to be prognostic in DLBCL, NOS. SNPs involving loci at 5q23.2 and 6q21 have been associated with event-free survival in patients with DLBCL treated with R-CHOP {1351}.

Therapy
The standard of care for the treatment of advanced-stage DLBCL, NOS, is R-CHOP. Other regimens exist, but it is unclear whether these provide an overall survival benefit {3611}. Attempts to improve the survival of ABC DLBCLs, are currently being made with the addition of novel agents to an R-CHOP backbone {1057,2562,2902,2903,2932,4334,4419}.

T-cell/histiocyte-rich large B-cell lymphoma

Ott G.
Delabie J.
Gascoyne R.D.
Campo E.
Stein H.
Jaffe E.S.

Definition

T-cell/histiocyte-rich large B-cell lymphoma (THRLBCL) is characterized by a limited number of scattered, large B cells embedded in a background of abundant T cells and histiocytes. THRLBCL may arise de novo; however, more recent data suggest the possibility of a closer relationship with progression forms of nodular lymphocyte predominant Hodgkin lymphoma (NLPHL) than previously thought, indicating that NLPHL may proceed to or contain areas indistinguishable from THRLBCL. In small biopsies in particular, differentiating between a progression form of NLPHL (i.e. NLPHL with THRLBCL-like transformation) and de novo THRLBCL may be difficult, if not impossible.

ICD-O code   9688/3

Synonyms

T-cell–rich B-cell lymphoma; B-cell lymphoma rich in T cells and simulating Hodgkin disease; histiocyte-rich/T-cell–rich large B-cell lymphoma; T-cell–rich large B-cell lymphoma; T-cell–rich/histiocyte-rich large B-cell lymphoma; histiocyte-rich large B-cell lymphoma

Epidemiology

THRLBCL mainly affects middle-aged men. It accounts for < 10% of all DLBCLs.

Localization

THRLBCL mainly affects the lymph nodes, but bone marrow, liver, and spleen involvement is frequently found at diagnosis.

Clinical features

Patients present with fever, malaise, splenomegaly, and/or hepatomegaly. At diagnosis, almost half of cases are at an advanced Ann Arbor stage, with an intermediate-risk to high-risk International Prognostic Index (IPI) score (Table 13.24). The disease is often refractory to the chemotherapy regimens currently in use.

Imaging

Because of the important differential

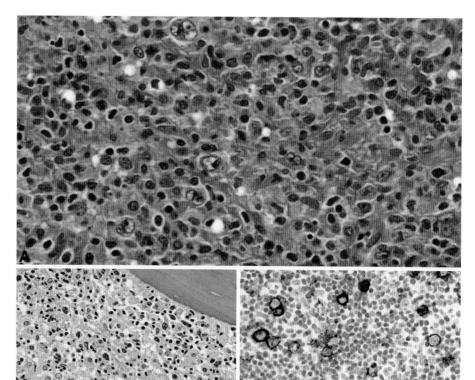

Fig. 13.108 T-cell/histiocyte-rich large B-cell lymphoma. **A** Lymph node. **B** Bone marrow. **C** CD20 stain highlights the large neoplastic B cells.

diagnosis with NLPHL, clinical staging procedures (including imaging analyses) are important. NLPHL usually affects one or two regions, whereas THRLBCL frequently manifests as systemic disease. Because THRLBCL is more PET-avid than is NLPHL, staging procedures such as FDG-PET and CT may facilitate the differential diagnosis {246}.

Microscopy

THRLBCL has a diffuse or less commonly vaguely nodular growth pattern replacing most of the normal lymph node parenchyma. It is composed of scattered, single large B cells embedded in a background of small T cells and variable numbers of histiocytes. The tumour cells are always dispersed and do not form aggregates or sheets. These cells may mimic the neoplastic lymphocyte predominant

(LP) cells of NLPHL, but usually show greater variation in size and, in some cases, may resemble centroblasts or more pleomorphic cells, mimicking Reed–Sternberg or Hodgkin cells {19,3299}. They are typically found within clusters of bland-looking non-epithelioid histiocytes that may not be obvious on conventional examination. These histiocytes are a main and distinctive component of THRLBCL and are useful for the diagnosis {1448}. Nearly all of the background lymphocytes are of T-cell lineage, with typically only very few scattered B cells. Meshworks of follicular dendritic cells are absent. Eosinophils and plasma cells are not found. De novo THRLBCLs are usually diffuse and do not show the typical small B-cell background of NLPHL. However, there are cases of NLPHL in which the small B cells are diminished in number, and in which nodular very T-cell rich areas can be seen. Follow-up data suggest that these variant histologies may negatively affect prognosis {1572}, and there are some cases of histological progression in NLPHL, in which the process is entirely diffuse and the histological appearance is virtually indistinguishable from that of de novo THRLBCL, constituting THRLBCL-like transformation. More recent genetic and gene expression data suggest that the relationship between de novo THR-LBCL and secondary THRLBCL may be closer than previously thought.

In cases predominantly affecting the spleen, there is a multifocal or micronodular involvement of the white pulp; in the liver, the lymphomatous foci are localized in the portal tracts {1014}. In these extranodal locations as well as in the bone marrow, the lymphoma is characterized by the same composition as in the lymph node.

On recurrence, the number of atypical cells may increase, resulting in a picture of DLBCL, which portends an inferior outcome {19}.

Several studies have recognized cases with similar morphology but without histiocytes. Whether these cases constitute the same entity as typical THRLBCL is not yet clear. Studies including cases rich in T cells with and without histiocytes have defined a more heterogeneous group of large B-cell lymphomas, which probably include more than one entity {13,1448, 2118,2330,3299}. Further studies should clarify the relationship between these lymphomas. Although cases lacking significant numbers of histiocytes may currently be included in the THRLBCL category, the paucity or absence of histiocytes should be noted. Lymphomas

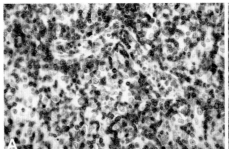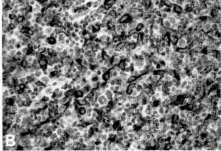

Fig. 13.109 T-cell/histiocyte-rich large B-cell lymphoma. **A** Small lymphocytes correspond to CD3-positive T cells. **B** A large proportion of histiocytes stained for CD68.

containing B cells with a spectrum of cell size, morphology, and distribution (clusters or sheets of medium-sized to large B cells) should not be included within the category of THRLBCL, and may be considered a subtype of DLBCL, NOS.

Immunophenotype

The large atypical cells express pan–B-cell markers such as CD19, CD20, and CD79a. BCL6 is also positive. A variable number stain for BCL2 and EMA, and no expression of CD15, CD30, or CD138 is found. The background is composed of variable numbers of CD68+ and CD163+ histiocytes and CD3+ and CD5+ T cells. T-cell rosettes around the tumour cells and remnants of B-cell follicles or clusters of small B lymphocytes are absent in de novo THRLBCL {2822}. CD279/PD1 rosettes are a feature of NLPHL, and may be seen in cases progressing to a diffuse pattern resembling THRLBCL. However, the presence or absence of CD279/PD1+ T cells is not specific for NLPHL. Lack of residual IgD+ mantle cells and lack of follicular dendritic cell meshworks are of further diagnostic help in differentiating de novo THRLBCL from NLPHL {18,1240}. There are aggressive B-cell lymphomas, rich in reactive T cells, in which the neoplastic cells are sparse and EBV-positive. In some cases, the neoplastic cells exhibit a Hodgkin-like morphology. Such cases should not be classified as THRLBCL, and should be considered within the spectrum of EBV-positive DLBCL {2330,2867}.

Postulated normal counterpart

A germinal centre B cell

Genetic profile

The tumour B cells harbour clonally rearranged IG genes carrying high numbers of somatic mutations and intraclonal diversity indicating derivation from germinal centre cells {487}.

Limited karyotypic studies failed to show recurrent abnormalities. Comparative genomic hybridization on microdissected tumour cells demonstrated more imbalances in NLPHL than in THRLBCL {1246}. However, more recent array comparative genomic hybridization studies showed that the number of genomic aberrations was higher in THRLBCL than in typical and THRLBCL-like variants of NLPHL {1571}. Gains of 2p16.1 and losses of 2p11.2 and 9p11.2 were recurrent aberrations in both typical and THRLBCL-like variants of NLPHL, as well as in THRLBCL. Expression of the REL protein was observed at similar frequencies in NLPHL and THRLBCL. Gene expression profiling has identified a subgroup of DLBCL characterized by a host immune response and a very bad prognosis {2719}, which includes most of the cases diagnosed as THRLBCL. Microdissected histiocytes from NLPHL and THRLBCL showed similar gene expression profiles, expressing genes related to proinflammatory and regulatory macrophage activity. Unlike histiocytes of NLPHL, those from THRLBCL strongly expressed metal-binding proteins {1576}. Overall, more recent expression profiling and genetic studies have revealed similarities between NLPHL and THRLBCL that suggest that these entities may constitute a pathobiological continuum with various clinical presentations {1570, 1576}.

Prognosis and predictive factors

THRLBCL is considered an aggressive lymphoma, although clinical heterogeneity is described. Cases with histiocytes are reported to define a more homogeneous group of patients with a very aggressive lymphoma and frequent failure of current therapies. The IPI score is the only known parameter of prognostic significance {19,428}.

Table 13.24 T-cell/histiocyte-rich large B-cell lymphoma

Median patient age	12–61 years
Male	75%
Stage III–IV	64%
Liver involvement	13–70%
Spleen involvement	33–67%
Bone marrow involvement	17–60%

Data based on 277 cases of patients with T-cell/histiocyte-rich large B-cell lymphoma in the literature {8A,428,429A,1240,2384A,2437A, 3362A,4000A,4070A,4249A}.

Primary diffuse large B-cell lymphoma of the CNS

Kluin P.M.
Deckert M.
Ferry J.A.

Definition

Primary diffuse large B-cell lymphoma (DLBCL) of the CNS is defined as DLBCL arising within the brain, spinal cord, leptomeninges or eye. Excluded are lymphomas of the dura, intravascular large B-cell lymphomas, lymphomas with evidence of systemic disease or secondary lymphomas, and all immunodeficiency-associated lymphomas.

ICD-O code   9680/3

Synonyms

Primary CNS lymphoma; primary intraocular lymphoma; lymphomatosis cerebri (no longer recommended)

Epidemiology

CNS DLBCL accounts for <1% of all non-Hodgkin lymphomas and 2.4–3% of all brain tumours {3556}. The overall annual incidence rate of CNS DLBCL is 0.47 cases per 100 000 population {4196}. This lymphoma can affect patients of any age, with a peak incidence in the fifth to seventh decade of life, a median patient age of 56 years, and a male-to-female ratio of 3:2. In the past two decades, an increased incidence has been reported among patients aged >60 years {821,4196}.

Etiology

In immunocompetent individuals, the etiological factors are unknown. Viruses, including EBV, HHV6 {3114}, HHV8 {2708}, and the polyomaviruses SV40 and BK virus {2705,2795}, do not play a role. Pathogenically, expression or absence of chemokines and chemokine receptors or cytokines may contribute to the specific localization {3706}. Tumour cells and endothelial cells may interact via activation of IL4 to create a favourable microenvironment for tumour growth {3443}.

Tumour cells of CNS DLBCL recognize proteins present in the CNS via their poly-reactive B-cell receptor, and thus have the capacity to stimulate B-cell receptor signalling. This interaction between CNS antigens and the lymphoma

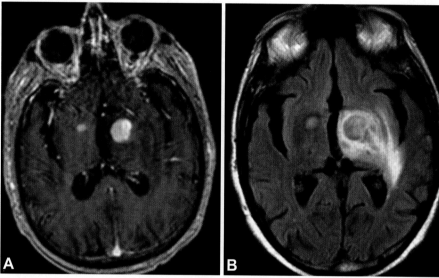

Fig. 13.110 Primary diffuse large B-cell lymphoma of the CNS. Nuclear MRI. T1-weighted image after gadolinium injection (**A**) and FLAIR sequences (**B**). There are two enhancing mass lesions in the basal ganglia.

cells may also contribute to organ restriction {2710}. Upon relapse, CNS DLBCLs show a restricted homing to the main immune sanctuaries (i.e. the brain, eyes, and testes) {416,1552,1828,3289}, and primary testicular and intraocular lymphomas frequently spread to the CNS {4205}, suggesting that the tumour cells need to hide in an immune sanctuary. Many DLBCLs of the CNS and testis show decreased or absent expression of HLA class I and II proteins, allowing the tumour cells to further escape from immune attack {415,3355}.

Localization

About 60% of CNS DLBCLs involve the supratentorial space, including the frontal lobe (affected in 15% of cases), temporal lobe (in 8%), parietal lobe (in 7%), occipital lobe (in 3%), basal ganglia and periventricular brain parenchyma (in 10%), and corpus callosum (in 5%). Less frequently affected sites include the posterior fossa (affected in 13% of cases) and spinal cord (in 1%) {919}. A single tumour is present in 60–70% of cases, with the remainder presenting as multifocal disease {919}. The leptomeninges may be involved, but exclusive meningeal manifestation is unusual. Approximately 20% of patients present with or develop intraocular lesions, and 80–90% of patients with intraocular DLBCL develop contralateral tumours

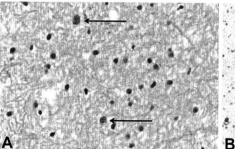
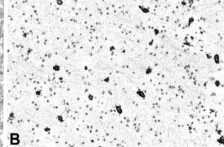

Fig. 13.111 Primary diffuse large B-cell lymphoma of the CNS. **A** Histology of a case with very scarce lymphoma cells (arrows). **B** CD20 immunohistochemistry highlights the neoplastic cells.

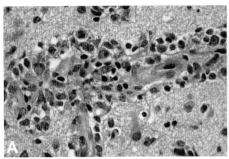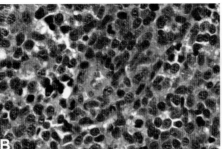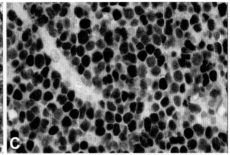

Fig. 13.112 Primary diffuse large B-cell lymphoma of the CNS. **A** Accumulation of tumour cells within the perivascular space. **B** More-solid pattern, still with some accumulation in the perivascular space. **C** Numerous tumour cells are strongly IRF4 / MUM1-positive.

and parenchymal CNS lesions. Dissemination to extraneural sites, including the bone marrow, is very rare; in these cases, preferential spread to the testis has been noted {416,1552,1828,3289}.

Clinical features
Patients more frequently present with cognitive dysfunction, psychomotor slowing, and focal neurological symptoms than with headache, seizures, and cranial nerve palsies. Blurred vision and eye floaters are symptoms of ocular involvement {293,2084,3128}.

Imaging
MRI is the most sensitive technique for detecting CNS DLBCL, which is hypointense on T1-weighted and isointense to hyperintense on T2-weighted images, typically appearing densely enhancing on postcontrast images. Peritumoural oedema is relatively limited, and less extensive than in malignant gliomas and metastases {2084}. Meningeal involvement may present as foci of abnormal contrast enhancement {2161}. With steroid therapy, lesions may vanish within hours {919}.

Macroscopy
As observed in postmortem examination, CNS DLBCL occurs as single or multiple masses in the brain parenchyma, most frequently in the cerebral hemispheres. The masses are often deep-seated and adjacent to the ventricular system. The tumours can be firm, friable, granular, haemorrhagic, and greyish-tan or yellow, with central necrosis or virtually indistinguishable from the adjacent neuropil. Demarcation from surrounding parenchyma is variable. Some tumours appear well delineated, like metastases. When diffuse borders and architectural effacement are present, the lesions resemble gliomas. Like malignant gliomas, the tu-

mours may diffusely infiltrate large areas of the hemispheres without forming a distinct mass. Meningeal involvement may resemble meningitis or meningioma, but can also be grossly inconspicuous.

Microscopy
CNS DLBCLs are usually highly cellular, diffusely growing tumours. Centrally, large areas of geographical necrosis are common, which may harbour viable perivascular lymphoma islands. At the periphery, this perivascular infiltration pattern is frequent. Infiltration of cerebral blood vessels causes fragmentation of the argyrophilic fibre network. From these perivascular cuffs, tumour cells invade the neural parenchyma, either with a well-delineated invasion front with small clusters or with single tumour cells diffusely infiltrating the tissue; this is accompanied by a prominent astrocytic and microglial activation and a reactive inflammatory infiltrate consisting of mature T cells and B cells and sometimes also many foamy histiocytes. In some cases, a distinct tumour mass is difficult to identify on imaging and the biopsy may have been taken from the periphery, resulting in the finding of an entirely interstitial pattern with isolated tumour cells intermingled between astrocytes. In such cases, immunohistology with CD20 or other B-cell markers is necessary to identify the lymphoma cells. Cytomorphologically, CNS DLBCL consists of atypical cells with medium-sized to large round, oval, irregular, or pleomorphic nuclei and distinct nucleoli, corresponding to centroblasts or immunoblasts. Some cases show a relatively monomorphic cell population with intermingled macrophages, mimicking Burkitt lymphoma.
Stereotactic biopsy is the gold standard for establishing the diagnosis and classification of CNS lymphomas. It is impor-

tant to withhold corticosteroids before biopsy, because they induce rapid tumour shrinkage. Corticosteroids have been shown to prevent diagnosis in as many as 50% of patients {485}.

Immunophenotype
The tumour cells are mature B cells with a PAX5+, CD19+, CD20+, CD22+, CD79a+ phenotype. IgM and IgD, but not IgG, are expressed on the cell surface {2713}, with either kappa or lambda light chain restriction. Most cases express BCL6 (60–80% of cases) as well as IRF4/MUM1 (90% of cases), whereas plasma cell markers (CD38 and CD138) are usually negative. CD10 is expressed by < 10% of these lymphomas {918}, but is more frequent in systemic DLBCL; therefore, CD10 positivity in a CNS lymphoma with DLBCL characteristics should prompt an intense search for systemic DLBCL that has disseminated to the CNS.
HLA-A, HLA-B, HLA-C, and HLA-DR are variably expressed, with approximately 50% of CNS DLBCLs having lost major histocompatibility complex (MHC) class I and/or II expression {415,3356}.
BCL2 expression is common, but not related to t(14;18)(q32;q21) {774}. About 82% of all cases of CNS DLBCL have a BCL2-high, MYC-high phenotype {478}. Mitotic activity is brisk; the Ki-67 (MIB1) proliferation index is usually >70% and can even be >90% {478}. Except in rare cases, there is no evidence of EBV infection {2709}; the presence of EBV should prompt evaluation for an underlying immunodeficiency.

Postulated normal counterpart
A late germinal centre exit B cell arrested in terminal B-cell differentiation that shares genetic characteristics with both activated B cells and germinal centre B cells {2706}

Genetic profile

Because the tumour cells correspond to late germinal centre exit B cells with blocked terminal B-cell differentiation, they carry rearranged and somatically mutated IG genes with evidence of ongoing somatic hypermutation {2709, 3127,3990}. Consistent with the ongoing germinal centre programming, they show persistent BCL6 activity {478}. The process of somatic hypermutation is not confined to its physiological targets (IG and *BCL6* genes), but extends to other genes that have been implicated in tumorigenesis, including *BCL2*, *MYC*, *PIM1*, *PAX5*, *RHOH* (also called *TTF*), *KLHL14*, *OSBPL10*, and *SUSD2* {482,2715,4163}. The fixed IgM/IgD phenotype of the tumour cells is in part due to miscarried IG class-switch rearrangements during which the S-mu region is deleted {2713}. *PRDM1* mutations also contribute to impaired IG class-switch recombination {825}.

Translocations recurrently affect the IG genes (in 38% of cases) and *BCL6* (in 17–47%), whereas *MYC* translocations are rare and *BCL2* translocations are absent {478,519,2716}. FISH and genome-wide SNP analyses have revealed recurrent gains of genetic material most frequently affecting 18q21.33-23 (in 43% of cases), including the *BCL2* and *MALT1* genes; chromosome 12 (in 26%); and 10q23.21 (in 21%) {3595}.

Loss of genetic material most frequently involves 6q21 (in 52% of cases), 6p21 (in 37%), 8q12.1-12.2 (in 32%), and 10q23.21 {3595}. Heterozygous deletions, homozygous loss, or copy-neutral LOH of chromosomal region 6p21.32 affects 73% of CNS DLBCLs; the 6p21 region harbours the MHC class II encoding genes *HLA-DRB*, *HLA-DQA*, and *HLA-DQB* {1883, 3355,3595}. Approximately 50% of CNS DLBCLs have lost expression of HLA class I and II gene products {415,3356}. The *MYD88* L265P mutation is highly recurrent: present in more of half of the cases {2707}. Other pathways involving the B-cell receptor, the toll-like receptor, and the NF-kappaB pathway are frequently activated due to genetic alterations affecting the genes *CD79B* (in 20% of cas-

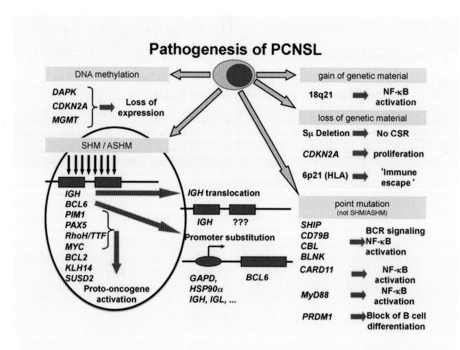

Fig. 13.113 Pathogenesis of primary diffuse large B-cell lymphoma of the CNS (PCNSL). ASHM, aberrant somatic hypermutation; BCR, B-cell receptor; CSR, class-switch recombination; SHM, somatic hypermutation.

es), *INPP5D* (also called *SHIP*; in 25%), *CBL* (in 4%), *BLNK* (in 4%), *CARD11* (in 16%), *MALT1* (in 43%), and *BCL2* (in 43%), which may foster proliferation and prevent apoptosis {665,1403,2097,2707, 2712,2714,3595}.

Epigenetic changes may also contribute to CNS DLBCL pathogenesis, including gene silencing by DNA methylation. Hypermethylation of *DAPK1* (seen in 84% of cases), *CDKN2A* (in 75%), *MGMT* (in 52%), and *RFC* (in 30%) may be of potential therapeutic relevance {753,774,1194, 3595}.

Prognosis and predictive factors

Patients with CNS DLBCL have a remarkably worse outcome than do patients with systemic DLBCL. Older patient age (> 65 years) is a major negative prognostic factor and is associated with reduced survival as well as an increased risk of neurotoxicity related to therapy {14,2084}. High-dose methotrexate-based polychemotherapy is currently the treatment of choice {2084}. The inclusion of whole-brain irradiation may improve outcome, but carries the risk of neurotoxicity re-

sulting in severe cognitive, motor, and autonomic dysfunction, particularly in elderly patients {14}. Most protocols report a median progression-free survival of about 12 months and an overall survival of approximately 3 years. In a subgroup of elderly patients with methylated *MGMT* within the lymphoma cells, temozolomide monotherapy appeared to be therapeutically effective {2144}.

On biopsy, the presence of reactive perivascular CD3+ T-cell infiltrates has been associated with improved survival {3213}. LMO2 protein expression by the tumour cells has been associated with prolonged overall survival {2394}. BCL6 expression has been suggested as a prognostic marker, although conflicting favourable versus unfavourable conclusions have been reported {2694,3237, 3308,3727}. Del(6)(q22) has been associated with inferior overall survival {519, 1403}.

With improvement of outcome, some sporadic systemic relapses have been observed; these can involve any organ, but relatively frequently involve the testis and breast {1828}.

Primary cutaneous diffuse large B-cell lymphoma, leg type

Willemze R.
Vergier B.
Duncan L.M.

Definition
Primary cutaneous diffuse large B-cell lymphoma (PCLBCL), leg type, is a PCLBCL composed exclusively of centroblasts and immunoblasts, most commonly arising in the leg.

ICD-O code   9680/3

Epidemiology
PCLBCL, leg type, accounts for 4% of all primary cutaneous lymphomas and 20% of all primary cutaneous B-cell lymphomas {1530,4320}. It typically occurs in elderly patients, in particular women, with a male-to-female ratio of 1:3–4. The median patient age is in the seventh decade of life {4189}.

Localization
These lymphomas preferentially affect the lower legs, but 10–15% of cases arise at other sites {2062,3623,4499}.

Clinical features
PCLBCL, leg type, presents with red or bluish-red, often rapidly growing tumours on one or both of the lower legs {1421, 2062,4189,4499}. These lymphomas frequently disseminate to extracutaneous sites.

Microscopy
These lymphomas are composed of a monotonous, diffuse, non-epidermotropic infiltrate of confluent sheets of centroblasts and immunoblasts {1421,4189}. Mitotic figures are frequently observed. Small B cells and CD21+/CD35+ follicular dendritic cell meshworks are absent. Reactive T cells are relatively few and are often confined to perivascular areas.

Immunophenotype
The neoplastic B cells express monotypic immunoglobulin, CD20, and CD79a. Unlike primary cutaneous follicle centre lymphomas, PCLBCLs, leg type, usually strongly express BCL2, IRF4/MUM1, FOXP1, MYC, and cIgM, with coexpression of IgD in 50% of cases {953,1318, 1409,1424,1653,1654,2062,2065,2066}. However, BCL2 and IRF4/MUM1 expression are absent in approximately 10% of the cases. {2062,3623}. The proliferation rate is high. BCL6 is expressed by most cases, but may be dim, whereas CD10 staining is usually negative {1654}.

Postulated normal counterpart
A peripheral B cell of post–germinal centre origin

Genetic profile
PCLBCL, leg type, has many genetic similarities with diffuse large B-cell lymphomas arising at other sites, but shows marked differences from primary cutaneous follicle centre lymphoma. PCLBCL, leg type, has the gene expression profile of the ABC subtype of DLBCL {1653}. Interphase

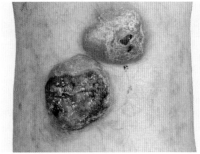

Fig. 13.114 Primary cutaneous diffuse large B-cell lymphoma, leg type. Typical clinical presentation with tumours on a leg.

FISH analysis frequently shows translocations involving *MYC* or *BCL6*, and IGH genes in PCLBCL, leg type {1524}. High-level DNA amplifications of 18q21.31-21.33, including the *BCL2* and *MALT1* genes, are detected in 67% of cases by array comparative genomic hybridization and FISH analyses {986}. Amplification of *BCL2* may well explain the strong BCL2 expression in these cases, particularly given that t(14;18) is not found {986,1525}. Loss of the *CDKN2A* and *CDKN2B* gene loci on chromosome 9p21.3, due to either gene deletion or promoter methylation, has been reported in as many as 67% of PCLBCLs, leg type, and correlates with an adverse prognosis {986,3625}. *MYD88* L265P mutation, found in 60% of cases, and mutations in various components of the B-cell receptor signalling pathway, including *CARD11* (in 10% of

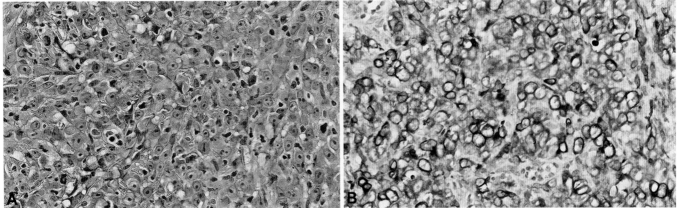

Fig. 13.115 Primary cutaneous diffuse large B-cell lymphoma, leg type. **A** Note the large transformed cells with prominent nucleoli. **B** Strong cytoplasmic staining for IgM.

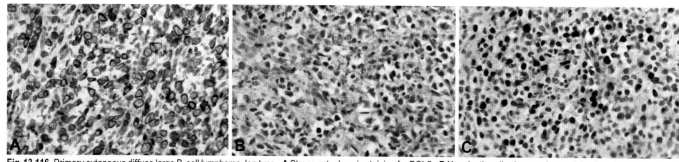

Fig. 13.116 Primary cutaneous diffuse large B-cell lymphoma, leg type. **A** Strong cytoplasmic staining for BCL2. **B** Neoplastic cells show nuclear staining for BCL6. **C** Neoplastic cells show nuclear staining for IRF4/MUM1.

cases), *CD79B* (in 20%), and *TNFAIP3* (encoding TNFAIP3, also called A20; in 40%), strongly suggest constitutive NF-kappaB activation in PCLBCL, leg type {2067,3163,3165}. The similarities in gene expression profile and cytogenetic alterations, including translocations and NF-kappaB activating mutations, underscore that PCLBCL, leg type, may be considered a cutaneous counterpart of activated B-cell subtype diffuse large B-cell lymphoma {3165}.

Prognosis and predictive factors
Earlier studies reported a 5-year survival rate of approximately 50% {1421,1422, 4189}. However, recent studies have reported a significantly better clinical outcome for patients when rituximab is added to a multiagent chemotherapy (CHOP or CHOP-like) regimen {1423,1530}. Multiple skin lesions at diagnosis, inactivation of *CDKN2A*, and *MYD88* L265P mutation have been reported to be associated with an inferior prognosis {986,1421,1422, 3162,3623,3625}.

EBV-positive diffuse large B-cell lymphoma, not otherwise specified (NOS)

Nakamura S.
Jaffe E.S.
Swerdlow S.H.

Definition
EBV-positive diffuse large B-cell lymphoma (DLBCL), NOS, is an EBV-positive clonal B-cell lymphoid proliferation {780, 1017,2701,2867,2957,3018,3019,3063, 3661}. Excluded from this category are cases of lymphomatoid granulomatosis, cases with evidence of acute or recent EBV infection, other well-defined lymphomas that may be EBV-positive (such as plasmablastic lymphoma and DLBCL associated with chronic inflammation), and EBV-positive mucocutaneous ulcer (localized EBV-driven proliferations affecting cutaneous or mucosal sites).
This disease was formerly designated as EBV-positive DLBCL of the elderly, but the restriction to elderly patients has been removed; although the disease usually occurs in individuals aged >50 years, it can present over a wide age range {326, 781,1675,2867,3661}. The NOS designation has been added to emphasize the exclusion of the more specific types of EBV-positive lymphoma. Although many cases have a distinctive histological appearance, routine EBV testing is required for all cases to be identified. The clinical outcome is variable {165,1017,1018,2867, 3018,3019}.

ICD-O code
9680/3

Synonyms
EBV-positive diffuse large B-cell lymphoma of the elderly; senile EBV-associated B-cell lymphoproliferative disorder; age-related EBV-positive lymphoproliferative disorder

Epidemiology
EBV-positive DLBCL accounts for <5–15% of DLBCLs among Asian and Latin American patients and <5% among western patients, with no documented predisposing immunodeficiency {325,1017,1367,1674,2405,2701,2956, 2957,3018,3019,3063}. Most cases occur in patients over age 50, with a peak in the eighth decade {3661}. However, cases also occur in younger patients sporadically, with a second smaller peak in the third decade {2867}. EBV-positive DLBCL is more common in males, with a male-to-female ratio of 1.2–3.6:1 {1017, 1675,2867,3018,3019,3661}.

Etiology
The increased incidence of EBV-positive DLBCL in older patients is believed to be related to immunosenescence {1017, 2746,3018,3019}. Alterations in the immune microenvironment may play a role at any patient age {668,2867}.

Localization
Nodal or extranodal sites can be involved. The most common extranodal sites are the lungs and gastrointestinal tract {1017,

3018,3019}. In young patients (aged < 45 years), the disease is predominantly nodal, with only about 10% of cases showing extranodal involvement {2867,4087}. Approximately 5–10% of patients have both nodal and extranodal involvement.

Clinical features

The clinical features at presentation are variable {1017,1663,2867,3018,3019}. More than half of the patients have a high or high-intermediate International Prognostic Index (IPI) score. Most patients have detectable EBV DNA in serum or whole blood, but this can also be seen in patients with EBV-negative DLBCL {2316,2961}.

Microscopy

The histological features overlap with those of other EBV-related lymphoid proliferations, including EBV-positive classic Hodgkin lymphoma. The neoplastic component most often consists of a variable number of large transformed cells/immunoblasts and Hodgkin/Reed–Sternberg-like cells. There is a variable component of reactive elements, including small lymphocytes, plasma cells, histiocytes, and epithelioid cells. The rich background of small lymphocytes and histiocytes may resemble T-cell/histiocyte-rich large B-cell lymphoma, also referred to as the polymorphic pattern in some studies {2867,4087}. This is the most common pattern in young patients. Other cases are more monomorphic, and may be difficult to distinguish from EBV-negative DLBCL without ancillary studies {165, 780,1017,1018,2701,3018,3019}. Large areas of geographical necrosis and angioinvasion are other characteristic findings, but they are not always present.

Immunophenotype

The neoplastic cells are usually positive

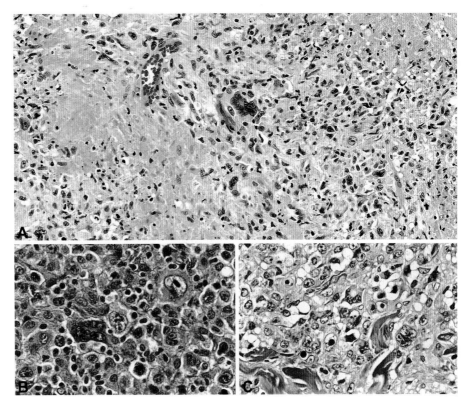

Fig. 13.117 EBV-positive diffuse large B-cell lymphoma. **A** This polymorphic lesion shows geographical necrosis. **B** There is a mixed proliferation of immunoblasts and medium-sized lymphoid cells, as well as small reactive lymphocytes. **C** Monotonous proliferation of immunoblast-like or Hodgkin/Reed–Sternberg–like cells with prominent central nucleoli.

for the pan–B-cell antigens CD19, CD20, CD22, CD79a, and PAX5, and have an activated–B-cell immunophenotype, being positive for IRF4/MUM1 and negative for CD10 and commonly BCL6 {1017, 2867,3018,3019}. CD30 is frequently positive and CD15 is sometimes coexpressed, but other phenotypic features typical of classic Hodgkin lymphoma are usually lacking {668,1017,2867}. Light chain restriction may be difficult to demonstrate. EBNA2 and LMP1 are expressed in 7–36% and > 90% of cases, respectively, indicating type III and (more often) type II EBV latency {2867}. The

tumour cells often express PDL1 and PDL2, providing a mechanism for immune escape {668,2867,4431}.

In situ hybridization for EBV-encoded small RNA (EBER) is mandatory for the diagnosis of EBV-positive DLBCL, NOS. With EBER in situ hybridization, more than 80% of the atypical cells are positive. Small numbers of EBER-positive cells may be present as bystander B-cells in EBV-negative B-cell or T-cell lymphomas {2867,2960,3821}.

Postulated normal counterpart

A mature B cell, transformed by EBV

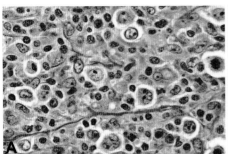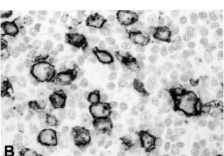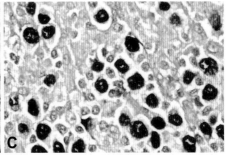

Fig. 13.118 EBV-positive diffuse large B-cell lymphoma with a T-cell/histiocyte-rich large B-cell lymphoma–like pattern. **A** Scattered large tumour cells are observed in a lymphohistiocytic microenvironment. **B** Scattered large tumour cells are positive for CD20. **C** In situ hybridization for EBV-encoded small RNA (EBER) highlights scattered tumour cells.

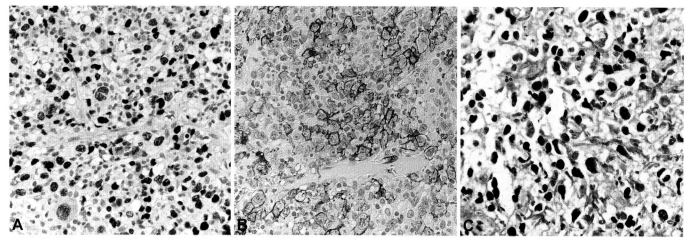

Fig. 13.119 EBV-positive diffuse large B-cell lymphoma. **A** The nuclei of the large lymphoid cells are EBNA2-positive. **B** More than 50% of the large lymphoid cells are CD20-positive. **C** In situ hybridization for EBV-encoded small RNA (EBER) reveals many positive cells.

Genetic profile

Clonality of the IG genes and EBV can usually be detected by molecular techniques, and is helpful for distinguishing polymorphous cases from reactive hyperplasia and infectious mononucleosis {2867,3018,3019}. Restricted/clonal T-cell receptor responses can be seen in some cases {1018,2867}, but can also be present in other EBV-associated lymphoproliferations such as infectious mononucleosis {2447}. IG translocations are uncommon (seen in ~15% of cases). The presence of an IGH/*MYC* translocation or variants should suggest a diagnosis of plasmablastic lymphoma {2365, 4110}. Mutations in *CD79B, CARD11*, and *MYD88*, which are often found in the activated B-cell type of DLBCL, are absent {1316}. Chromosomal gains at 9p24.1 may contribute to increased expression of PDL1 and PDL2 {4431}. Gene expression profiling shows activation of the JAK/STAT and NF-kappaB pathways {1958,2956}.

Prognosis and predictive factors

With an age cut-off point of 45 years, the prognosis of EBV-positive DLBCL differs significantly between elderly and young patients (*P* <0.0001) {1017,2867,3019}. The disease is aggressive, with a median survival of about 2 years in elderly patients, even when treated with rituximab immunochemotherapy {1017,3019,3527, 3820}, but younger patients appear to have an excellent prognosis, with long-term complete remission in >80% {2867, 4087}. Cases with the T-cell/histiocyte-rich large B-cell lymphoma–like or polymorphic pattern appears to have a better prognosis than do monomorphic EBV-positive DLBCL in young patients {1017, 1018,2867}. Positivity for CD30 {2956} and EBNA2 {3820} may have an adverse prognostic impact. In elderly patients, B symptoms and age >70 years appear to be adverse prognostic factors {3019}; patients with neither, one, or both of these factors have median overall survival times of 56, 25, and 9 months, respectively.

EBV-positive mucocutaneous ulcer

Gaulard P.
Swerdlow S.H.
Harris N.L.
Sundström C.
Jaffe E.S.

Definition

EBV-positive mucocutaneous ulcer (EBVMCU) is a newly recognized clinico-pathological entity occurring in patients with age-related or iatrogenic immuno-suppression, often with Hodgkin-like features and a typically indolent course, with spontaneous regression in some cases {1018}. It presents in cutaneous or mucosal sites. The most common site of involvement is the oral cavity, including gingiva. The outgrowth of the EBV-positive cells may be related to local trauma or inflammation.

ICD-O code   9680/1

Epidemiology

The incidence of EBVMCU has not been established {498,971,1017,1018,2010, 3852,4408}. EBVMCU occurs in a variety of clinical settings associated with defective surveillance for EBV, including advanced age in a high proportion of cases, but also in patients with iatrogenic immunosuppression, such as those receiving methotrexate, azathioprine, cyclosporine, or tumour necrosis factor inhibitors for autoimmune diseases, and in solid organ transplant recipients {1565}. Similar cases have been reported in allogeneic transplant recipients and HIV-infected patients {498,2847}. The disease has a mild male predominance and a median patient age >70 years {1018}. As would be expected, iatrogenically immuno-suppressed patients with EBVMCU are younger on average than those with age-related EBVMCU.

Etiology

The disease is uniformly associated with EBV and occurs in patients with various forms of immunosuppression {1018}. At least in elderly patients, alterations in T-cell responses, with the accumulation of clonal or oligoclonal restricted CD8+ T cells with diminished functionality, likely play a role in the pathogenesis of this EBV-associated lymphoproliferative disorder {1017}. The lesions often arise in locations subjected to local tissue damage or inflammation, such as in the intestine in patients with inflammatory bowel disease {2132}.

Localization

EBVMCU presents with ulcerated lesions, usually in the oral mucosa (tonsils, tongue, buccal mucosa, and palate), skin, and gastrointestinal tract (oesophagus, large bowel, rectum, and perianal region) {498,971,1017,1018,2010,3852}. Regional isolated lymphadenopathy is rarely seen, but there is no evidence of systemic lymphadenopathy, hepatosplenomegaly, or bone marrow involvement. Regional lymph nodes may show reactive hyperplasia.

Clinical features

The symptoms are related to the ulcerated lesion, whether in the oral cavity, skin, or intestine. Systemic symptoms are rare.

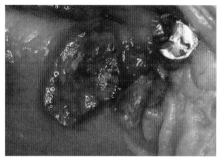

Fig. 13.120 EBV-positive mucocutaneous ulcer. A sharply circumscribed ulcer involves the palate in an 85-year-old man.

Macroscopy

Patients with EBVMCU present with sharply circumscribed, isolated, indurated mucosal or cutaneous ulcers.

Microscopy

The mucosal or cutaneous surface is ulcerated, sometimes with pseudoepitheliomatous hyperplasia of the adjacent intact epithelium. Beneath the ulcer, there is a dense polymorphic infiltrate with a variable number of plasma cells, histiocytes, and eosinophils, as well as a substantial number of large transformed cells, resembling either atypical immunoblasts or Hodgkin/Reed–Sternberg–like cells. Scattered apoptotic cells are often seen. Angioinvasion and necrosis can be present in addition to surface ulceration {1017,1018}. The lymphocytes in the background are abundant, many with angulated and medium-sized nuclei.

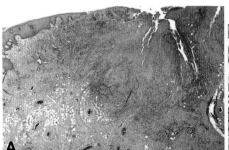 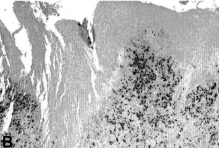 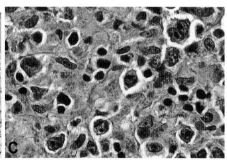

Fig. 13.121 EBV-positive mucocutaneous ulcer in the palate. **A** The squamous epithelium is ulcerated, with an underlying atypical lymphoid infiltrate. The lesion is circumscribed at the base, with underlying reactive lymphocytes. **B** In situ hybridization for EBV-encoded small RNA (EBER) reveals scattered EBV-positive cells superficially, with reactive lymphocytes at the base. **C** The atypical lymphoid cells are large, with prominent basophilic nucleoli. Admixed lymphocytes and histiocytes are abundant.

Some cases resemble diffuse large B-cell lymphoma or a polymorphic post-transplant lymphoproliferative disorder; others show Hodgkin-like morphology, with the distinction from classic Hodgkin lymphoma sometimes very difficult. However, the diagnosis of classic Hodgkin lymphoma in the skin or in mucosa should be rendered only with extreme caution. The deepest margin of the lesion usually contains a band-like infiltrate of mature lymphocytes. These cells are mainly T cells negative for EBV.

Immunophenotype

The large transformed immunoblasts and Hodgkin/Reed–Sternberg–like cells are B cells that in most cases have CD20 expression ranging from strong to weak and heterogeneous. These cells are positive for PAX5 and OCT2, with variable expression of BOB1. They have an activated–B-cell phenotype, being negative for CD10 and BCL6 and positive for IRF4/MUM1, and are CD30-positive. CD15 is expressed in about half of the cases. CD79a is often positive. EBV is consistently positive, with transformed cells commonly positive for LMP1. Positivity for EBV-encoded small RNA (EBER) parallels expression of most B-cell antigens, and is found in a range of cell sizes, from small lymphocytes to immunoblasts and cells with Hodgkin/Reed–Sternberg cell morphology. The background consists mainly of T cells, with numerous CD8+ T cells. A dense rim of CD3+ lymphocytes is present between the lesion and adjacent soft tissue.

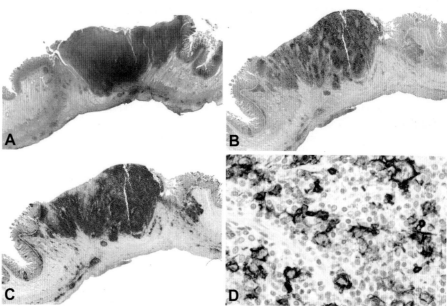

Fig. 13.122 EBV-positive mucocutaneous ulcer in the intestine, post-transplant. **A** This case is associated with iatrogenic immunosuppression. Note the sharply circumscribed base. **B** The EBV-positive cells are strongly positive for CD30. **C** Numerous CD3+ T cells are admixed with the EBV-positive cells. **D** The atypical cells are strongly positive for CD20.

Postulated normal counterpart

An EBV-transformed post–germinal centre B cell

Genetic profile

Fewer than half of all EBVMCUs show clonal IG gene rearrangements. Studies of TR gene rearrangement often reveal an oligoclonal or restricted pattern by PCR {971,1017,1018}.

Prognosis and predictive factors

Case reports and series suggest a benign natural history, with nearly all reported cases responding to reduction of immunosuppressive therapy. In patients in whom immunosuppression cannot be reversed, responses to rituximab, local radiation, and chemotherapy have been observed. Spread to distant sites is rare, but local progression may be seen. The outcome is superior to that to other immunodeficiency-associated EBV-driven lymphoproliferative disorders {1017, 1565,2597,3852,4408}. However, rare cases of relapses or progression to more widespread disease {2721} have been reported.

Diffuse large B-cell lymphoma associated with chronic inflammation

Chan J.K.C.
Aozasa K.
Gaulard P.

Definition

Diffuse large B-cell lymphoma (DLBCL) associated with chronic inflammation is a lymphoid neoplasm occurring in the setting of longstanding chronic inflammation and showing association with EBV. Most cases involve body cavities or narrow spaces. Pyothorax-associated lymphoma (PAL) is the prototypical form, developing in the pleural cavity of patients with longstanding pyothorax.

ICD-O code   9680/3

Synonym

Pyothorax-associated lymphoma

Epidemiology

PAL develops in patients with a 20 to 64-year (median: 37-year) history of pyothorax resulting from artificial pneumothorax for treatment of pulmonary or pleural tuberculosis {121,1797,2818,2827,3150}. Patient age at diagnosis ranges from the fifth to eighth decade of life (median: 65–70 years) {2818,2827}. The male-to-female ratio is 12:1 versus nearly equal in chronic pyothorax, suggesting that males are more susceptible to this type of lymphoma than are females {1797}. Although most cases of PAL have been reported in Japan, this lymphoma has also been described in the west {166,2518,3150}.

For DLBCLs arising in other settings of chronic suppuration or inflammation, such as chronic osteomyelitis, metallic implant insertion, surgical mesh implantation, and chronic skin venous ulcer, the interval between the predisposing event and malignant lymphoma is usually > 10 years (range: 1.2–57 years) {696, 804,1263}.

Etiology

Artificial pneumothorax, used in the past as a form of surgical therapy for pulmonary tuberculosis, is the only significant risk factor for development of PAL among patients with chronic pyothorax {120, 1679}. PAL is strongly associated with EBV, with expression of EBNA2 and/or LMP1 together with EBNA1 (i.e. usually

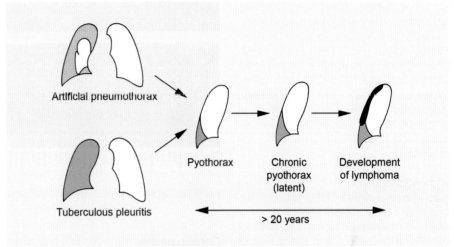

Fig. 13.123 Development of pyothorax-associated lymphoma.

type III EBV latency) {1264,2949,3150, 3525,3873,3874}. Chronic inflammation at the local site probably plays a role in the proliferation of EBV-transformed B cells by enabling them to escape from the host immune surveillance through production of IL10 (an immunosuppressive cytokine) and by providing autocrine to paracrine growth via IL6 and IL6R {1925,1928}.

DLBCLs associated with chronic inflammation that occur in other settings similarly harbour EBV, likely facilitated by so-called local immunodeficiency resulting from longstanding chronic suppuration or inflammation in a confined space {696, 804}.

Localization

The most common sites of involvement

are the pleural cavity (PAL), bone (especially femur), joints, and periarticular soft tissue {696}. In more than half of all PAL cases, the tumour mass is > 10 cm {121}. There is direct invasion of adjacent structures, but the tumour is often confined to the thoracic cavity at the time of diagnosis, with about 70% of patients presenting with clinical stage I or II disease {2818}. PAL differs from primary effusion lymphoma, which is characterized by lymphomatous serous effusions in the absence of tumour mass formation and is HHV8+.

Clinical features

Patients with PAL present with chest pain, back pain, fever, or tumorous swelling in the chest wall, or with respiratory symptoms such as productive cough, haemoptysis, and dyspnoea. Radiologi-

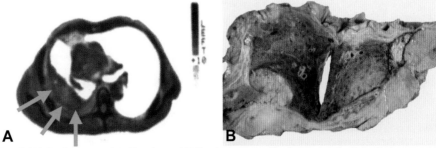

Fig. 13.124 Pyothorax-associated lymphoma. **A,B** Massive tumour proliferation surrounding the entire lung.

cal examination reveals a tumour mass in the pleura (in 80% of cases), pleura and lung (in 10%), or lung near the pleura (in 7%). The serum lactate dehydrogenase level is commonly elevated {2818,3150}. Patients who develop lymphoma in the bone, joint, periarticular soft tissue, or skin usually present with pain or mass lesion. The involved bone typically shows lytic lesions on radiological examination.

Microscopy
The morphological features are the same as those of DLBCL, NOS. Most cases show centroblastic or immunoblastic morphology, with round nuclei and large single or multiple nucleoli. Massive necrosis and angiocentric growth may be present.

Immunophenotype
Most cases express CD20 and CD79a. However, a proportion of cases may show plasmacytic differentiation, with loss of CD20 and/or CD79a, and expression of IRF4/MUM1 and CD138. The lymphoma has an activated B-cell phenotype. CD30 can be expressed. Occasional cases also express one or more T-cell markers (CD2, CD3, CD4, and/or CD7), causing problems in lineage assignment {2734, 2818,3150,4022}.

In situ hybridization for EBV-encoded small RNA (EBER) shows positive labelling of the lymphoma cells. Type III EBV latency (i.e. positivity for LMP1 and EBNA2) is characteristic {1263,3150}.

Postulated normal counterpart
An EBV-transformed post–germinal centre B cell

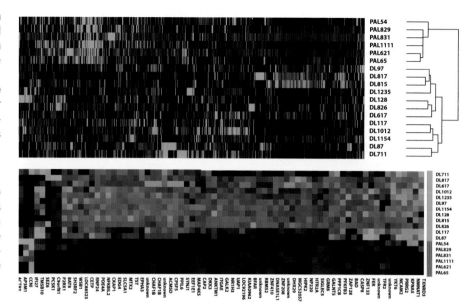

Fig. 13.125 The patterns of gene expression in pyothorax-associated lymphoma (PAL) and nodal diffuse large B-cell lymphoma (DL) are significantly different. Modified from Nishiu M et al. {2882}.

Genetic profile
IG genes are clonally rearranged and hypermutated, but lack ongoing mutations {2680,3875}. TP53 mutations are found in about 70% of cases, usually involving dipyrimidine sites, which are known to be susceptible to mutagenesis induced by ionizing radiation {1679}. MYC gene amplification is common {4412}, and TNFAIP3 (also called A20) is deleted in a proportion of cases {100}. Cytogenetic studies show complex karyotypes with numerous numerical and structural abnormalities {3874}. The gene expression profile of PAL is distinct from that of nodal DLBCL, which may be attributable to the presence of EBV {2882}. One of the most differentially expressed genes is IFI27, which is known to be induced in B lymphocytes by stimulation of interferon alpha, consistent with the role of chronic inflammation in this condition. Downregulation of HLA class I expression, which is essential for efficient induction of host cytotoxic T lymphocytes, and mutations of cytotoxic T-lymphocyte epitopes in EBNA3B, an immunodominant antigen for cytotoxic T-lymphocyte responses, might also contribute to escape of PAL cells from host cytotoxic T lymphocytes {1926,1927}.

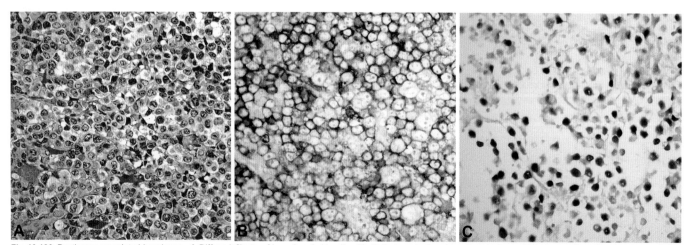

Fig. 13.126 Pyothorax-associated lymphoma. **A** Diffuse infiltrate of large lymphoid cells with distinct nucleoli and ample cytoplasm. **B** Tumour cells uniformly express CD20. **C** In situ hybridization for EBV-encoded small RNA (EBER) reveals positive signals for EBV in the nucleus of tumour cells.

Prognosis and predictive factors

DLBCL associated with chronic inflammation is an aggressive lymphoma. For PAL, the 5-year overall survival rate is 20–35% {2818,2827}. For patients achieving complete remission with chemotherapy and/or radiotherapy, the 5-year survival rate is 50% {2818}. Complete tumour resection (pleuropneumonectomy with or without resection of adjacent involved tissues) has also been reported to give good results {2809}. Poor performance status; high serum levels of lactate dehydrogenase, alanine transaminase (also called glutamic-pyruvic transaminase), or urea; and high clinical stage are unfavourable prognostic factors {119,2827}.

Fibrin-associated diffuse large B-cell lymphoma

An unusual form of diffuse large B-cell lymphoma associated with chronic inflammation is not mass-forming and does not directly produce symptoms, but is discovered incidentally on histological examination of surgical pathology specimens excised for various pathologies other than lymphoma. The specimens typically contain fibrinous materials, such as in the walls of pseudocysts (having been reported in splenic false cyst, renal pseudocyst, adrenal pseudocyst, paratesticular pseudocyst, and pseudocyst in ovarian teratoma), hydrocoele, lesions or materials located in the cardiovascular system (having been reported in cardiac myxoma, cardiac prosthesis, cardiac fibrin thrombus, and synthetic tube graft), wear debris (associated with metallic implants), and chronic subdural haematoma {36,418,1479,1907,2388,2663,4114, 4115}. Suggestions have been made to rename this group of lymphomas fibrin-associated EBV+ large B-cell lymphoma {440A}.

Histologically, single and small aggregates of large lymphoma cells are found in only small foci within the fibrinous or

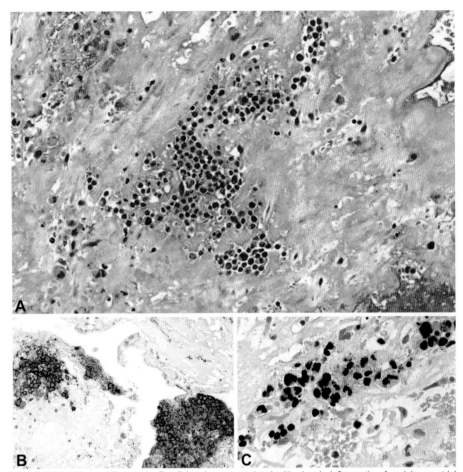

Fig. 13.127 Incidental diffuse large B-cell lymphoma associated with chronic inflammation found in an atrial myxoma. **A** Clusters of large lymphoma cells are visible within the fibrinous material that overlies an atrial myxoma. **B** Immunostaining for CD20 highlights the clusters of lymphoma cells within the fibrinous material. **C** The lymphoma cells show nuclear staining for EBNA2, indicating type III EBV latency.

amorphous material. The lymphoma cells show irregular nuclear foldings, coarse chromatin, distinct nucleoli, and amphophilic cytoplasm. Mitotic figures are easily found, and admixed apoptotic bodies are prominent. Chronic inflammatory cell infiltration in the background or vicinity is usually not prominent. The immunophenotypic features are similar to those of pyothorax-associated lymphoma, with expression of B-cell lineage markers and an activated B-cell phenotype. EBV is positive, with type III latency (typically EBNA2-positive).

Unlike in pyothorax-associated lymphoma, the clinical outcome is highly favourable, even with surgical excision alone. However, one report raised the possibility of progression to an infiltrative tumour; an incidental diffuse large B-cell lymphoma associated with chronic inflammation arising in a chronic subdural haematoma was accompanied by brain parenchymal infiltration {1907}.

Lymphomatoid granulomatosis

Pittaluga S.
Wilson W.H.
Jaffe E.S.

Definition

Lymphomatoid granulomatosis (LYG) is an angiocentric and angiodestructive lymphoproliferative disease involving extranodal sites, composed of EBV-positive B cells admixed with reactive T cells, which usually predominate. The lesion has a spectrum of histological grade and clinical aggressiveness, which is related to the proportion of large B cells.

ICD-O codes

Lymphomatoid granulomatosis
    Grade 1 or 2   9766/1
    Grade 3   9766/3

Synonym

Angiocentric immunoproliferative lesion (obsolete)

Epidemiology

LYG is a rare condition. It usually presents in adulthood, but may be seen in children with immunodeficiency disorders. It affects males more often than females, with a male-to-female ratio of ≥2:1 {1965, 3726}. It appears to be more common in western countries than in Asia.

Etiology

LYG is an EBV-driven lymphoproliferative disorder. Individuals with underlying immunodeficiency are at increased risk {1490,1544}. Predisposing conditions include allogeneic organ transplantation, Wiskott–Aldrich syndrome (eczema–thrombocytopenia–immunodeficiency syndrome), HIV infection, and X-linked lymphoproliferative syndrome. Patients presenting without evidence of underlying immunodeficiency usually manifest reduced immune function on careful clinical or laboratory analysis {3733,4332}.

Localization

Pulmonary involvement occurs in >90% of patients and is usually present at initial diagnosis. Other common sites of involvement include the brain, kidneys, liver, and skin. Involvement of the upper respiratory tract or gastrointestinal tract is relatively uncommon {841,1966,3726}.

The lymph nodes and spleen are very rarely involved {1823,1965,1966,2087, 2604,3726}.

Clinical features

Patients frequently present with signs and symptoms related to the respiratory tract, such as cough, dyspnoea, and chest pain. Constitutional symptoms are also common, including fever, malaise, weight loss, neurological symptoms, arthralgias, myalgias, and gastrointestinal symptoms. Patients with CNS disease may be asymptomatic or have varied presentations depending on the site of involvement, such as hearing loss, diplopia, dysarthria, ataxia, and/or altered mental status {1966, 3107,3726}. Few patients present with asymptomatic disease {1823}.

Macroscopy

LYG most commonly presents as pulmonary nodules that vary in size. The lesions are most often bilateral in distribution, involving the mid- and lower lung fields. Larger nodules frequently exhibit central necrosis and may cavitate. Nodular lesions are found in the kidneys and brain, usually associated with central necrosis {1966,3726}. Skin lesions are extremely diverse in appearance. Nodular lesions are found in the subcutaneous tissue. Dermal involvement may also be seen, sometimes with necrosis and ulceration. Cutaneous plaques or a maculopapular rash are less common cutaneous manifestations {309,1823,1965,2604}.

Microscopy

LYG is characterized by an angiocentric and angiodestructive polymorphous lymphoid infiltrate {1965,1966,2087, 3726}. Lymphocytes predominate and are admixed with plasma cells, immunoblasts, and histiocytes. Neutrophils and eosinophils are usually inconspicuous. The background small lymphocytes may show some atypia or irregularity, but do not appear overtly neoplastic. LYG is composed of a variable but usually small number of EBV-positive B cells admixed with a prominent inflammatory

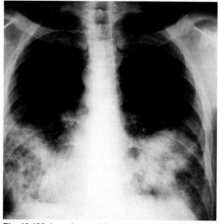

Fig. 13.128 Lymphomatoid granulomatosis. Chest radiograph identifies multiple nodules, mainly affecting the lower lung fields.

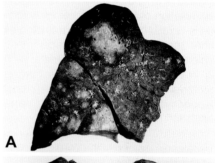

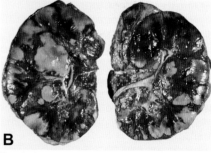

Fig. 13.129 Lymphomatoid granulomatosis. **A** Involved lung. Large nodules show central cavitation. **B** Large necrotic nodules are also found in the kidney.

background {1490,1966,1967}. The EBV-positive cells usually show some atypia. They may resemble immunoblasts or less commonly have a more pleomorphic appearance reminiscent of Hodgkin cells. Multinucleated forms may be seen. Classic Reed–Sternberg cells are generally not present; if seen, they should raise the possibility of Hodgkin lymphoma. Well-formed granulomas are typically absent in the lungs and most other extranodal sites {2357}. However, skin lesions often exhibit a prominent granulomatous reaction in subcutaneous tissue {309}.

Vascular changes are prominent in LYG. Lymphocytic vasculitis, with infiltration of the vascular wall, is seen in most cases. The vascular infiltration may compromise vascular integrity, leading to infarct-like tissue necrosis. More direct vascular damage, in the form of fibrinoid necrosis, is also common, and is mediated by chemokines induced by EBV {3943}.

LYG must be distinguished from nasal-type extranodal NK/T-cell lymphoma, which often has an angiodestructive growth pattern and is also associated with EBV {1819,3726}.

Immunophenotype

The EBV-positive B cells usually express CD20 {1491,1966,3726,3899,4332}. The cells are variably positive for CD30, but negative for CD15. LMP1 may be positive in the larger atypical and more pleomorphic cells. EBNA2 is frequently positive, consistent with latency type III {3726}. Stains for cytoplasmic immunoglobulin are frequently non-informative, although in rare cases monotypic cytoplasmic immunoglobulin expression may be seen, particularly in cells showing plasmacytoid differentiation {3726,4332}. The background lymphocytes are CD3+ T cells, with CD4+ cells more frequent than CD8+ cells {3726}.

Postulated normal counterpart

A mature B cell, transformed by EBV

Grading

The grading of LYG relates to the proportion of EBV-positive B cells relative to the reactive lymphocyte background {1491, 1966,2357,3726}. It is most important to distinguish grade 3 from grade 1 or 2. A uniform population of large atypical EBV-positive B cells without a polymorphous background should be classified as EBV-positive, diffuse large B-cell lymphoma, NOS and is beyond the spectrum of LYG as currently defined.

Grade 1 lesions contain a polymorphous lymphoid infiltrate without cytological atypia. Large transformed lymphoid cells are absent or rare, and are better appreciated by immunohistochemistry. When present, necrosis is usually focal.

By in situ hybridization for EBV-encoded small RNA (EBER), only infrequent EBV-positive cells are identified (< 5 per high-power field) {4332}. In some cases, EBV-positive cells may be absent; in this setting, the diagnosis should be made with caution, with studies to rule out other inflammatory or neoplastic conditions.

Grade 2 lesions contain occasional large lymphoid cells or immunoblasts in a polymorphous background. Small clusters can be seen, in particular with CD20 staining. Necrosis is more commonly seen. In situ hybridization for EBV readily identifies EBV-positive cells, which usually number 5–20 per high-power field. Variation in the number and distribution of EBV-positive cells can be seen within a nodule or among nodules, and occasionally as many as 50 EBV-positive cells per high-power field can be observed.

Grade 3 lesions still show an inflammatory background, but contain large atypical B cells that are readily identified by CD20 and can form larger aggregates. Markedly pleomorphic and Hodgkin-like cells are often present, and necrosis is usually extensive. By in situ hybridization, EBV-positive cells are extremely numerous (> 50 per high-power field), and focally may form small confluent sheets. It is important to take into consideration that in situ hybridization for EBV can be unreliable when large areas of necrosis

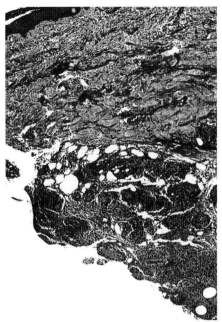

Fig. 13.130 Lymphomatoid granulomatosis. Cutaneous manifestation showing subcutaneous infiltration, with fat necrosis and a granulomatous response.

are present, due to poor RNA preservation; additional molecular studies for EBV may be helpful {3726}.

Genetic profile

In most cases of grade 2 or 3 disease, clonality of the IG genes can be demonstrated by molecular genetic techniques {1490,2604}. In some cases, different

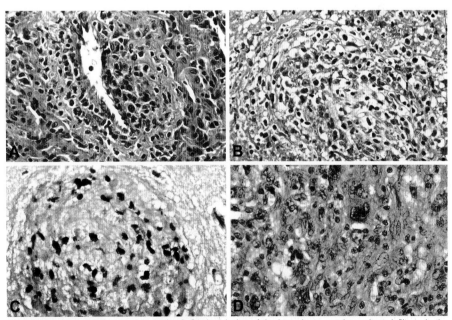

Fig. 13.131 Lymphomatoid granulomatosis. **A** Grade 1 lesion of the lung shows a polymorphous infiltrate in the vascular wall. **B** Grade 3 lesion of the brain contains numerous large transformed lymphoid cells. **C** Grade 3 lesion. The cells are positive for EBV by in situ hybridization for EBV-encoded small RNA (EBER). **D** Large pleomorphic cells may be seen, most commonly in grade 3 lesions and rarely in grade 2 lesions.

clonal populations may be identified in different anatomical sites {2678,4332}. Southern blot analysis may also show clonality of EBV {2607}. Demonstration of clonality in grade 1 cases is less consistent, an observation that may be related to the relative rarity of the EBV-positive cells in these cases. Alternatively, some cases of LYG may be polyclonal {3726}. TR gene analysis shows no evidence of monoclonality {2604,2607,3726}. Alterations of oncogenes have not been identified.

Genetic susceptibility
Genetic susceptibility includes Wiskott–Aldrich syndrome (eczema–thrombocytopenia–immunodeficiency syndrome), X-linked lymphoproliferative syndrome, and conditions linked to immunodeficiency.

Prognosis and predictive factors
The clinical behaviour of LYG varies widely; the disease ranges from an indolent process to an aggressive large B-cell lymphoma. In its most indolent form, LYG presents with pulmonary nodules in an otherwise asymptomatic patient, which can wax and wane and rarely resolve. A more typical course is characterized by symptoms and multiorgan involvement. In the largest retrospective series reported, from 1979, 63.5% of patients died, most within the first year of diagnosis, and the median overall survival was 14 months {1965}. Historically, corticosteroids and chemotherapy were the most common treatments, with most patients eventually succumbing to disease-related complications, including EBV-positive diffuse large B-cell lymphomas. More recently, the use of chemoimmunotherapy with dose-adjusted EPOCH-R and/or interferon has resulted in a 5-year overall survival rate of 70% {3406,4332}.

Primary mediastinal (thymic) large B-cell lymphoma

Gaulard P.
Harris N.L.
Pileri S.A.
Stein H.
Kovrigina A.M.
Jaffe E.S.
Möller P.
Gascoyne R.D.

Definition
Primary mediastinal (thymic) large B-cell lymphoma (PMBL) is a mature aggressive large B-cell lymphoma (LBCL) of putative thymic B-cell origin arising in the mediastinum, with distinctive clinical, immunophenotypic, genotypic, and molecular features. Cases that arise outside the mediastinum are probably very uncommon, and cannot be confidently recognized without gene expression profiling studies.

ICD-O code   9679/3

Synonyms
Primary mediastinal clear cell lymphoma of B-cell type (obsolete); mediastinal diffuse large cell lymphoma with sclerosis (no longer recommended)

Epidemiology
PMBL accounts for about 2–3% of non-Hodgkin lymphomas. Unlike most other mature aggressive B-cell lymphomas, it occurs predominantly in young adults (median patient age: ~35 years) and has a female predominance, with a female-to-male ratio of about 2:1 {1,589,3535,4498}.

Localization
The vast majority of patients with PMBL present with a localized anterosuperior mediastinal mass in the thymic area. The mass is often bulky (> 10 cm in 60–70% of patients) and frequently invades adjacent structures, such as the lungs, pleura, and pericardium. Regional involvement of supraclavicular and cervical lymph nodes can occur. At progression, dissemination to distant extranodal sites, such as the kidneys, adrenal glands, liver, and CNS, is relatively common; however, bone marrow involvement is usually absent {279, 589,2234}. Leukaemia is not observed. Uncommon cases of PMBL at non-mediastinal sites, and without evident

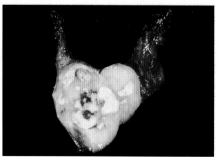

Fig. 13.132 Primary mediastinal large B-cell lymphoma. Cut surface showing fleshy tumour with necrosis.

mediastinal disease, have been identified, in particular by gene expression profiling {672,3412,3538,4452}. Most of these cases are missed in routine practice, because gene expression profiling is not a routine clinical test.

Clinical features
Symptoms are related to the mediastinal mass, frequently with superior vena cava syndrome. B symptoms may be present. Pleural or pericardial effusion is present in one third of cases {4498}. The absence of distant lymph node and bone marrow involvement is important to help exclude a systemic diffuse LBCL (DLBCL) with secondary mediastinal involvement. About 80% of cases are stage I–II at the time of diagnosis {4498}.

Microscopy
PMBL shows wide morphological/cytological variation from case to case {3112}. The growth pattern is diffuse, and it is commonly associated with compartmentalizing, alveolar fibrosis {279,589,2628,2799, 3112,3179}. The stromal component is frequently absent in involved lymph nodes. The neoplastic cells are usually medium-sized to large, with abundant pale cyto-

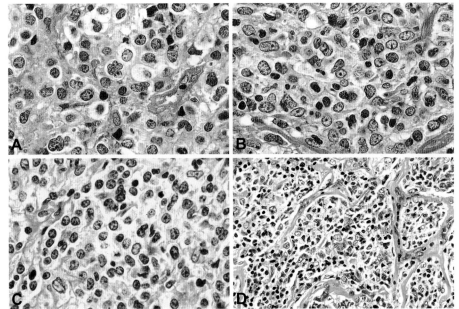

Fig. 13.133 Primary mediastinal large B-cell lymphoma. **A** Nuclei are round (centroblast-like) or sometimes multilobated. **B** Sheets of large cells with abundant pale cytoplasm, separated by collagenous fibrosis. **C** Medium-sized cells with abundant pale cytoplasm. **D** Classic clear-cell appearance of the tumour cells, with associated delicate interstitial fibrosis.

plasm and relatively round or ovoid nuclei. In some cases, the lymphoma cells have pleomorphic and/or multilobated nuclei and may resemble Reed–Sternberg cells, raising suspicion of Hodgkin lymphoma {3112,4047}. Rarely, there are so-called grey-zone lymphomas combining features of PMBL and classic Hodgkin lymphoma (CHL); these are separately designated as B-cell lymphoma, unclassifiable, with features intermediate between DLBCL and CHL. Examples of composite PMBL and nodular sclerosis CHL have also been described, and PMBL can occur either before or at relapse of nodular sclerosis CHL {4047,4333}.

Immunophenotype

PMBL expresses B-cell–lineage antigens such as CD19, CD20, CD22, and CD79a, but commonly lacks immunoglobulin despite a functional IG gene rearrangement and expression of the transcription factors PAX5, BOB1, OCT2, and PU1 {1915, 2379,3179,4274}. Flow cytometric studies may demonstrate surface IG in a subset of cases {4274}. CD30 is present in >80% of cases; however, staining is usually weak and heterogeneous compared to that in CHL {1633,3179}. CD15 may be expressed in a minority of cases {2800}. EBV is almost always absent {589}. The neoplastic cells are frequently positive for IRF4/MUM1; present in 75% of cases,

and have variable expression of BCL2, present in 55–80% of cases, and BCL6, in 45–100%; CD10 positivity is less common, seen in 8–32% of cases {899,3179}. CD11c is positive in about 40% of cases {3364}. Unlike most cases of DLBCL, approximately 70% of PMBL express CD23, MAL antigen, and programmed

cell death ligands PDL1 and PDL2 {524, 803,805,1327A,3179}. MYC can be expressed, sometimes on >30% of cells, independently of *MYC* gene alteration {2303}. Aberrant expression of TNFAIP2 is a frequent feature, in common with CHL but rarely found in other types of DLBCL {2080}. PMBL is also positive for CD54 and FAS (also known as CD95), and coexpresses TRAF1 and nuclear REL {3384,4460}. It often lacks HLA class I and/or class II molecules {2799,2800}.

Postulated normal counterpart

A thymic medullary, asteroid, activation-induced cytidine deaminase–positive B cell

Genetic profile

Antigen receptor genes

Immunoglobulin genes are rearranged and may be class switched, with a high load of somatic hypermutations without ongoing mutation activity {2262}.

Gene expression profiling

PMBL has a unique transcriptional signature that is distinct from those of other LBCLs, but shares similarities with CHL {3412,3538}.

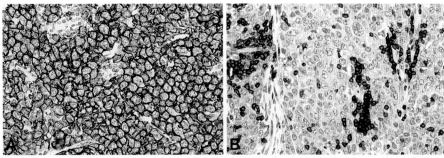

Fig. 13.134 Primary mediastinal large B-cell lymphoma. **A** All large cells express CD20 on the membrane. **B** Nests of CD3+ lymphocytes are present, with a perivascular distribution.

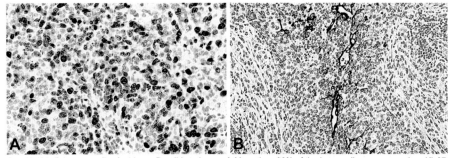

Fig. 13.135 Primary mediastinal large B-cell lymphoma. **A** More than 60% of the large cells express nuclear Ki-67. **B** Thymic remnants infiltrated by tumour cells; the epithelial component is positive for cytokeratin.

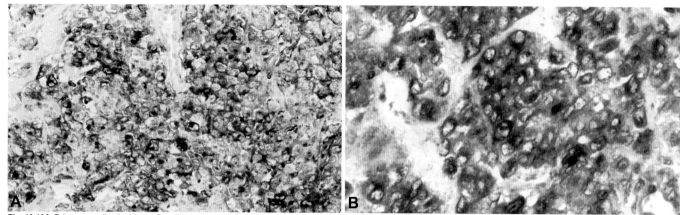

Fig. 13.136 Primary mediastinal large B-cell lymphoma. **A** Most tumour cells express CD23. **B** Tumour cells also express MAL, with a cytoplasmic accentuation in the Golgi region.

Cytogenetic abnormalities and oncogenes

Rearrangements of *BCL2*, *BCL6*, and *MYC* are absent or rare {3548,4067}. Rearrangements or mutations in the class II major histocompatibility complex (MHC) transactivator *CIITA* at 16p13.13 have been reported in as many as 53% of PMBLs, resulting in downregulated MHC class II molecules, creating an immune-privileged phenotype in PMBL. Translocations involving *CIITA* occur with *CD274* (also called *PDCD1LG1* or *PDL1*) and *PDCD1LG2* (also called *PDL2*); *CD274* and *PDCD1LG2* are also reported to fuse with partners other than *CIITA* in some cases {2763,3779, 4081}. Together with gains and amplifications at chromosome 9p24.1, including the *JAK2/PDCD1LG2/PDCD1LG1* locus (in as many as 75% of cases) {344,1881,2624, 4300}, these aberrations in the PDL locus likely explain the common overexpression of PDL1 and PDL2 in PMBL {668,3645}. This profile, with *CIITA* alterations and also copy-number gains and high-level amplification of the PDL locus (in 29–70% of cases), occurs almost exclusively in PMBL; it is unique among the LBCLs but shows similarities to what is found in CHL {1436, 3779,4081}.

The genomic profile also typically contains gains in chromosome 2p16.1 (seen in ~50% of cases), where candidate genes *REL* and *BCL11A* are amplified in a proportion of cases, leading to a frequent, albeit inconsistent, nuclear accumulation of their proteins {3384,4296,4297}. Gains involving chromosomes Xp11.4-21, Xq24-26, 7q22, 12q31, and 9q34 {344} are also seen in approximately one third of PMBLs. PMBL has a constitutively activated NF-kappaB pathway {1208}, which might be due to deleterious mutations in the *TNFAIP3* gene, present in as many as 60% of PMBLs {1049,3572A}. These tumours also have a constitutively activated JAK/STAT signalling pathway, also found in CHL, that seems to be frequently related to inactivating mutations of *SOCS1* {2624,3777,4073,4297}. Mutations affecting the *STAT6* DNA-binding domain and in *PTPN1*, a negative regulator of JAK/STAT signalling, are also common, found in in as many as 72% and 25% of PMBLs, respectively, but are almost absent in DLBCL {1049,1495,2280, 2504,3363}. The genetic landscape of PMBL suggests activation-induced cytidine deaminase–mediated aberrant somatic hypermutation as the mutational

mechanism {2763}, with *BCL6* mutations detected in about half of the cases {2477}. The landscape also includes truncating immunity pathway, *ITPKB*, *MFHAS1*, and *XPO1* mutations {1049}.

Genetic susceptibility

Exome sequencing of a family with three siblings with PMBL suggested *KMT2A* (previously called *MLL*) as a candidate predisposition gene, but these findings warrant replication {3465}.

Prognosis and predictive factors

Variations in microscopic appearance do not predict differences in survival {3112}. PMBL should be distinguished from B-cell lymphoma, unclassifiable, with features intermediate between DLBCL and CHL, which is more aggressive {4047}. Response to intensive chemotherapy, with or without radiotherapy, is usually good. PMBL is associated with a more favourable survival than are the germinal centre B-cell and activated B-cell subtypes of DLBCL, and recently developed chemotherapy protocols have shown high cure rates in adults and children {1058,2667,3412,4346}. Extension into adjacent thoracic viscera, pleural or pericardial effusion, and poor performance status are associated with inferior outcome {115,589,2233,2234,3535,3538}. FDG-PET predicts survival after chemo-immunotherapy {605,2514}.

Intravascular large B-cell lymphoma

Nakamura S.
Ponzoni M.
Campo E.

Definition

Intravascular large B-cell lymphoma is a rare type of extranodal large B-cell lymphoma characterized by the selective growth of lymphoma cells within the lumina of vessels, in particular capillaries, and with the exception of larger arteries and veins.

ICD-O code 9712/3

Synonyms

Malignant angioendotheliomatosis; angioendotheliomatosis proliferans syndrome; intravascular lymphomatosis; angioendotheliotropic lymphoma (all obsolete)

Epidemiology

This tumour occurs in adults, with a median age of 67 years (range: 13–85 years) and a male-to-female ratio of 1.1:1. The frequency and clinical presentation differ according to patients' geographical origin (West vs Far East) {1196,2789,3214, 3215,3655}.

Localization

This lymphoma is usually widely disseminated in extranodal sites, including the bone marrow, and may present in virtually any organ. However, the lymph nodes are usually spared.

Clinical features

Two major patterns of clinical presentation have been recognized: a so-called classic form (mostly present in western countries) characterized by symptoms related to the main organ involved, predominantly neurological or cutaneous, and a haemophagocytic syndrome–associated form, originally documented as an Asian variant, in which patients present with multiorgan failure, hepatosplenomegaly, and pancytopenia {1196,2789,3214,3215, 3655}. Exceptions to these geographical distributions may occur. B symptoms, in particular fever, are very common, occurring in 55–76% of patients, in both types of presentation. An isolated cutaneous variant has also been identified, invariably

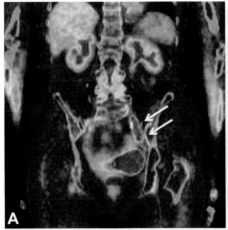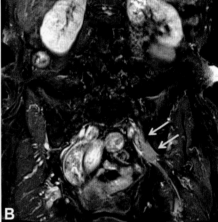

Fig. 13.137 Neurolymphomatosis as the relapse of intravascular large B-cell lymphoma. **A** FDG-PET/CT studies demonstrate hyperintense FDG uptake in the left lumbar plexus (white arrows), representing lymphoma invasion of the sciatic nerve. **B** A thin-sliced coronal image from gadolinium-enhanced T1-weighted MRI of the lumbosacral plexus also reveals the enhanced and enlarged left sciatic nerve (yellow arrows). Reprinted with permission from: Matsue K, Hayama BY, Iwama K, et al. {2570}

in western females; it is characterized by restriction of the tumour to the skin and is associated with a better prognosis {1193, 3214}. Conventional staging procedures are generally associated with a high proportion of false negatives due to the lack of detectable tumour masses. A random skin biopsy of normal-appearing skin and transbronchial lung biopsy are often helpful to make the diagnosis. Tumour cells are often seen in subcutaneous tissue irrespective of the absence of skin eruption, even in the haemophagocytic syndrome–associated form {2569}.

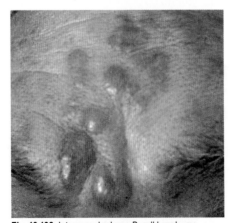

Fig. 13.138 Intravascular large B-cell lymphoma. Skin involvement.

Microscopy

The neoplastic lymphoid cells are mainly lodged in the lumina of small or intermediate sized vessels in many organs. Fibrin thrombi, haemorrhage, and necrosis may be observed in some cases. The tumour cells are large, with prominent nucleoli and frequent mitotic figures. Rare cases have cells with anaplastic features or smaller size {3215}. Minimal extravascular location of neoplastic cells may be seen. In the CNS, recurrences may be associated with extravascular brain masses {1642,3657}. Sinusoidal involvement occurs in the liver, spleen, and bone marrow. Malignant cells are occasionally detected in peripheral blood {3215}.

Immunophenotype

Tumour cells express mature B-cell–associated antigens. CD5 and CD10 coexpression is seen in 38% and 13% of the cases, respectively. Almost all CD10-negative cases are positive for IRF4/MUM1. An increasing number of intravascular NK/T-cell lymphomas with EBV-positive tumour cells {1317,4241} and rarely intralymphatic anaplastic large cell lymphomas, ALK-negative {2644, 3871}, have been reported, but they should be considered different entities.

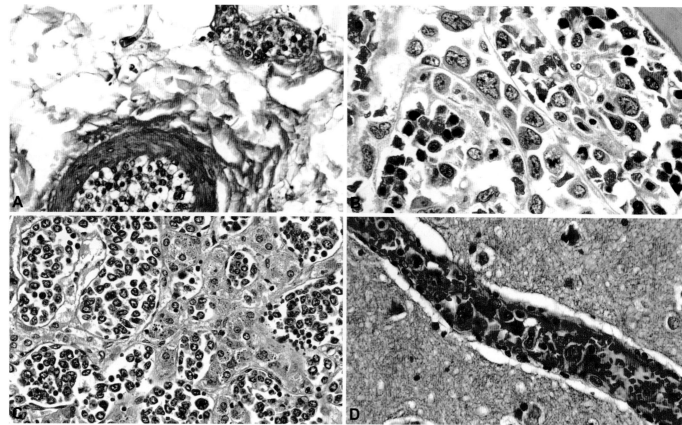

Fig. 13.139 Intravascular large B-cell lymphoma. **A** The large lymphoma cells fill the vein (lower left) and capillary (upper right). **B** The large tumour cells are present in the sinuses of the bone marrow, with abundant cytoplasm surrounding a more-or-less irregular nucleus. **C** The large lymphoma cells fill the vascular channels in the adrenal gland. **D** The large tumour cells are present in the lumen of small vessels in the CNS.

The intravascular growth pattern has been hypothesized to be secondary to a defect in homing receptors on the neoplastic cells {1204}, such as the lack of CD29 (integrin beta-1) and CD54 (ICAM1) adhesion beta-molecules {3212}.

Postulated normal counterpart
A transformed peripheral B cell

Genetic profile
Immunoglobulin genes are clonally rearranged. Karyotypic abnormalities have been described, but too few cases have been studied to demonstrate recurrent abnormalities {3655,3656}.

Prognosis and predictive factors
Intravascular large B-cell lymphoma is generally aggressive, except for the cases with disease limited to the skin {3655}. The poor prognosis is due in part to the delay of timely and accurate diagnosis related to the protean presentation of this lymphoma. Chemotherapeutic regimens with rituximab have significantly improved the clinical outcomes of these patients, with a 3-year overall survival rate of 60–81% {1195,1197,3655,3656}. However, CNS relapse, which occurs in ~25% of cases {3657} and neurolymphomatosis {2570} are serious complications in the rituximab era. Neither the clinical type of presentation nor clinical parameters predict CNS relapse.

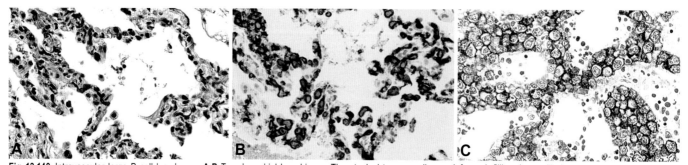

Fig. 13.140 Intravascular large B-cell lymphoma. **A,B** Transbronchial lung biopsy. The atypical tumour cells are deformed, filling the capillaries in the lung. CD20 staining highlights the deformed tumour cells in the alveolar capillaries. **C** Bone marrow biopsy. The tumour cells are highlighted by staining for CD20.

ALK-positive large B-cell lymphoma

Campo E.
Gascoyne R.D.

Definition
ALK-positive large B-cell lymphoma (LBCL) is an aggressive neoplasm of ALK-positive monomorphic large immunoblast-like B cells, which usually have a plasma cell phenotype.

ICD-O code
9737/3

Synonyms
Large B-cell lymphoma expressing the ALK kinase and lacking the t(2;5) translocation; ALK-positive plasmablastic B-cell lymphoma (both obsolete)

Epidemiology
This lymphoma is very rare, accounting for < 1% of diffuse LBCLs. It seems to occur more frequently in young men, with a male-to-female ratio of 5:1, but spans all age groups, with a patient age range of 9–85 years (median: 43 years). One third of cases occur in the paediatric age group {2230,3333}. There is no association with immunosuppression.

Localization
The tumour mainly involves lymph nodes {22,951,1307,1790,3333,3763} or presents as a mediastinal mass {907,1348}. Extranodal involvement has also been reported, at sites such as the nasopharynx {2976}, tongue {907}, stomach {2601}, bone {2976}, soft tissue {713}, liver, spleen, and skin {2230}.

Clinical features
Most patients present with generalized lymphadenopathy, and 60% present in advanced stage III/IV. Bone marrow is infiltrated in 25% of cases {2230}.

Microscopy
The lymph nodes show a marked diffuse infiltrate, frequently with a sinusoidal growth pattern. The infiltrate is composed of monomorphic large immunoblast-like cells with round pale nuclei containing a large central nucleolus and abundant amphophilic cytoplasm. Some cases show plasmablastic differentiation {951,

1307}. Atypical multinucleated neoplastic giant cells may be seen.

Immunophenotype
Lymphoma cells are strongly positive for the ALK protein, with most demonstrating a restricted granular cytoplasmic staining pattern highly indicative of the expression of the CLTC-ALK fusion protein. Few cases show cytoplasmic, nuclear, and nucleolar ALK staining associated with the NPM1-ALK fusion protein. *ALK* translocations with other partners may be associated with a cytoplasmic staining pattern. The tumours also characteristically strongly express EMA and plasma cell markers such as CD138, VS38, PRDM1 (also known as BLIMP1), and XBP1, and are negative or only positive in occasional cells for B-cell lineage-associated antigens (CD20, CD79a, and PAX5). IRF4/MUM1 is also positive {951,3763,4111}. CD45 is weak or negative {951,1307,2230}. CD30 is negative {951}, although focal and weak staining has been reported in a few cases {3763}. Most tumours express cytoplasmic immunoglobulin (usually IgA, more rarely IgG) with light chain restriction {951}. As described in some plasma cell tumours,

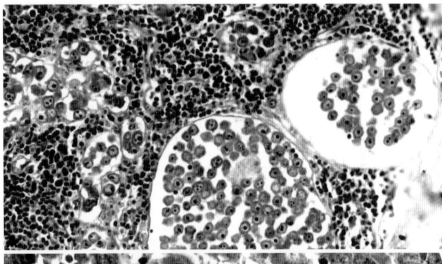

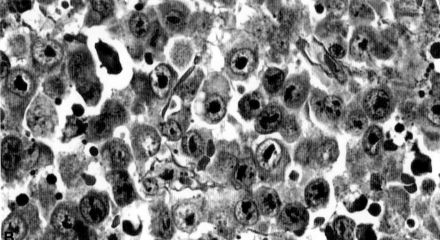

Fig. 13.141 ALK-positive large B-cell lymphoma. **A,B** Neoplastic cells show immunoblastic and plasmablastic features.

occasional cases are positive for cytokeratin, which may lead (in addition to EMA positivity, weak or negative staining for CD45, and the morphological features of cohesiveness and sinusoidal infiltration of the cells) to the mistaken diagnosis of carcinoma {2230}. The tumours are negative for T-cell markers but may be positive for CD4, CD57, CD43, and perforin {2230,3763}. All cases are EBV-negative and HHV8-negative {2230,4111}. These tumours should be distinguished from ALK-positive anaplastic large cell lymphoma, which is of T-cell origin; from other LBCLs with a sinusoidal growth pattern that are ALK-negative, may be CD30-positive, and express pan–B-cell antigens; and from other immunoblastic-appearing or plasmablastic lymphomas that are ALK-negative {785}.

Postulated normal counterpart
A post–germinal centre B cell with plasmablastic differentiation

Genetic profile
The IG genes are clonally rearranged {713,1307}. The key oncogenic factor of this tumour is ALK overexpression due to the fusion protein generated by the translocation of the *ALK* locus on chromosome 2. The most frequent abnormality is t(2;17)(p23;q23), responsible for a CLTC-ALK fusion protein. Few cases are associated with the t(2;5)(p23.2-23.1;q35.1)translocation, as described in ALK-positive anaplastic large cell lymphoma {22,2976}. A cryptic insertion of three *ALK* gene sequences into chromosome 4q22-24 has also been reported. *ALK* may also be fused to *SQSTM1*, *SEC31A*, or other uncommon fusion partners. These transloca-

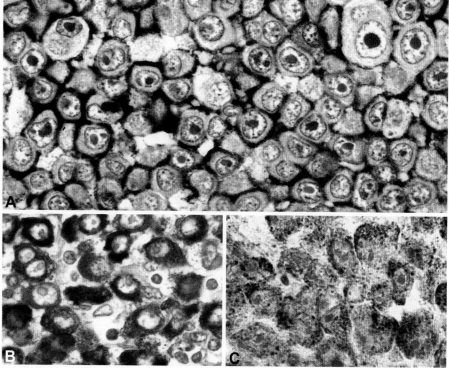

Fig. 13.142 ALK-positive large B-cell lymphoma. Tumour cells are positive for **A** EMA with a cytoplasmic membranous pattern, **B** for IgA, and (**C** for ALK with a restricted granular cytoplasmic pattern, highly indicative of the expression of the CLTC-ALK fusion protein.

tions are typically detected in the context of complex karyotypes {713,907,1307, 1348,1790,2230,2601,3333,3763,4111}. ALK protein oncogenic mechanisms include activation of the STAT3 pathway; concordantly, ALK-positive LBCLs express high phospho-STAT3 {4111}. MYC is also expressed in the absence of *MYC* translocations or amplifications, probably due to transcriptional activation downstream of STAT3 {4111}. Oncogenic *Alk* activation in murine B cells generates plasmablastic B-cell tumours {709}.

Prognosis and predictive factors
In one study, the reported median overall survival of patients with stage III/IV disease was 11 months {3333}. Longer survival (> 156 months) has been reported in children {951,2976}. These tumours are usually negative for CD20 antigen, and are thus unlikely to be sensitive to rituximab. Patients presenting with localized disease (stage I–II) have been found to have significantly longer survival {2230}.

Plasmablastic lymphoma

Campo E.
Stein H.
Harris N.L.

Definition

Plasmablastic lymphoma (PBL) is a very aggressive lymphoma with a diffuse proliferation of large neoplastic cells, most of which resemble B immunoblasts or plasmablasts, that have a CD20-negative plasmacytic phenotype. It was originally described in the oral cavity and frequently occurs in association with HIV infection, but it may also occur in other sites, predominantly extranodal, and in association with other causes of immunodeficiency {785,936}. Some cases, particularly in the oral cavity (i.e. the oral mucosa type), look most like a diffuse large B-cell lymphoma (LBCL); other cases have morphologically recognizable plasmacytic differentiation. Other subtypes of LBCLs with a plasmablastic immunophenotype (e.g. ALK-positive LBCL and HHV8-associated lymphoproliferative disorders) are not included in this category.

ICD-O code 9735/3

Epidemiology

This lymphoma occurs predominantly in adults with immunodeficiency, most commonly due to HIV infection but also in the setting of iatrogenic immunosuppression (transplantation and autoimmune diseases) and in elderly patients with presumptive immunosenescence.

PBL also occurs in children with immunodeficiency, mainly due to HIV infection {417,578,785,936,2365}.

Etiology

Immunodeficiency, due to various causes, predisposes individuals to the development of PBL. The tumour cells are EBV-infected in most patients {417,785, 936,1023}.

Localization

PBL most frequently presents as a mass in extranodal regions of the head and neck, in particular the oral cavity, with the gastrointestinal tract being the next most common site. Other extranodal localizations reported in > 1% of cases include the skin, bone, genitourinary tract, nasal cavity and paranasal sinuses, CNS, liver, lungs, and orbits. Nodal involvement is found in < 10% of cases overall, but in 30% of post-transplant cases {578,785, 936,1023}.

Clinical features

Disseminated stage III/IV disease, including bone marrow involvement, is found at presentation in 75% of HIV-positive patients and 50% of post-transplant patients, but in only 25% of patients without apparent immunodeficiency {578}. Most patients have an intermediate-risk or high-risk International Prognostic Index

(IPI) score. CT and PET show disseminated bone involvement in 30% of patients {3942}. A paraprotein may be detected in some cases {3865}. Tumours with features of PBL may occur in patients with prior plasma cell neoplasms, including plasma cell myeloma. Such cases should be considered plasmablastic transformation of myeloma and distinguished from primary PBL.

Microscopy

PBLs show a morphological spectrum varying from a diffuse and cohesive proliferation of cells resembling immunoblasts to cells with more obvious plasmacytic differentiation, which may resemble cases of plasmablastic plasma cell myeloma. Mitotic figures are frequent. Apoptotic cells and tingible body macrophages may be present. Cases with monomorphic plasmablastic cytology are most commonly seen in the setting of HIV infection and in the oral, nasal, and paranasal sinus areas (i.e. the oral mucosal type). Conversely, cases with plasmacytic differentiation tend to occur more commonly in other extranodal sites, as well as in lymph nodes {785,936}.

The differential diagnosis of cases with plasmacytic differentiation may include anaplastic or plasmablastic plasma cell myeloma. A history of immune deficiency and the presence of EBV by in

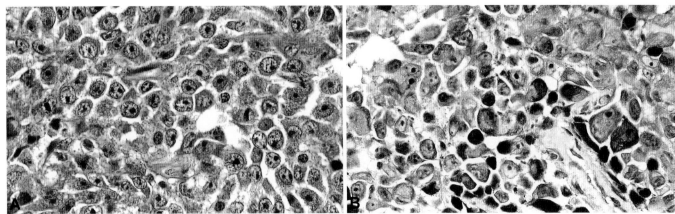

Fig. 13.143 Plasmablastic lymphoma (PBL). **A** PBL of the oral mucosa with a monomorphic proliferation of large, immunoblastic cells with prominent nucleoli. **B** PBL with plasmacytic differentiation. Many of the tumour cells are large, with round nuclei and variably prominent nucleoli and showing coarse chromatin. Smaller cells with plasmacytic differentiation are also present.

situ hybridization for EBV-encoded small RNA (EBER) are useful in establishing the diagnosis of PBL. However, some cases occurring in HIV-positive patients have overlapping features with plasma cell myeloma, such as lytic bone lesions and monoclonal serum immunoglobulins {3865,3942}. In some cases, a definite distinction cannot be made, and a descriptive diagnosis, such as 'plasmablastic neoplasm, consistent with PBL or anaplastic plasmacytoma', may be acceptable. LBCLs with plasmablastic features may occur as transformation of small B-cell lymphoid neoplasms. These cases have a morphology and phenotype similar to those of PBL, but immunodeficiency does not seem to play a role and EBV infection and *MYC* translocation are only rarely seen {2531}.

Immunophenotype

The neoplastic cells express a plasma cell phenotype, including positivity for CD138, CD38, VS38c, IRF4/MUM1, PRDM1 (also called BLIMP1), and XBP1. CD45, CD20, and PAX5 are either negative or sometimes weakly positive in a minority of cells. CD79a is positive in approximately 40% of cases {578,2699, 4111}. Cytoplasmic immunoglobulin is commonly expressed, most frequently IgG and either kappa or lambda light chain. CD56 is detected in 25% of cases. It is usually negative in the oral mucosal type, but may be seen in cases with plasmacytic differentiation. EMA and CD30 are frequently expressed. The Ki-67 proliferation index is usually very high (>90%). BCL2 and BCL6 expression is usually absent, whereas CD10 is expressed in 20% of cases. Cyclin D1 is negative. Some cases express the T-cell associated markers CD43 and CD45RO {578,785,936,1023,4164}. Reactive infiltrating T cells are usually very scarce. Some LBCLs may have marked morphological plasmablastic features but strongly express CD20, CD79a, and PAX5 {3682}. These cases should not be considered PBL and are better classified as diffuse LBCL, NOS.

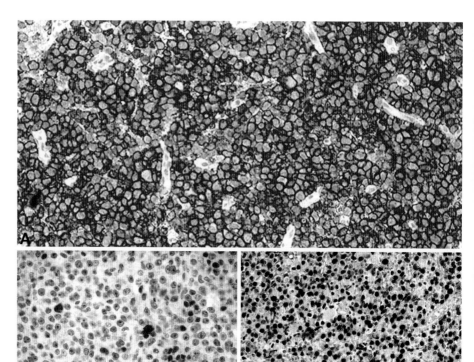

Fig. 13.144 Plasmablastic lymphoma (PBL). The PBL cells are strongly positive for CD138 (**A**) but negative for CD20 (**B**). In situ hybridization for EBV-encoded small RNA (EBER) reveals infection of all PBL cells by EBV (**C**).

In situ hybridization for EBER is positive in 60–75% of cases, but LMP1 is rarely expressed. PBL is more frequently EBV-positive in HIV-positive and post-transplant patients than in HIV-negative patients {578,2755}. HHV8 is consistently absent.

Postulated normal counterpart

A plasmablast (i.e. a blastic proliferating B cell that has switched its phenotype to the plasma cell gene expression programme)

Genetic profile

Clonal IGH rearrangement is demonstrable, even when immunoglobulin expression is not detectable, and IGHV may have somatic hypermutation or be unmutated with a germline configuration {1273}.

Genetic studies have revealed frequent complex karyotypes. *MYC* translocation

has been identified in approximately 50% of cases, more frequently in EBV-positive tumours (74%) than in EBV-negative tumours (43%), and it is associated with MYC protein expression {400,3865,4110, 4111}. The rearrangement usually occurs with IG genes {4110}.

Prognosis and predictive factors

The prognosis is generally poor; more than three quarters of patients die of the disease, with a median survival of 6–11 months {578,2755}. Newer therapies and better treatment of HIV infection may be associated with a better prognosis, but the results are not consistent across studies {578}. Evaluation of prognostic parameters has not yielded consistent results. However, *MYC* translocation has been associated with a worse outcome in two studies {578,2755}.

Primary effusion lymphoma

Said J.
Cesarman E.

Definition
Primary effusion lymphoma (PEL) is a large B-cell neoplasm usually presenting as serous effusions without detectable tumour masses. It is universally associated with the human herpesvirus 8 (HHV8), also called Kaposi sarcoma–associated herpesvirus. It most often occurs in the setting of immunodeficiency. Some patients with PEL secondarily develop solid tumours in adjacent structures such as the pleura. Rare HHV8-positive lymphomas indistinguishable from PEL present as solid tumour masses, and have been termed extracavitary PEL.

ICD-O code   9678/3

Synonym
Body cavity–based lymphoma (obsolete)

Epidemiology
Most cases arise in young or middle-aged men who have sex with men and who have HIV infection and severe immunodeficiency {2803,3479}. There is frequent coinfection with monoclonal EBV {623,2803,3479}. PEL has also been reported in recipients of solid organ transplants {1030,1875,2417}. The disease also occurs in the absence of immunodeficiency, usually in elderly patients, both men and women {3946}. In these patients, the lymphoma cells contain HHV8 and may lack EBV {775,3478}.

Etiology
The neoplastic cells are positive for HHV8 (Kaposi sarcoma-associated herpesvirus or KSHV) in all cases. Most cases are co-infected with EBV {110,157,1683,3479}, but EBV has restricted gene expression and is not required for the pathogenesis. HHV8 encodes > 10 homologues of cellular genes that provide proliferative and anti-apoptotic signals {116,156,172,1895}. HHV8-encoded proteins and microRNAs include LANA1, vIRF3, vFLIP, and miR-K1 {116,156,172,1895,4090}. HHV8 IL6 prevents apoptosis by suppressing proapoptotic cathepsin D {670}. HHV8-encoded vFLIP activates NF-kappaB by

binding IKBKGG/NEMO and prevents death-receptor induced apoptosis. PELs also express vIRF3, which inhibits HLA transactivators, resulting in inefficient recognition and killing by T cells {3468}. Secretome analysis has revealed proteins involved in inflammation, immune response, and cell cycle and growth; structural proteins; and other proteins {1385}.

Localization
The most common sites are the pleural, pericardial, and peritoneal cavities. Typically only a single body cavity is involved {308,955,3006}. PEL has also been reported in unusual cavities, such as an artificial cavity related to the capsule of a breast implant {3478}. Most cases of PEL remain restricted to the body cavity of origin, but subsequent dissemination can occur. Extracavitary tumours with morphological and phenotypic characteristics similar to those of PEL can occur in extranodal sites including the gastrointestinal tract, skin, lungs, and CNS, or can involve the lymph nodes {631,824, 955}.

Clinical features
PELs occur mainly in males. The median patient age at presentation is 42 years in HIV-infected individuals and 73 years in the general population. Male homosexual contact is the most common risk

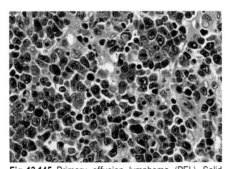

Fig. 13.145 Primary effusion lymphoma (PEL). Solid tissue mass from the mediastinum of an HIV-positive patient with PEL presenting with pleural effusions. The cells are large and pleomorphic, with eosinophilic macronucleoli and abundant cytoplasm. Many cells have an anaplastic or plasmacytoid appearance.

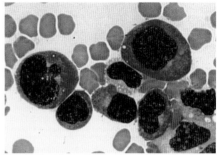

Fig. 13.146 Primary effusion lymphoma. Pleural fluid cytology. There is marked pleomorphism, with prominent nucleoli and a plasmacytoid appearance in the cytoplasm (Wright stain).

factor, followed by injection drug use. PELs also occur in HIV-seronegative men and women who have been exposed to HHV8. Patients typically present with effusions in the absence of lymphadenopathy or organomegaly. Approximately one third to half of the patients have pre-existing or develop Kaposi sarcoma {110}, and the CD4+ cell count is generally low. Occasional cases are associated with multicentric Castleman disease {3946}. PEL should be distinguished from the rare HHV8-negative effusion-based lymphoma morphologically similar to PEL that has been described in patients with fluid overload states {59,1753,2891, 3386,4378}, as well as from the EBV-associated HHV8-negative large B-cell lymphomas also occurring with chronic suppurative inflammation (diffuse large B-cell lymphoma associated with chronic inflammation), such as pyothorax-associated lymphoma {121,804}. Cases of extracavitary PEL occur in lymph nodes or extranodal sites without lymphomatous effusions during the course of the disease. These cases are similar to PEL in their clinical presentation occurring in HIV-positive men and morphology {3044}. Other lymphomas, including Burkitt lymphoma, can present with a malignant effusion and are unrelated to PEL.

Microscopy
In cytocentrifuge preparations, the cells exhibit a variety of appearances, ranging from large immunoblastic or plasma-

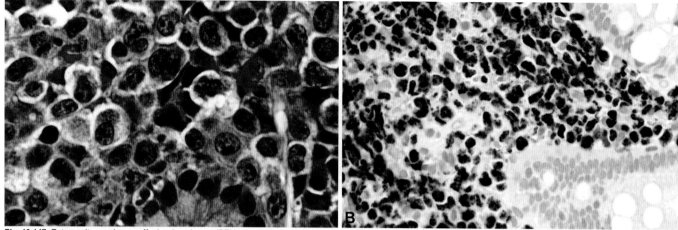

Fig. 13.147 Extracavitary primary effusion lymphoma (PEL) presenting initially as a mass in the large intestine of an HIV-positive patient. **A** Plasmablastic/anaplastic cells infiltrating between the glands of a large bowel mass. **B** The nuclei are strongly positive for HHV8 with an antibody to LANA1 (also called ORF73).

blastic cells to cells with more-anaplastic morphology. Nuclei are large and round to more irregular in shape, with prominent nucleoli. The cytoplasm can be abundant and is deeply basophilic, with vacuoles in occasional cells. A perinuclear hof consistent with plasmacytoid differentiation may be seen. Some cells resemble Hodgkin or Reed–Sternberg cells. Mitotic figures are numerous. The cells often appear more uniform in histological sections than in cytospin preparations {110, 955,2803}.

The histological features of extracavitary PELs include an immunoblastic to anaplastic morphology similar to that seen in effusions. There may be lymph node sinus involvement, and staining for HHV8 may be helpful in differentiating these cases from anaplastic large cell lymphoma {826}. Pleomorphic large cells may have a Hodgkin-like appearance, necessitating differentiation from classic Hodgkin lymphoma. There may be involvement of endothelial-lined lymphatic or vascular channels, and cases resembling intravascular lymphoma have been reported {826}.

Immunophenotype

The lymphoma cells usually express CD45 but lack pan–B-cell markers such as CD19, CD20, and CD79a {2054,2803}. Surface and cytoplasmic immunoglobulin is absent. BCL6 is usually absent. Activation and plasma cell–related markers and a variety of non–lineage associated antigens such as HLA-DR, CD30, CD38, VS38c, CD138, and EMA are often demonstrable. Levels of immunoglobulin expression are usually undetectable or low. The cells usually lack T/NK-cell antigens, although aberrant expression of T-cell markers may occur, and may be more frequent in cases of extracavitary PEL {308,431,826,3044,3477}. The nuclei of the neoplastic cells are positive for the HHV8-associated latent protein LANA1 (also called ORF73) {1065}. This is very useful in establishing a diagnosis. Despite the usual positivity for EBV by in situ hybridization for EBV-encoded small RNA (EBER), EBV LMP1 is absent {110,775,1683,3946}. EBV-negative PELs usually occur in elderly HIV-negative patients from HHV8-endemic areas such as the Mediterranean {3725}. Solid tumours constituting the extracavitary variant of PEL have a phenotype similar to that of PEL but express B-cell associated antigens and immunoglobulins slightly more frequently {631}. They may have lower expression of CD45 but higher expression of CD20 and CD79a, as well as aberrant expression of T-cell markers {3044}.

Postulated normal counterpart

Post-germinal centre B cell with plasmablastic differentiation

Genetic profile

Immunoglobulin genes are clonally rearranged and hypermutated, indicating a B-cell derivation {2565,4234}. Some cases also have rearrangement of TR genes in addition to IG genes (so-called genotypic infidelity) {1667,3477}. Rare cases diagnosed as T-cell PEL have been reported, as well as a case with monoclonal TR and IGH pseudomonoclonality due to extremely low numbers of B cells {824,2245}. Such cases should not be diagnosed as PEL. Nearly all cases of PEL contain clonal EBV; the exceptions are in the non–HIV infected population, which may be EBV-negative. No recurrent chromosomal abnormalities have been identified. HHV8 viral genomes are present in all cases. Gene expression profiling of AIDS-related PEL shows a distinct profile, with features of both plasma cells and EBV-transformed lymphoblastoid cell lines {2040}. PELs lack structural alterations in the *MYC* gene but have deregulated MYC protein due to the activity of HHV8 encoded latent proteins {4017}. They also lack mutations in the RAS family of genes and *TP53*, as well as rearrangements of *CCND1*, *BCL2*, and *BCL6*. A subset have mutations involving *BCL6* {1271}. They have complex karyotypes with numerous abnormalities, including trisomy 12, trisomy 7, and abnormalities of 1q21-25 {1271}. Comparative genomic analysis has revealed gains in chromosomes 12 and X {2780}.

Prognosis and predictive factors

The clinical outlook is extremely unfavourable, and median survival is <6 months. Rare cases have responded to chemotherapy and/or immune modulation {1357}.

HHV8-associated lymphoproliferative disorders

Said J.
Isaacson P.G.
Campo E.
Harris N.L.

Definition

In addition to causing Kaposi sarcoma, which may involve the lymph nodes, the human herpesvirus HHV8 (also called Kaposi sarcoma–associated herpesvirus) is responsible for a spectrum of lymphoproliferative disorders. These include HHV8-positive multicentric Castleman disease (MCD); HHV8-positive diffuse large B-cell lymphoma (DLBCL), NOS, which frequently arises in the background of MCD; and germinotropic lymphoproliferative disorder (GLPD). Except for GLPD, these disorders are most commonly seen in the setting of HIV infection and in HHV8-endemic areas, but they can also occur in other immunosuppressed states, including following transplantation {2238}. GLPD is most commonly seen in immunocompetent individuals. Primary effusion lymphoma (PEL) and extracavitary PEL are also caused by HHV8, but are discussed elsewhere (see *Primary effusion lymphoma*, p. 323).

Associated conditions

Kaposi sarcoma is frequently present in patients with MCD and HHV8-positive DLBCL, NOS, arising in MCD. PEL and its extracavitary counterpart may complicate HHV8-positive MCD.

Other HHV8-positive lymphoproliferative disorders

Although most cases of HHV8-positive lymphoproliferative disorders fall within the spectrum defined above, individual cases have been reported in which there are overlapping features. For example, cases arising in the background of MCD intermediate between HHV8-positive DLBCL and GLPD have been reported in HIV-positive and HIV-negative patients {1404A}. They may resemble HHV8-positive DLBCL, NOS, but are also positive for EBV-encoded small RNA (EBER) {3052,3616}. Although GLPD tends not to progress, one reported case evolved to a high-grade HHV8-positive, EBV-positive lymphoma {826}. The differential between HHV8-positive DLBCL, NOS, and extracavitary PEL may be problematic, but

most cases of PEL are EBV-positive, lack cytoplasmic immunoglobulins, express activation and plasma cell-associated antigens, including CD30, CD38, CD138, and EMA, and arise from a terminally differentiated rather than a naïve B cell.

Rare cases of other HHV8-positive lymphomas have been described, including a case with a Hodgkin-like appearance in an immunocompetent patient and cases resembling intravascular large B-cell lymphoma {834,1206}. Node-based HHV8-positive B-cell lymphomas with anaplastic large cell morphology have also been reported, and may constitute an anaplastic variant of HHV8-positive DLBCL, NOS {558,1721}.

Multicentric Castleman disease

Definition

Multicentric Castleman disease (MCD) is a clinicopathological entity that encompasses a group of systemic polyclonal lymphoproliferative disorders in which there is a proliferation of morphologically benign lymphocytes, plasma cells, and vessels, due to excessive production of cytokines, in particular IL6 {556, 1133}. Activation of the IL6R signalling pathway by the virus plays a key role in the development of HHV8-infected B-cell lymphoproliferative lesions, including MCD {1048}. In patients with HIV, MCD is almost always HHV8-related. In the absence of HIV, MCD is HHV8-related in as many as 50% of cases, and usually occurs in HHV8-endemic areas {1029}.

Table 13.25 Key features of HHV8-positive multicentric Castleman disease (MCD); diffuse large B-cell lymphoma (DLBCL), NOS; and germinotropic lymphoproliferative disorder (GLPD)

Feature	HHV8-positive MCD	HHV8-positive DLBCL, NOS	HHV8-positive GLPD
Clinical presentation	Generalized lymphadenopathy Splenomegaly Constitutional symptoms	Large lymph node Splenic mass Extranodal sites Peripheral blood	Localized or sometimes multifocal lymph node involvement
Microscopy	Abnormal follicles Plasmablasts predominantly in mantle zones Interfollicular plasma cell hyperplasia	Sheets of large plasmablastic cells	Retention of architecture with germinal centres containing variable numbers of plasmablasts sometimes replacing follicles
Phenotype	B-cell antigens +/– cIgM lambda + IRF4[a] + CD138 –	B-cell antigens +/– cIgM lambda + IRF4[a] + CD138 –	B-cell antigens – Monotypic kappa or lambda Any heavy chain CD138 – CD30 +/–
Clonality	Polyclonal	Monoclonal	Polyclonal or oligoclonal
HHV8 LANA1	+	+	+
EBER	–	–	+
HIV status	+/–	+/–	–
Prognosis	Poor but improved with new therapies	Poor	Usually responds to treatment

EBER, EBV-encoded small RNA.

[a] Also known as MUM1.

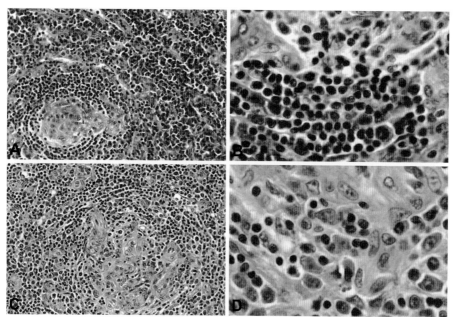

Fig. 13.148 HHV8-positive multicentric Castleman disease. **A** B-cell follicle with a regressed, partially hyalinized germinal centre. **B** The mantle zone contains scattered plasmablasts. **C** B-cell follicle showing partial hyalinization of the germinal centre, with an attenuated mantle zone. **D** Germinal centre containing numerous plasmablasts.

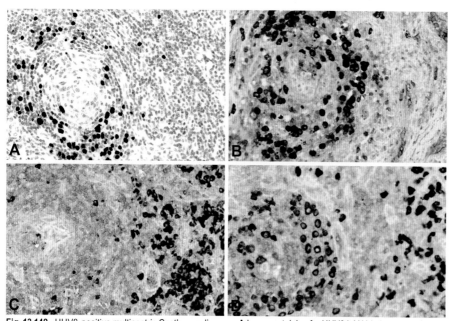

Fig. 13.149 HHV8-positive multicentric Castleman disease. **A** Immunostaining for HHV8 LANA1 shows localization in the plasmablasts present in the mantle zones. **B** Staining for IgM shows localization within the cytoplasm of the plasmablastic cells **C** Plasmablasts are negative for kappa light chains. The interfollicular reactive plasma cells stain positively. **D** Plasmablasts stained for lambda light chains show lambda light chain restriction.

MCD is idiopathic in HHV8-negative and HIV-negative patients. Idiopathic HIV- and HHV8-negative multicentric Castleman disease (iMCD) is a systemic disease with constitutional symptoms, laboratory abnormalities, and multicentric lymphadenopathy characterized by polytypic plasmacytosis and variably prominent hypervascular or regressed germinal centres {1132A,3475A,4450A}. The diagnosis requires exclusion of infectious, neoplastic, and autoimmune diseases that may have similar clinical presentations. In this syndrome, the hypercytokinaemia may be driven by inflammatory disease or inflammatory gene mutations, autoantibodies, ectopic cytokine secretion, as seen in paraneoplastic syndromes, or viral signalling by a non-HHV8 virus {1133}.

Epidemiology

HHV8-positive MCD occurs worldwide in immunosuppressed patients, particularly in association with HIV/AIDS. It may also affect immunocompetent individuals in HHV8-endemic areas (e.g. sub-Saharan Africa and Mediterranean countries) {425}. In HIV-infected patients, there is a strong association with sexual transmission, and men are predominantly affected.

Etiology

MCD is a heterogeneous group of disorders thought to arise from excessive hypercytokinaemia, most notably of IL6 {1133}. In HHV8-positive MCD, the plasmablastic cells are infected with HHV8, which produces viral IL6. In addition, HHV8-encoded proteins and microRNAs provide proliferative and anti-apoptotic signals contributing to the pathogenesis. These include LANA1, LANA2, IL10, vFLIP, and miR-K1 {116,156,172,1895, 4090}. HHV8-encoded vGPCR induces expression of proinflammatory and angiogenic factors contributing to the inflammatory and hyperproliferative nature of the lesions, and also constitutively activates the nuclear factor of activated T cells {3097}.

Localization

HHV8-positive MCD usually presents with generalized lymphadenopathy and splenomegaly.

Clinical features

Patients with HHV8-positive MCD present with constitutional symptoms, enlarging lymph nodes, and splenomegaly. Constitutional symptoms include fever, night sweats, fatigue, weight loss, and respiratory symptoms {440}. Kaposi sarcoma is commonly also present {1064, 2968}. In addition to lymphadenopathy, patients may have hepatosplenomegaly and a skin rash {556}. Laboratory findings include anaemia, thrombocytopenia, hypoalbuminaemia, hypergammaglobulinaemia, and elevated C-reactive protein {556}.

Microscopy

The B-cell follicles of lymph nodes and spleen show varied degrees of involution and hyalinization of their germinal centres, with prominent mantle zones that may intrude into the germinal centres and completely efface them. Follicles may show onion skinning or widened concentric rings of mantle zone lymphocytes, and prominent penetrating venules typical of Castleman disease. Among these mantle zone cells and adjacent interfollicular regions, there are variable numbers of medium-sized to large plasmablastic cells with amphophilic cytoplasm and vesicular, often eccentrically placed nuclei containing one or two prominent nucleoli. The blasts may be single in the intrafollicular and perifollicular areas, or may form small clusters or aggregates. Sheets of mature plasma cells expand the interfollicular region, including cells with cytoplasmic inclusions (Russell bodies) and crystalline forms. As the disease progresses, the plasmablasts may coalesce to form clusters {1064,1404A}. There may be clonal expansion of these clusters to form sheets of lymphoma cells effacing the architecture, with progression to HHV8-positive diffuse large B-cell lymphoma, NOS (see below).

Immunophenotype
The plasmablasts in MCD show stippled nuclear staining for HHV8 LANA1 and strong cIgM expression, with lambda light chain restriction. A proportion of the plasmablasts are positive for viral IL6. Plasmablasts have a CD20+/–, CD79a–/+, CD138–, PAX5–, CD38–/+, CD27– phenotype and are negative for EBV-encoded small RNA (EBER) {2968}. The interfollicular plasma cells are typically cIgM-negative and cIgA-positive, express polytypic light chains, and do not show nuclear expression of LANA1 antigen.

Postulated normal counterpart
A naïve B cell

Genetic profile
Despite the constant expression of monotypic IgM lambda by the plasmablasts in HHV8-positive MCD, careful molecular studies have shown that they constitute a polyclonal population {1048}. The plasmablastic aggregates that can develop during the progression of MCD may be monoclonal or oligoclonal.

Prognosis and predictive factors
Prognosis has been poor, related to the lymphoid proliferation and underlying

immune disorder. However, multitarget treatment strategies including rituximab, antiherpesvirus therapy, and targeted therapy against IL6 have improved outcome {556,1133,2064,4090}.

HHV8-positive diffuse large B-cell lymphoma, NOS

Definition
HHV8-positive diffuse large B-cell lymphoma (DLBCL), NOS, usually arises in association with HHV8-positive multicentric Castleman disease (MCD). However, similar lymphomas (HHV8-positive, EBV-positive, with lambda light chain restriction) have been reported in the absence of MCD {1108}. The lymphoma is characterized by a monoclonal proliferation of HHV8-infected lymphoid cells resembling plasmablasts expressing IgM lambda. It is usually associated with HIV infection. The cells may morphologically resemble plasmablasts and have abundant cytoplasmic immunoglobulin; however, they correspond to a naïve, IgM-producing B cell without IG somatic hypermutations. This lymphoma must be distinguished from plasmablastic lymphomas presenting in the oral cavity or other extranodal sites that frequently show class-switched and hypermutated IG genes. HHV8-positive DLBCLs, NOS,

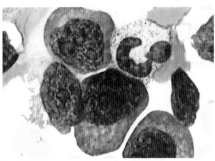

Fig. 13.150 Leukaemic HHV8-positive diffuse large B-cell lymphoma, NOS, arising in multicentric Castleman disease. Wright-Giemsa–stained tumour cells in the peripheral blood.

differ from primary effusion lymphoma (PEL) in that they are EBV-negative, do not have IG gene mutations, and are thought to arise from naïve IgM lambda–positive B cells rather than terminally differentiated B cells.

ICD-O code
9738/3

Epidemiology
Among patients with HIV and MCD, the risk of developing non-Hodgkin lymphoma is 15 times that within the general HIV-positive population {2700,2968}. In a series of 60 patients with HIV-positive MCD, 6 patients developed HHV8-positive DLBCL with a plasmablastic appearance {2968}.

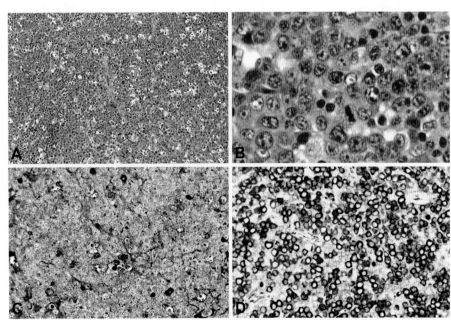

Fig. 13.151 HHV8-positive diffuse large B-cell lymphoma, NOS, arising in multicentric Castleman disease. **A** Sheets of plasmablasts efface normal lymph node architecture. **B** High magnification showing sheets of neoplastic plasmablasts. **C** Tumour cells are negative for immunoglobulin kappa light chain. **D** Tumour cells are positive for lambda light chain indicating lambda light chain restriction.

Etiology

By definition, the large lymphoid/plasmablastic cells in all cases are positive for HHV8. The molecular mechanisms involved in this lymphoma seem similar to those of the other HHV8-positive entities {116,156,172,1895}.

Localization

HHV8-positive DLBCL, NOS, characteristically involves the lymph nodes and/or spleen, but can disseminate to other viscera, including the liver, lungs, and gastrointestinal tract, and can also manifest as a leukaemia, with involvement of the peripheral blood {1064,2968}.

Clinical features

HHV8-positive DLBCL, NOS, usually arises in patients with clinical features of HHV8-positive MCD. HHV8-positive DLBCL, NOS, usually manifests with profound immunodeficiency, enlarging lymph nodes, and massive splenomegaly. There may also be manifestations of Kaposi sarcoma {1064,2968}. More rarely, HHV8-positive DLBCL, NOS, may arise in the absence of MCD {826,1108,1404A}.

Microscopy

The emergence of frank lymphoma is heralded by expansion of the small confluent sheets of HHV8 LANA1–positive plasmablasts to efface the lymph node and splenic architecture, often with massive splenomegaly. The large plasmablastic cells have vesicular, often eccentrically placed nuclei containing one or two prominent nucleoli and amphophilic cytoplasm. Infiltrates can also be present in the liver, lungs, and gastrointestinal tract, and in some cases there is involvement of the bone marrow and peripheral blood by HHV8-positive IgM lambda plasmablasts {1064,2968,2969}. Distinction from extracavitary PEL may be difficult, but EBV is usually positive in extracavitary PEL and there may be kappa or lambda light chain restriction.

Immunophenotype

The malignant large plasmablastic lymphoid cells show stippled nuclear staining for LANA1, and like the plasmablasts in HHV8-positive MCD, strongly express cIgM with lambda light chain restriction {2968}. They have a CD20+/–, CD79a–, CD138–, CD38–/+, CD27– phenotype, and are negative for EBV-encoded small RNA (EBER).

Postulated normal counterpart

A naïve B cell

Genetic profile

Frank HHV8-positive DLBCLs, NOS, are monoclonal. The IG genes are unmutated, unlike in PEL and extracavitary PEL, in which IG genes are clonally rearranged and hypermutated.

Prognosis and predictive factors

HHV8-positive DLBCL, NOS, is an extremely aggressive disorder.

HHV8-positive germinotropic lymphoproliferative disorder

Definition

HHV8-positive germinotropic lymphoproliferative disorder (GLPD) is a monotypic HHV8-positive lymphoproliferative lesion that usually occurs in HIV-negative individuals {1047,1404A}. HHV8-positive

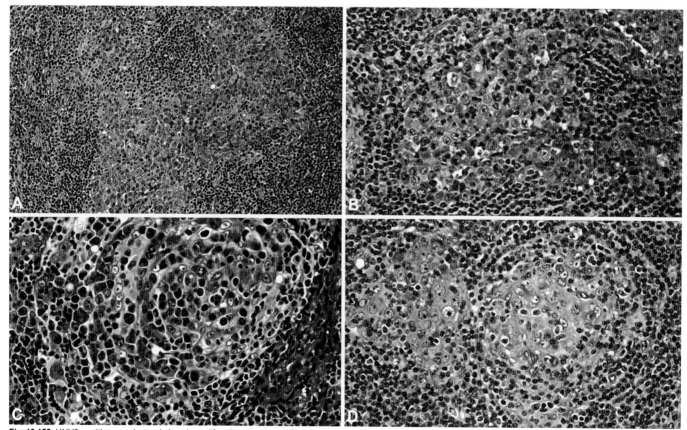

Fig. 13.152 HHV8-positive germinotropic lymphoproliferative disorder. **A** Germinal centre replaced by confluent sheets of plasmablasts. **B** Germinal centre largely replaced by plasmablasts. **C** Plasmablasts are seen within a hyperplastic germinal centre. **D** Clusters of plasmablasts within hyperplastic germinal centres.

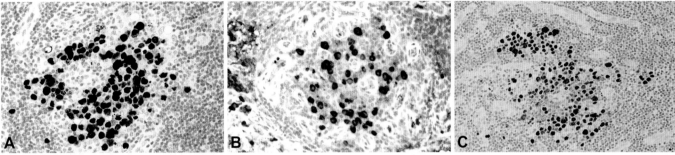

Fig. 13.153 HHV8-positive germinotropic lymphoproliferative disorder. **A** Plasmablasts stained for HHV8 LANA1. **B** Plasmablasts stain for lambda light chains. **C** Plasmablasts are positive for EBV-encoded small RNA (EBER).

plasmablasts partially or completely replace germinal centres {1047,2938, 3904}. The plasmablasts show either kappa or lambda light chain restriction but are polyclonal or oligoclonal. Coinfection with EBV is characteristic.

ICD-O code   9738/1

Epidemiology
GLPD mainly affects immunocompetent individuals, but occasional cases have been described in HIV-positive patients {1404A}. There is no known epidemiological association.

Etiology
The large plasmablastic cells are positive for HHV8 in all cases. Unlike in MCD and HHV8-positive DLBCL, NOS, in GLPD, the large cells are also positive for EBV-encoded small RNA (EBER). The contribution of EBV to the pathogenesis is uncertain. Occasional EBV-negative cases have been described {1404A}.

Localization
GLPD involves the lymph nodes.

Clinical features
The disorder presents with localized and sometimes multifocal lymph node involvement in otherwise healthy individuals.

Microscopy
There is overall retention of nodal architecture. The lymphoid proliferation is characterized by medium-sized to large lymphoid cells resembling plasmablasts that involve or replace germinal centres. In some nodes, there may be atrophic follicles resembling those seen in multicentric Castleman disease.

Immunophenotype
Plasmablastic cells are negative for CD20, CD79a, CD138, BCL6, and CD10, and negative or positive for CD30. Occasional cases may co-express CD3 in the absence of other T-cell markers {1404A}. They may be positive for IRF4/MUM1 and may show monotypic kappa or lambda light chain, unlike the cells in multicentric Castleman disease, which are always lambda-positive. In some cases, immunoglobulin expression cannot be demonstrated. They are positive for HHV8 LANA1 and EBER. Cases are negative for the EBV latency proteins LMP-1, EBNA2, and BZLF-1 indicating latency 1 {366A}.

Postulated normal counterpart
A germinal centre B cell {1047}

Genetic profile
Despite the constant expression of monotypic immunoglobulin, HHV8-positive GLPD has a polyclonal or oligoclonal pattern of IG gene rearrangements. There may be somatic mutation and intraclonal variation in the rearranged IG genes {1047}.

Prognosis and predictive factors
In most cases, there is a favourable response to chemotherapy or radiation {1047}. However, there are rare cases with features of both GLPD and HHV8-positive diffuse large B-cell lymphoma, NOS; one reported case in an HIV-negative patient progressed from GLPD to HHV8-positive EBV-positive diffuse large B-cell lymphoma, NOS, suggesting that there can be overlap between these conditions {826,3616,1404A}.

Burkitt lymphoma

Leoncini L.
Campo E.
Stein H.
Harris N.L.
Jaffe E.S.
Kluin P.M.

Definition

Burkitt lymphoma (BL) is a highly aggressive but curable lymphoma that often presents in extranodal sites or as an acute leukaemia. It is composed of monomorphic medium-sized B cells with basophilic cytoplasm and numerous mitotic figures, usually with a demonstrable *MYC* gene translocation to an IG locus. The frequency of EBV infection varies according to the epidemiological subtype of BL. No single parameter, such as morphology, genetic analysis, or immunophenotyping, can be used as the gold standard for diagnosis of BL; a combination of several diagnostic techniques is necessary.

ICD-O code   9687/3

Synonyms

Burkitt tumour (obsolete); malignant lymphoma, undifferentiated, Burkitt type (obsolete); malignant lymphoma, small noncleaved, Burkitt type (obsolete); Burkitt cell leukaemia (9826/3)

Epidemiology

Three epidemiological variants of BL are recognized, which mainly differ in their geographical distribution, clinical presentation, subtle morphological aspects, molecular genetics, and biological features.

Endemic BL occurs in equatorial Africa and in Papua New Guinea, with a distribution that overlaps with regions endemic for malaria. In these areas, BL is the most common childhood malignancy, with an incidence peak among children aged 4–7 years and a male-to-female ratio of 2:1 {503,4369}.

Sporadic BL is seen throughout the world, mainly in children and young adults. The incidence is low, accounting for only 1–2% of all lymphomas in western Europe and in the USA. In these countries, BL accounts for approximately 30–50% of all childhood lymphomas. The median age of the adult patients is 30 years, but there is also an incidence peak in elderly patients {2590}. The male-to-female ratio is 2–3:1. In some parts of the world (e.g.

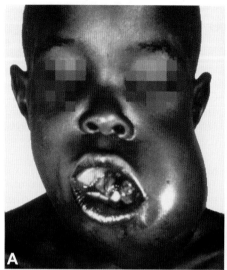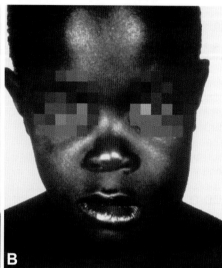

Fig. 13.154 Endemic Burkitt lymphoma. **A** This patient from the malaria belt region in Uganda presented with a large jaw tumour. **B** The mass underwent rapid shrinkage with subsequent complete remission after treatment with high dose cyclophosphamide therapy.

South America and northern Africa), the incidence of BL is intermediate between that of sporadic BL in developed countries and endemic BL {2441,3258}.

Immunodeficiency-associated BL is more common in the setting of HIV infection than in other forms of immunosuppression. In HIV-infected patients, BL appears early in the progression of the disease, when CD4+ T-cell counts are still high {2332,3309}. The increased risk of developing BL seems to have persisted among HIV-infected patients over time, across the pre- and post-HAART eras {1370}.

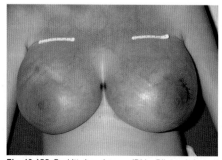

Fig. 13.155 Burkitt lymphoma (BL). Bilateral breast involvement may be the presenting manifestation during pregnancy and puberty. BL cells have prolactin receptors.

Etiology

In all patients with endemic BL, the EBV genome is present in >95% of the neoplastic cells. There is also a strong epidemiological link with holoendemic malaria. Therefore, EBV and *Plasmodium falciparum* are thought to be responsible for endemic BL {915,1870}. Recent data have provided new insight into how these two human pathogens interact to cause the disease, supporting the emerging concepts of polymicrobial disease pathogenesis {688,2692,2937,3285,3368}. Malaria and EBV are ubiquitous within the lymphoma belt of Africa, suggesting that other etiological agents may also be involved, including arboviruses, schistosomiasis, and plant tumour promoters {4121,4122,2486}. A recent study using RNA sequencing found herpesviruses in 12 of 20 cases (60%) of endemic BL, in particular HHV5 and HHV8, and confirmed their presence by immunohistochemistry in the adjacent non-neoplastic tissue {8}. The polymicrobial nature of endemic BL is further supported by the status of B-cell receptor, which carries the signs of antigen selection due to chronic antigen stimulation {84,3171}.

In sporadic BL, EBV can be detected in

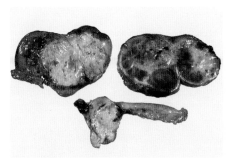

Fig. 13.156 Sporadic Burkitt lymphoma with bilateral ovarian tumours.

approximately 20 30% of cases; however, low socioeconomic status and early EBV infection are associated with a higher prevalence of EBV-positive cases {2441}. The proportion of EBV-positive sporadic BL appears to be much higher in adults than in children {3531}. In immunodeficiency-associated cases, EBV is identified in only 25–40% of cases {1531,3396}. The variation in EBV association among the different forms of BL and among different countries makes it difficult to determine the role of the virus in BL pathogenesis. EBV may impact host cell homeostasis in various ways by encoding its own genes

and microRNAs and by interfering with cellular microRNA expression {85,1982, 2283,3173,4181}. However, recent studies have shown that the mutation landscape and viral landscape of BL is more complex than previously reported. In fact, a distinct latency pattern of EBV involving the expression of LMP2 along with that of lytic genes has been demonstrated {8, 158,4003}. These results confirm recent evidence that LMP2A cooperates in reprogramming normal B-lymphocyte function and increases *MYC*-driven lymphomagenesis through activation of the PI3K pathway, crucial cooperating mechanisms of *MYC* transformation {1008,1221, 3509}. However, expression of the latency pattern in BL is heterogeneous, not only from case to case, but also within a given case from cell to cell, suggesting that the tumour is under selective pressure and needs alternative mechanisms to survive and proliferate.

Localization

Extranodal sites are most often involved, with some variation among the epidemiological variants. However, in all three

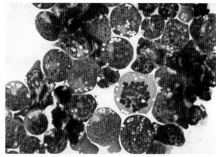

Fig. 13.157 Burkitt lymphoma. Touch imprint. The deeply basophilic cytoplasm can be appreciated, as can abundant lipid vacuoles in the cytoplasm.

variants, patients are at risk for CNS involvement. In endemic BL, the jaws and other facial bones (e.g. the orbit bones) are the site of presentation in about 50–70% of cases. The distal ileum, caecum, omentum, gonads, kidneys, long bones, thyroid, salivary glands, and breasts are frequently involved. Bone marrow involvement may be present, but may not be associated with leukaemic expression {503,2912}. In sporadic BL, tumours in facial structures, in particular the jaws, are very rare. Most cases present with abdominal masses. The ileocaecal region

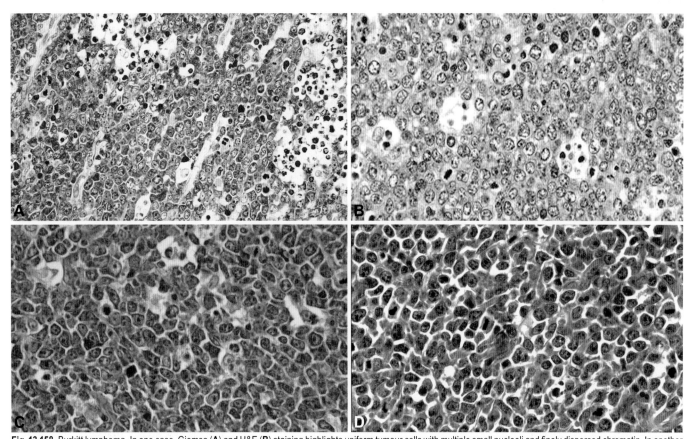

Fig. 13.158 Burkitt lymphoma. In one case, Giemsa (**A**) and H&E (**B**) staining highlights uniform tumour cells with multiple small nucleoli and finely dispersed chromatin. In another case, Giemsa (**C**) and H&E (**D**) staining highlights greater nuclear irregularity.

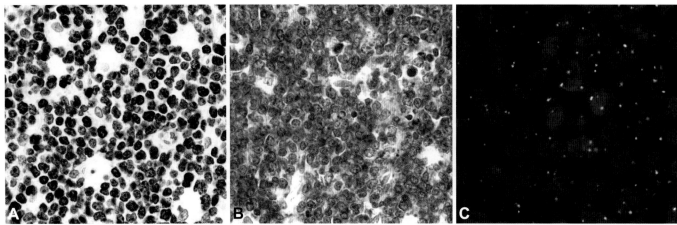

Fig. 13.159 Burkitt lymphoma. Immunohistochemistry shows strong and homogeneous positivity for Ki-67 by MIB1 antibody staining (**A**) and for CD10 (**B**). Break-apart FISH for *MYC* (**C**) shows one allele with colocalization of both probes (red and green) and one allele with separation of the probes. From: Haralambieva E, et al. {1550}.

is the most frequent site of involvement. Like in endemic BL, the ovaries, kidneys, and breasts may also be involved {4369}. Breast involvement, often bilateral and massive, has been associated with onset during puberty, pregnancy, or lactation. Retroperitoneal masses may result in spinal cord compression with paraplegia. Lymph node presentation is unusual, but more common in adults than in children. Waldeyer ring or mediastinal involvement is rare. In immunodeficiency-associated BL, nodal localization and bone marrow involvement are frequent {3396}.

Clinical features

Patients often present with bulky disease and high tumour burden due to the short doubling time of the tumour. In the typical paediatric cases, the parents of affected children usually report symptoms of only a few weeks' duration. Specific clinical manifestations at presentation may vary according to the epidemiological subtype and the site of involvement.
Paediatric BL cases are staged according to the system proposed by Murphy and Hustu {2793}. A revised international paediatric non-Hodgkin lymphoma staging system has been recently proposed {3417}. Localized-stage (I or II) disease and advanced-stage (III or IV) disease are found in approximately 30% and 70% of patients, respectively, at presentation. Upon initiation of therapy, a tumour lysis syndrome can occur due to rapid tumour cell death.

Burkitt leukaemia variant
A leukaemic phase can be observed in patients with bulky disease, but only rare cases, typically in males, present purely

as leukaemia with peripheral blood and bone marrow involvement {2443,2444, 3741}. Burkitt leukaemia tends to involve the CNS at diagnosis or early in the disease course. Its high and immediate chemosensitivity easily leads to an acute tumour lysis syndrome. Involvement of the bone marrow or presentation as acute leukaemia is uncommon in endemic BL {2442}.

Macroscopy

Involved organs are replaced by masses with a fish-flesh appearance, often associated with haemorrhage and necrosis. Adjacent organs or tissues are compressed and/or infiltrated. Nodal involvement is rare in endemic and sporadic BL, but more frequent in immunodeficiency-associated BL. Even when nodal involvement is not present, uninvolved lymph nodes may be surrounded by tumour.

Microscopy

The prototype of BL is observed in endemic BL, in a high proportion of sporadic BL cases, in particular in children, and in many cases of immunodeficiency-related BL. The tumour cells are medium-sized and show a diffuse monotonous pattern of growth. The cells appear to be cohesive but often exhibit squared-off borders of retracted cytoplasm in formalin-fixed material. The nuclei are round, with finely clumped chromatin, and contain multiple basophilic medium-sized, paracentrally located nucleoli. The cytoplasm is deeply basophilic and usually contains lipid vacuoles, which are better seen in imprint preparations or fine-needle aspiration cytology. The tumour has an extremely high proliferation rate, with

many mitotic figures, as well as a high rate of spontaneous cell death (apoptosis). A so-called starry sky pattern is usually present, which is due to the presence of numerous tingible body macrophages. Some cases have a florid granulomatous reaction that may cause difficulties in the recognition of the tumour. These cases typically present with limited stage disease and have an especially good prognosis {1549,1666}.
Some cases of BL may show greater nuclear pleomorphism despite clinical, immunophenotypic, and molecular features characteristics of typical BL. In such cases, the nucleoli may be more prominent and fewer in number. In other cases, particularly in adults with immunodeficiency, the tumour cells exhibit plasmacytoid differentiation, with eccentric basophilic cytoplasm and often a single central nucleolus {3396}. These morphological features are consistent with gene expression profile studies suggesting that the morphological spectrum of BL is broader than previously thought {1732}.

Immunophenotype

The tumour cells typically express moderate to strong membrane IgM with light chain restriction, B-cell antigens (CD19, CD20, CD22, CD79a, and PAX5), and germinal centre markers (CD10 and BCL6). CD38, CD77, and CD43 are also frequently positive {280,2190,2826}. Almost all BLs have strong expression of MYC protein in most cells {3902}. The proliferation rate is very high, with nearly 100% of the cells positive for Ki-67. The characteristic cytoplasmic lipid vesicles can also be demonstrated by immunohistochemistry on paraffin-embedded tissue

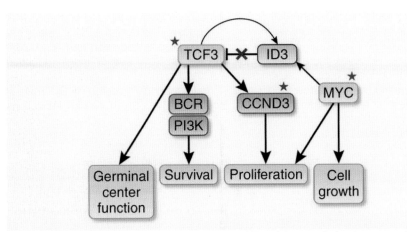

Fig. 13.160 Burkitt lymphoma (BL), molecular pathogenesis. TCF3 modulates germinal centre genes and is preferentially expressed in the highly proliferative area of this structure, recognized histologically as the dark zone (DZ). TCF3 also regulates survival and proliferation of lymphoid cells through the BCR and PI3K signalling pathway and by modulating cell cycle regulators such as CCND3. TCF3 also induces its own inhibitor, ID3, creating an autoregulatory loop that may attenuate this programme and facilitate the transition of the germinal centre cells to the light zone (LZ). MYC is not normally expressed in cells of the DZ and is upregulated in the LZ. Its induction of ID3 may contribute to the attenuation of the TCF3 pathway in the normal germinal centre. Burkitt lymphoma frequently harbours mutations in *ID3*, *TCF3* and *CCND3* that activate the TCF3 pathway. The t(8;14) translocation present in BL dysregulates MYC. Cooperation of these two pathways plays a crucial role in BL, in which virtually all cells are proliferating. From Campo E {540A}.

sections using a monoclonal antibody against adipophilin {86}. There are very few infiltrating T cells. TCL1 is strongly expressed in most paediatric BLs {321, 3385}. The neoplastic cells are usually negative for CD5, CD23, CD138, BCL2, and TdT. The immunophenotype may be more variable in sporadic BLs in older patients {280}. Aberrant phenotypes, such as CD5 expression, lack of CD10, or weak BCL2 expression in a variable number of cells, have been described in these cases {1547,2339,2543}. However, high BCL2 expression should suggest the presence of an additional *BCL2* breakpoint consistent with high-grade B-cell lymphoma with *MYC* and *BCL2* and/or *BCL6* rearrangements. Several scoring systems have been proposed to facilitate the differential diagnosis between BL and similar lymphomas {1547,2826}.

Unlike in B-lymphoblastic leukaemia, the blasts of Burkitt leukaemia have a phenotype similar to that of typical BL. However, approximately 2% of otherwise classic paediatric Burkitt leukaemias with a t(8;14)(q24;q32) or variant translocation involving *MYC* have a phenotype of precursor B cells, with expression of TdT and sometimes CD34, and absence of CD20 and surface immunoglobulin expression {2844}. The reason for this aberrant phenotype is unknown.

Postulated normal counterpart

A germinal centre B cell

Genetic profile

Antigen receptor genes

The tumour cells show clonal IG rearrangements with somatic hypermutation and intraclonal diversity {84}.

Cytogenetic abnormalities

The molecular hallmark of BL is the translocation of *MYC* at band 8q24.2 to the IGH region on chromosome 14q32, t(8;14)(q24;q32), or less commonly to the IGK locus on 2p12 [t(2;8)] or the IGL locus on 22q11 [t(8;22)]. Most breakpoints originate from aberrant somatic hypermutation mediated by the activity of activation-induced cytidine deaminase, in contrast to the previous assumption that they derived from aberrant VDJ gene recombination, and the translocation primarily involves the switch regions of the IGH locus. In sporadic and immunodeficiency-associated BL, most breakpoints are nearby or within *MYC*, whereas in endemic cases most breakpoints are dispersed over several hundred kilobases further upstream of the gene {2093}. *MYC* translocations are not specific for BL, and may occur in other types of lymphoma. Additional chromosomal abnormalities may also occur in BL, including gains of 1q, 7, and 12 and losses of 6q, 13q32-34, and 17p, that may play a role in the progression of the disease {195, 2507,3579,4036}.

Approximately, 10% of classic BL cases lack an identifiable *MYC* rearrangement {1550,1732,1827,2282}. However, none of the techniques currently used to diagnose genetic changes can unambiguously rule out all *MYC* translocations {1827}, in particular due to very distant breakpoints or insertions of the *MYC* gene in an IG locus or vice versa. The expression of MYC mRNA and protein in these cases suggests that there are also alternative mechanisms deregulating MYC {2282,2979,3579}. In these cases, strict clinical, morphological, and phenotypic criteria should be used to exclude lymphomas that can mimic BL. At least some of these cases constitute the new provisional entity Burkitt-like lymphoma with 11q aberration.

Gene expression profile

Gene and microRNA expression profiling can identify molecular signatures that are characteristic of BL and different from those of other lymphomas (e.g. diffuse large B-cell lymphoma) {877,1732,2275, 3171}. Slight differences in the expression profiles have been identified between the endemic and sporadic BL subtypes {2275,3171}. In addition, molecularly defined BLs do include some cases that are best not diagnosed as BL, and some cases of BL may have a gene expression profile intermediate between those of BL and diffuse large B-cell lymphoma.

Next-generation sequencing

Next-generation sequencing analysis has revealed the importance of the B-cell receptor signalling pathway in the pathogenesis of BL. Mutations of the transcription factor *TCF3* (also known as *E2A*) or its negative regulator *ID3* have been reported in about 70% of sporadic BL cases. These mutations activate B-cell receptor signalling, which sustains BL cell survival by engaging the PI3K pathway {2401,3354,3509,3573}. Other recurrent mutations, in *CCND3*, *TP53*, *RHOA*, *SMARCA4*, and *ARID1A*, occur in 5–40% of BLs {1381,2112,2401,3354,4225}. Both the number of mutations overall and the proportion of cases with mutations in *TCF3* or *ID3* are lower in endemic than sporadic BL {8,3573}. An inverse correlation between EBV infection and the number of mutations has been observed, suggesting that these mutations may serve in place of the virus for the activation of the B-cell receptor signalling {8,1381}.

Genetic susceptibility

Individuals with X-linked lymphoproliferative syndrome (also known as 'Duncan disease') associated with *SH2D1A* mutations are at greatly increased risk of developing BL.

Prognosis and predictive factors

BL is a highly aggressive but potentially curable tumour; intensive chemotherapy leads to long-term overall survival in 70–90% of cases, with children doing better than adults. However, there are several adverse prognostic factors: advanced-stage disease, bone marrow and CNS involvement, unresected tumour > 10 cm in diameter, and high serum lactate dehydrogenase levels. Relapse, if it occurs, is usually seen within the first year after diagnosis. The overall survival rate in endemic BL has improved from < 10–20% to almost 70% due to the introduction of the International Network for Cancer Treatment and Research (INCTR) protocol INCTR 03-06 in African institutions {2861}.

Burkitt-like lymphoma with 11q aberration

Leoncini L.
Campo E.
Stein H.
Harris N.L.

Jaffe E.S.
Kluin P.M.

Definition

Burkitt-like lymphoma with 11q aberration is a subset of lymphomas identified by several recent studies that resemble Burkitt lymphoma (BL) morphologically, to a large extent phenotypically, and in terms of microRNAs and gene expression profile, but that lack *MYC* rearrangements. Instead, they have a chromosome 11q alteration characterized by proximal gains and telomeric losses: specifically, interstitial gains including a minimal region of gain in 11q23.2-23.3 and losses of 11q24.1-ter {195,3175,3490}. These lymphomas lack the 1q gain frequently seen in BL and have more-complex karyotypes than BL. They also have a certain degree of cytological pleomorphism, occasionally a follicular pattern, and frequently a nodal presentation {3490,4454}. The clinical course seems to be similar to that of BL, but only a limited number of cases have been reported. Very similar cases have also been reported in the post-transplant setting {1191}.

ICD-O code   9687/3

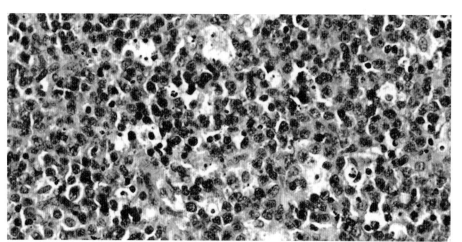

Fig. 13.161 Burkitt-like lymphoma with 11q aberration. The tumour cells are medium-sized to large, with a high mitotic index. A starry-sky pattern is usually seen.

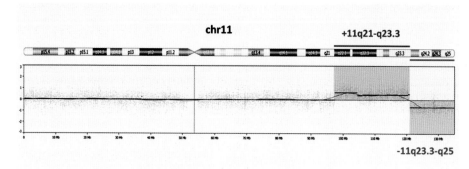

Fig. 13.162 Burkitt-like lymphoma with 11q aberration. Chromosomal view of chromosome 11 analysed by OncoScan array, depicting gains of 11q21-23.3 in blue and terminal losses of 11q23.3-25 in red.

High-grade B-cell lymphoma

Kluin P.M.
Harris N.L.
Stein H.
Leoncini L.

Campo E.
Jaffe E.S.
Gascoyne R.D.
Swerdlow S.H.

Definition

High-grade B-cell lymphoma (HGBL) is a group of aggressive, mature B-cell lymphomas that for biological and clinical reasons should not be classified as diffuse large B-cell lymphoma (DLBCL), NOS, or as Burkitt lymphoma (BL). There are two categories of HGBL {1547,3846}. The first category, HGBL with *MYC* and *BCL2* and/or *BCL6* rearrangements, encompasses all B-cell lymphomas (except some rare follicular lymphomas and B-lymphoblastic leukaemia/lymphomas) that have a *MYC* (8q24.2) rearrangement in combination with a *BCL2* (18q21.3) and/or a *BCL6* (3q27.3) rearrangement, i.e. the so-called double-hit and triple-hit lymphomas. Morphologically, these cases typically either resemble DLBCL, NOS, or can have features of both BL and DLBCL (referred to in the 2008 WHO classification as B-cell lymphoma, unclassifiable, with features intermediate between DLBCL and BL). Less commonly, they have a blastoid appearance, morphologically mimicking lymphoblastic lymphoma or the blastoid variant of mantle cell lymphoma.

The second category, HGBL, NOS, encompasses cases that either have features intermediate between DLBCL and BL or appear blastoid, but by definition do not harbour a genetic double hit as defined above. This category excludes cases with the morphology of DLBCL, which should be diagnosed as such, even if they have a high proliferative fraction.

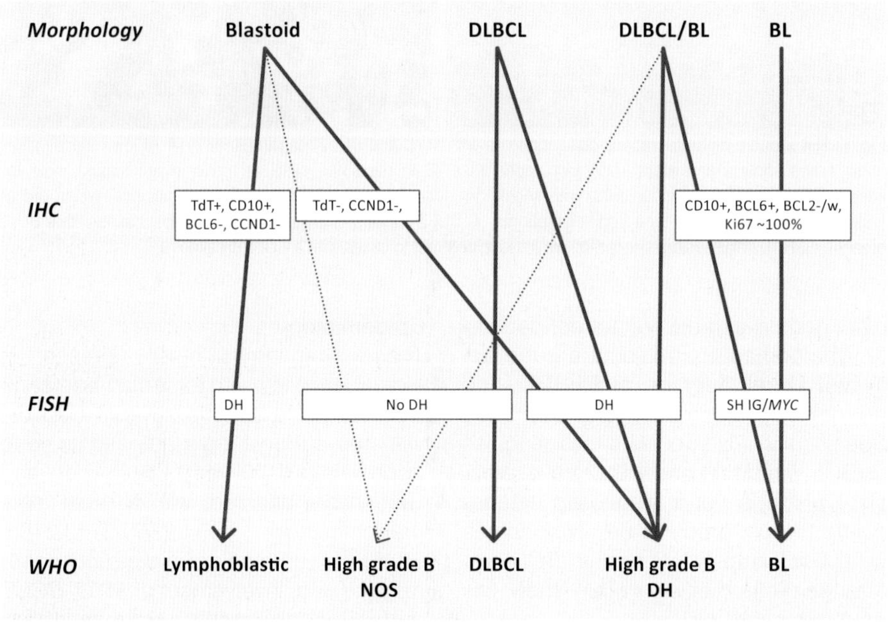

Synonym

B-cell lymphoma, unclassifiable, with features intermediate between diffuse large B-cell lymphoma and Burkitt lymphoma (no longer recommended)

High-grade B-cell lymphoma with MYC and BCL2 and/or BCL6 rearrangements

Definition

High-grade B-cell lymphoma (HGBL) with *MYC* and *BCL2* and/or *BCL6* rearrangements is an aggressive mature B-cell lymphoma that harbours a *MYC* rearrangement at chromosome 8q24.2 and a rearrangement in *BCL2* (at chromosome 18q21.3) and/or in *BCL6* (at chromosome 3q27.3). These lymphomas are often called double-hit lymphomas, or triple-hit lymphomas if there are both *BCL2* and *BCL6* rearrangements in addition to the *MYC* rearrangement. The term "double-hit" as defined for this category refers only to the co-occurrence of *MYC* and *BCL2* and/or *BCL6* translocations. Lymphomas with two oncogenic translocations other than *MYC* (e.g. concomitant *BCL2* and *BCL6* translocations without a *MYC* breakpoint) or other gene translocations associated with *MYC* translocations (e.g. *CCND1* translocations) are not included in this category.

Fig. 13.163 Diagnostic algorithm useful in the differential diagnosis of the high-grade B-cell lymphomas. This scheme is intended to help pathologists classify many of the aggressive B-cell lymphomas, using the morphology seen on an H&E-stained slide as the starting point. The various morphologies are listed in the top row. "Blastoid" morphology means that the case looks like a lymphoblastic lymphoma; this term is also used for some aggressive variants of mantle cell lymphoma. "DLBCL" morphology means that the case is a B-cell lymphoma with the morphological features of a diffuse large B-cell lymphoma (DLBCL), NOS. "DLBCL/ BL" morphology means that the case has morphological features of both DLBCL and Burkitt lymphoma (BL), with a relatively monotonous appearance with or without a starry-sky pattern; in the 2008 edition of the WHO classification, such cases were designated as B-cell lymphoma, unclassifiable, with features intermediate between DLBCL and BL. Please note that while some cases of BL have a somewhat atypical morphological appearance that might suggest DLBCL/BL, finding a typical Burkitt lymphoma phenotype (CD10+, BCL2-) and an isolated IGH/MYC translocation cannot be used by themselves to make a definitive diagnosis of BL in a case with a DLBCL/BL morphologic appearance if the morphologic or other features are considered to be too atypical. The current WHO diagnostic categories are listed in the bottom row; differential diagnoses not included in this chapter are not shown. Only the minimum immunohistochemical (IHC) and molecular requirements are shown. Prognostic tests are not included.

DH, double hit (i.e. rearrangement of *MYC* and *BCL2* and/or *BCL6*); FISH, FISH or a comparable method; FL, follicular lymphoma; High grade B, high-grade B-cell lymphoma; Lymphoblastic, proven B-lymphoblastic leukaemia/lymphoma, de novo or progressed from an antecedent or synchronously diagnosed FL; SH IG/MYC, single hit with IG/MYC translocation but no translocations involving *BCL2*, *BCL6*, or *CCND1*. As discussed in the section on Burkitt lymphoma, some cases of molecular BL, in particular post-transplant BL, lack a *MYC* rearrangement but have specific 11q abnormalities. These cases are best considered to be a Burkitt-like lymphoma with 11q aberration.

Except for proven follicular lymphoma and rare cases of B-lymphoblastic leukaemia/lymphoma, NOS, all other lymphomas and leukaemias with these molecular features should be included in this category. The category therefore includes (1) double-hit cases previously classified as B-cell lymphoma, unclassifiable, with features intermediate between diffuse large B-cell lymphoma (DLBCL) and Burkitt lymphoma (BL); (2) blastoid cases with a double hit; and (3) cases with a DLBCL, NOS, morphology that upon evaluation have rearrangements of MYC and BCL2 and/or BCL6. Grade 3B follicular lymphomas with a double hit that are completely follicular should still be diagnosed as follicular lymphoma, with a comment indicating the cytogenetic findings; however, if there is an associated DLBCL with a double hit, the diagnosis of a follicular lymphoma and HGBL with MYC and BCL2 and/or BCL6 rearrangements should be rendered. Given the possibility of prognostic implications, the morphological appearance of the HGBL with MYC and BCL2 and/or BCL6 rearrangements should be noted in a diagnostic comment.

Rare cases of B-lymphoblastic leukaemia/lymphoma with MYC and BCL2 translocations, sometimes transformed from an antecedent or synchronous follicular lymphoma, are not included in this category, and should be classified as B-lymphoblastic leukaemia/lymphoma with the translocations specified in a comment. Patients with such findings are usually treated like patients with lymphoblastic leukaemia {896,1349,2061,2121,4446}.

Rearrangements of MYC, BCL2, and BCL6 should be detected by a cytogenetic/molecular method such as FISH. The presence of only copy-number increase/amplification or somatic mutations, without an underlying rearrangement, is insufficient to qualify a case for this category. There are indications that such cases are also aggressive, similar to the double-hit lymphomas, but there are insufficient data to justify the inclusion of such cases in this category.

Although so-called double-expresser DLBCLs that show immunohistochemical overexpression of MYC and BCL2 protein also have a relatively poor prognosis, overexpression cannot be used as a surrogate marker for double-hit cytogenetic status. Most double-hit lymphomas are also double-expressers, but

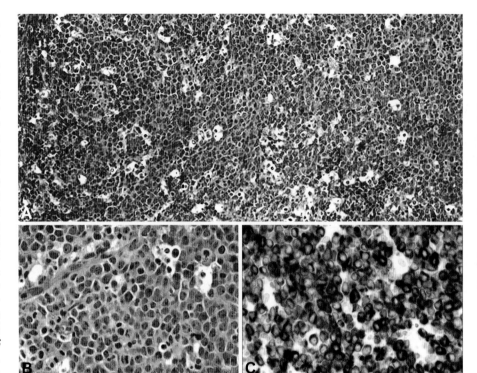

Fig. 13.164 Double-hit high-grade B-cell lymphoma with MYC and BCL2 rearrangements. **A** At low magnification, many cases show a prominent starry-sky appearance. **B** In the same case, at higher magnification, note the intermediate size of the tumour cells, with slightly irregular contours and relatively large nucleoli, which are all features somewhat atypical for a Burkitt lymphoma. **C** BCL2 staining of the same case. In most cases with a BCL2 breakpoint, BCL2 expression is very high, which is in contrast to cases with a BCL6 breakpoint.

most double-expressers are not double-hit lymphomas; the majority are the activated B-cell subtype of DLBCL, and do not harbour translocations {3846}. Specifically, it is important to distinguish DLBCL with MYC and BCL2 co-expression, which is not a diagnostic category, from high grade B-cell lymphomas with MYC and BCL2 and/or BCL6 rearrangements that also often show this double-expression

This classification is primarily applicable to de novo cases; lymphomas with a proven history of a pre-existing or co-existent indolent lymphoma (of follicular or other type) should be diagnosed as such (e.g. HGBL with MYC and BCL2 rearrangements, transformed from follicular lymphoma).

ICD-O code   9680/3

Synonyms

(Subset of) B-cell lymphoma, unclassifiable, with features intermediate between diffuse large B-cell lymphoma and Burkitt lymphoma (no longer recommended); (subset of) diffuse large B-cell lymphoma; double or triple-hit lymphoma

Epidemiology

These lymphomas mostly present in elderly patients, with a median age at diagnosis in the sixth to seventh decade; with the youngest reported patients aged approximately 30 years. Both men and women are affected, with a slight male predominance {194,2350,3143,3183, 3846}. In one study of triple-hit lymphomas (i.e. with involvement of MYC, BCL2, and BCL6), all patients were men {4254}.

Etiology

By definition, these mature B-cell lymphomas harbour two or more recurrent cytogenetic events, and in almost all cases, classic cytogenetic analysis also shows many additional abnormalities (complex karyotype). It is likely that the rearrangement of MYC is a secondary event, but this has only been proven for the combination of BCL2 and MYC rearrangements in patients who first had a follicular lymphoma and later developed a MYC rearrangement, and in patients with de novo disease in which two subclones with and without the MYC rearrangement are present. Although it might be envisaged that all lymphomas with both *MYC* and *BCL2* rearrangements are the result of transformation from an antecedent indolent lymphoma, this is found in only half of the cases.

Localization

More than half of all patients present with widespread disease, including involvement of the lymph nodes. There can also be involvement of more than one extranodal site (occurring in 30–88% of cases), the bone marrow (in 59–94%), and even the CNS (in as many as 45%) {2350, 3158,3523}.

Clinical features

Most patients (70–100%) present with advanced disease (stage IV according to the Ann Arbor classification), more than one extranodal localization, a high International Prognostic Index (IPI), and elevated lactate dehydrogenase levels {2350,3158,3523,3846}. Extranodal localizations include the bone marrow and CNS. Double-hit HGBLs are particularly enriched in patients diagnosed with DLBCL who do not respond well to induction therapy with the CHOP chemotherapy regimen plus rituximab (R-CHOP) or who have early relapses after complete remission {843}.

Microscopy

Double-hit HGBLs have variable morphology. The specific morphological appearance should be stated in a diagnostic comment. Although the incidence differs between studies, most authors conclude that approximately half of the cases have the morphology of a DLBCL, NOS {193, 194,1820,1865,2304,3158,3523,3712}. This is due to the fact that DLBCL is by far the most frequent lymphoma subtype, and approximately 4–8% of all DLBCLs are double-hit lymphomas. In a recent study, 69% of the *MYC* and *BCL2* double-hit lymphomas and 85% of the *MYC* and *BCL6* double-hit lymphomas had DLBCL morphology {2304}. The differences between individual studies may be due to referral bias, inclusion bias, and the variable morphological criteria {2720A,3712}. The growth pattern is completely diffuse, often with relatively few small lymphocytes. Some fibrosis may be present. Starry-sky macrophages may be present, sometimes only focally. The numbers of mitotic figures and apoptotic figures are highly variable, with some cases having a low number of mitotic figures and also a low Ki-67 pro-

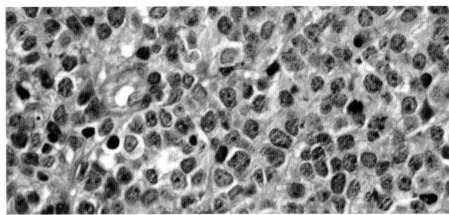

Fig. 13.165 Triple-hit high-grade B-cell lymphoma with *MYC*, *BCL2*, and *BCL6* rearrangements. This case shows the morphology of a diffuse large B-cell lymphoma, NOS, with large tumour cells with abundant cytoplasm, large nuclei, and prominent nucleoli.

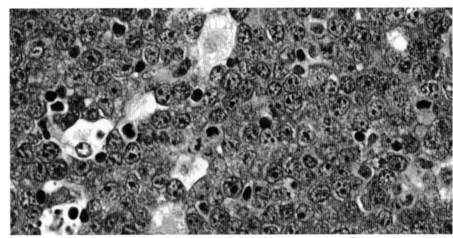

Fig. 13.166 Double-hit high-grade B-cell lymphoma with *MYC* and *BCL6* rearrangements. This case shows monomorphic tumour cells with indistinct cell borders, relatively large nuclei (somewhat larger than those of macrophages) and prominent, often single nucleoli.

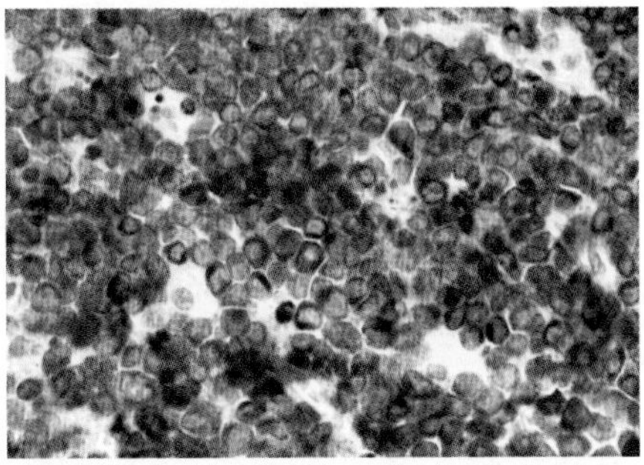

liferation index (see below). Therefore, a low proliferation rate does not exclude this type of lymphoma. The nuclei have a variable size and contour, with some cases showing nuclei that are 3–4 times the size of normal lymphocytes (much larger than BL cells). The cytoplasm is usually more abundant and less basophilic than in BL.

Because these lymphomas can be indistinguishable from other DLBCL, a double-hit status should be investigated in all DLBCLs, NOS, using cytogenetic or molecular cytogenetic studies. Some pathologists may prefer to look for evidence of a double-hit only after immunohistochemical or other pre-selection (see below).

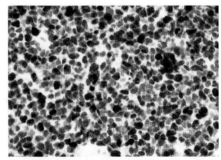

Fig. 13.167 Double-hit high-grade B-cell lymphoma with *MYC* and *BCL6* rearrangements. The intensity of BCL2 staining is variable in such cases, and can be negative.

Fig. 13.168 Double-hit high-grade B-cell lymphoma with *MYC* and *BCL2* rearrangements. The Ki-67 proliferation index is ~90%.

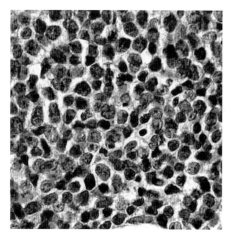

Fig. 13.169 Double-hit high-grade B-cell lymphoma with *MYC* and *BCL2* rearrangements, blastoid morphology. As is typical in blastoid cases, this patient had a history of follicular lymphoma. The lymphoma cells are monotonous and mimic lymphoblasts, with overlapping nuclei, finely dispersed chromatin, and inconspicuous nucleoli. However, in this case they are mature B cells with expression of CD20, CD10, and BCL2 but negative for BCL6. TdT was negative. The Ki-67 proliferation index was 70%.

Another subset (also accounting for ~50% of cases) shows a morphology that mimics that of BL, or has features intermediate between DLBCL and BL {193,194,3143, 3712,3846}. Approximately 50% of cases with this morphologic appearance have a double-hit status. They show a diffuse proliferation of medium-sized to large cells with very few admixed small lymphocytes and no stromal reaction or fibrosis. Starry-sky macrophages are generally present, along with many mitotic figures and prominent apoptosis. The cellular morphology varies. Some cases are relatively monomorphic, very closely resembling BL. Others exhibit more variation in nuclear size and nucleolar features than is gene-

rally seen in BL. The cytoplasm is usually less basophilic than in BL, a feature best appreciated on Giemsa-stained imprints. In most cases, cytoplasmic vacuoles are absent. In cases that closely mimic BL, the diagnosis of BL can be excluded on the basis of an aberrant clinical presentation, immunophenotype (typically strong BCL2 expression), and molecular genetic findings (see below).

Other cases may have a blastoid cytomorphology, with medium-sized cells often resembling small centroblasts. Nucleoli are inconspicuous. The chromatin has a finely granular texture. The cells have a small rim of cytoplasm. Thus, they closely mimic true lymphoblasts, and staining for TdT should be performed in all cases {1914,4097}. Because the blastoid variant of mantle cell lymphoma shares many of these features, cyclin D1 staining should also be performed. These tumour cells are CD10+ and BCL6+ mature B cells. In many of these cases, an antecedent or synchronous follicular lymphoma is present; such cases should be diagnosed as double-hit HGBL transformed from a follicular lymphoma.

Lymphomas with a similar blastoid or lymphoblastic morphology but a phenotype of precursor B cells with expression of nuclear TdT should not be included in this category.

Immunophenotype

These lymphomas are mature B-cell lymphomas with expression of CD19, CD20, CD79a, and PAX5 and lack of TdT. Some double-hit HGBL cases lack surface immunoglobulin expression as detected by flow cytometry, which may be related to the involvement of multiple IG loci

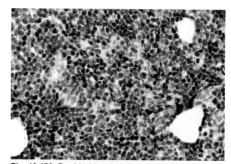

Fig. 13.170 Double-hit high-grade B-cell lymphoma with *MYC* and *BCL2* rearrangements. MYC staining (Y69 antibody). Patient with prior follicular lymphoma and progression to double-hit lymphoma with blastoid morphology (*MYC* and *BCL2* breakpoints, no IGH/*MYC* colocalization; IGK and IGL not tested).

by translocations {2101}. This absence should not be interpreted as proof of a precursor B-cell phenotype.

CD10 and BCL6 expression is found in most of these lymphomas (75–90%), and IRF4/MUM1 is expressed in approximately 20% of the cases {193,3846}. Almost all cases with a *BCL2* (18q21.3) breakpoint have strong cytoplasmic BCL2 positivity, in contrast to the absent or weak expression of BCL2 in BLs.

It has been suggested that immunostaining for CD10, BCL6, IRF4/MUM1, and BCL2 or gene expression analysis of paraffin-embedded materials could be used to select cases of DLBCL to be tested by *MYC* FISH {3117,3601,3846}. However, the less-frequent double-hit lymphomas with *MYC* (8q24.2) and *BCL6* (3q27.3) rearrangements without a concomitant *BCL2* (18q21.3) breakpoint variably express BCL2 and CD10 and express IRF4/MUM1 more commonly than do the other double-hit lymphomas {2304,3183,

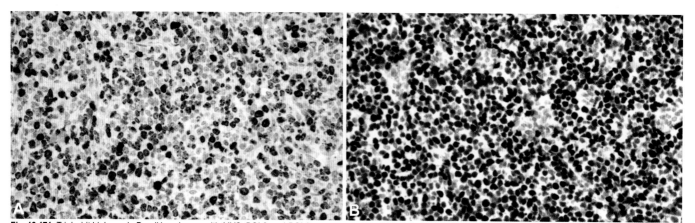

Fig. 13.171 Triple-hit high-grade B-cell lymphoma, with *MYC*, *BCL2*, and *BCL6* rearrangements. **A** Note the low and heterogeneous Ki-67 proliferation index of ~40%. This case illustrates that Ki-67 staining cannot be used for selecting diffuse large B-cell lymphoma cases for FISH analysis. **B** In the same case, homogeneous and strong p53 staining is highly suggestive of a *TP53* mutation.

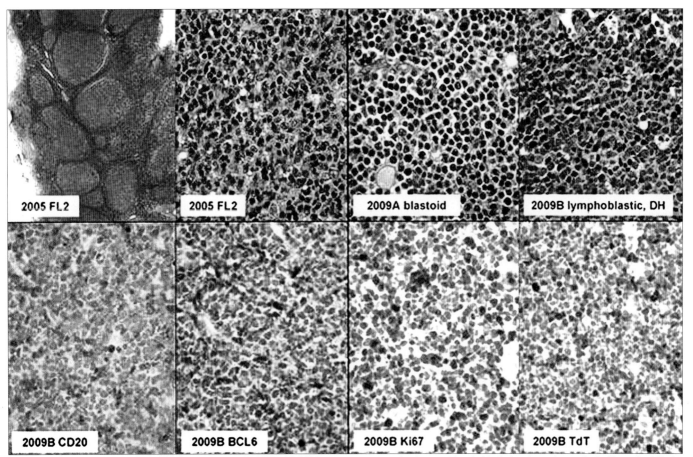

Fig. 13.172 Double-hit (DH) high-grade B-cell lymphoma with *MYC* and *BCL2* rearrangements and subsequent lymphoblastic lymphoma in a patient with a prior follicular lymphoma. A 66-year-old man presented with grade 2 follicular lymphoma (FL2) in 2005 and a histologically documented relapse in 2006. In 2009, he presented with an abdominal mass and extensive bone marrow involvement. The 2005 biopsies showed a classic phenotype: CD20+, CD10+, BCL6+, and BCL2+. The bone marrow biopsy in 2009 (2009A) showed a diffuse infiltration of blastoid cells. Immunohistochemistry revealed a persistent mature phenotype, with expression of CD20 and BCL6 and absence of TdT. The Ki-67 proliferation index was ~60%. Flow cytometry confirmed this phenotype and showed expression of surface IgG without detectable light chains. The simultaneously obtained needle biopsy of the para-iliac abdominal mass (2009B) showed a blastoid/lymphoblastic morphology, with loss of both CD20 and BCL6 expression, strong CD10 and BCL2 expression, a Ki-67 proliferation index of ~90%, and expression of TdT in ~30% of the cells. By FISH analysis, rearrangements of both *MYC* and *BCL2* were identified, the *MYC* rearrangement without colocalization of the IGH locus (IGK and IGL were not tested).

4077} and therefore could be missed by such a selection procedure.

Ki-67 immunohistochemistry shows variable results. In cases that mimic BL, the Ki-67 proliferation index is 80–95%. However, in cases with DLBCL morphology, the index may be deceptively low (<30%). Therefore, the Ki-67 proliferation index cannot be used to select cases for *MYC* FISH {2564,4113}.

Similarly, MYC protein expression cannot be used to select cases for FISH either. Although there is consensus that high expression (in >80% of nuclei) is present in most cases of BL with an IG/*MYC* translocation, there is much more variability in the double-hit lymphomas; most authors have concluded that MYC staining is not reliable enough to be used for the selection of cases that should have cytogenetic or molecular/cytogenetic testing {722,

1439,1440,1866,3143,4085}. Nevertheless, some authors suggest performing FISH studies only in cases with >30% or >40% MYC-positive tumour cells.

Postulated normal counterpart

The limited gene expression data available and the applied immunohistochemical algorithms suggest that almost all cases with *MYC* and *BCL2* rearrangements originate from mature germinal centre B cells, whereas the cell of origin for cases with *MYC* and *BCL6* rearrangements is more variable {802,3601}.

Genetic profile

By definition, these lymphomas have a *MYC* (8q24.2) rearrangement as detected by classic cytogenetics, FISH, or other molecular genetic tests. In approximately 65% of cases, *MYC* is juxtaposed

to one of the IG genes (usually IGH, less frequently IGK or IGL); in the other cases, *MYC* has a non-IG partner, such as at 9p13 (gene unknown), 3q27.3 (*BCL6*), or other loci {193,3118}. Some reports suggest that an IG/*MYC* translocation confers a poor outcome compared with cases in which *MYC* has a non-IG partner {193,802,1865,3118}, but the clinical impact of the individual non-IG partners is not fully established. Identification of an IGK/*MYC* or IGL translocation requires the use of dual fusion probes, because the identification of *MYC* and IGK or IGL rearrangements using only break-apart probes does not exclude the possibility of two separate unrelated translocations {802}.

In addition to *MYC* rearrangement, all cases contain a *BCL2* rearrangement at 18q21.3 and/or a *BCL6* rearrangement

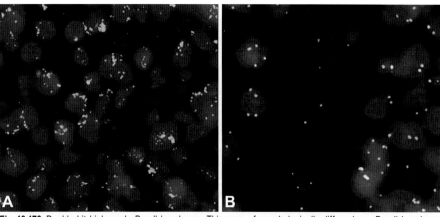

Fig. 13.173 Double-hit high-grade B-cell lymphoma. This case of morphologically diffuse large B-cell lymphoma had *MYC* and *BCL6* rearrangements as well as gain/amplification of *BCL2* at 18q21.3. **A** *BCL2* FISH. The local concentration of dual signals in the nuclei suggests amplification rather than gain by aneusomy. Note that isolated single-coloured signals are absent, indicating the absence of a rearrangement. **B** *BCL6* FISH. The same case shows *BCL6* in a break-apart assay, with two normal copies (with colocalization) and one separate green signal, strongly suggesting a rearrangement/breakpoint (see two cells in the upper left; in other cells, only isolated green signals are seen). This suggests loss of the telomeric part of chromosome 3q, with a break 5' of *BCL6*, likely within the alternative breakpoint region of the gene.

at 3q27.3. Other infrequent recurrent combinations with *MYC* rearrangement, such as rearrangement of *BCL3* at 19q13 and of an unknown gene at 9p13, are also recognized, but there have been no systematic studies of these lymphomas; therefore, such cases should not be included in this category {194}. Cases with a combination of *MYC* and *CCND1* (at 11q13) breakpoints constitute aggressive mantle cell lymphoma with the acquisition of a secondary *MYC* breakpoint and should not be included in this category either {734,933,1069,3628}.

Lymphomas can show a combination of a chromosomal rearrangement of one gene and copy-number increase or amplification of other genes, for example, a *MYC* (8q24.2) rearrangement with gain or amplification of *BCL2* (18q21.3) or vice versa. In the current classification, such a combination is not sufficient to classify a case as a double-hit HGBL. Notably, the definitions of amplification and copy-number increase differ across publications, and in some clinically oriented papers, these phenomena are lumped with rearrangements {2307, 2344}. High-level amplification at 8q24.2 may occur together with a rearrangement {2527}, and in combination with a *BCL2* rearrangement, it likely has a similar clinical impact as the classic double-hit configuration {4113}. In contrast, the biological and clinical impact of a small increase in copy number (mostly caused by aneusomy) in DLBCL is controver-

sial {2307,2404,4113}. Therefore, until more data are available, cases with only gains or amplification without a proven rearrangement should not be included in this category, but rather in the category of DLBCL or HGBL, NOS.

Double-hit HGBLs often have complex karyotypes, with many other structural and numerical abnormalities {193}. Sequencing studies reveal frequent *TP53* mutations (especially frequent in the *MYC* and *BCL2* double-hit cases {1314}) and few *MYD88* mutations {1315}. Whereas *TCF3* mutations and in particular homozygous mutations or deletion of its inhibitor, *ID3*, are frequent in BL, hemizygous mutations of *ID3* may be present in double-hit HGBL as well {193,1313,2401, 2693,3573}.

Prognosis and predictive factors

With R-CHOP or comparable therapies, the complete response rate is relatively low, and overall survival is short, with median survivals of 4.5–18.5 months {269, 1055,1865,2237,2304,2306,3712,4019, 4020}. Clinical trials are under way to test other polychemotherapy modalities and new drugs that may improve the outcome of these patients {778,1055,1709}. Several clinical and biological factors, including the tumour morphology, the *MYC* partner, and extent of the disease, may influence survival and warrant further studies {541}. A small subset of patients with no risk factors may have a favourable outcome {1865,3158}.

High-grade B-cell lymphoma, NOS

Definition

High-grade B-cell lymphoma (HGBL), NOS, is a heterogeneous category of clinically aggressive mature B-cell lymphomas that lack *MYC* plus *BCL2* and/or *BCL6* rearrangements and do not fall into the category of diffuse large B-cell lymphoma (DLBCL), NOS, or Burkitt lymphoma (BL). However, they do share some morphological, immunophenotypic, and genetic features with these lymphomas. These cases are rare; the diagnosis should be made sparingly, and only when the pathologist is truly unable to confidently classify a case as DLBCL or BL.

In the 2008 edition of the WHO classification, these cases were included in the category of B-cell lymphoma, unclassifiable, with features intermediate between DLBCL and BL {3848}, which also included cases now classified as HGBL with *MYC* and *BCL2* and/or *BCL6* rearrangements. Because the double-hit and triple-hit HGBLs have now been classified as a distinct category of their own, the category of HGBL, NOS, represents the remaining cases of the previous classification system. This category also includes cases of blastoid-appearing mature B-cell lymphomas (not of mantle cell type), which in the past might have

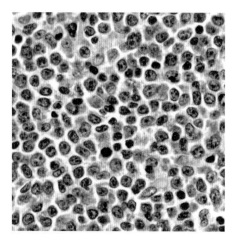

Fig. 13.174 High-grade B-cell lymphoma, NOS, with blastoid morphology. There was no antecedent or synchronous follicular lymphoma. The tumour cells have relatively small nuclei with a slightly irregular contour, containing small nucleoli and fine but not very dense chromatin. The tumour cells expressed CD20, BCL6, and BCL2 but were negative for CD5, cyclin D1, TdT, CD10, and IRF4/MUM1). The Ki-67 proliferation index was > 70%. FISH analysis revealed an IGH/*MYC* fusion without *BCL2* or *BCL6* rearrangement.

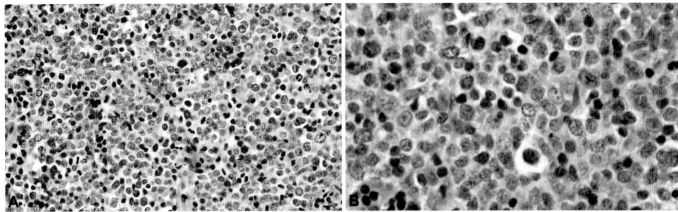

Fig. 13.175 High-grade B-cell lymphoma, NOS, with some features of Burkitt lymphoma. **A** The tumour cells show a squared-off cytoplasm, but no distinct starry-sky pattern. Immunohistochemistry showed expression of CD20, CD10, BCL6, and BCL2. The Ki-67 proliferation index showed a heterogeneous staining of ~50%. Strong and homogeneous p53 staining suggested *TP53* mutation. FISH analysis revealed a *BCL2* rearrangement but no rearrangements of *MYC* or *BCL6*. **B** Same case at higher magnification. Despite the impression at low magnification, the cytological appearance is blastoid: the nuclei show a finely granular chromatin pattern and absence of nucleoli.

been included among the DLBCLs. Cases of otherwise typical DLBCL, NOS, harbouring an isolated *MYC* translocation should still be classified as DLBCL, NOS. Some paediatric lymphomas also share features of both DLBCL and BL, and more than half of such cases harbour a *MYC* rearrangement in combination with a relatively simple karyotype. They often have a molecular Burkitt or intermediate gene expression profile and show an excellent prognosis. It is therefore recommended that these cases be classified as BL or DLBCL, and not as HGBL, NOS {2038}.

ICD-O code   9680/3

Epidemiology
Few epidemiological data are available for this category, because in most reports these lymphomas and the double-hit HGBLs with a similar morphology are described together. In general, elderly patients are affected, with incidence increasing with age. Men and women are affected almost equally.

Microscopy
Most cases have a morphology that mimics that of BL more closely than that of DLBCL. They show a diffuse proliferation of medium-sized to large cells with very few admixed small lymphocytes and no stromal reaction or fibrosis. Starry-sky macrophages may be present, along with many mitotic figures and prominent apoptosis. The cellular morphology varies. Some cases are relatively monomorphic, resembling BL; others exhibit more variation in nuclear size and nucleolar

features than is generally seen in BL. The cytoplasm is usually less basophilic than in BL, a feature best appreciated on Giemsa-stained sections or imprints. In most cases, cytoplasmic vacuoles are absent. In cases that closely mimic BL, the diagnosis of BL can be excluded on the basis of an aberrant clinical presentation, immunophenotype, and/or molecular genetic findings (see below).

Rare mature (CD20+ and TdT−) B-cell lymphomas with a blastoid appearance that do not constitute a blastoid variant of mantle cell lymphoma and that lack a double hit (*MYC* rearrangement in combination with *BCL2* and/or *BCL6* rearrangement) are also included in this category.

Immunophenotype
The immunophenotype is not well described, due to the heterogeneous nature of these lymphomas and the fact that most cases were previously included in reports that also included cases with double or triple translocations, or were classified as DLBCL. All cases are CD20-positive, mature B-cell lymphomas. Most show expression of BCL6, but CD10 expression is variable. In most cases, expression of IRF4/MUM1 is absent. Ki-67 positivity is also variable. MYC expression is variable, partially dependent on the presence of a *MYC* rearrangement.

Genetic profile
Molecular/cytogenetic data have been systematically analysed in few studies. By definition, the presence of a *BCL2* and/or a *BCL6* rearrangement in combination with a *MYC* rearrangement should be excluded. Approximately 20–35% of cases

have a *MYC* rearrangement, with or without increased copy numbers or, rarely, amplification of 18q21.3 involving *BCL2*. Cases with a *BCL2* rearrangement and increased copy number or high-level amplification of *MYC* have also been identified {2307,2344,3143}. Among the so-called blastoid cases, 40% of 24 cases studied lacked rearrangements in both *MYC* and *BCL2* {1914,4097}; in another study, none of the 8 cases studied contained such rearrangements {725}.

Prognosis and predictive factors
Patients with HGBL, NOS, have a poor outcome, although it may be slightly better than that of patients with double-hit HGBL {794,2344,3143}. A relatively poor outcome in HGBL, NOS, with amplification of *MYC*, with or without rearrangement of *BCL2* (or vice versa) has been reported. However, in most studies, this aspect was analysed mainly or exclusively in patients with DLBCL {2307,2344, 2404,3143,4113}. In general, clinical correlates from studies on HGBL, NOS, are hampered by their retrospective nature, by the lumping together of these cases with other lymphoma types, and by small cohort sizes.

B-cell lymphoma, unclassifiable, with features intermediate between diffuse large B-cell lymphoma and classic Hodgkin lymphoma

Jaffe E.S.
Stein H.
Swerdlow S.H.
Campo E.
Pileri S.A.
Harris N.L.

Definition
B-cell lymphoma, unclassifiable, with features intermediate between diffuse large B-cell lymphoma (DLBCL) and classic Hodgkin lymphoma (CHL) is a B-cell–lineage lymphoma that demonstrates overlapping clinical, morphological, and/or immunophenotypic features between CHL and DLBCL, especially primary mediastinal (thymic) large B-cell lymphoma (PMBL). These lymphomas are most commonly associated with mediastinal disease, but similar cases have been reported in peripheral lymph node groups as the primary site. Mediastinal cases are often referred to as mediastinal grey-zone lymphoma (MGZL) and non-mediastinal cases as grey-zone lymphoma (GZL), avoiding the cumbersome nomenclature of the official diagnosis.

ICD-O code   9596/3

Synonyms
Mediastinal grey-zone lymphoma; Hodgkin-like anaplastic large cell lymphoma (obsolete)

Epidemiology
MGZL is most common in young men, usually presenting in patients aged 20–40 years {1297,4047}. It has been re-ported rarely in children {2995}. Mediastinal presentations are infrequent among elderly patients {1077,1121}. Most cases have been reported from western countries. Like CHL, these tumours are less common in Black and Asian populations.

Etiology
The etiology is unknown, but gene expression profiling studies and genetic studies have revealed close links to PMBL and CHL {1059}.

Localization
The most common presentation is with a large anterior mediastinal mass, with or without involvement of supraclavicular lymph nodes {1297,4047}. Peripheral and intra-abdominal lymph nodes are less commonly involved. There may be spread to lung by direct extension, as well as spread to liver, spleen, and bone marrow. Non-lymphoid organs are rarely involved, unlike in PMBL.

Clinical features
Most patients have bulky mediastinal masses, sometimes leading to superior vena cava syndrome or respiratory distress. Supraclavicular lymph nodes may be involved. Non-mediastinal GZL more often presents in older patients, and shows less of a male predominance {1077,1121}. Cases of composite CHL and PMBL and cases of sequential development of CHL and PMBL in the same patient are not strictly accepted as examples of MGZL, but are thought to be biologically related phenomena {1402, 3140}. When seen sequentially, CHL is more often the initial presentation, followed by PMBL {4463}.

Microscopy
A characteristic feature is the broad spectrum of cytological appearances within a given tumour; some areas more closely resemble CHL and others resemble PMBL. There is also variation across different cases, with some examples being more Hodgkin-like and others more closely resembling either PMBL or diffuse large cell lymphoma. As discussed below (see *Immunophenotype*), discordance between the cytological appearance and the immunophenotype is common. Tumour cell density is high, often with sheet-like growth of pleomorphic tumour cells in a diffusely fibrotic stroma {1297,4047}. Focal fibrous bands may be seen in some cases. The cells are larger and more pleomorphic than is typical in PMBL, although some centroblast-like cells may be present. There is usually a

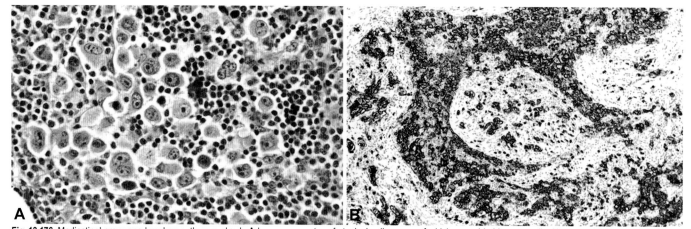

Fig. 13.176 Mediastinal grey-zone lymphoma, thymus gland. **A** Large aggregates of atypical cells, some of which resembled lacunar cells. However, CD20 was strongly and uniformly positive. **B** The neoplastic cells are strongly and uniformly positive for CD20.

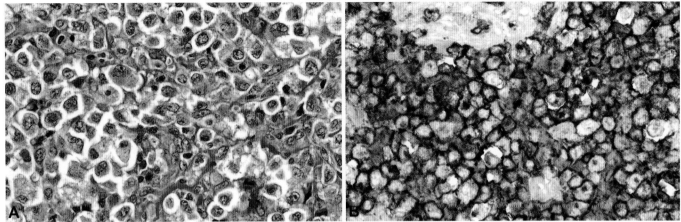

Fig. 13.177 B-cell lymphoma, unclassifiable, with features intermediate between DLBCL and CHL. Mediastinal mass. **A** The lymphoma is composed of sheets of cells with clear cytoplasm and fine sclerosis. The appearance resembles that of primary mediastinal large B-cell lymphoma. However, CD20 and CD79a are both negative. **B** The tumour cells are strongly CD15-positive and also CD30-positive (not shown).

sparse inflammatory infiltrate, although eosinophils, lymphocytes, and histiocytes may be present focally. Necrosis is frequent, but unlike in CHL, the necrotic areas do not contain neutrophilic infiltrates. Due to the variations in histological pattern in different portions of the tumour, diagnosing these lymphomas on a core needle biopsy is challenging and not recommended.

Immunophenotype

The lymphoma cells exhibit an aberrant immunophenotype, making the distinction between CHL and PMBL difficult {1297,4047}. Neoplastic cells typically express CD45. Cases in which the cytological appearance might suggest CHL show preservation of the B-cell programme, with strong and uniform positivity for CD20 and CD79a. CD30 is usually positive, and CD15 may be expressed. Cases in which the histological appearance on H&E staining might suggest PMBL show loss of B-cell antigens but positivity for CD30 and CD15. Surface or cytoplasmic immunoglobulin is absent. The transcription factors PAX5, OCT2, and BOB1 are usually expressed. BCL6 is variably positive but CD10 is generally negative. ALK is consistently negative. The background lymphocytes are predominantly positive for CD3 and CD4, as seen in CHL.

Weak or variable positivity for CD20 in a tumour otherwise compatible with a diagnosis of nodular sclerosis CHL should not lead to a diagnosis of B-cell lymphoma, unclassifiable, with features intermediate between DLBCL and CHL. Particularly with antigen-retrieval techniques, nodular sclerosis CHL may be positive for CD20, usually with variable intensity. Additionally, CD30 may be expressed in a subset of DLBCLs, and should not lead to a diagnosis of MGZL by itself. Notably, PMBL is frequently positive for CD30 {1633}.

MAL, a marker associated with PMBL, is expressed in at least a subset of the cases presenting with mediastinal disease {805,4047}. Supporting a relationship to PMBL, nuclear REL/p65 protein has been identified in the cases tested {1300, 3384}. IRF4/MUM1 is usually positive, but is not useful in differential diagnosis, because it is positive in most cases of CHL and PMBL. In one series, p53 was expressed in most cases {1300}. Expression of cyclin E and p63 in most cases has also been reported {1077}. Most cases of MGZL are negative for EBV; positivity for EBV-encoded small RNA (EBER) or LMP1 should prompt suspicion for EBV-positive DLBCL, especially in elderly patients. However, rare cases of MGZL have been EBV-positive {2867}.

In instances of composite or metachronous lymphomas, the various components exhibit a phenotype characteristic of that entity, either CHL or PMBL.

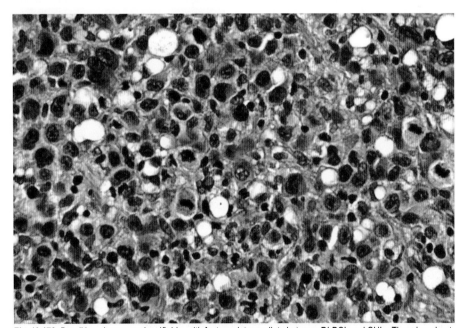

Fig. 13.178 B-cell lymphoma, unclassifiable, with features intermediate between DLBCL and CHL. There is a sheet-like growth of pleomorphic lymphoid cells. Some binucleated cells are present, but there is marked variation in cell size and shape. The biopsy was taken from a 28-year-old man with a mediastinal mass and supraclavicular lymph node involvement.

Postulated normal counterpart

The postulated cell of origin for cases arising in the mediastinum is a thymic B cell {4047}; cases arising in the peripheral lymph nodes are thought to arise from a non-thymic B cell.

Genetic profile

Clonal rearrangement of the IG genes is positive by PCR in most cases, presumably due to the high content of tumour cells in comparison with CHL. Many of the genetic aberrations identified by FISH are similar to those observed in PMBL {1077}. Gains and amplification of the *JAK2* and *PDCD1LG2* (also called *PDL2*) loci at 9p24.1 are common, seen in >50% of cases. Increased expression of CD274 (PD-L1) may occur as a result. Also frequent are gains/amplification at 2p16.1 involving *REL*. Breaks in the *CIITA* locus at 16p13.13 have been reported in approximately one third of cases {1077}. Gains in *MYC* have been observed in 20–30% of cases. The aberrations above are seen in both mediastinal and non-mediastinal cases, although gains/amplification at 9p24.1 are more common in patients with mediastinal than non-mediastinal presentations, occurring in 61% and 38% of such cases, respectively {1077}.

Prognosis and predictive factors

MGZLs generally have a more aggressive clinical course and poorer outcome than do either CHLs or PMBLs {1060}. Combined modality treatment appears to be required in most cases, and systemic multiagent chemotherapy followed by radiation to the mediastinal mass produces event-free survival in a majority of patients {4333}. Consistent with the strong expression of CD20, the addition of rituximab appears to be of benefit. Regimens effective in the treatment of CHL, such as ABVD chemotherapy (i.e. doxorubicin, bleomycin, vinblastine, and dacarbazine), have been reported to be less effective than regimens used for treating DLBCLs {1121}. Like in CHL, a decrease in the absolute lymphocyte count has

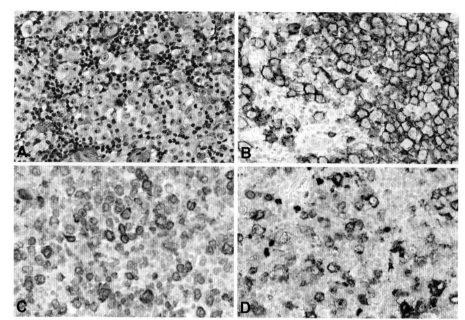

Fig. 13.179 B-cell lymphoma, unclassifiable, with features intermediate between DLBCL and classic HL. **A** Sheets of tumour cells resembling lacunar cells are present, with a minimal inflammatory background. **B** In the same case, the tumour cells are strongly positive for CD20. **C** CD79a is uniformly positive. **D** CD15 is positive, but the sheet-like growth and strong staining for CD20 and CD79a favour mediastinal grey-zone lymphoma.

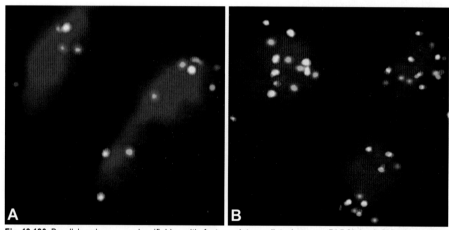

Fig. 13.180 B-cell lymphoma, unclassifiable, with features intermediate between DLBCL and CHL. Mediastinal mass. **A** Rearrangement of the *PDL1/PDL2* locus is demonstrated by FISH using a break-apart probe with a split green signal suggesting the presence of an inversion within this region. **B** Amplification of the *PDL1/PDL2* locus, which shows multiple fusion signals (69% with more than 6 signals, 20% with 3–4 signals, and 11% with <2 copies/cell). In both panels *PDL1/PDL2* are red/green and CEP 9 is aqua. Figure contributed by Pack S.

been associated with a worse outcome {4333}. In one study, a high content of DC-SIGN–positive dendritic cells was associated with an adverse prognosis {4333}. This association may be comparable to the association between a high content of tumour-associated macrophages and adverse outcome in CHL {3778}.

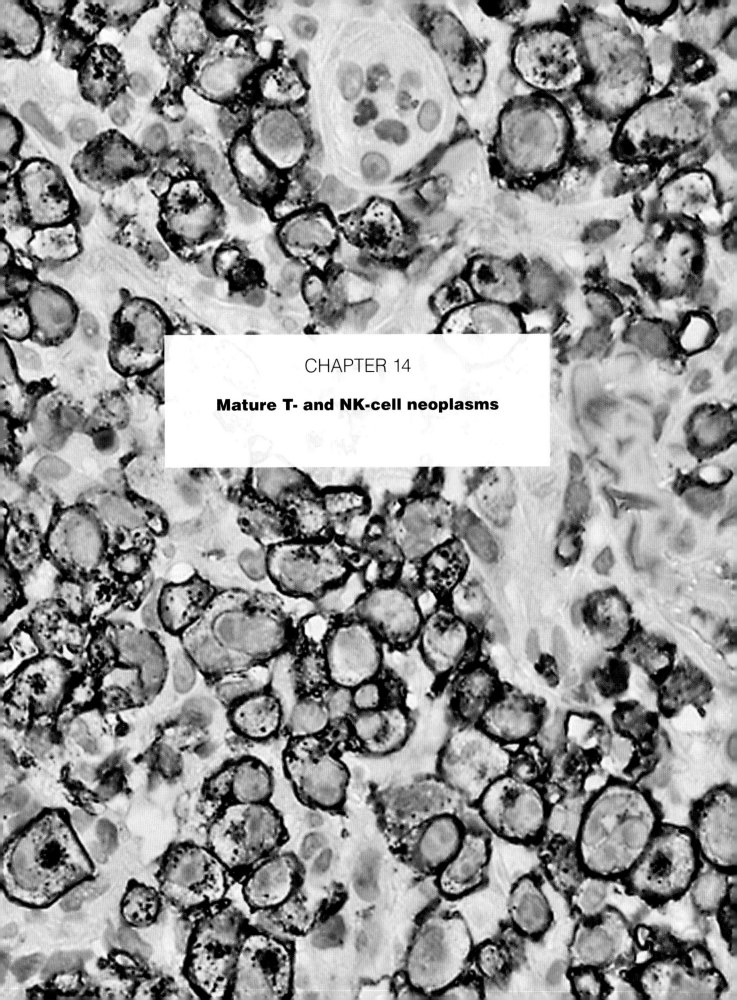

CHAPTER 14

Mature T- and NK-cell neoplasms

T-cell prolymphocytic leukaemia

Matutes E.
Catovsky D.
Müller-Hermelink H.K.

Definition

T-cell prolymphocytic leukaemia (T-PLL) is an aggressive T-cell leukaemia characterized by the proliferation of small to medium-sized prolymphocytes with a mature post-thymic T-cell phenotype, involving the peripheral blood, bone marrow, lymph nodes, liver, spleen, and skin.

ICD-O code   9834/3

Synonym

Prolymphocytic leukaemia, T-cell type

Epidemiology

T-PLL is rare, accounting for approximately 2% of cases of mature lymphocytic leukaemias in adults aged >30 years {2575}; the median patient age is 65 years (range: 30–94 years). It is very infrequent among individuals aged <30 years.

Localization

Leukaemic T cells are found in the peripheral blood, bone marrow, lymph nodes, spleen, liver, and sometimes skin.

Clinical features

Most patients present with hepatosplenomegaly and generalized lymphadenopathy. Skin infiltration is seen in 20% of cases, and serous effusions in a minority {2575}. Anaemia and thrombocytopenia are common, and the lymphocyte count is usually $> 100 \times 10^9$/L. Serum immunoglobulins are normal. Serology for HTLV-1 is negative.

Microscopy

Peripheral blood and bone marrow

The diagnosis is made on peripheral blood films, which show a predominance of small to medium-sized lymphoid cells with non-granular basophilic cytoplasm; round, oval, or markedly irregular nuclei, and visible nucleoli. In 25% of cases, the cell size is small and the nucleolus may not be visible by light microscopy (small-cell variant) {2577}. In 5% of cases, the nuclear outline is very irregular and can even be cerebriform (cerebriform variant) {3115}. Irrespective of the nuclear features, a common morphological feature is cytoplasmic protrusions or blebs. The bone marrow is diffusely infiltrated, but the diagnosis is difficult to make on the basis of bone marrow histology alone.

Other tissues

Cutaneous involvement consists of perivascular and periadnexal or more diffuse dermal infiltrates, without epidermotropism {2472,2575}. The spleen contains a dense red pulp infiltrate, which invades the spleen capsule, blood vessels, and atrophic white pulp {3004}. In lymph nodes, the involvement is diffuse and tends to predominate in the para-

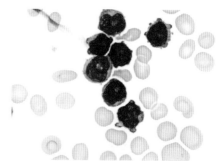

Fig. 14.01 T-cell prolymphocytic leukaemia, small-cell variant. Small lymphocytes showing a regular or irregular nuclear outline and cytoplasmic blebs.

cortical areas, sometimes with sparing of follicles. Prominent high endothelial venules may be numerous and are often infiltrated by neoplastic cells.

Cytochemistry

T-cell prolymphocytes stain strongly with alpha-naphthyl acetate esterase and acid phosphatase, with a dot-like pattern {2576}. However, cytochemistry is rarely used for routine diagnosis.

Immunophenotype

T-cell prolymphocytes are peripheral T cells that are negative for TdT and CD1a, and positive for CD2, CD5, CD3, and CD7; the membrane expression of CD3 may be weak. CD52 is usually expressed at high density, and can be used as a target of therapy {916}.

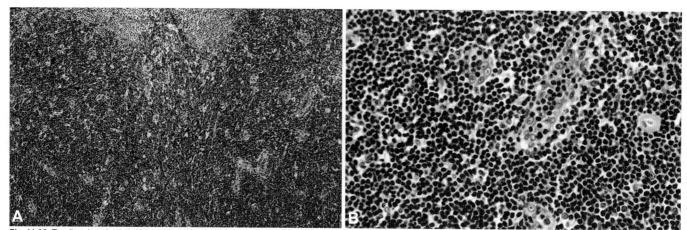

Fig. 14.02 T-cell prolymphocytic leukaemia. **A** Lymph node involvement showing infiltration of the paracortex with sparing of primary follicles. **B** Lymphocytes infiltrate high endothelial venules.

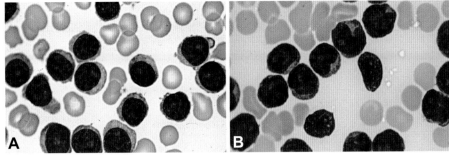

Fig. 14.03 T-cell prolymphocytic leukaemia. **A,B** Peripheral blood films from typical cases.

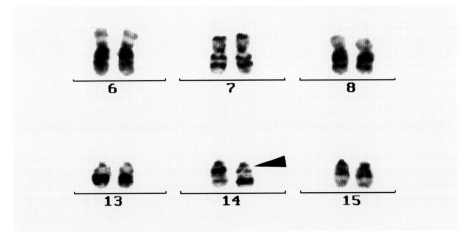

Fig. 14.04 T-cell prolymphocytic leukaemia. Partial karyotype showing inv(14)(q11.2q32.1).

In 60% of cases, the cells are CD4-positive and CD8-negative. In 25%, they coexpress CD4 and CD8, a feature which is almost exclusive to T-PLL; other post-thymic T-cell malignancies rarely coexpress these antigens. The other 15% of cases are CD4-negative and CD8-positive {2575}. Overexpression of the oncoprotein TCL1 can be demonstrated by immunohistochemistry or flow cytometry {1616}, which is useful for detecting residual T-PLL after therapy. Expression of S100 has been documented in 30% of cases {29}.

Postulated normal counterpart

The postulated normal counterpart is an unknown T cell with a mature (post-thymic) immunophenotype. Strong expression of CD7, coexpression of CD4 and CD8, and weak membrane expression of CD3 may suggest that T-PLL arises from a T cell at an intermediate stage of differentiation between a cortical thymocyte and a mature T lymphocyte.

Genetic profile

Antigen receptor genes
TR genes (TRB and TRG) are clonally rearranged.

Cytogenetic abnormalities and oncogenes
The most frequent chromosome abnormality in T-PLL involves inversion of chromosome 14 with breakpoints in the long arm at q11.2 and q32.1, seen in 80% of patients and described as inv(14)(q11.2q32.1). In 10%, there is t(14;14)(q11.2;q32.1) {457,2470}. These translocations juxtapose the TRA locus with the oncogenes *TCL1A* and *TCL1B* at 14q32.1, which are activated through the translocation {3121}. The t(X;14)(q28;q11.2) translocation is less common, but it also involves the TRA locus, at 14q11.2 with the *MTCP1* gene, which is homologous to *TCL1A/B* at Xq28 {3797}. Both *TCL1A/B* and *MTCP1* have oncogenic properties; both can induce a T-cell leukaemia (CD4–, CD8+) in transgenic mice {1467,4198}. The oncoprotein TCL1 inhibits activation-induced death in the neoplastic T cells, further contributing to the neoplastic process {961}. Rearrangements of *TCL1A/B* or *MTCP1* are initiating events but are probably not sufficient to drive leukaemogenesis.
Abnormalities of chromosome 8, idic(8)(p11), t(8;8)(p11-12;q12), and trisomy 8q are seen in 70–80% of cases {3121}, and gains in the *MYC* gene have been

documented by FISH in some cases {1713}. Deletions at 12p13 and 22q and amplification of 5p are also a feature of T-PLL on FISH and/or SNP array {493, 1631,2901}. Molecular and FISH studies also show deletions at 11q22.3 (the locus for *ATM*), and mutation analysis has shown missense mutations at the *ATM* locus in T-PLL {3803,4215}. T-PLL is not an uncommon neoplasm in patients with ataxia-telangiectasia {457}. Abnormalities of chromosomes 6 (present in 33% of cases) and 17 (in 26%) have also been identified in T-PLL by conventional karyotyping and comparative genomic hybridization {457,818}. The *TP53* gene (at 17p13.1) is deleted, with overexpression of p53, in some cases {458}.
Whole-exome and targeted sequencing studies have shown recurrent alterations in genes of the JAK/STAT signalling pathway. Mutations of *JAK3* have been documented in 30–42% of cases, of *JAK1* in about 8%, and of *STAT5B* in 21–36% {322,349,2007,3794}. These mutations, which are largely mutually exclusive, lead to constitutive activation of the STAT signalling pathway. In addition, although more rarely, genes encoding epigenetic modifiers, such as *EZH2* and *BCOR*, have been described to be recurrently mutated in T-PLL {2007,3794}.

Genetic susceptibility

Patients with ataxia-telangiectasia may be at increased risk for the development of T-PLL.

Prognosis and predictive factors

The disease course is aggressive, with a median survival of 1–2 years. Cases with a more chronic course have also been reported {1296}, but such cases may progress after 2–3 years. The best responses have been reported with the monoclonal antibody alemtuzumab (anti-CD52) {917, 1978}. Autologous or allogeneic stem cell transplantation should be considered for eligible patients who achieve remission following immunotherapy {1488, 2116}. The findings of mutation activation of the JAK/STAT signalling pathway may provide opportunities to develop novel therapies with inhibitors targeting this pathway. High levels of expression of both TCL1 and AKT1 have been identified as poor prognostic markers {1617}, and more recently, *STAT5B* mutations have been documented to have a negative prognostic impact {3794}.

T-cell large granular lymphocytic leukaemia

Chan W.C.
Foucar K.
Morice W.G.
Matutes E.

Definition

T-cell large granular lymphocytic leukaemia (T-LGLL) is a heterogeneous disorder characterized by a persistent (>6 months) increase in the number of peripheral blood large granular lymphocytes (LGLs), usually to $2–20 \times 10^9$/L, without a clearly identified cause.

ICD-O code   9831/3

Synonyms

T-cell large granular lymphocytosis; CD8+ T-cell chronic lymphocytic leukaemia (obsolete); T-cell lymphoproliferative disease of granular lymphocytes; T-gamma lymphoproliferative disease (obsolete)

Epidemiology

T-LGLL accounts for 2–3% of mature small lymphocytic leukaemias. There is an approximately equal male-to-female ratio, with no clearly defined age peak. The disease is rare in individuals aged <25 years, with <3% of cases occurring in this age group; most cases (73%) occur in individuals aged 45–75 years.

Etiology

The underlying pathophysiological mechanisms of T-LGLL are not well understood, and this disorder is fairly unique in that the clonal T-cell LGLs (T-LGLs) retain many phenotypic and functional properties of normal cytotoxic T lymphocyte effector memory cells {377}. One theory is that T-LGLL arises in a setting of sustained immune stimulation. The frequent association of T-LGLL with autoimmune disorders supports this hypothesis {377,4343}. The absence of homeostatic apoptosis is also a feature of the T-LGLs; these cells express high levels of FAS and FASL, leading investigators to propose activation of prosurvival pathways in T-LGLs, which prevents activation-induced cell death {1112,3549}. FASL levels are elevated in the sera of many patients, and this elevation is postulated to be important in the pathogenesis of neutropenia {2368}. Other pathways

reported to be dysregulated include the MAPK, PI3K/AKT, NF-kappaB, and JAK/STAT signalling pathways {3791}. About one third of the cases carry *STAT3* mutations, which affect the SH2 domain of *STAT3* {1854,2086}. Rarely, mutations affecting the SH2 domain of *STAT5B* are observed {3288}. There is evidence that these are activating mutations that may contribute to the pathogenesis of the disease by providing prosurvival and growth signals {1854,2086}. It is possible that T-LGLL starts as an immune response to a chronic persistent stimulus, with clonal selection and eventually the acquisition of an oncogenic mutation that allows the further expansion and establishment of a monoclonal population.

Localization

T-LGLL involves the peripheral blood, bone marrow, liver, spleen, and rarely skin. Lymphadenopathy is very rare.

Clinical features

Most cases have an indolent clinical course. Severe neutropenia (with or without anaemia) is frequent, whereas thrombocytopenia is not; 60% of patients are symptomatic at presentation {650,967, 2203,3046}. The lymphocyte count is usually $2–20 \times 10^9$/L. There is disagreement about the level of lymphocytosis required for the diagnosis of T-LGLL {3620}, but a T-LGL count of $>2 \times 10^9$/L is frequently associated with a large clonal proliferation. However, cases that have LGL counts of $<2 \times 10^9$/L but meet

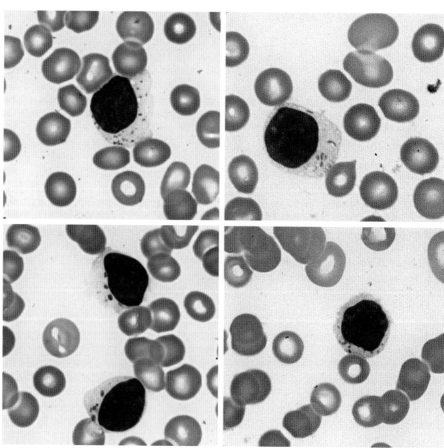

Fig. 14.05 T-cell large granular lymphocytic leukaemia. The various morphological variants of large granular lymphocyte in the peripheral blood (Wright stain).

all other criteria are consistent with this diagnosis. Cases with low counts of LGLs in the blood and low bone marrow infiltration generally have small clonal populations; their designation as T-LGLL is questionable, and other names have been proposed {3687}. A pitfall in diagnosis is the frequent development of oligoclonal T-cell populations following allogeneic bone marrow transplantation as lymphocyte reconstitution occurs {1253, 2552,3687}. Severe anaemia due to red blood cell hypoplasia has been reported in association with T-LGLL {2203}. Moderate splenomegaly is the main physical finding. Rheumatoid arthritis, the presence of autoantibodies, circulating immune complexes, and hypergammaglobulinaemia are also common {650,2203, 3001}. Oligoclonal or clonal expansions of T-LGLs can be observed in a variety of situations. For example, rare cases of T-LGLL have been observed as a form of post-transplant lymphoproliferative disorder {151,186,2829}. Clonal populations of T-LGLs are also seen in association with low-grade B-cell malignancies, including hairy cell leukaemia and chronic lymphocytic leukaemia, and in particular following immunochemotherapy {151,2529}. Cases that are CD4-positive have been reported to be frequently (i.e. in 30% of cases) associated with an underlying haematological or (less often) non-haematological malignancy {2335}.

Morbidity and mortality are mostly due to the accompanying cytopenias or other accompanying diseases. There is no difference in survival between cases with and without STAT3 mutation, although

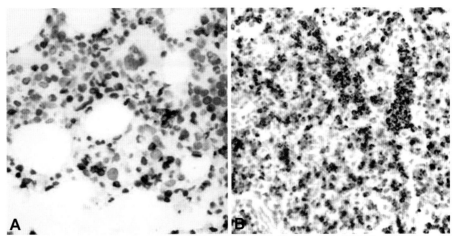

Fig. 14.06 Immunohistochemical staining for TIA1 of bone marrow (**A**) and spleen (**B**). In the spleen the cells accumulate in the sinusoids and cords.

mutation seems to be associated with more-symptomatic disease and shorter time to treatment failure {1854,2086}. The rare finding of STAT5B mutations appears to be associated with more-aggressive disease {3288}.

Microscopy

The predominant lymphocytes in blood and bone marrow films are LGLs with moderate to abundant cytoplasm and fine or course azurophilic granules {464, 650,2599}. The granules in the LGLs often exhibit a characteristic ultrastructural appearance described as parallel tubular arrays {2599} and contain a number of proteins that play a role in cytolysis, such as perforin and granzyme B. Despite the cytopenias, the bone marrow is normocellular or hypocellular in about 50% of cases; in the other 50%, the mar-

row is slightly hypercellular {2741,3003}. The granulocytic series often shows left-shifted maturation, and mild to moderate reticulin fibrosis is present {650}. The extent of bone marrow involvement is variable, and usually constitutes <50% of the cellular elements, with interstitial/intrasinusoidal infiltrates that are difficult to identify by morphological review {2741}. Non-neoplastic nodular lymphoid aggregates containing many B cells surrounded by a rim of CD4+ T cells are also frequently present {3003}.

Splenic involvement is characterized by infiltration and expansion of the red pulp cords and sinusoids by T-LGLs, with sparing of the often hyperplastic white pulp {3004}.

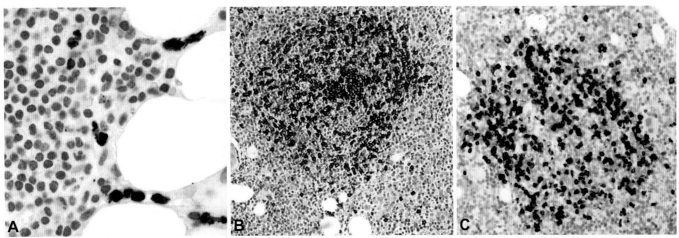

Fig. 14.07 T-cell large granular lymphocytic leukaemia. Bone marrow findings. **A** Neoplastic cells infiltrate interstitially, as demonstrated by staining for TIA1. **B,C** Reactive lymphoid aggregates. Lymphoid nodules in the bone marrow immunostained with anti-CD20 (B) and anti-CD3 (C). B cells in the nodule are admixed with CD3+ T cells that predominate at the periphery.

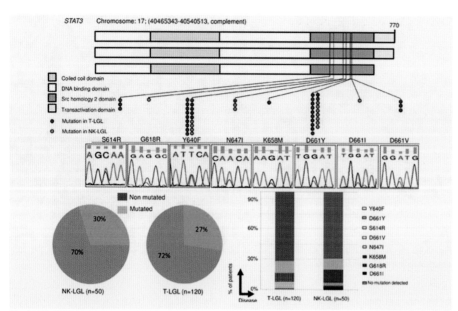

Fig. 14.08 *STAT3* mutations in large granular lymphocytic leukaemia (LGL). From: Jerez A et al. {1854}

Variant

Cases that morphologically resemble T-LGLL but have an NK-cell immunophenotype, i.e. that are negative for surface CD3 (sCD3) and T-cell receptor (TCR) expression, are classified with the NK-cell disorders.

Cytochemistry

The granules are positive for acid phosphatase and beta-glucuronidase. Enzyme cytochemical studies are rarely performed for routine diagnosis.

Immunophenotype

T-LGLL is typically a disorder of mature CD2+, CD3+, CD8+, CD57+, and alpha beta TCR–positive cytotoxic T cells {650,3046}. Uncommon variants include CD4+ / alpha beta TCR–positive cases and gamma delta TCR–positive cases; approximately 60% of the latter express CD8, and the remainder are CD4/CD8-negative {650,2335,3046,3504,3620}. Abnormally diminished or lost expression of CD5 and/or CD7 is common in T-LGLL {2416, 2740}. CD57 and CD16 are expressed in >80% of cases {2203,2740}. Expression of CD94/NKG2 family and killer-cell immunoglobulin-like receptor (KIR) family members, which are major histocompatibility complex (MHC) class I receptors, can be detected in ≥50% of T-LGLLs, but expression of CD56 is infrequent. KIR–positive cases usually show uniform expression of a KIR–family member, and this finding can serve as a surrogate indicator of clonality

similar to the restricted expression of TCR-beta family members {2416,2740}. T-LGLs express the cytotoxic effector proteins TIA1, granzyme B, and granzyme M. Bone marrow core biopsy immunohistochemistry can confirm the diagnosis by highlighting the interstitial and intrasinusoidal T-LGL infiltrates and revealing the non-neoplastic nature of the nodular aggregates {2738,2741,3003}.

Cell of origin

A subset of CD8+ alpha beta T cells for the common type and a subset of gamma delta T cells for the rare type expressing the gamma delta TCR

Genetic profile

Antigen receptor genes

As a rule, cases classified as T-LGLL are clonal as documented by TR gene rearrangement studies {2203}. The TRG gene is rearranged in all cases, regardless of the type of TCR expressed. TRB is rearranged in cases expressing the alpha beta TCR, but the TRB gene may be in germline configuration in gamma delta TCR cases {4194}. Deep sequencing of the TRB CDR3 has demonstrated that the dominant clonotypes in the CD8+ LGLs tend to be private and not commonly shared in the CDR3 repertoire seen in normal individuals {768}.

Cytogenetic abnormalities and oncogenes

STAT3 mutations have been found in

about one third of cases. These activating somatic mutations affect the SH2 domain of *STAT3*; the vast majority are heterozygous, and they most frequently affect codon Y640 or D661 {1854,2086}. Very rarely, *STAT5B* SH2 domain mutations have been documented, and the N642H mutation may be associated with more-aggressive disease {3288}.

There is no recurrent karyotypic abnormality, but numeric and structural chromosomal abnormalities have been described in a small number of cases {2203}.

Prognosis and predictive factors

The lymphoproliferation is typically indolent and non-progressive, and some investigators feel that this entity is better regarded as a clonal disorder of uncertain significance than as a leukaemia. Morbidity is associated with the cytopenias (especially neutropenia), but mortality due to this cause is uncommon. In a series of 68 cases, the actuarial median survival was 161 months {967}. There appears to be no difference in survival between cases with and without *STAT3* mutation, although mutation seems to be associated with more-symptomatic disease and shorter time to treatment failure {1854,2086}. The rare finding of *STAT5B* mutations appears to be associated with more aggressive disease {3288,1327,4025}. Rare cases have undergone transformation to a peripheral T-cell lymphoma composed of large cells {2585}. Some of the aggressive cases may represent peripheralization of a peripheral T-cell lymphoma. Conversely, rare cases with spontaneous remission have also been reported {4338}. Patients who require treatment may benefit from cyclosporine, cyclophosphamide, and corticosteroids or low-dose methotrexate, which has been reported to induce clinical remission in as many as 50% of patients {650,2203,3005}. Some patients have benefited from pentostatin {3005}. Splenectomy has been performed in patients with a large spleen, but does not correct the cytopenia. In light of the discovery of activation of the STAT3 or STAT5B pathway in patients with (and possibly also patients without) activating mutations {1854}, inhibiting this pathway could be an option for the treatment of T-cell and NK-cell LGL proliferations.

Chronic lymphoproliferative disorder of NK cells

Villamor N.
Morice W.G.
Chan W.C.
Foucar K.

Definition

Chronic lymphoproliferative disorders of NK cells (CLPD-NKs) are rare and heterogeneous. They are characterized by a persistent (>6 months) increase in the peripheral blood NK-cell count (usually to $\geq 2 \times 10^9$/L) without a clearly identified cause. It is difficult to distinguish between reactive and neoplastic conditions without highly specialized techniques. CLPD-NK is a proliferation of NK cells associated with a chronic clinical course, and is considered a provisional entity.

ICD-O code   9831/3

Synonyms

Chronic NK-cell lymphocytosis; chronic NK large granular lymphocyte lymphoproliferative disorder; NK-cell large granular lymphocyte lymphocytosis; indolent large granular NK-cell lymphoproliferative disorder; indolent leukaemia of NK cells

Epidemiology

CLPD-NK occurs predominantly in adults, with a median patient age of 60 years and no sex predominance {2204,2336,3274}. Unlike in EBV-associated aggressive NK-cell leukaemia, there is no racial or genetic predisposition.

Etiology

A transient increase in circulating NK cells can be encountered in many conditions, such as autoimmune disorders and viral infections {2204,3274}. NK-cell activation due to an unknown stimulus, presumably viral, is postulated to play a role in the early pathogenesis of CLPD-NKs by selecting and expanding NK-cell clones, although no evidence of direct NK-cell infection has been observed {1113,2336, 2398,3274,3605,4456,4457}. The tyrosine kinase inhibitor dasatinib produces a sustained increase in NK cells that can be monoclonal {2113,2796}. One third of cases have activating mutations in the *STAT3* SH2 domain {1163,1854}.

Localization

The peripheral blood and bone marrow are the predominant sites.

Clinical features

Most patients are asymptomatic, but some present with systemic symptoms and/or cytopenia (mainly neutropenia and anaemia). Lymphadenopathy, hepatomegaly, and cutaneous lesions are infrequent {260,2336,3001,3274}. CLPD-NKs may occur in association with other medical conditions, such as solid and haematological tumours, vasculitis, splenectomy, neuropathy, and autoimmune disorders {2336,3001,3075,3274}. CLPD-NK is distinguished from NK-cell lymphoproliferative disorders involving the gastrointestinal tract, designated as NK-cell enteropathy or lymphomatoid gastropathy of NK-cell type {2489A; 3882A}.

Microscopy

The circulating NK cells are typically intermediate in size, with round nuclei with condensed chromatin and moderate amounts of slightly basophilic cytoplasm containing fine or coarse azurophilic granules. These large granular lymphocytes are monotonous, and features of lymphocyte activation are not apparent. Lymphocytosis may be apparent on bone marrow aspirate smears, but large granular lymphocyte morphology is often subtle. The bone marrow biopsy is characterized by intrasinusoidal and interstitial infiltration by cells with small, minimally irregular nuclei and modest amounts of pale cytoplasm. These infiltrates are difficult to detect without immunohistochemistry.

Immunophenotype

CLPD-NK shows a distinctive profile by flow cytometric immunophenotyping. Surface CD3 is negative, whereas cCD3-epsilon is often positive. CD16 is positive, and weak CD56 expression is frequently observed {2336,2738,2739,2740,3075, 4259}. Cytotoxic markers (including TIA1,

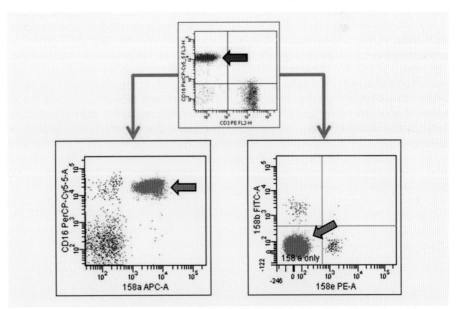

Fig. 14.09 Chronic lymphoproliferative disorder of NK cells (CLPD-NK). Peripheral-blood flow-cytometric immunophenotyping reveals an increase in CD16+/CD3− NK cells (upper panel, red arrow). Selective gating on these cells reveals that they uniformly express the killer-cell immunoglobulin-like receptor isoform CD158a (lower-left panel, orange arrow) and lack expression of the isoforms CD158b and CD158e (lower-right panel, orange arrow). This restricted pattern of killer-cell immunoglobulin-like receptor expression by NK cells is abnormal and supports the diagnosis of CLPD-NK.

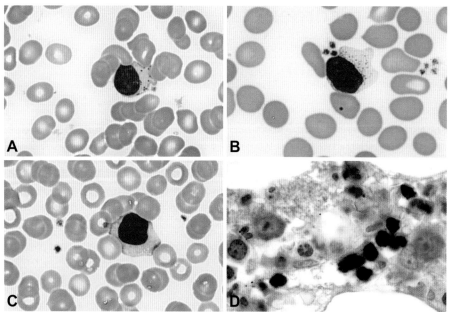

Fig. 14.10 Chronic lymphoproliferative disorder of NK cells. **A–C** Peripheral blood films show a lymphocyte with coarse azurophilic granulation (A), a lymphocyte with numerous fine granulations (B), and a lymphocyte with scarce granulation at the limit of visibility (C). **D** Intrasinusoidal marrow infiltration by cells positive for granzyme B. Note the bland nuclear cytology of the antigen-positive cells.

granzyme B, and granzyme M) are positive. There may be diminished or lost expression of CD2, CD7, and CD57, and abnormal uniform expression of CD8 {2735,2740}. Expression of the killer-cell immunoglobulin-like receptor (KIR) family of NK-cell receptors is abnormal in CLPD-NK; either restricted KIR isoform expression or a complete lack of detectable KIRs may be seen {1113,1661,2740, 3075,4456,4459}. KIR-positive cases preferentially express activating receptor isoforms {1113,4456}. Other abnormalities of NK-cell receptors include uniform, bright CD94/NKG2A heterodimer expression and diminished CD161 expression {2336,2740,3605,4259}.

Postulated normal counterpart
A mature NK cell

Genetic profile
The karyotype is normal in most cases {3001,3274,3925}. Activating mutations in the *STAT3* SH2 domain are present in 30% of cases, and the finding of this mutation excludes non-neoplastic NK-cell proliferations {1163}. There are no rearrangements of the IG and TR genes, as expected for NK cells. In female patients, it is possible to use X-chromosome inactivation as an indirect marker of clonality. A skewed ratio of X-chromosome inactivation restricted to NK cells is indicative of a clonal population.

With such methodologies, clonality is found in some patients {1981,2336,2831}. Unlike in aggressive NK-cell leukaemia, EBV is negative {2204,2398,4457}.

Genetic susceptibility
A genetic susceptibility may be linked to haplotypes containing higher numbers of activating KIR genes {1113,3605,4456}.

Prognosis and predictive factors
In most patients, the clinical course is indolent over a prolonged period, and no therapy is needed. In general, the management of CLPD-NKs is similar to that of T-cell large granular lymphocytic leukaemia {2205}. Disease progression with increasing lymphocytosis and worsening of cytopenias is observed in some cases. Cytopenias, recurrent infections, and comorbidity may be harbingers of a worse prognosis. Rare cases with either spontaneous complete remission {2336, 3001,3274,4458} or transformation to an aggressive NK-cell disorder have been described {1722,2948,3427}. Cytogenetic abnormalities may imply a worse prognosis and could be associated with the rare transformations reported in the literature {2948}.

Aggressive NK-cell leukaemia

Chan J.K.C.
Jaffe E.S.
Ko Y.-H.

Definition
Aggressive NK-cell leukaemia is a systemic neoplastic proliferation of NK cells frequently associated with EBV and an aggressive clinical course.

ICD-O code   9948/3

Synonym
Aggressive NK-cell leukaemia/lymphoma

Epidemiology
This rare form of leukaemia is much more prevalent among Asians than in other ethnic populations {3460}. Patients are most commonly young to middle-aged adults, with a median age of 40 years and two incidence peaks, in the third and fifth decades of life {1786,2297,3062, 3728,3840}. There is no definite sex predilection {640,647,1756,2155,2157,2297, 2999,3460,3462,3728,3840}.

Etiology
Little is known about the etiology of aggressive NK-cell leukaemia, but the strong association with EBV suggests a pathogenetic role of the virus. In younger patients, the leukaemia may evolve from chronic active EBV infection {1788,1789, 3062}.

Localization
The most commonly involved sites are the peripheral blood, bone marrow, liver, and spleen, but any organ can be involved.

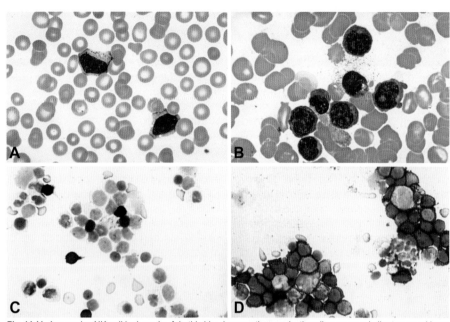

Fig. 14.11 Aggressive NK-cell leukaemia. **A** In this blood smear, the neoplastic cells are very similar to normal large granular lymphocytes. **B** In the peripheral blood, the neoplastic cells in this case have basophilic cytoplasm and nuclei with more open chromatin and distinct nucleoli. Azurophilic granules can be seen in the cytoplasm. **C** The neoplastic cells are negative for surface CD3, whereas the normal T lymphocytes are stained. **D** Neoplastic cells show strong immunoreactivity for CD56.

There can be overlap with extranodal NK/T-cell lymphoma showing multiorgan involvement; it is unclear whether aggressive NK-cell leukaemia is the leukaemic counterpart of extranodal NK/T-cell lymphoma {640}.

Clinical features
Patients usually present with fever, constitutional symptoms, and a leukaemic blood picture. The number of circulating leukaemic cells may be low or high (a few per cent to >80% of all leukocytes); anaemia, neutropenia, and thrombocytopenia are common. Serum lactate dehydrogenase levels are often markedly elevated. Hepatosplenomegaly is common, sometimes accompanied by lymphade-

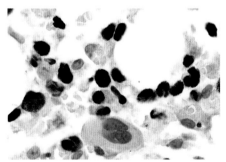

Fig. 14.12 Aggressive NK-cell leukaemia. In situ hybridization for EBV-encoded small RNA (EBER) highlights the neoplastic cells in the bone marrow biopsy. The nuclear atypia in this example is striking.

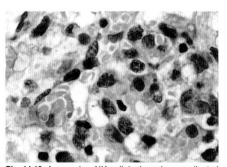

Fig. 14.13 Aggressive NK-cell leukaemia complicated by haemophagocytic syndrome. The marrow biopsy shows neoplastic cells with substantial nuclear pleomorphism and irregular nuclear foldings. There are admixed histiocytes with phagocytosed red blood cells.

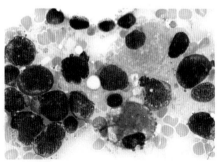

Fig. 14.14 Aggressive NK-cell leukaemia. The neoplastic cells in this marrow aspirate smear show substantial nuclear pleomorphism. Histiocytes with phagocytosed red blood cells are apparent.

nopathy, but skin lesions are uncommon. Effusions are common. The disease may be complicated by coagulopathy, haemophagocytic syndrome, or multiorgan failure {647,1756,2157,2297,2733,2970, 3728,3840}. Rare cases may evolve from extranodal NK/T-cell lymphoma or chronic lymphoproliferative disorder of NK cells {1591,2948,3001,3722,4482}.

Microscopy

Circulating leukaemic cells can show a range of appearances, from cells indistinguishable from normal large granular lymphocytes to cells with atypical nuclei featuring enlargement, irregular foldings, open chromatin, or distinct nucleoli. There is ample pale or lightly basophilic cytoplasm containing fine or coarse azurophilic granules. The bone marrow shows massive, focal, or subtle infiltration by the neoplastic cells, and there can be intermingled reactive histiocytes with haemophagocytosis. In tissue sections, the leukaemic cells show diffuse or patchy destructive infiltrates. They often appear monotonous, with round or irregular nuclei, condensed chromatin, and small nucleoli, but they can sometimes show substantial nuclear pleomorphism. There are frequently admixed apoptotic bodies. Necrosis is common, and there may or may not be angioinvasion.

Immunophenotype

The neoplastic cells typically have a CD2+, surface CD3−, CD3-epsilon+, CD5−, CD56+ phenotype and are positive for cytotoxic molecules. Thus, the immunophenotype is identical to that of extranodal NK/T-cell lymphoma, except that CD16 is frequently (in 75% of cases) positive {3840}. Aberrant immunophenotypes can also occur, such as loss of expression of CD2, CD7, or CD45 {2297}. CD11b may be expressed, whereas CD57 is usually negative {640,2999}. The neoplastic cells express FASL, and high levels can be found in the serum of affected patients {1960,2452,3891}.

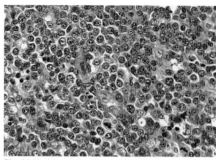

Fig. 14.15 Aggressive NK-cell leukaemia. Lymph node. The neoplastic cells appear monotonous and have round nuclei. There are many interspersed apoptotic bodies.

Cell of origin
An activated NK cell

Genetic profile
TR genes are in germline configuration. EBV is reported to be positive in 85–100% of cases, and EBV is present in a clonal episomal form {647,1564,1971}. The EBV-negative subset of cases occur *de novo* or evolve from chronic lymphoproliferative disorder of NK cells, and have clinicopathological features similar to those of EBV-positive cases; however, it is unclear whether the clinical outcome is similar {1773,2057,2866A,3062,3139, 3840}.

Various clonal cytogenetic abnormalities have been reported, such as del(6) (q21q25) and 11q deletion {3462}. An array comparative genomic hybridization study identified significant differences in genetic changes between aggressive NK-cell leukaemia and extranodal NK/T-cell lymphoma: losses in 7p and 17p as well as gains in 1q are frequent in the former but not the latter; deletions in 6q are common in the latter but rare in the former {2817}.

Prognosis and predictive factors
Most cases have a fulminant clinical course, frequently complicated by multiorgan failure, coagulopathy, and haemophagocytic syndrome. The median survival is <2 months {640,2297,3462, 3728,3840,4482}. Response to chemotherapy is usually poor, and relapse is common in patients who achieve remission with or without bone marrow transplantation {2297,3840}.

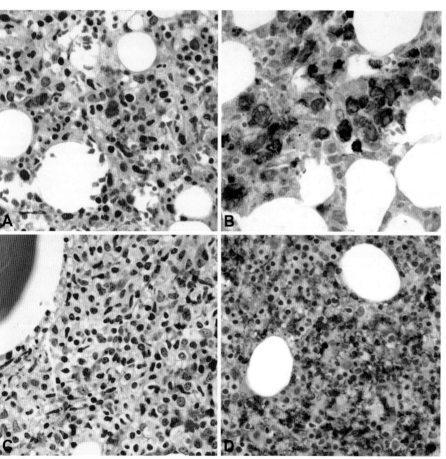

Fig. 14.16 Aggressive NK-cell leukaemia. Bone marrow biopsy. **A** Patchy involvement by neoplastic cells with substantial nuclear pleomorphism. **B** Immunostaining for CD3 highlights the neoplastic population and accentuates the nuclear irregularities. **C** Extensive bone marrow involvement by a monotonous population of uniform-looking cells. **D** The neoplastic cells stain positively for CD56.

EBV-positive T-cell and NK-cell lymphoproliferative diseases of childhood

Quintanilla–Martinez L.
Ko Y.-H.
Kimura H.
Jaffe E.S.

EBV-associated T-cell and NK-cell lymphoproliferative disorders in the paediatric age group can be categorized into two major groups: systemic EBV-positive T-cell lymphoma of childhood and chronic active EBV infection. Both occur with increased frequency in Asians and in Native Americans from Central and South America and Mexico. Systemic EBV-positive T-cell lymphoma of childhood has a very fulminant clinical course, usually associated with a haemophagocytic syndrome. Chronic active EBV infection of T- and NK-cell type shows a broad range of clinical manifestations, from indolent, localized forms such as hydroa vacciniforme–like lymphoproliferative disorder and severe mosquito bite allergy to more systemic disease characterized by fever, hepatosplenomegaly, and lymphadenopathy, with or without cutaneous manifestations diseases. Additionally, significant overlap in the morphological features of the following conditions is present. Therefore, correlation with clinical features is critical for accurate diagnosis.

Systemic EBV-positive T-cell lymphoma of childhood

Definition
Systemic EBV-positive T-cell lymphoma of childhood is a life-threatening illness of children and young adults, characterized by a clonal proliferation of EBV-infected T cells with an activated cytotoxic phenotype. It can occur shortly after primary acute EBV infection or in the setting of chronic active EBV infection (CAEBV). It has rapid progression, with multiorgan failure, sepsis, and death, usually within a timeframe of days to weeks. A haemophagocytic syndrome is nearly always present. This entity has some clinicopathological features overlapping with those of aggressive NK-cell leukaemia.

ICD-O code   9724/3

Synonyms and historical terminology
Historically, this process has been de-

Table 14.01 Classification of EBV-positive T-cell and NK-cell proliferations

Diagnosis	Usual patient age group(s)
EBV-positive haemophagocytic lymphohistiocytosis (benign, may be self-limited)	Paediatric, adolescent
Systemic CAEBV	Paediatric, adolescent
Cutaneous CAEBV, hydroa vacciniforme–like lymphoproliferative disorder	Paediatric, adolescent
Cutaneous CAEBV, severe mosquito bite allergy	Paediatric, adolescent
Systemic EBV-positive T-cell lymphoma	Paediatric, adolescent
Aggressive NK-cell leukaemia	Adult
Extranodal NK/T-cell lymphoma, nasal type	Adult
Nodal peripheral T-cell lymphoma, EBV-positive[a]	Adult
CAEBV, chronic active EBV infection.	

[a] Included within the category of peripheral T-cell lymphoma, NOS.

scribed using a variety of terms, including fulminant EBV-positive T-cell lymphoproliferative disorder of childhood {3269}, sporadic fatal infectious mononucleosis, fulminant haemophagocytic syndrome in children (in Taiwan, China) {3822}; fatal EBV-associated haemophagocytic syndrome (in Japan) {2011}; and severe CAEBV {2025,2963,3838}. The term fulminant or fatal haemophagocytic syndrome was used to describe a systemic disease secondary to acute primary EBV infection affecting previously healthy children, but the disease has since been shown to be a monoclonal CD8+ T-cell EBV-associated lymphoproliferative dis-

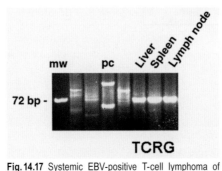

Fig. 14.17 Systemic EBV-positive T-cell lymphoma of childhood. PCR for TR gamma rearrangement demonstrates an identical T-cell clone in liver, spleen, and lymph nodes.

order, and is therefore now considered equivalent to systemic EBV-positive T-cell lymphoma of childhood {3269}. The term CAEBV was coined to describe an infectious mononucleosis–like syndrome persisting for at least 6 months and associated with high titres of IgG antibodies against EBV viral capsid antigen and early antigen, with no association with malignancy, autoimmune diseases, or immunodeficiency {3809}. Because the earliest described cases, which were found in western populations, showed EBV predominantly in B cells {779,3809}, CAEBV was originally thought to be a disorder affecting B cells, but has since been shown to affect primarily T cells and NK cells {780,2025,2026}. Progression to EBV-positive T-cell lymphoma is not unusual {1877,1918,2026,3269}. A more severe form of CAEBV, characterized by high fever, hepatosplenomegaly, extensive lymphadenopathy, haemophagocytic syndrome, and pancytopenia, has been described in patients in Japan {2025,2028,3838}. These patients had higher viral copy numbers in peripheral blood, as well as monoclonal expansion of EBV-infected T cells or NK cells. Severe CAEBV with monoclonal EBV-positive T-cell proliferation is part of the

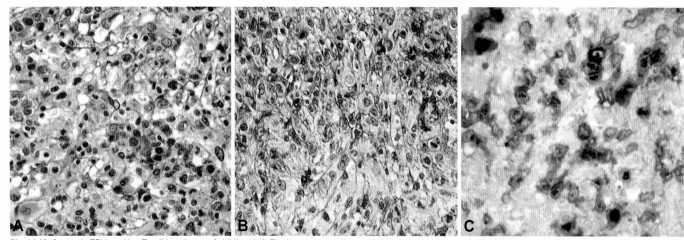

Fig. 14.18 Systemic EBV-positive T-cell lymphoma of childhood. **A** The bone marrow shows histiocytic hyperplasia with a lymphoid infiltrate composed of relatively large cells with bland nuclei and inconspicuous nucleoli. **B** CD8 is positive in the large lymphoid cells. **C** Double staining demonstrates that many of the CD8+ lymphocytes (brown) are also positive for EBV-encoded small RNA (EBER) (black).

spectrum of systemic EBV-positive T-cell lymphoma of childhood {2951,3269}; to avoid confusion, it should not be referred to as CAEBV.

Epidemiology
Systemic EBV-positive T-cell lymphoma of childhood is most prevalent in Asia, primarily in Japan and Taiwan, China {2011, 2025,3822,3838}. It has been reported in Mexico and in Central and South America, and is reported rarely in non-indigenous populations in western countries {3269}. It occurs most often in children and young adults. There is no sex predilection.

Etiology
Although the etiology of systemic EBV-positive T-cell lymphoma of childhood is unknown, its association with primary EBV infection and its racial predisposition strongly suggest a genetic defect in the host immune response to EBV {2011, 2025,3269,3822,3838}.

Localization
This is a systemic disease. The most commonly involved sites are the liver and spleen, followed by the lymph nodes, bone marrow, skin, and lungs {2011,2025, 3269,3822,3838}.

Clinical features
Previously healthy patients present with acute onset of fever and general malaise suggestive of an acute viral respiratory illness. Within a period of weeks to months, patients develop hepatosplenomegaly and liver failure, sometimes accompanied by lymphadenopathy. Laboratory tests show pancytopenia, abnormal liver function, and often abnormal EBV serology, with low or absent IgM antibodies against viral capsid antigen. The disease is usually complicated by haemophagocytic syndrome, coagulopathy, multiorgan failure, and sepsis {3269}. Some cases occur in patients with a well-documented history of CAEBV {1877,1918}. A disorder that is probably related but presents mainly with lymphadenopathy and high lactate dehydrogenase levels has recently been reported in children from Peru {3388}.

Spread
The disease is systemic, with the potential to involve all organ systems. However, involvement of the CNS is less often seen.

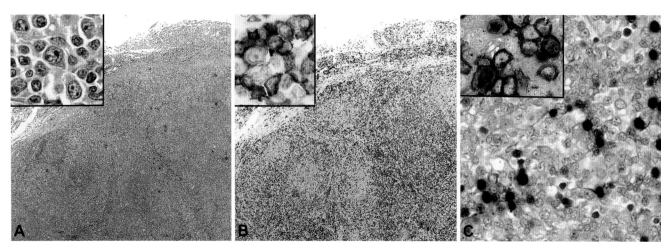

Fig. 14.19 Systemic EBV-positive T-cell lymphoma of childhood. Lymph node. **A** The lymph node shows partial preservation of the architecture with residual regressive follicles and expanded interfollicular area. Inset: The interfollicular infiltrate is polymorphic with some relatively large cells with irregular nuclei and prominent nucleoli. **B** The infiltrating lymphocytes are CD8-positive. Inset: The atypical cells are CD8-positive **C** Many cells are positive for EBV-encoded small RNA (EBER). Inset: Double staining demonstrates that the EBER-positive cells (black) are positive for CD8 (brown).

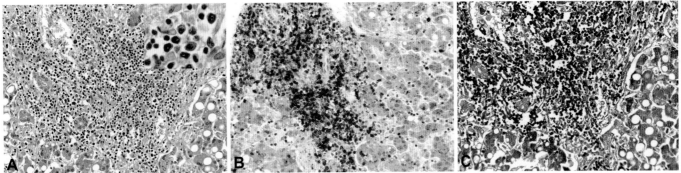

Fig. 14.20 Systemic EBV positive T-cell lymphoma of childhood. **A** The liver shows a dense lymphoid infiltrate in the portal tract with sinusoidal extension. Inset: The lymphoid cells are medium-sized with irregular nuclei. **B** The infiltrating lymphocytes are CD8-positive. **C** In situ hybridization for EBV-encoded small RNA (EBER) shows that the CD8+ cells are also positive for EBV RNA.

Microscopy

The infiltrating T cells are usually small and lack substantial cytological atypia {3269}. However, cases with pleomorphic medium-sized to large lymphoid cells, irregular nuclei, and frequent mitoses have been described {3838}. The liver and spleen show mild to marked sinusoidal infiltration, with striking haemophagocytosis. The splenic white pulp is depleted. The liver has prominent portal and sinusoidal infiltration, cholestasis, steatosis, and necrosis. The lymph nodes usually show preserved architecture with open sinuses. The B-cell areas are depleted, whereas the paracortical areas may be expanded and show a subtle to dense infiltration and a broad cytological spectrum ranging from small or medium-sized lymphocytes to large atypical lymphocytes with hyperchromatic and irregular nuclei. The more advanced the disease, the more depleted the lymph nodes look. A variable degree of sinus histiocytosis with erythrophagocytosis is present. Bone marrow biopsies show histiocytic hyperplasia with prominent erythrophagocytosis.

Immunophenotype

The neoplastic cells most typically have a CD2+, CD3+, CD56–, TIA1+ phenotype. Most cases secondary to acute primary EBV infection are CD8-positive {1952, 3269,3822}, whereas cases occurring in the setting of severe CAEBV are CD4-positive {1877,1918,3269}. Rare cases show both CD4+ and CD8+ EBV-infected T cells {3269}. EBV-encoded small RNA (EBER) is positive.

Postulated normal counterpart

A cytotoxic CD8+ T cell or activated CD4+ T cell

Genetic profile

The cells have monoclonally rearranged TR genes. All cases harbour EBV in a clonal episomal form {1877,2011,2025, 3838}. All cases analysed carry type A EBV, with either wildtype or the 30 bp–deleted product of the *LMP1* gene {1952, 3269,3838}. In situ hybridization for EBER shows that most of the infiltrating lymphoid cells are positive. No consistent chromosomal aberrations have been identified {675,2025,3707}.

Prognosis and predictive factors

Most cases have a fulminant clinical course resulting in death, usually within days to weeks of diagnosis. The disease is usually complicated by haemophagocytic syndrome. Few cases have been reported to respond to an etoposide- and dexamethasone-based regimen followed by allogeneic haematopoietic stem cell transplantation (the HLH-2004 protocol) {178,1611,1882,2026,3707}. The rapidly progressive clinical course is similar to that of aggressive NK-cell leukaemia.

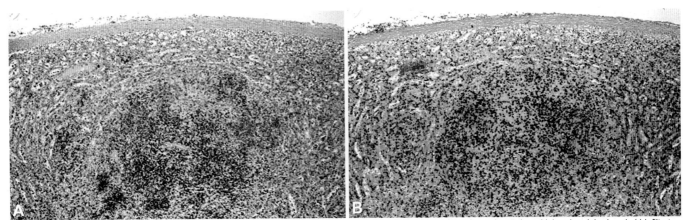

Fig. 14.21 Systemic EBV-positive T-cell lymphoma of childhood. **A** The spleen shows depletion of the white pulp and prominent sinusoidal and nodular lymphoid infiltrates. The nodules are composed predominantly of CD4+ cells. **B** In situ hybridization for EBV-encoded small RNA (EBER) shows that the CD4+ cells are also positive for EBV RNA.

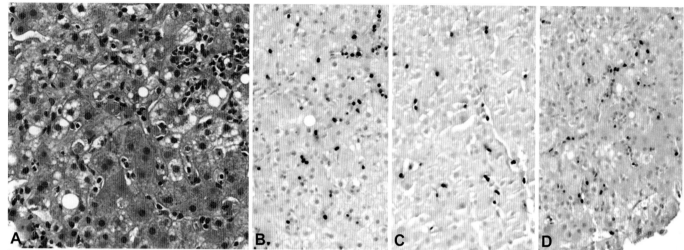

Fig. 14.22 Chronic active EBV infection of T-cell type in the liver. Sequential liver biopsies demonstrating stable disease without progression. **A** Liver biopsy shows single cell necrosis and a sinusoidal lymphocytic infiltrate. Lymphocytes (CD3+) do not show cytological atypia. **B,C,D** EBER in situ hybridization of sequential biopsies obtained over a period of four years shows no increase in EBER-positive cells over time.

Chronic active EBV infection of T- and NK-cell type, systemic form

Definition

Chronic active EBV infection (CAEBV) of T-cell or NK-cell type is a systemic EBV-positive polyclonal, oligoclonal, or (often) monoclonal lymphoproliferative disorder characterized by fever, persistent hepatitis, hepatosplenomegaly, and lymphadenopathy, which shows varying degrees of clinical severity depending on the host immune response and the EBV viral load. The revised diagnostic criteria for CAEBV include infectious mononucleosis–like symptoms persisting for >3 months, increased EBV DNA (> $10^{2.5}$ copies/mg) in peripheral blood, histological evidence of organ disease, and demonstration of EBV RNA or viral protein in affected tissues in patients without known immunodeficiency, malignancy, or autoimmune disorders.

Synonym

Systemic chronic active EBV infection of T-cell and NK-cell type

Epidemiology

Systemic CAEBV of T- and NK-cell type has a strong racial predisposition, with most cases reported from Asia, primarily in Japan {1954,2025,2026,2951, 3838}; the Republic of Korea {1676}; and Taiwan, China {4244}. It has also been reported in Latin America and rarely in western {3422,3592,3730} and African populations {3353}. It occurs most often in children and adolescents. Adult-onset disease is rare and appears to be rapidly progressive and more aggressive {124, 1792}. There is no sex predilection.

Etiology

Although the etiology is unknown, the strong racial predisposition for the development of CAEBV of T- and NK-cell type in immunocompetent individuals strongly suggests that genetic polymorphisms in

genes related to the EBV immune response are responsible for the development of this disease {780,2023}. EBV-specific cytotoxic T lymphocyte activity is impaired in patients with CAEBV {780,3829,4071}.

Localization

This is a systemic disease. The most commonly involved sites are the liver, spleen, lymph nodes, bone marrow, and skin. The lungs, kidneys, heart, CNS, and gastrointestinal tract can also be involved {2025,2026,3062}.

Clinical features

Approximately 50% of patients present with infectious mononucleosis–like illness, including fever, hepatosplenomegaly, and lymphadenopathy. Accompanying symptoms include skin rash (occurring in 26% of cases), severe mosquito bite allergy (in 33%), hydroa vacciniforme–like eruptions (in 10%), diarrhoea (in 6%), and uveitis (in 5%). Laboratory tests reveal pancytopenia and abnormal

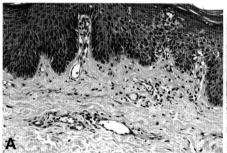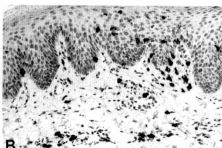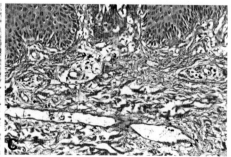

Fig. 14.23 Chronic active EBV infection in skin. **A** Skin biopsy shows a discrete lymphoid infiltrate without atypia in the dermis surrounding blood vessels, extending to the epidermis. **B** The lymphoid cells are positive for CD8. **C** The relatively discrete lymphoid infiltrate is positive for EBV as demonstrated by in situ hybridization for EBV-encoded small RNA (EBER).

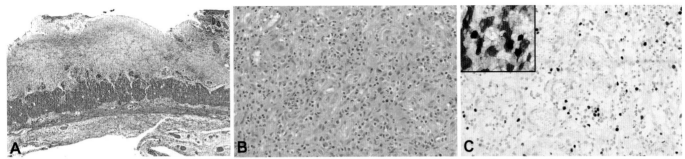

Fig. 14.24 Chronic active EBV infection of probable NK-cell type in the intestine of a 4-year-old girl with recurrent bowel perforation and NK-cell lymphocytosis. **A** Colon resection with ulceration of the mucosa. **B** The submucosa shows granulation tissue and a subtle lymphoid infiltrate without atypia. **C** In situ hybridization for EBV-encoded small RNA (EBER) shows scattered positive cells. Inset: Double staining shows that the EBER+ cells (brown) are CD3-positive (red). CD56 was positive in fewer cells (not shown).

liver function. In most patients, EBV serology reveals high titres of IgG antibodies against EBV viral capsid antigen and early antigen. All patients have increased levels of EBV DNA ($> 10^{2.5}$ copies/mg) in the peripheral blood. The clinical course varies but is usually protracted, with some patients surviving for many years without disease progression. The severity of CAEBV is probably related to the immunological response of the individual and to the EBV viral load. The clinical course also varies depending on the predominant infected cell type in the peripheral blood {2024,2025}. Patients with T-cell CAEBV have a shorter survival time than patients with NK-cell disease. Patients with T-cell CAEBV often present with prominent systemic symptoms and high titres of EBV-specific antibodies and have rapid disease progression. In contrast, patients with NK-cell disease, in addition to mild systemic symptoms, often have severe mosquito bite allergy, rash, and high levels of IgE, and do not always have elevated EBV-specific antibody titres. Life-threatening complications include haemophagocytic syndrome (which occurs in 24% of cases), coronary artery aneurysm (in 9%), hepatic failure (in 15%), interstitial pneumonia (in 5%), CNS involvement (in 7%), gastrointestinal perforation (in 11%), and myocarditis (in 4%). Due to the variety of the clinical presentations, diagnosis is often delayed. Progression to NK/T-cell lymphoma or aggressive NK-cell leukaemia occurs in 16% of cases {1676,2026,2028,2951}.

Microscopy

The infiltrating cells do not show changes suggestive of a neoplastic lymphoproliferation. The liver shows sinusoidal and portal infiltration suggestive of viral hepatitis. The spleen shows atrophy of the white pulp with congestion of the red pulp. The lymph nodes exhibit variable morphology, including paracortical and follicular hyperplasia, focal necrosis, and small epithelioid granulomas. Bone marrow biopsies usually appear normal. In cases complicated by haemophagocytic syndrome, sinus histiocytosis with erythrophagocytosis is present {2026}.

Immunophenotype

The immunophenotype of the EBV-infected cells varies; it includes T cells in 59% of cases, NK cells in 41%, and both T and NK cells in 4%. CAEBV of B-cell phenotype is seen in only 2% of cases. Unlike the T cells in systemic EBV-positive T-cell lymphoma of childhood, the T cells in CAEBV are predominantly CD4-positive, and less often show a cytotoxic CD8+ phenotype {780,2026}. EBV-encoded small RNA (EBER) is positive.

Cell of origin

The postulated cells of origin are CD4+ T cells, NK cells, cytotoxic CD8+ lymphocytes, and (rarely) gamma delta T cells.

Genetic profile

Chromosomal aberrations are detected in a minority of cases {2026}. One series reported monoclonally rearranged TR genes in 84% of cases, oligoclonally rearranged TR genes in 11%, and polyclonal TR genes in only 5% of cases {2026}. However, this report includes cases of 'severe CAEBV', which might be

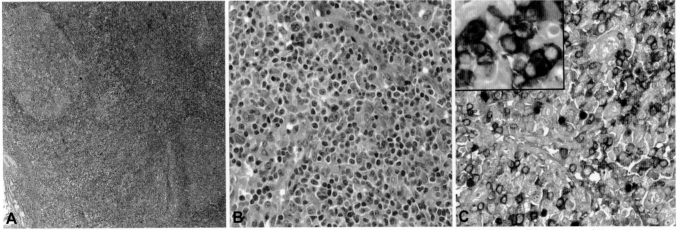

Fig. 14.25 Chronic active EBV infection in lymph node. **A** The lymph node shows follicular and paracortical hyperplasia. **B** At high magnification, the interfollicular areas show a polymorphic infiltrate lacking cytological atypia. **C** In situ hybridization for EBV-encoded small RNA (EBER) shows scattered positive cells. Inset: Double staining shows that the EBER+ cells (black) are CD4-positive (brown).

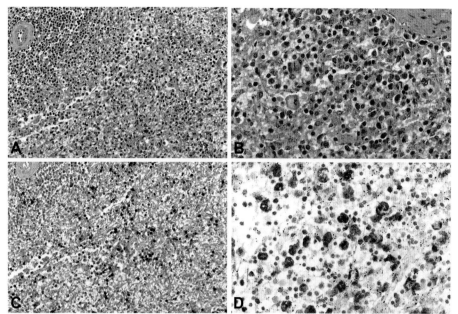

Fig. 14.26 Chronic active EBV infection of NK-cell type in spleen. Haemophagocytic syndrome. **A** The spleen shows white pulp atrophy with congestion of the red pulp. **B** Higher magnification shows that the red pulp is congested with a subtle lymphoid infiltrate and numerous histiocytes, some with erythrophagocytosis. **C** In situ hybridization for EBV-encoded small RNA (EBER) shows scattered positive cells. **D** CD4 staining highlights the abundant histiocytes with erythrophagocytosis. Note that most of the lymphoid cells are CD4-negative.

reclassified as systemic EBV+ T-cell lymphoma using the current WHO system. Somatic mutation of the perforin gene has been reported in one case {1956}.

Prognosis and predictive factors

The prognosis is variable, with some cases following an indolent clinical course and others constituting rapidly progressive disease. Patient age >8 years at onset of disease and liver dysfunction are risk factors for mortality. Adult patients with CD4+ T-cell infection may have more-aggressive disease. The 5-year survival rates associated with cases of T-cell type and NK-cell type, respectively, are 59% and 87%. Monoclonality of the proliferating cells does not correlate with increased mortality and does not warrant a diagnosis of lymphoma. Patients who undergo bone marrow transplantation have a better prognosis {2024,2025, 2026}. A specific classification of CAEBV based on cytology and clonality of the proliferating cells has been proposed {2951}. A1 cases are polymorphic and polyclonal; A2 cases are polymorphic and monoclonal; A3 cases are monomorphic and monoclonal; and B cases are monomorphic and monoclonal but with a fulminant course. The A1–A3 categories are thought to represent a continuous spectrum of CAEBV from lymphoproliferative disorder (A1–A2) to overt lymphoma (A3), whereas the B category is equivalent to systemic EBV-positive T-cell lymphoma of childhood.

Hydroa vacciniforme–like lymphoproliferative disorder

Definition

Hydroa vacciniforme (HV)–like lymphoproliferative disorder is a chronic EBV-positive lymphoproliferative disorder of childhood, associated with a risk of developing systemic lymphoma. HV-like lymphoproliferative disorder is a primarily cutaneous disorder of polyclonal or (most often) monoclonal T cells or NK cells, with a broad spectrum of clinical aggressiveness and usually a long clinical course. As the disease progresses, patients develop severe and extensive skin lesions and systemic symptoms including fever, hepatosplenomegaly, and lymphadenopathy. Classic HV, severe HV, and HV-like T-cell lymphoma constitute a continuous spectrum of EBV-associated HV-like lymphoproliferative disorder.

ICD-O code   9725/1

Synonyms and historical terminology

In western countries, classic HV was orig-

inally described as a benign photodermatosis characterized by light-induced vesicles that evolve to crusts and leave varicelliform scars after healing. It was noted that systemic symptoms were not observed and that the disease usually remitted spontaneously in adolescence {1395,1498,3731}. Because these cases were rarely biopsied, their clonality and EBV status were not thoroughly investigated. Subsequent studies in Asian populations showed that classic HV was an EBV-associated disorder {1806,1807}. A condition that clinically mimics classic HV was recognized in children and young adults who were mainly from Asia {1805} and Latin America {3456}. Patients with the condition present with marked facial oedema, vesicles, crusts, and large ulcers, sometimes with severe scarring and disfigurement. Unlike in classic HV, the skin lesions are not limited to sun-exposed areas and are not associated with light hypersensitivity; sun protection does not prevent the development of HV-like eruption. Because later studies demonstrated that these lesions are also associated with EBV infection {1807,2440} and often show monoclonal rearrangement of the TR genes {274}, the term HV-like lymphoma was suggested and was included in the 2008 WHO classification. However, given the broad clinical spectrum of the disease and the lack of reliable morphological or molecular criteria to predict its clinical behaviour (classic HV vs HV-like lymphoma), the term HV-like lymphopro-

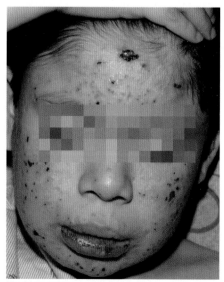

Fig. 14.27 Hydroa vacciniforme–like lymphoproliferative disorder. Sun-exposed areas of the skin exhibit a papulovesicular eruption. Many of the lesions are ulcerated, with a haemorrhagic crust.

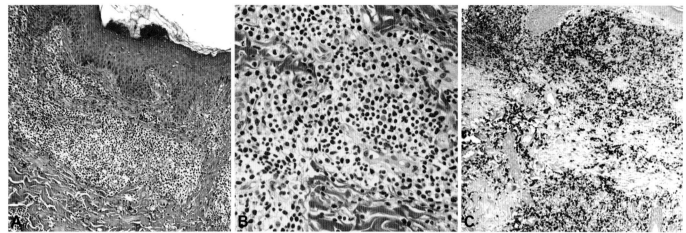

Fig. 14.28 Hydroa vacciniforme–like lymphoproliferative disorder. **A** The infiltrate is concentrated in the superficial dermis, but often extends to the subcutaneous tissue. **B** Neoplastic cells, which can be of T-cell or NK-cell lineage, are predominantly small, without marked atypia. **C** The lymphoid cells are positive for EBV, as demonstrated by in situ hybridization for EBV-encoded small RNA (EBER).

liferative disorder has been proposed, to encompass the various manifestations of the EBV-associated HV-like skin lesions {3271}. In the past, this disease has also been referred to as oedematous, scarring vasculitic panniculitis {3456}; angiocentric cutaneous T-cell lymphoma of childhood {2440}; hydroa-like cutaneous T-cell lymphoma {274}; and severe HV {1806}.

Epidemiology
This condition is seen mainly in children and adolescents from Asia {731,1805, 1806,2883,4397}, and in Native Americans from Central {1012} and South {274, 3389,3512} America and Mexico {2439, 3271}. The median patient age at diagnosis is 8 years (range: 1–15 years). The male-to-female ratio is slightly elevated (2.3:1). It is rare in adults {731,3512}.

Etiology
The etiology is unknown. The geographical and ethnic distribution indicate that, like in other EBV-positive T-cell and NK-cell lymphomas, genetic predisposition plays a major role.

Localization
This is a cutaneous condition that affects sun-exposed and non-exposed skin areas. In the early phases, it affects mainly the face, dorsal surface of the hands, and earlobes; in advanced stages, it can be generalized {3271}.

Clinical features
It is characterized by a papulovesicular eruption that generally proceeds to ulceration and scarring. The severity of the skin lesions and the clinical pre-

sentation varies between patients, with a broad spectrum. Some cases present with a very indolent course, with localized skin lesions in sun-exposed areas and no systemic symptoms (classic HV). Spontaneous remission and clearing after photoprotection can occur, but most cases show a long clinical course, with remissions and recurrences that may finally progress to more-severe disease {732}. There is seasonal variation, with increased recurrences in spring and summer. In more-severe cases, in addition to extensive skin lesions, systemic symptoms (including fever, wasting, lymphadenopathy, and hepatosplenomegaly) may be present, in particular late in the course of the disease {1806,2026, 3271,3512}. Some patients develop severe mosquito bite allergy {1639,3271}. A rare clinical presentation with primarily periorbital swelling has been reported in children from Bolivia {3206}.

Macroscopy
In addition to prominent swelling of the face, lips, and eyelids, multiple vesiculopapules with umbilication and crust are characteristic.

Microscopy
The characteristic histological feature of HV is epidermal reticular degeneration leading to intraepidermal spongiotic vesiculation. The lymphoid infiltrate predominates in the dermis but may extend deep into the subcutaneous tissue. The infiltrate is mainly located around adnexa and blood vessels, often with angiodestructive features. The intensity of the infiltrate and atypia of the lymphocytes

varies. The neoplastic cells are generally small to medium-sized, without significant atypia. In severe cases, the overlying epidermis is frequently ulcerated {3271}.

Immunophenotype
The cells have a cytotoxic T-cell phenotype, mostly CD8-positive, with few cases being CD4-positive. One third of the cases show an NK-cell phenotype, with expression of CD56 {1919,4484,2026, 3271,3389}. Clonal expansion of gamma delta T cells has been documented in the peripheral blood in most cases {1639, 2026,4224}, but only in rare cases in the infiltrating lymphocytes in the skin {2439, 3271,4224}. CCR4 is expressed in the gamma delta T cells {1917}. CD30 is often expressed in the infiltrating EBV-positive T cells. LMP1 is usually negative {3271}.

Postulated normal counterpart
The postulated normal counterpart is a skin-homing cytotoxic T cell or NK cell. Gamma delta T cells have been hypothesized to play a central role in the formation of HV-like eruptions {1972}.

Genetic profile
Most cases have clonal rearrangements of the TR genes. Some cases of NK-cell derivation do not show TR gene rearrangement {2026,3271}. In situ hybridization for EBV-encoded small RNA (EBER) is positive, but the number of positive cells varies from case to case. EBV is monoclonal by terminal repeat analysis. Although LMP1 is negative by immunohistochemistry, it can be detected in most cases by PCR in peripheral blood, indicating type II EBV latency {1804}.

Prognosis and predictive factors

The clinical course is variable, and patients may have recurrent skin lesions for as long as 10–15 years before progression to systemic involvement. With systemic spread, the clinical course is much more aggressive {1805}. T-cell clonality, the amount of EBV-positive cells, and/or the density of the infiltrate do not predict which patients will eventually progress to systemic disease or develop a systemic lymphoma. No standard treatment has been established. The disease is resistant to conventional chemotherapy, and treated patients often die of infectious complications {274,3512}. In indolent cases, a conservative approach is recommended, whereas haematopoietic stem cell transplantation has been introduced as a curative therapy in more advanced cases {2026,3271}.

Severe mosquito bite allergy

Definition

Severe mosquito bite allergy is an EBV-positive NK-cell lymphoproliferative disorder characterized by high fever and intense local skin symptoms, including erythema, bullae, ulcers, skin necrosis, and deep scarring following mosquito bites. Patients have NK-cell lymphocytosis in the peripheral blood and an increased risk of developing haemophagocytic syndrome and progressing into overt NK/T-cell lymphoma or aggressive NK-cell leukaemia in the longstanding clinical course.

Synonym

Hypersensitivity to mosquito bites

Epidemiology

Severe mosquito bite allergy is very uncommon. Most cases have been reported in Japan {1788,2025,2026,4016}, with a few cases from Taiwan, China {1158}; the Republic of Korea {730}; and Mexico {3024,3456}. The patient age at onset ranges from birth to 18 years (mean: 6.7 years) {4015}. There is no sex predilection.

Etiology

The etiology is unknown. Genetic background and environmental factors may play a role. Severe mosquito bite allergy is due to CD4+ T-cell proliferation in response to mosquito salivary gland secretions and plays a key role in the reactivation of EBV in NK cells inducing the expression of LMP1 {161}. LMP1 expression induces NK-cell proliferation and may be responsible for the development of aggressive NK-cell leukaemia {162, 4072}.

Localization

This is primarily a cutaneous condition.

Clinical features

Severe mosquito bite allergy is characterized by local skin symptoms including erythema, bullae, ulcers, necrosis, and scarring. High fever and general malaise are common symptoms. Patients have a high level of serum IgE, a high EBV DNA load in the peripheral blood, and NK-cell lymphocytosis. Lymphadenopathy, hepatosplenomegaly, hepatic dysfunction, haematuria, and proteinuria are occasionally seen in the clinical course. After recovering, patients are asymptomatic until the next mosquito bite. Common complications are progression to

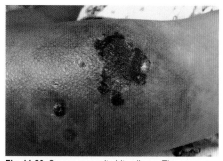

Fig. 14.29 Severe mosquito bite allergy. The upper arm shows extreme oedema and erythema with necrosis and haemorrhagic crust after a mosquito bite.

systemic chronic active EBV infection of NK-cell type, haemophagocytic syndrome, aggressive NK-cell leukaemia, and nasal-type extranodal NK/T-cell lymphoma {160,2025,2026}.

Microscopy

The skin biopsy at the bite site shows epidermal necrosis and ulceration or intraepidermal bullae. The dermis shows oedema and a dense infiltrate extending into the subcutaneous tissue. There is angioinvasion and angiodestruction. The infiltrate is polymorphic, with small lymphocytes, large atypical cells, histiocytes, and abundant eosinophils. The morphological characteristics are similar to those of hydroa vacciniforme–like lymphoproliferative disorder.

Immunophenotype

The infiltrating cells have an NK-cell phenotype, including positivity for CD3-epsilon and CD56, with expression of the cytotoxic molecules TIA1 and granzyme B. Reactive T cells, both CD4-positive and CD8-positive, are found at various intensities. LMP1 is rarely positive. CD30 is often positive in the EBV-infected cells.

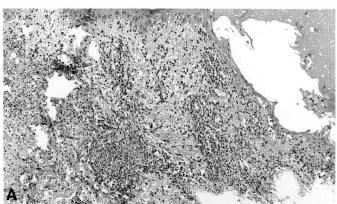
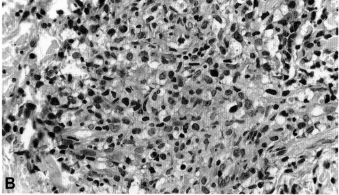

Fig. 14.30 Severe mosquito bite allergy. **A** Skin biopsy with a subepidermal bulla with a dense infiltrate in the dermis, mainly surrounding blood vessels. **B** Higher magnification. The infiltrate is polymorphic but mainly composed of relatively large cells with bland nuclei, inconspicuous nucleoli, and abundant cytoplasm.

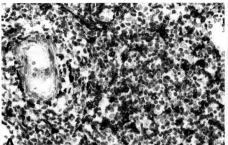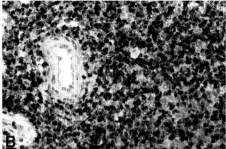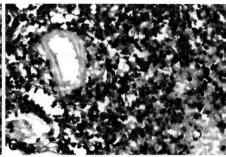

Fig. 14.31 Severe mosquito bite allergy. **A** CD56 is positive in a subset of the lymphoid cells. **B** The infiltrating lymphocytes are TIA1-positive. The infiltrate is composed of both NK and T cells. **C** The infiltrating lymphocytes are positive for EBV-encoded small RNA (EBER). The high density of EBER-positive cells raises concern for progression to lymphoma; clinical correlation is essential.

Postulated normal counterpart
Mature activated NK cell

Genetic profile
NK cells are infected with monoclonal EBV as demonstrated by terminal repeat analysis, indicating clonal expansion of NK cells. Rarely, monoclonal TR gene rearrangement has been documented {2025}. Chromosomal alterations are rarely identified {2026}. In situ hybridization for EBV-encoded small RNA (EBER) is positive in a fraction of the NK cells. LMP1 is detected by PCR in peripheral blood, indicating type II EBV latency {1804}.

Prognosis and predictive factors
Patients usually have a long clinical course, with an increased risk of developing haemophagocytic syndrome and aggressive NK-cell leukaemia after 2–17 years (median: 12 years). Patients with chromosomal aberrations appear to have a higher risk of developing lymphoma/leukaemia {2026,4015}.

Adult T-cell leukaemia/lymphoma

Ohshima K.
Jaffe E.S.
Yoshino T.
Siebert R.

Definition
Adult T-cell leukaemia/lymphoma (ATLL) is a mature T-cell neoplasm most often composed of highly pleomorphic lymphoid cells. The disease is usually widely disseminated and is caused by the human retrovirus HTLV-1. Most ATLL patients present with widespread lymph node involvement as well as involvement of peripheral blood. The histology shows remarkable pleomorphism, with several morphological variants having been described. The leukaemic cells often show a multilobed appearance of so-called flower cells. Neoplastic cells show monoclonal integration of HTLV-1 and express T-cell–associated antigens (CD2, CD3, CD5), but usually lack CD7. Most cases are CD4-positive and CD8-negative. ATLL most often occurs in regions endemic for HTLV-1, and the frequency is estimated to be 2.5% among HTLV-1 carriers. ATLL occurs only in adults, with an average patient age of 58 years. The male-to-female ratio is 1.5:1. ATLL is a systemic disease, and the prognosis is poor (Fig. 14.45, p. 367).

ICD-O code   9827/3

Synonyms
Adult T-cell lymphoma/leukaemia; adult T-cell leukaemia

Epidemiology
ATLL is endemic in several regions of the world, in particular south-western Japan, the Caribbean basin, and parts of central Africa. The distribution of the disease is closely linked to the prevalence of HTLV-1 in the population.
The disease has a long latency, and affected individuals are usually exposed to the virus very early in life. The virus may be transmitted in breast milk, as well as through exposure to peripheral blood and blood products. The cumulative incidence of ATLL is estimated to be 2.5% among HTLV-1 carriers in Japan {3869}. Sporadic cases have been described,

Table 14.02 Clinical spectrum of HTLV-1–associated diseases

Neoplastic disorders
Adult T-cell leukaemia/lymphoma
    Smouldering
    Chronic
    Acute
    Lymphomatous

Non-neoplastic disorders {2521}
   - HTLV-1–associated myelopathy
    (tropical spastic paraparesis)

   - HTLV-1–associated infective dermatitis

   - Other HTLV-1 inflammatory disorders
    Uveitis
    Thyroiditis
    Pneumonitis
    Myositis

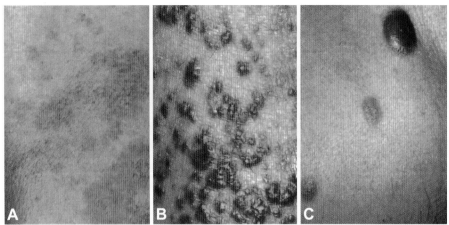
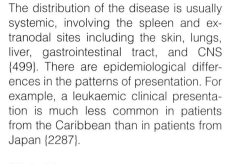

Fig. 14.32 Adult T-cell leukaemia/lymphoma. Macroscopic findings of cutaneous lesions have been classified as **A** erythema, **B** papules, and **C** nodules.

but the affected patients often derive from an endemic region of the world. ATLL occurs only in adults, and the patient age at onset ranges from the third to the ninth decade of life, with an average patient age of 58 years. The male-to-female ratio is 1.5:1 {4405}.

Etiology

HTLV-1 is causally linked to ATLL, but HTLV-1 infection alone is not sufficient to result in neoplastic transformation of infected cells. HTLV-1 enters cells mainly through cell-to-cell contact via three cellular molecules: heparan sulfate proteoglycan, neuropilin 1, and the glucose transporter GLUT1 {1352}. Neuropilin 1 appears to function as the viral receptor. The p40 tax viral protein leads to transcriptional activation of many genes in HTLV-1–infected lymphocytes {1241}. In addition, the HTLV-1 basic leucine zipper

factor (HBZ) is thought to be important for T-cell proliferation and oncogenesis {3532}. However, additional genetic alternations acquired over time may result in the development of a malignancy. Hypermethylation is associated with disease progression {3528}. HTLV-1 can also indirectly cause other diseases (Table 14.02), such as HTLV-1–associated myelopathy / tropical spastic paraparesis {3880}.

Localization

Most patients present with widespread lymph node involvement and involvement of the peripheral blood. The number of circulating neoplastic cells does not correlate with the degree of bone marrow involvement. This suggests that circulating cells are recruited from other organs, such as the skin, which is the most common extralymphatic site of involvement (involved in >50% of cases).

The distribution of the disease is usually systemic, involving the spleen and extranodal sites including the skin, lungs, liver, gastrointestinal tract, and CNS {499}. There are epidemiological differences in the patterns of presentation. For example, a leukaemic clinical presentation is much less common in patients from the Caribbean than in patients from Japan {2287}.

Clinical features

Several clinical variants have been identified: acute, lymphomatous, chronic, and smouldering (see Table 14.03) {3660}. The acute variant is most common and is characterized by a leukaemic phase, often with a markedly elevated white blood cell (WBC) count, skin rash, and generalized lymphadenopathy. Hypercalcaemia, with or without lytic bone lesions, is a common feature. Patients with acute ATLL have systemic disease accompanied by hepatosplenomegaly, constitutional symptoms, and elevated lactate dehydrogenase. Leukocytosis and eosinophilia are common. Many patients have an associated T-cell immunodeficiency, with frequent opportunistic infections such as *Pneumocystis jirovecii* pneumonia and strongyloidiasis.

The lymphomatous variant is characterized by prominent lymphadenopathy but without peripheral blood involvement. Most patients present with advanced-stage disease similar to the acute form, although hypercalcaemia is seen less often.

Cutaneous lesions are common in both the acute and the lymphomatous forms

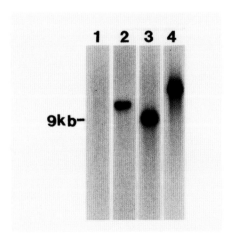

Fig. 14.33 Adult T-cell leukaemia/lymphoma. Southern blot analysis. Lanes 2-4 each display a single proviral HTLV-1 DNA band. The difference in band sizes (different cases) illustrates the difference in integration sites.

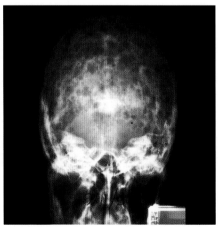

Fig. 14.34 Adult T-cell leukaemia/lymphoma. A radiograph shows extensive lytic bone lesions.

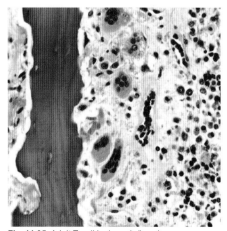

Fig. 14.35 Adult T-cell leukaemia/lymphoma. Bone marrow infiltrate is sparse. Osteoclastic activity surrounding the bone trabeculae is prominent.

of ATLL. They are clinically diverse and include erythematous rashes, papules, and nodules. Larger nodules may show ulceration.

The chronic variant is frequently associated with an exfoliative skin rash. An absolute lymphocytosis may be present, but atypical lymphocytes are not numerous in the peripheral blood. Hypercalcaemia is absent.

In the smouldering variant, the WBC count is normal with >5% circulating neoplastic cells. ATLL cells are generally small, with a normal appearance. Patients frequently have skin or pulmonary lesions, but there is no hypercalcaemia. Progression from the chronic or smouldering variant to the acute variant occurs in 25% of cases, usually after a long duration {3660}.

Imaging

In patients with hypercalcaemia, imaging studies may show lytic bone lesions. FDG-PET/CT is usually positive in sites of disease activity {582}.

Macroscopy

Macroscopic findings of the skin have been classified as erythema, papules, and nodules. Rare cases show tumour-like lesions or erythroderma as seen in Sézary syndrome.

Microscopy

ATLL is characterized by a broad spectrum of cytological features {2950}. Several morphological variants have been described, reflecting this varied cytology and referred to as pleomorphic small, medium, and large cell types, anaplastic, and a rare form resembling angioimmunoblastic T-cell lymphoma {2950}. The use of these variants is optional but they call attention to the spectrum of morphological appearances.

Table 14.03 Diagnostic criteria for clinical subtypes of adult T-cell leukaemia/lymphoma. Modified, from Shimoyama M {3660}

Clinical manifestation	Smouldering	Chronic	Acute
Lymphocytosis	No	Yes	Yes
Blood abnormal lymphocytes	>5%	Increased	Increased
Lactate dehydrogenase	Normal	Slightly increased	Increased
Calcium	Normal	Normal	Variable
Skin rash	Erythema, papules	Variable	Variable
Lymphadenopathy	No	Mild	Variable
Hepatosplenomegaly	No	Mild	Variable
Bone marrow infiltration	No	No	Variable

Some cases exhibit a leukaemic pattern of infiltration, with preservation or dilation of lymph node sinuses that contain malignant cells. The inflammatory background is usually sparse, although eosinophilia may be present. The neoplastic lymphoid cells are typically medium-sized to large, often with pronounced nuclear pleomorphism. The nuclear chromatin is coarsely clumped with distinct, sometimes prominent, nucleoli. Blast-like cells with transformed nuclei and dispersed chromatin are present in variable proportions {3660}. Giant cells with convoluted or multilobed nuclear contours may be present. Rare cases may be composed predominantly of small lymphocytes, with irregular nuclear contours. Cell size does not correlate with the clinical course {1818}, with the exception of the chronic and smouldering forms, in which the lymphocytes have a more normal appearance.

Lymph nodes in some patients in an early phase of adult T-cell lymphoma/leukaemia may exhibit a Hodgkin lymphoma–like histology {2953}. The lymph nodes have expanded paracortical areas containing a diffuse infiltrate of small to medium-sized lymphocytes with mild nuclear irregularities, indistinct nucleoli, and scant cytoplasm. EBV-positive B lymphocytes with Hodgkin-like features are interspersed in this background. The expansion of EBV-positive B cells is thought to be secondary to the underlying immunodeficiency seen in patients with ATLL.

In the peripheral blood, the multilobed appearance of the neoplastic cells has led to the term 'flower cells'. These cells have deeply basophilic cytoplasm, most readily observed with Giemsa staining of air-dried smears. Marrow infiltrates are usually patchy, ranging from sparse to moderate. Osteoclastic activity may be prominent, even in the absence of bone marrow infiltration by neoplastic cells.

Skin lesions are seen in >50% of patients with ATLL. Epidermal infiltration with Pautrier-like microabscesses is common {2950}. Dermal infiltration is mainly perivascular, but larger tumour nodules with extension to subcutaneous fat may be observed.

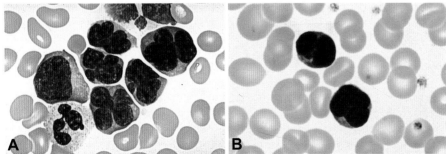

Fig. 14.36 Adult T-cell leukaemia/lymphoma (ATLL). Peripheral blood films. **A** In the acute variant, the leukaemic cells are medium-sized to large lymphoid cells with irregular nuclei and basophilic cytoplasm. The characteristic ATLL cells have been described as 'flower cells', with many nuclear convolutions and lobes. **B** ATLL cells in the chronic variant are generally small, with slight nuclear abnormalities such as notching and indentations.

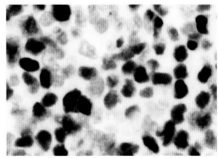

Fig. 14.37 Adult T-cell leukaemia/lymphoma cells frequently express FOXP3. The coexpression of FOXP3 and CD25 is characteristic of T regulatory (Treg) cells.

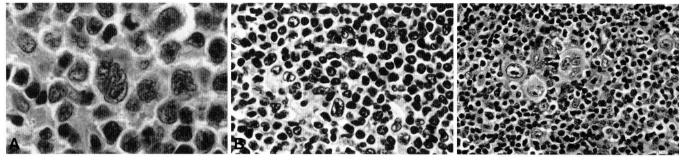

Fig. 14.38 Adult T-cell leukaemia/lymphoma (ATLL). **A** The pleomorphic (medium-sized and large cell) type shows a diffuse proliferation of atypical medium-sized to large lymphoid cells with irregular nuclei, intermingled with cerebriform giant cells (centre). **B** The lymph nodes in the pleomorphic small-cell type show a diffuse proliferation of atypical medium-sized to small lymphoid cells. **C** The presence of pleomorphic tumour cells and background eosinophilia may simulate classic Hodgkin lymphoma.

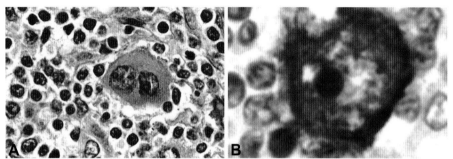

Fig. 14.39 Adult T-cell leukaemia/lymphoma (ATLL). **A** The lymph nodes in Hodgkin-like ATLL show Reed–Sternberg–like giant cells of B-cell (not T-cell) lineage, which (**B**) react with CD30 antibody and are EBV-positive (not shown).

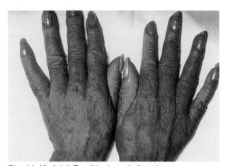

Fig. 14.40 Adult T-cell leukaemia/lymphoma, smouldering variant. Diffuse exfoliative skin rash.

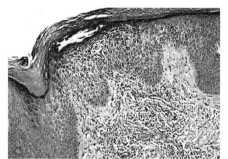

Fig. 14.41 Adult T-cell leukaemia/lymphoma, smouldering variant. A sparse infiltrate in the skin is seen with minimal cytological atypia.

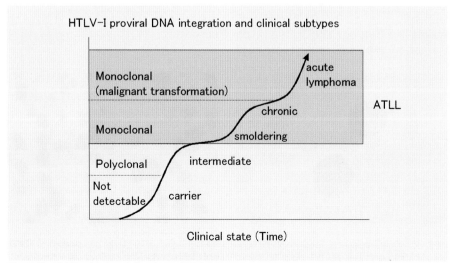

Fig. 14.42 Adult T-cell leukaemia/lymphoma (ATLL). HTLV-1 proviral DNA integration and clinical subtypes.

Diffuse infiltration of many organs is indicative of the systemic nature of the disease and of the presence of circulating malignant cells.

Immunophenotype

Tumour cells express T-cell–associated antigens (CD2, CD3, CD5), but usually lack CD7. Most cases are CD4-positive and CD8-negative, but a few are CD4-negative and CD8-positive or double-positive for CD4 and CD8. CD25 is strongly expressed in nearly all cases. The large transformed cells may be positive for CD30, but are negative for ALK {3882} and cytotoxic molecules. Tumour cells frequently express the chemokine receptor CCR4. FOXP3, a feature of T regulatory (Treg) cells, is expressed in a subset of cases {1948,3398}, but often only in a subset of the neoplastic cells.

Postulated normal counterpart

The postulated normal counterpart is a peripheral CD4+ T cell. It has been hypothesized that the CD4+, CD25+, FOXP3+ Treg cells are the closest normal counterparts {1948}, which would be consistent with the disease's characteristic association with immunodeficiency.

Grading

There is no formal grading system for ATLL. However, the four clinical variants – acute (leukaemic), lymphomatous, chronic, and smouldering – vary in their clinical course and cytological atypia {3660}. In the chronic and smouldering forms the neoplastic cells are small, and can have minimal cytological atypia. Pronounced cytological atypia is seen in the acute and lymphomatous forms.

Genetic profile
Antigen receptor genes
TR genes are clonally rearranged {2952}.

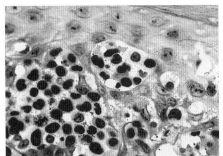

Fig. 14.43 Adult T-cell leukaemia/lymphoma. Neoplastic cells infiltrate the epidermis, producing Pautrier-like microabscesses.

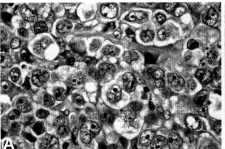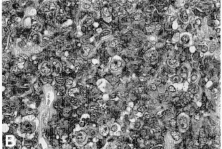

Fig. 14.44 Adult T-cell leukaemia/lymphoma. **A** In this case, the infiltrate consists of large cells with anaplastic features. **B** The cells are strongly CD30-positive, raising the differential diagnosis of anaplastic large cell lymphoma.

Oncogenes and other molecular changes

Neoplastic cells show monoclonal integration of HTLV-1. No clonal integration is present in healthy carriers {4075}. Tax, encoded by the HTLV-1 pX region, is a critical non-structural protein that plays a key role in leukaemogenesis and activates a variety of cellular genes {3126}. Enhancement of cAMP response element-binding transcription factor (CREB) phosphorylation by Tax appears to play a role in leukaemogenesis {2022}. CREB is highly phosphorylated in a panel of HTLV-1–infected human T-cell lines, and Tax is responsible for promoting elevated levels of CREB phosphorylation. However, Tax is not critical to sustained tumour cell growth and is inactivated in a high proportion of cases of ATLL {1957}. *HBZ* also appears to play a critical role in tumorigenesis {4487}. *HBZ* is the only gene that is consistently expressed in all ATLL cases; it modulates a variety of cellular signalling pathways that are related to cell growth, immune response, and T-cell differentiation. In whole-transcriptome sequencing, *CCR4* mutations have been detected in one quarter of cases, and are associated with gain of function and increased PI3K signalling {2808}.

A recent study ({1957}, reviewed in {4193}) provided an integrated genomic and transcriptomic analysis of >400 ATLL cases. The authors identified a single viral integration site in most cases of ATLL, confirming the clonal nature of the disease. Transcriptome analysis confirmed the critical role of *HBZ*, which is expressed at high levels in all cases. ATLL showed considerable genomic instability, with a high number of structural variations per case. A total of 50 genes were recurrently mutated. Among the most frequently mutated genes were *PLCG1*, *PRKCB*, *VAV1*, *IRF4*, *FYN*, *CARD11*, and *STAT3*, some

of which are involved in T-cell receptor signalling. This study also confirmed a high incidence of *CCR4* mutations and identified mutations in *CCR7* in some other cases. The additional mutations identified affect the NF-kappaB pathway and genes involved in T-cell signalling. Whole-genome sequencing identified intragenic deletions involving *TP73*, a homologue of *TP53*. These deletions resulted in mutant p73, lacking the transactivation domain (TAD). Recurrent splice-site mutations were found in *GATA3*, *HNRNPA2B1*, and *FAS*.

ATLL genomes demonstrated prominent CpG island DNA hypermethylation, leading to transcriptome silencing of many genes, including genes encoding major histocompatibility complex (MHC) class I, death receptors, and immune checkpoints, providing a mechanism for immune escape of the tumour cells {1957}.

Prognosis and predictive factors

Clinical subtype, patient age, performance status, and serum calcium and lactate dehydrogenase levels are major prognostic factors {4410}. The survival time for the acute and lymphomatous variants ranges from 2 weeks to > 1 year. Death is often caused by infectious complications, including *P. jirovecii* pneumonia, cryptococcal meningitis, disseminated herpes zoster, and hypercalcaemia {3660}. The chronic and smouldering forms have a more protracted clinical course and better survival, but can progress to an acute phase with an aggressive course in approximately 25% of patients {1961,2954}.

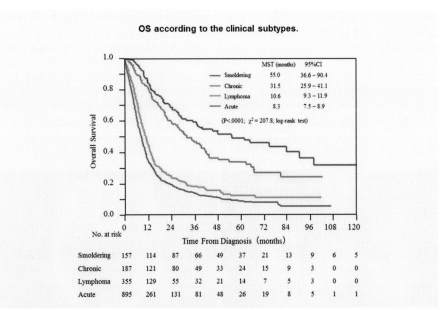

Fig. 14.45 Adult T-cell leukaemia/lymphoma. Overall survival (OS) of 1665 patients diagnosed between 2000 and 2009 in Japan. A total of 227 patients underwent allogeneic bone marrow transplantation; 25% of those patients had long survival. MST, median survival time. Data from Katsuya H et al. {1961}.

Extranodal NK/T-cell lymphoma, nasal type

Chan J.K.C.
Quintanilla-Martinez L.
Ferry J.A.

Definition

Extranodal NK/T-cell lymphoma, nasal type, is a predominantly extranodal lymphoma of NK-cell or T-cell lineage, characterized by vascular damage and destruction, prominent necrosis, cytotoxic phenotype, and association with EBV. It is designated an NK/T-cell lymphoma because although most cases appear to be genuine NK-cell neoplasms, some cases are of cytotoxic T-cell lineage.

ICD-O code   9719/3

Synonyms

Angiocentric T-cell lymphoma (obsolete); malignant reticulosis, NOS (obsolete); malignant midline reticulosis (obsolete); polymorphic reticulosis (obsolete); lethal midline granuloma (obsolete); T/NK-cell lymphoma

Epidemiology

Extranodal NK/T-cell lymphoma is more prevalent in Asians and the indigenous populations of Mexico, Central and South America {187,640,2232,3266,3949}. It occurs most often in adults, with a reported median patient age of 44–54 years {189,647,704,1484,1858,2305,3062, 3210}. It is more common in males than in females.

Etiology

The very strong association with EBV, irrespective of the ethnic origin of the patients, suggests a pathogenic role of the virus {133,647,649,1091,1916,3266, 4133}. EBV is present in a clonal episo-

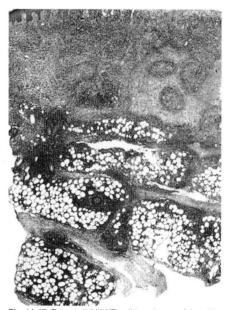

Fig. 14.47 Extranodal NK/T-cell lymphoma of the skin. The lymphomatous infiltrate involves the epidermis, dermis, and subcutaneous tissue. Necrosis is prominent in the dermal component.

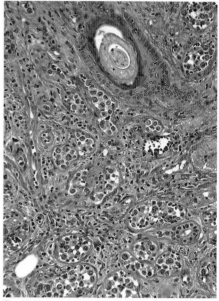

Fig. 14.48 Extranodal NK/T-cell lymphoma of the skin, intravascular variant. Neoplastic cells are confined to vascular spaces. Note the uninvolved hair follicle and glandular structures.

mal form {133,649,1091,1646,1916,2607, 3266,3842,4133} with type II latency (EBNA1+, EBNA2–, LMP1+), and commonly shows a 30 bp deletion in the *LMP1* gene {708,1000,1091,2139,3868}. Most studies show that the EBV is almost always of subtype A {275,1091,1484,3120, 3842,4023}. The disease activity can be monitored by measuring circulating EBV DNA; a high titre is correlated with extensive disease, unfavourable response to therapy, and poor survival {188,4257}. Extranodal NK/T-cell lymphomas can occur in the setting of immunosuppres-

sion, including following transplantation {1702,2156}.

Localization

Extranodal NK/T-cell lymphoma almost always has an extranodal presentation. The upper aerodigestive tract (nasal cavity, nasopharynx, paranasal sinuses, and palate) is most commonly involved, with the nasal cavity being the prototypical site of involvement. Preferential sites of extranasal involvement include the skin, soft tissue, gastrointestinal tract, and testes. Some cases may be accompanied by secondary lymph node involvement {640, 647,1996,2154,3154,4023}. Rare cases with features of intravascular lymphoma have been reported, involving sites such as the skin and CNS {2138,2372,2810, 4385}.

Primary EBV-positive nodal T-cell or NK-cell lymphomas have been reported {178, 718, 1901}. These usually have a monomorphic pattern of infiltration and lack the angiodestruction and necrosis seen in extranodal NK/T-cell lymphoma. They are more common in elderly patients, or

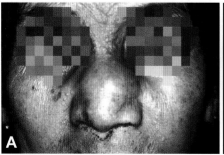
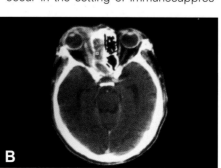

Fig. 14.46 Extranodal NK/T-cell lymphoma, nasal type. **A** Expansion of the nasal bridge. **B** CT. The tumour in the nasal cavity extends upwards into the orbit, resulting in proptosis.

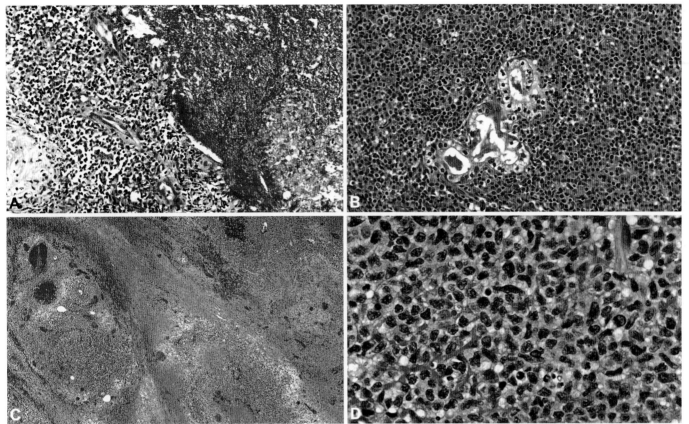

Fig. 14.49 Extranodal NK/T-cell lymphoma, nasal type. **A** Prominent ulceration and necrosis in the nasal mucosa. **B** The nasal mucosa is diffusely infiltrated and expanded by an abnormal lymphoid infiltrate. The mucosal glands commonly show a peculiar clear-cell change. **C,D** Nasal-type NK/T-cell lymphoma in the testis. There is a diffuse dense lymphoid infiltrate, with prominent coagulative necrosis (C). The neoplastic cells appear monotonous and are medium-sized (D).

in the setting of immune deficiency. They are considered a variant of peripheral T-cell lymphoma, NOS, and seem distinct from cases with primary extranodal presentations.

Clinical features

Patients with nasal involvement present with symptoms of nasal obstruction or epistaxis due to the presence of a mass lesion, or with extensive destructive midfacial lesions (lethal midline granuloma). The lymphoma can extend to adjacent tissues, such as the nasopharynx, paranasal sinuses, orbits, oral cavity, palate, and oropharynx. The disease is often localized to the upper aerodigestive tract at presentation, and bone marrow involvement is uncommon {4356}. The disease may disseminate to various sites (e.g. the skin, gastrointestinal tract, testes, and cervical lymph nodes) during the clinical course. Some cases may be complicated by haemophagocytic syndrome {704, 2154}.

Extranodal NK/T-cell lymphomas occurring outside of the upper aerodigestive tract (often referred to as extranasal NK/T-cell lymphomas) have variable presentations, depending on the major site of involvement. Skin lesions are commonly nodular, often with ulceration. Intestinal lesions often manifest as perforation or gastrointestinal bleeding. Other involved sites present as mass lesions. The patients commonly have high stage disease at presentation, with involvement of multiple extranodal sites. Systemic symptoms such as fever, malaise, and weight loss can be present {647,1996,4357}. Lymph

nodes can be involved as part of disseminated disease. Marrow and peripheral blood involvement can occur, and such cases may overlap with aggressive NK-cell leukaemia.

Microscopy

The histological features of extranodal NK/T-cell lymphoma are similar irrespective of the site of involvement. Mucosal sites often show extensive ulceration. The lymphomatous infiltrate is diffuse and permeative. Mucosal glands often

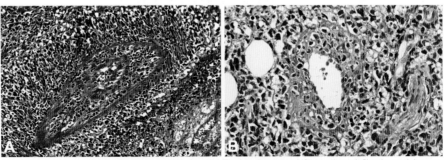

Fig. 14.50 Extranodal NK/T-cell lymphoma, nasal type. **A** The lymphomatous infiltrate shows infiltration and destruction of an artery. **B** In this case involving the skin, the lymphomatous infiltrate has an angiocentric angiodestructive quality.

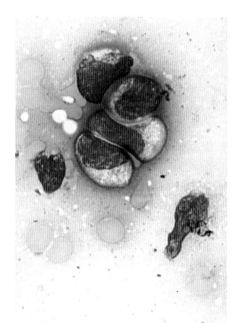

Fig. 14.51 Extranodal NK/T-cell lymphoma, nasal type. Touch preparation of a nasal tumour (Giemsa stain). Azurophilic granules are evident in the pale cytoplasm of the lymphoma cells.

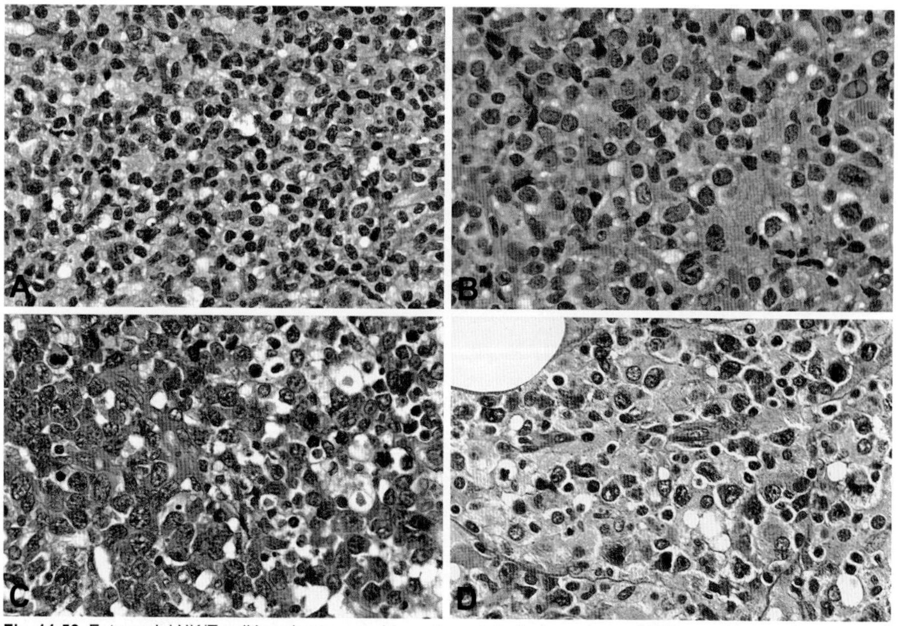

Fig. 14.52 Extranodal NK/T-cell lymphoma, nasal type: the cytological spectrum. **A** This nasal tumour is composed predominantly of small cells with irregular nuclei. **B** Medium-sized cells with pale cytoplasm. **C** Large cells. **D** Nasal-type extranodal NK/T-cell lymphoma of skin, with pleomorphic large cells admixed with smaller cells.

become widely spaced or are lost. An angiocentric and angiodestructive growth pattern is frequently present, and fibrinoid changes can be seen in the blood vessels even in the absence of angioinvasion. Coagulative necrosis and admixed apoptotic bodies are common findings. These have been attributed to vascular occlusion by lymphoma cells, but other factors (e.g. chemokines and cytokines) have also been implicated {3943}.

The cytological spectrum is very broad. Cells may be small, medium-sized, large, or anaplastic. In most cases, the lymphoma is composed of medium-sized cells or a mixture of small and large cells. The cells often have irregularly folded nuclei, which can be elongated. The chromatin is granular, except in the very large cells, which may have vesicular nuclei. Nucleoli are generally inconspicuous or small. The cytoplasm is moderate in amount and often pale to clear. Mitotic figures are easily found, even in small cell–predominant lesions. On Giemsa-stained touch preparations, azurophilic granules are commonly detected. Ultrastructurally, electron-dense membrane-bound granules are present.

Extranodal NK/T-cell lymphomas, particularly those in which small-cell or mixed-cell populations predominate, and those accompanied by a heavy admixture of inflammatory cells (small lym-

phocytes, plasma cells, histiocytes, and eosinophils), may mimic an inflammatory process {640,1591}. The lymphoma can sometimes be accompanied by florid pseudoepitheliomatous hyperplasia of the overlying epithelium {2355}.

Immunophenotype

The most typical immunophenotype of extranodal NK/T-cell lymphoma is: CD2+, CD5–, CD56+, surface CD3– (as demonstrated on fresh or frozen tissue), and cCD3-epsilon+ (as demonstrated on fresh, frozen, or fixed tissues) {640,648, 1814,1819,3266,4069}. CD56, although a highly useful marker for NK cells, is not specific for extranodal NK/T-cell lymphoma, and can be expressed in some peripheral T-cell lymphomas. CD43 and CD45RO are often positive, and CD7 is

variably expressed. Other T-cell–associated and NK-cell–associated antigens, including CD4, CD8, CD16, and CD57, are usually negative. The subset of cases of cytotoxic T-cell lineage may express CD5, CD8, and T-cell receptor (gamma delta or alpha beta) {1858,3210,4407}. Cytotoxic molecules (e.g. granzyme B, TIA1, and perforin) are positive {1091}. HLA-DR, CD25, FAS (also known as CD95), and FASL are commonly expressed {2858,2955}. CD30 is positive in about 30% of cases {189,1484,2021, 2139,2305}. Nuclear expression of megakaryocyte-associated tyrosine kinase (MATK) is common {3210,3890}.

Lymphomas that demonstrate a CD3-epsilon+, CD56– immunophenotype are also classified as extranodal NK/T-cell lymphomas if both cytotoxic molecules

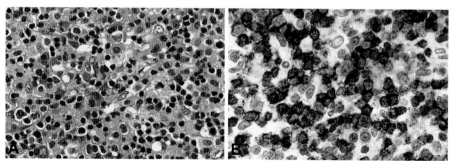

Fig. 14.53 Extranodal NK/T-cell lymphoma, nasal type. **A** This example is difficult to diagnose because the neoplastic cells are practically indistinguishable from normal small lymphocytes. There are many admixed plasma cells. **B** The presence of large numbers of cells staining for CD56 supports a diagnosis of lymphoma.

and EBV are positive, because these cases show a similar clinical disease as cases with CD56 expression {2859}. On the other hand, nasal or other extranodal lymphomas that are CD3+ and CD56– but negative for EBV and cytotoxic molecules should be diagnosed as peripheral T-cell lymphoma, NOS.

The diagnosis of extranodal NK/T-cell lymphoma should be considered with scepticism if EBV is negative {518,649, 1091,2139,2859,3850,3868}. On the other hand, EBV can occasionally occur in other T-cell lymphoma types, so EBV positivity does not always equate with a diagnosis of extranodal NK/T-cell lymphoma {3850}. In situ hybridization for EBV-encoded small RNA (EBER) is the most reliable way to demonstrate the presence of EBV, with virtually all lymphoma cells being labelled. Immunostaining for EBV LMP1 is often negative, consistency with EBV latency type 1.

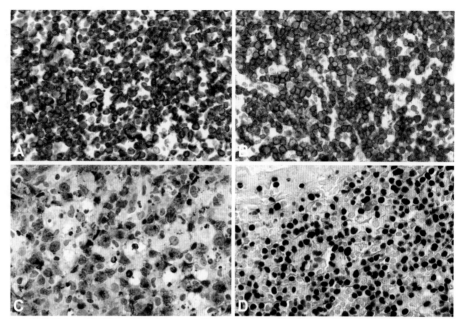

Fig. 14.54 Extranodal NK/T-cell lymphoma, nasal type. The neoplastic cells show strong staining for cCD3-epsilon (**A**) and CD56 (**B**). **C** The neoplastic cells show strong granular staining for granzyme B. **D** In situ hybridization for EBV-encoded small RNA (EBER). In this nasal tumour, virtually all the neoplastic cells show nuclear labelling.

Postulated normal counterpart
Activated NK cells and (less commonly) cytotoxic T cells

Grading
The prognostic importance of cytological grade is controversial; some studies suggest that tumours composed predominantly of small cells are less aggressive, but other studies have not shown this feature to be of significance on multivariate analysis {275,704,1645,2139,2305, 3210}. The International Peripheral T-cell Lymphoma Project reports that the presence of > 40% transformed cells predicts worse overall survival in nasal (but not extranasal) cases {189}.

Genetic profile
Antigen receptor genes
TR and IG genes are in germline configuration in most cases. Clonal TR gene rearrangements are reported in 10–40% of cases, presumably the cases of cytotoxic T lymphocyte derivation {189,1858,2058, 2305,2859,3210,3868}.

Gene expression profiling
The gene expression profiles of all extranodal NK/T-cell lymphomas cluster together, irrespective of NK-cell or gamma delta T-cell lineage {1728,1773}. Non-hepatosplenic gamma delta T-cell lymphomas show very similar gene expression profiles.

Cytogenetic abnormalities and oncogenes
A variety of cytogenetic aberrations have been reported, but so far no specific chromosomal translocations have been identified. The commonest cytogenetic abnormality is del(6)(q21q25) or i(6)(p10), but it is unclear whether this is a primary or progression-associated event {3688, 3689,4002,4359}. Comparative genomic hybridization studies show that the commonest aberrations are gain of 2q and loss of 1p36.23-36.33, 6q16.1-27, 4q12, 5q34-35.3, 7q21.3-22.1, 11q22.3-23.3, and 15q11.2-14 {2817}.

Recurrent mutations, deletions, and hypermethylation have been found in the genes encoding RNA helicase *DDX3X*, members of the JAK/STAT signalling pathway (*STAT3*, *STAT5B*, *JAK3*, and *PTPRK*) and other signalling pathways (*KIT* and *CTNNB1*), tumour suppressors (*TP53*, *MGA*, *PRDM1*, *ATG5*, *AIM1*, *FOXO3*, and *HACE1*), oncogenes (the RAS family of genes and *MYC*), epigenetic modifiers (*KMT2D/MLL2*, *ARID1A*, *EP300*, and *ASXL3*), cell-cycle regulators (*CDKN2A*, *CDKN2B*, and *CDKN1A*), and apoptosis regulators (*FAS*) {429,686, 1678,1727,1859,1946,2027,2083,2158, 2159,2160,3062,3268}.

Prognosis and predictive factors
The prognosis of nasal NK/T-cell lymphoma is variable, with some patients responding well to therapy and others dying of disseminated disease despite aggressive therapy. Historically, the survival rate has been poor (30–40%), but the survival has improved in recent years with more intensive therapy including upfront radiotherapy {275,704,705, 719,841,2058,2154,2317}. Significant unfavourable prognostic factors include advanced-stage disease (stage III or IV), unfavourable International Prognostic Index (IPI), invasion of bone or skin, high circulating EBV DNA levels, presence of EBV-positive cells in bone marrow, and a high Ki-67 proliferation index (> 40–65%) {189,705,719,1724,1860,2018,2251, 2859,3210}.

Extranasal NK/T-cell lymphoma is highly aggressive, with short survival and poor response to therapy {189,640,647,1858, 3210}. However, rare cases of primary cutaneous NK/T-cell lymphoma may pursue a protracted clinical course {655,740, 1791}.

Intestinal T-cell lymphoma

Introduction

Jaffe E.S.
Chott A.
Ott G.
Chan J.K.C.

Bhagat G.
Tan S.Y.
Stein H.
Isaacson P.G.

Recent data have led to changes in the categorization of intestinal T-cell lymphomas. It has become apparent that the two subtypes formerly designated as variants of enteropathy-associated T-cell lymphoma (EATL) are distinct {178,3850}. Type I EATL, now simply designated as EATL, is closely linked to coeliac disease, and is primarily a disease of individuals of northern European origin. Type II EATL, now formally designated as monomorphic epitheliotropic intestinal T-cell lymphoma (MEITL), shows no association with coeliac disease, and appears relatively increased in incidence in Asian and Hispanic populations. EATL generally has a polymorphic cellular composition and wide range in cytology, whereas MEITL is monomorphic, is usually positive for CD8 and CD56, and expresses megakaryocyte-associated tyrosine kinase (MATK). Gains in chromosome 8q24.2 involving *MYC* are seen in a high proportion of cases of MEITL but not EATL. Many cases of MEITL are derived from gamma delta T cells, but exceptions exist; some cases are T-cell receptor–silent and some cases express the alpha beta T-cell receptor. Likewise, most cases of EATL express the alpha beta T-cell receptor, but gamma delta variants exist. Mutations in *STAT5B* and *SETD2* have been associated with gamma delta MEITL, but investigations of classic EATL or alpha beta cases are limited {2160,2869A}. Both forms of intestinal T-cell lymphoma are clinically aggressive and almost always occur in adults. They are negative for EBV, which is strongly associated with nasal-type extranodal NK/T-cell lymphoma; this disease can present with intestinal disease {3210}. There remains a small group of intestinal T-cell lymphomas that do not meet the criteria for EATL or MEITL as currently defined {178}. These should be designated as intestinal T-cell lymphoma, NOS. They are clinically aggressive, usually have a cytotoxic phenotype, and may present in either the small or large bowel. Such cases often manifest other extra-nodal sites of disease, so it may be difficult to confirm the intestine as the primary site. They generally lack the epitheliotropism seen in EATL and MEITL.

A new provisional entity is also included within the broad group of intestinal T-cell neoplasms. Indolent T-cell lymphoproliferative disorder of the gastrointestinal tract is a clonal T-cell disorder that can involve multiple sites in the gastrointestinal tract, but is most common in the small bowel {3145}. In this condition, the mucosa is infiltrated by a monotonous population of small mature-appearing lymphocytes. Most cases express CD8, with fewer cases reported positive for CD4 {2506}. The clinical course is indolent, although rare cases progressing to more aggressive disease have been described.

Enteropathy-associated T-cell lymphoma

Bhagat G.
Jaffe E.S.
Chott A.
Ott G.

Chan J.K.C.
Tan S.Y.
Stein H.
Isaacson P.G.

Definition

Enteropathy-associated T-cell lymphoma (EATL), previously designated type I EATL, is a neoplasm of intraepithelial T cells that occurs in individuals with coeliac disease and exhibits varying degrees of cellular pleomorphism. It commonly presents as a tumour composed of medium-sized to large lymphocytes, often accompanied by a component of chronic inflammatory cells. The adjacent small intestinal mucosa shows villous atrophy, crypt hyperplasia, and increased intraepithelial lymphocytes. Lymphomas composed of monomorphic medium-sized cells (formerly called type II EATL) are now considered to constitute a distinct entity (monomorphic epitheliotropic intestinal T-cell lymphoma).

ICD-O code   9717/3

Synonyms

Enteropathy-type intestinal T-cell lymphoma; classic enteropathy-associated T-cell lymphoma; malignant histiocytosis of the intestine (obsolete)

Epidemiology

EATL is the most common subtype of primary intestinal T-cell lymphoma in western countries, accounting for almost two thirds of all cases {932}. It is uncommon in many Asian countries due to the low population frequency of coeliac HLA risk alleles. EATL characteristically occurs in the sixth and seventh decades of life and shows a slight male predominance, with a male-to-female ratio of 1.04–2.8:1 {932,1276,2456,3675,4177}. It is seen with greater frequency in areas with a high prevalence of coeliac disease, such as Europe (0.05–0.14 cases per 100 000 population) {583,3675,

Table 14.04 Comparison of enteropathy-associated T-cell lymphoma (EATL) and monomorphic epitheliotropic intestinal T-cell lymphoma (MEITL)

Feature	EATL	MEITL
Ethnicity (excess incidence)	Northern European	Asian, Hispanic
Risk factors	Coeliac disease, HLA-DQ2/DQ8	None recognized
Morphology	Polymorphic	Monomorphic
Usual immunophenotype	CD3+, CD5–, CD4–, CD8–, CD56–, CD103+, CD30+/–, cytotoxic +	CD3+, CD5–, CD4–, CD8+, CD56+, CD103+/–, CD30–, cytotoxic +
T-cell receptor expression	Alpha beta > gamma delta	Gamma delta > alpha beta
Localization	Small intestine	Small intestine

4177} and the USA (0.016 cases per 100 000 population) {3637}.

The prevalence of EATL in the coeliac population is 0.22–1.9 cases per 100 000 population {171,814,823,1295}.

Etiology

EATL is a recognized complication of coeliac disease or gluten-sensitive enteropathy {1437,2913,3857}. The association of EATL with coeliac disease is borne out by the detection of anti-endomysial (or anti-tissue transglutaminase 2) antibodies, the presence of HLA-DQ2 or HLA-DQ8 alleles, clinical findings such as dermatitis herpetiformis, and demonstration of gluten sensitivity in EATL patients, and a protective effect of gluten-free diet on EATL development {171,814, 1438,1672,1708,2913,3676}.

Coeliac disease may be diagnosed prior to (20–73%) or concomitant with (10–58%) EATL, and occasionally only at autopsy, because some individuals might have lifelong so-called 'silent' gluten sensitivity {876,1276,2456,2899,3675}. Risk factors for EATL include homozygosity for the HLA-DQ2 allele {49} and advanced age {2456}.

Localization

The small intestine is involved in >90% of EATLs, most commonly the jejunum and ileum {932,1276,2456,3675}, and multifocal lesions are observed in 32–54% of cases {1276,2456}. Other common gastrointestinal sites include the large intestine and stomach {932}. EATL might oc-

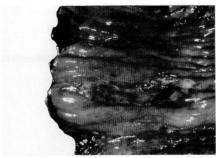

Fig. 14.55 Enteropathy-associated T-cell lymphoma. Jejunum showing circumferentially oriented ulcers.

casionally present at extragastrointestinal sites (e.g. the skin, lymph nodes, spleen, or CNS) {932,1389,2456,4080}, usually in cases evolving from type 2 refractory coeliac disease {2454,2456,4186}.

Clinical features

EATL most commonly presents with abdominal pain (65–100%) and gluten-insensitive malabsorption or diarrhoea (40–70%) in individuals without prior symptoms, or recurrence of symptoms in those with a history of adult-onset (or occasionally childhood-onset) coeliac disease and prior response to a gluten-free diet {599,876,932,1081,1276,2456, 2899,3675}. Other presentations include weight loss (50–80%), anorexia, fatigue or early satiety and nausea or vomiting due to intestinal obstruction, and (not infrequently) intestinal perforation (25–50%) or haemorrhage {599,876,932, 1081,1276,2456,2899,3675}.

B symptoms, besides weight loss, are present in less than one third of patients {876,1276,2899}. The duration of symptoms prior to diagnosis varies widely {1276}, but is <3 months in most cases {3675}. Elevated lactate dehydrogenase levels are observed in 25–62%, low serum albumin in 76–88%, and low haemoglobin in 54–91% of patients {932,1276, 2456,3675}. In a proportion, there is a prodromal period of refractory coeliac disease, which is sometimes accompanied by intestinal ulceration (ulcerative jejunitis) {169,223}. A haemophagocytic syndrome occurs in 16–40% of patients {90,2456}.

Imaging

Endoscopy is used to visualize sites of EATL involvement within the gastrointestinal tract. Double balloon enteroscopy and wireless capsule endoscopy are useful when ulceration, strictures, or large masses are present.

CT is the standard imaging modality for staging EATL. FDG-PET and MRI enteroclysis are useful in screening for the development of EATL in patients with refractory coeliac disease and for assessment of treatment response {1507,1660,4144}.

Spread

Common sites of disease dissemination include the intra-abdominal lymph nodes (affected in 35% of cases), bone marrow (in 3–18%), lungs or mediastinal lymph nodes (in 5–16%), liver (in 2–8%), and skin (in 5%) {932,2456,3675}. The CNS may be involved in occasional cases {352}.

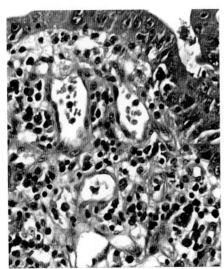

Fig. 14.56 Enteropathy-associated T-cell lymphoma. Only rare large neoplastic lymphocytes are present within the epithelium.

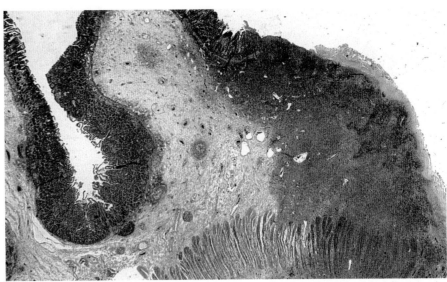

Fig. 14.57 Enteropathy-associated T-cell lymphoma. The overlying mucosa is ulcerated and the infiltrate invades the muscularis propria.

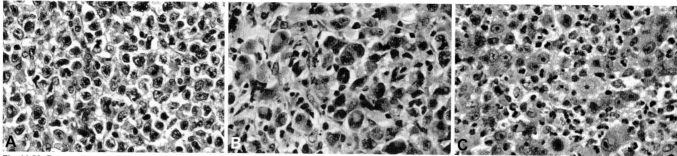

Fig. 14.58 Enteropathy-associated T-cell lymphoma. **A** Tumour cells are characterized by moderate amounts of eosinophilic cytoplasm and round or angulated nuclei with prominent nucleoli. **B** Anaplastic variant. **C** There is a heavy infiltrate of eosinophils between the tumour cells.

Staging

The Ann Arbor staging system, with or without the modification proposed by Rohatiner et al. {3394}, is frequently used for staging EATL. High stage disease is detected in 43–90% of patients at diagnosis {932,1276,2456,3675}.

Macroscopy

The tumour may form ulcerating nodules, plaques, strictures, or (less commonly) a large exophytic mass. The uninvolved mucosa can be thin and can show loss of mucosal folds. The mesentery and mesenteric lymph nodes are commonly involved. Occasionally, lymph node infiltration by EATL occurs in the absence of macroscopic evidence of intestinal disease.

Microscopy

The neoplastic lymphocytes exhibit a wide range of cytological appearances {2456,4370}. Most lymphomas show pleomorphic medium-sized to large cells with round or angulated vesicular nuclei, prominent nucleoli, and moderate to abundant pale-staining cytoplasm. As many as 40% of cases exhibit predominant large cell or anaplastic cytomorphology {2456}. Angiocentricity and angioinvasion, as well as extensive areas of necrosis, are frequently observed. Most tumours have an admixture of inflammatory cells, including large numbers of histiocytes and eosinophils, which may obscure the relatively small number of neoplastic cells in some cases. Intraepithelial spread of tumour cells may be striking, but sometimes only single scattered atypical lymphocytes are observed in the epithelium. The intestinal mucosa

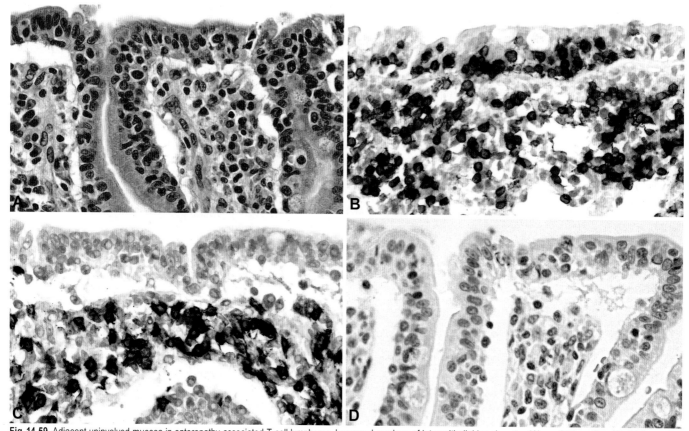

Fig. 14.59 Adjacent uninvolved mucosa in enteropathy-associated T-cell lymphoma. Increased numbers of intraepithelial lymphocytes (**A**) are CD3-positive (**B**), CD8-negative (**C**), and CD56-negative (**D**).

adjacent to EATL, especially in the jejunum, usually shows features of coeliac disease, i.e. villous atrophy, crypt hyperplasia, intraepithelial lymphocytosis, and increased lymphocytes and plasma cells within the lamina propria {746,747}. However, these alterations are highly variable. Sometimes only an increase in intraepithelial lymphocytes is noted, and occasionally the jejunum appears near-normal {223}.

The mesenteric lymph nodes can show intrasinusoidal and/or paracortical infiltration by EATL. However, some cases display various degrees of necrosis in the absence of morphologically recognizable lymphoma. Abdominal (and extra-abdominal) lymph nodes may also show a spectrum of degenerative changes, including dissolution of the node and replacement with lymph fluid (so-called lymph node cavitation) {1706,2573}.

Immunophenotype

The neoplastic lymphocytes are usually CD3+, CD5–, CD7+, CD4–, CD8–, and CD103+, and they express cytotoxic granule–associated proteins (e.g. TIA1, granzyme B, and perforin). However, variability in the immunophenotype is observed. CD8 may be expressed by 19–30% of cases, overall {746,2456, 2794}, with a higher frequency (50%) reported in patients without a history of refractory coeliac disease, type II {2456}. In a minority of cases, the lymphoma cells express cytoplasmic T-cell receptor (TCR) beta {746,2794} or TCR gamma {178,644} chains, or rarely both. The frequency of CD30 expression varies in the different cytomorphological variants, but almost all EATLs manifesting large cell morphology are CD30+ {2456}. The immunophenotype of the intraepithelial lymphocytes in uninvolved areas may be normal in de novo EATLs, but in most cases preceded by type 2 refractory coeliac disease, the intraepithelial lymphocytes exhibit an aberrant phenotype similar to that of the EATL.

Postulated normal counterpart

Small intestinal intraepithelial T cells have been postulated to be the normal counterparts of EATL cells, on the basis of shared immunophenotypic features {2456,3748}. Most EATL cells correspond to conventional intraepithelial T cells (type A), expressing the CD8 alpha beta heterodimer.

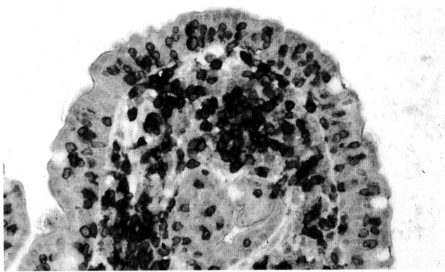

Fig. 14.60 Refractory coeliac disease. Small intestinal mucosa immunostained sequentially for CD3 (alkaline phosphatase, blue) and CD8 (peroxidase, brown). Most intraepithelial lymphocytes are CD3+, CD8–.

Grading
Precursor lesions

EATL may be preceded by refractory coeliac disease, also referred to as refractory sprue, which is defined as persistent gastrointestinal symptoms and abnormal small intestinal mucosal architecture with increased intraepithelial lymphocytes despite a strict gluten-free diet for ≥6–12 months {3446}. The diagnosis of refractory coeliac disease requires exclusion of coeliac disease–related conditions (e.g. bacterial overgrowth, microscopic colitis, and lymphoma) and other small intestinal disorders (e.g. common variable immunodeficiency and autoimmune enteropathy) {2914}. Refractory coeliac disease can be primary (lack of response to gluten-free diet at diagnosis) or secondary (symptom onset after a variable duration of a gluten-free diet).

The range of reported prevalence rates of refractory coeliac disease is wide (1.5–10%) {140,2256,2914,3416,3445}. However, a recent epidemiological survey suggests a much lower prevalence in the community (0.31% in coeliacs) {1755}. Similar to in EATL, the duration and dose of gluten exposure are considered risk factors, based on the high frequency of HLA-DQ2 homozygosity {49,2454} and older patient age (majority > 50 years) {1755,2454,3445}.

Refractory coeliac disease is considered to be a biologically heterogeneous entity {50,2454,3416,3445}, and it is currently categorized into two types based on immunophenotypic and molecular criteria {874}.

Type 1 refractory coeliac disease

The small intestinal intraepithelial lymphocytes have a normal phenotype, i.e. they express CD8 and surface CD3 and TCR. Polyclonal products are detected on TR gene rearrangement analysis. Small intestinal histology is similar to that observed in uncomplicated coeliac disease. Type 1 refractory coeliac disease accounts for 68–80% of all refractory coeliac disease cases {50,875,1755, 2454,3416,3445}. Surreptitious gluten ingestion is thought to sustain intestinal inflammation in many cases {1669}, and transition to an autoimmune state is suspected in a minority {2458}. No genetic or molecular alterations have been identified in this disease subtype. The symptoms are milder than those of type 2 refractory coeliac disease {2454}. The 5-year survival rate is high (80–96%), and the risk for developing EATL is low (3–14% in 4–6 years) {50,1755,2454,3445}.

Type 2 refractory coeliac disease

The small intestinal intraepithelial lymphocyte immunophenotype is aberrant, i.e. CD8, surface CD3, and TCR expression is absent. However, CD8 expression may be detected on a subset of intraepithelial lymphocytes by flow cytometry in as many as one third of cases {601}. The intraepithelial lymphocytes usually do not express CD5, and variable downregulation or loss of other T-cell antigens can be seen. CD30 expression is considered to indicate transformation to EATL {1162}. Clonal products are detected on TR gene rearrangement analysis. The degree of

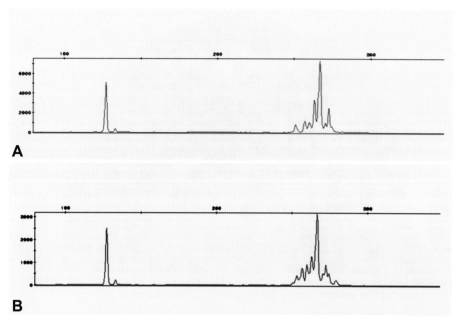

Fig. 14.61 Enteropathy-associated T-cell lymphoma (EATL). **A** Capillary gel electrophoresis showing a clonal TRB gene rearrangement product (dominant peak on the right) in a duodenal biopsy sample from an individual with type 2 refractory coeliac disease. **B** Capillary gel electrophoresis showing a similar clonal TRB gene rearrangement in an EATL that arose in the stomach a couple of years later.

villous atrophy is usually severe (subtotal or total). The intraepithelial lymphocytes lack significant cytological atypia, but they can be widely distributed throughout the gastrointestinal tract {599,2454, 4186}. Small aggregates of lymphocytes are seen in the lamina propria in approximately half of the cases {4178}. Some cases exhibit ulcerated mucosa associated with variable degrees of chronic inflammation and a relative paucity of intraepithelial lymphocytes (ulcerative jejunitis) {169,223,599}.

The identification of TR gene rearrangements of similar size in biopsies exhibiting features of type 2 refractory coeliac disease and concurrent or subsequent EATL helped establish that the aberrant intraepithelial lymphocytes are precursors of EATL in a proportion of cases and that they constitute a neoplastic population (low-grade lymphoma of intraepithelial T lymphocytes, EATL in situ, or cryptic EATL) {169,223,562,599,4371}.

In most cases, the aberrant intraepithelial lymphocytes are considered to be of alpha beta TCR lineage. However, recent studies have suggested that some cases might derive from gamma delta TCR T cells or possibly immature T/NK-cell precursors (innate immune cells), and that the maturational state of the cell of origin could impact the risk of extraintestinal dissemination and transformation to

EATL {3571,3864}. Disruption of intestinal immune homeostasis by deregulated expression of IL15 contributes to disease pathogenesis {7,1747,2635,2639}. IL15 also increases survival of the aberrant intraepithelial lymphocytes {2457}, which can facilitate genomic instability and acquisition of genetic abnormalities.

Recurrent gains of chromosome 1q22-44 are detected in type 2 refractory coeliac disease in common with EATL {297,937, 2454,4187,4471}. This finding suggests early acquisition of chromosome 1q abnormalities in the evolution of EATL. Loss of p16 protein, in the absence of LOH at chromosome 9p21, is observed in 40% of type 2 refractory coeliac disease cases exhibiting features of ulcerative jejunitis, and aberrant nuclear p53 expression can be detected in 57% of cases in the absence of molecular lesions of TP53 {2923}.

Most patients have severe symptoms and they usually have profound malnourishment (body mass index < 18) due to protein-losing enteropathy {1755,2454, 3445}. Large ulcers or stenotic areas are frequently observed on endoscopy {2454}. As systemic dissemination of aberrant intraepithelial lymphocytes occurs in a high proportion of cases (44–60%), patients may present with extraintestinal symptoms or disorders (e.g. skin lesions) {2454,4178,4186}. The 5-year survival

rate is low (44–58%), with 30–52% of patients developing EATL over the course of 4–6 years {50,1755,2454,3445}. The current chemotherapy and bone marrow transplantation regimens used for EATL are ineffective in eradicating the aberrant clonal intraepithelial lymphocytes {445, 2455,3446}.

Genetic profile

TRB or TRG genes are clonally rearranged in virtually all cases {169,2456, 2794}. Unlike primary nodal peripheral T-cell lymphoma, most EATLs (~80%) either display gains of the 9q34 region, which harbours known proto-oncogenes (e.g. NOTCH1, ABL1, and VAV2) or, alternatively, show deletions of 16q12.1 {297, 596,937,4471}. Similar changes are also observed in monomorphic epitheliotropic intestinal T-cell lymphoma. However, EATLs frequently display chromosomal gains of chromosomes 1q and 5q, which are less common in monomorphic epitheliotropic intestinal T-cell lymphoma {937,4471}.

Losses at 9p are detected in 18% of EATLs; however, LOH at 9p21, targeting the cell-cycle inhibitor CDKN2A/B is observed in 56% of cases, accompanied by loss of p16 protein expression {2923, 4471}. Loss of the 17p12-13.2 region, containing the TP53 tumour suppressor gene, is noted in 23% of EATLs, but aberrant nuclear p53 expression can be seen in 75% of cases {937,2923}. Recent studies have reported recurrent mutations in constituents of the JAK-STAT signalling pathway in EATL {2869A}. Additionally, the detection of JAK1 and STAT3 mutations in type 2 refractory coeliac disease implicates deregulation of JAK-STAT signalling to be an early event in disease pathogenesis {1116A}.

Genetic susceptibility

Coeliac disease, or gluten-sensitive enteropathy, predisposes to EATL. Coeliac disease is a polygenic disorder with various risk loci associated, including the HLA locus. EATL is associated with the HLA-DQA1*0501 and HLA-DQB1*0201 genotypes {49}. More than 90% of EATL patients carry HLA-DQ2.5 heterodimers encoded by HLA-DQA1*05 and HLA-DQB1*02 alleles, either in cis or trans configuration {1708}.

Prognosis and predictive factors

The prognosis of EATL patients is poor, due to the usually multifocal nature of the disease and a high rate of intestinal recurrence {743}. The median survival is 7 months, and 1-year and 5-year overall survival rates are 31–39% and 0–59%, respectively {50,876,1081,1276,2456, 2899}. Better outcomes have been reported for patients receiving intensive chemotherapy and autologous stem cell transplantation (with 5-year overall and progression-free survival rates of 60% and 52%, respectively) {3675}. However, an Eastern Cooperative Oncology Group (ECOG) score > 1 is noted in 88% of patients, and many have a poor performance status, making them poor candidates for chemotherapy {1276,3675}. Moreover, response to most current chemotherapy regimens is suboptimal.

Prognostic factors are not well established for EATL. Disease stage and the International Prognostic Index (IPI) are not useful in predicting survival. Chemotherapy and surgical resection are associated with prolonged survival, and low serum albumin with an adverse outcome {2456}. Malnutrition, which is common in EATL patients with prior type 2 refractory coeliac disease, is considered responsible for their markedly lower 5-year survival rate (0–8%) {50,2456}. The Prognostic Index for T-cell Lymphoma (PIT) has been shown to be useful in predicting survival of EATL patients {932}. Recently, an EATL prognostic index (EPI) has been developed that can distinguish three risk groups and reportedly performs better than the IPI and PIT {888}.

Monomorphic epitheliotropic intestinal T-cell lymphoma

Jaffe E.S.
Chott A.
Ott G.
Chan J.K.C.
Bhagat G.
Tan S.Y.
Stein H.
Isaacson P.G.

Definition

Monomorphic epitheliotropic intestinal T-cell lymphoma (MEITL) is a primary intestinal T-cell lymphoma derived from intraepithelial lymphocytes. Unlike in the classic form of enteropathy-associated T-cell lymphoma (EATL), there is no clear association with coeliac disease {3850}. The neoplastic cells have medium-sized

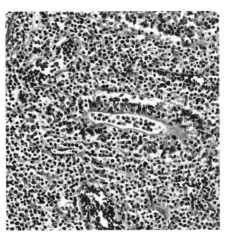

Fig. 14.62 Monomorphic epitheliotropic intestinal T-cell lymphoma. The mucosa is diffusely infiltrated by medium-sized lymphoid cells with round nuclei and dispersed chromatin.

round nuclei with a rim of pale cytoplasm. There is usually florid infiltration of intestinal epithelium. An inflammatory background is absent, and necrosis is usually less evident than in classic EATL. Based on distinctive pathological and epidemiological features, and to facilitate distinction from EATL, this disease is no longer referred to as type II EATL.

ICD-O code 9717/3

Synonym
Type II enteropathy-associated T-cell lymphoma

Epidemiology
MEITL has a worldwide distribution. There is no clear association with coeliac disease. It accounts for the vast majority of cases of primary intestinal T-cell lymphoma occurring in Asia, and also appears to occur with increased frequency in individuals of Hispanic origin {644, 1299,3832}. Males are affected more often than females; the male-to-female ratio is approximately 2:1.

Localization
The disease most often presents in the small intestine, with the jejunum affected more often than the ileum. Tumour masses, with or without ulceration, are common. Diffuse spread within the intestinal mucosa is often seen. Involvement of mesenteric lymph nodes is common. There can also be involvement of the stomach (occurring in 5% of cases) or the large bowel (in 16%) {4070}. With dissemination, multiple extranodal sites may be affected.

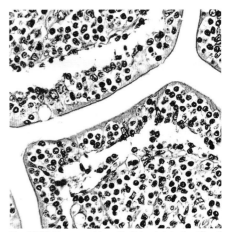

Fig. 14.63 Monomorphic epitheliotropic intestinal T-cell lymphoma. The neoplastic cells have clear cytoplasm. Note the prominent epitheliotropism by tumour cells.

Clinical features
The tumour presents with symptoms referable to the intestinal lesions, such as abdominal pain, obstruction or perforation, weight loss, diarrhoea, and gastrointestinal bleeding {644,4070}. A history of malabsorption is generally absent.

Spread
Diffuse spread of tumour cells in the adjacent mucosa is common. There is risk of dissemination to many extranodal sites, as well as regional lymph nodes.

Microscopy
The neoplastic lymphocytes are generally medium in size {747}. The nuclei are round and regular in appearance, with finely dispersed chromatin and inconspicuous nucleoli. There is a generous rim of pale cytoplasm. Within a given tumour the nuclear appearance is

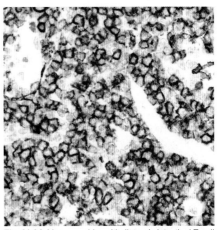

Fig. 14.64 Monomorphic epitheliotropic intestinal T-cell lymphoma. CD56 staining is diffusely positive.

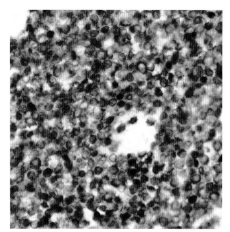

Fig. 14.65 Monomorphic epitheliotropic intestinal T-cell lymphoma. This case was positive for T-cell receptor gamma expression.

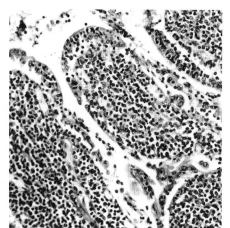

Fig. 14.66 Monomorphic epitheliotropic intestinal T-cell lymphoma. The villi are markedly widened and infiltrated by tumour cells.

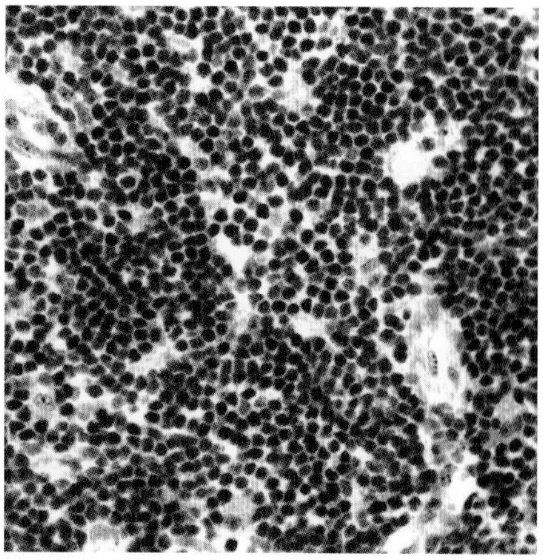

Fig. 14.67 Monomorphic epitheliotropic intestinal T-cell lymphoma. MATK shows strong nuclear expression in nearly all tumour cells, a helpful feature in the differential with enteropathy-associated T-cell lymphoma.

generally uniform, although the disease shows variation in cell size between patients. The tumour cells show prominent epitheliotropism. The villous architecture is distorted, and broadly expanded villi may be present. Unlike in classic EATL (formerly type I EATL), an inflammatory background is absent. Areas of necrosis are uncommon.

Immunophenotype

MEITL has a distinctive immunophenotype, being positive for CD3, CD8, and CD56 in the vast majority of cases {746}. Most tumours lack CD5, a feature suggesting a gamma delta T-cell derivation. Expression of T-cell receptor (TR) gamma is often positive, although some cases express TR beta {178,3889}. In a minority of cases, the tumour cells are TR-silent, or rarely both TR gamma and TR beta are expressed {644}. One study reported a high incidence of CD8 alpha homodimers (CD8 alpha alpha) {3889}. The cytotoxic granule–associated protein TIA1 is usually positive, but expression of other cytotoxic molecules (including granzyme B and perforin) is less consistent {4021}. Approximately 20% of cases show aberrant expression of CD20 {3889}. Most cases express MATK, a marker helpful in the distinction from EATL {3890} if present in > 80% of tumour cells.

Cell of origin

MEITL arises from an intraepithelial T cell, which can be of either gamma delta or alpha beta derivation. These intestinal intraepithelial cells have a distinct ontogeny and function {1593,3255}.

Grading

All cases are clinically aggressive, irrespective of cell size.

Genetic profile

Clonal rearrangement of the TR genes is seen in > 90% of cases. Extra signals for *MYC* at 8q24.2 are commonly seen {937}. Gains at 9q34.3 may be identified by FISH and copy-number analysis, and are the most common genetic change, seen in > 75% of cases {937,2056, 4021}. Other aberrations include gains at 1q32.3, 4p15.1, 5q34, 7q34, 8p11.23, 9q22.31, 9q33.2, 8q24.2 (*MYC* locus), and 12p13.31 and losses of 7p14.1 and 16q12.1 {2807,4021}. Compared with classic EATL, gains at 1q32.2-41 and 5q34-35.5 are seen less often {2807}.

Activating mutations in *STAT5B* have been identified in a high proportion of cases {2160}; in one study, 63% of cases had mutations in *STAT5B* when examined by whole-exome sequencing {2807}. Moreover, mutations in *STAT5B* were seen in cases of both gamma delta and alpha beta derivation. *JAK3* and *GNAI2* are also mutated in some cases. These findings implicate activation of the *JAK/STAT* and G protein-coupled receptor signalling pathways {2807}. The most commonly mutated gene is *SETD2*, in one study mutated in > 90% of cases {3368A}. EBV is negative; if positive, it suggests a diagnosis of extranodal NK/T-cell lymphoma. As in other forms of T-cell lymphoma, EBV may sometimes be identified in background reactive B cells.

Genetic susceptibility

Unlike in EATL, there is no association with the *HLA-DQA1*0501* and *HLA-DQB1*0201* genotypes.

Prognosis and predictive factors

The clinical outcome of patients with MEITL is poor, with a median survival of 7 months. The five year overall and complete response rates are poor: 46% and 48%, respectively. In one study, good performance status was associated with better overall survival (*P* = 0.03), and response to initial treatment led to better overall survival and progression-free survival (*P* < 0.001) {4070}.

Intestinal T-cell lymphoma, NOS

Jaffe E.S.
Chott A.
Ott G.
Chan J.K.C.

Bhagat G.
Tan S.Y.
Stein H.
Isaacson P.G.

Definition

This category is used for T-cell lymphomas arising in the intestines, or sometimes other sites in the gastrointestinal tract, that do not conform to either classic enteropathy-associated T-cell lymphoma or monomorphic epitheliotropic intestinal T-cell lymphoma. Sometimes this diagnosis is made based on an inadequate biopsy in which the mucosal surface cannot be evaluated or immunophenotypic data are incomplete. It is not considered a specific disease entity. At a recent workshop of the European Association for Haematopathology, most cases assigned to this category involved the colon {178}. The cases were heterogeneous in their morphology and immunophenotype; 4 of the 5 cases with evaluable data were T-cell receptor–silent, but most had a cytotoxic phenotype. Several of the cases had widespread disease, so the intestines may not have been the primary site. All cases were clinically aggressive.

ICD-O code   9717/3

Indolent T-cell lymphoproliferative disorder of the gastrointestinal tract

Jaffe E.S.   Bhagat G.
Chott A.   Tan S.Y.
Ott G.   Stein H.
Chan J.K.C.   Isaacson P.G.

Definition
Indolent T-cell lymphoproliferative disorder of the gastrointestinal tract is a clonal T-cell lymphoproliferative disorder that can involve the mucosa in all sites of the gastrointestinal tract, but is most common in the small intestine and colon. The lymphoid cells infiltrate the lamina propria but usually do not show invasion of the epithelium. The clinical course is indolent, but most patients do not respond to conventional chemotherapy. A subset of cases progress to a higher-grade T-cell lymphoma with spread beyond the gastrointestinal tract.

ICD-O code   9702/1

Epidemiology
The disease presents in adulthood, more frequently in men than in women. Rare cases have been reported in children. No ethnic or genetic factors have been identified for increased risk. However, some patients have a history of Crohn disease {3145}.

Localization
Most patients present with disease affecting the small bowel or colon {3145, 3305}. However, all sites in the gastrointestinal tract can be involved, including the oral cavity and oesophagus {1082}. The bone marrow and peripheral blood are usually not involved.

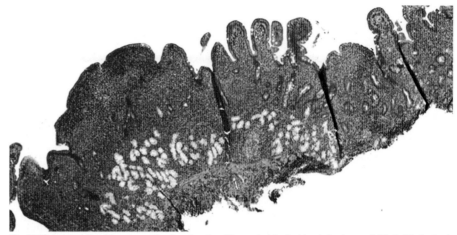

Fig. 14.68 Indolent T-cell lymphoproliferative disorder of the gastrointestinal tract, duodenum. Infiltrate fills the lamina propria and focally extends beyond the muscularis mucosae. However, glands are largely intact.

Clinical features
Presenting symptoms include abdominal pain, diarrhoea, vomiting, dyspepsia, and weight loss {561,3145}. The clinical course is chronic, but progression to disseminated disease has been reported infrequently. Peripheral lymphadenopathy is not present, but a subset of patients exhibit mesenteric lymphadenopathy {2506}.

Spread
Multiple sites in the gastrointestinal tract are involved, with a chronic relapsing clinical course. A subset of patients are at risk for disease progression and more widespread disease, usually after many years {561,2506}.

Macroscopy
The mucosa of affected sites in the gastrointestinal tract is thickened, with prominent folds or nodularity. In some cases, the infiltrate produces intestinal polyps resembling lymphomatous polyposis {1640,1794}. The mucosal surface can be hyperaemic, with superficial erosions.

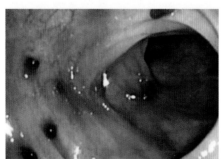

Fig. 14.69 Indolent T-cell lymphoproliferative disorder of the gastrointestinal tract. Small polypoid lesions are hyperaemic. Reprinted from Perry AM et al. {3145}.

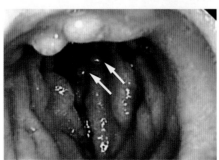

Fig. 14.70 Indolent T-cell lymphoproliferative disorder of the gastrointestinal tract. The mucosa displays multiple small polyps (arrows). From Perry AM et al. {3145}.

Microscopy
The lamina propria is expanded by a dense, non-destructive lymphoid infiltrate {3145}. Infiltration of the muscularis mucosae and submucosa may be seen focally. The mucosal glands are displaced by the infiltrate but not destroyed. However, epitheliotropism is occasionally seen. The infiltrate is monotonous, composed of small, round, mature-appearing lymphocytes. Admixed inflammatory cells are rare, but epithelioid granulomas may be focally present {563,2506}. Some of the histological changes may resemble those of Crohn disease; whether some of these patients truly have preceding inflammatory bowel disease remains uncertain.

Immunophenotype
The cells have a mature T-cell phenotype, positive for CD3. Most reported cases have been positive for CD8 {3145}, but CD4 has been expressed in a significant number {561,2506,3305}. The CD8+ cases express TIA1, but granzyme B is generally negative. Other

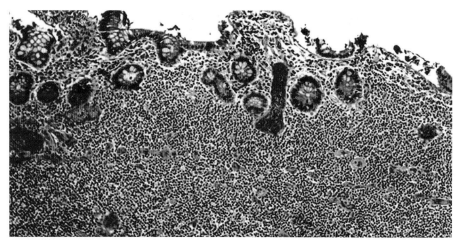

Fig. 14.71 Indolent T-cell lymphoproliferative disorder of the gastrointestinal tract, ileum. The lamina propria is diffusely infiltrated by small lymphoid cells.

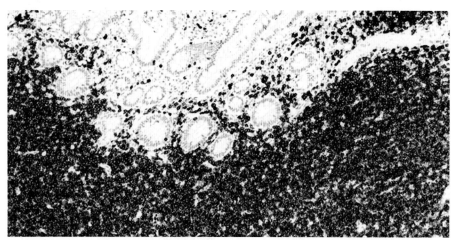

Fig. 14.72 Indolent T-cell lymphoproliferative disorder of the gastrointestinal tract, ileum. Lymphocytes are positive for CD3.

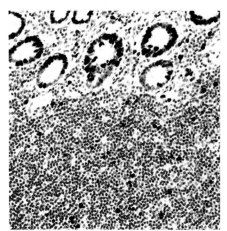

Fig. 14.73 Indolent T-cell lymphoproliferative disorder of the gastrointestinal tract. The Ki-67 proliferation index is extremely low.

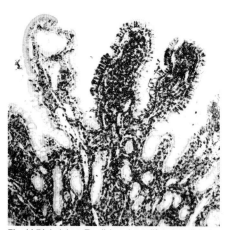

Fig. 14.74 Indolent T-cell lymphoproliferative disorder of the gastrointestinal tract. CD8, duodenal biopsy. Glands are largely intact, but some epitheliotropism is seen.

mature T-cell markers are also positive, including CD2 and CD5, with variable expression of CD7. All reported cases have expressed the alpha beta T-cell receptor, with no cases positive for T-cell receptor gamma. CD56 is negative but expression of CD103 has been reported in some cases. The proliferation rate is extremely low, with a Ki-67 proliferation index < 10% in all cases studied. Rare cases have phenotypic aberrancy, such as double-negativity for CD4 and CD8; this phenotype is associated with a more aggressive clinical course, and may constitute a different entity.

Cell of origin

The postulated cell of origin is a mature peripheral T cell

Genetic profile

All reported cases have had clonal rearrangements of TR genes, either TRG or TRB {2506,3145}. Recurrent mutations or translocations have not been identified. In limited studies, activating mutations of *STAT3* were absent. In situ hybridization for EBV-encoded small RNA (EBER) was negative in all cases studied.

Prognosis and predictive factors

Most patients have a chronic relapsing clinical course. Response to conventional chemotherapy is poor, but patients have prolonged survival with persistent disease. The presence of an aberrant T-cell phenotype in a small subset may indicate potential for more-aggressive clinical behaviour. Additionally, cases expressing CD4 rather than CD8 appear to be at higher risk for progression, although data are limited {561,2506}.

Hepatosplenic T-cell lymphoma

Gaulard P.
Jaffe E.S.
Krenacs L.
Macon W.R.

Definition

Hepatosplenic T-cell lymphoma (HSTL) is an aggressive subtype of extranodal lymphoma characterized by a hepatosplenic presentation without lymphadenopathy and a poor outcome. The neoplasm results from a proliferation of cytotoxic T cells, usually of gamma delta T-cell receptor type. It is usually composed of medium-sized lymphoid cells, demonstrating marked sinusoidal infiltration of spleen, liver, and bone marrow.

ICD-O code   9716/3

Epidemiology

HSTL is a rare form of lymphoma, reported in both western and Asian countries. It accounts for 1–2% of all peripheral T-cell lymphomas {904,4217}. Peak incidence occurs in adolescents and young adults (median patient age at diagnosis: ~35 years), with a male predominance {178,319,797}.

Etiology

As many as 20% of HSTLs arise in the setting of chronic immune suppression, most commonly during long-term immunosuppressive therapy for solid organ transplantation or prolonged antigenic stimulation {319,4168,4375}. In this setting, HSTL is regarded as a late-onset post-transplant lymphoproliferative disorder of host origin. A number of HSTL cases have been reported in patients (especially children) treated with azathioprine and infliximab for Crohn disease {922, 3414}. Rare cases have been reported in patients with psoriasis or rheumatoid arthritis receiving tumour necrosis factor inhibitors and immunomodulators {3825}.

Localization

Patients present with marked splenomegaly and usually hepatomegaly, but without lymphadenopathy. The bone marrow is almost always involved {178, 319,797,4166}.

Clinical features

HSTL typically presents with hepatosplenomegaly and systemic symptoms. Patients usually manifest marked thrombocytopenia, often with anaemia and leukopenia. Peripheral blood involvement is uncommon at presentation but may

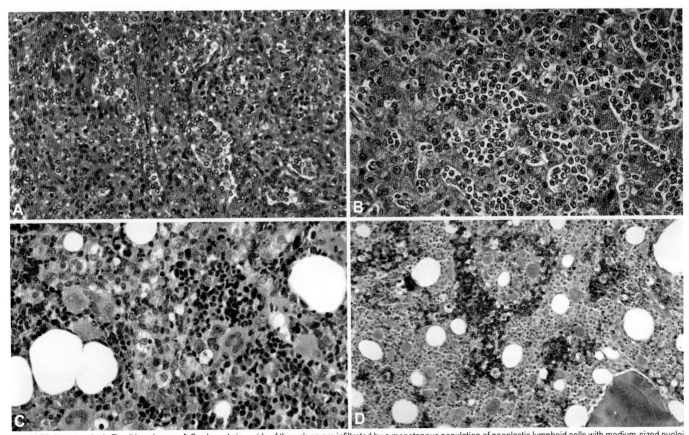

Fig. 14.75 Hepatosplenic T-cell lymphoma. **A** Cords and sinusoids of the spleen are infiltrated by a monotonous population of neoplastic lymphoid cells with medium-sized nuclei and a moderate rim of pale cytoplasm. **B** The neoplastic cells diffusely infiltrate the hepatic sinusoids. **C** The bone marrow is usually hypercellular, with neoplastic cells infiltrating sinusoids. **D** Neoplastic cells in the bone marrow are highlighted with immunohistochemistry for CD3.

occur late in the clinical course {178,319, 4166}. Given the almost constant bone marrow involvement, virtually all patients have Ann Arbor stage IV disease. HSTL is easily distinguishable from other gamma delta T-cell lymphomas that involve extranodal localizations (i.e. the skin and subcutaneous tissue, intestines, or nasal region) {150,1299}, but may be more difficult to differentiate clinically from some cases of T-cell large granular lymphocytic leukaemia with a gamma delta phenotype {178}.

Macroscopy
The spleen is enlarged, with diffuse involvement of the red pulp but no gross lesions. Diffuse hepatic enlargement is also present.

Microscopy
Histopathologically, the cells of HSTL are monotonous, with medium-sized nuclei and a rim of pale cytoplasm. The nuclear chromatin is loosely condensed, with small inconspicuous nucleoli. Some pleomorphism may occasionally be seen. The neoplastic cells involve the cords and sinuses of the splenic red pulp, with atrophy of the white pulp. The liver shows a predominant sinusoidal infiltration. Neoplastic cells are almost constantly present in the bone marrow, with a predominantly intrasinusoidal distribution. This may be difficult to identify without the aid of immunohistochemistry or flow cytometry. Cytological atypia, with large cell or blastic changes may be seen, especially with disease progression {178,319,4166}.

Immunophenotype
The neoplastic cells are CD3+ and usually gamma delta T-cell receptor+, alpha beta T-cell receptor–, CD56+/–, CD4–, CD8–/+, and CD5–. Most gamma delta cases express the V delta 1 chain {319, 3243}. A minority of cases appear to be of alpha beta type, which is considered a variant of the more common gamma delta form of the disease {2431,4168}. The determination of the alpha beta or gamma delta phenotype is now possible in formalin-fixed, paraffin-embedded tissues {1299,3850}. The cells express the cytotoxic granule–associated proteins TIA1 and granzyme M, but are usually negative for granzyme B and perforin {797,2109,3850}. They often show aberrant coincident expression of multiple killer-cell immunoglobulin-like receptor isoforms along with dim or absent CD94 {2742}. Therefore, the cells appear to be mature, non-activated cytotoxic T cells with phenotypic aberrancy. This contrasts with T-cell large granular lymphocytic leukaemia, in which the cells have a more mature lymphocytic appearance; have a CD8+, often CD57+ phenotype with granzyme B expression; and disclose a subtle, diffuse interstitial infiltrate in the marrow, with minimal (not prominent) infiltration of sinuses {178,4168}.

Postulated normal counterpart
Peripheral gamma delta (or less commonly alpha beta) cytotoxic T cells of the innate immune system with a memory phenotype, recirculating between spleen, bone marrow, and liver {1816, 2109}

Genetic profile
Cases of gamma delta origin have rearranged TRG genes and show a biallelic rearrangement of TRD genes. TRB genes are rearranged in alpha beta cases; however, unproductive rearrangements of TRB genes have been reported in some gamma delta cases.

Isochromosome 7q is present in most cases, and with disease progression, a variety of FISH patterns equivalent to 2–5 copies of i(7)(q10) or numerical and structural aberrations of the second chromosome 7 have been detected {4340}. Ring chromosomes leading to 7q amplification have also been reported. The common gained region, which has been mapped at 7q22, is associated with increased expression of several genes, including the gene encoding the multidrug resistance glycoprotein ABCB1 {1214}. Trisomy 8 may also be present. In situ hybridization for EBV is generally negative. Recent gene expression profiling studies have shown that HSTL discloses a distinct molecular signature unifying alpha beta and gamma delta cases {4048}. Missense mutations in *STAT5B* and more rarely *STAT3* have been found in about 40% of HSTLs {2160,2869}, consistent with the significant enrichment in genes of the JAK/STAT pathway in the gene expression profile {4048}. Chromatin-modifying genes, including *SETD2*, *INO80*, and *ARID1B*, are commonly mutated in HSTL, affecting 62% of cases {2600A}.

Prognosis and predictive factors
The course is aggressive. Patients may respond initially to chemotherapy, but relapses are seen in the vast majority of cases. The median survival is <2 years {319,1135}. Platinum–cytarabine {319} and pentostatin have been shown to be active agents {807}. Early use of high-dose therapy followed by haematopoietic stem cell transplantation (especially allogeneic transplantation) may improve survival {4220}.

Subcutaneous panniculitis-like T-cell lymphoma

Jaffe E.S.
Gaulard P.
Cerroni L.

Definition

Subcutaneous panniculitis-like T-cell lymphoma (SPTCL) is a cytotoxic T-cell lymphoma that preferentially infiltrates subcutaneous tissue. It is composed of atypical lymphoid cells of varying size, typically with prominent apoptotic activity of tumour cells and associated fat necrosis. Cases expressing the gamma delta T-cell receptor are excluded, and are instead classified as primary cutaneous gamma delta T-cell lymphoma. SPTCL has a very wide patient age distribution, with cases seen in both children and adults. The prognosis is generally good, especially compared with other forms of peripheral T-cell lymphoma.

ICD-O code   9708/3

Epidemiology

SPTCL is a rare form of lymphoma, accounting for < 1% of all non-Hodgkin lymphomas. It is slightly more common in females than in males and has a broad patient age range {2133}. Approximately 20% of patients are aged < 20 years (median: 35 years) {4321}, and the disease can also present in infancy {1737}. As many as 20% of patients may have associated autoimmune disease, most commonly systemic lupus erythematosus {4321}. The differential diagnosis with lupus panniculitis may be challenging.

Etiology

Autoimmune disease may play a role in some cases. The lesions may show features overlapping with those of lupus panniculitis, and a diagnosis of systemic lupus erythematosus has been documented in some cases {2445,2550}. In some patients, the early lesions may closely mimic lobular panniculitis. Whether a benign lobular panniculitis precedes the development of SPTCL in patients

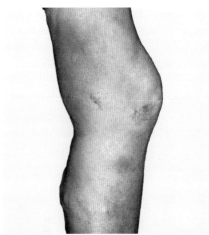

Fig. 14.76 Subcutaneous panniculitis-like T-cell lymphoma. Multiple subcutaneous nodules are common on the extremities. The overlying epidermis may show mild to moderate erythema.

without systemic lupus erythematosus is unclear. EBV is absent {2133}.

Localization

Patients present with multiple subcutaneous nodules or plaques, usually in the absence of other extracutaneous sites of disease. The most common sites of localization are the extremities and trunk. The nodules range in size from 0.5 cm to several centimetres in diameter. Larger nodules may become necrotic, but ulceration is rare {2133,4321}. It is rare for patients to present with only a single skin lesion.

Clinical features

Clinical symptoms are primarily related to the subcutaneous nodules. Systemic symptoms may be seen in as many as 50% of patients. Laboratory abnormalities, including cytopenias and elevated liver function tests are common, and a frank haemophagocytic syndrome is seen in 15–20% of cases {1401}. In such cases, hepatosplenomegaly may be present. Lymph node involvement is usually absent. Bone marrow involvement has been reported rarely, with involvement of fat cells within the marrow space {2133}.

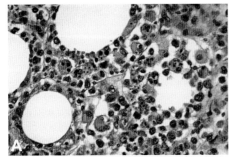
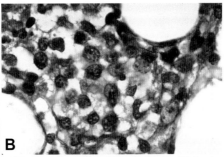

Fig. 14.77 Subcutaneous panniculitis-like T-cell lymphoma. **A** Tumour cells are associated with abundant histiocytes containing apoptotic debris. **B** Neoplastic cells have round to oval hyperchromatic nuclei with inconspicuous nucleoli and abundant pale cytoplasm.

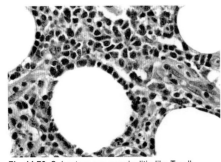
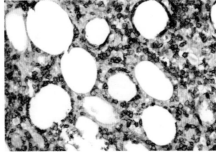

Fig. 14.78 Subcutaneous panniculitis-like T-cell lymphoma. Neoplastic cells rim fat spaces. They are usually medium-sized, with coarse chromatin. Mitotic figures are evident.

Fig. 14.79 Subcutaneous panniculitis-like T-cell lymphoma. CD8 staining highlights the atypical cells rimming fat spaces.

Table 14.05 Differential diagnosis of neoplasms expressing T-cell and NK-cell markers with frequent cutaneous involvement

Disease	Clinical features	CD3	CD4	CD8	Cytotoxic molecules[a]	CD56	EBV	TR genes	Lineage
SPTCL	Tumours (extremities and trunk)	+	–	+	+	–	–	R	T-cell
PCGD-TCL	Tumours, plaques, ulcerated nodules	+	–	–/+	+	+	–	R	T-cell
Extranodal NK/TCL	Nodules, tumours	+	–	–/+	+	+	+	G	NK-cell, sometimes T-cell
Primary C-ALCL[b]	Superficial nodules with epidermal involvement	+	+	–	–	–	–	R	T-cell
Mycosis fungoides	Patches, plaques, tumours late in course	+	+	–	–	–	–	R	T-cell
Blastic PDC neoplasm	Nodules, tumours	–	+	–	–	+	–	G	Precursor of PDC

C-ALCL, cutaneous anaplastic large cell lymphoma; G, in germline configuration; PCGD-TCL, primary cutaneous gamma delta T-cell lymphoma; PDC, plasmacytoid dendritic cell; R, rearranged; SPTCL, subcutaneous panniculitis-like T-cell lymphoma; TCL, T-cell lymphoma; TR, T-cell receptor.

[a] Cytotoxic granule–associated protein(s) TIA1, granzyme B, and/or perforin.
[b] Marked variation in T-cell antigens, including frequent antigen loss of CD3, CD2, and CD5 (see p. 396).

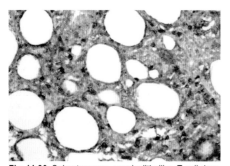

Fig. 14.80 Subcutaneous panniculitis-like T-cell lymphoma. CD4 is negative in tumour cells but positive in macrophages, which may be abundant.

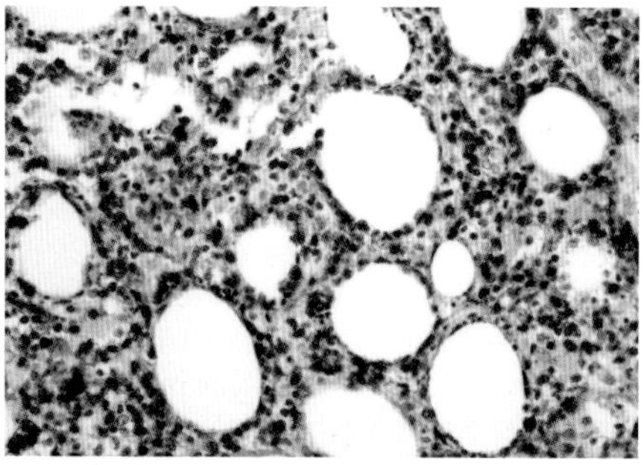

Fig. 14.81 Subcutaneous panniculitis-like T-cell lymphoma. The neoplastic cells stain for beta F1, indicative of origin from alpha beta T cells.

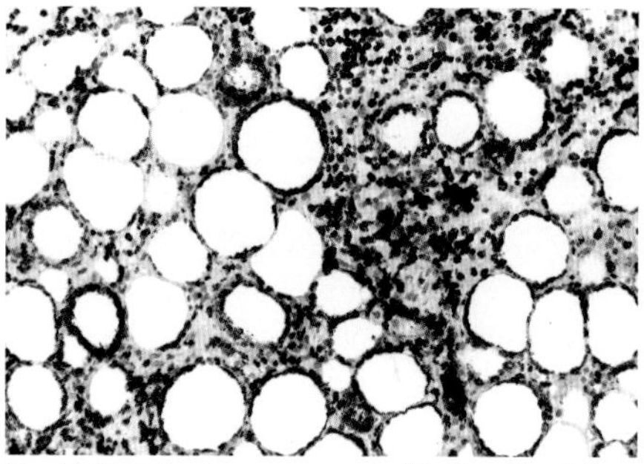

Fig. 14.82 Subcutaneous panniculitis-like T-cell lymphoma. Tumour cells have a cytotoxic phenotype and express granzyme B as well as other cytotoxic molecules.

Microscopy

The infiltrate involves the fat lobules, usually with sparing of septa. The overlying dermis and epidermis are typically uninvolved. The neoplastic cells range in size, but in any given case, cell size is relatively consistent. The neoplastic cells have irregular and hyperchromatic nuclei. The lymphoid cells have a rim of pale-staining cytoplasm. A helpful diagnostic feature is the rimming of the neoplastic cells surrounding individual fat cells. Admixed reactive histiocytes are frequently present, in particular in areas of fat infiltration and destruction. The histiocytes are frequently vacuolated, due to ingested lipid material. Other inflammatory cells are typically absent, notably plasma cells and plasmacytoid dendritic cells, which are both common in lupus panniculitis {2320,3189}. Vascular invasion may be seen in some cases, and necrosis and karyorrhexis are common {2551}. Karyorrhexis is helpful in the differential diagnosis from other lymphomas involving skin and subcutaneous tissue {2133}. Cutaneous gamma delta T-cell lymphomas may show panniculitis-like features, but commonly involve the dermis and epidermis, and may show epidermal ulceration.

Immunophenotype

The cells have a mature alpha beta T-cell phenotype, usually CD8-positive, with expression of cytotoxic molecules including granzyme B, perforin, and TIA1 (Table 14.05) {2133,3495}. The cells express beta F1 and are negative for CD56,

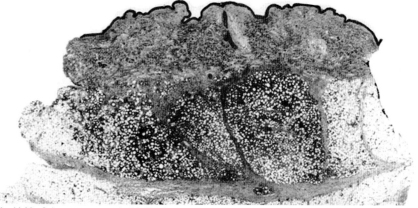

Fig. 14.83 Subcutaneous panniculitis-like T-cell lymphoma. The infiltrate is confined to the subcutaneous tissue with no involvement of the overlying dermis or epidermis. Note the predominant lobular growth pattern and relative sparing of septa.

facilitating the distinction from primary cutaneous gamma delta T-cell lymphoma {150,4030}. CD123 is generally negative, whereas this marker frequently identifies increased plasmacytoid dendritic cells in lupus panniculitis {426}.

Postulated normal counterpart
A mature cytotoxic alpha beta T cell

Genetic profile
The neoplastic cells show rearrangement of TR genes and are negative for EBV sequences. No specific cytogenetic features or mutation patterns have been reported.

Prognosis and predictive factors
Dissemination to lymph nodes and other organs is rare {1401,2071,3495}. The median 5-year overall survival rate is 80%; however, if a haemophagocytic syndrome is present, the prognosis is poor {2551,2998,4321}. Combination chemotherapy has traditionally been used, but some studies suggest that more conservative immunosuppressive regimens (cyclosporine A, prednisone) may be effective {1485,1869,2805,4074}. The distinction from cutaneous gamma delta T-cell lymphomas is important, because SPTCL has a much better prognosis {4031,4321}.

Mycosis fungoides

Cerroni L.
Sander C.A.
Smoller B.R.
Willemze R.
Siebert R.

Definition
Mycosis fungoides is an epidermotropic, primary cutaneous T-cell lymphoma characterized by infiltrates of small to medium-sized T lymphocytes with cerebriform nuclei. The term mycosis fungoides should be used only for classic cases, characterized by the evolution of patches, plaques, and tumours, or for variants with a similar clinical course.

ICD-O code   9700/3

Epidemiology
Mycosis fungoides is the most common type of cutaneous T-cell lymphoma and accounts for almost 50% of all primary cutaneous lymphomas {4320}. Most patients are adults/elderly, but the disease can also be observed in children and adolescents {395,1218}. The male-to-female ratio is 2:1 {4320}. Worldwide, the incidence is about 10 cases per one million population, with marked regional variation {2085} and a higher incidence in Black populations {1636}. An elevated risk of mycosis fungoides has been associated with several professions, including crop and vegetable farming, painting, woodworking, and carpentry. These findings suggest possible environmental cofactors in the pathogenesis of the disease {167}. Studies have shown increased risk for individuals in the petrochemical, textile, and metal industries {776}. Certain lifestyle factors have also been associated with increased risk: obesity and a smoking history of ≥40 years {167}. It has been speculated that mycosis fungoides might be associated with certain retroviruses, but no such association has been identified through high-throughput sequencing {956}.

Localization
The disease is generally limited to the skin, with variable distribution, for a protracted period. Extracutaneous dissemination may occur in advanced stages, mainly to the lymph nodes, liver, spleen, lungs, and blood {892}. Involvement of the bone marrow is rare {4320}.

Clinical features
Mycosis fungoides has an indolent clinical course, with slow progression over years or sometimes decades from patches to more-infiltrated plaques and eventually tumours. In early stages, the

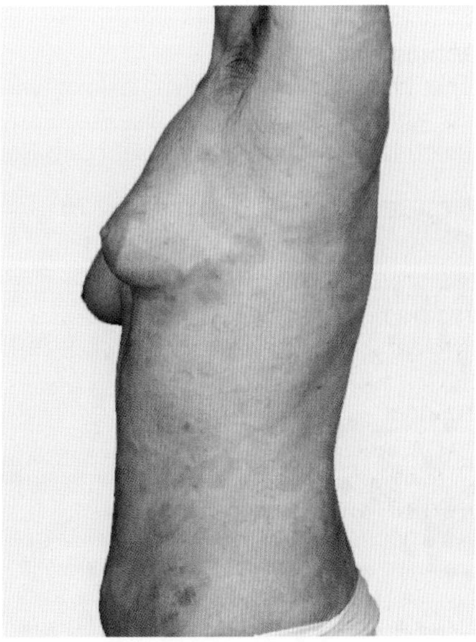

Fig. 14.84 Early mycosis fungoides. Generalized patches and thin plaques (stage IB).

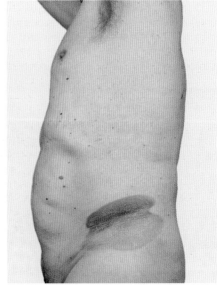

Fig. 14.85 Early mycosis fungoides. A localized patch/thin plaque covering < 10% of the body surface (stage IA).

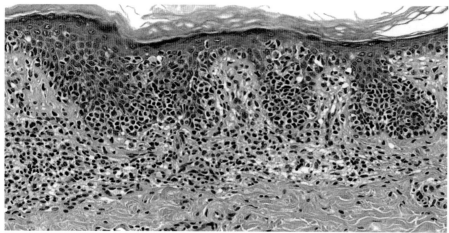

Fig. 14.86 Early mycosis fungoides. Band-like lymphoid infiltrates with several epidermotropic lymphocytes. Fibrosis of the papillary dermis is common.

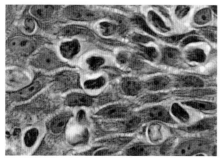

Fig. 14.87 Early mycosis fungoides. Detail of cerebriform epidermotropic lymphocytes.

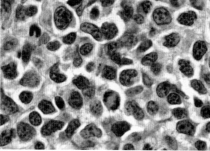

Fig. 14.88 Mycosis fungoides. Histological transformation to a large cell lymphoma.

lesions are often confined to sun-protected areas. Patients with tumour-stage mycosis fungoides characteristically show a combination of patches, plaques, and tumours, which often show ulceration {4320}. Uncommonly, patients present with or develop an erythrodermic stage of disease that lacks the haematological criteria for Sézary syndrome. Besides the clinicopathological variants discussed in detail later in this chapter, several other clinical (and histopathological) variants of the disease have been described, such as hypopigmented and hyperpigmented variants {605A}.

Staging
See Table 14.06 (p. 387) and Table 14.07 (p. 390).

Microscopy
The histology of the skin lesions varies with the stage of the disease. Early patch lesions show superficial band-like or lichenoid infiltrates, mainly consisting of lymphocytes and histiocytes. Atypical cells with small to medium-sized, highly indented (cerebriform) nuclei are few and mostly confined to the epidermis, where they characteristically colonize the epidermal basal layer, often as haloed cells, either singly or in a linear distribution {2549}. In typical plaques, epidermotropism is more pronounced. Intraepidermal collections of atypical cells (Pautrier microabscesses) are a highly characteristic feature, but are observed in only a minority of cases {2549}. With progression to tumour stage, the dermal infiltrates become more diffuse, and epidermotropism may be lost. The tumour cells increase in number and size, showing variable proportions of small, medium-sized, and large cerebriform cells with pleomorphic or blastoid nuclei {4320}. Histological transformation, defined by the presence of > 25% large lymphoid cells in the dermal infiltrates, may occur, mainly in the tumour stage {609,1898,4184}. These large cells may be CD30-negative or CD30-positive. Enlarged lymph nodes from patients with mycosis fungoides frequently show dermatopathic lymphadenopathy with paracortical expansion due to the large number of histiocytes and interdigitating cells with abundant, pale cytoplasm. The International Society for Cutaneous Lymphomas (ISCL) / European Organisation for Research and Treatment of Cancer (EORTC) staging system for clinically abnormal lymph nodes (> 1.5 cm) in mycosis fungoides and Sézary syndrome recognizes three categories: N1, reflecting no involvement; N2, early involvement (with no architectural effacement); and N3, overt involvement (with partial or complete architectural effacement)

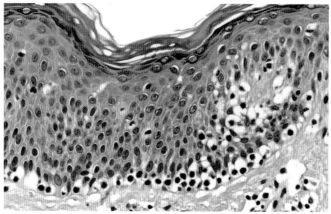

Fig. 14.89 Early mycosis fungoides. A case showing epidermotropic lymphocytes aligned along the basal layer of the epidermis.

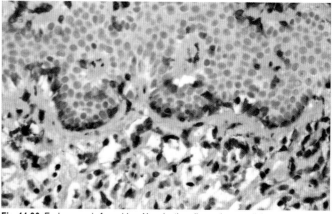

Fig. 14.90 Early mycosis fungoides. Neoplastic cells can be seen lining up in the basal layer, referred to as a string-of-pearls pattern (CD3 stain).

Table 14.06 Staging of mycosis fungoides and Sézary syndrome according to the International Society for Cutaneous Lymphomas (ISCL) and the European Organisation for Research and Treatment of Cancer (EORTC). From: Olsen et al. Blood 110:1713–22 (2007) {2972}

Skin	
T1	Limited patches[a], papules, and/or plaques[b] covering < 10% of the skin surface. May further stratify into T1a (patch only) vs T1b (plaque ± patch)
T2	Patches, papules, or plaques covering > 10% of the skin surface. May further stratify into T2a (patch only) vs T2b (plaque ± patch)
T3	≥ 1 tumour[c] (≥ 1 cm in diameter)
T4	Confluence of erythema covering ≥ 80% of the body surface area

Lymph nodes (see also Table 14.07, p. 390)	
N0	No clinically abnormal peripheral lymph nodes[d]; biopsy not required
N1	Clinically abnormal peripheral lymph nodes; histopathology Dutch grade 1 or NCI LN0–2 　　N1a: Clone-negative[e] 　　N1b: Clone-positive[e]
N2	Clinically abnormal peripheral lymph nodes; histopathology Dutch grade 2 or NCI LN3 　　N2a: Clone-negative[e] 　　N2b: Clone-positive[e]
N3	Clinically abnormal peripheral lymph nodes; histopathology Dutch grade 3–4 or NCI LN4; clone-positive or clone-negative
Nx	Clinically abnormal peripheral lymph nodes; no histological confirmation

Viscera	
M0	No visceral organ involvement
M1	Visceral organ involvement (must have pathology confirmation[f]; organ involved should be specified)

Blood	
B0	Absence of significant blood involvement: ≤ 5% of peripheral blood lymphocytes are atypical (Sézary) cells[g] 　　B0a: Clone-negative[e] 　　B0b: Clone-positive[e]
B1	Low blood tumour burden: > 5% of peripheral blood lymphocytes are atypical (Sézary) cells, but criteria for B2 are not met 　　B1a: Clone-negative[e] 　　B1b: Clone-positive[e]
B2	High blood tumour burden: Sézary cell count ≥ 1000/μL, clone-positive[e]

Stage					
IA	T1, N0, M0, B0–1	IB	T2, N0, M0, B0–1		
II	T1–2, N1–2, M0, B0–1	IIB	T3, N0–2, M0, B0–1		
III	T4, N0–2, M0, B0–1	IIIA	T4, N0–2, M0, B0	IIIB	T4, N0–2, M0, B1
IVA1	T1–4, N0–2, M0, B2	IVA2	T1–4, N3, M0, B0–2	IVB	T1–4, N0–3, M1, B0–2

[a] For skin, the term "patch" means a skin lesion of any size without significant elevation or induration; the presence or absence of hypo- or hyperpigmentation, scale, crusting, and/or poikiloderma should be noted.

[b] For skin, the term "plaque" means a skin lesion of any size that is elevated or indurated; the presence or absence of scale, crusting, and/or poikiloderma should be noted; histological features such as folliculotropism and large-cell transformation (> 25% large cells), CD30 positivity or negativity, and clinical features such as ulceration are important to document.

[c] For skin, the term "tumour" means a solid or nodular lesion ≥ 1 cm in diameter with evidence of depth and/or vertical growth; note the total number of lesions, total volume of lesions, largest size of lesion, and region of body involved; also note whether there is histological evidence of large-cell transformation; phenotyping for CD30 is recommended.

[d] For nodes, the term "abnormal peripheral lymph node" means any palpable peripheral node that on physical examination is firm, irregular, clustered, fixed, or ≥ 1.5 cm in diameter; node groups examined on physical examination include cervical, supraclavicular, epitrochlear, axillary, and inguinal; central nodes, which are not generally amenable to pathological assessment, are not considered in the nodal classification unless used to establish N3 histopathologically.

[e] A T-cell clone is defined by PCR or Southern blot analysis of the TR gene.

[f] Spleen and liver involvement can be diagnosed on the basis of imaging criteria.

[g] Sézary cells are defined as lymphocytes with hyperconvoluted cerebriform nuclei; if Sézary cells cannot be used to determine tumour burden for B2, then one of the following modified ISCL criteria along with a positive clonal rearrangement of the TR gene can be used instead:
(1) expanded CD4+ T cells with a CD4:CD8 ratio of ≥ 10, (2) expanded CD4+ T cells with abnormal immunophenotype including loss of CD7 or CD26.

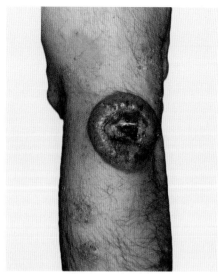

Fig. 14.91 Mycosis fungoides. Ulcerated tumour surrounded by patches and plaques.

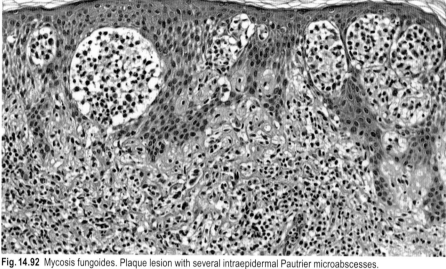

Fig. 14.92 Mycosis fungoides. Plaque lesion with several intraepidermal Pautrier microabscesses.

{2972}. Recognition of the early infiltrates can be difficult and can be facilitated by PCR for clonal TR rearrangement analysis {2972}. N3 lymph nodes may simulate peripheral T-cell lymphoma, NOS, or Hodgkin lymphoma.

Variants

Folliculotropic mycosis fungoides

Folliculotropic mycosis fungoides is characterized by infiltrates of atypical (cerebriform) CD4+ T lymphocytes involving hair follicles, often with sparing of the epidermis {608}. Many cases show mucinous degeneration of the hair follicles (follicular mucinosis), but mucin deposition can be absent {1222,4131}. The lesions preferentially involve the head and neck area and often present with grouped follicular papules and plaques associated with alopecia {4131}. Due to the deep

localization of the neoplastic infiltrate, folliculotropic mycosis fungoides is less accessible to skin-targeted therapies. The 5-year disease-specific survival rate is approximately 70–80%, which is significantly worse than that seen in classic plaque-stage mycosis fungoides {4131}.

Pagetoid reticulosis

Pagetoid reticulosis is characterized by patches or plaques with an intraepidermal proliferation of neoplastic T cells {1516}. The term should only be used for the localized type (Woringer–Kolopp type) and not for the disseminated type (Ketron–Goodman type), because most cases corresponding to the latter category would instead be classified as aggressive epidermotropic CD8+ cytotoxic T-cell lymphoma or cutaneous gamma delta T-cell lymphoma {4320}. The atypi-

cal cells have medium-sized or large cerebriform nuclei and either a CD4–/CD8+ phenotype or (less commonly) a CD4+/CD8– phenotype. CD30 is often expressed. Unlike with classic mycosis fungoides, neither extracutaneous dissemination nor disease-related deaths have ever been reported {4320}.

Granulomatous slack skin

Granulomatous slack skin is an extremely rare subtype of cutaneous T-cell lymphoma characterized clinically by the development of bulky, pendulous skin folds in the flexural areas (axillae, groin), and histologically by a granulomatous infiltrate within the dermis and subcutaneous tissues, with clonal CD4+ T cells, abundant macrophages with many multinucleated giant cells, and loss of elastic fibres {1989,2241}. Most reported cases

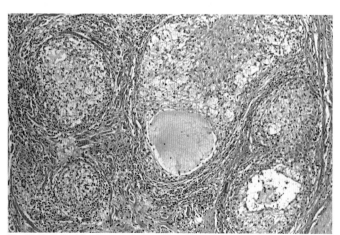

Fig. 14.93 Folliculotropic mycosis fungoides. Hyperplastic hair follicles surrounded and infiltrated by lymphocytes.

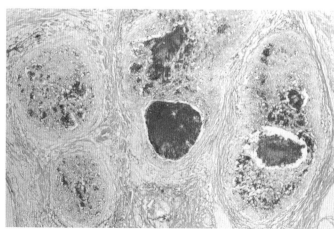

Fig. 14.94 Folliculotropic mycosis fungoides. Colloidal iron staining shows marked deposition of mucin in all follicles.

have been associated with mycosis fungoides {2241}, but in some cases the disease was concomitant with Hodgkin lymphoma. Granulomatous slack skin is characterized by an indolent clinical course {2241}.

Immunophenotype

The typical phenotype is CD2+, CD3+, TR beta+, CD5+, CD4+, CD8−, TR gamma−. Cases with a cytotoxic phenotype (CD8+ and/or TR gamma+) are well recognized {2547,3390}. Such cases have the same clinical behaviour and prognosis as CD4+ cases, and should not be considered a separate entity {2547}. A CD8+ phenotype has been reported more commonly in paediatric mycosis fungoides. Expression of CD56 has been observed in otherwise conventional mycosis fungoides. A lack of CD7 is frequent in all stages of the disease. Cutaneous lymphocyte antigen (CLA), associated with lymphocyte homing to the skin, is expressed in most cases. Other alterations in the expression of T-cell antigens may be seen, but mainly occur in the advanced (tumour) stages. Partial expression of CD30 by neoplastic cells may be found in all stages, in particular in plaques and tumours of the disease. Cytotoxic granule–associated proteins are uncommonly expressed in the early patch/plaque lesions, but may be positive in neoplastic cells in more-advanced lesions {4188}.

Cell of origin

A mature skin-homing CD4+ T cell

Genetic profile

TR genes are found to be clonally rearranged in most cases when sensitive techniques (e.g. BIOMED-2) are used {3211}. Complex karyotypes are present in many patients, in particular in the advanced stages. Somatic copy-number

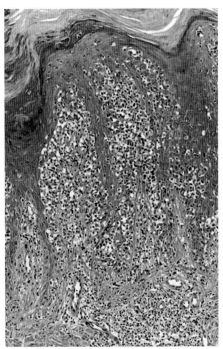

Fig. 14.95 Pagetoid reticulosis. Hyperplastic epidermis infiltrated by numerous lymphocytes.

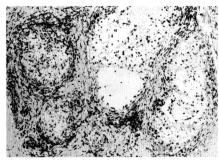

Fig. 14.96 Folliculotropic mycosis fungoides. Staining for CD5 highlights intraepithelial lymphocytes.

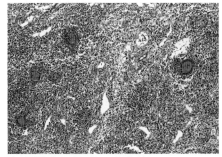

Fig. 14.97 Granulomatous slack skin. Diffuse lymphoid infiltrates admixed with histiocytes and with several large, multinucleated giant cells.

variants constitute the vast majority of all driver mutations, including mutations in multiple components of the TR and IL2 signalling pathways, in genes that drive T helper 2 (Th2) cell differentiation, in genes that facilitate escape from TGF-beta–mediated growth suppression, and in genes that confer resistance to tumour necrosis factor receptor superfamily (*TNFRSF*)–mediated apoptosis {736,2598,4039,4091,4134}. Constitutive activation of *STAT3* and inactivation of *CDKN2A* (also called *p16INK4a*) and *PTEN* have been identified and may be associated with disease progression {3547}.

Prognosis and predictive factors

The single most important prognostic factor in mycosis fungoides is the extent of cutaneous and extracutaneous disease, as reflected by the clinical stage. Patients with limited disease generally have an excellent prognosis, with a similar survival as the general population {27,958,3256, 4132}. Large Pautrier microabscesses and dermal atypical lymphocytes in early lesions have been associated with progression to advanced stage {4212}. In advanced stages, the prognosis is poor, in particular in patients with skin tumours and/or extracutaneous dissemination {337,4132}. Failure to achieve complete remission after the first treatment, patient age > 60 years, and elevated lactate dehydrogenase are adverse prognostic parameters {27,973}, as is histological transformation with increase in blast cells (> 25%) {155,609}.

Sézary syndrome

Whittaker S.J.
Cerroni L.
Willemze R.
Siebert R.

Definition

Sézary syndrome (SS) is defined by the triad of erythroderma, generalized lymphadenopathy, and the presence of clonally related neoplastic T cells with cerebriform nuclei (Sézary cells) in skin, lymph nodes, and peripheral blood. In addition, one or more of the following criteria are required: an absolute Sézary cell count ≥ 1000/μL, an expanded CD4+ T-cell population resulting in a CD4:CD8 ratio of ≥ 10, and loss of one or more T-cell antigens. SS and mycosis fungoides are closely related neoplasms, but are considered separate entities on the basis of differences in clinical behaviour and cell of origin {4211}.

ICD-O code   9701/3

Synonym
Sézary disease

Epidemiology

This is a rare disease, accounting for < 5% of all cutaneous T-cell lymphomas {4320}. It occurs in adults, characteristically presents in patients aged > 60 years, and has a male predominance.

Localization

As a leukaemia, SS is by definition a generalized disease. Any visceral organ can be involved in advanced stages, but the most common sites are the oropharynx, lungs, and CNS. Bone marrow involvement is variable.

Clinical features

Patients present with erythroderma and generalized lymphadenopathy. Other features are pruritus, alopecia, ectropion, palmar or plantar hyperkeratosis, and onychodystrophy. An increased prevalence of secondary cutaneous and systemic malignancies has been reported in SS and attributed to the immunoparesis associated with skewing of the normal T-cell repertoire and loss of normal circulating CD4+ cells {1720}.

Table 14.07 Histopathological staging for clinically abnormal lymph nodes (> 1.5 cm) in mycosis fungoides and Sézary syndrome

ISCL/EORTC {2972}	Dutch system {3552A}	NCI classification {3532A}
N1	Category 1: DL, no atypical CMCs	LN 0: No atypical lymphocytes
		LN 1: Occasional, isolated atypical lymphocytes
		LN 2: Clusters (3–6 cells) of atypical lymphocytes
N2[a]	Category 2: DL with early involvement and scattered atypical CMCs	LN 3: Aggregates of atypical lymphocytes, but architecture preserved
N3	Category 3: Partial effacement of architecture, with many CMCs	LN 4: Partial or complete effacement of architecture, with many atypical lymphocytes
	Category 4: Complete effacement of architecture	

CMC, cerebriform mononuclear cell with nuclei > 7.5 μm; DL, dermatopathic lymphadenopathy; EORTC, European Organisation for Research and Treatment of Cancer; ISCL, International Society for Cutaneous Lymphomas; NCI, United States National Cancer Institute.

[a] N2 is divided into two categories:
N2a (without clonally rearranged T cells) and N2b (with clonally rearranged T cells).

Staging

Staging of mycosis fungoides and SS is performed according to the International Society for Cutaneous Lymphomas (ISCL) / European Organisation for Research and Treatment of Cancer (EORTC) system (Table 14.06, p. 387) {2972}. SS patients are erythrodermic (T4) and have peripheral blood involvement, which requires demonstration of clonal TR gene rearrangement (preferably the same clone in skin and peripheral blood)

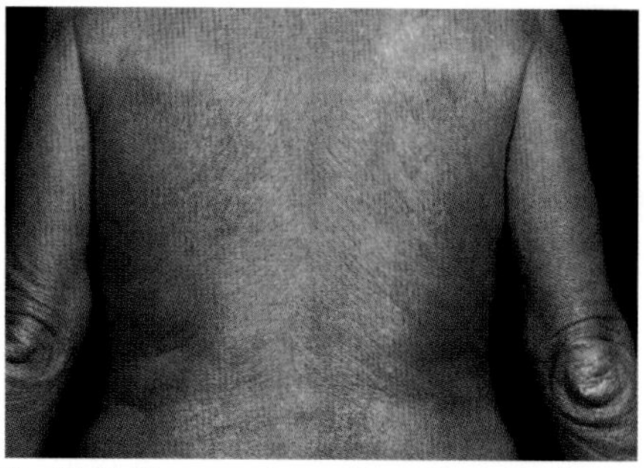

Fig. 14.98 Sézary syndrome. Generalized skin disease with erythroderma.

in combination with (1) a total Sézary cell count ≥ 1000/μL, (2) an expanded CD4+ T-cell population with a CD4:CD8 ratio of ≥ 10, or (3) an expanded CD4+ T-cell population with abnormal immunophenotype including loss of CD7 or CD26 {2972}. For determination of the Sézary cell count, Sézary cells are defined as lymphocytes with hyperconvoluted cerebriform nuclei. SS cases are stage IVA1, IVA2, or IVB according to the ISCL/ EORTC system.

Microscopy

The histological features in SS may be similar to those in mycosis fungoides. However, the cellular infiltrates in SS are more often monotonous, and epidermotropism may sometimes be absent. In as many as one third of biopsies from patients with otherwise classic SS, the histological picture may be non-specific {4062}. Involved lymph nodes characteristically show a dense, monotonous infiltrate of Sézary cells with effacement of the normal lymph node architecture {3553}. Bone marrow may be involved, but the infiltrates are often sparse and mainly interstitial {3669}.

Immunophenotype
The neoplastic T cells have a CD3+, CD4+, CD8– phenotype; characteristically lack CD7 and CD26; and express PD1 (also known as CD279) in almost all cases {625}. Sézary cells express cutaneous lymphocyte antigen (CLA) and the skin-homing receptor CCR4 {1213}, as well as CCR7 {2825}. Flow cytometry analysis of peripheral blood lymphocytes shows a CD4+/CD7– (> 30%) or CD4+/CD26– (> 40%) T-cell population {356, 3718}.

Postulated normal counterpart
The normal counterparts of Sézary cells are circulating central memory T cells (CD27+, CD45RA–, CD45RO+); this is in contrast to the tumour cells of mycosis fungoides, which derive from skin-resident memory T cells {539}.

Genetic profile
TR genes are clonally rearranged {3211, 4308,4309}. A characteristic gene expression signature consists of overexpression of *PLS3*, *DNM3*, *TWIST1*, and *EPHA4* and underexpression of *STAT4* {1519,1941,4130}.
Recurrent balanced chromosomal translocations have not been detected in SS, but complex numerical and structural alterations are common and similar to those in mycosis fungoides {294,552,2491}, including losses of 1p, 6q, and 10q and gains of 8q, with isochromosome 17q as a recurrent feature of SS {4190}. High-throughput sequencing techniques have revealed a markedly heterogeneous pattern of novel gene mutations and focal copy-number variants, indicating a high rate of genomic instability {736,2005, 4091,4150}. Recurrent gain-of-function mutations affecting genes involved in T-cell receptor signalling, including *PLCG1*,

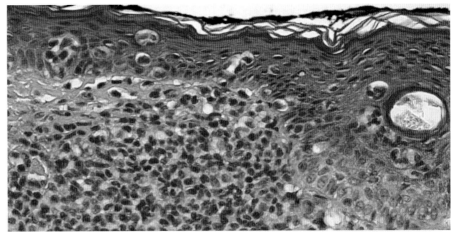

Fig. 14.99 Sézary syndrome. Skin infiltrates with epidermotropic infiltrates of atypical, cerebriform lymphocytes.

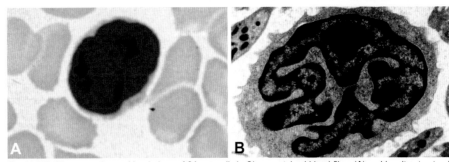

Fig. 14.100 Sézary syndrome. Morphology of Sézary cells in Giemsa-stained blood films (**A**) and by ultrastructural examination (**B**).

CD28, and *TNFRSF1B*, may explain the constitutive activation of NF-kappaB in SS. *RHOA* mutations described in other mature T-cell lymphomas are also present in SS. Recurrent loss-of-function aberrations also target epigenetic modifiers, including *ARID1A*, in which functional loss from nonsense and frameshift mutations and/or targeted deletions is observed in around 40% of SS cases {2005}. Both single nucleotide mutations and copy-number variants affecting genes encoding members of the JAK/STAT pathway may also explain the constitutive activation of *STAT3* in tumour cells. Mutations affecting chromatin-modifying genes such as *DNMT3A* are also present in SS, as are frequent inactivating mutations of *TP53* {736} and deletions of *CDKN2A* (also called *p16INK4a*) {2843,

3546}. Hypermethylation and inactivation of genes involved in the FAS-dependent apoptotic pathway is common {1873}.

Prognosis and predictive factors
SS is an aggressive disease, with a median survival of 32 months and a 5-year overall survival rate of 10–30%, depending on stage {4320}. Most patients die of opportunistic infections. Lymph node involvement (stage IVA2) and visceral involvement (stage IVB) indicate a worse prognosis {343}. The degree of peripheral blood involvement at diagnosis may have an impact on prognosis {2041,4213}, but the prognostic relevance of bone marrow involvement is unknown.

Primary cutaneous CD30-positive T-cell lymphoproliferative disorders

Willemze R.
Paulli M.
Kadin M.E.

Definition

Primary cutaneous CD30+ lymphoproliferative disorders are the second most common group of cutaneous T-cell lymphomas, accounting for approximately 30% of cases. This group includes lymphomatoid papulosis, primary cutaneous anaplastic large cell lymphoma (C-ALCL), and borderline cases.

These diseases form a spectrum and may show overlapping histopathological, phenotypic, and genetic features {4171, 4223,4320}. The clinical appearance and course are therefore critical for the definite diagnosis. The term 'borderline' refers to cases in which, despite careful clinicopathological correlation, a definite distinction between lymphomatoid papulosis and C-ALCL cannot be made. However, clinical examination during follow-up will generally disclose whether such patients have lymphomatoid papulosis or C-ALCL {314}. Clinicopathological correlation is not only required to differentiate between lymphomatoid papulosis and C-ALCL, but is also essential for differentiating these primary cutaneous CD30+ lymphoproliferative disorders from a wide variety of infectious and inflammatory skin diseases and other types of cutaneous T-cell lymphomas (in particular, mycosis fungoides) that contain significant numbers of CD30+ cells {1986}.

Lymphomatoid papulosis

Definition

Lymphomatoid papulosis (LyP) is a chronic, recurrent, self-healing skin disease that combines a usually benign clinical course with histological features suggestive of a cutaneous T-cell lymphoma.

ICD-O code   9718/1

Synonym

Primary cutaneous CD30+ T-cell lymphoproliferative disorder

Epidemiology

LyP most often occurs in adults (median patient age: 45 years), but children may also be affected. The male-to-female

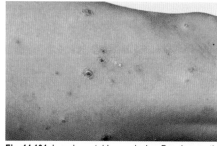

Fig. 14.101 Lymphomatoid papulosis. Papulonecrotic skin lesions at various stages of evolution.

ratio is 2–3:1 {314,1088,2367,4138}.

Localization

LyP is a skin-limited disease that most frequently affects the trunk and extremities {314}. In rare cases, concurrent oral mucosal lesions can be present {3597}.

Clinical features

LyP is characterized by papular, papulonecrotic, and/or nodular skin lesions at various stages of development {314}. The number of lesions may vary from a few to more than a hundred. Individual skin

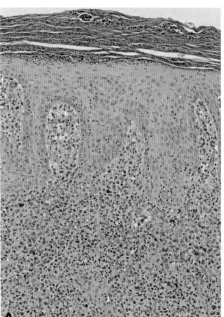
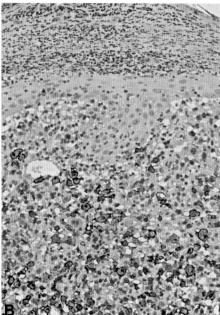
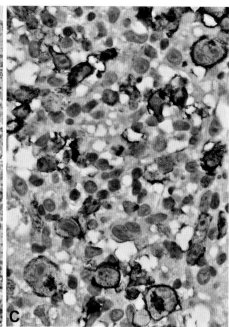

Fig. 14.102 Lymphomatoid papulosis type A. **A** Mixed inflammatory infiltrate with scattered large atypical cells. **B** Staining for CD30 shows scattered large atypical cells. **C** Scattered large anaplastic cells expressing CD30.

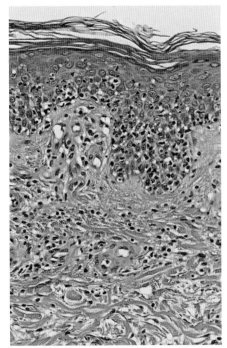

Fig. 14.103 Lymphomatoid papulosis, type B. Epidermotropic infiltrate of small to medium-sized atypical lymphocytes simulating early-stage mycosis fungoides.

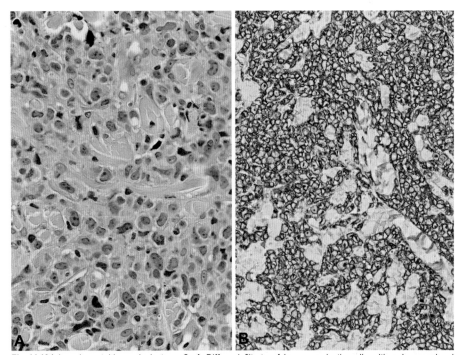

Fig. 14.104 Lymphomatoid papulosis type C. **A** Diffuse infiltrate of large anaplastic cells with only occasional admixed inflammatory cells. This histological picture is indistinguishable from that of cutaneous anaplastic large cell lymphoma, and clinicopathological correlation is required to make a definite diagnosis. **B** Staining for CD30.

lesions disappear within 3–12 weeks and may leave behind superficial scars. The duration of the disease may vary from several months to >40 years. In as many as 20% of patients, LyP may be preceded by, associated with, or followed by another type of malignant lymphoma, generally mycosis fungoides, cutaneous anaplastic large cell lymphoma, or Hodgkin lymphoma {314,910}.

Microscopy

The histological picture of LyP is extremely variable, and in part correlates with the age of the biopsied skin lesion. Several histological subtypes of LyP have been described.

Type A LyP is the most common type (>80%) and is characterized by scattered or small clusters of large atypical (sometimes multinucleated or Reed–Sternberg–like) CD30+ cells intermingled with numerous inflammatory cells, including small lymphocytes, neutrophils, and/or eosinophils {314}.

LyP, Type B is uncommon (<5%) and is characterized by a predominantly epidermotropic infiltrate of small atypical CD30+ or CD30– cells with cerebriform nuclei, histologically simulating early-stage mycosis fungoides {314}.

LyP, Type C lesions (~10%) demonstrate a monotonous population or cohesive sheets of large CD30+ T cells with relatively few admixed inflammatory cells, very similar to cutaneous anaplastic large cell lymphoma {314}.

LyP, Type D lesions (<5%) are characterized by a strongly epidermotropic, sometimes pagetoid infiltrate of atypical small to medium-sized CD8+, CD30+ pleomorphic T cells, mimicking primary cutaneous aggressive epidermotropic CD8+ cytotoxic T-cell lymphoma {3473}.

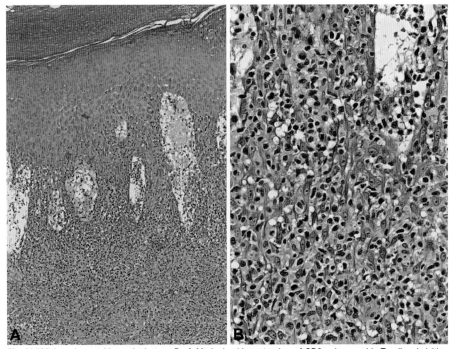

Fig. 14.105 Lymphomatoid papulosis type D. **A** Marked epidermotropism of CD8+ pleomorphic T cells mimicking cutaneous aggressive epidermotropic CD8+ cytotoxic T-cell lymphoma. **B** Extensive epidermotropism of small to medium-sized pleomorphic T cells.

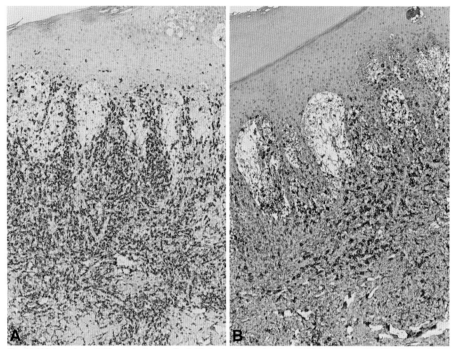

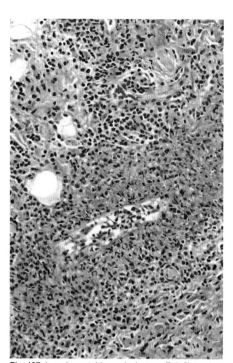

Fig. 14.106 Lymphomatoid papulosis type D. **A** Marked epidermotropism of CD8+ pleomorphic T cells mimicking cutaneous aggressive epidermotropic CD8+ cytotoxic T-cell lymphoma. **B** Expression of CD30 by epidermal and dermal T cells.

Fig. 107 Lymphomatoid papulosis, type E. Infiltrate has an angiodestructive growth pattern

Some of these cases may have a gamma delta T-cell phenotype {3390}.

Type E LyP (<5%) is characterized by angiocentric and angiodestructive infiltrates of small to medium-sized CD8+, CD30+ pleomorphic T cells {1988}. Vascular occlusion, haemorrhages, extensive necrosis, and ulceration may be present. Clinically, patients present with a few papulonodular lesions that rapidly ulcerate and evolve into large necrotic eschar-like lesions.

LyP with 6p25.3 rearrangement (<5%) is characterized by chromosomal rearrangements involving the *DUSP22-IRF4*

locus on 6p25.3 {1938}. Patients are older adults and often present with localized skin lesions. Histologically, skin lesions show extensive epidermotropism by weakly CD30+ small to medium-sized T cells with cerebriform nuclei and strongly CD30+ medium-sized to large blast cells in the dermis, simulating transformed mycosis fungoides.

Other rare histological variants have also been described, including folliculotropic, syringotropic, and granulomatous LyP {1986,1987}. Different subtypes of LyP may occur in separate but concurrent le-

sions, and a single LyP lesion may show histological features of multiple subtypes. Recognition of these different subtypes of LyP is important, to avoid misdiagnosis of other, often more aggressive, types of cutaneous T-cell lymphoma (see Table 14.08). However, the subtypes have no therapeutic or prognostic implications.

Immunophenotype

The large atypical cells in the lesions of type A and type C LyP have the same phenotype as the tumour cells in cutaneous anaplastic large cell lymphoma.

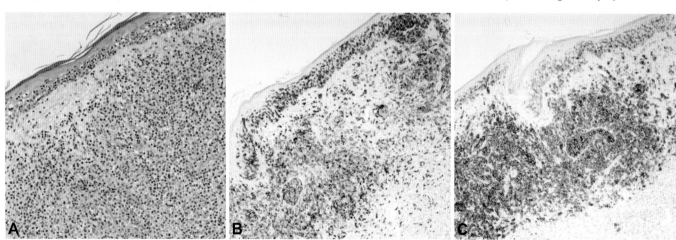

Fig. 14.108 Lymphomatoid papulosis with *DUSP22-IRF4* rearrangement. **A** Diffuse dermal infiltrate of medium-sized to large atypical lymphocytes. Intraepidermal infiltrate of small atypical lymphocytes with hyperchromatic nuclei. **B** Diffuse dermal infiltrate of medium-sized to large atypical lymphocytes. Expression of CD8 by both intraepidermal and dermal atypical T cells. **C** Diffuse dermal infiltrate of medium-sized to large atypical lymphocytes. CD30 expression by both intraepidermal and dermal atypical lymphocytes.

Table 14.08 Lymphomatoid papulosis: histological subtypes and differential diagnosis

Subtype	Relative frequency	Predominant phenotype	Main differential diagnoses
Type A	>80%	CD4+, CD8−	C-ALCL Tumour-stage MF Hodgkin lymphoma
Type B	<5%	CD4+, CD8−	Plaque-stage MF
Type C	~10%	CD4+, CD8−	C-ALCL Transformed MF (CD30+)
Type D	<5%	CD4−, CD8+	CD8+ aggressive epidermotropic TCL
Type E	<5%	CD4−, CD8+	Extranodal NK/TCL
With *DUSP22-IRF4* rearrangement	<5%	CD4−, CD8+ or CD4−,CD8−	Tumour-stage MF

C-ALCL, cutaneous anaplastic large cell lymphoma; MF, mycosis fungoides; TCL, T-cell lymphoma.

The atypical cells are predominantly CD4-positive in LyP types A–C, CD8-positive in types D and E, and either CD8-positive or double negative for CD4 and CD8 in *DUSP22-IRF4*–translocated cases. The expression of CD56 has also been sporadically reported {316,1223}.

Postulated normal counterpart

An activated skin-homing T cell

Genetic profile

Antigen receptor genes
Clonally rearranged TRG genes have been detected in most cases of LyP {748, 887,3789}. Identical rearrangements have been demonstrated in LyP lesions and associated lymphomas {748,887}.

Cytogenetic abnormalities
No consistent abnormalities have been described. The t(2;5)(p23.2-23.1;q35.1) translocation or its variants, leading to activation of the ALK kinase, are not detected in LyP {920}. Rearrangements of the *DUSP22-IRF4* locus on chromosome 6p25.3 are found in a small subset of LyP cases, which show distinctive clinico-pathological features {1938,4223}.

Prognosis and predictive factors

LyP has an excellent prognosis. In two large studies, together including 242 patients, only 2% of LyP patients died of associated lymphomas {314,910}. However, because the risk factors for the development of a systemic lymphoma are unknown, long-term follow-up is recommended.

Primary cutaneous anaplastic large cell lymphoma

Definition

Cutaneous anaplastic large cell lymphoma (C-ALCL) is composed of large cells with an anaplastic, pleomorphic, or immunoblastic cytomorphology, the majority (>75%) of which express the CD30 antigen {4320}. Patients with C-ALCL should not have clinical evidence or history of mycosis fungoides; in this setting a diagnosis of mycosis fungoides with large cell transformation, which may be CD30-positive or CD30-negative, is more likely {337}. The disease must also be distinguished from systemic anaplastic large cell lymphoma with cutaneous involvement, which is a separate disease with different cytogenetics, clinical features, and outcome {4389}.

ICD-O code   9718/3

Synonyms

Primary cutaneous CD30+ large T-cell lymphoma (obsolete); primary cutaneous

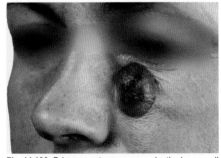

Fig. 14.109 Primary cutaneous anaplastic large cell lymphoma with an ulcerated skin tumour.

CD30+ T-cell lymphoproliferative disorder; regressing atypical histiocytosis (obsolete)

Epidemiology

C-ALCL is the second most common type of cutaneous T-cell lymphoma {4320}. The median patient age is 60 years. Children are sporadically affected {314}. The male-to-female ratio is 2–3:1 {314}.

Localization

This is a skin-limited disease that most frequently affects the trunk, face, and extremities {338,4361}.

Clinical features

Most patients present with solitary or localized nodules or tumours, and sometimes papules, and often show ulceration {314,2367}. Multifocal lesions are seen in about 20% of patients. The skin lesions may show partial or complete spontaneous regression, as is seen in lymphomatoid papulosis. These lymphomas frequently relapse in the skin. Extracutaneous dissemination occurs in about 10% of patients, and mainly involves the regional lymph nodes {314,4320}.

Microscopy

Histology shows diffuse infiltrates with cohesive sheets of large CD30+ tumour cells. Epidermotropism may be present, and is particularly marked in cases carrying a *DUSP22-IRF4* rearrangement {2975}. In most cases, the tumour cells have the characteristic morphology of anaplastic cells, with round, oval, or irregularly shaped nuclei; prominent eosinophilic nucleoli; and abundant cytoplasm {4320}. Less commonly (20–25%), they have a non-anaplastic (pleomorphic or immunoblastic) appearance {314,2548, 3111}. Reactive lymphocytes are often present at the periphery of the lesions. Ulcerating lesions may show a lymphomatoid papulosis–like histology, with an abundant inflammatory infiltrate of reactive T cells, histiocytes, eosinophils, neutrophils, and relatively few CD30+ cells. In such cases, epidermal hyperplasia may be prominent. The inflammatory background is especially prominent in the rare neutrophil-rich (pyogenic) variant {500}. Rare cases of intralymphatic C-ALCL have been reported {3500}.

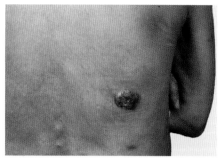

Fig. 14.110 Primary cutaneous anaplastic large cell lymphoma presenting with a solitary tumour on the back.

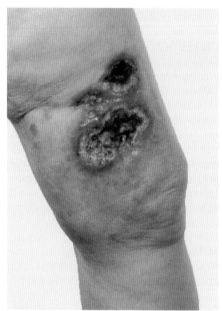

Fig. 14.111 Primary cutaneous anaplastic large cell lymphoma presenting with a large ulcerating tumour on the left leg.

Immunophenotype

The neoplastic cells show an activated CD4+ T-cell phenotype with variable loss of CD2, CD5, and/or CD3 and frequent expression of cytotoxic proteins (e.g. granzyme B, TIA1, and perforin) {432, 2136,4320}. Some cases may have a CD4–/CD8+ or CD4+/CD8+ T-cell phenotype or a null-cell phenotype {2545}. CD30 is by definition expressed by the majority (>75%) of the neoplastic cells {4320}. Unlike systemic anaplastic large cell lymphomas, most C-ALCLs express the cutaneous lymphocyte antigen (CLA), but do not express EMA or ALK {891, 920,3940}. CD15 is expressed in approximately 40% of cases, whereas staining for IRF4/MUM1 is positive in almost all cases {336,4262}. Unlike Hodgkin lymphomas, C-ALCLs do not express PAX5 and are negative for EBV. Coexpression of CD56 is observed in rare cases, but does not appear to be associated with an unfavourable prognosis {2839}.

Postulated normal counterpart

A transformed/activated skin-homing T cell

Genetic profile

Antigen receptor genes
Most cases show clonal rearrangement of the TR genes {2425}. However, T-cell receptor proteins are often not expressed {413}.

Cytogenetic abnormalities and oncogenes
Unlike systemic anaplastic large cell lymphomas, the vast majority of C-ALCLs do not carry translocations involving the *ALK* gene at chromosome 2 {920}. However, unusual cases of ALK-positive C-ALCL, including cases showing strong nuclear and cytoplasmic staining characteristic of the t(2;5) chromosomal translocation and cases expressing cytoplasmic ALK protein (indicative of a variant *ALK* translocation), have been reported {178,1900,2996,3267}. Many of these cases had an excellent prognosis. Rearrangements of the *DUSP22-IRF4* locus on chromosome 6p25.3 are found in approximately 25% of C-ALCLs and in a small subset of lymphomatoid papulosis {3166,4223}. Frequent chromosomal aberrations affecting almost half of the patients are gains of 7q31 and losses on 6q16-21 and 13q34 {2185,4135}. Unlike in tumour-stage mycosis fungoides and peripheral T-cell lymphoma, NOS, loss of 9p21.3 harbouring the *CDKN2A* tumour suppressor gene is rarely observed in C-ALCL {2870}. A recurrent *NPM1-TYK2* gene fusion resulting in constitutive STAT signalling has been described in both C-ALCL and lymphomatoid papulosis {4171}. *TYK2* breaks were found in 15% of primary cutaneous CD30+ lymphoproliferative disorder cases. *TP63* rearrangements have been observed in rare C-ALCL cases with an unusually aggressive clinical behaviour {4161}.

Gene expression profiling showed high expression of the skin-homing chemokine receptor genes *CCR10* and *CCR8* in C-ALCLs, which may explain their affinity for the skin and their low tendency to disseminate to extracutaneous sites {4135}.

Prognosis and predictive factors

The prognosis is usually favourable, with a 10-year disease-specific survival rate of approximately 90% {314,2367}. Patients presenting with multifocal skin lesions and patients with involvement of regional lymph nodes have a prognosis similar to that of patients with only skin lesions {314}. No differences in clinical presentation, clinical behaviour, or prognosis have been found between cases with an anaplastic morphology and cases with a non-anaplastic (pleomorphic or immunoblastic) morphology {338,2367, 4361}.

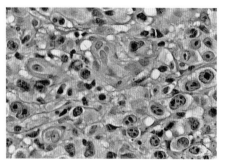

Fig. 14.112 Primary cutaneous anaplastic large cell lymphoma with confluent sheets of large cells with anaplastic morphology.

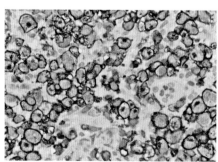

Fig. 14.113 Primary cutaneous anaplastic large cell lymphoma with cohesive sheets of CD30+ anaplastic cells.

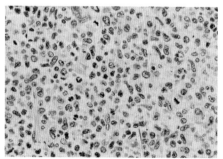

Fig. 14.114 Primary cutaneous anaplastic large cell lymphoma with a diffuse proliferation of medium-sized pleomorphic cells.

Primary cutaneous peripheral T-cell lymphomas, rare subtypes

Introduction

Gaulard P.
Berti E.
Willemze R.
Petrella T.
Jaffe E.S.

Peripheral T-cell lymphomas commonly involve the skin, either as primary or secondary manifestations of disease. Within this group, three rare provisional entities were delineated in the WHO-EORTC classification for cutaneous lymphomas {4320}: primary cutaneous gamma delta T-cell lymphoma, primary cutaneous aggressive epidermotropic CD8+ cytotoxic T-cell lymphoma, and primary cutaneous CD4+ small/medium T-cell lymphoma. The last two entities are still considered provisional, and altered terminology is proposed for the CD4+ small/medium proliferations. A diagnosis of mycosis fungoides must be ruled out by complete clinical examination and an accurate clinical history. A new provisional entity has been added: primary cutaneous acral CD8+ T-cell lymphoma.

Primary cutaneous gamma delta T-cell lymphoma

Gaulard P.
Berti E.
Willemze R.
Petrella T.
Jaffe E.S.

Definition

Primary cutaneous gamma delta T-cell lymphoma (PCGD-TCL) is a lymphoma, involving primarily the skin, composed of a clonal proliferation of mature, activated gamma delta T cells with a cytotoxic phenotype. This group includes cases previously called subcutaneous panniculitis-like T-cell lymphoma with a gamma delta phenotype. Gamma delta T-cell lymphomas presenting primarily in mucosal sites

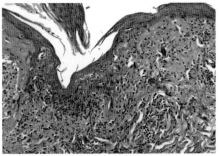

Fig. 14.115 Primary cutaneous gamma delta T-cell lymphoma. The epidermis is necrotic.

(in the past referred to as mucocutaneous gamma delta T-cell lymphoma) are likely unrelated conditions belonging to other site-dependent peripheral T-cell lymphoma entities {150,1299,3850}. The gamma delta T-cell receptor (TR) may also be expressed by rare cases of otherwise classic mycosis fungoides and lymphomatoid papulosis, which have the same indolent clinical course as cases with an alpha beta T-cell phenotype {2533,2547, 3390}. Such cases should be diagnosed as mycosis fungoides or lymphomatoid papulosis, irrespective of TR expression.

ICD-O code 9726/3

Epidemiology

PCGD-TCLs are rare, accounting for approximately 1% of all cutaneous T-cell lymphomas {4031,4320,4321}. Most cases occur in adults. There is no sex predilection.

Etiology

The distribution of disease reflects the localization of normal gamma delta T cells, which are believed to play a role in host mucosal and epithelial immune responses. Impaired immune function associated with chronic antigen stimulation may predispose individuals to the development of PCGD-TCL {150,3850}.

Localization

PCGD-TCLs often present with generalized skin lesions, preferentially affecting the extremities {4031,1493}.

Clinical features

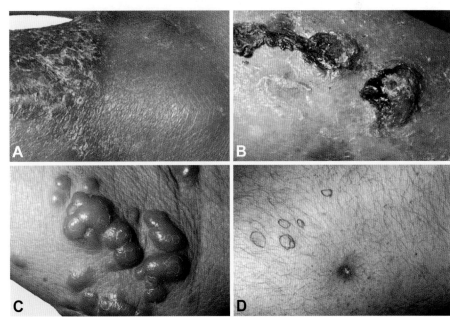

Fig. 14.116 Primary cutaneous gamma delta T-cell lymphoma. Lesions are clinically diverse, and consist of plaques, without ulceration (**A**) or with ulceration (**B**), or tumours (**C**). The lesion may consist of an indurated plaque with subcutaneous infiltration (**D**).

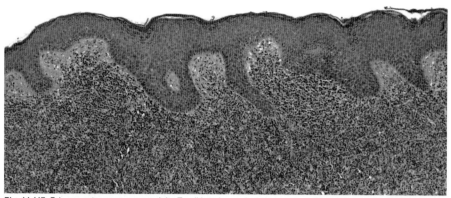

Fig. 14.117 Primary cutaneous gamma delta T-cell lymphoma. In this case, the infiltrate is primarily dermal.

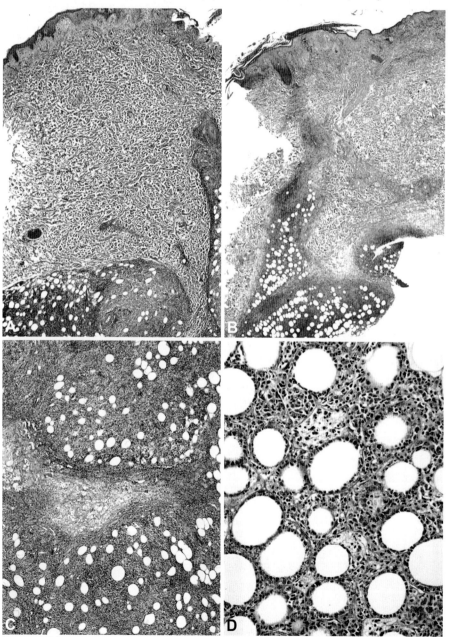

Fig. 14.118 Primary cutaneous gamma delta T-cell lymphoma. Histological patterns are diverse. **A** Dermal infiltration is usually present, and, as seen in **B**, the infiltrate may extend from the epidermis to the subcutis. **C,D** Panniculitis-like pattern may be seen.

The clinical presentation of patients with PCGD-TCL is variable. The disease may be predominantly epidermotropic and present with patches/plaques. Some patients may present with deep dermal or subcutaneous tumours, with or without epidermal necrosis and ulceration {359, 4031,4321}. The lesions are most often present on the extremities, but other sites may also be affected {4031,4321}. Dissemination to mucosal and other extranodal sites is frequently observed, but involvement of lymph nodes, spleen, or bone marrow is uncommon. A haemophagocytic syndrome is common, in particular in patients with panniculitis-like tumours {4031,4321}. B symptoms, including fever, night sweats, and weight loss, occur in most patients.

Imaging
Abnormal PET and/or CT findings are common in sites of active disease {1493}.

Microscopy
Three major histological patterns of involvement can be present in the skin: epidermotropic, dermal, and subcutaneous. Often more than one histological pattern is present in the same patient in different biopsy specimens or within a single biopsy specimen {359,4031,4321}. Epidermal infiltration may occur as mild epidermotropism to marked pagetoid reticulosis–like infiltrates {359}. Subcutaneous cases may show rimming of fat cells, similar to subcutaneous panniculitis-like T-cell lymphoma of alpha beta origin, but usually show dermal and/or epidermal involvement in addition {4031,4321}. The neoplastic cells are generally medium-sized to large, with coarsely clumped chromatin {4031}. Large blastic cells with vesicular nuclei and prominent nucleoli are infrequent. Apoptosis and necrosis are common, often with angioinvasion {4031,4321}.

Immunophenotype
The tumour cells characteristically have a gamma delta TR–positive, beta F1-negative, CD3+, CD2+, CD5−, CD7+/−, CD56+ phenotype with strong expression of cytotoxic proteins, including granzyme B, perforin, and TIA1 {1821, 3495,4031,4321}. Most cases lack both CD4 and CD8, although CD8 may be expressed in some cases {4031,4321}. The gamma delta T-cell phenotype (TR gamma–positive, beta F1–negative) can

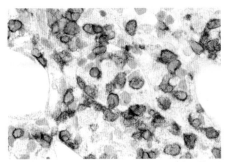

Fig. 14.119 Primary cutaneous gamma delta T-cell lymphoma. Neoplastic cells infiltrate the subcutis and are positive for T-cell receptor gamma by immunohistochemistry.

now be assessed on formalin-fixed, paraffin-embedded tissue sections in most instances {1299,3850}. Coexpression of TR gamma and beta F1 has been reported in some cases {1310A,3390}.

Postulated normal counterpart
Functionally mature and activated cytotoxic gamma delta T cells of the innate immune system

Genetic profile
The cells show clonal rearrangement of the TRG and TRD genes. TRB may be rearranged or deleted, but is not expressed. PCGD-TCLs usually express V delta 2, consistent with the prevalence of V delta 2 gamma delta T cells residing in the skin {3243}. EBV is negative {150,3850,4031}. In common with other tumours of gamma delta T-cell origin, some cases have activating mutations in STAT5B and rarely in STAT3.
Activation of the JAK/STAT pathway is common to many cytotoxic T-cell malignancies {2160}.

Prognosis and predictive factors
PCGD-TCLs are usually resistant to multiagent chemotherapy and/or radiation and have a poor prognosis, with a median survival of approximately 15 months {4031,4321}. Patients with subcutaneous fat involvement tend to have a more unfavourable prognosis than do patients with epidermal or dermal disease only {4031}. However, rare cases with an indolent clinical course have been reported {178,1104, 1493,3267}. In one recent large series, median survival was 31 months {1493}.

Primary cutaneous CD8+ aggressive epidermotropic cytotoxic T-cell lymphoma

Berti E.
Gaulard P.
Willemze R.
Petrella T.
Jaffe E.S.

Definition
This provisional entity is a cutaneous T-cell lymphoma characterized by proliferation of epidermotropic CD8+ cytotoxic T cells and aggressive clinical behaviour. Differentiation from other types of cutaneous T-cell lymphomas with a CD8+ cytotoxic T-cell phenotype is based on the clinical presentation, clinical behaviour, and certain histological features, such as marked epidermotropism with epidermal necrosis.

ICD-O code   9709/3

Epidemiology
This disease is rare, accounting for < 1% of all cutaneous T-cell lymphomas {30, 361,4320}. It occurs mainly in adults. There are no known predisposing factors.

Localization
Most patients present with generalized skin lesions.

Clinical features
Clinically, these lymphomas are characterized by localized ulcerated nodules, tumours, or plaques, or (more commonly) by disseminated eruptive papules, nodules, and tumours showing central ulceration and necrosis {361,3377,3518}. These lymphomas may disseminate to

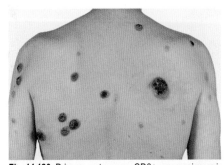

Fig. 14.120 Primary cutaneous CD8+ aggressive epidermotropic cytotoxic T-cell lymphoma. Lesions are often haemorrhagic, and are associated with ulceration and epidermal necrosis.

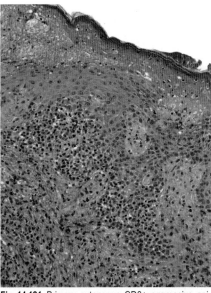

Fig. 14.121 Primary cutaneous CD8+ aggressive epidermotropic cytotoxic T-cell lymphoma. The atypical lymphoid cells infiltrate in the superficial dermis and extend into the epidermis in a pagetoid fashion.

other visceral sites (lungs, testes, CNS, oral mucosa), but lymph nodes are often spared {361,2535,3267,3377}.

Microscopy
The histological appearance is very variable, ranging from a lichenoid pattern with marked, pagetoid epidermotropism and subepidermal oedema (disseminated variant) to deeper, more-nodular and less-epidermotropic infiltrates (localized variant). The epidermis may be acanthotic or atrophic, often with necrosis, ulceration, and blister formation {30, 361,3377}. Invasion and destruction of adnexal skin structures are commonly seen. Angiocentricity and angioinvasion may be present {2546,3377}. Tumour cells are small-medium or medium-large, with pleomorphic or blastic nuclei {361}.

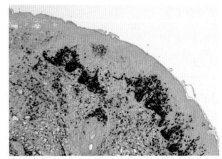

Fig. 14.122 Primary cutaneous CD8+ aggressive epidermotropic cytotoxic T-cell lymphoma. Skin section stained for CD8, highlighting the marked epidermotropism, with most of the neoplastic cells localized to the epidermis.

Immunophenotype

The tumour cells characteristically have a beta F1–positive, CD3+, CD8+, CD4–, granzyme B–positive, perforin-positive, TIA1+, CD45RA+, CD45RO– phenotype. Most cases lack CD5 and CD2, with variable expression of CD7 {30,317,361, 2546,3267,3377,3518}. Most cases are CD30-negative {3267,3377}.

Primary cutaneous aggressive epidermotropic CD8+ cytotoxic T-cell lymphoma may be histopathologically and phenotypically indistinguishable from a variant of lymphomatoid papulosis (type D) characterized by self-healing papules and nodules (necrotic lesions) with spontaneous resolution {3473}. Clinical information is also important, to differentiate from other CD8+ cutaneous T-cell lymphomas, including CD8+ mycosis fungoides {3267}.

Postulated normal counterpart

A skin-homing, CD8+, cytotoxic T cell of alpha beta type

Genetic profile

The neoplastic T cells show clonal TR gene rearrangements. Specific genetic abnormalities have not been described. EBV is negative {317,2546,3377}.

Prognosis and predictive factors

These lymphomas have an aggressive clinical course, with a median survival of 12 months in a recent series {3377}. There is no difference in survival between cases with small or large cell morphology {317}, or between cases with localized or diffuse lesions {3377}.

Primary cutaneous acral CD8+ T-cell lymphoma

Petrella T.
Gaulard P.
Berti E.
Willemze R.
Jaffe E.S.

Definition

Primary cutaneous acral CD8+ T-cell lymphoma is a rare cutaneous tumour characterized by skin infiltration of clonal atypical medium-sized cytotoxic lymphocytes {3156}. The tumour is clinically characterized by preferential involvement of acral sites (in particular the ears) and by a good prognosis.

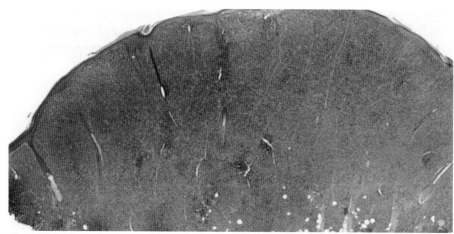

Fig. 14.123 Primary cutaneous acral CD8+ T-cell lymphoma. Dense and monotonous dermal and hypodermal infiltrate of the helix.

ICD-O code 9709/3

Synonym

Indolent cutaneous CD8+ lymphoid proliferation

Epidemiology

The disease affects adults; no paediatric cases have been reported. The median patient age is 53 years, and there is a male predominance, with a male-to-female ratio of 3.2:1 {324,1331,1515,2302, 2311,3156,3828,3856,4345,4468}.

Etiology

There are currently no clues as to the etiology of primary cutaneous acral CD8+ T-cell lymphoma. A local trigger agent may be suspected by analogy to *Helicobacter pylori* in gastric MALT lymphoma or *Borrelia burgdorferi* and *Chlamydia psittaci* in skin MALT lymphoma {1198}, but to date no infectious or toxic candidate has been identified.

Clinical features

Cutaneous lesions are most often an isolated reddish papule or nodule measuring from several millimetres to 3–4 cm, with a history of slow growth over several weeks or months. The most frequent site is the ear (61%), generally the helix or the conch, rarely the lobe. The nose is the second most frequent (22%) site followed by the foot (8%). Other skin sites (eyelids, hands, leg) are anecdotally reported. Occasionally, lesions are multiple {1446}, and in particular bilateral on the ears {324,3156} and the feet {4345}. Local recurrence after treatment is possible. In rare cases, recurrence may occur at other cutaneous sites {2302,4345}.

Microscopy

The tumours are composed of a monotonous dermal proliferation of atypical medium-sized lymphocytes with irregular and frequently folded nuclei and small nucleoli {3156}. A case with signet ring cells has been reported {2311}. Mitoses and apoptotic figures are absent or very rare. Reactive B-cell lymphoid aggregates of follicles may be seen within the atypical infiltrate. Plasma cells, histiocytes, neutro-

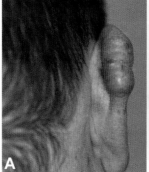 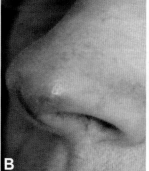 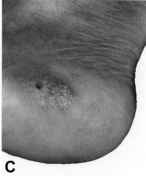

Fig. 14.124 Primary cutaneous acral CD8+ T-cell lymphoma. **A** Nodule of the right helix. **B** Nodule of the nose. **C** Nodule/plaque of the left foot.

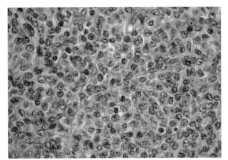

Fig. 14.125 Primary cutaneous acral CD8+ T-cell lymphoma. At high power, the infiltrate is monomorphic and composed of atypical lymphoid cells, with some nuclear irregularity and fine chromatin.

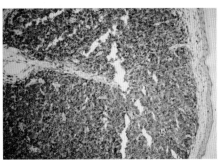

Fig. 14.126 Primary cutaneous acral CD8+ T-cell lymphoma. Diffuse CD8 positivity in the dermis, with a grenz zone.

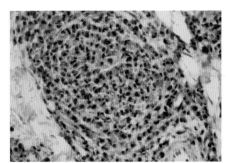

Fig. 14.127 Primary cutaneous acral CD8+ T-cell lymphoma. TIA1 shows Golgi dot–like immunostaining.

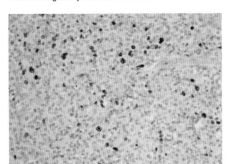

Fig. 14.128 Primary cutaneous acral CD8+ T-cell lymphoma. Fewer than 10% of the tumour cells are positive for Ki-67.

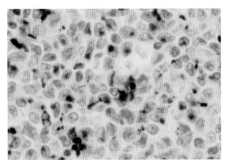

Fig. 14.129 Primary cutaneous acral CD8+ T-cell lymphoma. Several atypical cells show Golgi dot–like staining for CD68 (PGM1), besides normally stained reactive histiocytes.

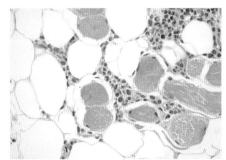

Fig. 14.130 Primary cutaneous acral CD8+ T-cell lymphoma. Infiltration of cutaneous fat tissue and nasal ala muscle.

phils, and eosinophils are absent or very rare. The epidermis is most often spared, with a grenz zone. Occasionally, minimal insignificant epidermotropism may be seen {1446,1515}. Skin appendages are always spared, and angiotropism, angiodestruction, and necrosis are never seen. The proliferation frequently involves the underlying fat tissue.

Immunophenotype
The tumoural infiltrate is composed of T cells that express CD3, CD8, TIA1, and beta F1. TIA1 displays Golgi dot–like staining. CD4 is always negative. CD2, CD5, and CD7 are regularly positive but one or more of them can be lost or weak. Granzyme B and perforin are generally negative but may occasionally be positive. CD56, CD57, CD30, and TdT are always negative, as are the T follicular helper (TFH) cell markers (CD10, BCL6, PD1, and CXCL13) {1446}. CD68 is frequently positive, displaying as does TIA1, Golgi dot–like staining {4345}. In the vast majority of cases, the Ki-67 proliferation index is very low (< 10%). A few typical cases with a high proliferation index have been reported {4468}; however, when the proliferation index is > 50%, other

CD8+ cutaneous lymphomas should be carefully considered {3377}. Staining for B-cell markers (CD20, CD79a) might reveal reactive B-cell aggregates or follicles. LMP1 and EBV-encoded small RNA (EBER) are negative.

Postulated normal counterpart
The postulated normal counterpart is a skin-homing CD8+ T cell. However, cases that are very similar in terms of morphology, phenotype, and clinical outcome have also been recently described in the gastrointestinal tract {3145} and genital tract {3863}, suggesting a new lymphoma entity arising from tissue-resident CD8+ memory T cells.

Genetic profile
The neoplastic T cells show clonal TRG gene rearrangements. Specific genetic abnormalities have not yet been described. EBV is negative.

Prognosis and predictive factors
The tumour has a very good prognosis. Complete remission after surgical excision or radiotherapy is the rule. Local or extra-site skin recurrence may occur. There is no evidence of dissemination

to other organs or lymphoid tissue. No chemotherapy is needed. It is important to recognize this disease to avoid overtreatment.

Primary cutaneous CD4+ small/medium T-cell lymphoproliferative disorder

Gaulard P.
Berti E.
Willemze R.
Petrella T.
Jaffe E.S.

Definition
Primary cutaneous CD4+ small/medium T-cell lymphoproliferative disorder is characterized by a predominance of small to medium-sized CD4+ pleomorphic T cells, and by presentation with a solitary skin lesion in almost all cases, without evidence of the patches and plaques typical of mycosis fungoides. Because these cases have the same clinicopathological features and benign clinical course as cutaneous pseudo–T-cell lymphomas with a nodular growth pattern {323,626,3267}, the term

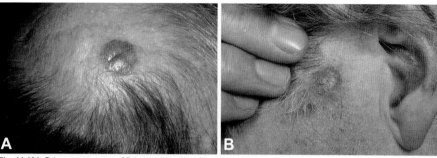

Fig. 14.131 Primary cutaneous CD4+ small/medium T-cell lymphoproliferative disorder. **A** Typical presentation as a solitary lesion on the scalp. **B** The lesion is usually a single raised erythematous nodule.

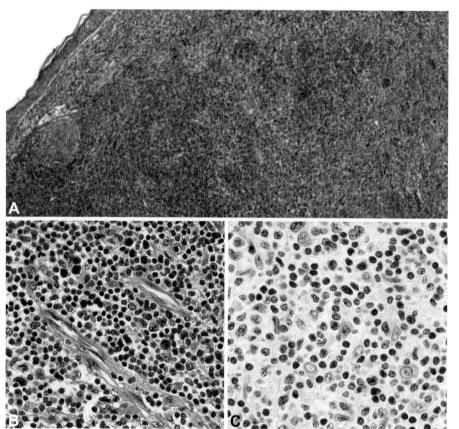

Fig. 14.132 Primary cutaneous CD4+ small/medium T-cell lymphoproliferative disorder. **A** Atypical lymphoid cells form a dense infiltrate in the dermis, but do not extend into the epidermis. **B** Atypical lymphoid cells form a dense infiltrate in the dermis. **C** The lymphoid cells are small to medium-sized, with mild pleomorphism. Admixed histiocytes or plasma cells may be present, and histiocytes can be abundant in some cases.

'primary cutaneous CD4+ small/medium T-cell lymphoproliferative disorder' is preferred, rather than 'primary cutaneous CD4+ small/medium T-cell lymphoma'. Rare cases presenting with widespread skin lesions, large rapidly growing tumours, >30% large pleomorphic T cells, and/or a high proliferative fraction do not belong to this group {1298,1471}. Such cases usually have a more aggressive clinical behaviour and are better classified as peripheral T-cell lymphoma, NOS.

ICD-O code 9709/1

Synonym
Primary cutaneous CD4+ small/medium T-cell lymphoma (no longer used)

Epidemiology
This is a rare disease, accounting for 2% of all cutaneous T-cell lymphomas {4320}.

Localization
These lesions usually present as a solitary plaque or nodule, most commonly on the face, neck, or upper trunk {317, 323,626,1298,1471,1832,3267}.

Clinical features
Patients are asymptomatic; a single slow-growing skin lesion is the sole manifestation of disease. In rare cases, multiple lesions are present {323,626}. By definition, there should be no patches typical of mycosis fungoides.

Microscopy
These lymphomas show dense, diffuse, or nodular infiltrates within the dermis, with a tendency to infiltrate the subcutis. Epidermotropism may be present focally, but if epidermotropism is conspicuous, the diagnosis of mycosis fungoides should be considered. There is a predominance of small/medium-sized pleomorphic T cells {317,323,626,1298,1471, 1832,3267,3391}. A small proportion (<30%) of large pleomorphic cells may be present {320}. In almost all cases, the atypical CD4+ T cells are admixed with small reactive CD8+ T cells, B cells, plasma cells, and histiocytes (including multinucleated giant cells) {323,626,3391}.

Immunophenotype
By definition, these proliferations have a CD3+, CD4+, CD8–, CD30– phenotype. Loss of pan–T-cell antigens (except for CD7) is uncommon, and cytotoxic proteins are not expressed {323,626,1471, 3391}. Atypical CD4+ T cells express PD1, BCL6 (variable), and CXCL13, suggesting T follicular helper (TFH) cell derivation {626,3391}. CD10 is usually negative. The Ki-67 proliferation index is low (typically 5%, and at most 20%).

Postulated normal counterpart
A skin-homing CD4+ T cell with TFH-cell characteristics

Genetic profile
TR genes are clonally rearranged in most cases {626,3391}. Specific genetic abnormalities have not been described. EBV is negative.

Prognosis and predictive factors
Patients have an excellent prognosis. Intralesional steroids, surgical excision, and radiotherapy are preferred modes of treatment {323,626,1471}. Spontaneous remission after biopsy has been reported {626, 1471,1832}. Local recurrences are rare.

Peripheral T-cell lymphoma, NOS

Pileri S.A.
Weisenburger D.D.
Sng I.
Nakamura S.
Müller-Hermelink H.K.
Chan W.C.
Jaffe E.S.

Definition

Peripheral T-cell lymphoma (PTCL), NOS, is a heterogeneous category of nodal and extranodal mature T-cell lymphomas that do not correspond to any of the specifically defined entities of mature T-cell lymphoma in the current classification (Table 14.09). Excluded from this category are tumours with a T follicular helper (TFH) cell phenotype, as defined by the expression of at least two (ideally three) of the following markers: CD10, BCL6, PD1, CXCL13, CXCR5, ICOS, and SAP {34,2231,2496}. PTCL, NOS, nearly always presents in adults, and has an aggressive clinical course.

ICD-O code   9702/3

Synonyms

T-cell lymphoma, NOS; peripheral T-cell lymphoma, pleomorphic small cell; peripheral T-cell lymphoma, pleomorphic medium and large cell; peripheral T-cell lymphoma, large cell; lymphoepithelioid lymphoma; Lennert lymphoma

Table 14.09 Differential diagnosis of nodal peripheral T-cell lymphoma, NOS

Disease	Immunophenotypic features
Peripheral T-cell lymphoma, NOS	CD4 > CD8; antigen loss frequent (CD7, CD5, CD4/CD8, CD52); GATA3–/+; TBX21–/+; cytotoxic granules–/+; CD30–/+; CD56–/+; rare cases EBV+
Angioimmunoblastic T-cell lymphoma	CD4+; expression of at least two (preferably three) of the following TFH-cell markers: CD10, BCL6, PD1, CXCL13, CXCR5, ICOS, SAP; hyperplasia of FDCs (CD21+) and HEVs (MECA79+); EBV+ CD20+ B blasts
Nodal peripheral T-cell lymphoma with TFH phenotype	Expression of at least two (preferably three) of the following TFH-cell markers: CD10, BCL6, PD1, CXCL13, CXCR5, ICOS, SAP; no hyperplasia of FDCs or HEVs
Adult T-cell leukaemia/lymphoma	CD4+; CD25+; CD7–; CD30–/+; CD15–/+; FOXP3–/+
ALK+ anaplastic large cell lymphoma	CD30+; ALK+; EMA+; CD25+; cytotoxic granules+/–, CD4+/–; CD3–/+; CD43+
ALK– anaplastic large cell lymphoma	CD30+; EMA+; CD25+; cytotoxic granules+/–; CD4+/–; CD3–/+; CD43+; PAX5/BSAP–
T-cell/histiocyte-rich large B-cell lymphoma	Large CD20+ blasts in background of reactive T cells with complete phenotypic profile
T-zone hyperplasia	Expansion of T cells with complete phenotypic profile and mixed CD4/CD8, variable CD25 and CD30; scattered CD20+ B cells

+, nearly always positive; +/–, majority positive; –/+, minority positive; –, negative
FDC, follicular dendritic cell; HEV: high endothelial venule; TFH, T follicular helper

Epidemiology

These tumours account for approximately 30% of PTCLs in western countries {3365}. Most patients are adults. These lymphomas are very rare in children. The male-to-female ratio is 2:1.

Etiology

The infection of neoplastic cells by EBV is reported in a small number of cases, in which the virus plays a pathogenetic role {178,1068,1505,4298}. More commonly, EBV may be found in background B cells.

Localization

Most patients present with peripheral lymph node involvement, but any site can be affected. Advanced-stage disease is common, with secondary involvement of the bone marrow, liver, spleen, and extranodal tissues {3365}. The peripheral blood is sometimes involved, but leukaemic presentation is uncommon {3365}.

Extranodal presentations can occur, most commonly in the skin and gastrointestinal tract {3365}. In this setting, the diagnosis of PTCL, NOS, should be made only after more specific entities have been excluded. Other less frequently involved sites include the lungs and CNS {2632}.

Clinical features

Patients most often present with lymph node enlargement, and most have

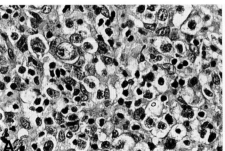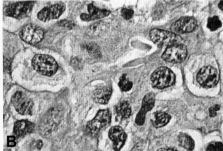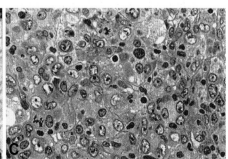

Fig. 14.133 Peripheral T-cell lymphoma, NOS, with prominent clear-cell features (**A,B**) or large lymphoid cells with vesicular, immunoblast-like nuclei (**C**).

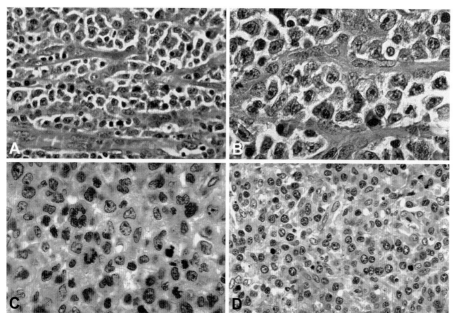

Fig. 14.134 Peripheral T-cell lymphoma, NOS. **A** Diffuse infiltrates of large lymphoid cells with pleomorphic, irregular nuclei and prominent nucleoli. **B** Between the neoplastic cells, there are scattered eosinophils and numerous vessels. **C** Nuclei are markedly pleomorphic and multilobed. **D** In some cases, nuclei are round and monomorphic in appearance.

advanced disease with B symptoms {3365}. Paraneoplastic features such as eosinophilia, pruritus, or (rarely) haemophagocytic syndrome may be seen {3365}.

Microscopy

In the lymph node, these lymphomas show paracortical or diffuse infiltrates with effacement of the normal architecture. The cytological spectrum is extremely broad, from polymorphous to monomorphic. Most cases consist of numerous medium-sized and/or large cells with irregular, pleomorphic, hyperchromatic, or vesicular nuclei; prominent nucleoli; and many mitotic figures {1557,1816}. Clear cells and Reed–Sternberg–like cells can also be seen. Rare cases have a pre-dominance of small lymphoid cells with atypical, irregular nuclei. Hyperplasia of high endothelial venules and/or follicular dendritic cells and the open marginal sinuses characteristic of angioimmunoblastic T-cell lymphoma (AITL) are not usually seen {1557,1816}. An inflammatory background is often present, including small lymphocytes, eosinophils, plasma cells, large B cells (which may be clonal irrespective of EBV infection) {4258}, and clusters of epithelioid histiocytes. Epithelioid histiocytes are particularly numerous in the lymphoepithelioid variant. Extranodal involvement takes the form of diffuse infiltrates composed of similar cells. In the skin, the lymphomatous population tends to infiltrate the dermis and subcutis, often producing nodules, which may undergo central necrosis {3110}. Epidermotropism, angiocentricity, and adnexal involvement are sometimes seen {3110}. In the spleen, the pattern is variable, from solitary or multiple fleshy nodules to diffuse white pulp involvement with colonization of the periarteriolar sheaths or, in some cases, predominant infiltration of the red pulp {641}.

Variants

Lymphoepithelioid lymphoma
This variant, also known as Lennert lymphoma, shows diffuse or (less commonly) interfollicular growth. Cytologically, it consists predominantly of small cells with slight nuclear irregularities; numerous and sometimes confluent clusters of epithelioid histiocytes; and some larger, more atypical, proliferating blasts. There can be admixed inflammatory cells and scattered Reed–Sternberg–like B cells (usually EBV-positive). High endothelial venules are not prominent. In most cases, the neoplastic cells are CD8-positive and have a cytotoxic profile {34,1321,1569, 4411}. This variant may have a somewhat better prognosis than do other forms of PTCL, NOS.

Other variants
The follicular variant included within the PTCL, NOS, category in the 2008 edition of the WHO classification has been moved to the category of AITL and other nodal lymphomas of T follicular helper cell origin in this update.
The same is true for a proportion of cases previously designated as the T-zone variant, because they usually have a TFH-cell phenotype {34}. Thus, the growth of atypical small T lymphocytes around florid reactive germinal centres {3463,4258} is no longer considered to be a variant of PTCL, NOS, but rather a non-specific

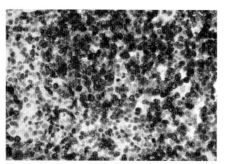

Fig. 14.135 Peripheral T-cell lymphoma, NOS. Neoplastic cells express CD3.

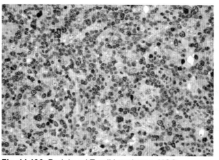

Fig. 14.136 Peripheral T-cell lymphoma, NOS. Neoplastic cells express T-cell receptor beta as assessed by beta F1 monoclonal antibody staining.

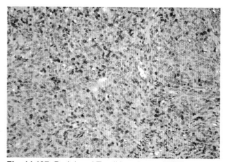

Fig. 14.137 Peripheral T-cell lymphoma, NOS. Neoplastic cells lack CD5 expression. Note the presence of some reactive T lymphocytes, which serve as an internal control.

morphological pattern. This pattern may sometimes be mistaken for benign paracortical hyperplasia.

Primary EBV-positive nodal T-cell or NK-cell lymphomas have been reported {178,718,1505,1901}. These usually have a monomorphic pattern of infiltration and lack the angiodestruction and necrosis seen in extranodal NK/T-cell lymphoma. They are more common in elderly patients, or in the setting of immune deficiency. For the time being, they are considered a variant of peripheral T-cell lymphoma, NOS, but may be designated as a separate entity with more data.

Immunophenotype

PTCL, NOS, is usually characterized by an aberrant T-cell phenotype with frequent downregulation of CD5 and CD7 {4298} (see Table 14.09, p. 403). A CD4+/ CD8– phenotype predominates in nodal cases. CD4/CD8 double-positivity or double-negativity is sometimes seen, as is CD8, CD56, and cytotoxic granule expression (e.g. TIA1, granzyme B, and perforin) {4298}. T-cell receptor beta (beta F1) is usually expressed, facilitating the distinction from gamma delta T-cell lymphomas and NK-cell lymphomas. CD15 may be positive, and may be coexpressed with CD30 in rare cases {277}. Such cases may show features overlapping with those of ALK-negative (ALK–) anaplastic large cell lymphoma (ALCL), but are classified as PTCL, NOS, under the current guidelines. CD15 expression is associated with an adverse prognosis {4298}.

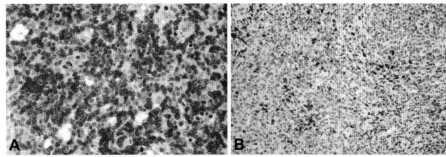

Fig. 14.138 Peripheral T-cell lymphoma, NOS. **A** Neoplastic cells express CD4. **B** In the same case, neoplastic cells lack CD8 expression. Note the presence of some reactive T lymphocytes, which serve as an internal control.

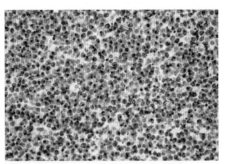

Fig. 14.139 Peripheral T-cell lymphoma, NOS. Neoplastic cells express the cytotoxic marker TIA1.

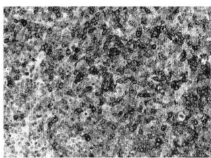

Fig. 14.140 Peripheral T-cell lymphoma, NOS. Neoplastic cells show partial and variable expression of CD30.

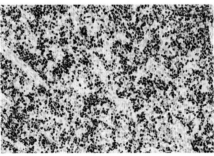

Fig. 14.141 Peripheral T-cell lymphoma, NOS. Most neoplastic cells express TBX21.

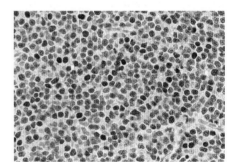

Fig. 14.142 Peripheral T-cell lymphoma, NOS. Most neoplastic cells express GATA3.

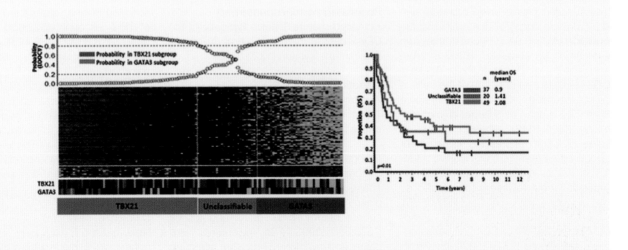

Fig. 14.143 Peripheral T-cell lymphoma (PTCL), NOS. Gene expression profiling identifies two main subgroups of PTCL, NOS, characterized by overexpression of TBX21 and GATA3, respectively. The former is associated with a more favourable clinical course, with longer overall survival (OS).

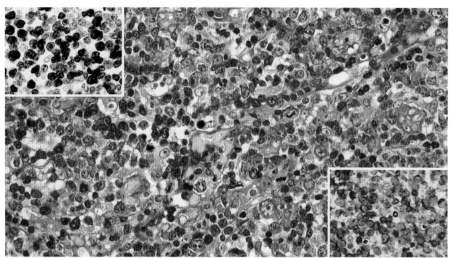

Fig. 14.144 Peripheral T-cell lymphoma, NOS. Note the marked pleomorphism of the neoplastic population. Upper inset: High Ki-67 labelling. Lower inset: Beta F1 staining.

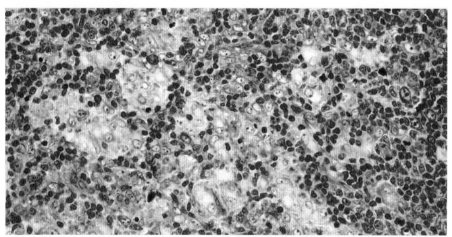

Fig. 14.145 Peripheral T-cell lymphoma, NOS, lymphoepithelioid variant. Neoplastic cells are admixed with prominent epithelioid histiocytic clusters, which tend to obscure the lymphomatous growth (Giemsa stain).

The expression of TBX21 (also known as T-BET) and GATA3 may be relevant for the subclassification of PTCL, NOS (see also *Genetic profile* and *Prognosis and predictive factors*) {1775,4253}. The expression of a single TFH-cell marker can sometimes be observed. CD52 is present in 40% of cases {656,3170,3383}. CD30 is detected in > 25% of the cells in half of the cases {427,3467} and in some instances is used as a target of immunotoxins {2965,4442}, although the cut-off value of CD30 expression required for effective treatment remains elusive {1160, 1701}. PTCL, NOS, with high CD30 expression does not seem to respond as well as does ALK– ALCL {3172,3536}. Aberrant expression of CD20 and/or CD79a, as well as of CD15, is occasionally encountered {277,4258,4298}. Proliferation is usually high, and a Ki-67 prolif-

eration index > 70% is associated with a worse prognosis {4298}.

Postulated normal counterpart
Activated mature T cells, typically of the CD4+ central memory type of the adaptive immune system {1320,3169}

Genetic profile
Antigen receptor genes
TR genes are clonally rearranged in most cases {3365}.

Cytogenetic abnormalities and oncogenes
These are usually highly aberrant neoplasms with complex karyotypes and recurrent chromosomal gains and losses {1573,3365,3992,4472}. Genomic imbalances have been reported, affecting several regions containing members of NF-kappaB signalling and genes involved

in cell-cycle control {1573}. The genetic aberrations observed in PTCL, NOS, differ from those of other T-cell lymphomas, such as AITL and ALCL {3992,4472}. Gene expression profiling and microRNA profiling studies have revealed distinctive signatures distinct from those of AITL and ALK+ and ALK– ALCL {31,243,842,905,1774, 1775,2184,2364,2617,3169,3172,3202}. Gene expression profiling has also allowed the identification of groups of PTCL, NOS, cases characterized by the expression of TBX21 (also known as T-BET) or GATA3 {1775}. The former group includes some cases with a cytotoxic profile {1775}. Although TBX21 and GATA3 are transcription factors that are master regulators of gene expression profiles in T helper (Th) cells, skewing Th cell polarization into Th1 cell and Th2 cell differentiation pathways, respectively {900,1775}, further studies are needed to confirm them as definitive markers of Th1-cell–derived and Th2-cell–derived neoplasms. Immunohistochemical surrogate markers have been used in lieu of gene expression profiling studies, and may have prognostic significance {4253} (see *Prognosis and predictive factors*). In comparison to normal T lymphocytes, PTCL, NOS, is characterized by the recurrent deregulation of genes involved in relevant cell functions (e.g. matrix deposition, cytoskeleton organization, cell adhesion, apoptosis, proliferation, transcription, and signal transduction) {3169}. The products of these genes might have therapeutic relevance {842,3169}. For example, overexpression of PDGFRA (likely due to an autocrine loop) can herald sensitivity to tyrosine kinase inhibitors {2192,3174}. Although recurrent mutations have been reported in AITL and other nodal PTCLs of TFH-cell origin {523,900,1010A,2264, 3040,3176,3395,3485,4238,4428,4429}, it is still unclear whether similar alterations are seen in PTCL, NOS. Two publications based on small series of PTCL, NOS, cases {3552,3683} reported different recurrent mutations, findings that do not allow a firm conclusion as to the mutational landscape of the tumour. Two recent studies reported activating mutations or translocations of *VAV1* in 10–15% of cases of PTCL, NOS {7A,396A}

Differential diagnosis
Now that the PTCLs with TFH-cell phenotype are excluded from this category, the distinction of PTCL, NOS, from AITL is less of a problem. More problematic

remains the distinction from ALK– ALCL. In fact, CD30 is highly expressed by a subset of PTCL, NOS {427,3467}. On morphological and immunohistochemical grounds, the simultaneous occurrence of hallmark cells (with kidney-shaped or horseshoe-shaped nuclei), strong and uniform CD30 positivity, EMA positivity, and cytotoxic marker expression is characteristic of ALK– ALCL and not observed in PTCL, NOS {1775,3172}. The gene and microRNA signatures of ALK– ALCL are much closer to those of ALK+ ALCL than to those of PTCL, NOS {31,1774,1775,2364,3202}. Importantly, ALK– ALCL carries genomic aberrations

(e.g. *DUSP22* and *TP63* rearrangement) that to date have not been reported in PTCL, NOS {402,836,3069}.

Prognosis and predictive factors

These are highly aggressive lymphomas with a poor response to therapy, frequent relapses, and low 5-year overall survival and failure-free survival rates (20–30%) {3365}. The only factors consistently associated with prognosis are stage and International Prognostic Index (IPI) score {3365}. New scoring systems have recently been developed {1282, 4298}. Involvement of the bone marrow and a Ki-67 proliferation index > 70%

have been proposed as negative prognostic factors, but further confirmation is needed. EBV positivity, NF-kappaB pathway deregulation, a high proliferation signature by gene expression, transformed cells > 70%, a GATA3 or cytotoxic profile, and CD30 expression in most or all cells have been found to correlate with a poor prognosis {164,842,1068,2184, 3172,3536,4217,4283,4298}. Upfront autologous stem cell transplantation seems to significantly improve both overall and relapse-free survival {855}.

Angioimmunoblastic T-cell lymphoma and other nodal lymphomas of T follicular helper cell origin

Dogan A.
Gaulard P.
Jaffe E.S.
Müller-Hermelink H.K.
de Leval L.

Since the recognition of T follicular helper (TFH) cells as a unique physiological subset of T helper (Th) cells with a characteristic phenotype, it has been discovered that a subset of peripheral T-cell lymphomas have phenotypic features of TFH cells. These lymphomas are thought to constitute the neoplastic counterpart of TFH cells {905,1470}. The best-studied of these is angioimmunoblastic T-cell lymphoma, in which the neoplastic cells have a TFH-cell gene expression signature and express many of the TFH-cell–associated markers, such as CD10, CXCL13, BCL6, ICOS, CXCR5, SAP, MAF (also called c-MAF), and (in most cases) CD200 {177,1028,1067,1470,2108,2496, 3399}. Additionally, a number of nodal peripheral T-cell lymphomas previously classified within the peripheral T-cell lymphoma, NOS, category have recently been shown to have a TFH-cell phenotype {179,906,1010A,1729}. Such cases, including so-called follicular T-cell lymphoma, show some morphological, immunophenotypic, genetic, and clinical overlap with angioimmunoblastic T-cell lymphoma but also have a number of unique, distinctive features as discussed

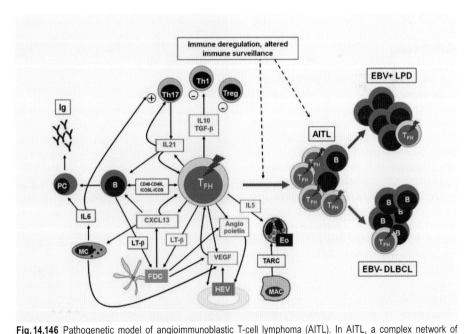

Fig. 14.146 Pathogenetic model of angioimmunoblastic T-cell lymphoma (AITL). In AITL, a complex network of interactions take place between the tumour cells and the various cellular components of the reactive microenvironment, the molecular mediators of which have been partly deciphered. Various factors released by T follicular helper (TFH) cells are involved in B-cell recruitment, activation, and differentiation (CXCL13); in the modulation of other T-cell subsets (IL21, IL10, TGF-beta); and in promoting vascular proliferation (VEGF, angiopoietin), and may also act as autocrine factors. CXCL13 may also attract mast cells (MCs), which are a source of IL6, promoting T helper 17 (Th17) cell differentiation. EBV reactivation occurs in the context of a deregulated immune response, which also favours the expansion of both TFH cells and B cells. TGF-beta is a mediator of follicular dendritic cell (FDC) differentiation and proliferation, and FDCs, in turn, are a source of CXCL13 and VEGF.

below. For these reasons, in this update, they have been included under the broader category of nodal lymphomas of TFH-cell origin with angioimmunoblastic T-cell lymphoma, but are summarized separately. Cutaneous T-cell lymphomas and lymphoproliferative disorders expressing TFH-cell markers are excluded from this group of neoplasms.

Angioimmunoblastic T-cell lymphoma

Definition

Angioimmunoblastic T-cell lymphoma (AITL) is a neoplasm of mature T follicular helper (TFH) cells characterized by systemic disease and a polymorphous infiltrate involving lymph nodes, with a prominent proliferation of high endothelial venules (HEVs) and follicular dendritic cells (FDCs). EBV-positive B cells are nearly always present, and in some cases constitute a significant part of the cellular infiltrate. Recent studies using next-generation sequencing have identified recurrent mutations that help to unify AITL with other T-cell neoplasms derived from TFH cells. The disease is clinically aggressive and seen mainly in older adults.

ICD-O code   9705/3

Synonyms and historical terminology

Peripheral T-cell lymphoma, angio-immunoblastic lymphadenopathy with dysproteinaemia; (obsolete); immuno-blastic lymphadenopathy (obsolete); lym-phogranulomatosis X (obsolete)

AITL, previously designated as angio-immunoblastic lymphadenopathy, was thought to be an atypical reactive process, with an increased risk of progression to lymphoma. Overwhelming evidence now indicates that AITL arises de novo as a peripheral T-cell lymphoma (PTCL) {901,1013}.

Epidemiology

AITL occurs in middle-aged and elderly individuals, with a higher incidence in males than in females {901}. It is one of the most common specific subtypes of PTCL, accounting for 15–30% of non-cutaneous T-cell lymphomas and 1–2% of all non-Hodgkin lymphomas {904, 3464,4217}.

Etiology

The strong association with EBV infection suggests a possible role for the virus in the etiology, possibly through antigen drive {1061}. However, the neoplastic T cells are EBV-negative.

Localization

The primary site of disease is the lymph node, and virtually all patients present with generalized lymphadenopathy. The spleen, liver, skin, and bone marrow are also frequently involved {901,1013,1169, 2767}.

Clinical features

AITL typically presents with advanced-stage disease, generalized lymphadenopathy, hepatosplenomegaly, systemic symptoms, and polyclonal hypergam-maglobulinaemia {1013,2181,2767,3674}. Skin rash, often with pruritus, is frequently present. Other common findings are pleural effusion, arthritis, and ascites. Laboratory findings include circulating immune complexes, cold agglutinins with haemolytic anaemia, positive rheu-matoid factor, and anti–smooth muscle antibodies.

Patients exhibit immunodeficiency secondary to the neoplastic process. In most cases (75%), expansion of EBV-positive B cells is seen, which is thought to be a consequence of underlying immune dysfunction {92,938,4288}.

Microscopy

AITL is characterized by partial or total effacement of the lymph node architecture, often with perinodal infiltration but sparing of the peripheral cortical sinuses. Cytologically, the neoplastic T cells of AITL are small to medium-sized lymphocytes, with clear to pale cytoplasm, distinct cell membranes, and minimal cytological atypia. They frequently form small clusters, often adjacent to HEVs. Vascularity is often prominent, with arborization of HEVs in the paracortex. The neoplastic cells are present in a polymorphous inflammatory background containing variable numbers of reactive lymphocytes, histiocytes, plasma cells, and eosinophils. The cellular density varies, and in

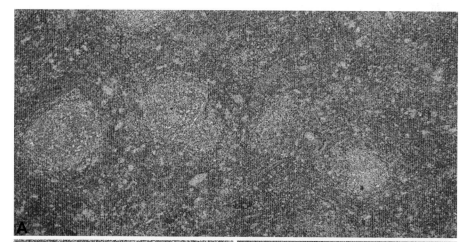
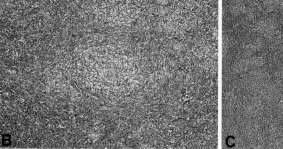

Fig. 14.147 Histological patterns of angioimmunoblastic T-cell lymphoma (AITL). **A** Early involvement by AITL characterized by bare, hyperplastic follicles with paracortical expansion and marked vascular proliferation associated with perifollicular or atypical lymphoid cells (pattern 1). **B** Case with depleted/atrophic follicles reminiscent of Castleman disease and marked perifollicular expansion of clear cells (pattern 2). **C** Classic morphology with effacement of normal architecture and marked vascular proliferation associated with aggregates of atypical lymphoid cells (pattern 3).

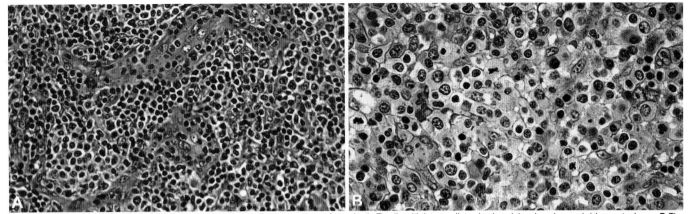

Fig. 14.148 Angioimmunoblastic T-cell lymphoma. **A** Pattern 3. Typical cytology of neoplastic T cells with intermediate-sized nuclei and copious pale/clear cytoplasm. **B** The infiltrate is composed of medium-sized to large lymphoid cells with abundant clear cytoplasm.

some cases there is amorphous interstitial precipitate, producing a hypocellular appearance.

Three overlapping patterns are recognized {177}. In pattern 1, the neoplastic cells surround hyperplastic follicles with well-formed germinal centres, but often lacking well-defined mantle cuffs {3328}. Pattern 1 is difficult to distinguish from reactive follicular hyperplasia, and immunohistochemical stains are necessary to highlight the neoplastic T cells with their characteristic TFH-cell phenotype. In pattern 2, remnants of follicles remain but show regressive changes. The neoplastic cells are more readily identified in the expanded paracortex. In pattern 3, the architecture is totally or subtotally effaced; remnants of regressed follicles may be seen in the outer cortex, displaced by the expanded paracortex. Progression from pattern 1 to pattern 3 in consecutive biopsies has been reported {3387}.

In advanced cases, the inflammatory component may be diminished, and the proportion of clear cells and large cells may increase (so-called tumour cell–rich AITL), which may simulate a PTCL, NOS. In such cases, demonstration of a TFH-cell immunophenotype and the presence of expanded FDC meshworks are helpful in diagnosis {178}. In some cases, there may be a prominent infiltrate of reactive epithelioid histiocytes, mimicking a granulomatous reaction and resembling lymphoepithelioid lymphoma {34,178}. The polymorphic infiltrate is frequently associated with increased extrafollicular FDC meshworks, which are most prominent around the HEVs. The neoplastic cells are often arranged in clusters, surrounded by dendritic processes and highlighted by CD21.

Variable numbers of B immunoblasts are usually present in the paracortex, which may be positive or negative for EBV by in situ hybridization for EBV-encoded small RNA (EBER). EBV-positive B cells are present in 80–95% of cases. They range in size, and expansion of B immunoblasts may be prominent {4288,4470}. The EBV-positive B immunoblastic proliferation may progress, either composite with AITL or at relapse, to EBV-positive diffuse large B-cell lymphoma {182,4470}. EBV-positive Reed–Sternberg–like cells of B-cell lineage may be present and may simulate classic Hodgkin lymphoma {178,3265}. In rare cases, EBV-negative Reed–Sternberg–like cells of B-cell lineage may be present {2868}. Plasma cells may be very abundant, in rare cases obscuring the neoplastic T cells {238A, 1736A}. The plasma cells are usually polyclonal, but may be monoclonal in some cases. The expansion of normal B cells and plasma cells in the lesions has been linked to the functional properties of the neoplastic TFH cells {1061}.

Immunophenotype

The neoplastic T cells express most pan–T-cell antigens (e.g. CD3, CD2, and CD5) and in the vast majority of cases are positive for CD4. Surface CD3 may be reduced or absent by flow cytometry {679,3684}. Variable numbers of reactive CD8+ T cells are present. Characteristically, the tumour cells show the immunophenotype of normal TFH cells, expressing CD10, CXCL13, ICOS, BCL6, and PD1 (CD279) in 60–100% of cases {177, 905,1026,1470,3399}. This phenotype is helpful in distinguishing AITL from atypical paracortical hyperplasia and other PTCLs {1067,1469}, as well as in diagnosing extranodal dissemination {180, 284,2993}. None of these markers is TFH cell–specific, and conversely, although several TFH-cell markers can usually be detected in the neoplastic cells, both

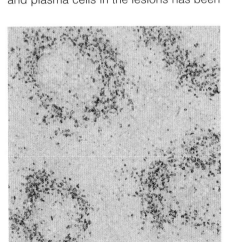

Fig. 14.149 Angioimmunoblastic T-cell lymphoma, pattern 1. CD10 staining highlights neoplastic T cells surrounding the hyperplastic germinal centres.

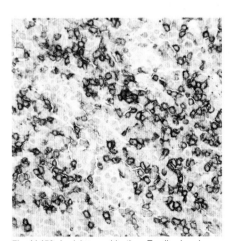

Fig. 14.150 Angioimmunoblastic T-cell lymphoma, pattern 3, expressing PD1.

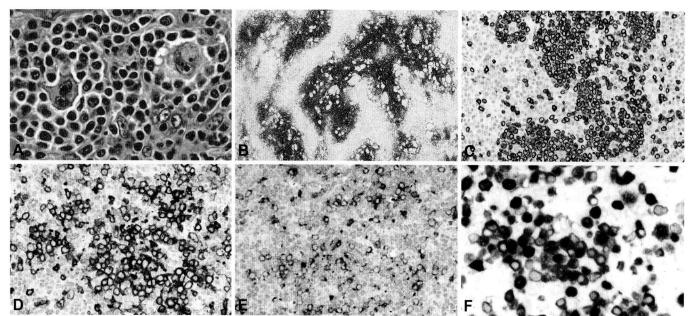

Fig. 14.151 Angioimmunoblastic T-cell lymphoma (AITL). **A** Multinucleated cells resembling Reed–Sternberg cells. **B** Low-power view of CD21 immunostaining highlighting marked follicular dendritic cell proliferation entrapping high endothelial venules (pattern 3). **C–E** The characteristic phenotype of tumour cells expressing CD3 (C), CD10 (D), and CXCL13 (E) (pattern 3). **F** EBV-positive B-cell proliferation in AITL double stained for CD79a (brown, cytoplasmic staining) and EBV-encoded small RNA (EBER) (blue, nuclear staining).

the extent and the intensity of staining are variable. An inverse correlation tends to be observed between sensitivity and specificity of individual markers, with CXCL13 and CD10 being among the most specific and PD1 and ICOS being more sensitive. B immunoblasts and plasma cells are polytypic; however, secondary EBV-positive B-cell proliferations, including diffuse large B-cell lymphoma, classic Hodgkin lymphoma, and plasmacytoma, may be seen {182, 901,3887}. FDC meshworks expressing CD21, CD23, and CD35 are expanded with an extrafollicular pattern, usually surrounding the HEVs.

Postulated normal counterpart
A CD4+ TFH cell

Genetic profile
TR genes show clonal rearrangements in 75–90% of cases {179,901,3887}. Clonal IG gene rearrangements are found in about 25–30% of cases {179,3887} and correlate with expanded EBV-positive B cells. Most EBV-infected B cells show ongoing mutation activity while carrying hypermutated IG genes with destructive mutations, suggesting that in AITL, alternative pathways operate to allow the survival of these mutating so-called 'forbidden' (immunoglobulin-deficient) B cells.

At the gene expression level, the molecular profile of AITL is dominated by a strong microenvironment imprint, including overexpression of B-cell–related and FDC-related genes, chemokines and chemokine receptors, and genes related to extracellular matrix and vascular biology. The signature contributed by the neoplastic cells, although quantitatively minor, shows features of normal TFH cells {905,1010A}.

By conventional cytogenetic analysis, clonal aberrations (most commonly trisomies of chromosomes 3, 5, and 21; gain of X; and loss of 6q) have been reported in as many as 90% of cases {1013,3558}. Comparative genomic hybridization has shown recurrent gains of 22q, 19, and 11q13 and losses of 13q, whereas trisomies 3 and 5 were identified in only a small number of cases {3992}.

Classic and more recently next-generation sequencing studies have identified frequent mutations of genes encoding epigenetic modifiers such as *IDH2* (20–30%), *TET2* (50–80%), and *DNMT3A* (20–30%), as well as the small GTPase *RHOA* (60–70%) {523,2264,2928,3040,3485, 4238,4429}. Among these, *IDH2* R172 mutations appear to be specific for AITL, but the others can be seen in other PTCLs, in particular those with a TFH-cell–like immunophenotype. The hotspot *RHOA* mutation in AITL results in a

Gly17Val-mutant, dominant-negative variant of the enzyme {3485,4429}. Several genes encoding components of the T-cell receptor signalling pathway, such as *FYN*, *PLCG1*, and *CD28*, have been found to be mutated in 5–10% of the cases {2254, 2488}. Moreover, fusion genes encoding a CTLA4-CD28 hybrid protein consisting of the extracellular domain of CTLA4 and the cytoplasmic region of CD28, likely capable of transforming inhibitory signals into stimulatory signals for T-cell activation, have been identified in >50% of AITLs, and other PTCLs as well {4428}. Rare cases carry t(5;9)(q33.3;q22.2), which results in *ITK-SYK* gene fusion, an alteration initially recognized in association with follicular PTCL {181,3814}.

Prognosis and predictive factors
The course of AITL is variable, but overall the prognosis is poor, with a median survival of <3 years in most studies, even when treated aggressively {2767,4217}. No well-defined prognostic factors have been identified. The International Prognostic Index (IPI) and Prognostic Index for T-cell Lymphoma (PIT) are of limited value {901}. Histological features and genetic findings have not been shown to affect clinical course. In multivariate analysis, only male sex, mediastinal lymphadenopathy, and anaemia adversely affected overall survival {2767}.

Fig. 14.152 Follicular T-cell lymphoma with a follicular lymphoma–like growth pattern showing a nodular growth pattern.

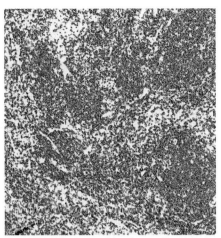

Fig. 14.153 Follicular T-cell lymphoma with a follicular lymphoma–like growth pattern. CD3 staining highlights the nodular growth pattern.

Follicular T-cell lymphoma

Definition
Follicular T-cell lymphoma (FTCL) is a lymph node–based neoplasm of T-follicular helper (TFH) cells, with a predominantly follicular growth pattern and lacking characteristic features of angioimmunoblastic T-cell lymphoma (AITL) such as proliferation of high endothelial venules or extrafollicular follicular dendritic cells {34,213,906,1729}.

ICD-O code   9702/3

Epidemiology
Like AITL, FTCL is seen in middle-aged and elderly individuals, with a slightly higher incidence in males than in females {1729}. It is a rare neoplasm; the true incidence is unknown, but it likely accounts for < 1% of all T-cell neoplasms.

Localization
FTCL is a lymph node–based neoplasm, sometimes involving the skin and bone marrow.

Clinical features
The presenting clinical syndrome resembles that of AITL and other nodal peripheral T-cell lymphomas, characterized by advanced-stage disease, generalized lymphadenopathy, splenomegaly, B symptoms, and skin rash. In a subset of patients, laboratory findings typical of AITL (e.g. hypergammaglobulinaemia, eosinophilia, or a positive Coombs test) can be seen {1729}. However, a few patients with localized disease and/or no B symptoms have also been reported {1729}.

Microscopy
The lymph node architecture is partially or completely effaced by a nodular/follicular proliferation of intermediate-sized monotonous lymphoid cells with round nuclei and abundant pale cytoplasm {906, 1729}. Two distinct growth patterns are recognized: one that mimics follicular lymphoma and one that mimics progressive transformation of germinal centres {1729}. In the follicular lymphoma–like pattern, the neoplastic cells are arranged into well-defined nodules that lack morphological features of normal follicular B cells. In the progressive transformation of germinal centres–like pattern, the neoplastic cells are seen in well-defined aggregates surrounded by numerous small IgD+ mantle zone B cells arranged into large irregular nodules. The interfollicular areas lack the polymorphic infiltrates and vascular proliferation characteristic of AITL. However, scattered immunoblasts can be seen. In a subset of cases, Hodgkin/Reed–Sternberg–like cells, often surrounded by neoplastic T cells, are present {2750}.

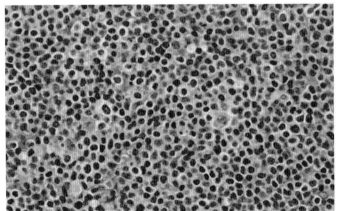

Fig. 14.154 Follicular T-cell lymphoma, cytological features. The lymph node contains an infiltrate of monotonous lymphoid cells with round nuclei and pale, so-called "monocytoid" cytoplasm.

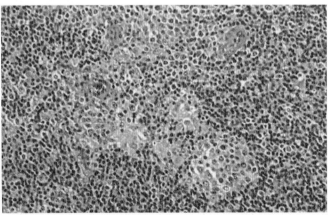

Fig. 14.155 Follicular T-cell lymphoma with a progressive transformation of germinal centres (PTGC)–like growth pattern showing nodules with nests of neoplastic cells reminiscent of follicle centre B cells in PTGCs.

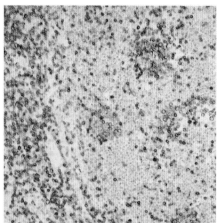

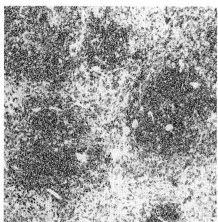

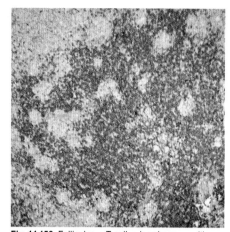

Fig. 14.156 Follicular T-cell lymphoma with a progressive transformation of germinal centres–like growth pattern. CD3 staining highlights nests of neoplastic T cells surrounded by mantle zone B cells.

Fig. 14.157 Follicular T-cell lymphoma with a follicular lymphoma–like growth pattern. The neoplastic cells express PD1.

Fig. 14.158 Follicular T-cell lymphoma with a progressive transformation of germinal centres–like growth pattern. IgD staining highlights mantle zone B cells surrounding the nests of neoplastic T cells.

In a limited number of cases in which consecutive biopsies from different time points were studied, change of morphology from FTCL to typical AITL or vice versa has been observed, suggesting that these two entities may constitute different morphological representations of the same biological process {1729}.

Immunophenotype
The neoplastic T cells express the pan–T-cell antigens CD2, CD3, and CD5 (with frequent loss of CD7) and have a CD4+ T helper (Th) cell phenotype. Consistent with a TFH-cell origin, multiple TFH-cell markers (e.g. PD1, CXCL13, BCL6, CD10, and ICOS) are expressed {1729}. Like in AITL, interfollicular CD20+ B immunoblasts, often with EBV reactivity, are present in half of the cases. When Hodgkin/Reed–Sternberg–like large cells are present, they may show phenotypic features of classic Hodgkin lymphoma, expressing CD30, CD15, PAX5 (weakly), and frequently EBV, but lacking other B-cell markers {2868}. Such cells should not be diagnosed as classic Hodgkin lymphoma in the absence of a typical classic Hodgkin lymphoma background. CD21, CD23, and CD35 staining often reveals a retained follicular dendritic cell meshwork structure underlying the follicular lymphoma–like or progressive transformation of germinal centres–like nodular growth pattern.

Genetic profile
FTCLs show clonal TR gene rearrangements in most cases. About 20% of cases carry a t(5;9)(q33.3;q22.2) translocation, leading to *ITK-SYK* fusion {1729, 3814}. This translocation appears to be specific for FTCL; it has not been seen in other peripheral T-cell lymphomas, except in a rare case of AITL {181}. Comprehensive genomic profiling of FTCL cases has not been specifically performed, but it is likely that some cases of peripheral T-cell lymphoma with TFH-cell–like immunophenotype showing mutations of *TET2*, *RHOA*, and *DNMT3A* are FTCLs {2264}.

Prognosis and predictive factors
The clinical course is not well characterized, due to the rarity of the lesion and the retrospective nature of most studies. The disease appears to have an aggressive course, with half of the patients dying within 24 months of diagnosis {1729}.

Nodal peripheral T-cell lymphoma with T follicular helper phenotype

Definition
It has been recognized that a subset of the peripheral T-cell lymphomas classified as NOS have a T follicular helper (TFH) cell phenotype (i.e. positive for CD4, PD1, CD10, BCL6, CXCL13, and ICOS) and some pathological features of angioimmunoblastic T-cell lymphoma (AITL). The minimum criteria for assignment of TFH-cell phenotype is not very well established, but the detection of at least two (ideally three) of the TFH-cell markers in addition to CD4 is suggested to assign a TFH-cell phenotype to a nodal CD4+ T-cell lymphoma. These neoplasms frequently show a diffuse infiltration pattern without a prominent polymorphic inflammatory background, vascular proliferation, or expansion of follicular dendritic cell meshworks. In some cases, a so-called T-zone pattern may be evident {34}. Genetic studies show that these cases share some of the genetic alterations seen in AITL, including mutations of *TET2*, *DNMT3A*, and *RHOA* {2264,3485}. These phenotypic and genetic characteristics suggest that such cases may be related to AITL and may constitute a tumour cell–rich variant of AITL {178}. However, until further evidence showing that they are biologically and clinically within the spectrum of AITL, it is recommended that such cases are classified as peripheral T-cell lymphoma with a TFH-cell phenotype.

ICD-O code   9702/3

Anaplastic large cell lymphoma, ALK-positive

Falini B.
Lamant-Rochaix L.
Campo E.
Jaffe E.S.
Gascoyne R.D.
Stein H.
Müller-Hermelink
H.K.
Kinney M.C.

Definition

ALK-positive (ALK+) anaplastic large cell lymphoma (ALCL) is a T-cell lymphoma consisting of lymphoid cells that are usually large and have abundant cytoplasm and pleomorphic, often horseshoe-shaped nuclei, with a chromosomal translocation involving the *ALK* gene and expression of ALK protein and CD30. ALCL with comparable morphological and phenotypic features, but lacking *ALK* rearrangement and the ALK protein, is considered to be a separate category: ALK-negative (ALK–) ALCL. ALK+ ALCL must also be distinguished from primary cutaneous ALCL and from other subtypes of T-cell or B-cell lymphoma with anaplastic features and/or CD30 expression.

ICD-O code   9714/3

Synonym

Ki-1 lymphoma (obsolete)

Epidemiology

ALK+ ALCL accounts for approximately 3% of adult non-Hodgkin lymphomas and 10–20% of childhood lymphomas {3782}. ALK+ ALCL is most frequent in the first three decades of life {335,1151} and shows a male predominance, with a male-to-female ratio of 1.5:1.

Localization

ALK+ ALCL frequently involves both lymph nodes and extranodal sites. The most commonly involved extranodal sites include the skin, bone, soft tissue, lungs, and liver {475,1151,1543,3782}. Involvement of the gut or CNS is rare. Mediastinal disease is less frequent than in classic Hodgkin lymphoma. The estimated incidence of bone marrow involvement is approximately 10% when investigated using H&E staining, but higher (30%) when immunohistochemical stains are used {1239}, because bone marrow involvement is often subtle. The small-cell variant of ALK+ ALCL may have a leukaemic presentation with peripheral blood involvement {301,2031,3752}.

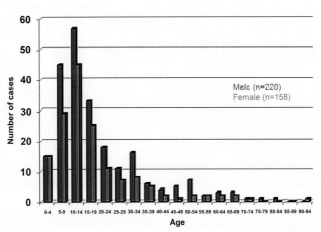

Fig. 14.159 Anaplastic large cell lymphoma, ALK-positive. Distribution by patient age and sex (N = 386).

A few cases of indolent ALK+ ALCL restricted to the skin have been reported {2996}. Clinical history and staging are required to distinguish such lesions from the aggressive, poor-prognosis secondary cutaneous involvement by systemic ALK+ ALCL.

Clinical features

Most patients (70%) present with advanced (stage III–IV) disease with peripheral and/or abdominal lymphadenopathy, often associated with extranodal infiltrates and involvement of the bone marrow {475,1151,1543}. Most patients (75%) have B symptoms, especially high fever {475,1151}. Rare cases of skin and satellite lymph node involvement by ALK+ ALCL following insect bites have been reported {2200}. The significance remains unclear. Possibly, ALK+ ALCL cells home to these sites of inflammation.

Microscopy

ALK+ ALCLs show a broad morphological spectrum {335,643,949,1138,2031, 3181}. However, all cases contain a variable proportion of cells with eccentric, horseshoe-shaped, or kidney-shaped nuclei, often with an eosinophilic region

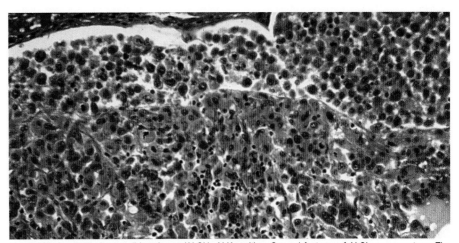

Fig. 14.160 Anaplastic large cell lymphoma (ALCL), ALK-positive. General features of ALCL, common type. The lymph node architecture is obliterated by malignant cells, and intrasinusoidal cells are observed.

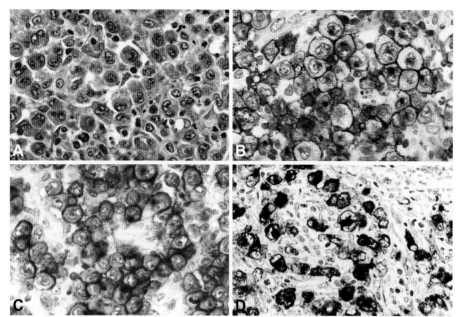

Fig. 14.161 Anaplastic large cell lymphoma (ALCL), ALK-positive. General features of ALCL, common pattern. **A** Predominant population of large cells with irregular nuclei. Note the large hallmark cells showing eccentric kidney-shaped nuclei. All malignant cells are strongly positive for CD30 (**B**), EMA (**C**), and granzyme B (**D**).

near the nucleus. These cells have been referred to as hallmark cells because they are present in all morphological variants {335}. The hallmark cells are typically large, but smaller cells with similar cytological features may also be seen and can greatly facilitate accurate diagnosis {335}. Depending on the plane of section, some cells may appear to contain nuclear inclusions; however, these are not true inclusions but rather invaginations of the nuclear membrane. Cells with these features have been referred to as doughnut cells.

Morphologically, ALK+ ALCLs range from small-cell neoplasms to the opposite extreme in which very large cells predominate. Several morphological patterns can be recognized.

The so-called common pattern accounts for 60% of cases {335,1138}. The tumour

cells have abundant cytoplasm that may appear clear, basophilic, or eosinophilic. Multiple nuclei may occur in a wreath-like pattern and may give rise to cells resembling Reed–Sternberg cells. The nuclear chromatin is usually finely clumped or dispersed, with multiple small, basophilic nucleoli. In cases composed of larger cells, the nucleoli are more prominent, but eosinophilic, inclusion-like nucleoli are rarely seen. When the lymph node architecture is only partially effaced, the tumour characteristically grows within the sinuses and thus may resemble a metastatic tumour.

The lymphohistiocytic pattern (10%) is characterized by tumour cells admixed with a large number of reactive histiocytes {335,1138,3181}. The histiocytes may mask the malignant cells, leading to an incorrect diagnosis of a reactive

lesion. The neoplastic cells are usually smaller than in the common pattern, but often cluster around blood vessels and can be highlighted by immunostaining using antibodies to CD30 and/or ALK. Occasionally, the histiocytes show evidence of erythrophagocytosis.

The small-cell pattern (5–10%) shows a predominant population of small to medium-sized neoplastic cells with irregular nuclei {335,1138,2031}. In some cases, most of the cells have pale cytoplasm and centrally located nucleus; these are referred to as fried-egg cells. Signet ring–like cells may also be seen rarely {335}. Hallmark cells are always present and are often concentrated around blood vessels {335,2031}. This morphological variant of ALCL is often misdiagnosed as peripheral T-cell lymphoma, NOS, by conventional examination. When the peripheral blood is involved, small atypical cells with folded nuclei reminiscent of flower-like cells in addition to rare large cells with blue, vacuolated cytoplasm can be noted in smear preparations.

The Hodgkin-like pattern (3%) is characterized by morphological features mimicking nodular sclerosis classic Hodgkin lymphoma {4162}.

In 15% of cases, more than one pattern can be seen in a single lymph node biopsy; this is called the composite pattern {335}. Relapses may have morphological features different than those seen initially {335,1650}. Other histological patterns include tumours showing cells with monomorphic, rounded nuclei, either as the predominant population or mixed with more-pleomorphic cells, and cases rich in multinucleated neoplastic giant cells or displaying sarcomatoid features {643}. Occasional cases may have a hypocellular appearance, with a myxoid or oedematous background {698}. Spindle cells may be prominent in such cases and may simulate sarcoma in cases presenting in soft tissue {1815}. In rare cases, malignant cells are exceedingly scarce, scattered in an otherwise reactive lymph node. Capsular fibrosis and fibrosis associated with tumour nodules may be seen, mimicking metastatic non-lymphoid malignancy.

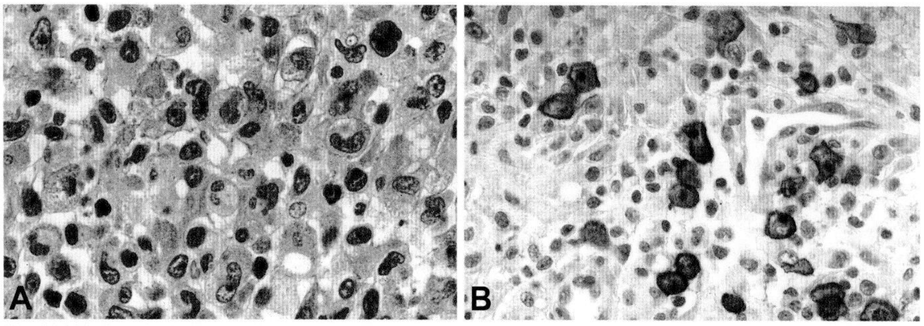

Immunophenotype

The tumour cells are positive for CD30 on the cell membrane and in the Golgi region {3787}. The strongest immunostaining is seen in the large cells. Smaller

Fig. 14.162 Anaplastic large cell lymphoma, lymphohistiocytic pattern. **A** Large cells (hallmark cells) are admixed with a predominant population of non-neoplastic cells, including histiocytes and plasma cells. **B** Malignant cells are highlighted by CD30 staining.

tumour cells may be only weakly positive or even negative for CD30 {335,1138}. In the lymphohistiocytic and small-cell patterns, the strongest CD30 expression is also present in the larger tumour cells, which often cluster around blood vessels {335,1138}. ALK expression is absent from all normal postnatal human tissues except rare cells in the brain {3250}. For this reason, immunohistochemistry with specific anti-ALK monoclonal antibodies has supplanted molecular tests for the diagnosis of ALK+ ALCL. In most cases that have the t(2;5) (*NPM1-ALK*) translocation, ALK staining of large cells is both cytoplasmic and nuclear {335,1138, 3782}. In the small-cell variant, ALK positivity is usually restricted to the nucleus of tumour cells {335,1138,3782}. In cases with variant translocations, i.e. fusion of *ALK* to partners other than *NPM1*, the ALK staining is usually cytoplasmic and rarely membranous {335,1138,1147, 3782}. Cases with the t(2;5) (*NPM1-ALK*) translocation show aberrant cytoplasmic expression of NPM1, whereas ALK+ ALCLs carrying variant translocations show the expected nuclear-restricted expression of NPM1 {1152}.

Most ALK+ ALCLs are positive for EMA, but in some cases only a proportion of malignant cells are positive {335,949}. The great majority of ALK+ ALCLs express one or more T-cell antigens {335}. However, due to loss of several pan–T-cell antigens, some cases may have an apparent so-called null-cell phenotype, but show evidence of a T-cell lineage at the genetic level {1237}. Because no other differences can be found in cases with a T-cell versus a null-cell phenotype, T-cell/null-cell ALK+ ALCL is considered a single entity {335,1557}. CD3 (the most widely used pan–T-cell marker) is negative in >75% of cases {335,413}. CD2, CD5, and CD4 are more useful and are positive in a significant proportion of cases (70%). Furthermore, most cases exhibit positivity for the cytotoxic antigens TIA1, granzyme B, and/or perforin {1237,2111}. CD8 is usually negative, but rare CD8+ cases exist, particularly those with variant morphology {12}. CD43 is expressed in two thirds of cases, but lacks lineage specificity. Tumour cells are variably positive for CD45 and CD45RO and strongly positive for CD25 {949}. In the rare cases in which CD15 expression is observed, only a small proportion of the neoplastic cells are stained {335}. Tumour cells are

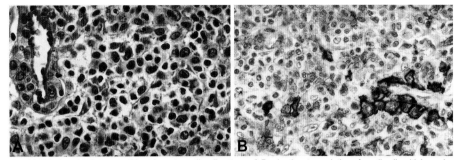

Fig. 14.163 Anaplastic large cell lymphoma, small-cell pattern. **A** Predominant population of small cells with irregular nuclei, associated with scattered hallmark cells. Note that large cells predominate around the vessel. **B** CD30 staining highlights the perivascular pattern. Large cells are strongly positive for CD30, whereas small and medium-sized malignant cells are weakly stained.

negative for the macrophage-restricted form of the CD68 antigen recognized by the PGM1 monoclonal antibody, but may show granular staining with other, less-specific anti-CD68 clones, such as KP1. ALK+ ALCLs are BCL2-negative {819}. ALCLs are also consistently negative for EBV, i.e. for EBV-encoded small RNA (EBER) and LMP1 {465}. A number of other antigens are expressed in ALCL but are not of diagnostic value; these include clusterin {4292}, SHP1 phosphatase {1682}, BCL6, CEBPB {3270}, SERPINA1 {2196}, and fascin.

Differential diagnosis

A rare, distinct diffuse large B-cell lymphoma with immunoblastic/plasmablastic features expressing the ALK protein may superficially resemble ALK+ ALCL due to frequent sinusoidal growth pattern. These lymphomas (ALK+ large B-cell lymphomas) express EMA (as do ALCLs) but lack CD30, and most cases show a characteristic cytoplasm-restricted granular staining for the ALK protein {951}.

Subsets of non-haematopoietic neoplasms, such as rhabdomyosarcoma

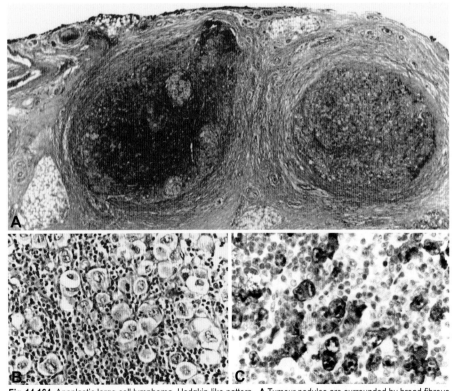

Fig. 14.164 Anaplastic large cell lymphoma, Hodgkin-like pattern. **A** Tumour nodules are surrounded by broad fibrous bands. **B** Numerous tumour cells are present, and some resemble lacunar Reed–Sternberg cells. **C** Tumour cells have cytoplasmic, nuclear, and nucleolar ALK staining, indicating the presence of the t(2;5)(p23.2-23.1;q35.1) translocation and the NPM1-ALK fusion protein.

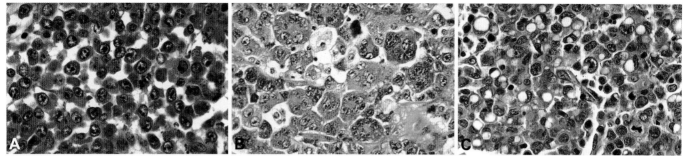

Fig. 14.165 Other histological patterns of anaplastic large cell lymphoma (ALCL), ALK positive. **A** ALCL showing monomorphic large cells with round nuclei. **B** ALCL consisting of pleomorphic giant cells. **C** ALCL rich in signet ring cells.

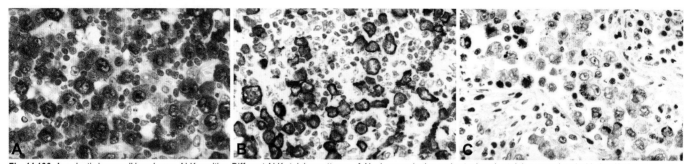

Fig. 14.166 Anaplastic large cell lymphoma, ALK-positive. Different ALK staining patterns. **A** Nuclear, nucleolar, and cytoplasmic staining associated with the t(2;5) translocation (expression of the NPM1-ALK fusion protein). **B** Strong membranous and cytoplasmic staining sparing the nucleus in a case associated with the t(1;2) translocation (expression of the TPM3-ALK fusion protein). **C** Finely granular cytoplasmic staining associated with the t(2;17) translocation (expression of the CLTC-ALK fusion protein).

{1138}, inflammatory myofibroblastic tumours {1459}, and neural tumours {2512}, can be positive for ALK but are morphologically distinguishable from ALCL and are negative for CD30. ALK+ ALCL must also be distinguished from a rare form of ALK+ systemic histiocytosis occurring in early infancy {646}. ALK+ histiocytosis is characterized by a proliferation of large histiocytes that look morphologically different from ALCL cells, are CD30-negative, and express the CD68 antigen {646}.

Postulated normal counterpart
An activated mature cytotoxic T cell

Genetic profile
Antigen receptor genes
Approximately 90% of ALK+ ALCLs show clonal rearrangement of the TR genes irrespective of whether they express T-cell antigens. The remainder show no rearrangement of TR or IG genes {1237}.

Cytogenetic abnormalities and oncogenes
The genes fused with *ALK* in various chromosomal translocations and the subcellular distribution of NPM1-ALK and ALK variant chimeric proteins are shown in Table 14.10. The most frequent genetic alteration is a translocation, t(2;5)(p23.2-23.1;q35.1), between the *ALK* gene on chromosome 2 and the *NPM1* gene on chromosome 5 {2199,2541,2753}. Variant translocations involving *ALK* and other partner genes on chromosomes 1, 2, 3, 17, 19, 22, and X also occur {801,1152, 1177,1623,2195,2197,2542,2608,3410,

3782,4033,4037,4059,4339}. FISH using an *ALK* break-apart probe or karyotyping is not mandatory in routine practice if ALK staining is positive {1138,3201}. RT-PCR is usually reserved for detection of minimal residual disease in blood or bone marrow {865}. All of these translocations result in upregulation and aberrant expression of ALK, but the subcellular distribution of ALK staining varies depending on the translocation partner {1147}.

The *ALK* gene encodes a tyrosine kinase receptor belonging to the insulin receptor superfamily, which is normally silent in lymphoid cells {2753}. In the t(2;5)(p23.2-23.1;q35.1) translocation, *NPM1* (a housekeeping gene encoding a nucleolar protein) fuses with *ALK* to produce a chimeric protein in which the N-terminal portion of NPM1 is linked to the intracytoplasmic

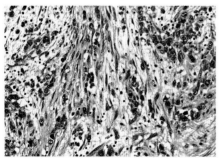

Fig. 14.167 Anaplastic large cell lymphoma showing sarcomatous features.

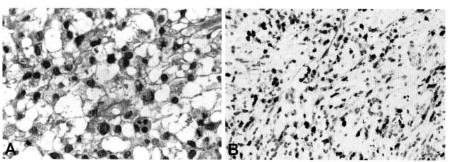

Fig. 14.168 A Hypocellular anaplastic large cell lymphoma. **B** Malignant cells are highlighted by ALK staining.

portion of ALK {2753}. In addition to cytoplasmic ALK positivity, cases with t(2;5) show nuclear and nucleolar ALK staining. The latter pattern is due to the transport of the NPM1-ALK fusion protein into the nucleus through formation of heterodimers between wildtype NPM1 and NPM1-ALK. On the other hand, the formation of NPM1-ALK homodimers using dimerization sites at the N-terminus of NPM1 mimics ligand binding and is responsible for the activation of the ALK catalytic domain and for the oncogenic properties of the ALK protein {3249}. *ALK* variant translocations also cause ALK activation through self-association and formation of homodimers. In turn, the activation of the ALK catalytic domain (mediated by all translocations) results in the activation of multiple signalling cascades, including the RAS-ERK, JAK/STAT, and PIK-AKT pathways {403}.

Comparative genomic hybridization analysis shows that ALK+ ALCLs carry frequent secondary chromosomal imbalances including losses of chromosomes 4, 11q, and 13q and gains of 7, 17p, and 17q {3488}. In addition, this study demonstrates that ALK+ and ALK− ALCLs have a different representation of secondary genetic alterations, supporting the concept that they constitute different biological entities.

Gene expression profiling
Supervised analysis by class comparison between ALK+ ALCL and ALK− ALCL tumours showed evidence for distinct molecular signatures {2196}. However, the gene expression profile also shows a common signature between the ALK+ and ALK− groups, which facilitates their distinction from other types of peripheral T-cell lymphoma. Some of the genes differentially expressed between the ALK+ and ALK− groups are related to ALK signalling {403}. Among the 117 genes overexpressed in ALK+ ALCL, *BCL6*, *PTPN12*, *SERPINA1*, and *CEBPB* were the four top genes, being overexpressed with the most significant *P* values. This overexpression was also confirmed at the protein level for CEBPB, BCL6, and SERPINA1. A robust classifier for ALK+ ALCL also included highly expressed transcripts related to STAT3 regulators (IL6, IL31RA) or targets, cytotoxic molecules, and T helper 17 (Th17) cell–associated molecules {1774}.

Table 14.10 Translocations and fusion proteins involving *ALK* at 2p23

Chromosomal anomaly	*ALK* partner	MW of ALK hybrid protein	ALK staining pattern	Percentage of cases
t(2;5)(p23.2-23.1;q35.1)	NPM1	80 kDa	Nuclear, diffuse cytoplasmic	84%
t(1;2)(q25;p23)	TPM3	104 kDa	Diffuse cytoplasmic with peripheral intensification	13%
inv(2)(p23q35)	ATIC	96 kDa	Diffuse cytoplasmic	1%
t(2;3)(p23;q12.2)[a]	TFG Xlong	113 kDa	Diffuse cytoplasmic	<1%
	TFG long	97 kDa	Diffuse cytoplasmic	
	TFG short	85 kDa	Diffuse cytoplasmic	
t(2;17)(p23;q23)	CLTC	260 kDa	Granular cytoplasmic	<1%
t(X;2)(q11-12;p23)	MSN	125 kDa	Membrane staining	<1%
t(2;19)(p23;p13.1)	TPM4	95 kDa	Diffuse cytoplasmic	<1%
t(2;22)(p23;q11.2)	MYH9	220 kDa	Diffuse cytoplasmic	<1%
t(2;17)(p23;q25)	RNF213	ND	Diffuse cytoplasmic	<1%
Others[b]	ND	ND	Nuclear or cytoplasmic	<1%

MW, molecular weight; ND, not determined.

[a] Three different fusion proteins (TFG-ALK$_{XL}$, TFG-ALK$_L$, and TFG-ALK$_S$) are associated with the t(2;3) (p23;q12.2) translocation that involves *TFG*.
[b] Unpublished series of 270 cases of ALK-positive anaplastic large cell lymphoma.

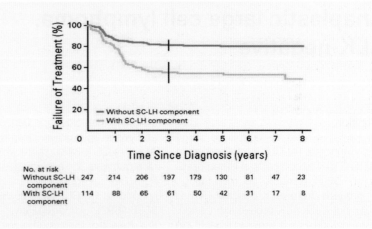

Fig. 14.169 Anaplastic large cell lymphoma (ALCL), ALK-positive. In a cohort of 361 patients, the time to treatment failure was shorter for patients with a small-cell (SC) or lymphohistiocytic (LH) component than for patients with ALK-positive ALCL, common type. From: Lamant L, et al. {2198}.

Prognosis and predictive factors
No differences have been found between *NPM1-ALK*–positive tumours and tumours showing ALK variant translocations {1152}. Concurrent *MYC* rearrangement could be associated with a more aggressive course {2318,2748}. Most cases with small-cell or lymphohistiocytic variant histology do not have the same favourable prognosis as the other ALK+ tumours, because these patients often present with disseminated disease at diagnosis {58,2198}. Risk stratification according to the International Prognostic Index (IPI) is important in assessing prognosis in ALK+ ALCL {1151,1543, 3536}. The long-term survival rate associated with ALK+ ALCL approaches 80%, and is better overall than that of ALK− ALCL {1151,1306,1543,3536,3662, 3670}. It appears that this difference may be ascribed to the fact that ALK+ ALCL

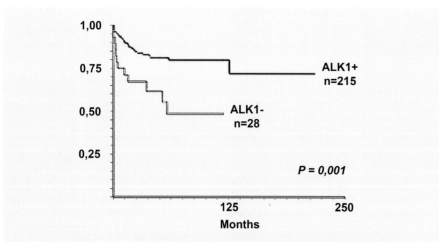

Fig. 14.170 Anaplastic large cell lymphoma. Overall survival of ALK-positive and ALK-negative patients.

occurs more frequently than ALK– ALCL at a younger patient age, rather than to the expression of ALK {1151,3670}. In fact, when analysis is restricted to patients aged <40 years, the outcomes in ALK+ ALCL and ALK– ALCL appear to be similar {1543,3536,3670}.

At least in children, the detection of minimal residual disease by qualitative PCR for *NPM1-ALK* in bone marrow and peripheral blood at diagnosis and an early positive minimal residual disease during treatment identify patients at risk of relapse {865}. This could be linked to a poor immune control of the disease, partly reflected by the anti-ALK antibody titre, which is inversely correlated to prognosis {39}.

Relapses often remain sensitive to chemotherapy; allogeneic bone marrow transplantation may be effective in refractory cases {2360}. Because ALK is essential for the proliferation and survival of ALK+ ALCL cells, it provides a unique therapeutic target. Promising clinical results have been obtained in small case series of relapsed ALK+ ALCL treated with small-molecule inhibitors of ALK kinase {1285}. CD30-targeting with antibody-drug conjugates is another appealing therapeutic approach for relapsed/refractory ALK+ ALCL {3241}.

Anaplastic large cell lymphoma, ALK-negative

Feldman A.L.
Harris N.L.
Stein H.
Campo E.
Kinney M.C.

Jaffe E.S.
Falini B.
Inghirami G.G.
Pileri S.A.

Definition

ALK-negative (ALK–) anaplastic large cell lymphoma (ALCL) is defined as a CD30+ T-cell neoplasm that is not reproducibly distinguishable on morphological grounds from ALK-positive (ALK+) ALCL, but lacks ALK protein expression. It was included as a provisional entity in the 2008 edition of the WHO classification, but is now considered an accepted entity. ALK– ALCL must be distinguished from primary cutaneous ALCL (C-ALCL), other subtypes of CD30+ T-cell or B-cell lymphoma with anaplastic features, and classic Hodgkin lymphoma (CHL).

ICD-O code   9715/3

Synonyms and historical terminology

ALK– ALCL was included in the 2008 edition of the WHO classification as a provisional entity distinct from ALK+ ALCL, on the basis of important clinical differences including the older median patient age and more-aggressive clinical course of ALK– ALCL {3848}. There were also valid arguments for excluding ALK– ALCL from the category of peripheral T-cell lymphoma (PTCL), NOS {913,1136,1815, 3536,3692}. Unfortunately, there are few detailed clinicopathological studies of ALK– ALCL {3939}, and although recurrent genetic events have been identified, their role in classification has not been established. Thus, the distinction between PTCL, NOS, and ALK– ALCL is not always straightforward.

Epidemiology

The peak incidence of ALK– ALCL is in adults (aged 40–65 years), unlike ALK+ ALCL, which occurs most commonly in children and young adults, although cases can occur at any age {1136,3782}. There is a modest male preponderance, with a male-to-female ratio of 1.5:1.

Localization

ALK– ALCL involves both lymph nodes and extranodal tissues (e.g. the bone, soft tissue, and skin), although extranodal sites are less commonly involved than in ALK+ ALCL. Cutaneous cases must be distinguished from primary C-ALCL, and cases that involve the gastrointestinal tract must be distinguished from CD30+ enteropathy-associated and other intestinal T-cell lymphomas. Conversely, if a single lymph node is suggestive of ALK– ALCL, clinical history of skin lesions should be sought, to exclude nodal involvement by primary C-ALCL {178,314}.

Clinical features

Most patients present with advanced (stage III–IV) disease, with peripheral and/or abdominal lymphadenopathy and B symptoms {3938}.

Microscopy

In most cases, the nodal or other tissue architecture is effaced by solid, cohesive sheets of neoplastic cells. When lymph node architecture is preserved, the neoplastic cells typically grow within sinuses or within T-cell areas, commonly showing a so-called cohesive pattern, which may mimic carcinoma. Absence of these features should suggest a diagnosis of PTCL, NOS {178}. Needle biopsies may be inadequate to assess these features. The overall features typically resemble the so-called common pattern described in ALK+ ALCL, and variant morphological patterns are not recognized. Features such as sclerosis and eosinophils may occur, but when present should raise suspicion for CHL. Cases with a confirmed T-cell origin that morphologically resemble CHL are usually best classified as PTCL, NOS {178}. Cases resembling CHL may also constitute nodal involvement by lymphomatoid papulosis {1078}.

The cytological features of the neoplastic cells show a similar spectrum to ALK+ ALCL, although the small tumour cells seen in the small-cell and lymphohistiocytic variants of ALK+ ALCL should not be prominent in ALK– ALCL. Biopsies typically show large pleomorphic cells, sometimes containing prominent nucleoli. Multinucleated cells, including wreathlike cells, may also be present, and mitotic figures are not infrequent. In addition, to a variable degree, hallmark cells with eccentric, horseshoe-shaped, or kidney-shaped nuclei are seen. In most cases of ALK– ALCL, the neoplastic cells are larger and more pleomorphic than those seen in classic ALK+ ALCL, and/or have a higher N:C ratio {1151,2814,3201,3662}. A higher N:C ratio may suggest a diagnosis of PTCL, NOS, but in that disorder, abnormal small to medium-sized lymphocytes are often admixed with a morphologically homogeneous neoplastic cell population, and the sheet-like or sinus pattern of infiltration typical of ALCL is absent. Of note, cases of ALK– ALCL with *DUSP22-IRF4* rearrangements tend to lack large pleomorphic cells and to have more so-called doughnut cells showing central nuclear pseudoinclusions than do cases lacking *DUSP22-IRF4* rearrangements {2029}.

Immunophenotype

All tumour cells are strongly positive for CD30, usually most strongly at the cell

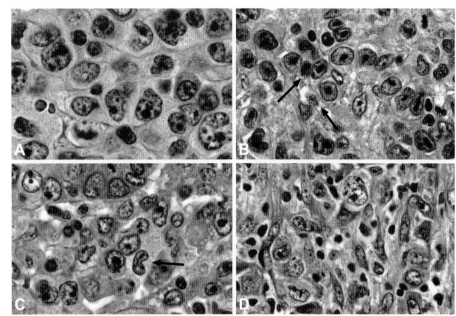

Fig. 14.171 Anaplastic large cell lymphoma (ALCL), ALK-negative. Morphological features of four cases. **A** Note the high N:C ratio. **B** Eosinophils (arrows) are present (often in clusters), but other features of Hodgkin lymphoma are absent. **C** Typical morphological and phenotypic features of ALCL, including a hallmark cell (arrow), that arose in the gastrointestinal tract. **D** A case with more cellular pleomorphism.

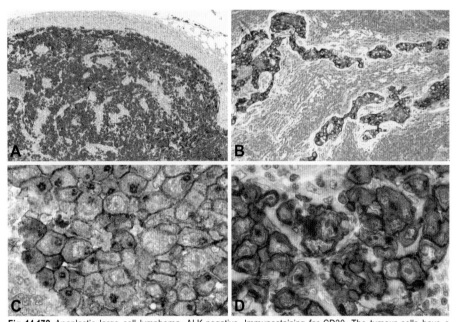

Fig. 14.172 Anaplastic large cell lymphoma, ALK-negative. Immunostaining for CD30. The tumour cells have a cohesive (**A**) and intrasinusoidal growth pattern (**B**). **C,D** CD30 shows strong membranous and Golgi positivity.

membrane and in the Golgi region, although diffuse cytoplasmic positivity is also common. Staining should be strong and of equal intensity in all cells, a feature that is important in distinguishing ALK– ALCL from other PTCLs, which can express CD30 in at least a proportion of the cells, and usually with variable intensity. By definition, ALK protein is undetectable.

Loss of T-cell markers occurs with greater frequency than is typically seen in PTCL, NOS. In this respect, ALK– ALCL is similar to ALK+ ALCL. However, more than half of all cases express one or more T-cell markers. CD2 and CD3 are found more often than CD5, and CD43 is almost always expressed. CD4 is positive in a significant proportion of cases, whereas CD8+ cases are rare. Many cases express the cytotoxic markers TIA1, granzyme B, and/or perforin.

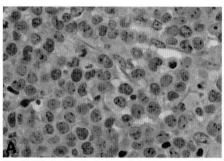
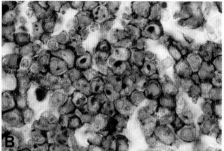

Fig. 14.173 Anaplastic large cell lymphoma, ALK-negative, with *DUSP22* rearrangement. **A** Densely packed monomorphic large cells. **B** Strong, uniform staining for CD30.

These markers tend to be absent in cases bearing *DUSP22* rearrangements {3069}; therefore, although desirable, their expression is not an absolute requirement for the diagnosis of ALK– ALCL. About 43% of cases are positive for EMA, on at least a proportion of malignant cells, a marker that is almost always seen in ALK+ ALCL but only occasionally in PTCL, NOS {3536}. Nuclear phospho-STAT3 is expressed in about 43% of cases {836}.

In cases that lack all T-cell/cytotoxic markers, CHL rich in neoplastic cells and other large cell malignancies (e.g. embryonal carcinoma) should be ruled out. In this regard, staining for PAX5 is useful, because CHL reveals weak expression of PAX5 in most cases; however, rare cases of ALCL (ALK– or ALK+) may express PAX5 {1175}. The demonstration of CD15

should raise suspicion for CHL. However, CD15 may be expressed in some cases of PTCL, NOS, and such cases are generally strongly CD30-positive {277}. Whether peripheral T-cell neoplasms expressing both CD30 and CD15 should be classified as ALK– ALCL or PTCL, NOS, remains to be determined. Notably, these cases have a very poor prognosis, clinically more closely resembling PTCL, NOS. ALK– ALCLs are consistently negative for EBV, i.e. for EBV-encoded small RNA (EBER) and LMP1, and the expression of these markers should strongly suggest the possibility of CHL.

ALK– ALCL and ALK+ ALCL lack T-cell receptor proteins, and in this respect tend to differ from PTCL, NOS {413,1322}. Clusterin is also commonly expressed in both ALK– and ALK+ ALCL, but rarely in PTCL, NOS {2183,2830,3470}; this mark-

er has not been examined extensively in CHL, but was negative in the cases studied {4292}.

Differential diagnosis
The principal differential diagnosis of ALK– ALCL is with PTCL, NOS, and CHL. Most cases referred to historically as Hodgkin-like ALCL are now considered to be tumour cell–rich forms of CHL. With complete immunophenotypic and genetic studies, ALK– ALCL can be distinguished from CHL in virtually all cases. In contrast, the distinction between PTCL, NOS, and ALK– ALCL is not always clear-cut, and even experts may disagree on this subject. In general, the WHO classification advocates a conservative approach, recommending the diagnosis of ALK– ALCL only if both the morphology and phenotype are very close to those of ALK+ cases, with the only distinction being the presence or absence of ALK. ALK– ALCL must also be distinguished from primary C-ALCL, which can have a similar phenotype and morphology. Clinical correlation with staging is of paramount importance in this differential. Primary C-ALCL has a much better prognosis than does ALK– ALCL.

Postulated normal counterpart
An activated mature cytotoxic T cell

Genetic profile
Most cases show clonal rearrangement of the TR genes, whether or not they express T-cell antigens.

A constellation of genetic findings, notably recurrent activating mutations of *JAK1* and/or *STAT3*, has been shown to lead to constitutive activation of the JAK/STAT3 pathway in ALK– ALCL {836}. Translocations involving tyrosine kinase genes other than *ALK* also lead to STAT3 activation in a small subset of systemic and cutaneous ALK– ALCLs {836,4171}. These genetic events in ALK– ALCL partially explain the biological and pathological similarities to ALK+ ALCL, in which ALK fusion proteins lead to constitutive STAT3 activation {710}, and may have therapeutic implications.

DUSP22 rearrangements, i.e. chromosomal rearrangements in or near the *DUSP22-IRF4* locus on 6p25.3, occur in about 30% of cases {3069}. These are associated with decreased expression of the *DUSP22* dual-specificity phosphatase

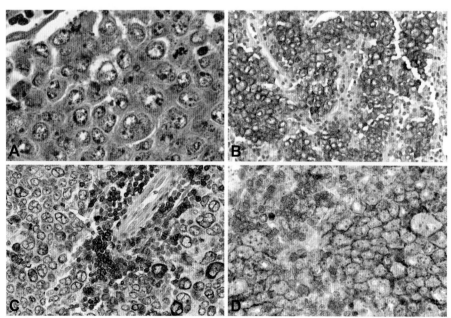

Fig. 14.174 Anaplastic large cell lymphoma, ALK-negative. **A** Some of the features raise a differential diagnosis with PTCL, NOS, expressing CD30, such as absence of hallmark cells. **B** CD30 is strongly expressed in all tumour cells. **C** Lymphoma cells express CD3. Note a vessel surrounded by normal, small CD3+ T cells. **D** Tumour cells express CD4.

gene, with no detectable alteration in expression of the neighbouring *IRF4* gene {1174}. The most common partner is the *FRA7H* fragile site on 7q32.3. Rearrangements of *TP63* occur in about 8% of cases and encode p63 fusion proteins, most commonly with TBL1XR1, as a result of inv(3)(q26.3q28) {3069,4161}. Rearrangement of *DUSP22* or *TP63* has not been reported in ALK+ ALCL, but can be seen in a fraction of other PTCLs.

Several studies have shown differences in copy-number abnormalities between ALK– ALCL and both PTCL, NOS, and ALK+ ALCL, including gains of 1q, 6p, 8q, and 12q and losses of 4q, 6q21 (encompassing the *PRDM1* gene, which encodes PRDM1, also known as BLIMP1), 13q, and 17p13.1 (*TP53*) {402,3488,4472}. Despite their biological and possible prognostic importance (see below), none of the aforementioned genetic abnormalities has an established diagnostic role in distinguishing ALK– ALCL from other entities.

Gene expression studies have shown that ALK– ALCL shares a common molecular signature with ALK+ ALCL, but also shows differential expression of some genes, including a subset related to ALK signalling in the latter entity {403,1774,2196,3991}. In addition, ALK– ALCL has a gene expression profile distinct from that of PTCL, NOS {31,243,1775,3172,3202}. As few as three genes (*TNFRSF8*, *BATF*, and *TMOD1*) could distinguish ALK– ALCL from PTCL, NOS, and cases reclassified from PTCL, NOS, to ALK– ALCL on the basis of molecular signature have been confirmed to be ALK– ALCL on pathological re-review {31,1775}.

Prognosis and predictive factors

In general, the clinical outcome of ALK– ALCL with conventional therapy is poorer than that of ALK+ ALCL; however, the findings have been variable and may relate in part to patient age, International Prognostic Index (IPI) score, and the genetic heterogeneity in ALK– ALCL {1151, 1306,1543,3536,3938}. A report by the International Peripheral T-cell Lymphoma Project {3536} also showed outcome differences between PTCL, NOS, and ALK– ALCL. The 5-year failure-free survival rate (36% vs 20%) and overall survival rate (49% vs 32%) were superior in ALK– ALCL compared with PTCL, NOS. Furthermore, restricting the analysis to cases of PTCL, NOS, with high CD30 expression (>80% of cells), which is the group most difficult to differentiate from ALK– ALCL, magnified the difference in 5-year failure-free survival rate and 5-year overall survival rate (19%) compared with ALK– ALCL. A recent study found that ALK– ALCL with *DUSP22* rearrangement was associated with a 5-year overall survival rate similar to that of ALK+ ALCL (90% vs 85%) {3069}. Conversely, the 5-year overall survival rate associated with ALK– ALCL with *TP63* rearrangement was only 17%, compared with 42% in ALK– ALCL with neither *DUSP22* nor *TP63* rearrangement. Loss of *PRDM1* (also known as *BLIMP1*) and/or *TP53* has been associated with poor outcome {402}.

Breast implant–associated anaplastic large cell lymphoma

Feldman A.L.
Harris N.L.
Stein H.
Campo E.
Kinney M.C.
Jaffe E.S.
Falini B.
Inghirami G.G.
Pileri S.A.

Definition

This provisional entity is a T-cell lymphoma with morphological and immunophenotypic features indistinguishable from those of ALK-negative anaplastic large cell lymphoma (ALCL), arising primarily in association with a breast implant.

ICD-O code   9715/3

Synonym

Seroma-associated anaplastic large cell lymphoma

Epidemiology

Breast implant–associated ALCL is very rare, with an estimated incidence of 1 case per 500 000 to 3 million women with implants {461}. Although a possible etiological relationship between implants and ALCL has been suggested, large studies have not identified an increased risk of lymphoma in women with breast implants {895,2220,2358,2672}.

Localization

The tumour cells may be localized to the seroma cavity or may involve the pericapsular fibrous tissue, sometimes forming a mass. Locoregional lymph nodes may be involved.

Clinical features

The mean patient age is 50 years {2235, 2672,3382}. Most patients present with stage I disease, usually with a peri-implant effusion and less frequently with a mass. As many as 29% of patients have axillary lymphadenopathy, but not all biopsied nodes are positive for tumour. Rare cases present with disseminated disease. The mean interval from implant placement to lymphoma diagnosis is 10.9 years, but the interval varies greatly. No association with the type of implant (silicone vs saline, textured vs smooth) or with breast cancer history has been established.

Microscopy

The tumour cells may be identified initially in cytology specimens from aspirated effusion fluid. At capsulectomy, the tumour cells often line the capsule and may show varying degrees of capsular infiltration. In some cases, they extend beyond the capsule to form a mass, which may be palpable in the specimen at the time of gross evaluation {51}. The tumour cells are typically large and pleomorphic, and the so-called hallmark cells seen in other forms of ALCL can usually be identified.

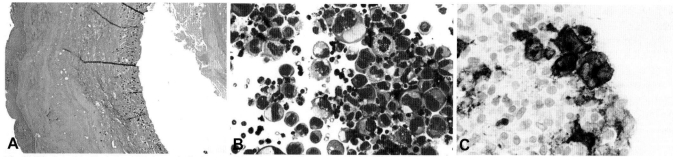

Fig. 14.175 Breast implant–associated anaplastic large cell lymphoma. **A** Section of the capsule surrounding the breast implant shows a fibrinous exudate, with atypical anaplastic cells in the fluid and exudate. **B** Seroma fluid contains pleomorphic tumour cells (Wright-Giemsa stain). **C** Tumour cells are strongly CD30-positive, and are confined to the surface of the exudate without invasion.

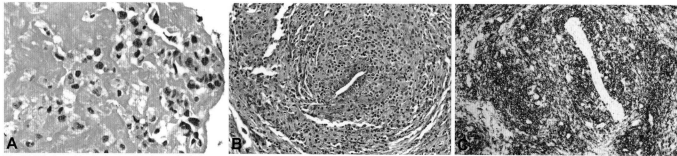

Fig. 14.176 Breast implant–associated anaplastic large cell lymphoma. **A** The tumour cells have pleomorphic nuclear features. This case had invasion of the capsule and underlying breast, shown in B and C. **B** Some tumours may show invasion of the breast, which is associated with a more aggressive clinical course. **C** Neoplastic cells with strong staining for CD30 surround a duct in the breast.

Immunophenotype

The phenotype is similar to that of ALK-negative ALCL {51,3382,3911}. Tumour cells show strong and uniform expression of CD30, are negative for ALK, and often show incomplete expression of pan–T-cell antigens.

Postulated normal counterpart

An activated mature cytotoxic T cell

Genetic profile

TR genes are clonally rearranged in most cases. Tumours may show complex karyotypes {2246}. Recurrent activating *JAK1* and *STAT3* mutations have been reported {391A}.

Prognosis and predictive factors

Most patients have excellent outcomes, often after excision alone. The median overall survival is 12 years {2672}. The most important adverse prognostic factor is the presence of a solid mass of tumour cells, which may indicate a need for systemic therapy {2229}. In cases restricted to the seroma cavity, the addition of chemotherapy does not appear to affect outcomes {2672}.

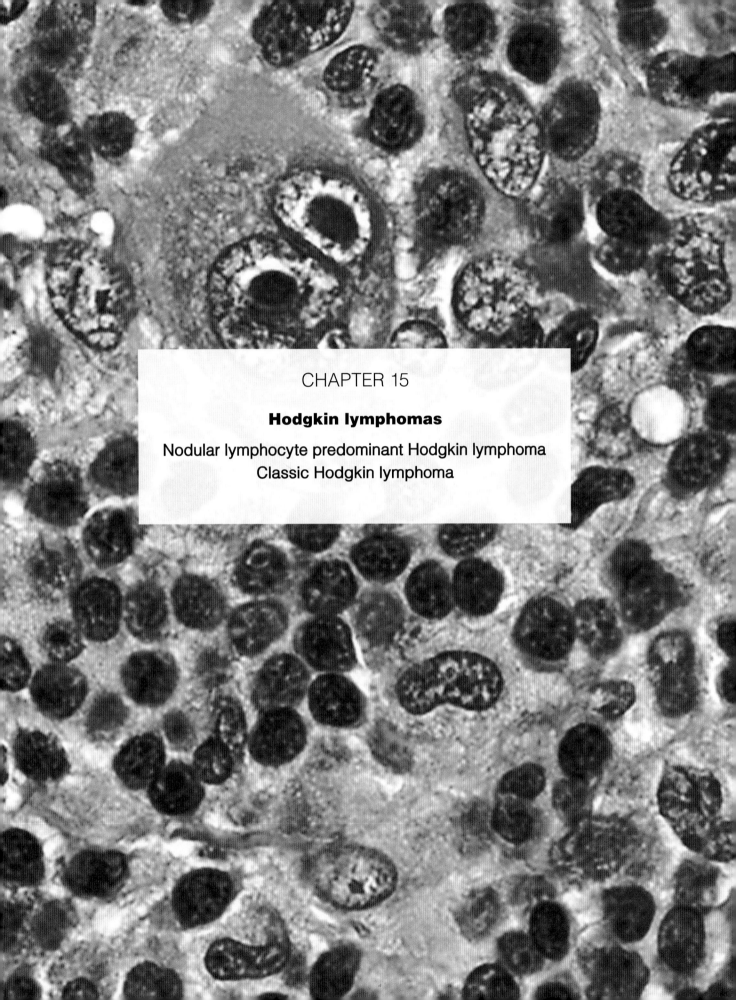

CHAPTER 15

Hodgkin lymphomas

Nodular lymphocyte predominant Hodgkin lymphoma
Classic Hodgkin lymphoma

Hodgkin lymphomas: Introduction

Stein H.
Pileri S.A.
Weiss L.M.
Poppema S.
Gascoyne R.D.
Jaffe E.S.

Definition

Hodgkin lymphomas (HLs) are lymphoid neoplasms usually affecting lymph nodes. They are composed of large dysplastic mononuclear and multinucleated cells surrounded by a variable mixture of mature non-neoplastic inflammatory cells. Abundant band-like and/or more diffuse collagen fibrosis may be present. The neoplastic cells are often ringed by T cells in a rosette-like manner. On the basis of the immunophenotype and morphology of the neoplastic cells and the cellular background, two major types of HL are recognized: nodular lymphocyte predominant HL (NLPHL) and classic HL (CHL).

NLPHL differs from CHL in that the B-cell programme is generally preserved, although there may be partial loss of the B-cell phenotype {477}. Both NLPHL and CHL are characterized by a paucity of neoplastic cells and a rich inflammatory background of non-neoplastic cells, mainly T cells. The features of NLPHL are more fully discussed in a subsequent section.

CHL accounts for approximately 90% of all HLs, with a peak incidence among individuals aged 15–35 years and a second peak in late life for subtypes other than nodular sclerosis. EBV infection plays a significant role in the pathogenesis of some subtypes, in particular mixed cellularity and lymphocyte-depleted forms. Patients usually present with peripheral lymphadenopathy, localized to one or two preferentially cervical lymph node–bearing areas. B symptoms consisting of fever, drenching night sweats, and significant body weight loss are present in as many as 40% of patients.

Histopathologically, mononuclear Hodgkin cells and multinucleated Reed–Sternberg cells are seen in a cellular background rich in lymphocytes, histiocytes, plasma cells, and/or eosinophils or neutrophils. In >98% of cases, neoplastic cells are derived from mature B cells at the germinal centre stage of differentiation and contain clonal IG gene rearrangements. Treatment advances have resulted in a 5-year survival rate of >90%. Four histological subtypes are distinguished: nodular sclerosis CHL (NSCHL), lymphocyte-rich CHL (LRCHL), mixed cellularity CHL (MCCHL), and lymphocyte-depleted CHL (LDCHL). These subtypes differ in the character of the microenvironment and the cytological features of the neoplastic cells. They also differ in their clinical features, risk factors, and association with EBV.

Epidemiology

Approximately 90% of HLs are of classic type, and only 10% are NLPHL {2230A}. The age peak of NLPHL patients lies in the fourth and fifth decades of life, but NLPHL is also common in children. It is more common in males than in females. The patient age distributions of the various types of CHL vary greatly. MCCHL has a bimodal age distribution, with a peak in young patients and a second peak in older adults. NSCHL has a peak among individuals aged 15–35 years. There is a male predominance for most CHL subtypes, with the exception of NSCHL, in which the incidence is slightly higher in females. Individuals with a history of infectious mononucleosis have a higher incidence of CHL, in particular the mixed cellularity subtype {2777}. Both

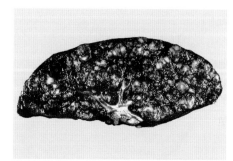

Fig. 15.01 Classic Hodgkin lymphoma. Spleen.

familial clustering and geographical clustering have been described {2777}. The age-adjusted annual incidence rate of HL is 2.8 cases per 100 000 population. Unlike that of non-Hodgkin lymphoma, the incidence of HL has not increased over the past decades.

Etiology

EBV has been postulated to play a role in the pathogenesis of CHL. EBV is found in only a proportion of cases, most frequently in MCCHL and LDCHL, but a search for other viruses has been unsuccessful. Loss of immune surveillance in immunodeficiency states, such as HIV infection, may predispose individuals to the development of EBV-associated CHL. In tropical regions and developing countries, as many as 100% of CHL cases are

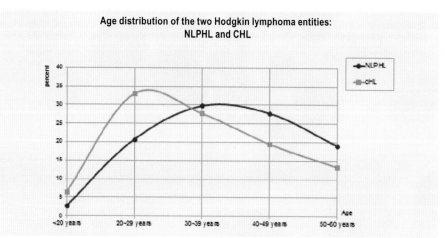

Fig. 15.02 Age distribution of the two Hodgkin lymphoma entities: nodular lymphocyte predominant Hodgkin lymphoma (NLPHL) and classic Hodgkin lymphoma (CHL). Individuals with a history of infectious mononucleosis have a higher risk for the development of CHL; both familial clustering and geographical clustering have been described. From: Mueller NE and Grufferman S {2777}.

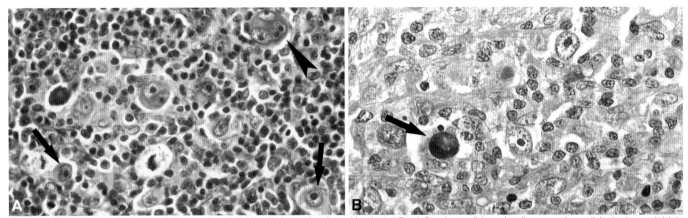

Fig. 15.03 Classic Hodgkin lymphoma. **A** Mononuclear Hodgkin cells (arrows) and a multinucleated Reed–Sternberg cell (arrowhead) are seen in a cellular background rich in lymphocytes and containing histiocytes and some eosinophils. **B** One mummified Hodgkin cell (arrow) and four vital Hodgkin cells can be seen.

EBV-positive {125,276,1190,2276,4277, 4278}. However, there are differences between urban and rural areas. For example, NSCHL is more common in urban areas, whereas EBV-positive MCCHL is more common in rural regions {1092}. Delayed exposure to childhood infections has been postulated to play a role {1383}. It is possible that EBV infection of a B cell replaces one of the genetic alterations necessary for the development of CHL. NLPHL is only rarely positive for EBV (< 5% of cases) {1736}.

Localization

CHL most often involves lymph nodes of the cervical region (75% of cases), followed by the mediastinal, axillary, and para-aortic regions. Non-axial lymph node groups, such as mesenteric and epitrochlear lymph nodes, are rarely involved. Primary extranodal involvement is rare. More than 60% of patients

have localized disease (stage I or II). Approximately 60% of patients, most with NSCHL, have mediastinal involvement. Splenic involvement is common (20%) and is associated with an increased risk of extranodal dissemination. Bone marrow involvement is much less common (5%). Because the bone marrow lacks lymphatics, bone marrow infiltration indicates vascular dissemination of the disease (stage IV). The anatomical distribution varies between the histological subtypes of CHL {3654}. NLPHL tends to spare axial lymph node groups, and is more common in peripheral lymph nodes. The mediastinum is uncommonly involved, but mesenteric lymph node involvement may be seen.

Clinical features

Patients with CHL usually present with peripheral lymphadenopathy, localized to one or two lymph node–bearing areas.

Mediastinal involvement is most frequently seen in the nodular sclerosis subtype, whereas abdominal involvement and splenic involvement are more common in mixed cellularity cases. B symptoms consisting of fever, drenching night sweats, and significant body weight loss are present in as many as 40% of patients. Most patients with NLPHL are asymptomatic and present with enlargement of peripheral lymph nodes; B symptoms are rare.

Macroscopy

Lymph nodes are enlarged and encapsulated, and show a fish-flesh tumour on cut section. In NSCHL, there is prominent nodularity, dense fibrotic bands, and a thickened capsule. Splenic involvement usually shows scattered nodules within the white pulp. Very large masses are sometime seen; these can demonstrate fibrous bands in the nodular sclerosis

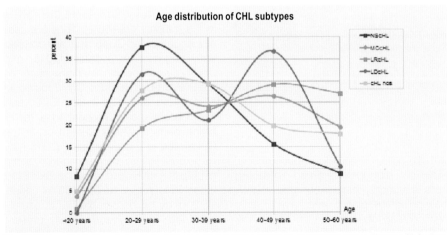

Fig. 15.04 Age distribution of classic Hodgkin lymphoma (CHL) subtypes. Individuals with a history of infectious mononucleosis have a higher risk for the development of CHL. LDCHL, lymphocyte-depleted CHL; LRCHL, lymphocyte-rich CHL; MCCHL, mixed cellularity CHL; NSCHL, nodular sclerosis CHL. From: Mueller NE and Grufferman S {2777}.

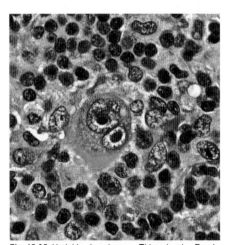

Fig. 15.05 Hodgkin lymphoma. This classic Reed–Sternberg cell is binucleated, with prominent eosinophilic nucleoli, producing the so-called owl's eye appearance.

Table 15.01 Differential diagnosis of Hodgkin lymphoma: comparative tumour cell immunophenotypes

Marker	NLPHL	THRLBCL	CHL	DLBCL	ALCL, ALK+	ALCL, ALK–
CD30	– [a]	– [a]	+	–/+ [b]	+	+
CD15	–	–	+/–	–	– [c]	– [c]
CD45	+	+	–	+	+/–	+/–
CD20	+	+	–/+ [d]	+	–	–
CD79a	+	+	–/+	+	–	–
CD75	+	+	–	+	–	–
PAX5	+	+	+ [e]	+	–	–
J chain	+/–	+/–	–	–/+	–	–
Ig	+/–	+/–	– [f]	+/–	–	–
OCT2	S+	S+	–/+ [g]	+	n/a	n/a
BOB1	+	+	– [h]	+	n/a	n/a
CD3	–	–	– [a]	–	–/+	–/+
CD2	–	–	– [a]	–	–/+	+/–
Perforin/ granzyme B	–	–	– [a]	–	+	+ [i]
CD43	–	–	–	–/+	+/–	+/–
EMA	+/–	+/–	– [j]	–/+ [k]	+/–	+/–
ALK	–	–	–	–	+	–
LMP1	–	–	+/–	–/+	–	–

+, All (or nearly all) cases positive; +/–, majority of cases positive; –/+, minority of cases positive; –, all (or nearly all) cases negative; ALCL, anaplastic large cell lymphoma; CHL, classic Hodgkin lymphoma; DLBCL, diffuse large B-cell lymphoma; Ig, immunoglobulin; n/a, not applicable; NLPHL, nodular lymphocyte predominant Hodgkin lymphoma; S, strong expression; THRLBCL, T-cell/histiocyte-rich large B-cell lymphoma.

---

[a] Positive in fewer than 10% of cases.
[b] Prominent expression in anaplastic variant and variable expression in mediastinal large B-cell subtype.
[c] Occasional cases may show focal positivity.
[d] Present in as many as 40% of cases, but usually expressed on a minority of tumour cells, with variable intensity.
[e] As many as 10% might be negative.
[f] The common positivity for IgG and both Ig light chains reflects uptake of these proteins by the tumour cells rather than synthesis.
[g] Strong expression found in ~10% of the cases.
[h] Rare cases (~10%) may show scattered weak positivity.
[i] Only a minority of cases are negative.
[j] Weak expression may be seen in tumour cells in 5% of cases.
[k] Most frequently positive in DLBCLs with anaplastic morphology.

subtype. CHL in the thymus can be associated with cystic degeneration and epithelial hyperplasia {2349}. Rare cases can be confined to the thymus.

Microscopy

In CHL, the lymph node architecture is effaced by variable numbers of Hodgkin/ Reed–Sternberg (HRS) cells admixed with a rich inflammatory background. Classic diagnostic Reed–Sternberg cells are large, have abundant slightly basophilic cytoplasm, and have at least two nuclear lobes or nuclei. The nuclei are large and often rounded in contour, with a prominent, often irregular, nuclear membrane; pale chromatin; and usually one prominent eosinophilic nucleolus, with perinuclear clearing (a halo), resembling a viral inclusion. Prototypical Reed–Sternberg cells have at least two nucleoli in two separate nuclear lobes: the so-called owl's eye appearance. Mononuclear variants are termed Hodgkin cells. Some HRS cells may have condensed cytoplasm and pyknotic reddish nuclei. These variants are known as mummified cells. Many of the neoplastic cells are not prototypical Reed–Sternberg cells. The lacunar Reed–Sternberg variant is characteristic of nodular sclerosis CHL.

The neoplastic cells typically constitute only a minority of the cellular infiltrate, amounting to 0.1–10%. The composition of the reactive cellular infiltrate varies according to the histological subtype.

Involvement of secondary sites (bone marrow and liver) is determined based on the identification of atypical mononuclear (CD30+ Hodgkin cells with or without CD15 expression in the appropriate inflammatory background); thus, diagnostic multinuclear Reed–Sternberg cells are not required in a patient with CHL diagnosed at another site {3311}.

The neoplastic cells of NLPHL are referred to as lymphocyte predominant (LP) cells. They have lobed nuclei, usually with smaller basophilic nucleoli than are seen in CHL. They have a rim of pale cytoplasm. The background differs from that of CHL in that it has a predominance of lymphocytes. Epithelioid histiocytes, sometimes in clusters, may be abundant, often around the nodules.

Immunophenotype

The HRS cells of CHL are positive for CD30 in nearly all cases {3590,3783, 3787} and for CD15 {1716,3787,3788} in the majority (75–85%). They are usually negative for CD45 and are consistently negative for J chain, CD75, and macrophage-specific markers such as the PGM1 epitope of the CD68 molecule {724,1143} (Table 15.01). Both CD30 and CD15 are typically present in a membrane pattern, with accentuation in the Golgi area of the cytoplasm; CD15 may be expressed by only a minority of the neoplastic cells and may be restricted to the Golgi region. In 30–40% of cases, CD20 may be detectable but is usually of varied intensity and usually present only on a minority of the neoplastic cells {3565,4504}. The B-cell–associated antigen CD79a is less often expressed. The B-cell nature of HRS cells is further

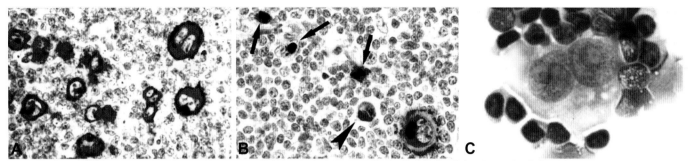

Fig. 15.06 Classic Hodgkin lymphoma. **A** The cytokine receptor CD30 is selectively expressed by the Hodgkin/Reed–Sternberg cells. **B** The typical membrane and perinuclear dot-like staining of a large Reed–Sternberg cell for CD15 is seen. The small binucleated Reed–Sternberg cell (arrowhead) shows only a very faint labelling. In addition, three neutrophil granulocytes (arrows) are strongly labelled. **C** Touch imprint of a binucleated Reed–Sternberg cell ringed by lymphocytes.

demonstrable in approximately 95% of cases by their expression of the B-cell–specific activator protein PAX5 (also called BSAP) {1238}. The immunostaining of HRS cells for PAX5 is usually weaker than that of reactive B cells, a feature that makes the PAX5+ HRS cells easily identifiable. The transcription factor IRF4/MUM1 is consistently positive in HRS cells, usually at high intensity. In one study, PRDM1 (also known as BLIMP1), the key regulator of plasma cell differentiation, was expressed in only a small proportion of HRS cells in 25% of CHLs {492}. The plasma cell–associated adhesion molecule CD138 is consistently absent {492}. EBV-infected HRS cells express LMP1 and EBNA1 without EBNA2, a pattern characteristic of type II EBV latency {950}. EBV-encoded LMP1 has strong transforming and antiapoptotic potential.

Membranous and less often globular cytoplasmic expression of one or more T-cell antigens by a minority of HRS cells may be encountered in some cases {862,4176}. However, this is often difficult to assess because of the T cells that usually surround the HRS cells. Most T-cell antigen–positive CHL cases have both PAX5 expression and IG gene rearrange-

ment in the HRS cells, so that the expression of T-cell antigens is either aberrant or artefactual {3614,4176}. Expression of EMA is rare and usually weak if present. A further characteristic finding is the absence of the transcription factor OCT2 (also known as POU2F2) in up to 90% of cases in some reports and the absence of its coactivator BOB1 (also known as POU2AF1) in the same proportion {2379}. The transcription factor PU1 is consistently absent from HRS cells {2379,4027}. Most HRS cells express the proliferation-associated nuclear antigen Ki-67 {1332}. CHL cases rich in neoplastic cells may resemble anaplastic large cell lymphoma (ALCL), a T-cell neoplasm. Their identification as CHL is facilitated by demonstrating positivity for PAX5 and absence of EMA and ALK protein {1238,3782}. The detection of EBV-encoded small RNA (EBER) or LMP1 favours CHL over ALCL {1731}. The most difficult differential diagnosis is with diffuse large B-cell lymphoma displaying anaplastic morphology and expressing CD30. There may be a true biological overlap between such cases and CHL, especially in cases with mediastinal disease.

Unlike CHL, NLPHL generally shows preservation of the B-cell programme.

The LP cells are positive for CD20, CD79a, PAX5, OCT2, and BOB1. EMA is sometimes positive, but often only in a fraction of the LP cells. IgD (but not IgM) is expressed in LP cells in a subset of cases, most commonly in young males {3231}. However, stains for immunoglobulin light chains are generally negative. CD30 may be weakly expressed in some cases, but CD15 is nearly always negative.

Cytokines and chemokines

CHL is associated with overexpression and an abnormal pattern of cytokines and chemokines and/or their receptors in HRS cells {1613,1751,1897,1899,1937, 4120}, which likely explains the abundant admixture of inflammatory cells {1876, 3944}, the fibrosis {1897}, and the predominance of T helper 2 (Th2) cells in the infiltrating T-cell population {4120}.

Postulated normal counterpart

Classic Hodgkin lymphoma (CHL)

The cellular origin of HRS was unknown for many years, because the cells lack the morphology and immunophenotype of any normal counterpart. However, IG gene rearrangement studies have provided convincing evidence that HRS

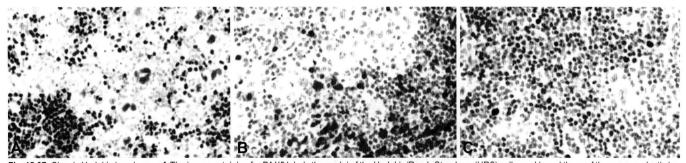

Fig. 15.07 Classic Hodgkin lymphoma. **A** The immunostaining for PAX5 labels the nuclei of the Hodgkin/Reed–Sternberg (HRS) cells weakly and those of the non-neoplastic bystander B cells strongly. **B** Immunostaining for BOB1 (the coactivator of the octamer-binding transcription factors OCT1 and OCT2) fails to stain the HRS cells in most instances. This is in contrast to the non-neoplastic bystander B cells and plasma cells, which show a moderately strong to strong labelling of their nuclei and in part of their cytoplasm. **C** Immunostaining for the octamer-binding transcription factor OCT2 is negative in the HRS cells, whereas the non-neoplastic bystander B cells show a nuclear positivity.

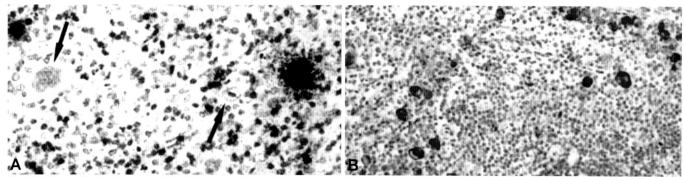

Fig. 15.08 Classic Hodgkin lymphoma. **A** Radiolabelled in situ hybridization for Igµ mRNA is negative in the Hodgkin/Reed–Sternberg cells (arrows), and the non-neoplastic bystander small B cells are moderately strongly positive. **B** Immunostaining for the antiapoptotic TRAF1 protein. The Hodgkin/Reed–Sternberg cells strongly overexpress TRAF1.

cells are clonal and derived from germinal centre B cells (GCBs) despite the frequent absence of B-cell markers other than PAX5. Thus, HRS cells are one of the most extreme examples of discordance between genotype and phenotype {1934,2495}.

The HRS cells of rare CHL cases have been reported to harbour clonally rearranged TR genes, indicating that exceptional cases with morphological features of CHL may be derived from T cells {2798,3614}. Because the neoplastic cells in some cases of peripheral T-cell lymphoma can have an appearance similar to that of HRS cells, the differential diagnosis is challenging. Additionally, some peripheral T-cell lymphomas express CD30 and CD15, making their distinction from CHL even more difficult {277}.

Nodular lymphocyte predominant Hodgkin lymphoma (NLPHL)

Due to their expression of B-cell markers, LP cells were more readily identified as B-cell derived {783,3192,3193}, and this origin was confirmed by rearrangement studies of the IGH gene. These studies

also showed that LP cells are clonal expansions of B cells with genotypic features of GCBs, indicating that LP cells constitute a neoplasm of this B-cell type.

Genetic profile

Antigen receptor genes

Rearrangement studies of antigen receptor genes of LP or HRS cells usually provide only reliable results for these cells when DNA of isolated single LP and HRS cells is investigated and not whole tissue DNA.

NLPHL

In all cases LP cells harbour a clonal immunoglobulin gene rearrangement with a high load of somatic mutations and signs of ongoing mutations in the variable (V) region. The rearrangements are usually functional and IG mRNA transcripts are detectable in the LP cells. Consistent with this finding, the transcription factor OCT2 and its coactivator BOB1, which are dominantly involved in the regulation of the expression of IG mRNA, are consistently expressed {3785}.

CHL

HRS cells contain clonal immunoglobulin gene rearrangements in more than 98% of cases. The rearranged IGHV genes harbour a high load of somatic hypermutations in the variable (V) region, usually without signs of ongoing mutations. However, the B-cell program is downregulated in CHL, and HRS cells do not express immunoglobulin transcripts. Experimental data from several studies partially explain this defect. In approximately 25% of cases of CHL nonsense mutations in the V region genes were identified, which were proposed to result in the failure of Ig secretion {1934}. A major contributory factor is the absent or decreased expression in most cases of CHL of the transcription factors (OCT2, BOB1) that regulate Ig expression {3785}. Finally, there is evidence of hypermethylation of multiple genes and pathways in CHL, which may further contribute to the damage to the B-cell programme {2180A}. These findings, in conjunction with the study of composite lymphomas consisting of CHL and follicular non-Hodgkin lymphoma, support the assumption that

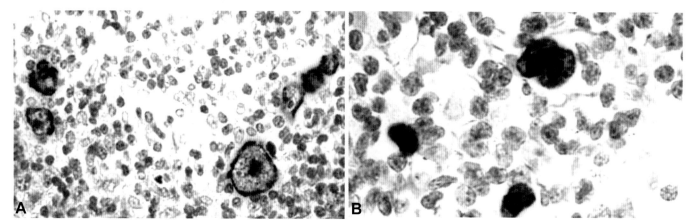

Fig. 15.09 Classic Hodgkin lymphoma. **A** EBV-infected Hodgkin/Reed–Sternberg cells strongly express the EBV-encoded latent membrane protein LMP1. **B** EBV-infected Hodgkin/Reed–Sternberg cells consistently show a strong expression of EBV-encoded small RNA (EBER) in their nuclei as revealed by in situ hybridization.

HRS cells of B-cell lineage are derived from a GCB {486,2494}.

Abnormal gene expression

Despite their derivation from GCBs, HRS cells have lost much of the B-cell–specific expression programme and have acquired B-cell–inappropriate gene products {1083,1838,2178,2498,2560,3594,3786}. In addition, deregulated transcription factors in CHL promote proliferation and abrogate apoptosis in the neoplastic cells. The transcription factor NF-kappaB is constitutively activated in HRS cells, and there is altered activity of the NF-kappaB target genes, which regulate proliferation and survival {1637,1638,1751}, the AP1 complex {2559,2560}, and the JAK/STAT signalling pathway {3693}. Mutations of the JAK regulator SOCS1 are associated with nuclear STAT5 accumulation in HRS cells, indicating a blockage of the negative feedback loop of the JAK/STAT5 pathway {1879,2625,4297}.

EBV infection

The prevalence of EBV in HRS cells varies according to the histological subtype and epidemiological factors. The highest prevalence (~75%) is found in MCCHL and LDCHL and the lowest (5%) in NLPHL {1731,1736}. NSCHL shows an intermediate range of EBV-positivity (10–25%). In resource-poor regions and in patients infected with HIV, EBV infection is more frequent, with prevalence approaching 100% in CHL {125,2276, 4277,4278}. The prevalent EBV strain also varies across geographical areas. In resource-rich countries, strain 1 prevails; in resource-poor countries, strain 2. Dual infection by both strains is more common in resource-poor countries {466,4277, 4278}.

It is possible that EBV infection of a B cell replaces one of the genetic alterations necessary for the development of CHL. Loss of immune surveillance in immunodeficiency settings, such as HIV infection, may predispose individuals to the development of EBV-associated CHL. In tropical regions, resource-poor regions, and patients infected with HIV, as many as 100% of CHL cases are EBV-positive {125,2276,4277,4278}. Most patients with AIDS-associated CHL are EBV-infected. In 1991–1995, AIDS-associated non-Hodgkin lymphomas were 30 times as frequent as were CHLs, but during the period of 2001–2005, the ratio of non-

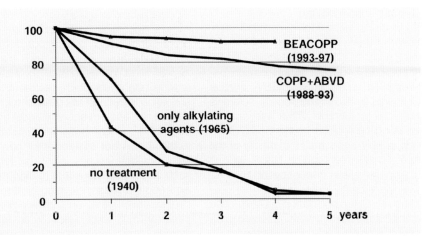

Fig. 15.10 Hodgkin lymphoma. Historical overview of progress in the treatment of advanced stage CHL since 1940.

Hodgkin lymphoma cases to CHL cases fell to 7:1. This change might have been influenced by the development of HAART. The risk for the development of CHL appears to be higher in patients with moderately decreased CD4 counts than in patients with very low CD4 counts {1391}.

Cytogenetic abnormalities and oncogenes in CHL

Despite their derivation from GCBs, the HRS cells lack much of the B-cell–specific expression programme, and express B-cell–inappropriate gene products, such as CD15, GATA3, TRAF1, ID2, ABF1, JUN, JUNB, AP1, FLIP (CFLAR), JAK/STAT, and STAT5 {1083,1838,2178, 2498,2560,3594}. In addition, deregulated transcription factors in CHL promote proliferation and abrogate apoptosis in the neoplastic cells. NF-kappaB–inducing kinase (NIK) is stably expressed in the HRS cells, indicating that NIK and the non-canonical NF-kappaB pathway are very prevalent in CHL {3307}. The transcription factor NF-kappaB is constitutively activated in HRS cells, and there is altered activity of the NF-kappaB target genes, which regulate proliferation and survival {1637,1638,1751}, the AP1 complex {2559,2560}, and the JAK/STAT signalling pathway {3693}. Mutations of SOCS1, a negative regulator of JAK, are associated with nuclear STAT5 accumulation in HRS cells, indicating a blockage of the negative feedback loop of the JAK/STAT5 pathway {1879,2625, 4297}. Despite the frequent overexpression of p53, mutations of TP53 are rare or absent in primary CHL tissue {2711}. CHL has a high incidence of aberra-

tions in the CD274 (also called PDL1) and PDCD1LG2 (also called PDL2) loci at 9p24.1, leading to increased expression of PD1 ligands {3391A}. The 9p24.1 region also includes the JAK2 gene {3453}. JAK2 amplification induces transcription and expression of the PD1 ligand {1436}.

Whole-exome sequencing of purified HRS cells has shown the inactivating B2M mutation to be the most frequently detected gene mutation in CHL. This mutation leads to loss of major histocompatibility complex (MHC) class I expression {3334}.

Conventional cytogenetic and FISH studies show aneuploidy and hypertetraploidy, consistent with the multinucleation of the neoplastic cells; however, these techniques fail to demonstrate recurrent and specific chromosomal changes in CHL {3524,3557}. However, comparative genomic hybridization reveals recurrent gains of the chromosomal subregions on chromosome arms 2p, 9p, and 12q and distinct high-level amplifications on chromosome bands 4p16, 4q23-24, and 9p23-24 {1880}. The translocations t(14;18) and t(2;5) are absent from HRS cells {1427,2199}, but t(14;18) may occur in CHL arising in follicular lymphoma {2811}. One study using interphase cytogenetics found breakpoints in the IGH locus in HRS cells in 17% of CHL cases {2526}. Array comparative genomic hybridization identified copy number alterations in > 20% of cases {3780}. Gains in 2p, 9p, 16p, 17q, 19q, and 20q were noted, as were losses of 6q, 11q, and 13q. The affected gene segments harbour genes involved in NF-kappaB signalling, such as REL, IKBKB, CD40, and MAP3K14.

Genetic susceptibility

Some novel gene loci have been identified as being linked to risk for the development of CHL, irrespective of EBV status {1867,4092}. The association between SNP rs6903608 and EBV-negative CHL was limited to the nodular sclerosis histological subtype. Other associations involving HLA class I have been identified in EBV-positive CHLs, mainly of the mixed cellularity subtype {1867}. In one study, the allele frequency of HLA-A2 was significantly decreased in the EBV-positive CHL population {1726}. Two class II associations were observed to be specific for the EBV-negative population, with an increase of HLA-DR2 and HLA-DR5. HLA-B5 was significantly increased and HLA-DR7 significantly decreased in the total CHL patient population compared with controls. These observations confirm the relevance of histological subtyping of CHL, and in particular the differences between EBV-positive and EBV-negative cases.

Prognosis and predictive factors

CHL

With modern polychemotherapy protocols such as ABVD (i.e. doxorubicin, bleomycin, vinblastine, and dacarbazine) and escalated BEACOPP (bleomycin, etoposide, doxorubicin, cyclophosphamide, vincristine, procarbazine, and prednisone), and with improvements in radiotherapy, CHL is now curable in >85% of cases {790,979}. Patients receive stage-adapted treatment after allocation to defined risk groups (early, intermediate, and advanced stages) on the basis of the extent of disease (according to the Ann Arbor system) and the presence or absence of clinical risk factors such as large mediastinal (bulky) mass, extranodal disease, elevated erythrocyte sedimentation rate, and involvement of three (or four) nodal areas. In advanced stages, the International Prognostic Score (IPS), consisting of seven risk factors, correlates with prognosis {1581, 2683}. In recent years, interim FDG-PET has been recognized as a valid tool to distinguish between good-risk patients and poor-risk patients requiring more-intensive treatment {70,1281,1581,1744, 1886}. In addition to conventional chemotherapy, novel targeted treatment approaches using the histological properties of CHL have become available. The CD30-directed antibody–drug conjugate brentuximab vedotin has already been approved for the treatment of patients with relapsed/refractory CHL, and its combination with conventional chemotherapy is under evaluation {4443}. Anti-PD1 antibodies have also been investigated in clinical studies, with promising initial results in patients with relapsed disease {113}. Studies using gene expression profiling have identified a signature associated with tumour-infiltrating macrophages associated with an adverse prognosis {3778}. In the same study, the authors enumerated macrophages positive for CD68 and correlated the results with clinical outcome. A high content of CD68+ cells correlated with reduced progression-free survival. The significance of macrophage content has been confirmed in some studies {4034,4084}, but not in others {38,204,600}, and macrophage content is not routinely used as a measure to guide therapy or for prognosis. Notably, a high content of tumour-infiltrating macrophages is a feature of some aggressive forms of CHL, such as the lymphocyte-depleted subtype.

NLPHL

Historically, the treatment of NLPHL has been based on treatment approaches used for CHL. However, approaches have more recently diverged on the basis of clinical observations and differences in underlying biology.

Nodular lymphocyte predominant Hodgkin lymphoma

Stein H.
Swerdlow S.H.
Gascoyne R.D.
Poppema S.
Jaffe E.S.
Pileri S.A.

Definition

Nodular lymphocyte predominant Hodgkin lymphoma (NLPHL) is a B-cell neoplasm usually characterized by a nodular or a nodular and diffuse proliferation of small lymphocytes with single scattered large neoplastic cells known as lymphocyte predominant (LP) or popcorn cells, formerly called L&H cells for lymphocytic and/or histiocytic Reed–Sternberg cell variants. The LP cells are ringed by PD1/CD279+ T cells in almost all instances. In typical cases, the LP cells reside in large nodular meshworks of follicular dendritic cell (FDC) processes that are filled with non-neoplastic lymphocytes (mainly B cells) and histiocytes. They can also grow in an extrafollicular distribution associated with a diffuse background of T cells. There is increasing evidence that NLPHL cases with a purely diffuse growth pattern overlap with T-cell/histiocyte-rich large B-cell lymphoma (THRLBCL).

ICD-O code   9659/3

Synonyms

Hodgkin lymphoma, lymphocyte predominance, nodular; Hodgkin paragranuloma, NOS (obsolete); Hodgkin paragranuloma, nodular (obsolete)

Epidemiology

NLPHL accounts for approximately 10% of all Hodgkin lymphoma {2230A}. Patients are predominantly male and most are aged 30–50 years.

Localization

NLPHL usually involves cervical, axillary, or inguinal lymph nodes. Mediastinal involvement is rare. Mesenteric lymph node involvement can be seen, unlike in classic Hodgkin lymphoma (CHL). Patients with advanced disease may have involvement of the spleen and bone marrow. Rare cases may have destructive lesions involving bone.

Clinical features

Most patients present with localized peripheral lymphadenopathy (stage I or II). Approximately 20% of patients present with advanced-stage disease {3654}.

Microscopy

The lymph node architecture is totally or partially replaced by a nodular, nodular and diffuse, or predominantly diffuse infiltrate consisting of small lymphocytes, histiocytes, epithelioid histiocytes, and intermingled LP cells. A detailed description of growth patterns observed in NLPHL has been given by Fan et al. {1159}. Six distinct immunoarchitectural patterns are recognized: pattern A is typical (B-cell–rich) nodular; pattern B is serpiginous nodular; pattern C is nodular with prominent extranodular LP cells; pattern D is T-cell–rich nodular; pattern E is THRLBCL-like, and pattern F is diffuse B-cell–rich. In NLPHLs of patterns A, B, C, and F, the architectural background is composed of variably large spherical meshworks of FDCs. A prominence of extranodular LP cells is associated with a propensity to develop a diffuse pattern, with a loss of FDC meshworks, resembling THRLBCL. Such progression to a process with features of THRLBCL is seen more frequently in patients with recurrence {1159}. For lesions that appear totally diffuse on H&E staining, immunostaining is needed to detect the presence of LP cells in association with small B-cells in residual follicular structures. The detection of one such area is sufficient to exclude THRLBCL.

LP cells are large and usually have one large nucleus and scant cytoplasm. The cells have been referred to as popcorn cells due to their nuclei, which are often folded or multilobed. The nucleoli are usually multiple, basophilic, and smaller than those seen in classic Hodgkin/Reed–Sternberg cells. However, some LP cells may contain one prominent nucleolus and/or have more than one nucleus, and thus may be indistinguishable from classic Hodgkin/Reed–Sternberg (HRS) cells on purely cytological grounds. Histiocytes and some polyclonal plasma cells can be found at the margin of the nodules containing LP cells. Neutrophils and

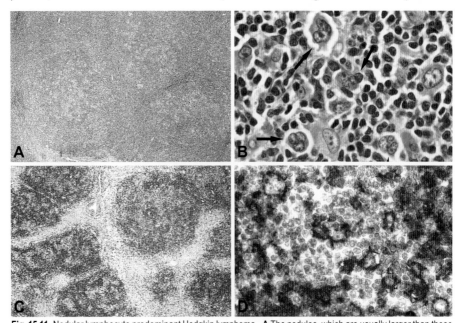

Fig. 15.11 Nodular lymphocyte predominant Hodgkin lymphoma. **A** The nodules, which are usually larger than those in follicular lymphoma and follicular hyperplasia, lack mantle zones. **B** Three lymphocyte predominant (LP) cells (arrows), also called popcorn cells, with the typically lobed nuclei, are visible in a background of small lymphoid cells and a few histiocytes. **C** CD20 staining reveals that the nodules consist predominantly of B cells. **D** At higher magnification, the strong membrane staining of the LP cells for CD20 is apparent.

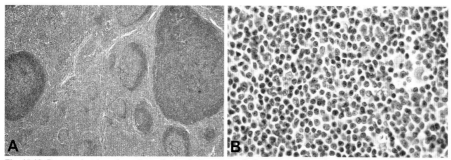

Fig. 15.12 Progressive transformation of germinal centres. **A** An enlarged lymph node with two progressively transformed germinal centres, with several normal germinal centres in between. **B** Higher magnification shows a predominance of small lymphocytes, with rare centroblasts and centrocytes. Lymphocyte predominant (LP) cells are absent.

eosinophils are seldom seen in either the nodular or the diffuse regions. Occasionally, there is reactive follicular hyperplasia (with or without progressive transformation of germinal centres) adjacent to the NLPHL lesions {91,1557}. It is uncertain whether the progressively transformed germinal centres are preneoplastic. However, the vast majority of patients with reactive hyperplasia and progressive transformation of germinal centres do not develop Hodgkin lymphoma {1207, 2994}. A rim of reactive lymphoid tissue may be seen peripherally to the dominant nodular lesion.

Sclerosis is infrequently present in primary biopsies (7%), but can be found more frequently in recurrences (44%). Remnants of small germinal centres are infrequently present in the nodules of NLPHL, a finding more typical of nodular lymphocyte-rich CHL {91,1159}.

Immunophenotype

LP cells are positive for CD20, OCT2, CD75, CD79a, BOB1, PAX5, and CD45 in all or nearly all cases {783,3192,3193, 3785}. Staining for OCT2 and CD75 is strong and highlights the presence of LP cells; admixed small mantle zone B cells are only weakly positive {472, 3785}. J chain is present in most cases and EMA in >50% {91,724,3218,3784} (Table 15.01, p.426). LP cells are positive for BCL6 {1139}, but CD10 is absent. Unlike the HRS cells in CHL, LP cells co-express OCT2, BOB1, and activation-induced cytidine deaminase {2762,3785}. Staining for immunoglobulin light and/or heavy chains is variable {3565,3566}. In 9–27% of cases, the LP cells are IgD-positive, but negative for IgM {1451,3231}. The expression of IgD is more common in young males {3231}. LP cells lack CD15 and CD30 in nearly all instances. However, CD30+ large cells, which usually constitute reactive immunoblasts unrelated to the LP cells, may be seen {91}. Infrequently, the LP cells show weak expression of CD30, and rare cases with CD15 positivity have been reported {4175}. As revealed by their nuclear positivity for Ki-67, LP cells are usually in cycle.

FDC meshworks highlighted by CD21 or other FDC-associated antigens are seen in the patterns A, B and C described by Fan et al. {1159}. The FDC meshworks are predominantly filled with small bystander B cells and a varying number of T cells of the TFH type typically expressing PD1/CD279 and/or CD57 {3219}. PD1+ T cells form rosettes around LP cells in all NLPHL cases with a nodular or a nodular and diffuse growth pattern, and to a lesser and variable extent in the diffuse areas {2822}. The rosette formation by PD1+ T cells can therefore serve as a useful additional diagnostic feature. The T cells in NLPHL express molecules such as MAF (also called c-MAF), BCL6, IRF4/MUM1, and CD134, consistent with a subset of germinal centre T cells, but they do not produce IL2 or IL4 {175}. Cells positive for TIA1 and CD40 ligand are usually absent, whereas T cells double-positive for CD4 and CD8 detected by flow cytometry are frequent {882,3281}. In diffuse growth patterns, the presence of CD4+CD8+/CD57+/PD1+ T cells favours NLPHL, whereas a total absence of small B cells, low numbers of CD57+ T cells, and a dominant presence of CD8+ cells and TIA1+

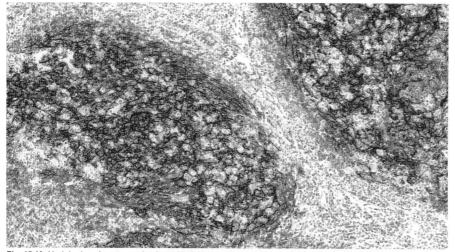

Fig. 15.13 Nodular lymphocyte predominant Hodgkin lymphoma. Immunostaining for CD21 highlights the expanded meshwork of follicular dendritic cells in the nodules of this lymphoma type.

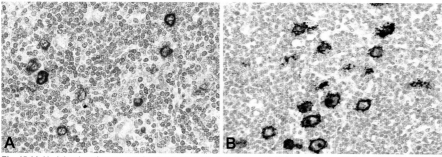

Fig. 15.14 Nodular lymphocyte predominant Hodgkin lymphoma. **A** Cytoplasmic positivity of the lymphocyte predominant (LP) cells, also called popcorn cells, for J chain. **B** Membrane and dot-like staining in the Golgi region for EMA.

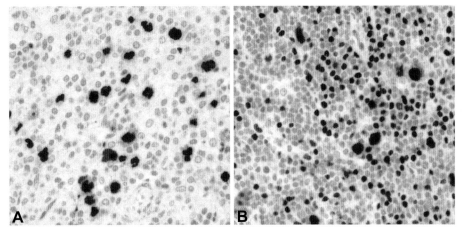

Fig. 15.15 Nodular lymphocyte predominant Hodgkin lymphoma with variant growth pattern, immunostained for OCT2. **A** Diffuse, T-cell–rich (T-cell/histiocyte-rich large B-cell lymphoma–like) area with few scattered lymphocyte predominant (LP) cells. **B** Tissue section of the same lymph node, showing a single area with LP cells in association with small B cells at the margin of the section.

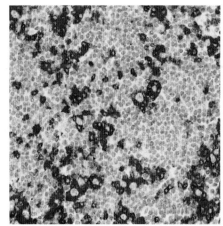

Fig. 15.16 Nodular lymphocyte predominant Hodgkin lymphoma. The PD1+ T cells form rosettes around lymphocyte predominant (LP) cells.

cells favour primary THRLBCL. Strongly stained LP cells in association with weakly stained B cells are best identified by OCT2 or PAX5 immunostaining.

Postulated normal counterpart
A germinal centre B cell at the centroblastic stage of differentiation

Genetic profile
LP cells harbour clonally rearranged IG (IGHV) genes {2493,2947}. The clonal rearrangements are usually not detectable in whole-tissue DNA but only in the DNA of isolated single LP cells. The IGHV genes carry a high load of somatic mutations, and also show signs of ongoing mutations. The rearrangements are usually functional, and IG mRNA transcripts are detectable in the LP cells of most cases {2493}. EBV infection detected by EBV-encoded small RNA (EBER) may be found in the LP cells in 3–5% of cases in both children and adults {1736}. EBV positivity might be higher in Asia {653}. EBV may also be present in bystander lymphocytes {91}. *BCL6* rearrangements (involving IG genes, IKAROS family genes, *ABR*, and other partner genes) are present in about half of NLPHLs {174,3343,4341}. Aberrant somatic hypermutations were found in 80% of NLPHL cases, most frequently in *PAX5*, but also in *PIM1*, *RHOH* (also called *TTF*), and *MYC* {2359}. Mutations of *SGK1*, *DUSP2*, and *JUNB* are also reported in about half of NLPHLs {1575}.

Relationship between NLPHL and THRLBCL
LP cells by gene expression profiling

are similar to the cells of THRLBCL and CHL {477}. They show partial loss of their B-cell phenotype, and deregulation of many apoptosis regulators and putative oncogenes. The only investigations that point to distinct pathogeneses of NLPHL and primary THRLBCL are two comparative genomic hybridization studies in which more and different genomic aberrations were identified in NLPHL than in THRLBCL {1246,1247}. Such different genetic patterns were not found in the gene expression profiling study of microdissected tumour cells of typical cases of NLPHL and THRLBCL {1570,1571}. These studies revealed, in addition to a common expression of BCL6, CD75, EMA, J chain, and PU1, an identical expression of *BAG6* (also called *BAT3*), *HIGD1A*, and *UBD* (also called *FAT10*) in the tumour cells of cases with a nodular, a nodular and diffuse, and a diffuse growth in NLPHL and primary THRLBCL, suggesting the possibility that THRLBCL may represent a variant or extension of NLPHL. This speculation is supported by the observation that NLPHL can show a THRLBCL-like transformation, which is indistinguishable from primary THRLBCL. It is likely that the distinction between NLPHL and THRLBCL does not lie in different genomic alterations and the immunophenotype of the tumour cells, but rather in the different cellular composition of the microenvironment as described above.

Genetic susceptibility
An increased familial risk of NLPHL has been noted in some families {3466}.

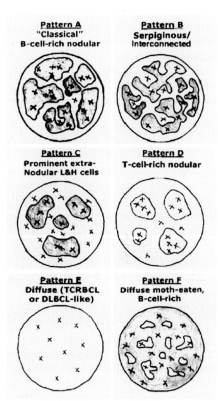

Fig. 15.17 Immunoarchitectural patterns in nodular lymphocyte predominant Hodgkin lymphoma {1159}. In this schematic illustration, the X's represent lymphocyte predominant (LP) cells, the grey background a B-cell–rich background, and the white background a T-cell–rich background. **Pattern A** So-called classic B-cell–rich nodular pattern. **Pattern B** Serpiginous nodular pattern. **Pattern C** Nodular pattern with many extranodular LP cells (formerly called L&H cells). **Pattern D** T-cell–rich nodular pattern. **Pattern E** Diffuse, T-cell–rich (TCRBCL-like) pattern. **Pattern F** (Diffuse), moth-eaten (B-cell–rich) pattern.
DLBCL, diffuse large B-cell lymphoma; TCRBCL, T-cell/histiocyte-rich large B-cell lymphoma.
From: Fan Z, Natkunam Y, Bair E, Tibshirani R, Warnke RA. *Am J Surg Pathol* (2003) {1159}.

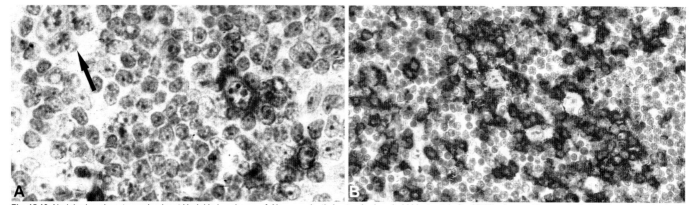

Fig. 15.18 Nodular lymphocyte predominant Hodgkin lymphoma. **A** Non-neoplastic bystander lymphoid blasts stain for CD30, whereas the neoplastic lymphocyte predominant (LP) cell (arrow), also called a popcorn cell, remains unlabelled. **B** Many non-neoplastic bystander T cells are labelled for CD57. These CD57+ cells may be involved in the rosette-like binding to the LP cells, which is particularly pronounced in the case illustrated here.

However, the specific genetic factors have not been identified. NLPHL has also been identified in patients with Hermansky–Pudlak syndrome type 2 {2391}.

The affected patients in that study exhibited NK-cell and T-cell defects. An increased risk is also seen in patients with autoimmune lymphoproliferative syndrome with mutations in *FAS* {3810}, which may also be linked to defective immune surveillance.

Prognosis and predictive factors

NLPHL in its nodular and its nodular and diffuse forms develops slowly, with fairly frequent relapses. It usually remains responsive to therapy and thus is rarely fatal. The prognosis of patients with stage I or II disease is very good, with a 10-year overall survival rate >80% {980, 2888}. It is not yet clear whether immediate therapy is necessary to achieve this favourable prognosis; in some countries (e.g. France), stage I disease (especially in children) is not treated after the resec-

tion of the affected lymph node {3125}. Histopathological variants characterized by LP cells outside B-cell nodules, B-cell depletion of the microenvironment, or THRLBCL-like transformation (patterns C, D, E and F as described by Fan et al., Figure 15.17) are associated more often with advanced disease and a higher relapse rate compared with that of typical NLPHL {1572}. Therefore, it is useful to note these variant features in the diagnostic report. Clinically recognized advanced stages have an unfavourable prognosis {980}. Progression to diffuse large B-cell lymphoma has been reported in approximately 3–5% of cases {723,1538,2660}. The neoplastic cells in such cases may resemble LP cells or may have centroblastic or immunoblastic features. However, they keep their typical immunophenotype (strong coexpression of CD20, OCT2, and CD75). In some cases, diffuse large B-cell lymphoma was found to precede NLPHL {1159}. The large B-cell lymphomas associated with NLPHL, if localized, generally have a good prognosis {1538}. A clonal relationship between NLPHL and the associated diffuse large B-cell lymphoma has been demonstrated {1452,1575,4310}. Bone marrow involvement is rare in NLPHL and raises the possibility of THRLBCL, or THRLBCL-like transformation, in particular if the characteristic microenvironment is absent. Cases of NLPHL with bone marrow involvement are clinically aggressive {2003}. Advanced-stage NLPHL responds poorly to the chemotherapy regimens traditionally used for CHL, but responds better to the CHOP chemotherapy regimen plus rituximab (R-CHOP), or regimens used for aggressive B-cell lymphomas {4387}.

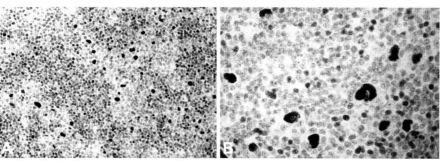

Fig. 15.19 Nodular lymphocyte predominant Hodgkin lymphoma. **A** Immunostaining for the transcription factor OCT2, which is involved in the regulation of immunoglobulin expression, produces strong nuclear staining of the lymphocyte predominant (LP) cells (also called popcorn cells), and weaker labelling of the bystander B cells; thus, OCT2 often highlights the presence and the nuclear atypia of LP cells. **B** Higher magnification.

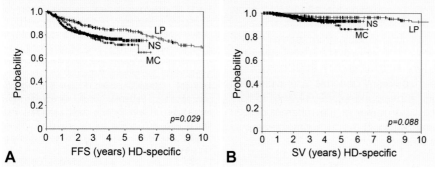

Fig. 15.20 Hodgkin lymphoma (HD)–specific survivals associated with the nodular lymphocyte predominant (LP), nodular sclerosis (NS), and mixed cellularity (MC) subtypes of classic Hodgkin lymphoma. **A** Failure-free survival (FFS). **B** Overall survival (SV). German Hodgkin Study Group (GHSG)

Classic Hodgkin lymphoma

Introduction

Jaffe E.S.
Stein H.
Swerdlow S.H.

Classic Hodgkin lymphoma (CHL) is a monoclonal lymphoid neoplasm derived from B cells, composed of mononuclear Hodgkin cells and multinucleated Reed–Sternberg cells in a background containing a variable mixture of non-neoplastic reactive immune cells, including small lymphocytes, eosinophils, neutrophils, histiocytes, and plasma cells. On the basis of the characteristics of the reactive infiltrate and to a certain extent the morphology of the Hodgkin/Reed–Sternberg (HRS) cells, four histological subtypes have been distinguished: nodular sclerosis CHL, lymphocyte-rich CHL, mixed cellularity CHL, and lymphocyte-depleted CHL. The HRS cells in all forms of CHL share similar immunophenotypic features, with reduced expression of most B-cell antigens (CD20, CD79a, PAX5) and positive staining for CD30 and CD15 in most cases. The association with EBV varies across subtypes, being most commonly positive (i.e. in as many as 75% of cases) in mixed cellularity CHL and lymphocyte-depleted CHL. The four subtypes of CHL also differ in their epidemiological features, clinical presentation, and prevalence of systemic symptoms, as discussed in the following text. These observations suggest potential differences in underlying biology and pathogenesis. It is customary to subclassify CHL as one of the four subtypes, but with limited biopsy material, precise subclassification is not always feasible, and the diagnosis of CHL, NOS, is sometimes made. It remains important to distinguish these cases from nodular lymphocyte predominant Hodgkin lymphoma.

ICD-O code
Classic Hodgkin lymphoma   9650/3

Nodular sclerosis classic Hodgkin lymphoma

Stein H.   Guenova M.
Pileri S.A.   Gascoyne R.D.
MacLennan K.A.   Jaffe E.S.
Poppema S.

Definition
Nodular sclerosis classic Hodgkin lymphoma (NSCHL) is a subtype of classic Hodgkin lymphoma (CHL) characterized by collagen bands that surround at least one nodule, and by HRS cells with lacunar-type morphology.

ICD-O code   9663/3

Synonyms
Hodgkin disease, nodular sclerosis, NOS; Hodgkin lymphoma, nodular sclerosis, grade 1 (9665/3); Hodgkin lymphoma, nodular sclerosis, grade 2 (9667/3); Hodgkin lymphoma, nodular sclerosis, cellular phase (9664/3)

Epidemiology
NSCHL accounts for approximately 70% of all CHLs in Europe and the USA. However, the rate varies greatly among other geographical regions; NSCHL is more common in resource-rich than in resource-poor areas, and the risk is highest among those with high socioeconomic status {762}. The incidence of NSCHL is similar in males and females, and peaks among individuals aged 15–34 years {184,2759}.

Localization
Mediastinal involvement occurs in 80% of cases, bulky disease in 54%, splenic and/or lung involvement in 8–10%, bone involvement in 5%, bone marrow involvement in 3%, and liver involvement in 2% {782,3654}.

Clinical features
Most patients present with Ann Arbor stage II disease. B symptoms are encountered in approximately 40% of cases {3654} and are more frequent with advanced-stage disease.

Macroscopy
The cut surface of lymph nodes typically shows a nodular configuration, with cellular nodules surrounded by dense fibrosis. With higher-grade lesions (grade 2), central areas of necrosis may be evident. Following therapy, a persistent mass lesion may be present, with diffuse fibrotic replacement and no viable involvement by Hodgkin lymphoma. Such lesions may persist radiologically, but should be negative by PET, confirming the absence of active disease.

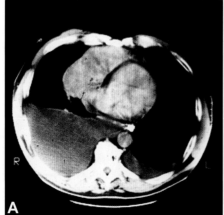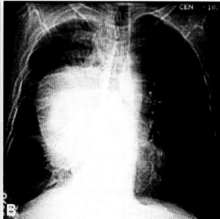

Fig. 15.21 Nodular sclerosis classic Hodgkin lymphoma. **A** CT shows a large anterior mediastinal mass. **B** Chest X-ray of the same patient shows a mediastinal mass exceeding one third of the chest diameter.

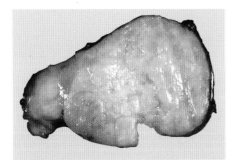

Fig. 15.22 Nodular sclerosis classic Hodgkin lymphoma. In this excised mediastinal mass, cellular nodules with a more yellowish-tan appearance are surrounded by dense fibrosis, which is white in colour.

Microscopy

The lymph nodes have a nodular growth pattern, with nodules surrounded by collagen bands (nodular sclerosis). The broad fibroblast-poor collagen bands surround at least one nodule. This fibrosing process is usually associated with a thickened lymph node capsule. The lymphoma contains a highly variable number of HRS cells, small lymphocytes, and other non-neoplastic inflammatory cells. The HRS cells tend to have more-segmented nuclei with smaller lobes, less prominent nucleoli, and a larger amount of cytoplasm than do HRS cells in other types of CHL. In formalin-fixed tissues, the cytoplasm of the HRS cells frequently shows retraction of the cytoplasmic membrane, so that the cells seem to be sitting in lacunae. These cells have therefore been designated lacunar cells. Lacunar cells may form cellular aggregates, which may be associated with necrosis and a histiocytic reaction, resembling necrotizing granulomas. When aggregates are very prominent, the term 'syncytial variant' has been used. Eosinophils, histiocytes, and (to a lesser extent) neutrophils are often numerous {3178}. Grading according to the proportion of HRS cells or the characteristics of the background infiltrate (e.g. the number of eosinophils) may predict prognosis in some settings, but is not

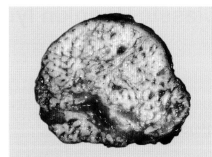

Fig. 15.23 Nodular sclerosis classic Hodgkin lymphoma (NSCHL). This lymph node was obtained following successful treatment for NSCHL. The lymph node shadow persisted on X-ray. Histological examination showed nodules composed of dense collagen, without evidence of Hodgkin/Reed–Sternberg cells. The internodular regions contained a scant inflammatory infiltrate of lymphocytes and plasma cells in an oedematous background.

necessary for routine clinical purposes {1630,2430,4141,4210}; it may serve a research purpose in protocol studies.

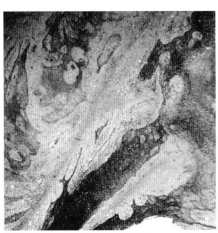

Fig. 15.24 Thymic cyst arising with thymic involvement by Hodgkin lymphoma. Cystic degeneration of the thymus gland is common with involvement by nodular sclerosis classic Hodgkin lymphoma.

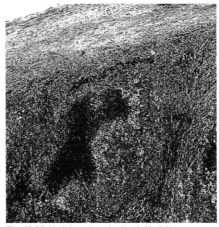

Fig. 15.25 Nodular sclerosis classic Hodgkin lymphoma, grade 2. Capsular fibrosis is present. Central areas of necrosis are noted in the nodular infiltrate.

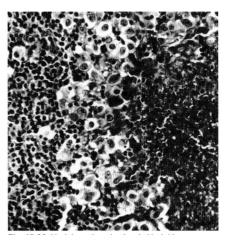

Fig. 15.26 Nodular sclerosis classic Hodgkin lymphoma, grade 2. Lacunar Hodgkin/Reed–Sternberg cells palisade around central necrotic area containing numerous neutrophils.

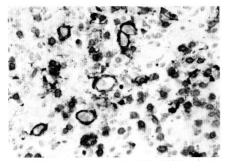

Fig. 15.27 Nodular sclerosis classic Hodgkin lymphoma with aberrant CD3. The neoplastic cells are positive for CD3. Expression of PAX5 (not shown) and negative studies for TR gene rearrangement helped to confirm the diagnosis.

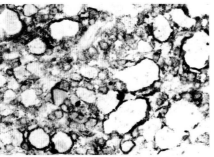

Fig. 15.28 Nodular sclerosis classic Hodgkin lymphoma. This case had aberrant expression of CD2, a finding usually seen in grade 2 disease. In this case, the CD2 antigen appears to be partially expressed on the outer surface of the cell membrane, suggestive of adsorption.

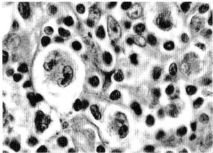

Fig. 15.29 Nodular sclerosis classic Hodgkin lymphoma. Lacunar cells show artificial retraction of the cytoplasm upon fixation. The nucleoli are often smaller than those seen in classic Reed–Sternberg cells.

Immunophenotype

The malignant cells exhibit a CHL phenotype; however, association with EBV as demonstrated by EBV-encoded small RNA (EBER) or the EBV-encoded LMP1 is less frequent (10–25%) than in mixed cellularity CHL {1612,1614,4285,4289}. CD30 is expressed in nearly all cases, but CD15 may be negative in 15–25% of cases. PAX5 is weakly positive in nearly all cases. CD20 may be variably expressed, but is usually weak and only on a subset of the neoplastic cells. CD79a is positive in approximately 10% of cases {4086}.

Approximately 5% of NSCHLs aberrantly express T-cell antigens {4083}, most commonly cases of high histological grade (grade 2). The T-cell antigens most often expressed are CD4 and CD2, and less commonly CD3; positive cases are associated with shorter overall and event-free survival compared with CHL negative for T-cell antigens {4176}. A pitfall in such cases is misdiagnosis as ALK-negative anaplastic large cell lymphoma. Nearly all cases (>90%) with aberrant T-cell antigen expression are positive for PAX5, consistent with a diagnosis of CHL. Gene rearrangement studies help to confirm the diagnosis, being negative for clonal rearrangement of TR genes and often positive for clonal rearrangements of IG. The basis for the aberrant T-cell antigen expression is unknown. In some cases, the aberrant T-cell antigen appears to be adsorbed to the surface of the neoplastic cells, but in other cases it appears to be a product of cell synthesis, and staining may also be observed in the Golgi region.

Grading

A grading system for NSCHL was proposed by the British National Lymphoma Investigation (BNLI). Two histological grades were proposed, which in some series show correlation with clinical features {2429,4313}. According to these criteria, nodular sclerosis is classified as grade 2 if >25% of the nodules show pleomorphic or reticular lymphocyte depletion; if >80% of the nodules show features of the fibrohistiocytic variant; or if >25% of the nodules show numerous bizarre, anaplastic-appearing Hodgkin cells without lymphocyte depletion. When these criteria are applied, approximately 15–25% of cases are classified as grade 2. In some older series, higher-grade cases of nodular sclerosis were referred to as the

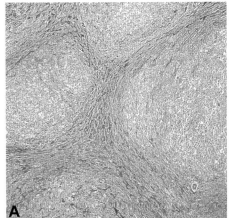
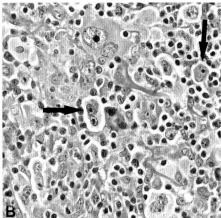

Fig. 15.30 Nodular sclerosis classic Hodgkin lymphoma. **A** Fibrous collagen bands divide the lymph node into nodules. **B** Several lacunar cells (arrows) are present.

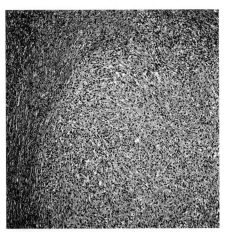

Fig. 15.31 Nodular sclerosis classic Hodgkin lymphoma, fibrohistiocytic variant. A paucicellular nodule contains abundant histiocytes and fibroblasts. Hodgkin cells are difficult to identify on H&E staining. The nodule is surrounded by a dense fibrous band.

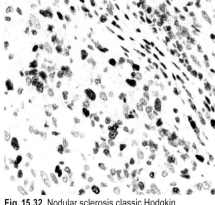

Fig. 15.32 Nodular sclerosis classic Hodgkin lymphoma, fibrohistiocytic variant. PAX5 is weakly positive in neoplastic cells. Some tumour cells are spindle-shaped, making them difficult to distinguish from histiocytes and fibroblasts.

lymphocyte-depleted subtype of nodular sclerosis {965}. Grading is not mandatory for clinical purposes, but has been investigated as a prognostic feature in some clinical trials. However, the importance of grading is declining due to advances in therapy, which obscure the differences seen in less-effectively treated patients {2539,4141}.

The fibrohistiocytic variant of NSCHL may mimic a reactive process or a mesenchymal neoplasm. Fibroblasts and histiocytes are abundant, and the HRS cells may be difficult to identify without immunohistochemical staining. In such cases, PAX5 and CD30 are valuable, because CD20 is typically negative.

In the syncytial variant of nodular sclerosis, the lacunar cells form cohesive nests in the centres of the nodules. Necrosis may or may not be present, but if prominent should prompt consideration

for grade 2 disease. The syncytial variant may prompt consideration for anaplastic large cell lymphoma or even a non-lymphoid neoplasm {588}. Positivity for PAX5 is helpful in ruling out anaplastic large cell lymphoma. However, some cases of CHL may have a cytotoxic phenotype {163}.

Prognosis and predictive factors

Overall, the prognosis of NSCHL is better than that of other types of CHL {70}. Massive mediastinal disease is an adverse prognostic factor {3745}. In the modern era, grading of NSCHL is less significant as an independent risk factor than in the past {4141}. However, grade may be more relevant in patients with advanced-stage disease, whereas it has little impact in patients with localized disease.

Lymphocyte-rich classic Hodgkin lymphoma

Anagnostopoulos I.
Piris M.A.
Isaacson P.G.
Jaffe E.S.
Stein H.

Definition
Lymphocyte-rich classic Hodgkin lymphoma (LRCHL) is a subtype of classic Hodgkin lymphoma (CHL) characterized by scattered Hodgkin/Reed–Sternberg (HRS) cells and a nodular or (less often) diffuse cellular background consisting of small lymphocytes, with an absence of neutrophils and eosinophils.

ICD-O code   9651/3

Synonyms
Hodgkin disease, lymphocytic–histiocytic predominance (obsolete); Hodgkin disease, lymphocyte predominance, diffuse (obsolete); Hodgkin disease, lymphocyte predominance, NOS (obsolete)

Epidemiology
LRCHL accounts for approximately 5% of all CHLs, occurring at a frequency slightly less than that of nodular lymphocyte predominant Hodgkin lymphoma (NLPHL). The median patient age is similar to that of NLPHL and significantly older than seen in other subtypes of CHL {980}. The male-to-female ratio is 2:1 {3654}.

Localization
Peripheral lymph nodes are typically involved. Mediastinal involvement and bulky disease are uncommon {980,3654}.

Clinical features
Most patients present with stage I or II disease. B symptoms are rare. The clinical features are similar to those of NLPHL, with the exception that multiple relapses seem to occur less frequently {980}. Patients are also older than those with NLPHL or the nodular sclerosis subtype.

Microscopy
There are two growth patterns: the common nodular pattern {91} and the rare diffuse pattern {91}. The nodules of the nodular variant encompass most of the involved tissue, so that the T-zone is attenuated. The nodules are composed of small

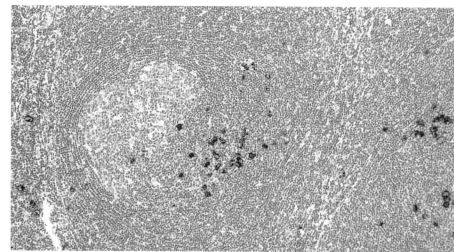

Fig. 15.33 Lymphocyte-rich classic Hodgkin lymphoma, nodular variant. CD30 staining highlights the presence of Hodgkin/Reed–Sternberg cells. They are located within or at the peripheral margin of the follicular mantles, but not within the germinal centres.

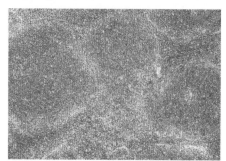

Fig. 15.34 Lymphocyte-rich classic Hodgkin lymphoma, nodular variant. Cellular nodules are composed of small lymphocytes surrounding regressed germinal centres.

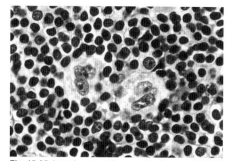

Fig. 15.35 Lymphocyte-rich classic Hodgkin lymphoma, nodular variant. Classic Reed-Sternberg cells are surrounded by small lymphocytes.

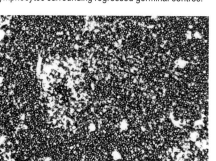

Fig. 15.36 Lymphocyte-rich classic Hodgkin lymphoma. CD20 immunostain identifies small lymphocytes and is negative in HRS cells.

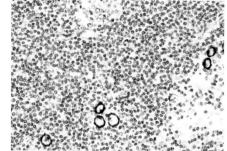

Fig. 15.37 Lymphocyte-rich classic Hodgkin lymphoma. HRS cells in perifollicular region are highlighted by CD30 immunostain.

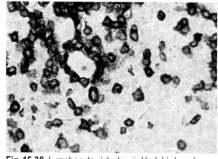

Fig. 15.38 Lymphocyte-rich classic Hodgkin lymphoma. CD3–positive T cells form a rosette around an HRS cell.

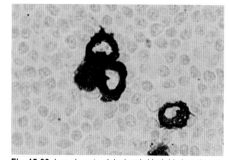

Fig. 15.39 Lymphocyte-rich classic Hodgkin lymphoma. CD15 immunostain of HRS cells.

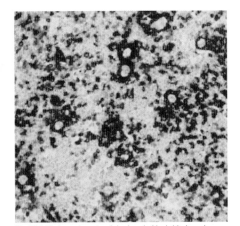

Fig. 15.40 Lymphocyte-rich classic Hodgkin lymphoma. Immunostaining for PD1 shows PD1+ T cells forming rosettes around HRS cells

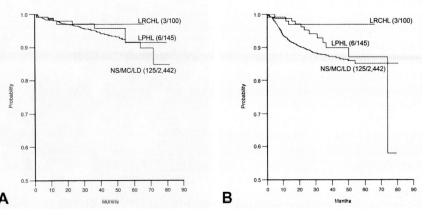

Fig. 15.41 Hodgkin lymphoma (HL). Overall survival (**A**) and overall event-free survival (**B**) by histological subtype {3654}. LD, lymphocyte-depleted classic HL; LPHL, lymphocyte predominant HL; LRCHL, lymphocyte-rich classic HL; MC, mixed cellularity classic HL; NS, nodular sclerosis classic HL. From: Shimabukuro-Vornhagen A, Haverkamp H, Engert A, et al. {3654}. Reprinted with permission. ©2005 American Society of Clinical Oncology. All rights reserved.

lymphocytes and may harbour germinal centres, which are usually eccentrically located and relatively small or regressed. The HRS cells are predominantly found within the nodules, but consistently outside of the germinal centres. A proportion of the HRS cells may resemble lymphocyte predominant (LP) cells or mononuclear lacunar cells. This subtype can easily be confused with NLPHL. In the past, approximately 30% of cases initially diagnosed as NLPHL were later found to be LRCHL {91}. The demonstration of an immunophenotype typical of classic HRS cells is essential in making this distinction. Eosinophils and/or neutrophils are absent from the nodules, or if present, are located in the interfollicular zones and are few in number. In rare instances, the LRCHL-typical nodules may be surrounded by fibrous bands associated with randomly distributed HRS cells in T-cell–rich zones. Typing of these cases as nodular

sclerosis CHL might be more appropriate. In some cases, sequential biopsies have shown nodular sclerosis CHL, implying a possible relationship between the two subtypes of CHL; this is further inferred by the finding of HRS cells within expanded follicular mantle zones in some cases of nodular sclerosis CHL {1780}. Coexistence of LRCHL and mixed cellularity CHL occurs but is rare.

In diffuse LRCHL cases, the small lymphocytes of the cellular background may be admixed with histiocytes with or without epithelioid features.

Immunophenotype

The immunophenotype of the neoplastic cells and their microenvironment display a mixture of features of NLPHL and CHL. The atypical cells in LRCHL show the same immunophenotype (CD30+, CD15+/−, IRF4/MUM1+, PAX5+/−, CD20−/+, J chain−, CD75−, PU1−, EBV/LMP1+ for EBV-har-

bouring cases) as the HRS cells in the other subtypes of CHL. Thus, the distinction of LRCHL from NLPHL is possible by immunophenotyping in nearly all instances {91}. The expression of B-cell transcription factors such as OCT2, BOB1, and BCL6 has been found to be more frequent in LRCHL than in the other CHL subtypes {2821}. Rosettes with a T follicular helper (TFH) cell immunophenotype (PD1/CD279+, CD57−/+) surrounding the neoplastic cells are present in as many as 50% of cases {2821}. The small lymphocytes in the nodules have the features of mantle cells (i.e. positivity for IgM and IgD). Thus, the nodules predominantly constitute expanded mantle zones. At least some of them contain eccentrically located, usually small, germinal centres, which are highlighted by a dense meshwork of CD21+ follicular dendritic cells. Because intact germinal centres are infrequent in NLPHL, this feature is helpful in differential diagnosis.

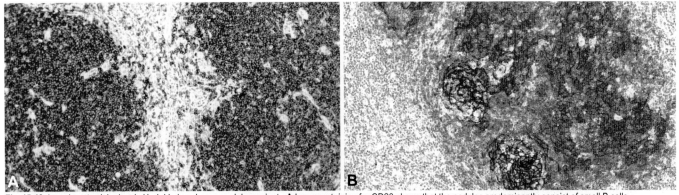

Fig. 15.42 Lymphocyte-rich classic Hodgkin lymphoma, nodular variant. **A** Immunostaining for CD20 shows that the nodules predominantly consist of small B cells. HRS cells, evident as holes in the B-cell rich background are negative. **B** Immunostaining for CD21 reveals that the nodules contain a meshwork of follicular dendritic cells, and demonstrates that they predominantly constitute follicular mantles, with occasional (usually regressed) germinal centres. The follicular dendritic cell meshwork is denser and more sharply defined in the germinal centres.

CD15+ granulocytes are absent from the expanded mantle zones but may be present in low numbers within the interfollicular zones. In the rare diffuse subtype, the lymphocytes are nearly all of T-cell type, with CD15+ granulocytes and eosinophils being absent. These features facilitate the differentiation of LRCHL from mixed cellularity CHL. EBV LMP1 expression is seen more frequently than in nodular sclerosis CHL but less frequently than in mixed cellularity CHL {91}.

Prognosis and predictive factors

With modern risk-adjusted treatment, overall and progression-free survival rates are slightly better than those of the other subtypes of CHL and similar to those of NLPHL, except that relapses are more common in NLPHL than in LRCHL {91,980,3654}.

Mixed cellularity classic Hodgkin lymphoma

Weiss L.M.
Poppema S.
Jaffe E.S.
Stein H.

Definition

Mixed cellularity Hodgkin lymphoma (MCCHL) is a subtype of classic Hodgkin lymphoma (CHL) characterized by classic Hodgkin/Reed–Sternberg (HRS) cells in a diffuse mixed inflammatory background. Fine interstitial fibrosis may be present, but fibrous bands are absent and capsular fibrosis is usually absent. This subtype of CHL is frequently (i.e. in ~75% of cases) associated with EBV.

ICD-O code   9652/3

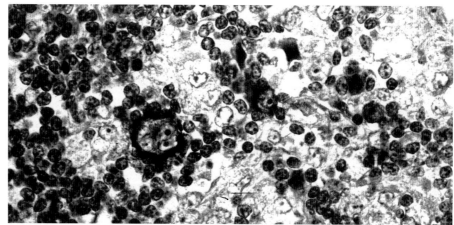

Fig. 15.44 Mixed cellularity classic Hodgkin lymphoma. CD30–negative histiocytes, with a pronounced epithelioid differentiation, forming clusters, predominate. CD30 immunostaining highlights the presence of a large Reed–Sternberg cell and a small mononuclear variant.

Synonym

Classic Hodgkin disease, mixed cellularity, NOS

Epidemiology

The mixed cellularity subtype accounts for approximately 20–25% of CHLs. MCCHL is more frequent in patients with HIV infection and in developing countries {374}. In the developing world, this form of CHL may be seen in the paediatric age group, and is frequently EBV-positive {3671,4489}. There is a second peak among elderly individuals, without special geographical distribution {1109}. The median patient age is 38 years, and approximately 70% of patients are male.

Localization

Peripheral lymph nodes are frequently involved, and mediastinal involvement is uncommon. The spleen is involved in 30% of cases, bone marrow in 10%, liver in 3%, and other organs in 1–3% {782}.

Clinical features

B symptoms are frequent.

Microscopy

The lymph node architecture is usually obliterated, although an interfollicular growth pattern may be seen. Interstitial fibrosis may be present, but the lymph node capsule is usually not thickened, and there are no broad bands of fibrosis as seen in nodular sclerosis CHL. The HRS cells are typical in appearance. The background cells consist of a mixture of cell types, the composition of which varies greatly. Eosinophils, neutrophils, histiocytes, and plasma cells are usually present. One of these cell types may predominate. The histiocytes may show pronounced epithelioid features, particularly in EBV-associated cases {950}, and may form granuloma-like clusters or granulomas.

Immunophenotype

The malignant cells exhibit the CHL immunophenotype; however, EBV-encoded LMP1 and EBV-encoded small RNA (EBER) are expressed much more frequently (i.e. in ~75% of cases) than in nodular sclerosis CHL or lymphocyte-rich CHL {91}.

Prognosis and predictive factors

Before the introduction of modern therapy, the prognosis of MCCHL was worse than that of NSCHL and better than that of lymphocyte-depleted CHL. With current regimens, these differences have largely vanished, although not entirely {70}.

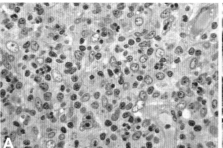
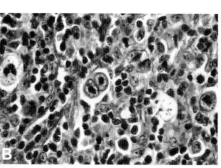

Fig. 15.43 Mixed cellularity classic Hodgkin lymphoma. A The mixed cellular infiltrate does not contain fibrotic bands. B A typical binucleated Reed–Sternberg cell in a mixed cellular infiltrate with lymphocytes, macrophages, and eosinophils is visible.

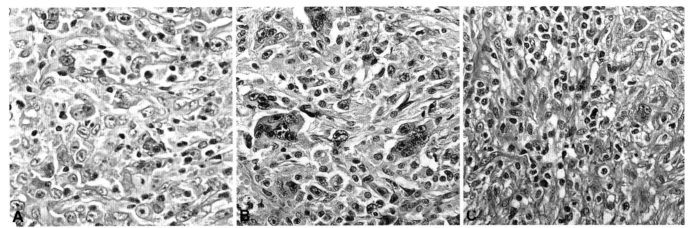

Fig. 15.45 Lymphocyte-depleted classic Hodgkin lymphoma. **A** Many Hodgkin cells with relatively few admixed lymphocytes are visible. **B** Many bizarre large and small Hodgkin/Reed–Sternberg cells are present in a cellular background rich in fibrillary matrix. **C** Scattered Hodgkin/Reed–Sternberg cells in a predominant fibrillary matrix with fibroblastic proliferation.

Lymphocyte-depleted classic Hodgkin lymphoma

Benharroch D.
Jaffe E.S.
Stein H.

Definition

Lymphocyte-depleted classic Hodgkin lymphoma (LDCHL) is a diffuse form of classic Hodgkin lymphoma (CHL) rich in Hodgkin/Reed–Sternberg (HRS) cells and/or depleted of non-neoplastic lymphocytes. Histiocytes are usually abundant. Prior to the introduction of modern immunohistochemical studies, LDCHL was often mistaken for other entities, mainly for aggressive forms of other B-cell or T-cell lymphomas {1930}. When stringent diagnostic criteria are applied, LDCHL accounts for < 2% of all Hodgkin lymphomas. It is more common in developing countries and is also seen with HIV infection. Like mixed cellularity CHL, it is frequently positive for EBV (i.e. in ~75% of cases). Most patients present with advanced-stage disease and B symptoms {2042}.

ICD-O code   9653/3

Synonyms

Hodgkin lymphoma disease, lymphocyte depletion, NOS; classic Hodgkin lymphoma, lymphocyte depletion, NOS; Hodgkin lymphoma, lymphocyte depletion, diffuse fibrosis (9654/3); Hodgkin lymphoma, lymphocyte depletion, reticular (9655/3)

Epidemiology

This is the rarest CHL subtype; it accounts for < 1% of cases in western countries {2042}, but may be more common in the developing world {334}. About 60–75% of patients are male and the age ranges from 30 to 71 years. Others have described LDCHL to an equal extent in women {3695}. This subtype is often associated with HIV infection. HIV prevalence was found in 3.8% of Hodgkin lymphoma patients, including 15.1% of LDCHL patients {3649}.

Localization

LDCHL has a predilection for the retroperitoneal lymph nodes, abdominal organs, and bone marrow. Peripheral lymphadenopathy may also be seen {2042}.

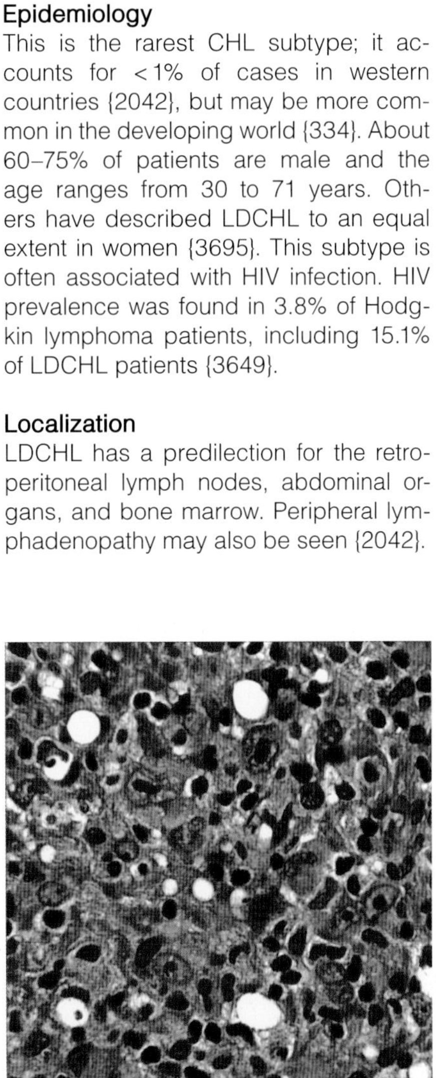

Clinical features

Widespread involvement (including of the subdiaphragmatic region and bone marrow at diagnosis), with B symptoms, supports an aggressive behaviour. However, peripheral lymph nodes are also affected {334,3695}.

Microscopy

Although the appearance of LDCHL is highly variable, a unifying feature is the relative predominance of HRS cells and the scarcity of background lymphocytes in relation to the neoplastic cells {2484}. Two patterns are seen. In one, there is diffuse fibrosis, in which prominent fibroblastic proliferation is seen. However, well-formed fibrous bands are absent. In this variant, the tumour microenvironment contains numerous histiocytes and some small lymphocytes, but usually

Fig. 15.46 Lymphocyte-depleted classic Hodgkin lymphoma. Hodgkin/Reed–Sternberg cells are readily seen in a background rich in histiocytes and some small lymphocytes.

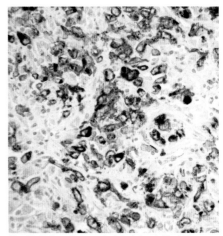

Fig. 15.47 Lymphocyte-depleted classic Hodgkin lymphoma. CD30 immunostaining.

lacks significant numbers of plasma cells or eosinophils. The second pattern is rich in neoplastic cells, often with anaplastic and pleomorphic features {3695}. These two variants correspond to the two subtypes initially described in the Lukes–Butler classification, diffuse fibrosis and reticular {2412}.

Immunophenotype
The immunophenotype is similar to that of other forms of CHL. EBV/LMP1 is frequently positive. Coexpression of CD30 and PAX5 helps to differentiate LDCHL from ALK-negative anaplastic large cell lymphoma. Either OCT2 or BOB1 may be expressed in HRS cells, but usually not both. CD79a is typically negative {3695}. Strong expression of B-cell markers such as CD20 and CD79a should prompt consideration for a diagnosis of EBV-positive diffuse large B-cell lymphoma, in which HRS–like cells may be seen.

Genetic profile
IGH gene rearrangement shows B-cell clonality, which can be more readily detected due to the paucity of normal B cells and relative abundance of tumour cells {3695}.

Prognosis and predictive factors
Patients with LDCHL have more adverse risk factors than do patients with other forms of CHL {1947,2042}. SEER data indicate a 5-year survival rate of 48.8% {65}. However, outcome has been less adverse in prospective clinical trials. Patients with LDCHL are more likely to have advanced-stage disease and B symptoms. However, with effective therapy, complete remission was achieved in 82% of patients with LDCHL, versus in 93% of patients with other Hodgkin subtypes {2042}. At 5 years, survival was significantly worse, with progression-free survival rates of 71% versus 85% ($P < 0.001$) and overall survival rates of 83% versus 92% respectively ($P = 0.0018$). Patients who underwent more-intensive therapy regimens appeared to fare better {2042}, suggesting that patients with LDCHL benefit from treatment with dose-intensive treatment strategies.

CHAPTER 16

Immunodeficiency-associated lymphoproliferative disorders

Lymphoproliferative diseases associated with primary immune disorders

van Krieken J.H.
Onciu M.
Elenitoba-Johnson K.S.J.
Jaffe E.S.

Definition

Lymphoproliferative diseases associated with primary immune disorders (PIDs) are lymphoid proliferations that arise in the setting of immune deficiency due to a primary immunodeficiency or immunoregulatory disorder. Because the pathology and pathogenesis of the >60 PIDs are heterogeneous, the manifestations of these lymphoproliferative diseases are highly variable. The PIDs most frequently associated with lymphoproliferative disorder are ataxia-telangiectasia (AT), Wiskott–Aldrich syndrome (WAS), common variable immunodeficiency (CVID), severe combined immunodeficiency (SCID), X-linked lymphoproliferative disease (XLP), Nijmegen breakage syndrome (NBS), hyper-IgM syndrome (HIgM), and autoimmune lymphoproliferative syndrome (ALPS).

Epidemiology

Patients with PIDs have an increased incidence of lymphomas {1878,3635}. Age-specific mortality rates for all neoplasms in patients with PIDs are 10–200 times the expected rates for the general population. However, given that PIDs are rare, the overall occurrence of PID-associated lymphoproliferative disorder is low, accounting for 2.4% of all paediatric lymphoma cases {144}. With the exception of CVID, these diseases present primarily in the paediatric age group. They are more common in males than in females, primarily because several of the primary genetic abnormalities are X-linked, for example, XLP, SCID, and HIgM {1871}. It should be kept in mind that children can present with a lymphoproliferation without the underlying immunodeficiency being known. Especially in polymorphous lesions, detection of EBV may indicate an underlying immune deficiency.

Etiology

The cause of the lymphoproliferative disorder is related to the underlying primary immune defect {2897}. EBV is involved in most PID-associated lymphoid proliferations {4136}. In these cases, defective

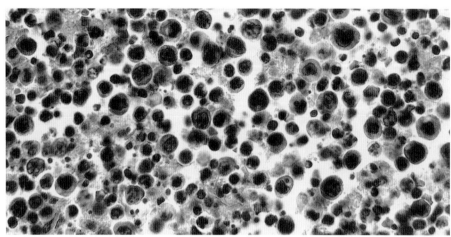

Fig. 16.01 Lymphoproliferative disease occurring in X-linked lymphoproliferative disease with features of fatal infectious mononucleosis. There is a proliferation of B cells with plasmacytoid and immunoblastic features. Note the prominent apoptosis.

T-cell immune surveillance to EBV is believed to be the primary mechanism {1628,3073,3251}. The absence of T-cell control may be complete (resulting in fatal infectious mononucleosis) or partial (resulting in other lymphoproliferative disorders) {1823}.

WAS is a complex immune disorder, with defects in function of T cells, B cells, neutrophils, and macrophages. T-cell dysfunction is significant, and tends to increase in severity during the course of the disease.

HIgM results from mutations in the gene for CD40 or CD40 ligand, which affect interactions between T cells and B cells and impair effective differentiation of B cells into class-switched plasma cells {1767}.

In ALPS, mutations in *FAS* or *FASLG* (and rarely other abnormalities) may contribute directly to lymphoid proliferations, through the accumulation of lymphoid cells that fail to undergo apoptosis, resulting in the accumulation of CD4– and CD8– cells in the peripheral blood and lymphoid tissues {2331,3711}. In ALPS, the severity of the apoptotic defect correlates directly with the risk of development of lymphoproliferative disorder {1822}. The importance of *FAS* mutations in causing lymphoproliferative disorder is supported by the fact that sporadic *FAS*

mutations are associated with lymphomas in the absence of immune abnormalities {1483}.

In AT, an abnormal DNA repair mechanism due to mutations of *ATM* can contribute to the development of lymphoma, leukaemia, and other neoplasms {1090}. In these cases, non-leukaemic T-cell clones that have translocations involving the TR genes similar to those seen in overt leukaemias can be detected in the peripheral blood. B-cell non-Hodgkin lymphoma, Hodgkin lymphoma, and lymphoblastic leukaemia occur at a high rate and earlier age than do carcinomas in AT. T-cell prolymphocytic leukaemias are rarer than initially reported. Prognosis is poor, but patients may benefit from treatment, with an improved survival {3823}.

NBS also results from defects in DNA repair due to mutations in the *NBN* gene (also called *NBS1*), resulting in many chromosomal breaks and translocations, including in antigen receptor genes. In patients with NBS, lymphoproliferative disorder is the most common neoplasm {565,2880,4158}. In patients with CVID, marked lymphoid hyperplasia may occur in the lungs and gastrointestinal tract {3507}, a setting in which more aggressive-lymphoproliferative disorder or overt lymphoma may develop {959}.

Table 16.01 Clinical features of the primary immune disorders (PIDs)

Type of PID	Frequency (among all PIDs)[a]	Genes or proteins implicated	Most common abnormalities	Most common associated lymphoproliferative disorders (percentage)[b]
Combined T-cell and B-cell immunodeficiencies	9–18%			
Severe combined immunodeficiency	1–5%	Gamma chain of IL2R, IL4R, IL7R, IL9R, IL15R, IL21R; JAK3 kinase; IL7R, CD45, CD3-delta or CD3-epsilon; RAG1/2, Artemis, ADA	Recurrent severe bacterial, fungal, and viral infections, including opportunistic infections; skin rash	EBV-associated lesions, fatal IM (nearly 100%)
CD40 ligand and CD40 deficiencies (hyper-IgM syndrome)	1–2%	CD40 ligand (CD40L, CD154) or CD40	Neutropenia, thrombocytopenia, haemolytic anaemia, biliary tract and liver disease, opportunistic infections	EBV-associated lesions (DLBCL, Hodgkin lymphoma), large granular lymphocytic leukaemia
Predominantly antibody PIDs	53–72%			
Common variable immunodeficiency	21–31%	Unknown	Bacterial infections (lung, gastrointestinal tract), autoimmune cytopenias, granulomatous disease (lung, liver)	EBV-associated lesions (DLBCL, Hodgkin lymphoma), extranodal marginal zone lymphoma, small lymphocytic lymphoma, lymphoplasmacytic lymphoma, PTCL (rare) (2–7%)
Other well-defined immunodeficiency syndromes	5–22%			
Wiskott–Aldrich syndrome	1–3%	WAS (also called WASP)	Thrombocytopenia, small platelets, eczema, autoimmune disease, bacterial infections	EBV-associated lesions (DLBCL, Hodgkin lymphoma, lymphomatoid granulomatosis) (3–9%)
Ataxia-telangiectasia	2–8%	ATM	Ataxia, telangiectasias, increased AFP, increased sensitivity to ionizing radiation	Non-leukaemic clonal T-cell proliferations, DLBCL, BL, T-PLL, T-ALL, Hodgkin lymphoma (10–30%)
Nijmegen breakage syndrome	1–2%	NBN (nibrin, also called NBS1)	Microcephaly, progressive mental retardation, sensitivity to ionizing radiation, predisposition to cancer	DLBCL, PTCL, T-ALL/LBL, Hodgkin lymphoma (28–36%)
Diseases of immune dysregulation	1–3%			
X-linked lymphoproliferative disease	<1%	SH2D1A	EBV-triggered abnormalities (fatal IM, hepatitis, aplastic anaemia), lymphoma	EBV-associated lesions (BL, DLBCL) (nearly 100%)
Autoimmune lymphoproliferative syndrome (Canale–Smith syndrome)	<1%	FAS (type 1a), FASLG (type 1b), CASP10 (caspase 10; type 2a), or CASP8 (caspase 8; type 2b)	Defective lymphocyte apoptosis, splenomegaly, adenopathy, autoimmune cytopenias, recurrent infections	NLPHL, CHL, DLBCL, BL, PTCL (rare) (CHL, DLBCL, and BL may be EBV+ or EBV−) (3–10%)

ADA, adenosine deaminase; AFP, alpha-fetoprotein; BL, Burkitt lymphoma; CHL, classic Hodgkin lymphoma; DLBCL, diffuse large B-cell lymphoma; IM, infectious mononucleosis; NLPHL, nodular lymphocyte predominant Hodgkin lymphoma; PTCL, peripheral T-cell lymphoma; T-ALL, T-lymphoblastic leukaemia; T-ALL/LBL, T-lymphoblastic leukaemia/lymphoma; T-PLL, T-cell prolymphocytic leukaemia.

[a] Data compiled from reports of several national and international registries.
[b] Percentages, where provided, indicate the approximate proportion of patients in whom lymphoproliferative disorder develops.

Localization

The presentation depends on the underlying disease. More often, lymphoproliferative disorders present in extranodal sites, most commonly the gastrointestinal tract, lungs, and CNS.

Clinical features

Patients often present with symptoms resembling those of infection or neoplasia (i.e. fever, fatigue, and infectious mononucleosis–like syndromes). In some diseases, such as ALPS and XLP, the lymphoid proliferation is the first sign of the underlying immune defect, but in most patients, the diagnosis of PID has already been established because of other manifestations (Table 16.01).

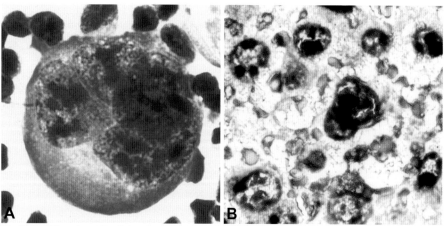

Fig. 16.02 Diffuse large B-cell lymphoma in a patient with longstanding common variable immunodeficiency syndrome. **A** Lymphoma cells are seen in ascites fluid and show marked pleomorphism. **B** Lymphoma cells are EBV-positive by in situ hybridization for EBV-encoded small RNA (EBER).

Microscopy

As in other immune deficiency states, lymphoid proliferations in patients with primary immunodeficiency include reactive hyperplasias, polymorphous lymphoid infiltrates similar to those seen in the post-transplant setting, and frank lymphomas that do not differ from those in immunocompetent hosts. The type and frequency of each lesion differ among the PIDs {4099} (see Table 16.01, p. 445).

Non-neoplastic lesions

Primary EBV infection in PID may result in fatal infectious mononucleosis, characterized by a highly polymorphous proliferation of lymphoid cells showing evidence of plasmacytoid and immunoblastic differentiation. Reed–Sternberg–like cells may be seen. This condition is primarily seen in patients with XLP (Duncan disease) {1372} and SCID {3251}. The abnormal B-cell proliferation is systemic,

involving both lymphoid and non-lymphoid organs, most commonly the terminal ileum. Haemophagocytic syndrome is frequent, and is most readily identified in bone marrow aspirates. In CVID, waxing and waning lymphoproliferations may occur in lymph nodes and extranodal sites, with variable morphology (including follicular hyperplasia) and paracortical expansion with many EBV-positive cells, often including large atypical cells that may resemble Reed–Sternberg cells. CVID is characterized by nodular lymphoid hyperplasia in the gastrointestinal tract; clonality testing may detect clonal B-cell populations that are a sign of more aggressive disease but may also be self-limited {2227,3507,4128}.

In ALPS, expansions of double-negative (CD4–/CD8–), alpha beta CD45RA+, CD45RO– T cells in peripheral blood, lymph nodes, spleen, and other tissues are the hallmark of the disease. T-cell

expansion can be very marked, and the T cells may have slightly immature chromatin, which can lead to a mistaken diagnosis of T-cell lymphoma, especially when (as is usual) the patient does not carry a pre-existing diagnosis of ALPS {2331}. Follicular hyperplasia is often prominent, and progressively transformed germinal centres may be seen {2331}.

HIgM is characterized by circulating peripheral blood B cells that bear only IgM and IgD. Germinal centres are absent in lymph nodes. IgM-producing plasma cells often accumulate, most commonly in extranodal sites, such as the gastrointestinal tract, liver, and gallbladder. These lesions may be so extensive as to be fatal, without progression to clonal lymphoproliferative disorder.

Lymphomas

Lymphomas occurring in patients with PIDs do not generally differ in their morphology from those occurring in immunocompetent hosts.

Lymphomatoid granulomatosis, an EBV-driven proliferation of B cells associated with a marked T-cell infiltration, is increased in frequency in patients with WAS {1754}. The most common sites of involvement are the lungs, skin, brain, and kidneys.

Diffuse large B-cell lymphoma is the most common type of lymphoma seen in PIDs in general; classic Hodgkin lymphoma and Burkitt lymphoma {4007}, as well as peripheral T-cell lymphoma {3146}, also occur. In AT, and to a lesser extent in NBS, T-cell lymphomas and leukaemias are more common than B-cell neoplasms {3910}. Rare cases of true peripheral T-cell lymphoma have been

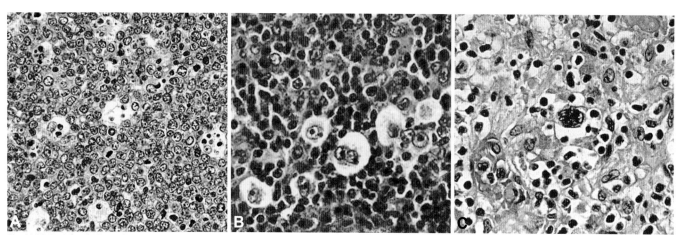

Fig. 16.03 Lymphomas in autoimmune lymphoproliferative syndrome. **A** Burkitt lymphoma. **B** Classic Hodgkin lymphoma, mixed-cellularity subtype. **C** T-cell/histiocyte-rich large B-cell lymphoma. Histologically, these lymphoma subtypes resemble those occurring sporadically, without predisposing immune abnormalities.

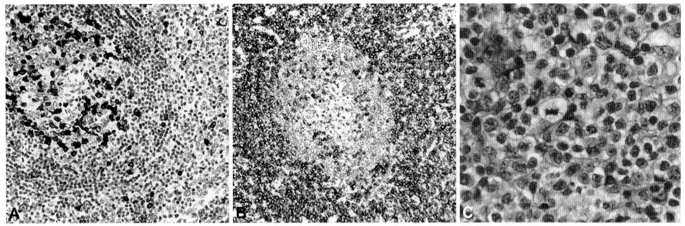

Fig. 16.04 Autoimmune lymphoproliferative syndrome, lymph node. Paracortical T cells are (**A**) CD45RO-negative and (**B**) CD3-positive. This phenotype is characteristic of naïve T cells. **C** Paracortical T cells show varying degrees of atypia, and mitotic figures may be frequent.

seen in patients with ALPS {3146,3810}. Both T-lymphoblastic leukaemia/lymphoma and T-cell prolymphocytic leukaemia have been reported in PIDs.

Hodgkin lymphoma

Hodgkin lymphoma–like lymphoproliferations resembling those seen in the setting of methotrexate therapy, as well as lymphoproliferative disorder with all morphological and phenotypic features of classic Hodgkin lymphoma, has been reported in patients with WAS or AT {1090,3476}. In ALPS, nodular lymphocyte predominant Hodgkin lymphoma, classic Hodgkin lymphoma, and T-cell/histiocyte-rich large B-cell lymphoma have been described {2331}.

Precursor lesions

The underlying PID is the principal precursor lesion leading to the development of lymphoproliferative disorder. This morphological spectrum is accompanied by an increasing dominant clonal population: from clearly polyclonal, to oligoclonal, to monoclonal. However, monoclonal expansions, particularly if they are minor clones, do not necessarily progress to major persistent clonal lesions {2227}. Nevertheless, the detection of a dominant clone indicates a more aggressive disease {4128}.

Immunophenotype

Non-neoplastic proliferations

In ALPS, there is expansion of a distinctive CD3+, CD4–, CD8–, CD45RA+, CD45RO– naïve T-cell population in the peripheral blood and bone marrow. The T cells may express CD57 but not CD25. Increased numbers of CD5+ polyclonal B cells may also be seen {2331}. HIgM is characterized by peripheral blood B cells that bear only IgM and IgD.

Neoplasms

Most of the lymphomas in patients with PID are of B-cell lineage, and thus express B-cell antigens corresponding to their differentiation stage. EBV infection of B cells often leads to downregulation of B-cell antigens. Thus, CD20, CD19, and CD79a may be negative or expressed on only some of the neoplastic cells in EBV-positive lymphoproliferative disorder. Similarly, EBV leads to the expression of CD30 in most cases. In patients with EBV-positive lymphoproliferative disorder resulting from defective immune surveillance, the latency genes including *LMP1* may be expressed. In cases showing evidence of plasmacytoid differentiation, monotypic cytoplasmic immunoglobulin may be identified. The immunophenotypes of the specific B-cell and T-cell lymphomas in PIDs do not differ from those of the same lymphomas in immunocompetent patients.

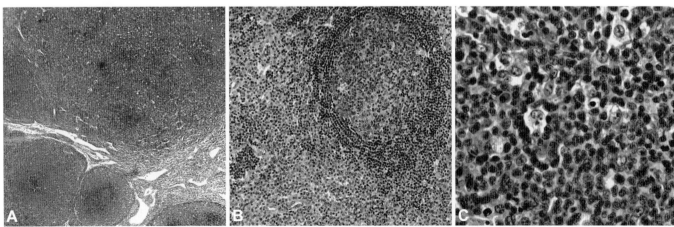

Fig. 16.05 Reactive lymph node from a patient with autoimmune lymphoproliferative syndrome. **A** There is prominent paracortical expansion. **B** Reactive germinal centres are present and the paracortex is expanded. **C** The cells are slightly larger than normal small lymphocytes, with dispersed chromatin.

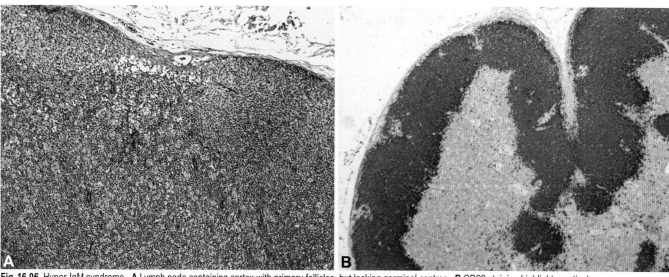

Fig. 16.06 Hyper-IgM syndrome. **A** Lymph node containing cortex with primary follicles, but lacking germinal centres. **B** CD20 staining highlights cortical areas.

Genetic profile

Antigen receptor genes

Because lymphoproliferative disorder in PID is a spectrum from reactive to aggressive lymphoproliferations, the proliferations can be polyclonal, oligoclonal, or monoclonal. Fatal infectious mononucleosis is generally polyclonal; overt lymphomas such as diffuse large B-cell lymphoma and Burkitt lymphoma have clonal IG heavy and light chain gene rearrangement {1090,2227,3507}. There is only limited experience with T-cell clonality tests in the setting of PIDs.

Cytogenetic abnormalities and oncogenes

Genetic alterations may be directly related to the primary immune defect, such as *FAS* mutation in patients with ALPS, mutations of the *SH2D1A* gene encoding for SAP/SLAM in XLP, and many chromosomal breaks in NBS {1371,3898}. Other abnormalities may occur in the course of lymphoproliferative disorder. In AT, in addition to mutations of *ATM*, inversions and translocations of the TR genes on chromosomes 7 and 14 are common. Consequently, these often show breakpoints at 14q11, 7q34 and 7p14.1 and chromosomal rearrangements/translocations including inv(7)(p13q35), t(7;7)(p13;q35), and t(7;14)(p13;q11), as well as t(14;14)(q11.2;q32.13), which can involve the IGH gene locus {3910}. Such translocations may also involve the *TCL1A* gene in 14q32.1 and other oncogenes leading to T-cell lymphoproliferative diseases, including T-cell prolymphocytic leukaemia and pre-T lymphoblastic leukaemia/lymphoma.

Prognosis and predictive factors

The prognosis is related to both the underlying PID and the type of lymphoproliferative disorder. The immunological status of the host is an important risk factor {547}. The lymphoid proliferations in ALPS are often self-limiting. Lymphoid hyperplasias in CVID may be indolent. Most of the other lymphoproliferative disorders in patients with PID are aggressive. However, given the wide variety of underlying conditions and ensuing lymphoproliferative disorders, the prognosis must be evaluated in each case individually, although clonality testing may be of additional value {4128}. In patients with EBV-driven infectious mononucleosis, a haemophagocytic syndrome may be the primary cause of death, usually associated with marked pancytopenia, liver dysfunction, coagulopathy, and further infectious complications.

Treatment is determined on the basis of both the nature of the neoplastic process and the underlying genetic defect. In general, less-aggressive therapy is needed than in patients without PID. Allogeneic bone marrow transplantation has been used in patients with WAS, SCID, and HIgM {1066,1508}. Because the EBV-driven B-cell expansion in lymphomatoid granulomatosis is often not autonomous, it may respond to immunoregulatory therapy using interferon alfa 2b {4332}; however, like in post-transplant lymphoproliferative disorder, anti-CD20 directed therapy is more important.

Lymphomas associated with HIV infection

Said J.
Cesarman E.
Rosenwald A.
Harris N.L.

Definition

Lymphomas that develop in HIV-positive patients are predominantly aggressive B-cell lymphomas. In a proportion of cases, they are considered AIDS-defining conditions and are the initial manifestation of AIDS. These disorders are heterogeneous and include lymphomas usually diagnosed in immunocompetent patients, as well as lymphomas seen much more often in the setting of HIV infection. The most common HIV-associated lymphomas include Burkitt lymphoma, diffuse large B-cell lymphoma (DLBCL; often involving the CNS), primary effusion lymphoma (PEL), and plasmablastic lymphoma. Classic Hodgkin lymphoma (CHL) is also increased in the setting of HIV infection.

Epidemiology

The incidence of all subtypes of non-Hodgkin lymphoma is increased 60–200 times in HIV-positive patients. Before HAART was available, primary CNS lymphoma and Burkitt lymphoma were increased approximately 1000 times in comparison with the general population {345,2285}. Since the introduction of HAART, the incidence of non-Hodgkin lymphoma has decreased by 50%, mainly due to decreased CNS lymphoma and the immunoblastic histological subtype {1107}. Moreover, the decreased incidence of most AIDS-associated non-Hodgkin lymphomas after HAART introduction is consistent with improved CD4 counts {363,373}. HAART is also associated with increased survival (with a 75% decrease in mortality), although lymphomas now account for a higher proportion of first AIDS-defining illnesses {974,1107}. In contrast, the risk of HIV-associated CHL has remained stable, and burden of disease has increased. The incidence of CHL is about 50 cases per 100 000 person-years among HIV-infected individuals, 5–20 times the incidence in the general population {3649}. Because CHL incidence is lower among patients with severe immunosuppression than among those with moderate immune defect,

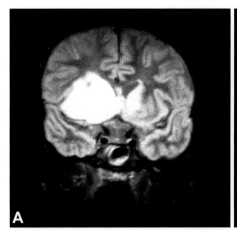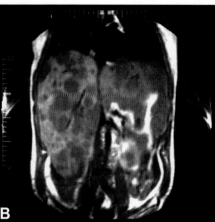

Fig. 16.07 Radiological findings in HIV-associated lymphoma. **A** Nuclear MRI of the brain showing a large tumour mass in the basal ganglia. **B** Multiple filling defects are seen in liver.

the relatively increased CHL incidence could be related to improvements in CD4 counts {374,770}. Lymphocyte predominant Hodgkin lymphoma can occur in HIV-infected individuals, but there is no known association.

Etiology

Lymphomas in HIV-infected patients are heterogeneous, reflecting several pathogenetic mechanisms: chronic antigen stimulation, genetic abnormalities, cytokine deregulation, and the role of EBV and HHV8 {555,557}. HIV-related lymphomas are consistently monoclonal and are characterized by a number of common genetic abnormalities of *MYC* and *BCL6*, as well as tumour suppressor genes {1272,4096}. The polyclonal or oligoclonal nature of some HIV-related lymphoid proliferations suggests a multistep

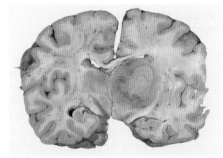

Fig. 16.08 HIV-associated diffuse large B-cell lymphoma involving the basal ganglia.

lymphomagenesis. B-cell stimulation, hypergammaglobulinaemia, and persistent generalized lymphadenopathy preceding the development of these lymphomas probably reflect the role of chronic antigenic stimulation and impaired immune response. Disruption of the cytokine network, leading to high serum levels of IL6 and IL10, is a feature of HIV-related lymphomas associated with EBV or HHV8. EBV is identified in the neoplastic cells of approximately 40% of HIV-related lymphomas, but the detection of EBV varies considerably with the site of presentation and the histological subtype. EBV infection is found in 80–100% of primary CNS lymphomas {536} and PELs, in 80% of DLBCLs with immunoblastic features, and in 30–50% of Burkitt lymphomas {1531}. Nearly all CHL cases in the setting of HIV infection are associated with EBV {191,3754}. HHV8 is specifically associated with PEL, which usually occurs in the late stages of the disease, in the setting of profound immunosuppression {623}.

Prevention

Despite the therapeutic advances with HAART, there is still no effective immunization or cure for HIV infection. Diversity caused by circulating recombinant viral forms is a major challenge, which has

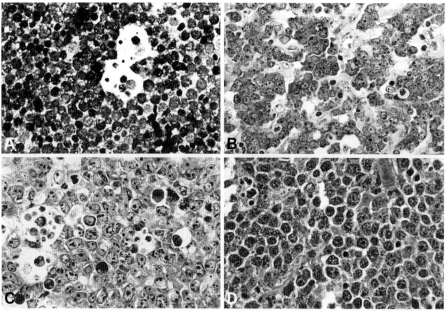

Fig. 16.09 Burkitt lymphoma associated with HIV infection. **A** Touch imprint reveals intermediate-sized cells with rim of blue cytoplasm and cytoplasmic vacuoles. There is a large tingible body phagocytic macrophage in the centre of the field. **B** The cell population is uniform. **C** In another case, the cells show much greater variation in the size and shape of the lymphoma cells. **D** Burkitt lymphoma with plasmacytoid differentiation. The cells have an eccentric rim of deeply stained cytoplasm.

been increased by the increasing ease of world travel {3912}.

Localization

HIV-related lymphomas display a marked propensity to involve extranodal sites, in particular the gastrointestinal tract, CNS (less frequently since HAART), liver, and bone marrow. The peripheral blood is rarely involved except in cases of Burkitt lymphoma, which may even present as acute leukaemia. Unusual sites such as the oral cavity, jaw, and body cavities are often involved. Other extranodal sites include lung, skin, testis, heart, and breast. Lymph nodes are involved in about one third of reported cases at presentation {365}, but since the HAART era, nodal involvement accounts for half of all cases {1643}.

Clinical features

Most patients present with advanced clinical stage; bulky disease with a high tumour burden is frequent. Lactate dehydrogenase is usually markedly elevated. There is a significant relationship between the subtype of lymphoma and the HIV disease status. DLBCL more often occurs in the setting of longstanding AIDS and is associated with a trend towards a higher rate of opportunistic infections and lower CD4+ T-cell counts

(mean: $< 100 \times 10^6$/L). In contrast, Burkitt lymphoma and Hodgkin lymphoma occur in less immunodeficient patients, with a shorter mean interval between the diagnosis of HIV seropositivity and lymphoma and significantly higher CD4+ T-cell counts ($> 200 \times 10^6$/L) {363,553}.

Microscopy

In HIV-positive patients, there is a spectrum of lymphoid proliferations, some of which resemble aggressive B-cell lymphomas that develop sporadically in the absence of HIV infection. Others, like the polymorphic lymphoid proliferations, may resemble those seen in other immunodeficiency states, including after transplantation. In addition, there are unusual lymphomas that occur more specifically (although not exclusively) in patients with AIDS.

Lymphomas also occurring in immunocompetent patients

Burkitt lymphoma

Burkitt lymphoma accounts for 20–30% of all HIV-associated lymphomas, and is more common in the setting of HIV infection than in other immunodeficiency states. The gastrointestinal tract is the most common site of presentation, but in patients with AIDS, Burkitt lymphoma can present in unusual sites including the

bone marrow. Burkitt lymphoma occurs in patients with CD4+ cell cut-offs above the threshold for AIDS, suggesting that onset may require functional CD4+ cells. There is a diffuse, monotonous, and cohesive proliferation of intermediate-sized cells with round nucleoli and basophilic cytoplasm, which appears vacuolated on imprints. Mitoses are frequent, as are tingible body macrophages imparting the starry-sky appearance, which is characteristic. {3310}. In some cases, there may be greater variation in cell size and shape, previously termed Burkitt-like lymphoma. In most HIV-related Burkitt lymphoma cases, the cells reveal plasmacytoid differentiation, which is peculiar to patients with AIDS. They are characterized by medium-sized cells with an eccentric nucleus, as many as four nucleoli, and a small rim of amphophilic cytoplasm. The cells may contain cytoplasmic immunoglobulin. EBV-encoded small RNA (EBER) is positive in about 30–50% of cases, whereas EBV LMP1 is negative {881}. Tumour cells have features of the small non-cleaved cells found in germinal centres, and are positive for CD20, CD10, and BCL6, but negative for BCL2. The Ki-67 proliferation index approaches 100%. The cells are positive for MYC with immunohistochemical stains, and the *MYC* translocation can usually be demonstrated by cytogenetics or FISH.

DLBCL

Patients with HIV-related DLBCL usually present with extranodal or disseminated disease; nodal presentation is less common than in the immunocompetent population. Most patients have high-stage disease (stage III or IV). The most common sites of extranodal disease are the CNS, gastrointestinal tract, bone marrow, and liver. There may be involvement of unusual sites, such as the heart or anorectal region. HIV-related DLBCL may be of the germinal centre B-cell type or the activated B-cell type, with the germinal centre B-cell type being more common. EBV is present in about 30% of cases, and together with expression of MYC, correlates with an impaired 2-year survival in patients with DLBCL treated in the HAART era {630,659,660,1056}. Most HIV-related DLBCLs consist of centroblasts, which are large cells with round or oval nuclei and two or more nucleoli, often aligned along the nuclear membrane. Mitoses may be frequent, but they usually

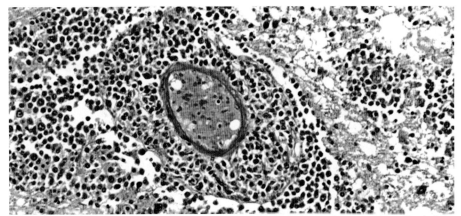

Fig. 16.10 HIV-associated diffuse large B-cell lymphoma involving the brain reveals perivascular cuffing by large immunoblastic cells.

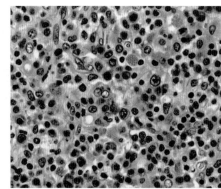

Fig. 16.11 Polymorphous lymphoid proliferation in HIV infection resembling post-transplant lymphoproliferative disorder, with a mixture of lymphoplasmacytoid cells including large immunoblasts.

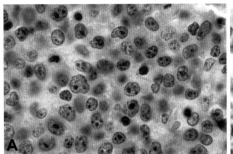
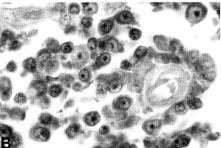
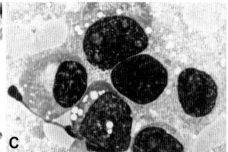

Fig. 16.12 HIV-associated diffuse large B-cell lymphoma (DLBCL). A Primary CNS DLBCL. B DLBCL, immunoblastic variant. The cells have prominent central nucleoli. C The cells exhibit marked plasmacytoid differentiation on touch imprint.

lack a starry-sky pattern. Immunoblastic lymphomas consist of larger cells with deeply basophilic or amphophilic cytoplasm, and may appear plasmacytoid with a perinuclear hof. The nuclei contain a prominent central nucleolus. Primary CNS lymphomas are usually of the immunoblastic type {536}. They are intracranial parenchymal tumours that may be deep-seated in the brain or may be multifocal. In addition to the cerebrum, they may be located in the basal ganglia and brain stem, and may involve the meninges. Lymphomas tend to follow vascular channels as perivascular cuffs, and there may be admixed small lymphocytes and glial cells. AIDS-related DLBCLs express B-cell–lineage antigens including CD19 and CD20, and have phenotypes similar to those of DLBCLs in the general population. Most have IG heavy and light chain gene rearrangements, and several proto-oncogenes may be involved in the pathogenesis, including *MYC*, *BCL2*, and *BCL6*. EBV infection is associated with expression of several tumour markers that are involved in the NF-kappaB pathway {659}.

Plasmablastic lymphoma
Plasmablastic lymphoma accounts for about 2% of all HIV-related lymphomas {554}. The blastoid morphology and immunophenotype suggest that these cells retain the blastoid appearance of immunoblasts or centroblasts, but have acquired the antigen profile of plasma cells. They may occur at all ages but are rare in paediatric patients. The median patient age at presentation is 38 years {577}. The cell or origin is considered to be an activated B cell after somatic hypermutation and class-switch recombination. About 60–70% of cases are positive for EBER in the absence of EBNA2 (compared with about 50% in immunocompetent patients with plasmablastic lymphoma) {2755}. There is expression of MYC in about 50% of cases, which correlates with *MYC* translocation or sometimes amplification. There are no translocations involving *BCL2*, *BCL6*, *MALT1*, or *PAX5*. EBV LMP1 is usually negative (type I EBV latency), although type III latency has been recorded {578}. Extranodal presentation is most frequent particularly in the oral cavity or jaw. For this reason, it is sometimes referred to as plasmablastic lymphoma of the oral

cavity type. Other sites of involvement include the gastrointestinal tract, skin, abdomen, retroperitoneum, and soft tissue of the extremities {578}. Patients do not usually have a monoclonal gammopathy, but may have advanced clinical stage, with B symptoms and bone marrow involvement. Histologically, plasmablastic lymphoma is characterized by sheet-like proliferation of large cells with immunoblastic or plasmablastic appearance, including central round or oval nuclei with prominent nucleoli and moderately abundant amphophilic cytoplasm. The nuclei may be eccentrically located with a perinuclear clearing or so-called hof. In the oral cavity, the cells may have a more centroblastic appearance but retain the plasmablastic phenotype {936}. There are frequent apoptotic cells, but a starry-sky pattern is rare. The neoplastic cells are negative or weakly positive for CD45 and usually negative for B-cell markers, including CD19, CD20, and PAX5, but most cases are positive for CD79a, IRF4 (also called MUM1), PRDM1 (also called BLIMP1), CD38, and CD138. Intracytoplasmic IgG may be detected in some patients. There may be aberrant expression of T-cell markers, including CD2 and

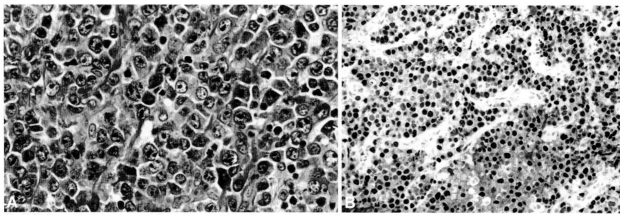

Fig. 16.13 Plasmablastic lymphoma. **A** Presenting as an oral cavity mass characterized by sheets of large plasmablastic cells with round or oval nuclei, prominent central nucleoli, and amphophilic cytoplasm. **B** Stained for IRF4 (also called MUM1).

CD4. The Ki-67 (MIB1) proliferation index is almost 100%.

Hodgkin lymphoma
The incidence of CHL may have increased since the introduction of HAART, suggesting that a threshold of CD4+ cells may be required for the pathogenesis, and that HAART does not provide protection from developing CHL {1657, 2218}. In the era before HAART, most cases were of the mixed-cellularity or lymphocyte-depleted subtypes. Likely due to improved immunity with anti-HIV therapy, nodular sclerosis CHL now accounts for nearly 50% of cases {3649}. HIV-associated CHL may have an atypical clinical presentation with advanced-stage bone marrow or liver involvement, as well as non-contiguous spread to multiple nodal groups. In HIV-related Hodgkin lymphoma, the Hodgkin/Reed–Sternberg cells are positive for EBER in 80–100% of cases; the cells express a type II EBV latency pattern in which expression of EBV-encoded genes is limited to EBNA1 and latent membrane proteins (LMP1 and LMP2) {1624}. Both these proteins have oncogenic potential, including the activation of the NF-kappaB pathway. In HIV-related CHL, there may be decreased nodal CD4+ T cells and lack of CD4+ rosetting around Hodgkin/Reed–Sternberg cells {1574}.

Other lymphomas
Cases of marginal zone lymphoma and lymphoma of mucosa-associated lymphoid tissue have been described in both paediatric and adult patients with HIV infection {1376,2593,3945}. Rare cases of NK/T-cell lymphomas have been reported, including mycosis fungoides, ana-

plastic large cell lymphoma, and nasal-type NK/T-cell lymphoma {159,365,501, 546,1266,1492,1667,1857,4008}. There is also an increased risk of lymphoplasmacytic lymphoma and lymphoblastic leukaemia {1370}.

Lymphomas occurring more specifically in HIV-positive patients
PEL, plasmablastic lymphoma, and HHV8-positive DLBCL, NOS, occur more specifically in HIV-positive patients.

Lymphomas occurring in other immunodeficient states
Polymorphic lymphoid proliferations resembling post-transplant lymphoproliferative disorder may be seen in adults and also in children, but are much less common than in the post-transplant setting, accounting for < 5% of HIV-associated lymphomas. The mean patient age at presentation is 38 years, similar to those of other HIV-related non-Hodgkin lymphomas. They may present in lymph nodes as well as extranodal sites. These conform to the criteria of polymorphic B-cell post-transplant lymphoproliferative disorder. The infiltrates contain a range of lymphoid cells, from small cells (often with plasmacytoid features) to immunoblasts, with scattered large bizarre cells expressing CD30. EBV is often present, but some cases are EBV-negative {2030, 2519,2804,3901}. A clonal B-cell population is present in most cases, and there may be an oligoclonal background, suggesting variable numbers of clonal cells within a polymorphic background. Clonal EBV infection has been demonstrated. They generally lack structural alterations in *MYC*, *BCL6*, the RAS family of genes, and *TP53* {2804}.

Prognosis and predictive factors
Before the HAART era, the outcome of patients with lymphoma and HIV infection was closely related to the severity of immunodeficiency {430}. HIV-directed therapy can now reduce the impact of HIV-related prognostic factors and allow curative therapy for most patients with aggressive lymphoma {278,2333,3580}. The achievement of complete remission is the most important prognostic factor with respect to survival {4351}. Expression of MYC in DLBCL from HIV-positive patients is associated with increased 2-year mortality {660}. In HIV-associated DLBCL, the stromal immune reaction may also influence patient survival {661}. Patients with HIV have reduced stromal CD4+ and FOXP3+ T cells, and increased density of stromal macrophages. A higher density of infiltrating CD8+ T cells may be associated with reduced mortality from lymphoma {661}. Plasmablastic lymphoma is associated with early relapses, and chemotherapy resistance with an inferior overall survival compared with DLBCL and Burkitt lymphoma {278, 578}. In Burkitt lymphoma, use of modified CODOX-M (cyclophosphamide, vincristine, doxorubicin, and high-dose methotrexate) regimens results in survival rates similar to those seen in studies that excluded HIV-positive patients {2906}. On the other hand, PEL usually has a very poor prognosis, with a low complete remission rate. CHL should be treated with curative intent, and has outcomes comparable to those in the non-HIV population {4089}. There is a need for increased supportive care and coincident HAART in the HIV-infected population {791}.

Post-transplant lymphoproliferative disorders

Swerdlow S.H.
Webber S.A.
Chadburn A.
Ferry J.A.

Definition

Post-transplant lymphoproliferative disorders (PTLDs) are lymphoid or plasmacytic proliferations that develop as a consequence of immunosuppression in a recipient of a solid organ or stem cell allograft. They constitute a spectrum ranging from usually EBV-driven polyclonal proliferations to EBV-positive or EBV-negative proliferations indistinguishable from a subset of B-cell or (less often) T/NK-cell lymphomas that occur in immunocompetent individuals. The monomorphic and classic Hodgkin lymphoma types of PTLD are further categorized as in non-immunosuppressed patients, according to the lymphoma they resemble. With the rare exception of EBV-positive MALT lymphomas, indolent B-cell lymphomas (e.g. follicular lymphoma and EBV-negative MALT lymphomas in allograft recipients) are designated as they are in the immunocompetent host and not considered a type of PTLD. The standardized incidence ratios for chronic lymphocytic leukaemia / small lymphocytic lymphoma, follicular lymphoma, mantle cell lymphoma, and splenic/nodal marginal zone lymphoma are not increased in solid organ transplant recipients, and those for lymphoplasmacytic lymphoma, marginal zone lymphoma, and mucosa-associated lymphoid tissue type lymphoma are only moderately elevated {763,2051}. The presence of rare EBV-positive cells in a lymphoid/plasmacytic proliferation, in the absence of other diagnostic features, is insufficient for the diagnosis of a PTLD. There are four major categories of PTLD, with all but the polymorphic group requiring further subcategorization (Table 16.02). Their criteria are summarized in Table 16.03. Patients may have more than one type of PTLD in a single site or at separate sites. Cases that fulfil the criteria for EBV-positive mucocutaneous ulcer should be separately designated. It is important to diagnose cases as PTLD and then indicate what type because of the prognostic and therapeutic implications. Given the intralesional heterogeneity of many PTLDs, the importance of

Table 16.02 Categories of post-transplant lymphoproliferative disorder (PTLD)

Non-destructive PTLDs
  Plasmacytic hyperplasia
  Infectious mononucleosis
  Florid follicular hyperplasia

Polymorphic PTLD

Monomorphic PTLDs[a]
(classify according to lymphoma they resemble)

  B-cell neoplasms
    Diffuse large B-cell lymphoma
    Burkitt lymphoma
    Plasma cell myeloma
    Plasmacytoma
    Other[b]

  T-cell neoplasms[a]
    Peripheral T-cell lymphoma, NOS
    Hepatosplenic T-cell lymphoma
    Other

Classic Hodgkin lymphoma PTLD[a]

---

[a] The ICD-O codes for these lesions are the same as those for the respective lymphoid or plasmacytic neoplasm.
[b] Indolent small B-cell lymphomas arising in transplant recipients are not included among the PTLDs, with the exception of EBV-positive marginal zone lymphomas (see text).

architectural features in their categorization, and the need in some cases for extensive ancillary studies, excisional biopsy is preferred over fine-needle aspiration or core needle biopsies whenever feasible.

Epidemiology

The characteristics of PTLD appear to differ somewhat across institutions, probably as a result of different patient populations, allograft types, and immunosuppressive regimens. A variety of risk factors have been identified {521,522, 2980}, but the most important risk factor for EBV-driven PTLD is EBV seronegativity at the time of transplantation {522,720, 4270}. Among adult and paediatric solid organ recipients, the frequency of PTLD correlates, in part, with the intensity and type of the immunosuppressive regimen, although no single immunosuppressive

agent is uniquely responsible. Among adults, patients receiving renal allografts have the lowest frequency of PTLD (generally < 1%); those with hepatic and cardiac allografts have an intermediate risk (approximately 1–5%); and those receiving heart–lung, lung, or intestinal allografts have the highest frequency (≥5%) {236,521,522,2980}. In children, for any given organ, the incidence is much higher {966,4271}, with most cases being associated with post-transplantation primary EBV infection {4271}. This is consistent with the finding of an increased incidence of PTLD among EBV-seronegative organ transplant recipients {720}. The incidence of PTLD is reported to rise again in patients aged > 50 years {1106,3262}. Lack of prior cytomegalovirus exposure is also a risk factor in some series. Additional host factors such as genetic polymorphisms may also impact the risk for PTLD {2756,3345}.
In general, stem cell allograft recipients have a low risk of PTLD (~1–2%); the risk of early-onset PTLD (< 1 year) is highest with unrelated or HLA-mismatched related donors, selective T-cell depletion of donor bone marrow, and use of anti-thymocyte globulin or anti-CD3 monoclonal antibodies. The risk of PTLD in these patients increases for those with two or more of these risk factors {851}. PTLD-like lesions are rare after autologous stem cell transplantation; they may be associated with additional high-dose immunosuppressive regimens and are best considered iatrogenic immunodeficiency-associated lymphoproliferative disorders rather than PTLD {2832}.

Etiology

Most PTLDs are associated with EBV infection, and appear to constitute EBV-induced monoclonal or, less often, polyclonal B-cell or monoclonal T-cell proliferations that occur in a setting of decreased T-cell immune surveillance {629, 767,1205,1245,2053,2819,3845}. EBV positivity is best demonstrated using in situ hybridization for EBV-encoded small RNA (EBER); EBV LMP1 immunostaining

Table 16.03 Criteria used in the categorization of post-transplant lymphoproliferative disorder (PTLD)

Pathological type of PTLD	Histopathology		Immunophenotype/ in-situ hybridization	Genetics	
	Architectural effacement	Major findings		IGH/TR clonal rearrangements	Cytogenetic/oncogene abnormalities
Plasmacytic hyperplasia	Absent	Predominantly small lymphocytes and plasma cells	Pcl B cells and admixed T cells; EBV+	Pcl or very small mcl B-cell population(s)	None
Infectious mononucleosis	Absent	Admixed small lymphocytes, plasma cells, and immunoblasts	Pcl B cells and admixed T cells; EBV+	Pcl or very small mcl B-cell population(s); may have clonal/ oligoclonal TR genes	Simple cytogenetic abnormalities rarely present
Florid follicular hyperplasia	Absent	Prominent hyperplastic germinal centres	Pcl B cells and admixed T cells; EBV±	Pcl or very small mcl B-cell population(s)	Non-specific simple cytogenetic abnormalities rarely present
Polymorphic	Present	Full spectrum of lymphoid maturation seen, not fulfilling criteria for NHL	Pcl ± mcl B cells and admixed T cells; most EBV+	Mcl B cells, non-clonal T cells	Some have BCL6 somatic hypermutations
Monomorphic	Usually present	Fulfils criteria for an NHL (other than one of the indolent B-cell neoplasms[a]) or plasma cell neoplasm	Varies based on type of neoplasm they resemble; EBV more variable than in other categories	Clonal B cells and/or T cells (except for rare NK-cell cases)	Variably present (see text)
CHL	Present	Fulfils criteria for CHL	Similar to other CHL; EBV+	IGH not easily demonstrated	Unknown

CHL, classic Hodgkin lymphoma; NHL, non-Hodgkin lymphoma; mcl, monoclonal; pcl, polyclonal.
Monoclonality and polyclonality are only inferred when finding monotypic or polytypic light chain expression.

[a] EBV-positive MALT lymphomas at least of skin/subcutaneous tissues should be considered a type of PTLD.

is less sensitive. Most EBV-positive cases exhibit a type III EBV latency pattern, but a moderate number show a type II pattern, and fewer show a type I pattern, although not all of the cells in a given case show the same pattern {1405,3011}. Evidence of lytic EBV infection can also be documented in more than half of the cases and has been associated with plasmacytic differentiation {1405}. About 20–40% of PTLDs are EBV-negative, with some series reporting an even higher proportion of cases. Approximately two thirds of the T-cell PTLDs are EBV-negative {47,385, 1205,2239,2756,2848,3845}. Furthermore, the proportion of EBV-negative PTLDs has increased since PTLDs were first being reported {2848}. EBV-negative PTLDs are more common in adults, tend to occur later after transplantation, and are more likely to be monomorphic compared with EBV-positive cases {1355, 2848}. Although data are limited, EBV-negative cases appear to have a gene expression profile similar to that of diffuse large B-cell lymphoma occurring in immunocompetent hosts {2754}. Differ-

ences in the regulation of BCL2 family proteins between EBV-positive and EBV-negative PTLD have also been reported {1354}. HHV8-associated PTLDs have been reported, including post-transplant primary effusion lymphoma {1030,1935, 2571}; however, the etiology of the vast majority of EBV-negative PTLDs is unknown. Some may be due to EBV that is no longer detectable {3760}, some due to other unknown viruses, and some due to chronic antigenic stimulation, including by the transplant itself {385}. Two gene expression profiling studies support a non-viral etiology for the EBV-negative cases, although other studies have failed to find differences between EBV-positive and EBV-negative PTLDs {832,2754, 4100}. The EBV-negative cases are still considered to represent PTLD, and some may respond to decreased immunosuppression {2848}.

The majority (>90%) of PTLDs in solid organ recipients are of host origin, and only a minority of donor origin. Donor-origin PTLDs appear to be most common in liver and lung allograft recipients,

and frequently involve the allograft {147, 632,2225,3756,4290}. In contrast, most PTLDs in stem cell allograft recipients are of donor origin, as would be expected, given that successful engraftment results in an immune system that is nearly exclusively of donor origin {4507}.

Localization

Involvement of lymph node, gastrointestinal tract, lungs, and liver is common, but disease can occur at almost any site in the body {1205,2819,3130,4271}. The CNS is involved uncommonly, either as the only site of disease or in association with multiorgan involvement {575,1119}. In solid organ transplant recipients, PTLD can involve the allograft, which can cause diagnostic confusion because rejection and infection can result in a similar clinical picture. Allograft involvement appears more frequently in early-onset, EBV-positive disease and is most common in lung and intestinal transplant recipients {236, 1355,2980,3296}. The non-destructive PTLDs often present with tonsil and/or adenoid involvement but can also occur at other sites. EBV-positive MALT lymphoma PTLDs most typically present in cutaneous or subcutaneous tissues {1368}. The plasmacytoma lesions may have nodal or, more commonly, extranodal presentations, usually without bone marrow involvement {1951,3352,4042}. Some cases have a myeloma-like presentation, including osteolytic bone lesions {1951,4042}. Overt bone marrow involvement by polymorphic PTLDs (P-PTLDs) and monomorphic PTLDs (M-PTLDs) is present in about 15–20% of cases, but peripheral blood is rarely involved {2697}. The presence of occasional small lymphoid aggregates or rare EBV-positive cells is not sufficient to diagnose PTLD in the marrow. Bone marrow allograft recipients tend to present with widespread disease involving nodal and extranodal sites, including liver, spleen, gastrointestinal tract, and lungs {3130,3636,4507}.

Clinical features

The clinical features of PTLD are highly variable and correlate to some extent with the type of allograft and morphologically defined categories. PTLD frequently presents in the first year after transplantation, especially in EBV-seronegative recipients who acquire early post-transplant EBV infection, often from the donor. This pattern of presentation is particularly common in children. However, the median time to PTLD in some studies, especially those of adult populations, is several years, and as many as 15–25% of cases occur > 10 years after the transplant {981,1122,2819,3130}. There is some evidence for an increase in prevalence of late-onset disease {720}, although this may in part reflect the ever-expanding population of patients at risk as the number of long-term survivors of transplantation increases. EBV-negative PTLD and T/NK-cell PTLD tend to present later (with median times to occurrence of 4–5 years and ~6 years, respectively), although T-cell PTLDs following haematopoietic stem cell or bone marrow transplantation occur significantly earlier {851,1625, 2239,2848,3845,3999}.

PTLD presentations vary greatly. Some PTLDs are found incidentally, some present with very vague non-specific symptoms such as fever and malaise, and some present with infectious mononucleosis–like findings. Others present with tonsil or adenoid enlargement, lymphadenopathy or tumorous mass-

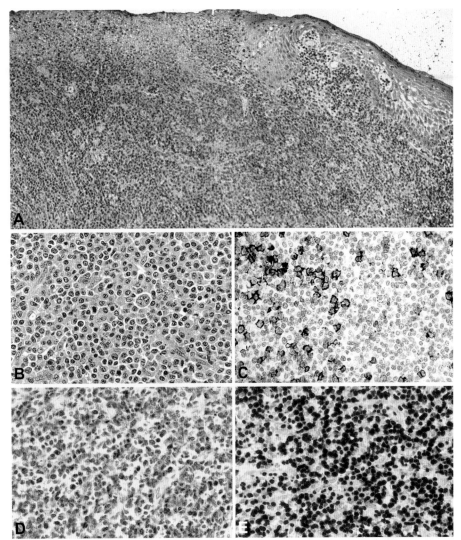

Fig. 16.14 Infectious mononucleosis post-transplant lymphoproliferative disorder in the tonsil of an 11-year-old renal allograft recipient. **A** There is preservation of overlying epithelium and crypts, but normal follicles are absent, and there is a diffuse lymphoid proliferation. **B** Polymorphic proliferation of immunoblasts, small lymphoid cells, and plasma cells. **C** CD20 staining showing scattered B cells. **D** In contrast, a stain for CD79a shows more-numerous positive cells, indicating plasmacytoid differentiation. **E** In situ hybridization identifies EBV-encoded small RNA (EBER) expression in most of the cells.

es, often at extranodal sites, sometimes with organ-specific dysfunction and occasionally with widely disseminated disease. A viral septic shock–like picture is another rare presentation.

Prognosis and predictive factors

Although overall mortality rates of 25–60% are still quoted {2756}, newer therapeutic strategies appear to be associated with a better overall outcome. The non-destructive PTLDs (previously termed early lesions) tend to regress with reduction in immune suppression; if this can be accomplished without graft rejection, the prognosis is excellent, particularly in children {2385,2849,4462}.

However, some infectious mononucleosis–like PTLDs can be fatal. P-PTLDs and even a significant minority of M-PTLDs may also regress with reduction in immune suppression {3346,3769,4271}. Some factors that have been reported to be associated with a lack of response to decreased immunosuppression include elevated lactate dehydrogenase, organ dysfunction, multiorgan involvement, advanced stage, bulky disease, and older patient age {3346,4066}. Clinical caution is required because rebound acute or chronic rejection is frequently observed during reduction of immunosuppression and can lead to graft loss and death {4271}. A proportion of P-PTLDs and

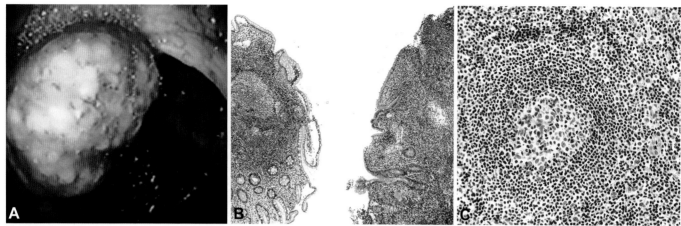

Fig. 16.15 Florid follicular hyperplasia post-transplant lymphoproliferative disorder in a 20-year-old man, 10 years after heart transplantation. The lesion, which had only rare EBV+ cells, regressed after the patient's immunosuppression was reduced and did not recur. **A** Endoscopic image of ileocaecal mass. **B,C** Biopsies showing a variably dense infiltrate composed of organized lymphoid tissue with scattered germinal centres, many small lymphocytes, some plasma cells, and infrequent transformed cells.

more-numerous M-PTLDs fail to regress, and require additional therapies such as monoclonal antibodies directed against B-cell antigens (most commonly anti-CD20), sometimes together with chemotherapy {741,742,1099,1404,1474}. The anti-CD30 antibody brentuximab vedotin has also been used, with mixed results {47,1634}. Surgical excision or sometimes radiation therapy are other important therapeutic modalities in localized cases. Adoptive T-cell immunotherapy is another therapeutic approach {1031, 1545,1629}. Although no comparative clinical trials have been reported for Burkitt lymphoma PTLDs, cessation of immunosuppression and immediate use of multidrug (immuno)chemotherapy likely offer the best outcomes for this aggressive PTLD {3168,4495}. Plasmacytoma-like PTLDs have a variable outcome, but many do well, sometimes with very limited therapy {981,3142,3205,3352,4042}. The myelomatous lesions and cases with osteolytic bone lesions are not expected to regress with decreased immunosuppression and have a poor prognosis, although they may respond to myeloma-type therapy {2053,4042}. T/NK-cell PTLDs are also typically aggressive, particularly those of hepatosplenic type, with the exception of those of large granular lymphocyte type, which typically do very well {3845,3999}. Nevertheless, some T-cell PTLDs do respond to reconstitution of the patient's immune system. Classic Hodgkin lymphoma PTLDs are generally treated with conventional classic Hodgkin lymphoma therapeutic regimens, with good results.

Risk factors for adverse outcome vary greatly across studies. Some of the reported factors that have been associated with an adverse prognosis include multiple sites of disease (perhaps not in children), advanced stage, involvement of the CNS, bone marrow and serous effusions, older patient age at diagnosis, elevated lactate dehydrogenase, and hypoalbuminaemia {522,741,981,1099, 1120,1356,2240,2435,4061,4271}. The combination of lytic EBV infection and type III EBV latency has also been associated with an adverse prognosis, as well as with early onset {1405}. Although EBV negativity in PTLD, and even among the T/NK-cell PTLDs, has been reported to be an adverse prognostic indicator, not all studies document a survival difference {741,3845}. PTLD of donor origin in solid organ transplant recipients and the overlapping group of PTLD localized to the allograft have better than average prognoses, although in T-cell PTLD, graft involvement has been reported to be an adverse prognostic indicator {3999}. PTLDs with oncogene abnormalities are also considered to be more aggressive. Whether P-PTLD does better than M-PTLD is controversial. Overall, the mortality of PTLD is much greater in bone marrow allograft recipients than in solid organ allograft recipients. It should also be remembered that, although uncommon, there may be progression from non-destructive to polymorphic and from polymorphic to monomorphic PTLD, sometimes with documented additional molecular abnormalities {3168,4377}.

Serial monitoring of EBV DNA levels in whole blood, peripheral blood mononuclear cell preparations, or plasma is often used to help predict the risk for PTLD and the onset of PTLD, as well as to follow PTLD, including to guide preemptive therapy in some patients. Its use appears most helpful in solid organ transplant recipients who are seronegative at transplantation, particularly children. However, it should be noted that EBV-positive PTLD can develop in the absence of high viral loads, high viral loads are not predictive in all settings, and a fall in load may not always predict treatment response. A rapid fall in EBV viral load is almost invariable when anti–B cell monoclonal antibodies are given as part of the treatment regimen, irrespective of long-term PTLD response {72,3451}. The lack of standardization of techniques and results for assessment of circulating viral load has been an additional complicating factor, although there is now an international WHO standard for determining EBV load {3451}.

Non-destructive post-transplant lymphoproliferative disorders

Definition

Non-destructive post-transplant lymphoproliferative disorders are defined as lymphoid proliferations in an allograft recipient characterized by architectural preservation of the involved tissue and an absence of features that would be diagnostic of a malignant lymphoma. In most cases, they form mass lesions. These PTLDs must be distinguished from lymphoid proliferations with other known explanations and from other non-specific chronic inflammatory processes.

Because cases of plasmacytic hyperplasia (PH) and florid follicular hyperplasia are histologically non-specific, the diagnosis requires the formation of a mass lesion and/or significant EBV positivity. This group of PTLDs were formerly known as early lesions; however, this term has been deleted due to confusion with the group of PTLDs that occur early after transplantation. In fact, a series of so-called early PTLDs from 2005–2007 were diagnosed at a median of 50 months after transplantation {2849}.

Clinical features
PH and infectious mononucleosis (IM) PTLDs tend to occur at a younger age than the other PTLDs, and are often seen in children or in adult solid organ recipients who have not had a prior EBV infection {629,2385,2849}. Cases of florid follicular hyperplasia PTLD also occur most commonly in children {2849,4101}. These non-destructive lesions involve lymph nodes or tonsils and adenoids more often than true extranodal sites {2848,2385}. They often regress spontaneously with reduction in immunosuppression or may be successfully treated by surgical excision; however, IM-like lesions can be fatal. In some cases, polymorphic or monomorphic PTLD may follow one of the non-destructive type lesions {2819, 4377}.

Microscopy
PH is characterized by numerous plasma cells, small lymphocytes, and generally infrequent bland-appearing immunoblasts, whereas IM PTLD has the typical morphological features of IM, with paracortical/interfollicular expansion and numerous immunoblasts in a background of T cells and plasma cells. Florid follicular hyperplasia is a mass lesion with marked follicular hyperplasia that does not suggest IM {4101}. Criteria for the distinction of these non-destructive PTLDs from other reactive lymphoid infiltrates are not well defined and rest on the extent of the proliferation, clinical correlation, and the presence or absence of EBV.

Immunophenotype
Immunophenotypic studies show an admixture of polytypic B cells, plasma cells, and T cells without phenotypic aberrancy. EBV is present in many of the reported cases of PH and florid follicular hyperplasia {2053,2849,4101}. These diagnoses should be made only with great caution in EBV-negative cases, due to the non-specificity of the histological/immunophenotypic findings. IM PTLDs are typically EBV+ with EBV LMP1+ immunoblasts {2385}.

Genetic profile
Clonally rearranged IG genes are not expected in PH, although small clonal populations may be demonstrated with Southern blot analysis using probes to the terminal repeat region of EBV. Some IM PTLDs may have small monoclonal or oligoclonal populations. The significance of oligoclonality or a small clonal band in these cases is unknown {2053,4377}. Florid follicular hyperplasia does not usually demonstrate clonal B cells but, as is also reported in IM PTLD, rarely demonstrates simple clonal cytogenetic abnormalities {2849,4101}.

Polymorphic post-transplant lymphoproliferative disorders

Definition
Polymorphic post-transplant lymphoproliferative disorders (P-PTLDs) are composed of a heterogeneous population of immunoblasts, plasma cells, and small and intermediate-sized lymphoid cells that efface the architecture of lymph nodes or form destructive extranodal masses and do not fulfil the criteria for any of the recognized types of lymphoma described in immunocompetent hosts. There are no established criteria for the proportion of transformed cells/immunoblasts that may be present in P-PTLD. Distinction from cases of infectious mononucleosis PTLD with marked architectural distortion may be difficult. More problematic is the distinction of some P-PTLDs from monomorphic PTLDs (M-PTLDs). The criteria for the distinction of P-PTLDs from M-PTLDs that have plasmacytic differentiation are not well defined. PTLDs that fulfil the criteria for T-cell/histiocyte-rich large B-cell lymphoma or EBV-positive diffuse large B-cell lymphoma, NOS, which may appear polymorphic, are best considered a form of M-PTLD, because they would be diagnosed as lymphoma in a non-transplant patient. Of great importance, cases of monomorphic T-cell PTLD, which can also appear very polymorphic, must not be confused with P-PTLD. Some PTLDs that appear polymorphic but fulfil the criteria for EBV-positive mucocutaneous ulcer should be so-designated (for a more detailed description, see *Other iatrogenic immunodeficiency-associated lymphoproliferative disorders*, p. 462) {1565}. The mucocutaneous ulcer type of PTLDs characteristically lack peripheral blood EBV DNA and do well with reduced/altered immunosuppression with or without rituximab {1565}.

ICD-O code   9971/1

Clinical features
The reported frequency of P-PTLDs varies widely, but they account for a minority of PTLDs in most studies. However, in children P-PTLD is generally more common and frequently follows post-transplantation primary EBV infection {4271}. The clinical presentation of P-PTLDs is not distinguishable from that of PTLDs in general, although they have been

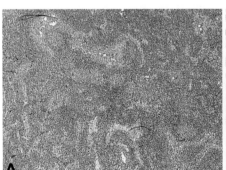
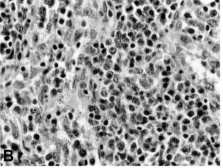

Fig. 16.16 Plasmacytic hyperplasia. **A** The normal architecture of the lymph node is intact. **B** Numerous plasma cells are present.

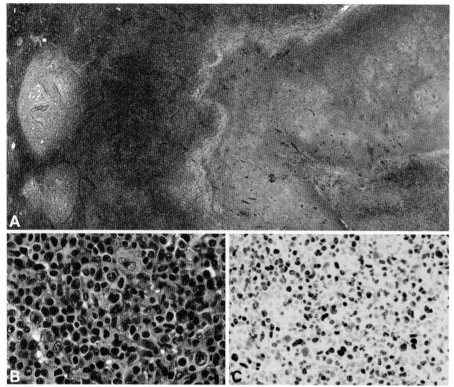

Fig. 16.17 Polymorphic post-transplant lymphoproliferative disorder. **A** Architectural effacement with large area of geographical necrosis. **B** Note the variably sized and shaped lymphoid cells, with one very large cell resembling a Reed–Sternberg variant. **C** Numerous CD30+ cells are also present.

reported to occur earlier than M-PTLD. Reduction in immunosuppression leads to regression in a variable proportion of cases; others may progress and require treatment for lymphoma {2053,2819, 3769,4271}.

Microscopy

Unlike the three types of non-destructive PTLD lesions, P-PTLDs show effacement of the underlying tissue architecture {1258,1541}. However, unlike many lymphomas, they show the full range of B-cell maturation, from immunoblasts to plasma cells, with small and medium-sized lymphocytes and cells with irregular nuclear contours, some of

which represent the typically prominent T-cell component. There may be areas of geographical necrosis and scattered large, bizarre cells that not infrequently resemble Reed–Sternberg cells (atypical immunoblasts). Numerous mitoses may be present. Some cases have areas that appear more monomorphic in the same or other tissues; thus, there may be a continuous spectrum between these lesions and M-PTLD. Other P-PTLDs have features that more closely resemble those of Hodgkin lymphoma. Some of these cases were previously referred to as Hodgkin-like. Variably sized, but usually small, lymphoid aggregates with or without plasma cell clusters are seen

in the bone marrow in some patients with P-PTLD {2068}. They are more common in children than in adults. The clinical significance of these aggregates, which are not always EBV-positive, is uncertain.

Immunophenotype

Immunophenotypic studies demonstrate B cells and a variable proportion of heterogeneous T cells that are usually moderately numerous and sometimes predominate {1062,2819}. Light chain class restriction does not exclude the diagnosis and, when present, may be focal, or with the presence of different clonal populations in the same or different sites {2819}. The presence of clear-cut light chain class restriction must be noted in the diagnostic report, because some of these cases could also be classified as monomorphic diffuse large B-cell lymphoma PTLD with plasmacytic differentiation or as plasma cell neoplasm with increased transformed cells. Prominent CD30 expression is common, but unlike in most cases of classic Hodgkin lymphoma, the CD30+ Reed–Sternberg–like cells are CD20+ and CD15– {694,4159}. Most cases of P-PTLD contain numerous cells positive for EBV-encoded small RNA (EBER). Detection of EBV by in situ hybridization for EBER is a useful tool in the differential diagnosis of PTLD versus rejection in allografts.

Genetic profile

P-PTLDs are expected to demonstrate clonally rearranged IG genes, although the clones are less predominant than in M-PTLD {766,1936,2053,2378}. EBV terminal repeat analysis is the most sensitive method for demonstrating clonal populations in the EBV-positive cases, but is not generally performed. In some reported cases, tumours at different sites in the same patient may be clonally distinct {628}. About 75% of P-PTLDs are reported to have mutated IGV genes without ongoing mutations, and the remainder are unmutated {550}. Significant T-cell clones are not expected. Clonal cytogenetic abnormalities may be present although less commonly detected than in B-cell M-PTLD {1010,4101}. Comparative genomic hybridization studies also demonstrate abnormalities in some P-PTLDs, including some recurrent abnormalities also seen in M-PTLD {3207}. *BCL6* somatic hypermutations are present in a subset of cases, as is aberrant promoter

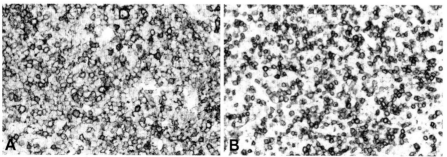

Fig. 16.18 Polymorphic post-transplant lymphoproliferative disorder, EBV-positive. There are (**A**) numerous variably sized CD20+ B cells as well as (**B**) many mostly small CD3+ T cells.

methylation, but other mutations are only uncommonly detected {550,622,4100}. Nevertheless, it has been reported that P-PTLD does not segregate from non–germinal centre M-PTLD based on gene expression profiling {4100}.

Monomorphic post-transplant lymphoproliferative disorders (B- and T/NK-cell types)

Introduction

Monomorphic post-transplant lymphoproliferative disorders (M-PTLDs), which make up about 60–80% of all PTLDs in most studies, fulfil the criteria for one of the B-cell or T/NK-cell neoplasms that are recognized in immunocompetent hosts and described elsewhere in this volume. The only exception to this is that the small B-cell lymphoid neoplasms are not designated as PTLD, except for the EBV-positive lymphoplasmacytic proliferations that typically occur in skin/subcutaneous tissue, which fulfil the criteria for extranodal marginal zone lymphoma of mucosa-associated lymphoid tissue (MALT lymphoma) {1368}.

The M-PTLDs should be designated as PTLD in the diagnostic line of the pathology report, and then further categorized based on the classification of lymphomas arising in immunocompetent hosts. Although the term monomorphic PTLD reflects the fact that many cases are composed of a monotonous proliferation of transformed lymphoid cells or plasmacytic cells, there may be significant pleomorphism, variability of cell size, and many admixed T cells within a given case. In addition, because polymorphic PTLD and M-PTLDs of B-cell origin form a spectrum, their distinction can become blurred, particularly with the recognition of pleomorphic EBV-positive diffuse large B-cell lymphomas that arise in the absence of primary or secondary immunodeficiency or in association with age-related immune senescence. A predominance of large transformed cells/immunoblasts and abnormalities in oncogenes and tumour suppressor genes favour the diagnosis of M-PTLD, but are not required findings {2053}. As noted above, cases that fulfil the criteria for EBV-positive mucocutaneous ulcer should be separately designated and not diagnosed as M-PTLD even if there are many atypical and transformed B cells and monoclonality {1565}.

M-PTLDs can be further categorized as either monomorphic B-cell PTLDs or monomorphic T/NK-cell PTLDs.

Monomorphic B-cell PTLD

Definition

The monomorphic B-cell PTLDs are monoclonal transformed B-lymphocytic or plasmacytic proliferations that fulfil the criteria for a diffuse large B-cell lymphoma, or less often a Burkitt lymphoma or a plasma cell neoplasm. The latter may have all the features of an extraosseous plasmacytoma with involvement of the gastrointestinal tract, lymph nodes, or other extranodal sites or much less often of plasma cell myeloma. EBV+ extranodal marginal zone lymphomas of mucosa-associated lymphoid tissue (MALT lymphomas) that typically present in the skin or subcutaneous tissues should also be considered a type of M-PTLD. These must be distinguished from the EBV– MALT lymphomas such as in the stomach or parotid that, like the other small B-cell lymphomas, would not be considered a type of PTLD. Although these EBV– MALT lymphomas may be somewhat more common in post-transplant individuals than in the general population, they are very much like the MALT lymphomas seen in immunocompetent hosts.

Clinical features

The clinical presentation of monomorphic B-PTLDs is not distinctive and is, in general, similar to the presentation of the lymphomas or plasma cell neoplasms that they resemble. The EBV+ MALT lymphoma M-PTLDs are distinctive, with a frequently cutaneous/subcutaneous presentation. They occur late after transplantation and are solitary, and the patients do well {2832A}.

Microscopy

Monomorphic B-PTLDs most commonly fulfil the conventional criteria for diffuse large B-cell lymphoma, with fewer cases of Burkitt lymphoma, plasmacytoma, or very rarely plasma cell myeloma PTLD. It is important to recognize that monomorphic B-PTLDs are not all monotonous proliferations of one cell type; there may be pleomorphism of the transformed cells, plasmacytic differentiation, and not infrequently Reed–Sternberg–like cells, all of which result in a more polymor-

phic appearance. Some cases resemble EBV+ diffuse large B-cell lymphoma, NOS. Nevertheless, many of these cases, with the exception of T-cell/histiocyte-rich forms, have a clear predominance of transformed B cells or sheets of plasma cells. Geographical necrosis may be present and is usually associated with EBV positivity. Cases diagnosed as plasmacytoma PTLD, which typically have sheets of plasma cells, may have occasional foci of lymphoid cells. Although many have mostly small plasma cells, some cases can have larger cells with nucleoli {3142}. A plasmablastic lymphoma PTLD must then be excluded. The EBV+ cutaneous/subcutaneous MALT lymphoma PTLDs resemble other MALT lymphomas that have plasmacytic differentiation, with many lymphoid cells with abundant pale cytoplasm, follicles with follicular colonization, and at least focally prominent plasma cells. Some cases have been diagnosed as plasmacytoma PTLD, consistent with the concept that plasmacytomas (immunocytomas) of skin are considered to represent MALT lymphomas. Rare cases at extracutaneous sites that might be otherwise similar have also been reported.

Immunophenotype

The lesions, other than those resembling plasma cell neoplasms, have B-cell–associated antigen expression (CD19, CD20, CD79a), sometimes with demonstrable monotypic immunoglobulin (often with expression of gamma or alpha heavy chain) in paraffin sections and more often if flow cytometric studies are performed. Many cases are CD30+, with or without anaplastic morphology. Most M-PTLDs are of non-germinal centre type based on immunohistochemistry. The EBV-positive cases usually have a non-germinal centre phenotype (CD10–, BCL6±, IRF4/MUM1+) even though only a minority are CD138+, whereas the EBV-negative cases are more likely to have a germinal centre type phenotype (CD10±, BCL6+, IRF4/MUM1–, CD138–; 60% of cases in one study). The Burkitt lymphoma PTLDs, which are often EBV-positive, however, are CD10+. The myeloma or plasmacytoma PTLDs, which may be EBV-positive or -negative, are phenotypically similar to those in immunocompetent patients. Although only a limited number of cases have been reported, the majority of the EBV+ MALT lymphoma PTLDs have been IgA+.

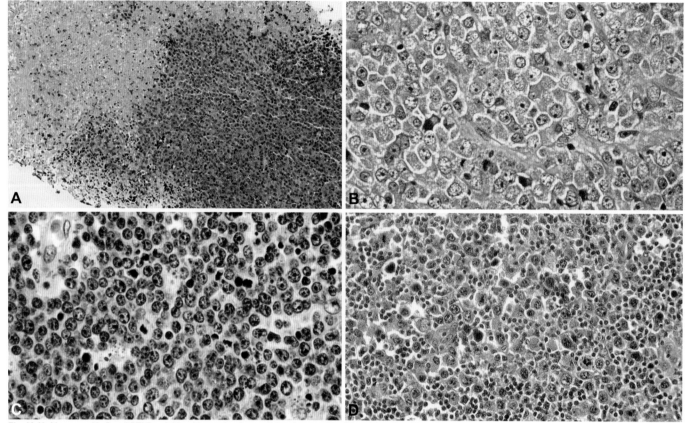

Fig. 16.19 Monomorphic B-cell PTLDs. **A** Liver biopsy showing partial replacement by diffuse large B-cell lymphoma, immunoblastic variant. **B** Diffuse large B-cell lymphoma, centroblastic variant, EBV-negative, showing large transformed cells, many of which have peripheral nucleoli, consistent with centroblasts. There are also admixed immunoblasts. **C** Burkitt lymphoma showing monotonous, medium-sized cells with multiple nucleoli, basophilic cytoplasm, and numerous mitoses. **D** Monomorphic B-cell PTLD with a polymorphic background. Note the admixture of many pleomorphic transformed cells with small lymphocytes and occasional plasma cells. The diagnosis of an M-PTLD is based on the very prominent light chain-restricted large transformed cells associated in part with many T cells.

Genetic profile

Clonal IG gene rearrangement is present in virtually all cases, and the majority contain EBV genomes, which, if present, are in clonal episomal form. PTLDs may have different clones at different sites, as well as when they relapse. Most cases have somatically mutated IGHV, with a minority showing ongoing mutations. However, some cases have IGHV, loci inactivation related to crippling mutations as seen in CHL. Caution in interpreting T-cell clonality studies is advised, because monoclonal T-cell receptor rearrangements in the absence of a T-cell neoplasm have been reported in about half of B-PTLDs, particularly when a prominent CD8+ T-cell population is present. Of interest, this finding was not observed in DLBCL associated with HIV or in immunocompetent hosts. Consistent with the phenotypic findings, EBV+ PTLDs are of activated B-cell type; in contrast, 45% of the EBV-negative cases are of germinal centre type. As in non-PTLD DLBCL, oncogene abnormalities (*RAS* mutations, *TP53* mu-

tations, and/or *MYC* rearrangements) may be found, and *BCL6* gene somatic hypermutation is common; however, *BCL6* translocations are uncommon. Aberrant promoter hypermethylation and aberrant somatic hypermutation also occur in M-PTLD. Cytogenetic abnormalities are common, and are more frequent than in the non-destructive or polymorphic PTLDs. Some recurrent abnormalities are reported in PTLD, such

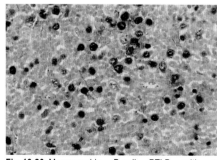

Fig. 16.20 Monomorphic B-cell PTLD with a polymorphic background (EBER ISH for EBV). The pleomorphic large cells and some smaller ones are EBER-positive.

as breaks involving the 1q11-q21 region, 8q24.1, 3q27, 16p13, 14q32 and 11q23-24, as well as trisomies 9, 11, 7, X, 2, and 12, but different studies find different common abnormalities. Comparative genomic hybridization and single nucleotide polymorphism (SNP) studies demonstrate additional gains and losses, although no individual abnormality is very common. Although some of these are shared with DLBCL in immunocompetent hosts, differences are observed as well. Differences from HIV-associated DLBCL are also observed {3361A}. EBV-negative monomorphic PTLDs frequently lack expression of the cyclin-dependent kinase inhibitor CDKN2A (p16INK4a). Although the majority of Burkitt lymphoma PTLDs do have IG/*MYC* translocations, 3 of 7 EBV-negative post-transplant molecularly defined Burkitt lymphomas had the same 11q abnormalities seen in the new provisional entity of Burkitt-like lymphoma with 11q aberration raising the possibility that these cases are more frequent in the post-transplant setting.

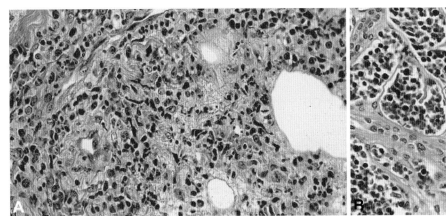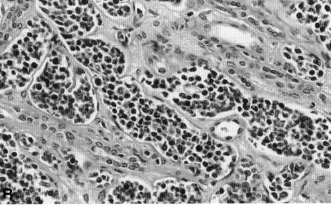

Fig. 16.21 Monomorphic T-cell PTLD. **A** Subcutaneous panniculitis-like T-cell lymphoma in an adult female renal allograft recipient, showing diffuse involvement of subcutaneous tissue. This case was EBV-negative. **B** Hepatosplenic gamma delta T-cell lymphoma (EBV-negative) in a 29-year-old male renal allograft recipient. There is infiltration of small blood vessels in the allograft.

Monomorphic T/NK-cell PTLD

Definition

Monomorphic T/NK-cell PTLDs (T/NK-PTLDs) include PTLDs that fulfil the criteria for any of the T- or NK-cell lymphomas. In North America and western Europe, these lesions constitute no more than 15% of PTLDs. They include almost the entire spectrum of T- and NK-cell neoplasms, with the largest group being peripheral T-cell lymphoma, NOS, followed by hepatosplenic T-cell lymphoma, which together make up slightly more than 10% of T-PTLDs. Other types of T/NK-cell PTLDs include T-cell large granular lymphocytic leukaemia; adult T-cell leukaemia/lymphoma (ATLL); extranodal NK/T cell lymphoma, nasal type; mycosis fungoides/Sézary syndrome; primary cutaneous anaplastic large cell lymphoma; other anaplastic large cell lymphomas; and even rare cases of T-lymphoblastic leukaemia/lymphoma. In some instances, T-cell PTLDs have occurred with, or subsequent to, other types of PTLDs. Very rarely, aggressive NK-cell PTLDs also occur.

Clinical features

Clinical presentation depends on the type of T/NK-cell neoplasm. Most cases present at extranodal sites, sometimes with associated lymphadenopathy. The more common sites of involvement include the peripheral blood or bone marrow, spleen, skin, liver, gastrointestinal tract, and lung.

Microscopy

The morphological features of T/NK-cell PTLDs do not differ from those of the same T/NK-cell lymphomas in immunocompetent hosts. It is critical to distinguish T-cell large granular lymphocytic leukaemias from the other T/NK-cell PTLDs.

Immunophenotype

T/NK-cell PTLDs show expression of pan–T-cell and sometimes NK-cell associated antigens. Depending on the specific type, they may express CD4 or CD8, CD30, ALK, and either alpha beta or gamma delta T-cell receptors. About one third of cases are EBV-positive. Cases of ATLL are associated with HTLV-1.

Genetic profile

Cases of T-cell origin have clonal T-cell receptor gene rearrangement. Caution is advised, because clonal or oligoclonal CD8+ T cells may be seen following bone marrow transplantation or in IM, and clonal T-cell rearrangements are also reported in M-PTLD of B-cell origin. Chromosomal abnormalities are common and similar to those seen in T/NK-cell neoplasms in the immunocompetent host, such as i(7)(q10) and +8 in most of the hepatosplenic T-cell lymphomas. Oncogene mutations, such as in *TP53*, are also reported in a high proportion of T/NK-cell PTLDs.

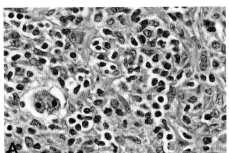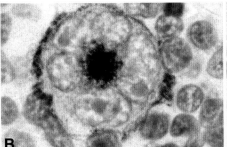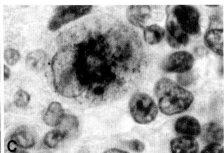

Fig. 16.22 Classic Hodgkin lymphoma post-transplant lymphoproliferative disorder in a 52-year-old man following renal transplant. The Reed–Sternberg cells were EBV-positive. **A** Reed–Sternberg cell surrounded by small lymphocytes and some eosinophils. **B,C** Reed–Sternberg cells with CD30 expression (B) and Golgi-type CD15 positivity (C).

Classic Hodgkin lymphoma post-transplant lymphoproliferative disorder

Definition

Classic Hodgkin lymphoma (CHL) post-transplant lymphoproliferative disorder (PTLD), the least common major form of PTLD, is almost always EBV-positive, and should fulfil the diagnostic criteria for CHL (see Chapter 15: *Hodgkin lymphomas*, p. 423). These lesions are usually of the mixed-cellularity type and have a type II EBV latency pattern as is typical in immunocompetent hosts. Because Reed–Sternberg–like cells may be seen in non-destructive, polymorphic, and some monomorphic PTLDs, the diagnosis of CHL must be based on both classic morphological and immunophenotypic features, preferably including both expression of both CD15 and CD30 {2820,3436}. Although CD15-negative CHLs occur, caution is advised in making the diagnosis of CHL PTLD, because these cases must be distinguished from the other types of PTLD that include Reed–Sternberg–like cells, which are most typically EBV+, CD45+, CD15–, and CD20+ and often present in association with small and intermediate-sized EBV+ lymphoid cells {694,1034,1417, 2820,3198,3304}. CHL PTLD is more likely to show B-cell antigen expression than is CHL in immunocompetent hosts {23}. Rare cases may follow other types of PTLD. Although the distinction of PTLD with some Hodgkin-like features, such as prominent Reed–Sternberg–like cells, from CHL PTLD may be difficult in some cases, cases that do not clearly fulfil the criteria for CHL are best classified as either polymorphic PTLD or monomorphic PTLD, depending on their overall morphological features {3198,3304}.

ICD-O code
9650/3

Other iatrogenic immunodeficiency-associated lymphoproliferative disorders

Gaulard P.
Swerdlow S.H.
Harris N.L.
Sundström C.
Jaffe E.S.

Definition

The other iatrogenic immunodeficiency-associated lymphoproliferative disorders are lymphoid proliferations or lymphomas that arise in patients treated with immunosuppressive drugs for autoimmune disease or conditions other than in the post-transplant setting. They constitute a spectrum ranging from polymorphic proliferations resembling polymorphic post-transplant lymphoproliferative disorders (PTLDs) to cases that fulfil the criteria for diffuse large B-cell lymphoma (DLBCL) or other B-cell lymphomas, such as EBV-positive DLBCL, peripheral T/NK-cell lymphoma, and classic Hodgkin lymphoma (CHL). EBV-positive mucocutaneous ulcer is a specific type of immunosuppression-associated lymphoproliferative disorder due to iatrogenic immunosuppression or age-related immune senescence that often has Hodgkin-like features and typically a self-limited, indolent course {1018}. Iatrogenically related lymphomas occurring in treated haematological malignancies are not covered here {16}.

Epidemiology

The frequency of these disorders is not well known, and it is difficult to determine how many are directly related to the iatrogenic immunosuppression rather than the underlying disorder or chance alone. However, their prevalence may be on the rise due to the increased number of patients receiving immunosuppression therapy. It is likely that the risk and type of lymphoproliferative disorders that develop in this setting vary depending on the type of immunosuppressive agent, the degree of immune deficiency, and the nature of the underlying disorder being treated, such as rheumatoid arthritis, inflammatory bowel disease, psoriasis and psoriatic arthritis, systemic lupus erythematosus, and other autoimmune disorders {528, 1478,1583,2636}. Complicating interpretation are the increased risk of non-Hodgkin lymphomas and/or CHL in patients with various autoimmune disorders in many studies {1155,1156,2636,3681} and the fact that many of these patients are on more than one immunomodulator. Most epidemiological studies have also highlighted the importance of disease severity and the degree of inflammatory activity {219,1665}. Methotrexate was the first reported immunosuppressive agent associated with lymphoproliferative disorders in this setting {1910,3109,3498}, predominantly in patients being treated for rheumatoid arthritis. Most studies have failed to show a significant increased lymphoma risk in patients with rheumatoid arthritis treated with tumour necrosis factor (TNF) inhibitors or receiving other biological response modifiers, although cases of large B-cell lymphoma and classic Hodgkin lymphoma have been reported in these patients {471,504,2387,2389,2510, 2673,4352,4355}. Although there is concern that patients with Crohn disease or inflammatory bowel disease treated with infliximab and/or other TNF antagonists (adalimumab and etanercept) are at increased risk for hepatosplenic T-cell lymphoma (HSTL), other studies have shown no increased risk {1054}, or an increased incidence only when patients were also receiving a thiopurine or in patients only receiving a thiopurine {1626,2091,2426, 3414,3824,4355}.

Etiology

Although some of these other iatrogenic lymphoproliferative disorders are associated with EBV, like in many PTLDs, the frequency of EBV infection is very variable {1703,3498}. Overall, about 40% of lymphoproliferative disorders in rheumatoid arthritis patients treated with methotrexate are EBV-positive, with EBV detected more frequently in Hodgkin lymphoma (~80%) than in DLBCL (~25–60%) or other B-cell lymphoma types {1752,2065,2673,4403}. EBV is almost always found in polymorphic lymphoproliferative disorders and in lymphoproliferative disorders that have been reported to have Hodgkin-like features in this setting {1703,1752,3498}. EBV is not seen in HSTL. The degree and duration of immunosuppression likely plays a role in the development of EBV-positive lymphoproliferative disorders. However, the degree of inflammation and/or chronic antigenic stimulation as well as the patient's genetic background may also be important determinants of the risk and type of lymphoproliferative disorder {219, 220}. For example, patients with rheumatoid arthritis are estimated to have a 2-fold to 20-fold increased risk of lymphoma even in the absence of methotrexate therapy {220,1155,3989}, a risk which might be increased in patients receiving methotrexate or tacrolimus and may have an altered EBV–host balance {527,1583}. Spontaneous regression of these lymphoproliferative disorders in some cases after drug withdrawal underscores the putative pathogenic role of methotrexate or other immunosuppressive drugs in these lymphoproliferative disorders {219}.

Table 16.04 Characteristics of methotrexate-associated lymphoproliferative disorders (LPDs), including EBV-positive mucocutaneous ulcer (EBVMCU), in 274 cases with details reported.
Compiled from the literature; see text for references.

Type	Total	EBV	Extranodal	Regress
B-cell lymphomas				
DLBCL	159	45/108	66/90	35/115
Polymorphic/lymphoplasmacytic infiltrates	27	12/17	6/6	10/14
Follicular lymphoma	11	2/10	2/5	3/8
Burkitt lymphoma	3	1/3	0/1	0/3
MZL/MALT lymphoma	3	0/3	3/3	1/1
Lymphoplasmacytic lymphoma	2	0/2	–	0/2
CLL/SLL	1	0/1	0/1	0/1
MCL	1	0/1	–	–
T-cell LPDs/lymphomas				
PTCL	7	0/4	0/1	3/5
Extranodal NK/T-cell lymphoma, nasal type	2	2/2	2/2	1/1
Other T-cell LPD	1	1/1	1/1	1/1
Hodgkin lymphoma	42	19/23	2/19	11/25
Hodgkin-like lesions[a]	6	6/6	3/5	6/6
EBVMCU[b]	9	9/9	9/9	5/6
Total	274	97/190	94/143	76/188

CLL/SLL, chronic lymphocytic leukaemia/ small lymphocytic lymphoma; DLBCL, diffuse large B-cell lymphoma; MALT, mucosa-associated lymphoid tissue; MCL, mantle cell lymphoma; MZL, marginal zone lymphoma; PTCL, peripheral T-cell lymphoma.

[a] Likely correspond to EBV-positive B-cell LPDs with Hodgkin-like cells, and may include EBV-positive cases presenting in oropharynx, skin, or gastrointestinal tract, which might represent the newly recognized EBVMCU.
[b] Only cases designated as EBVMCU occurring in patients receiving methotrexate are included here.

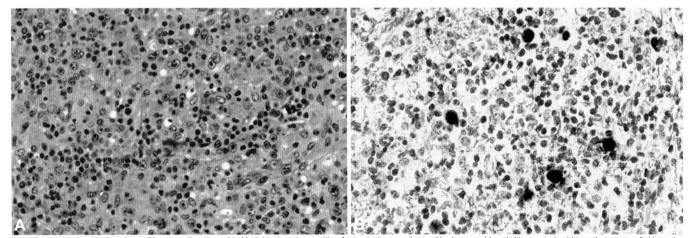

Fig. 16.23 Polymorphic lymphoproliferative disorder with Hodgkin lymphoma–like features in a patient with rheumatoid arthritis treated with methotrexate. **A** Note the polymorphous infiltrate, with lymphocytes, histiocytes, and Reed–Sternberg–like cells. **B** In situ hybridization for EBV-encoded small RNA (EBER) showing numerous positive large cells as well as many positive small lymphocytes.

Infliximab has been reported to induce clonal expansion of gamma delta T cells in patients with Crohn disease {1985}.

Localization

Of the cases reported in patients receiving methotrexate, 40–50% have been extranodal, occurring at sites such as the gastrointestinal tract, skin, liver and spleen, lung, kidney and adrenal gland, thyroid gland, bone marrow, CNS, gingiva, and soft tissue {74,1703,1787, 2065,2945,3498}. As is the case for HSTL in other settings, the spleen, liver, and bone marrow are the most common sites of involvement of HSTL in patients with Crohn disease receiving immunomodulators {2426,3414}.

Clinical features

The clinical features are the same as those seen in immunocompetent patients with similar-appearing lymphomas.

Microscopy

The distribution of histological types of iatrogenic lymphoproliferations in non-transplantation settings appears to differ from that seen in other immunodeficiency settings, with a probable increase in the frequency of Hodgkin lymphoma and lymphoid proliferations with Hodgkin-like features, such as EBV-positive mucocutaneous ulcer. Among patients treated with methotrexate, the reported cases are most commonly DLBCL (35–60%) and CHL (12–25%), with less frequent cases of follicular lymphoma (3–10%), Burkitt lymphoma, extranodal marginal zone lymphoma of mucosa-associated lymphoid tissue (MALT lymphoma), and peripheral T-cell lymphoma {1703,1752, 1908,2387,2509,3498}. Polymorphic or lymphoplasmacytic infiltrates resembling polymorphic PTLD have been described in as many as 20% of cases in this setting {1752}. Peripheral T-cell lymphomas occurring in this setting seem to have a common extranodal presentation, a cytotoxic profile, and may include extranodal NK/T-cell lymphomas {2079,3870}. Among CHLs, the mixed-cellularity subtype is more frequent than nodular sclerosis, with a significant proportion that cannot be further classified {2387}. Lesions containing Reed–Sternberg–like cells but not fulfilling the criteria for Hodgkin lymphoma, which in the past were referred to as Hodgkin-like lesions, have been reported {1911}, with some likely constitut-

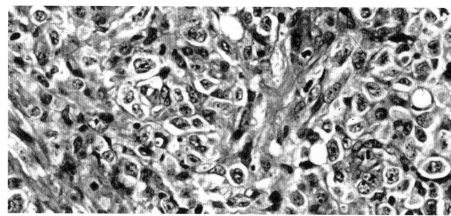

Fig. 16.24 EBV-positive large B-cell lymphoproliferation in a patient with rheumatoid arthritis treated with methotrexate. This lesion regressed following cessation of therapy.

ing the recently recognized EBV-positive mucocutaneous ulcer {1018} and others more closely resembling a polymorphic PTLD. HSTL in patients who have been treated with infliximab is indistinguishable from HSTL arising in immunocompetent or post-transplant patients.

Immunophenotype

The immunophenotype of the lymphoproliferative disorder does not appear to differ from that of the lymphomas in non-immunosuppressed hosts, which they resemble. Among methotrexate-associated DLBCLs, the majority have an activated–B-cell immunophenotype, especially EBV-positive cases. EBV-positive methotrexate-associated DLBCLs commonly express CD30 {2065,4403}. Immunophenotype is a useful tool in the distinction from lymphoproliferative disorders that may have some Hodgkin lymphoma–like features, but which should not be considered to represent CHL, the large cells most typically being CD20+/CD30+/CD15– and CD20–/CD30+/CD15+, respectively. EBV is variably positive, with type II latency (LMP1-positive and EBNA2-negative) more common than type III (LMP1-positive, EBNA2-positive) {1752,4403}.

Postulated normal counterpart

The postulated normal counterpart varies depending on the specific type of lymphoproliferative disorder.

Genetic profile

The genotype of these immunodeficiency-associated lymphoproliferative disorders does not appear to differ from those of lymphomas of similar histological types not associated with immunosuppression.

Prognosis and predictive factors

A significant proportion of patients with methotrexate-associated lymphoproliferative disorder have shown at least partial regression in response to drug withdrawal (Table 16.04). Although most responses have occurred in EBV-positive cases {1703,1752,1764,2387,3498,4403}, a proportion of EBV-negative cases also respond {1752,2065}. A variable proportion of DLBCLs (as many as ~40%) have regressed, while most require cytotoxic therapy. The proportion of polymorphic lymphoproliferative disorder patients with regression after withdrawal is higher. In recent studies of methotrexate-associated lymphoproliferative disorder in rheumatoid arthritis patients, the 5-year overall survival rate was >70%. Spontaneous regression following methotrexate withdrawal has been associated with EBV positivity and a non-DLBCL type of lymphoproliferative disorder, whereas patient age >70 years and DLBCL type are predictive of a shorter survival {1752, 4014}. Early lymphocyte recovery after methotrexate withdrawal may be predictive of good response {1764}. A moderate number of patients whose lymphoproliferative disorder initially regresses after discontinuation of methotrexate later relapse and then require chemotherapy {1703,1752}. Regression after discontinuation of drug seldom occurs in patients who develop lymphoproliferative disorder following the administration of TNF blockers. Like in individuals without overt immunodeficiency, cases of HSTL in patients treated with infliximab plus thiopurine have a very aggressive clinical course, with most survivors treated with allogeneic bone marrow transplantation {2426,3414}.

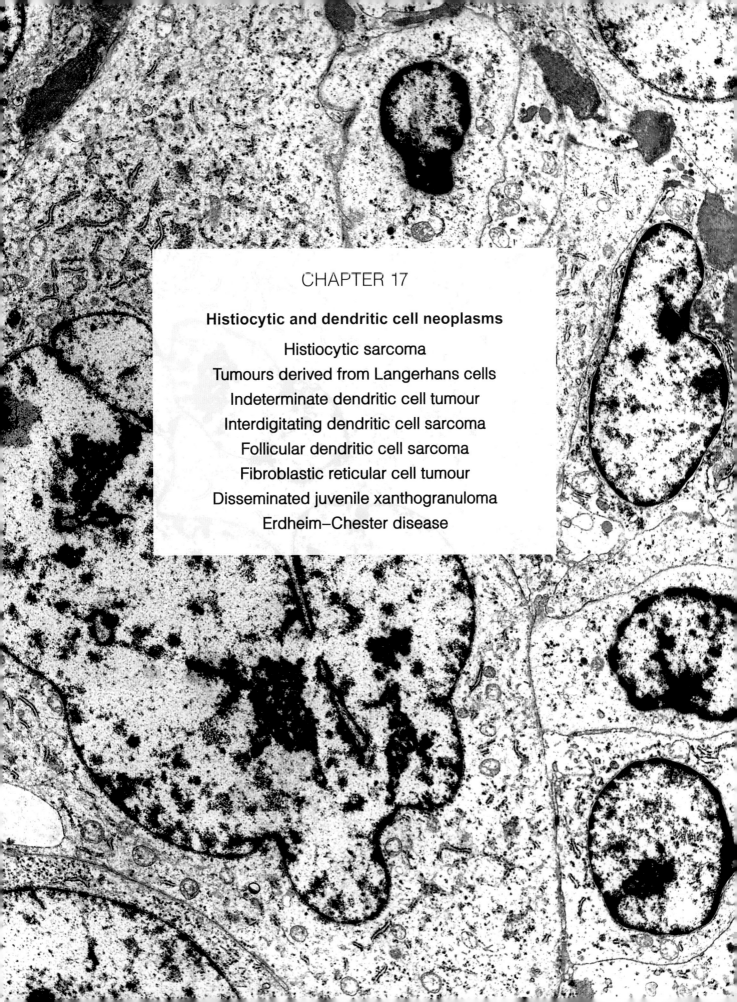

CHAPTER 17

Histiocytic and dendritic cell neoplasms

Histiocytic sarcoma

Tumours derived from Langerhans cells

Indeterminate dendritic cell tumour

Interdigitating dendritic cell sarcoma

Follicular dendritic cell sarcoma

Fibroblastic reticular cell tumour

Disseminated juvenile xanthogranuloma

Erdheim–Chester disease

Histiocytic and dendritic cell neoplasms

Introduction

Pileri S.A.
Jaffe R.
Facchetti F.
Jones D.M.
Jaffe E.S.

Definition

Histiocytic neoplasms are derived from mononuclear phagocytes (macrophages and dendritic cells) or histiocytes. Dendritic cell tumours are related to several lineages of accessory antigen-presenting cells (dendritic cells) that have a role in phagocytosis, processing, and presentation of antigen to lymphoid cells.

Epidemiology

Tumours of histiocytes are among the rarest tumours affecting lymphoid tissues, probably accounting for < 1% of tumours presenting in the lymph nodes or soft tissue {1165,3180}. Because several of these tumour types were poorly recognized until recently, their true incidence remains to be determined. Historically, some large cell lymphomas of B-cell or T-cell type were thought to be histiocytic or reticulum cell sarcomas on purely morphological grounds, but only a small number have proven to be of true macrophage or dendritic cell origin. Some of the regulatory disorders, such as macrophage activation and haemophagocytic syndromes, can have large numbers of histiocytes, but these are non-neoplastic. No sex, racial, or geographical predilection has been described (Table 17.01).

Histogenesis

The cellular counterparts of this group of neoplasms consist of myeloid-derived macrophages, myeloid-derived dendritic cells, and stromal-derived dendritic cells. The myeloid-derived macrophages and dendritic cells constitute divergent lines of differentiation from bone marrow precursors, although transdifferentiation or hybrid differentiation states likely occur. Histiocytic and dendritic cell neoplasms tend to reproduce the morphological, phenotypic, and ultrastructural charac-

teristics of terminally differentiated elements. In line with this, blastic plasmacytoid dendritic cell (PDC) neoplasm is excluded from this section on histiocytic and dendritic cell neoplasms, and is discussed after the acute myeloid leukaemias and related precursor neoplasms, because it stems from a cell that acquires terminal differentiation and dendritic appearance following activation (see Chapter 9, *Blastic plasmacytoid dendritic cell neoplasm, p. 173*).

Intriguingly, during the past few years, several publications have highlighted the fact that, irrespective of their supposed normal counterparts (myeloid-derived macrophages or myeloid-derived dendritic cells), some of these neoplasms are associated with or preceded by a malignant lymphoma (e.g. follicular lymphoma, chronic lymphocytic leukaemia, B-lymphoblastic leukaemia/lymphoma or T-lymphoblastic leukaemia/lymphoma, and peripheral T-cell lymphoma) {678, 859,860,1172,3313,3633}. Under these

circumstances, they carry the same TR or IG rearrangements and chromosomal aberrations as lymphoid neoplasms, consistent with transdifferentiation {678, 859,860,1172,3313,3633}. The histiocytic and lymphoid neoplasm may share a common progenitor {479}, but one that has already undergone IG rearrangement. To date, neither comprehensive gene expression profiling nor next-generation sequencing studies have been carried out, with the exception of studies based on canine models {399} and small series of follicular dendritic cell (FDC) sarcomas {1460,1569A,2184A,2383A}. A next generation sequencing study of 13 FDC sarcomas revealed recurrent loss-of-function alterations in tumour suppressor genes involved in the negative regulation of NF-kappaB activation (38% of cases) and cell-cycle progression (31% of cases) {1460}. The possible occurrence of BRAF V600E mutation has been reported in the setting of histiocytic sarcoma, Langerhans cell histiocytosis,

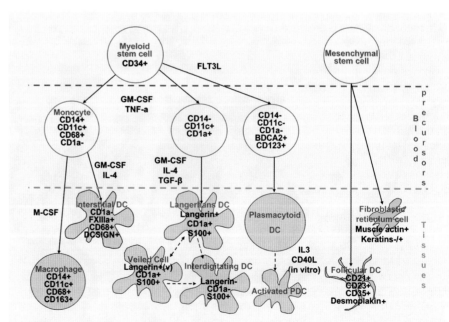

Fig. 17.01 Schematic diagram of the origin of histiocytic and dendritic cells. Macrophages and dendritic cells (DCs; antigen-presenting cells) are derived from a common bone marrow precursor. In contrast, follicular dendritic cells are thought to be of non-haematopoietic origin.

+, most (if not all) cells positive; –, all cells negative; –/+, a minority of cells positive; CLA, CD45 (note: monocytes are CD45+); v, variable intensity.

FDC sarcoma, and disseminated juvenile xanthogranuloma {1386}. In Erdheim–Chester disease, activating mutations in MAPK pathway genes, most notably BRAF V600E, as well as *NRAS* mutation, can be detected. Recurrent mutations in the PI3K pathway genes have also been described {71}.

Monocytes, macrophages, and histiocytes

Metchnikoff, considered the father of the macrophage, coined the term 'phagocytosis' in 1883, postulating a central role for the process in the body's innate defence against infection {1412,2648}. The histiocytes/macrophages are derived from bone marrow–derived monocytes. Following migration/maturation in tissues, they participate in the innate response with proinflammatory and anti-inflammatory cytokine effects, as well as in particulate removal and tissue reconstitution {1412,1413}. They are derived largely from the circulating peripheral blood monocyte pool that migrates through blood vessel walls to reach its site of action, but local proliferation also contributes {3303}. Histiocytic tumours are closely related to the monocytic tumours from which their precursors are derived. The distinction between a leukaemic infiltrate of monocytic origin and histiocytic sarcoma can sometimes be difficult on morphological grounds alone.

Macrophages display phagocytosis under some conditions of activation; at this stage, there is heightened expression of lysosomal enzymes that can be demonstrated by histochemistry, including non-specific esterases and acid phosphatase. Phagocytic activity is not a prominent feature of histiocytic malignancy but is a cardinal feature of the haemophagocytic syndromes. The haemophagocytic macrophage activation syndromes are an important group of non-neoplastic proliferative disorders that need to be differentiated from true histiocytic neoplasms, and are far more common. The haemophagocytic syndromes are the result of genetic or acquired disorders in the regulation of macrophage activation. The familial haemophagocytic lymphohistiocytosis is due to genetically determined inability to regulate macrophage killing by NK and/or T cells due to mutations in perforin or in its packaging, export, or release. Acquired or secondary causes of the haemophagocytic macrophage

activation syndromes follow certain infections, most notably by EBV and a wide variety of other infectious agents, as well as some malignancies, rheumatic disorders, and multiorgan failure {1834}. The characteristic cytopenias of the haemophagocytic syndromes are most likely

due to bone marrow suppression by the cytokine storm, because the bone marrow is often hypercellular at the outset.

Myeloid-derived dendritic cells

Dendritic cells or antigen-presenting cells are found in various sites and at different

Table 17.01 True histiocytic malignancy: a vanishing diagnosis

Original diagnosis	Currently considered
Histiocytic lymphoma, nodular and diffuse	Diffuse large B-cell lymphoma
	Follicular lymphoma, grade 3
	Peripheral T-cell lymphoma
	Histiocyte-rich variants of B-cell, T-cell, and Hodgkin lymphomas
	Anaplastic large cell lymphoma
Histiocytic medullary reticulosis	Haemophagocytic syndromes
Malignant histiocytosis	Anaplastic large cell lymphoma
	Haemophagocytic syndromes
Regressing atypical histiocytosis	Primary cutaneous CD30+ T-cell lymphoproliferative disorders
Intestinal malignant histiocytosis	Enteropathy associated T-cell lymphoma
Histiocytic cytopathic panniculitis	Subcutaneous panniculitis-like T-cell lymphoma with haemophagocytosis

Table 17.02 Immunophenotypic markers of non-neoplastic macrophages and dendritic cells. Expression is semi-quantitatively graded as 0 (−), low or varies with cell activity (−/+ and +/−), present (+), or high (++)

Marker	LC	IDC	FDC	PDC	Mø	DIDC
MHC class II	+c	++s	−	+	+	+/−
Fc receptors[a]	−	−	+	−	+	−
CD1a	++	−	−	−	−	−
CD4	+	+	+	+	+	+/−
CD21	−	−	++	−	−	−
CD35	−	−	++	−	−	−
CD68	+/−	+/−	−	++	++	+
CD123	−	−	−	++	−	−
CD163	−	−	−	−	++	−
Factor XIIIa	−	−	+/−	−	−/+	++
Fascin	−	++	+/++	−	−/+	+
Langerin	++	−	−	−	−	−
Lysozyme	+/−	−	−	−	+	−
S100	++	++	+/−	−	+/−	+/−
TCL1	−	−	−	+	−	−

c, Cytoplasmic; DIDC, dermal/interstitial dendritic cell; FDC, follicular dendritic cell; IDC, interdigitating dendritic cell; LC, Langerhans cell; MHC, major histocompatibility complex; Mø, macrophage; PDC, plasmacytoid dendritic cell; s, surface.

[a] Fc IgG receptors (these include CD16, CD32, and CD64 on some cells).

states of activation, and no single marker identifies all dendritic cell subsets {244, 3303,3790}. Langerhans cells are specialized dendritic cells in mucosal sites and skin that upon activation become specialized for antigen presentation to T cells, and then migrate to the lymph node through lymphatics. Lymph nodes also contain a paracortical dendritic cell type, the interdigitating dendritic cell, which may be derived in part from the Langerhans cell {1323}. This classic dendritic cell lineage is believed to give rise to Langerhans cell histiocytosis/sarcoma and to interdigitating dendritic cell sarcoma. A third, poorly defined subset of dendritic cells, dermal/interstitial dendritic cells, are found in the soft tissue, dermis, and most organs, and can be increased in some inflammatory states {244}.

PDCs (also known as plasmacytoid monocytes) are a distinct lineage of dendritic cells, which are believed to give rise to the blastic PDC neoplasm {1615}. The histogenetic origins of PDCs are controversial but are likely of myelomonocytic lineage. Interferon alpha–producing PDC precursors, which only acquire a dendritic appearance in cell culture, circulate in the peripheral blood and have the capacity to enter lymph nodes and tissue through high endothelial venules {2373}.

Stromal-derived dendritic cell types

FDCs, which are resident within primary and secondary B-cell follicles, trap and present antigen to B cells. FDCs can store antigen on the cell surface as immune complexes for long periods of time {4139}. FDCs appear to be closely related to bone marrow stromal progenitors with features of myofibroblasts {2436}. They are a non-migrating population that forms a stable meshwork within the follicle via cell-to-cell attachments and desmosomes.

Fibroblastic reticular cells are involved in maintenance of lymphoid integrity and in production and transport of cytokines and other mediators. In lymph nodes, they ensheath the postcapillary venules {1955,4165}. They are of mesenchymal origin and express SMA. Hyperplasia of fibroblastic reticular cells (i.e. stromal overgrowth) may be seen in Castleman disease {1808,2342}, and tumours of fibroblastic reticular cells arise in lymph nodes and have features of myofibroblastic tumours and closely related neoplasms {104}.

Prognosis and predictive factors

Because there are few phenotypic markers unique for dendritic cells, macrophages, or histiocytes, investigators should use a panel appropriate to the cell in question (Table 17.02, p. 467) and rigorously exclude other cell lineages (i.e. T-cell, B-cell, and NK-cell lineages, but also stromal, melanocytic, and epithelial lineages) by immunophenotypic and molecular means. It is also worth mentioning that some leukaemias and anaplastic large cell lymphomas can be accompanied in lymph nodes by an exuberant histiocytic response that may obscure the neoplastic cells.

Consistent with their rarity, the treatment of histiocytic and dendritic cell neoplasms is extremely variable, no specific trials being available {859,860,1021}. Excisional biopsies should be performed whenever possible, needle aspirates being indeed proscribed. Accurate staging is mandatory, because the distinction between localized and systemic forms impacts therapeutic decisions. Localized forms are usually surgically resected; the utility of radiotherapy and/or chemotherapy as adjuvant is debated {859,860, 1021}. The prognosis is relatively favourable, even in cases of relapse, which has been reported in at least one quarter of patients {859,860,1021}. In contrast, widespread disease requires chemotherapy and has a poor prognosis overall {859,860,1021}.

Histiocytic sarcoma

Weiss L.M.
Pileri S.A.
Chan J.K.C.
Fletcher C.D.M.

Definition

Histiocytic sarcoma is a malignant proliferation of cells showing morphological and immunophenotypic features of mature tissue histiocytes. Neoplastic proliferations associated with acute monocytic leukaemia are excluded.

ICD-O code   9755/3

Synonym

True histiocytic lymphoma (obsolete)

Epidemiology

Histiocytic sarcoma is a rare neoplasm, with only limited numbers of reported series of bona fide cases {806,860,1540, 1688,1909,3180,4216}. There is a wide patient age range, from infancy to old age; however, most cases occur in adults (median patient age: 52 years) {1688,3180, 4216}. A male predilection is found in some studies {3180,4216} but not others {1688}. Some cases are associated with prior or metachronous low-grade lymphoma, usually follicular lymphoma, but also chronic lymphocytic leukaemia/small lymphocytic lymphoma {1172,3633}.

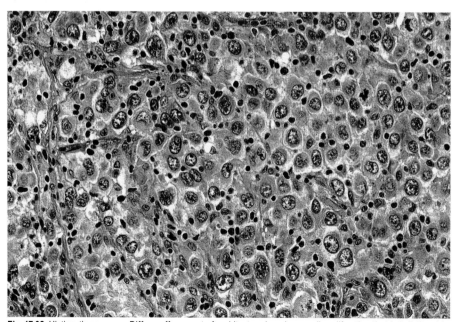

Fig. 17.02 Histiocytic sarcoma. Diffuse effacement of architecture by a large-cell proliferation that is indistinguishable from a diffuse large B-cell lymphoma by conventional histopathology.

Etiology

The etiology is unknown. A subset of cases occur in patients with mediastinal germ cell tumours, most commonly malignant teratoma, with or without a yolk sac tumour component {952}. Because teratocarcinoma cells may differentiate along haematopoietic lines in vitro {844}, histiocytic neoplasms may arise from pluripotent germ cells. Other cases may be associated with malignant lymphoma, either preceding or subsequent, or with myelodysplasia and leukaemia {1172, 1176,3180,4486}.

Localization

Most cases present in extranodal sites {1688,3180,4216}, most commonly the intestinal tract, skin, and soft tissue. Others present with lymphadenopathy. Rare patients have a systemic presentation, with multiple sites of involvement, sometimes referred to as malignant histiocytosis {585,3180,4331}.

Clinical features

Patients may present with a solitary mass, but systemic symptoms, such as fever and weight loss, are relatively common {1688,3180,4216}. Skin manifestations may range from a benign-appearing rash to solitary lesions to innumerable tumours on the trunk and extremities. Patients with intestinal lesions often present with intestinal obstruction. Hepatosplenomegaly and associated pancytopenia may occur. The bone may show lytic lesions {1688, 3180,4216}.

Microscopy

The tumour consists of a diffuse non-cohesive proliferation of large cells (>20 μm), but a sinusoidal distribution may be seen in the lymph nodes, liver, and spleen. The proliferating cells may be monomorphic or (more commonly) pleomorphic. The individual neoplastic

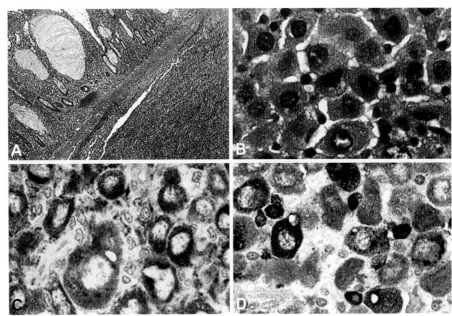

Fig. 17.03 Histiocytic sarcoma. **A** Histiocytic sarcoma involving the bowel. **B** Note the abundant cytoplasm, which stains strongly for CD68 (**C**) and lysozyme (**D**).

cells are usually large and round to oval in shape; however, focal areas of spindling (sarcomatoid areas) may be observed. The cytoplasm is usually abundant and eosinophilic, often with some fine vacuoles. Haemophagocytosis occurs occasionally in the neoplastic cells. The nuclei are generally large, round to oval or irregularly folded, and often eccentrically placed; large multinucleated forms are commonly seen. The chromatin pattern is usually vesicular, and atypia varies from mild to marked. Immunostaining is essential for distinction from other large cell neoplasms, such as large cell lymphoma, melanoma, and carcinoma. A variable number of reactive cells may be seen, including small lymphocytes, plasma cells, benign histiocytes, and eosinophils. Sometimes the neoplastic cells are obscured by a heavy inflammatory infiltrate including many neutrophils, mimicking an inflammatory lesion; this

feature is particularly common in histiocytic sarcoma involving the CNS {699}.

Ultrastructure

The neoplastic cells show abundant cytoplasm with numerous lysosomes. Birbeck granules and cellular junctions are not seen.

Immunophenotype

By definition, there is expression of one or more histiocytic markers, including CD163, CD68 (KP1 and PGM1), and lysozyme, with typical absence of Langerhans cell (CD1a, langerin), follicular dendritic cell (CD21, CD35), and myeloid cell (CD13, MPO) markers {1688,3180,4216}. Both CD68 and lysozyme show granular cytoplasmic staining. The lysozyme staining is accentuated in the Golgi region. CD163 staining is in the cell membrane and/or cytoplasm. Rarely, weak expression of CD15 occurs {3180}. In addition,

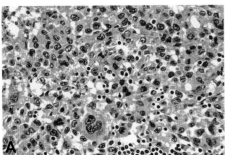 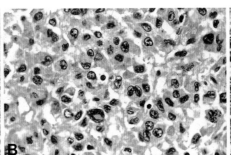 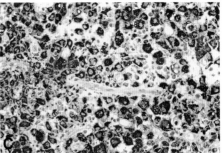

Fig. 17.04 Histiocytic sarcoma. **A** Note the multinucleated tumour cell. **B** The cytoplasm is relatively abundant, but the neoplasm is difficult to distinguish from a large B-cell lymphoma without immunohistochemical studies. **C** Diffuse staining for the lysosomal marker CD68.

CD45, CD45RO, and HLA-DR are usually positive. There may be expression of S100 protein, but this is usually weak and focal {3180}. There is no positivity for specific B-cell and T-cell markers. CD4 is often positive with cytoplasmic staining. These tumours are devoid of HMB45, EMA, and keratin. The Ki-67 proliferation index is variable {3180}.

Postulated normal counterpart

A mature tissue histiocyte

Genetic profile

A subset of cases of histiocytic sarcoma have clonal IG rearrangements {680}, particularly when there is an association with low-grade B-cell lymphoma, most likely constituting examples of transdifferentiation {1540,3294,4216}. In cases associated with t(14;18)-positive follicular lymphoma, identical chromosomal breakpoints in the BCL2 locus may be present in both neoplasms {1172}. In one study, 5 of 8 cases were found to have BRAF V600E mutations {1386}, although another study found the mutation to be absent in 3 cases {1553}. The rare cases arising in mediastinal germ cell tumour show isochromosome 12p, identical to the genetic change in the germ cell tumour {2865}.

Prognosis and predictive factors

Histiocytic sarcoma is usually an aggressive neoplasm, with poor response to therapy, although some exceptions have been reported {1688}. Most patients (60–80%) die of progressive disease, reflecting the high clinical stage at presentation (stage III/IV) in the majority (70%) of patients {3180,4216}. Patients with clinically localized disease and small primary tumours have a more favourable long-term outcome {1688,3180}.

Tumours derived from Langerhans cells

Weiss L.M.
Jaffe R.
Facchetti F.

Definition

Tumours derived from Langerhans cells (LCs) are divided into two main subgroups, according to the degree of cytological atypia and clinical aggressiveness: LC histiocytosis and LC sarcoma. Both subgroups maintain the phenotypic profile and ultrastructural features of LCs. Rare cases can be difficult to assign to one category or the other; these cases require further clinicopathological studies to clarify their nature.

Langerhans cell histiocytosis

Definition

Langerhans cell histiocytosis (LCH) is a clonal neoplastic proliferation of Langerhans-type cells that express CD1a, langerin, and S100 protein and show Birbeck granules by ultrastructural examination.

ICD-O codes

LCH, NOS	9751/1
LCH, monostotic	9751/1

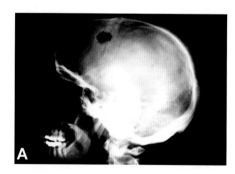

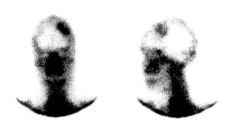

Fig. 17.05 Langerhans cell histiocytosis.
A Radiograph from a patient with eosinophilic granuloma of bone illustrates a discrete punched-out lesion. **B** Gallium scan shows high uptake in lytic bone lesion.

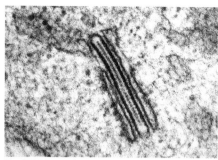

Fig. 17.06 Langerhans cell histiocytosis. Ultrastructure shows a typical Birbeck granule.

LCH, polystotic	9751/1
LCH, disseminated	9751/3

Synonyms

Langerhans cell granulomatosis; solitary lesion: histiocytosis X, eosinophilic granuloma (obsolete); multiple lesions: Hand–Schüller–Christian disease (obsolete); cases with disseminated or visceral involvement: Letterer–Siwe disease (obsolete); Langerhans cell histiocytosis, unifocal (9752/3) (obsolete); Langerhans cell histiocytosis, multifocal (9753/3) (obsolete); Langerhans cell histiocytosis, disseminated (9754/3) (obsolete)

Epidemiology

The annual incidence is about 5 cases per 1 million population, with most cases occurring in childhood. There is a male predilection, with a male-to-female ratio of 3.7:1 {3180}. The disease is more common in White populations of northern European descent and rare in Black populations. Primary LCH of the lung is almost always a disease of smokers {857}. Rare cases may be associated with follicular lymphoma {4302}.

Etiology

An IL1 loop model has been proposed for the pathogenesis, based on the finding of high levels of the tyrosine phosphatase SH1 in lesional tissues and increased levels of IL17A in peripheral blood and lesional tissues, particularly in patients with multiorgan disease {2787}.

Localization

The disease can be localized to a single site, can occur in multiple sites within a single system (usually bone), or can be more disseminated and multisystem {2668,4009}. The dominant sites of involvement in the solitary form are bone and adjacent soft tissue (skull, femur, vertebra, pelvic bones, and ribs) and,

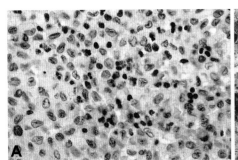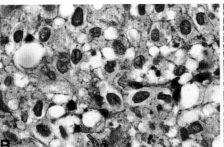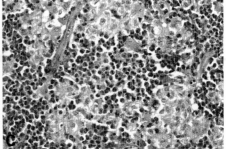

Fig. 17.07 Langerhans cell (LC) histiocytosis. **A** Numerous LCs are seen, with scattered eosinophils and small lymphocytes. **B** Note the typical cytological features of LCs, with many nuclei containing linear grooves. **C** Eosinophilic microabscess.

less commonly, lymph node, skin, and lung. Multifocal lesions are largely confined to bone and adjacent soft tissue. In multisystem disease, the skin, bone, liver, spleen, and bone marrow are the preferential sites of involvement. The gonads and kidney appear to be spared even in disseminated cases.

Clinical features

Patients with unifocal disease are usually older children or adults who most commonly present with a lytic bone lesion eroding the cortex. Solitary lesions at other sites present as mass lesions or enlarged lymph nodes. Patients with unisystem multifocal disease are usually young children who present with multiple or sequential destructive bone lesions, often associated with adjacent soft tissue masses. Skull and mandibular involvement is common. Diabetes insipidus follows cranial involvement. Patients with multisystem involvement are infants who present with fever, cytopenias, skin and bone lesions, and hepatosplenomegaly {142,2669}. Pulmonary disease in childhood is clinically variable {2927}.

There is an association between LCH and T-lymphoblastic leukaemia, with the leukaemia-associated TR gene rearrangement present in the LCH cells; this has been considered a transdifferentiation phenomenon {1173}.

Microscopy

The key feature is the LCH cells. These are oval; about 10–15 μm; and recognized by their grooved, folded, indented, or lobed nuclei with fine chromatin, inconspicuous nucleoli, and thin nuclear membranes. Nuclear atypia is minimal, but mitotic activity is variable and can be high without atypical forms. The cytoplasm is moderately abundant and slightly eosinophilic. Unlike epidermal Langerhans cells or dermal perivascular cells, LCH cells are oval in shape and devoid of dendritic cell processes. The characteristic milieu includes a variable number of eosinophils, histiocytes (both multinucleated LCH forms and osteoclast-type cells, especially in bone), neutrophils, and small lymphocytes. Plasma cells are usually sparse. Occasionally, eosinophilic abscesses with central necrosis, rich in Charcot–Leyden crystals, may be found. In early lesions, LCH cells predominate, along with eosinophils and neutrophils. In late lesions, the LCH cells are decreased in number, with increased foamy macrophages and fibrosis.

Involved lymph nodes have a sinus pattern with secondary infiltration of the paracortex. Spleen shows nodular red pulp involvement. Liver involvement has strong preference for intrahepatic biliary involvement with progressive sclerosing cholangitis. Bone marrow biopsy is preferred to aspiration for documentation of bone marrow involvement {2670}.

Large clusters or sheets of LCH cells accompanied by eosinophils can be found within other lesions (lymphomas and sarcomas). It remains to be determined whether these constitute a local reactive phenomenon or a transdifferentiation process {752}.

Ultrastructure

The ultrastructural hallmark is the cytoplasmic Birbeck granules, whose presence can be confirmed by langerin expression. The Birbeck granule has a tennis-racket shape, and is 200–400 nm long and 33 nm wide, with a zipper-like appearance.

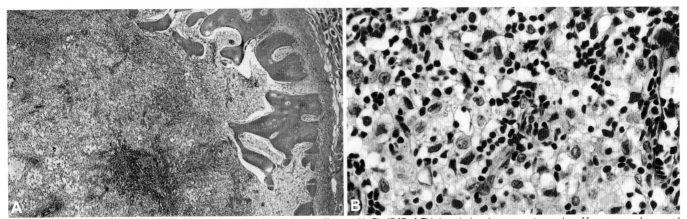

Fig. 17.08 Langerhans cell histiocytosis, at a later stage of evolution than the case illustrated in Fig 17.07. **A** This bony lesion shows a greater number of foamy macrophages and lymphocytes. **B** A greater number of foamy macrophages and lymphocytes are present, although nuclei with typical grooves are still discernible.

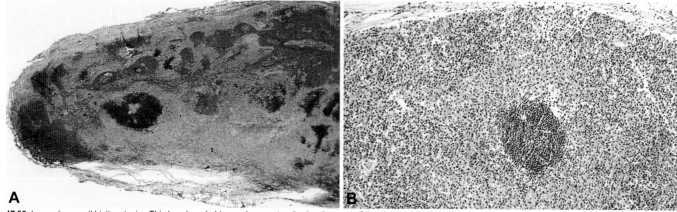

17.09 Langerhans cell histiocytosis. This lymph node biopsy shows extensive involvement of the sinuses (**A**) and paracortical regions (**B**).

Immunophenotype

LCH consistently expresses CD1a, langerin (also called CD207), and S100 protein {714,2110}. Langerin and CD1a staining may be particularly useful in detecting bone marrow involvement {2017}. In addition, the cells are positive for vimentin, CD68, and HLA-DR. CD45 expression and lysozyme content is low. B-cell and T-cell lineage markers (except for CD4), CD30, and follicular dendritic cell markers are absent. The Ki-67 proliferation index is highly variable {3180}. Expression of PDL1 is seen in many cases {1308}.

Postulated normal counterpart

A mature Langerhans cell

Genetic profile

LCH has been shown to be clonal by X-linked androgen receptor gene (HUMARA) assay, except in some adult pulmonary lesions {4330,4449, 4451}. About 30% of cases have detectable clonal IGH, IGK, or TR rearrangements, including some cases with both T-cell and B-cell gene rearrangements {681}. Approximately 50% of cases harbour *BRAF* V600E mutation {215,489}. *BRAF* V600E mutation has also been identified in 28% of pulmonary cases, suggesting that at least many of these cases constitute a clonal proliferation {3381}. In addition, about 25% of cases are associated with somatic *MAP2K1* mutations, almost always occurring in

BRAF germline cases {469,2852}. Other *BRAF* germline cases may have somatic *ARAF* mutations {2851}.

Genetic susceptibility

Familial clustering has shown a high concordance rate for identical twins but not dizygotic twins, and no vertical inheritance {145}. Rare familial cases are reported {141,143}. There is a suggestion that interferon gamma and IL4 polymorphisms affect susceptibility to LCH and might be responsible for some of the clinical variation {893}.

Prognosis and predictive factors

The clinical course is related to staging of the disease at presentation, with ≥99% survival for unifocal disease and 66% mortality for young children with multisystem involvement who do not respond promptly to therapy {1268,2668,4009}. Involvement of the bone marrow, liver, or lung is considered a high-risk factor {2668,4009}. Progression from initial focal disease to multisystem involvement can occur, most commonly in infants. Patient age, per se, is a less important indicator than is extent of disease {2668, 4009}. *BRAF* V600E mutation does not seem to affect prognosis {2612}. Systemic and (rarely) multifocal disease can be complicated by haemophagocytic syndrome {1166}.

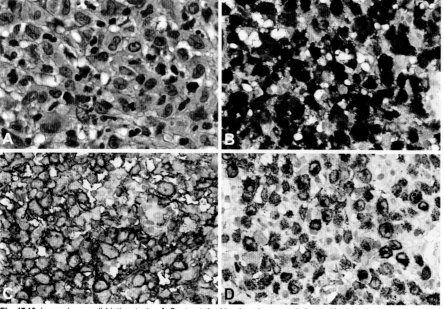

Fig. 17.10 Langerhans cell histiocytosis. **A** Contrast the bland nuclear morphology with that of the sarcoma (see Figs. 17.11 and 17.12). **B** Staining is both nuclear and cytoplasmic with S100. **C** CD1a uniformly stains the cell surface, with a perinuclear dot. **D** Langerin staining is more granular and cytoplasmic.

Langerhans cell sarcoma

Definition
Langerhans cell (LC) sarcoma is a high-grade neoplasm with overtly malignant cytological features and the LC phenotype.

ICD-O code
9756/3

Epidemiology
LC sarcoma is rare {327,401,3180}, and almost all reported cases are in adults. The median patient age is 41 years (range: 10–72 years). Rare cases may be associated with follicular lymphoma {4302}.

Etiology
Merkel cell polyomavirus sequences have been identified in a subset of cases {2786}.

Localization
The skin and underlying soft tissue are the most common sites of involvement. Multiorgan involvement can affect the lymph nodes, lung, liver, spleen, and bone {401,1202,3180}.

Clinical features
Most cases are extranodal (involving skin and bone) and multifocal; high-stage (III–IV) disease is seen in 44%. Only 22% of cases are primarily nodal. Hepatosplenomegaly is noted in 22% and pancytopenia in 11%.

Microscopy
The most prominent feature is the overtly malignant cytology of a pleomorphic tumour, and only the phenotype and/or ultrastructure reveal the LC derivation.

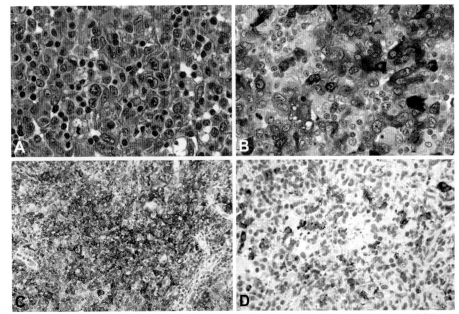

Fig. 17.11 Langerhans cell (LC) sarcoma. **A** Nuclear pleomorphism is not a feature of LC histiocytosis (LCH), but should raise the possibility of malignancy. **B** S100 is widely represented, nuclear and cytoplasmic, but variable in intensity. **C** Lesional cells express surface CD1a more variable than in LCH. **D** Langerin is demonstrable, though not as much as in LCH in this example.

Chromatin is clumped and nucleoli are conspicuous. Some cells may have the complex grooves of the LC histiocytosis cell, a key clue to the diagnosis. The mitotic rate is high, usually >50 mitoses per 10 high-power fields. Rare eosinophils may be admixed.

Ultrastructure
Birbeck granules are present, whereas desmosomes/junctional specializations are absent {3180}.

Immunophenotype
The immunophenotype is identical to that of LC histiocytosis, although staining for individual markers can be focal.

Postulated normal counterpart
A mature Langerhans cell

Genetic profile
At least one case has been found to harbour the *BRAF* V600E mutation {678}.

Prognosis and predictive factors
LC sarcoma is an aggressive, high-grade malignancy, with >50% mortality from progressive disease.

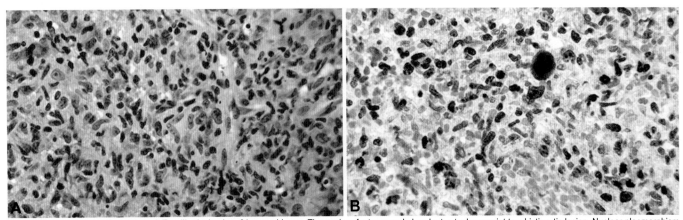

Fig. 17.12 Langerhans cell sarcoma. **A** Tonsillar lesion in a 31-year-old man. The nuclear features and abundant cytoplasm point to a histiocytic lesion. Nuclear pleomorphism and atypical mitoses indicate high-grade disease. **B** The Ki-67 proliferation index is high.

Indeterminate dendritic cell tumour

Weiss L.M.
Chan J.K.C.
Fletcher C.D.M.

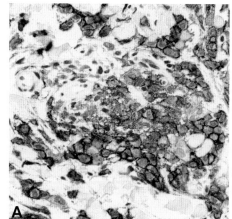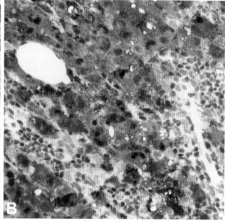

Fig. 17.13 Indeterminate dendritic cell tumour. The lesion is positive for CD1a (**A**) and S100 protein (**B**).

Definition

Indeterminate dendritic cell tumour, also known as indeterminate cell histiocytosis, is a neoplastic proliferation of spindled to ovoid cells with phenotypic features similar to those of normal indeterminate cells, the alleged precursor cells of Langerhans cells. These neoplasms are extraordinarily rare {104,360,412,651,2076, 3407,3672,4160,4174,4363,4374}. There may be an association with low-grade B-cell lymphoma {4160}.

ICD-O code   9757/3

Localization

Patients typically present with one or (more commonly) multiple generalized papules, nodules, or plaques on the skin. Less often, primary lymph node or splenic disease has been reported.

Clinical features

Systemic symptoms are usually not present.

Microscopy

The lesions are usually based in the dermis, but may extend into the subcutaneous fat. The infiltrate is diffuse, consisting of cells resembling Langerhans cells, with irregular nuclear grooves and clefts. Cytoplasm is typically abundant

and usually eosinophilic. Multinucleated giant cells may be present. In some cases, there may be spindling of the cells. The mitotic rate varies widely from case to case. An accompanying eosinophilic infiltrate is usually not present.

Ultrastructure

By definition, these cells lack Birbeck granules on ultrastructural examination. There can be complex interdigitating cell processes, but desmosomes are lacking.

Immunophenotype

The proliferating cells consistently express S100 protein and CD1a. Langerin is negative. They are negative for specific B-cell and T-cell markers, CD30, the histiocytic marker CD163, and the follicular dendritic cell markers CD21, CD23, and CD35. They are variably positive for CD45, CD68, lysozyme, and CD4. The Ki-67 proliferation index is highly variable.

Cell of origin

Normal indeterminate cells, the postulated precursors of Langerhans cells

Genetic profile

One case has been shown to be clonal by human androgen receptor gene assay {4374}. One case has been shown to harbour *BRAF* V600E mutation {2916}.

Prognosis and predictive factors

The clinical course has been highly variable, ranging from spontaneous regression to rapid progression. There are no known prognostic factors. One case was associated with the development of acute myeloid leukaemia {4174}.

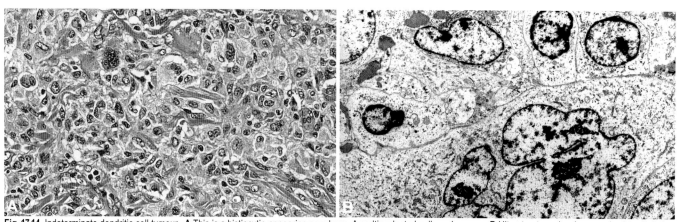

Fig. 17.14 Indeterminate dendritic cell tumour. **A** This is a histiocytic-appearing neoplasm. A multinucleated cell can be seen. **B** Ultrastructure showing complex interdigitating processes, but no Birbeck granules.

Interdigitating dendritic cell sarcoma

Weiss L.M.
Chan J.K.C.

Definition
Interdigitating dendritic cell (IDC) sarcoma is a neoplastic proliferation of spindle to ovoid cells with phenotypic features similar to those of IDCs.

ICD-O code   9757/3

Synonym
Interdigitating dendritic cell tumour

Epidemiology
IDC sarcoma is an extremely rare neoplasm, with most studies constituting single case reports or very small series {104, 1179, 2411, 2659, 2812, 2813, 3180, 3431, 4286}. The largest series to date have consisted of 4 cases {1269, 3180, 3186}. The reported cases have occurred predominantly in adults, although one paediatric series has been reported {3186}. There is a slight male predominance. Occasional cases have been associated with low-grade B-cell lymphoma, and rare cases have been associated with T-cell lymphoma {1172, 1269}.

Localization
The presentation can vary widely. Solitary lymph node involvement is most common, but extranodal presentations, in particular in the skin and soft tissue, have also been reported.

Clinical features
Patients usually present with an asymptomatic mass, although systemic symptoms, such as fatigue, fever, and night sweats, have been reported. Rarely, there may be generalized lymphadenopathy, splenomegaly, or hepatomegaly.

Microscopy
The lesional tissue in lymph nodes is present in a paracortical distribution with residual follicles. The neoplastic proliferation usually forms fascicles, a storiform pattern, and whorls of spindled to ovoid cells. Sheets of round cells are occasionally found. The cytoplasm of the neoplastic cells is usually abundant and slightly eosinophilic, and often has an indistinct border. The nuclei also appear spindled

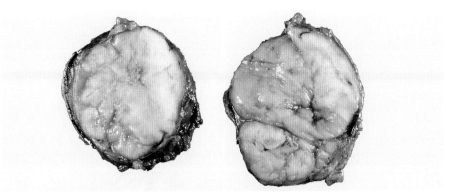

Fig. 17.15 Interdigitating dendritic cell sarcoma. The tumour is vaguely lobular in lymph node and firm in consistency.

to ovoid, and may show indentations; occasional multinucleated cells may be seen. The chromatin is often vesicular, with small to large, distinct nucleoli. Cytological atypia varies from case to case, although the mitotic rate is usually low (<5 mitoses per 10 high-power fields). Necrosis is usually not present. There are often numerous admixed lymphocytes, and less commonly, plasma cells. The histological appearance is sometimes indistinguishable from that of a follicular dendritic cell sarcoma, and phenotyping is necessary for precise diagnosis.

Ultrastructure
The neoplastic cells show complex interdigitating cell processes, but well-formed desmosomes are not present. Scattered lysosomes may be present, but Birbeck granules are not seen.

Immunophenotype
The neoplastic cells consistently express S100 protein and vimentin, with CD1a and langerin being negative. They are usually positive for fascin and (variably) weakly positive for CD68, lysozyme, and CD45. Strong nuclear staining for p53 may be present. They are negative for markers of follicular dendritic cells (CD21, CD23, and CD35), MPO, CD34, specific B-cell–associated and T-cell–associated antigens, CD30, EMA, and cytokeratins. The Ki-67 proliferation index is usually 10–20% (median: 11%) {1179}. The admixed small lymphocytes are almost always of T-cell lineage, with near absence of B cells.

Postulated normal counterpart
Interdigitating dendritic cell (IDC)

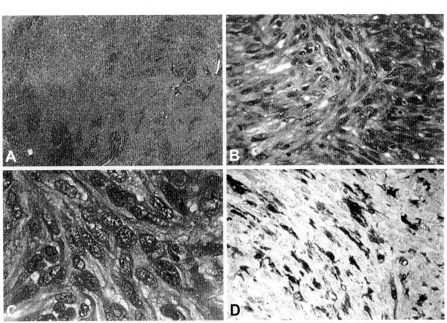

Fig. 17.16 Interdigitating dendritic cell sarcoma. **A** The tumour infiltrates the paracortex. Note the residual lymphoid tissue in one corner. **B** Sheets of spindled cells with a whorled pattern. **C** The cells show marked cytological atypia. **D** Staining for S100 protein is focally positive.

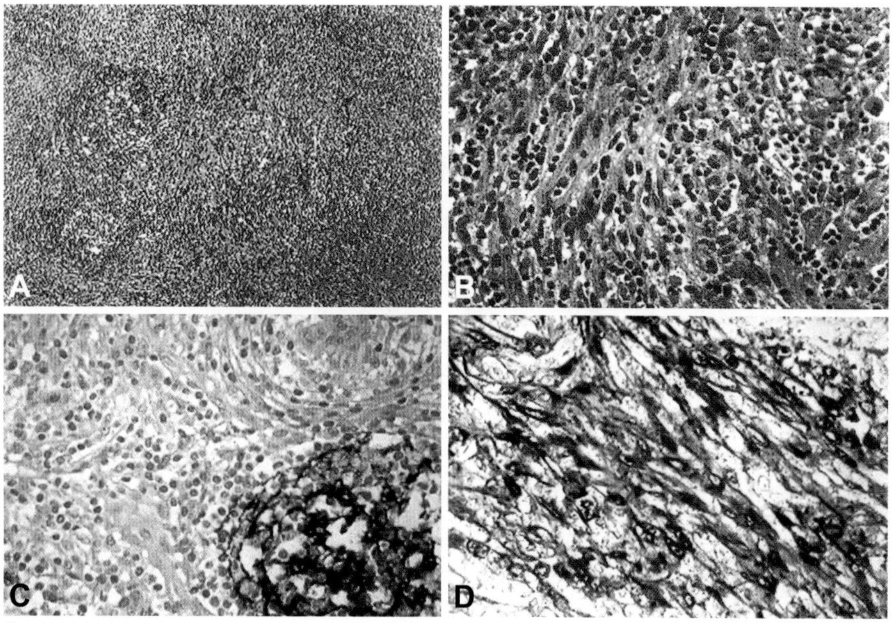

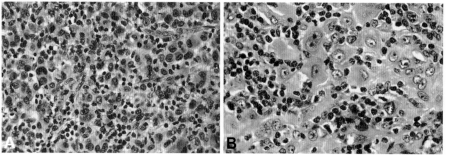

Fig. 17.17 Interdigitating dendritic cell sarcoma. **A** Note the paracortical pattern of tumour growth in the lymph node. **B** There are scattered small lymphocytes throughout the lesion. **C** The CD21 stain is negative on the tumour cells, but labels follicular dendritic cells in residual follicles. **D** In contrast, the stain for S100 protein is strongly positive in the tumour cells.

Fig. 17.18 Interdigitating dendritic cell sarcoma. **A** The cells are rounded, and the nuclei are relatively bland, but (**B**) have a vesicular chromatin pattern and a single medium-sized nucleolus.

Genetic profile

A subset of cases of IDC sarcoma have clonal IG rearrangements, particularly when there is an association with low-grade B-cell lymphoma, most likely constituting examples of transdifferentiation {680,1172}. In cases associated with t(14;18)-positive follicular lymphoma, identical chromosomal breakpoints affecting the *BCL2* locus are present in both neoplasms {1172}. The TR genes are in a germline configuration {4286}. At least one case has been shown to harbour somatic *BRAF* V600E mutation {2916}.

Prognosis and predictive factors

The clinical course is generally aggressive, with about half of all patients dying of the disease. Commonly affected visceral organs include the liver, spleen, kidney, and lung. Stage may be an important prognostic factor; however, histological features have not been correlated with clinical outcome.

Follicular dendritic cell sarcoma

Chan J.K.C.
Pileri S.A.
Fletcher C.D.M.
Weiss L.M.
Grogg K.L.

Definition

Follicular dendritic cell (FDC) sarcoma is a neoplastic proliferation of spindled to ovoid cells showing morphological and immunophenotypic features of FDCs.

ICD-O code   9758/3

Synonyms

Dendritic reticulum cell tumour (no longer recommended); follicular dendritic cell tumour

Epidemiology

FDC sarcoma is a rare neoplasm {104, 645,2695,3135,3180,4286}. There is a wide patient age range, with an adult predominance (median patient age: 50 years) {3180,3543}. The sex distribution is about equal {3180}.

Etiology

A proportion of cases appear to arise in the setting of hyaline-vascular Castleman disease, sometimes with a recognizable intermediary phase of FDC proliferation outside the follicles {638,645}. The Castleman disease lesion may be found concurrent with the FDC sarcoma, or may precede the latter by several years.

Localization

FDC sarcoma presents with lymph node disease in 31% of cases, extranodal disease in 58%, and both nodal and extranodal disease in 10% {3543}. Nodal disease most often affects the cervical nodes. A wide variety of extranodal sites can be affected, most commonly tonsil, gastrointestinal tract, soft tissue, mediastinum, retroperitoneum, omentum, and lung {1670,3543}. Common sites for metastasis include lymph nodes, lung, and liver {737}.

Clinical features

Patients most often present with a slow-growing, painless mass lesion, although patients with abdominal disease may present with abdominal pain. The tumours are often large, with a mean size of 7 cm {3543}. Most patients have localized disease at presentation {3543}. Systemic symptoms are uncommon. Rare patients have paraneoplastic pemphigus {2250,2536,4240}.

Microscopy

The neoplasm consists of spindled to ovoid cells forming fascicles, storiform arrays, whorls (sometimes reminiscent of the 360° pattern observed in meningioma), diffuse sheets, or vague nodules. The individual neoplastic cells generally show indistinct cell borders and a moderate amount of eosinophilic cytoplasm. The

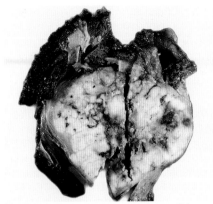

Fig. 17.19 Follicular dendritic cell sarcoma. This mass occurred in the soft tissue and has the appearance of a sarcoma.

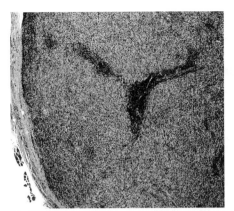

Fig. 17.20 Follicular dendritic cell sarcoma occurring in lymph node. The entire node is replaced by a spindle cell neoplasm. Perivascular cuffs of small lymphocytes are present.

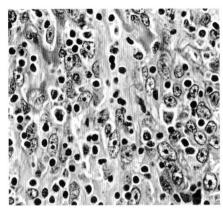

Fig. 17.21 Follicular dendritic cell sarcoma. Prototypical morphology. The plump spindly cells show indistinct cell borders, oval nuclei with vesicular chromatin, and distinct nucleoli. Focally, the nuclei appear clustered. There is a sprinkling of small lymphocytes throughout the tumour.

nuclei are oval or elongated, with vesicular or granular finely dispersed chromatin, small but distinct nucleoli, and a delicate nuclear membrane. The nuclei tend to be unevenly spaced, with areas showing clustering. Nuclear pseudoinclusions are common. Binucleated and multinucleated tumour cells are often seen. Although the cytological features are usually relatively bland, significant cytological atypia may be found in some cases. The mitotic rate is usually 0–10 mitoses per 10 high-power fields, although the more pleomorphic cases can show much higher mitotic rates (>30 mitoses per 10 high-power fields), easily found atypical mitoses, and coagulative necrosis.

The tumour is typically lightly infiltrated by small lymphocytes, which can sometimes be aggregated around the blood vessels as well {642}. Less common morphological features include epithelioid tumour cells with hyaline cytoplasm, clear cells, oncocytic cells, myxoid stroma, fluid-filled cystic spaces, prominent fibrovascular septa, and admixed osteoclastic giant cells {642,645,3135, 3136}. Uncommonly, there is a nodular growth pattern, with the large neoplastic cells scattered in a background of small B lymphocytes {2390}. Rare cases may also show jigsaw puzzle–like lobulation and perivascular spaces, mimicking thymoma or carcinoma showing thymus-like element {737}.

Ultrastructure
The neoplastic cells have elongated nuclei, often with cytoplasmic invaginations. There are characteristically numerous long, slender cytoplasmic process-

es, often connected by scattered, mature desmosomes. Birbeck granules and numerous lysosomes are not seen.

Immunophenotype
FDC sarcoma is positive for one or more of the FDC markers, such as CD21, CD35, and CD23 {2862}. CXCL13 and podoplanin (D2-40) are commonly positive, but are not entirely specific {4192, 4450}. Clusterin is often strongly positive, whereas this marker is usually negative or only weakly positive in other dendritic cell tumours {1472,1473}. The tumour is usually positive for desmoplakin, vimentin, fascin, EGFR, and HLA-DR {642,3833}, and variably positive for EMA, S100 protein, and CD68. Staining for cytokeratin, CD1a, lysozyme, MPO, CD34, CD3, CD79a, and HMB45 is negative. The Ki-67 proliferation index is 1–25% (mean: 13%). Positivity for the FDC secreted protein (FDCSP), serglycin (SRGN) and PD-L1 has recently been reported in FDC sarcoma {2184A,2383A}.

The admixed small lymphocytes can be predominantly B cells, predominantly

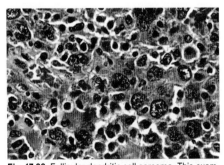

Fig. 17.22 Follicular dendritic cell sarcoma. This example shows significant nuclear atypia and pleomorphism.

T cells, or mixed B cells and T cells {645, 3180}. Rarely, there are abundant immature TdT+ T cells {2020,2944}, which may be associated with paraneoplastic pemphigus.

Postulated normal counterpart
Follicular dendritic cell (FDC) of the lymphoid follicle

Genetic profile
In one study, 3 of 8 cases of FDC sarcoma showed clonal rearrangements of the IG genes {680}, and thus the presence of antigen receptor gene rearrangements does not exclude a diagnosis of FDC sarcoma.

The limited cytogenetic data show complex karyotypes {3144}. A targeted next-generation sequencing study revealed recurrent loss-of-function alterations in tumour suppressor genes involved in negative regulation of NF-kappaB and cell-cycle progression {1460}. *BRAF* V600E mutation, a common genetic alteration in Langerhans cell histiocytosis, is reported in 0–19% of cases {1386,1460}.

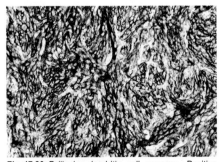

Fig. 17.23 Follicular dendritic cell sarcoma. Positive cell membrane staining for CD21 with an anastomosing pattern.

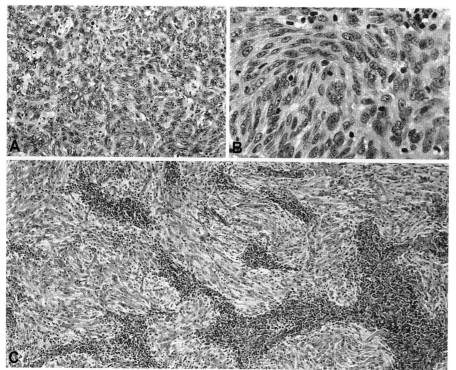

Fig. 17.24 Follicular dendritic cell sarcoma. **A** Spindle cell proliferation. **B** A 360° whorl is seen. Note the occasional multinucleated cells. **C** In this example, the small lymphocytes are aggregated around the blood vessels.

Two studies examining the transcriptional profile of FDC sarcoma have revealed (1) a peculiar immunological microenvironment enriched in T follicular helper (TFH) and T regulatory (Treg) cell populations, with special reference to the inhibitory immune receptor PD1 and its ligands PDL1 and PDL2, and (2) the highly specific expression of the genes encoding FDCSP and SRGN {1460B,1460C}.

Conventional FDC sarcomas are negative for EBV, whereas the inflammatory pseudotumour-like variant consistently shows EBV in the neoplastic cells {697}.

Prognosis and predictive factors

FDC sarcoma is usually treated by complete surgical excision, with or without adjuvant radiotherapy or chemotherapy. A pooled analysis of the literature showed local recurrence and distant metastasis rates of 28% and 27%, respectively {3543}, but the true figures are likely to be higher, because these adverse events are sometimes delayed many years. The 2-year survival rates for early, locally advanced, and distant metastatic diseases are 82%, 80%, and 42%, respectively {3543}. Some patients may die from refractory paraneoplastic pemphigus.

Large tumour size (≥6 cm), coagulative necrosis, high mitotic count (≥5 mitoses per 10 high-power fields), and significant cytological atypia are associated with a worse prognosis {645,3543}.

Inflammatory pseudotumour-like follicular/fibroblastic dendritic cell sarcoma

Inflammatory pseudotumour-like follicular/fibroblastic dendritic cell (FDC/FRC) sarcoma occurs predominantly in young to middle-aged adults, with a marked female predilection {697}. It typically involves the liver or spleen, but both sites may be simultaneously involved {134,697, 3619}. Rarely, it selectively involves the gastrointestinal tract in the form of a polypoid lesion {3042}. Patients are asymptomatic or present with abdominal distension or pain, sometimes accompanied by systemic symptoms {683,697,733}.

Histologically, the neoplastic spindled cells are dispersed within a prominent lymphoplasmacytic infiltrate. The nuclei usually show a vesicular chromatin pattern and small but distinct nucleoli. Nuclear atypia is highly variable; usually most cells are bland-looking, but some cells with enlarged, irregularly folded or hyperchromatic nuclei are almost always found. Some tumour cells may even resemble Reed–Sternberg cells {3619}. Necrosis and haemorrhage are often present, and may be associated with a histiocytic or granulomatous reaction. The blood vessels frequently show fibrinoid deposits in the walls. In occasional cases, the tumour may be masked by massive infiltrates of eosinophils or numerous epithelioid granulomas {2310}.

The neoplastic cells are often positive for follicular dendritic cell markers, such as CD21 and CD35, with the staining ranging from extensive to very focal. However, in some cases, they may be negative for follicular dendritic cell markers but express SMA, raising the possibility of fibroblastic reticular cell differentiation. Still other cases are positive for all these markers or lack these markers {129,697, 733,1399,2293}. Both FDC and FRC share a common mesenchymal origin, with plasticity in the immunophenotype. The neoplastic cells are consistently associated with EBV {134,697}, which is present in a monoclonal episomal form {3619}.Outcome data are limited, but

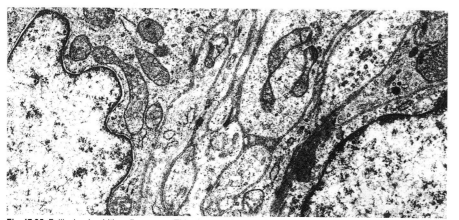

Fig. 17.25 Follicular dendritic cell sarcoma. This electron micrograph shows numerous cytoplasmic processes, with one well-formed desmosome present in the centre.

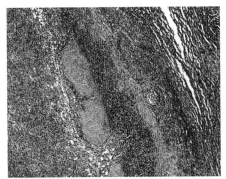

Fig. 17.26 Splenic inflammatory pseudotumour-like FDC/FRC sarcoma. Normal splenic tissue is seen in right, the tumour in left field.

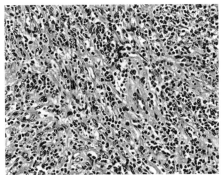

Fig. 17.27 Splenic inflammatory pseudotumour-like FDC/FRC sarcoma. The tumour shows an inflammatory pseudotumour pattern, with spindle cells admixed with many lymphocytes and plasma cells.

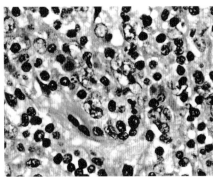

Fig. 17.28 Splenic inflammatory pseudotumour-like FDC/FRC sarcoma. Usually, some large cells with definite nuclear atypia can be found.

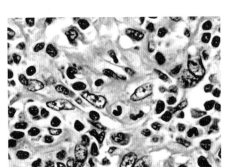

Fig. 17.29 Splenic inflammatory pseudotumour-like follicular dendritic cell sarcoma. Spindle cells with vesicular nuclei and distinct nucleoli are dispersed in a background of chronic inflammatory cells. They show minimal to mild atypia.

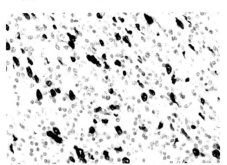

Fig. 17.30 Inflammatory pseudotumour-like follicular dendritic cell sarcoma. In situ hybridization for EBV-encoded small RNA (EBER) highlights the neoplastic spindle cells. Nuclear atypia in some neoplastic cells becomes easier to appreciate.

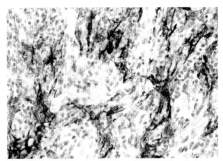

Fig. 17.31 Inflammatory pseudotumour-like follicular dendritic cell sarcoma. The atypical spindle cells focally exhibit immunoreactivity for CD21.

the tumour appears to be indolent, with a tendency to develop repeated intra-abdominal recurrences over many years {683,697}.

Fibroblastic reticular cell tumour

Weiss L.M.
Chan J.K.C.
Fletcher C.D.M.

Definition
Fibroblastic reticular cell tumour is very rare. Tumours diagnosed as cytokeratin-positive interstitial reticulum cell tumours probably constitute the same entity {104, 639}.

ICD-O code   9759/3

Synonyms
Cytokeratin-positive interstitial reticulum cell tumour; fibroblastic dendritic cell tumour

Localization
This tumour can occur in the lymph nodes, spleen, or soft tissue {104,639, 1415,1874}.

Microscopy
The tumour is histologically similar to follicular dendritic cell sarcoma or inter-

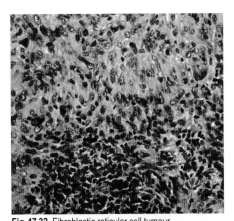

Fig. 17.32 Fibroblastic reticular cell tumour. This neoplasm features blunt spindle cells arranged in poorly formed whorls, with moderate cytological atypia. Stains for follicular and interdigitating dendritic cells were negative.

digitating dendritic cell sarcoma, but lacks the immunophenotypic profile of these tumour types. There are often interspersed delicate collagen fibres.

Ultrastructure
Ultrastructurally, the spindle cells show delicate cytoplasmic extensions and features similar to those of myofibroblasts (i.e. filaments with occasional fusiform densities, well-developed desmosomal attachments, rough endoplasmic reticulum, and basal lamina–like material).

Immunophenotype
The tumour cells are variably immunoreactive for SMA, desmin, cytokeratin (in a dendritic pattern), and CD68.

Prognosis and predictive factors
Available data regarding outcome are extremely limited. The clinical outcome is variable. Some patients die of the disease.

Disseminated juvenile xanthogranuloma

Brousse N.
Pileri S.A.
Haroche J.
Dagna L.
Jaffe R.
Fletcher C.D.M.
Jaffe E.S.
Harris N.L.

Definition

Disseminated juvenile xanthogranuloma (JXG) is characterized by a proliferation of histiocytes similar to those of the dermal JXG, commonly having a foamy (xanthomatous) component with Touton-type giant cells. There is evidence for clonality in some instances. Erdheim–Chester disease is distinguished from JXG in the current classification of histiocytic neoplasms {1101}.

Synonyms

Benign cephalic histiocytosis; progressive nodular histiocytosis; generalized (non-lipidaemic) eruptive histiocytosis (skin); xanthoma disseminatum (skin plus mucosa lesions)

Epidemiology

Solitary dermal JXG is vastly more common than other forms and does not progress to more-disseminated forms {925}. Most deep, visceral, and disseminated forms occur by the age of 10 years, half within the first year of life {1836}.

Etiology

There is a known association with neurofibromatosis type 1; patients with both are at slightly higher risk of juvenile myelomonocytic leukaemia {4508}. Patients with both Langerhans cell disease (i.e. Langerhans cell histiocytosis; LCH) and JXG are also encountered. To date, no cases of JXG bearing mutations of BRAF or other genes involved in the MAPK pathway have been described {634,1553}.

Localization

The skin and soft tissues are affected most commonly. Disseminated forms commonly affect the mucosal surfaces, in particular within the upper aerodigestive tract. When skin is involved, there seems to be a predilection for the head and neck region {925}. The CNS, dura, and pituitary stalk can be affected, as can eye, liver, lung, lymph node, and bone marrow. Retroperitoneal and peri-

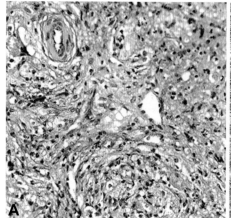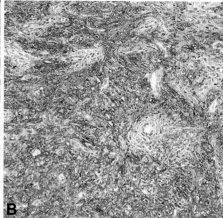

Fig. 17.33 Systemic juvenile xanthogranuloma involving liver. **A** The infiltrate is portal in nature but spares the bile duct. Few Touton cells are present. **B** There is diffuse factor XIIIa staining of the portal histiocytes.

aortic involvement is principally noted in Erdheim–Chester disease {925,1256, 1836}.

Clinical features

Skin lesions other than the common papular solitary form are small (1–2 mm) and multiple. Soft tissue lesions can be large, and the lesions present as mass effect. Optic lesions can cause glaucoma. Like in LCH, CNS and pituitary lesions can cause diabetes insipidus, seizures, hydrocephalus, and mental status changes {925,1256,1836}. Unlike in LCH, liver involvement does not target the biliary system or lead to sclerosing cholangitis {1826}. There is some capacity for lesions to slowly regress. JXG appears to be benign, but a concomitant macrophage activation syndrome can lead to cytopenias, liver damage, and (in the systemic forms) death.

Microscopy

The JXG cell is small and oval, sometimes slightly spindled with a bland round to oval nucleus without grooves and with pink cytoplasm. Touton cells are less common at non-dermal sites. The cells become progressively lipidized (xanthomatous). A mixed inflammatory component is invariable. Variants include epithelioid cells with glassy cytoplasm. The ultrastructural features are histiocytic, without distinguishing features {4465}.

Immunophenotype

In common with macrophages, cells express vimentin, surface CD14, CD68 (PGM1) in a coarse granular pattern, CD163 in a surface and cytoplasmic

pattern, and stabilin-1 (MS-1 antigen). Factor XIIIa staining is common but not universal. Fascin stains the cell cytoplasm and S100 is positive in < 20% of the cases. However, none of these markers is specific for JXG. CD1a and langerin are negative {654,2104,3513,4465}.

Cell of origin

The cell of origin is uncertain. Despite their macrophage phenotype, the cells of disseminated JXG have been postulated (on the basis of shared factor XIIIa and fascin immunostaining) to originate from a dermal/interstitial dendritic cell, but these characteristics have limited specificity {2104}.

Genetic profile

No consistent cytogenetic or molecular genetic change has been identified. IG and TR rearrangements are germline. There is evidence for clonality in some instances {1835}. Unlike in Erdheim–Chester disease, there are no reported cases of JXG bearing BRAF mutations {634, 1553}.

Genetic susceptibility

An association with neurofibromatosis type 1 is known in some cases.

Prognosis and predictive factors

All clinical forms are benign, although multiple lesions in brain, dura, or pituitary can cause local consequences and even death. Systemic forms that involve liver and bone marrow have been treated with LCH-type therapy.

Erdheim–Chester disease

Brousse N.
Pileri S.A.
Haroche J.
Dagna L.

Jaffe R.
Fletcher C.D.M.
Jaffe E.S.
Harris N.L.

Definition
Erdheim–Chester disease (ECD) is a clonal systemic proliferation of histiocytes, commonly having a foamy (xanthomatous) component, and containing Touton giant cells (considered to be a non–Langerhans cell histiocytosis). It was first described as lipoid granulomatosis in 1930 {693}. The name Erdheim–Chester disease was coined in 1972 to recognize the contribution to the discovery of the condition by Erdheim, who was Chester's mentor {693}. Diagnosis of ECD is based on clinical features, imaging, and histology {693,1101}.

ICD-O code   9749/3

Synonyms
Lipogranulomatosis; lipoid granulomatosis; lipid (cholesterol) granulomatosis; polyostotic sclerosing histiocytosis

Epidemiology
ECD is a rare condition. To date, < 1000 cases have been reported. The mean patient age at diagnosis is 55–60 years, but rare paediatric cases (i.e. in patients aged < 15 years) have also been reported. The male-to-female ratio is 3:1.

Localization
Virtually any organ or tissue can be infiltrated by ECD. Skeletal involvement occurs in >95% of cases. Cardiovascular involvement probably occurs in at least half of all patients, but is likely underdiagnosed. One third of patients have retroperitoneal involvement. CNS involvement, diabetes insipidus, and/or exophthalmos occur in 20–30% of patients. CNS involvement may occur due to tissue infiltration by histiocytes or degenerative alterations typically affecting the cerebellum, with involvement due to degenerative alterations being much more difficult to treat. Xanthelasma, generally involving the eyelids or periorbital spaces, is the most common cutaneous manifestation.

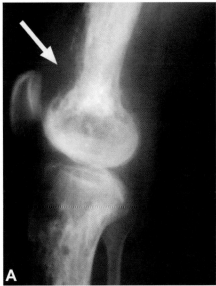

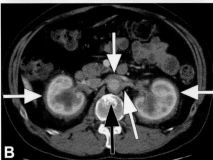

Fig. 17.34 Erdheim–Chester disease (ECD). **A** Radiograph showing a lytic and sclerotic lesion in the distal femur and the proximal tibia. There is destruction of the anterior femoral cortex, with an impacted pathological fracture through the lesion and an anterolateral soft tissue mass extending from the destroyed femur (arrow). Reprinted from Rosier RN and Rosenberg AE {3416A}. **B** Abdominal CT from a patient with ECD showing a soft tissue infiltrate surrounding the aorta and kidneys (white arrows). There is a sclerotic lesion in the vertebra (black arrow). Reprinted from Mills JA et al. {2665A}.

Clinical features
The clinical course of ECD depends on the extent and distribution of the disease. Some cases, with lesions limited to the bone, are asymptomatic; others, with multisystemic disease, may follow an aggressive, rapid clinical course. In one third of patients, bone involvement may cause mild pain that starts at any time during the course of the disease and usually affects the distal limbs. Cardiovascular involvement may be asymptomatic and detected incidentally by MRI or CT. The most common cardiovascular alteration corresponds to circumferential soft tissue sheathing of the thoracic and abdominal aorta and large arteries, infiltration of the right atrium or auricu-

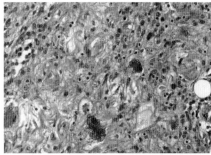

Fig. 17.35 Retroperitoneal Erdheim–Chester disease. The infiltrate is made up of foamy histiocytes and Touton cells admixed with scattered small lymphocytes in a fibrous tissue.

loventricular groove and diffuse pleural thickening. The clinical consequences are usually not severe, except for renovascular hypertension in a small number of cases, which may require stenting. Pericardial involvement can cause pericarditis, effusion, or even tamponade. Orbital infiltration, often bilateral, produces exophthalmos, pain, oculomotor nerve palsies, or blindness. Xanthelasmata of the eyelids or periorbital tissue are further ocular manifestations. Pituitary gland infiltration causes diabetes insipidus and (less frequently) hyperprolactinaemia, gonadotropin insufficiency, and hypotestosteronism. CNS involvement produces variable symptoms (cerebellar and pyramidal syndromes, seizures, headache, neuropsychiatric symptoms, cognitive impairment, sensory disturbances, and cranial nerve paralysis). The most serious neurological complication is neurodegenerative cerebellar disease, which is present in 15–20% of patients with ECD. In particular, CNS involvement is a major prognostic factor in ECD, constituting an independent predictor of death at survival analysis.

Imaging
Characteristic features on imaging studies are bilateral and symmetrical cortical osteosclerosis of the diaphyseal and metaphyseal parts of the long bones on X-ray and/or symmetrical and abnormally intense labelling of the distal ends of the long bones of the legs (and in some cases, arms) on ^{99}Tc bone scintigraphy. These findings are highly suggestive of ECD. Occasionally, osteolytic lesions are also seen. PET/CT has a high specificity for the diagnosis of bone involvement by ECD. Cardiovascular involvement manifests as circumferential sheathing of the thoracic or abdominal aorta (so-called

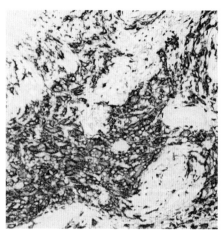

Fig. 17.36 Erdheim–Chester disease. The histiocytic infiltrate shows strong positivity for CD163.

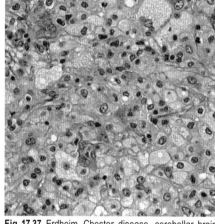

Fig. 17.37 Erdheim–Chester disease, cerebellar brain lesion. The atypical histiocytes have abundant foamy cytoplasm, resembling xanthoma cells.

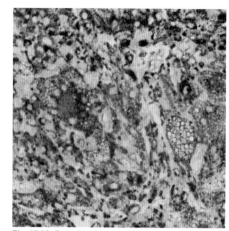

Fig. 17.38 Erdheim–Chester disease, cerebellar brain lesion. Histiocytes are positive for CD68 but negative for S100 (not shown).

coated aorta) and large arteries, pericardial effusion (sometimes leading to tamponade), infiltration of the right atrium or auriculoventricular groove, and diffuse pleural thickening. Retroperitoneal involvement may be prominent around the renal capsule (producing the characteristic so-called hairy kidney appearance) and ureters.

Microscopy

There is tissue infiltration by histiocytes, generally with single small nuclei and foamy (xanthomatous) cytoplasm. Other histiocytes, with compact eosinophilic cytoplasm, may also be present. A few multinucleated histiocytes with a central ring of nuclei (Touton cells) are frequently observed. Fibrosis is present in most cases and is sometimes abundant. Reactive small lymphocytes, plasma cells, and neutrophils are also frequently present. The infiltrate may easily be misdiagnosed as a reactive process.

Immunophenotype

ECD histiocytes express three molecules common to macrophages: CD14 (a monocyte or macrophage receptor that binds lipopolysaccharide), CD68 (a largely lysosomal macrosialin), and CD163 (a haemoglobin- and haptoglobin-scavenging receptor). In addition, the cells express factor XIIIa (a tissue transglutaminase) and fascin (an actin-bundling protein), both of which are typical of interstitial and interdigitating dendritic cells. The abnormal histiocytes lack

S100, CD1a, and langerin, which are all markers of Langerhans cells. However, cases focally positive for S100 have been reported {1101}. The characteristic immunophenotype is shared by all members of the xanthogranuloma family of histiocytoses. As many as 20% of patients with ECD also have Langerhans cell histiocytosis lesions, and infiltration by ECD and Langerhans cell histiocytosis may be present within the same biopsies {1101}. Cases of ECD with mutated *BRAF* are positive by immunohistochemistry with the VE1 monoclonal antibody to mutated BRAF protein {1101}.

Cell of origin

The postulated cell of origin is an interstitial dendritic cell, but this is the subject of some debate.

Genetic profile

In several cases, clonality has been identified by classic cytogenetics and other techniques. Activating mutations in MAPK pathway genes, most notably *BRAF* V600E (reported in >50% of cases), as well as *NRAS* mutation (recorded in ~4% of cases), can be detected in ECD {71,1553}. Recurrent mutations in *PI3KCA* have also been described in ~11% of cases {71}.

Molecular tests and differential diagnosis

Some cases of ECD may have dominant cutaneous manifestations, without other organ involvement, making the differen-

tial diagnosis with juvenile xanthogranuloma and some nonspecific inflammatory lesions challenging {71}. Molecular analysis of such cases may be useful, because characteristic genetic aberrations favour the diagnosis of ECD {1101}. Immunohistochemistry may be a useful diagnostic tool for the detection of mutated *BRAF*, in lieu of genetic studies.

Prognosis and predictive factors

ECD is a chronic disease. The disease outcome correlates with sites of involvement; patients with CNS disease or multisystemic disease have a worse outcome {149A,974A}. Disease activity is assessed by clinical examination, imaging, and C-reactive protein values, but no disease activity score has been established. PET scans are very useful for assessments of ECD activity {149C}. Histology is not predictive of evolution. ECD may respond to therapy with interferon alpha, but many cases are refractory, especially those with CNS and cardiovascular involvement {544A,1552A}. Vemurafenib, an inhibitor of BRAF that is approved for treating patients with metastatic melanoma and *BRAF* V600 mutations, has recently been used, with promising results {544A,1552A,1553A}. The reported 5-year overall survival rate of patients treated with interferon therapy is 68% {149B}. Older series, perhaps with less-effective therapy, reported 43% of patients alive after an average follow-up of 32 months {4192A}.

Contributors

Dr Cem AKIN [#]
Department of Internal Medicine
Division of Allergy and Immunology
University of Michigan
1150 West Medical Center Drive
5520-B, MSRB-1, Ann Arbor MI 48109-5600
USA
Tel. +1 734 647 6234; +1 734 936 5634
Fax +1 734 763 4151
cemakin@umich.edu; cakin@partners.org

Dr Ioannis ANAGNOSTOPOULOS
Institute of Pathology, Campus Mitte
Charité – Universitätsmedizin Berlin
Charitéplatz 1
10117 Berlin
GERMANY
Tel. +49 30 450 536 026
Fax +49 30 450 536 914
ioannis.anagnostopoulos@charite.de

Dr Katsuyuki AOZASA
Department of Pathology (C3)
Osaka University Graduate
School of Medicine
2-2 Yamadaoka
Suita, Osaka 565-0871
JAPAN
Tel. +81 6 6879 3710
Fax +81 6 6679 3713
aozasa@molpath.med.osaka-u.ac.jp

Dr Daniel A. ARBER [#]
Department of Pathology
University of Chicago
5841 S. Maryland Avenue,
S327, MC 3083
Chicago, IL 60637
USA
Tel. +1 773 702 0647
Fax +1 773 834 5414
darber@uchicago.edu

Dr Michele BACCARANI [#]
University of Bologna
GIMEMA CML Working Party
Via Adolfo Albertazzi 16/2
40137 Bologna
ITALY
Tel. +39 051 349845
Fax +39 051 349845
michele.baccarani@unibo.it

Dr Barbara J. BAIN
Department of Haematology
Imperial College Faculty of Medicine
St Mary's Hospital
Praed Street
London W2 1NY
UNITED KINGDOM
Tel. +44 20 3312 6806
Fax +44 20 3312 2390
b.bain@ic.ac.uk

Dr Tiziano BARBUI
Research Foundation
Ospedale Papa Giovanni XXIII
Piazza OMS 1
24127 Bergamo
ITALY
Tel. +39 35 267 5134
Fax +39 35 267 4926
tbarbui@asst-pg23.it

Dr Giovanni BAROSI
Center for the Study of Myelofibrosis
Fondazione IRCCS Policlinico San Matteo
27100 Pavia
ITALY
Tel. +39 0382 503636
Fax +39 0382 503917
barosig@smatteo.pv.it

Dr Irith BAUMANN
Gesundheitszentrum (MVZ)
Bunsenstrasse 120
71032 Böblingen
GERMANY
Tel. +49 7031 6682 2594
i.baumann@klinikverbund-suedwest.de

Dr Marie-Christine BÉNÉ [#]
Service d'Hématologie Biologique
Centre Hospitalier Universitaire (CHU) Nantes
9, Quai Moncousu
44000 Nantes
FRANCE
Tel. +33 2 40 08 41 89
Fax +33 3 83 44 60 22
mariecbene@gmail.com

Dr Daniel BENHARROCH
Department of Pathology
Soroka Medical Center
Ben Gurion University
Beer Sheva, 84101
ISRAEL
Tel. +972 8 640 0920
Fax +972 8 623 2770
benaroch@bgu.ac.il

Dr John M. BENNETT [#]
Departments of Medicine and Pathology
University of Rochester Medical Center
James P. Wilmot Cancer Center
601 Elmwood Avenue
Rochester NY 14642
USA
Tel. +1 585 275 4915
Fax +1 585 442 0039
john_bennett@urmc.rochester.edu

Dr Emilio BERTI
Department of Dermatology
Fondazione IRCCS Ca' Granda
Ospedale Maggiore Policlinico
Via Pace 9
20122 Milan
ITALY
Tel. +39 2 5503 5107; +39 2 5503 5200
Fax +39 2 5032 0779
emilio.berti@unimib.it; emilio.berti@gmail.com

Dr Govind BHAGAT
Division of Hematopathology
Department of Pathology and Cell Biology
Columbia University Medical Center
VC14-228, 630 West 168th Street
New York NY 10032
USA
Tel. +1 212 342 1323
Fax +1 212 305 2301
gb96@cumc.columbia.edu

Dr Gunnar BIRGEGÅRD [#]
Department of Hematology
Uppsala University Hospital
SE-751 85 Uppsala
SWEDEN
Tel. +46 18 61 14 412
Fax +46 18 50 92 97
gunnar.birgegard@medsci.uu.se

[#] Indicates disclosure of interests

Dr Clara D. BLOOMFIELD
Comprehensive Cancer Center
Ohio State University
C933 James Cancer Hospital
460 West 10th Avenue
Columbus OH 43210
USA
Tel. +1 614 293 7518
Fax +1 614 293 3132
clara.bloomfield@osumc.edu

Dr Michael J. BOROWITZ #
Department of Pathology and Oncology
Johns Hopkins Medical Institutions
401 North Broadway
Baltimore MD 21231
USA
Tel. +1 410 614 2889
Fax +1 410 502 1493
mborowit@jhmi.edu

Dr Nicole BROUSSE #
Department of Pathology
Necker University Hospital
149 Rue de Sèvres
75015 Paris
FRANCE
Tel. +33 1 44 49 40 00
nicole.brousse@nck.aphp.fr

Dr Richard D. BRUNNING
Department of Laboratory Medicine and
Pathology
University of Minnesota Hospital
420 Delaware Street South-east
Minneapolis MN 55455
USA
Tel. +1 612 332 8001
Fax +1 612 624 6662
brunn001@umn.edu

Dr Carlos BUESO-RAMOS
Division of Pathology and
Laboratory Medicine
UT MD Anderson Cancer Center
1515 Holcombe Boulevard, Unit 072
Houston TX 77030
USA
Tel. +1 713 563 1091
Fax +1 713 794 1800
cbuesora@mdanderson.org

Dr Elias CAMPO
Haematopathology Unit
Hospital Clínic de Barcelona
IDIBAPS, University of Barcelona
Villarroel 170
08036 Barcelona
SPAIN
Tel. +34 93 227 5450
Fax +34 93 227 5717
ecampo@clinic.ub.es

Dr Daniel CATOVSKY
Division of Molecular Pathology
Institute of Cancer Research
15 Cotswold Road, Brookes Lawley Building
Sutton, Surrey SM2 5NG
UNITED KINGDOM
Tel. +44 20 8722 4114
Fax +44 20 7795 0310
daniel.catovsky@icr.ac.uk

Dr Mario CAZZOLA
Department of Molecular Medicine
University of Pavia
Department of Hematology Oncology
Fondazione IRCCS Policlinico San Matteo
27100 Pavia
ITALY
Tel. +39 0382 526 263
Fax +39 0382 502 250
mario.cazzola@unipv.it

Dr Lorenzo CERRONI
Department of Dermatology
Medical University of Graz
Auenbruggerplatz 8
8036 Graz
AUSTRIA
Tel. +43 316 3851 2423
Fax +43 316 3851 2466
lorenzo.cerroni@medunigraz.at

Dr Ethel CESARMAN
Department of Pathology and Laboratory
Medicine
Weill Cornell Medical College
525 East 68th Street, Starr 715, Room C410
New York NY 10065
USA
Tel. +1 212 746 8838
Fax +1 212 746 4483
ecesarm@med.cornell.edu

Dr Amy CHADBURN #
Department of Pathology and Laboratory
Medicine
Weill Cornell Medical College
1300 York Avenue
New York NY 10065
USA
Tel. +1 212 746 6631
Fax +1 212 746 8173
achadbur@med.cornell.edu

Dr John K.C. CHAN
Department of Pathology
Queen Elizabeth Hospital
Wylie Road, Kowloon
Hong Kong SAR
CHINA
Tel. +852 2958 6830
Fax +852 2385 2455
jkcchan@ha.org.hk; jkcchan@netvigator.com

Dr Wing Chung CHAN #
Department of Pathology
City of Hope National Medical Center
1500 East Duarte Road
Familian Science Building, Room 1215
Duarte CA 91010
USA
Tel. +1 626 218 9158
Fax +1 626 218 9450
jochan@coh.org

Dr Andreas CHOTT
Department of Pathology and Microbiology
Wilhelminenspital
Montleartstrasse 37
A-1160 Vienna
AUSTRIA
Tel. +43 1 49 150 3201
Fax +43 1 49 150 3209
andreas.chott@wienkav.at

Dr James R. COOK #
Department of Laboratory Medicine
Cleveland Clinic
Main Campus, Mail Code L30
9500 Euclid Avenue
Cleveland OH 44195
USA
Tel. +1 216 444 4435
Fax +1 216 444 4414
cookj2@ccf.org

Dr Robert W. COUPLAND
Department of Pathology
Kelowna General Hospital
2268 Pandosy Street
Kelowna BC V1Y 1T2
CANADA
Tel. +1 250 980 6122
Fax +1 250 862 4337
robert.coupland@interiorhealth.ca

Dr Lorenzo DAGNA
Dep. of Medicine and Clinical Immunology
IRCCS San Raffaele Scientific Institute
Vita-Salute San Raffaele University
Via Olgettina 60
20132 Milan
ITALY
Tel. +39 2 9175 1545
Fax +39 2 2643 3787
lorenzo.dagna@unisr.it

Dr Daphne DE JONG #
Department of Pathology
VU University Medical Center
De Boelelaan 1117, ZH3E48
1081 HV Amsterdam
THE NETHERLANDS
Tel. +31 20 444 4978
Fax +31 20 444 4586
daphne.dejong@vumc.nl; d.dejong2@vumc.nl

Dr Laurence DE LEVAL
Institut Universitaire de Pathologie
de Lausanne
25 Rue du Bugnon
CH-1005 Lausanne
SWITZERLAND
Tel. +41 21 314 7194
laurence.deleval@chuv.ch

Dr Martina DECKERT
Department of Neuropathology
University of Cologne
Kerpener Strasse 62
D-50924 Cologne
GERMANY
Tel. +49 221 478 5265
Fax +49 221 478 7237
martina.deckert@uni-koeln.de

Dr Jan DELABIE
Department of Pathology
University Health Network and
University of Toronto
200 Elizabeth Street
Toronto ON M5G 2C4
CANADA
Tel. +1 416 340 5239
Fax +1 416 340 5543
jan.delabie@uhn.ca

Dr Ahmet DOGAN [#]
Departments of Pathology and
Laboratory Medicine
Memorial Sloan Kettering Cancer Center
Memorial Hospital
1275 York Avenue
New York NY 10065
USA
Tel. +1 212 639 2736
dogana@mskcc.org

Dr Hartmut DÖHNER
Department of Internal Medicine III
University Hospital Ulm
Albert-Einstein-Allee 23
89081 Ulm
GERMANY
Tel. +49 731 500 45501
Fax +49 731 500 45505
hartmut.doehner@uniklinik-ulm.de

Dr James R. DOWNING
St. Jude Children's Research Hospital
262 Danny Thomas Place
Memphis, TN 38105
USA
Tel. +1 901 595 3510
Fax +1 901 595 3749
james.downing@stjude.org

Dr Lyn M. DUNCAN
Dermatopathology Unit
Massachusetts General Hospital
55 Fruit Street, Warren 820
Boston MA 02114
USA
Tel. +1 617 726 8890
Fax +1 617 726 8711
duncan@helix.mgh.harvard.edu

Dr Kojo S.J. ELENITOBA-JOHNSON
Dept. of Pathology and Laboratory Medicine
Perelman School of Medicine,
University of Pennsylvania
Stellar-Chance Laboratories,
Office Suite 609A, 422 Curie Blvd.
Philadelphia, PA 19104
USA
Tel. +1 215 898 8198
kojo.elenitoba-johnson@uphs.upenn.edu

Dr Luis ESCRIBANO [#]
Servicio Central de Citometría
Dep. de Medicina Centro de Investigación del Cáncer
University of Salamanca
Campus Miguel de Unamuno, s/n
37007 Salamanca
SPAIN
Tel. +34 92 329 4811
Fax +34 92 329 4743
escribanomoraluis@gmail.com

Dr Fabio FACCHETTI
Department of Pathology
University of Brescia
Spedali Civili Brescia
Piazzale Spedali Civili 1
25123 Brescia
ITALY
Tel. +39 30 3995426
Fax +39 30 3995377
fabio.facchetti@unibs.it

Dr Brunangelo FALINI [#]
Institute of Hematology, Center for
Oncohematological Research (CREO)
University of Perugia
Santa Maria della Misericordia Hospital
06129 Perugia
ITALY
Tel. +39 75 57 83 896
Fax +39 75 57 83 834
brunangelo.falini@unipg.it

Dr Andrew L. FELDMAN [#]
Department of Laboratory
Medicine and Pathology
Mayo Clinic
200 First Street South-west
Rochester, MN 55905
USA
Tel. +1 507 284 4939
Fax +1 507 284 5115
feldman.andrew@mayo.edu

Dr Falko FEND [#]
Institute of Pathology,
University Hospital UKT
Eberhard Karls Universität Tübingen
Liebermeisterstrasse 8
72076 Tübingen
GERMANY
Tel. +49 707 1298 2266
Fax +49 707 1292 258
falko.fend@med.uni-tuebingen.de

Dr Judith A. FERRY
Pathology Department
Massachusetts General Hospital
55 Fruit Street, Warren 2
Boston, MA 02114
USA
Tel. +1 617 726 4826
Fax +1 617 726 7474
jferry@partners.org

Dr Christopher D.M. FLETCHER
Department of Pathology
Brigham and Women's Hospital
75 Francis Street
Boston, MA 02115
USA
Tel. +1 617 732 8558
Fax +1 617 566 3897
cfletcher@partners.org

Dr Kathryn FOUCAR
Department of Pathology
Hematopathology Division
UNM Health Sciences Center
1001 Woodward Place North-east
Albuquerque, NM 87102
USA
Tel. +1 505 938 8457
Fax +1 505 938 8414
kfoucar@salud.unm.edu

Dr Randy D. GASCOYNE [#]
Department of Pathology
Centre for Lymphoid Cancer
British Columbia Cancer Agency
675 West 10th Avenue
Vancouver BC V5Z 1L3
CANADA
Tel. +1 604 675 8025
Fax +1 604 675 8183
rgascoyn@bccancer.bc.ca

Dr Norbert GATTERMANN [#]
Department of Haematology,
Oncology and Clinical Immunology
Heinrich Heine University
Moorenstrasse 5
40225 Düsseldorf
GERMANY
Tel. +49 211 811 6500
Fax +49 211 811 8853
gattermann@med.uni-duesseldorf.de

Dr Philippe GAULARD
Department of Pathology
Henri Mondor Hospital, INSERM U841
51, Ave du Maréchal de Lattre de Tassigny
94010 Créteil
FRANCE
Tel. +33 1 49 81 27 43
Fax +33 1 49 81 27 33
philippe.gaulard@hmn.aphp.fr

Dr Ulrich GERMING #
Department of Haematology,
Oncology and Clinical Immunology
Heinrich Heine University
Moorenstrasse 5
40225 Düsseldorf
GERMANY
Tel. +49 211 811 7780
Fax +49 211 811 8853
germing@med.uni-duesseldorf.de

Dr Paolo GHIA #
Unit of B-cell Neoplasia
Università Vita-Salute San Raffaele
C/O DIBIT 1, Floor 1, Room 38 DX
Via Olgettina 58
20135 Milan
ITALY
Tel. +39 0226 434 797
Fax +39 0226 434 760
ghia.paolo@hsr.it

Dr Umberto GIANELLI
Haematopathology Service, Pathology Unit
Dep. of Pathophysiology & Transplantation,
Univ. of Milan, Fondazione IRCCS Ca' Granda
Ospedale Maggiore Policlinico
Via Francesco Sforza 35, 20132 Milan
ITALY
Tel. +39 255 035 875
Fax +39 255 034 608
umberto.gianelli@unimi.it

Dr Heinz GISSLINGER
Department of Internal Medicine I
Medical University of Vienna
Waehringer Guertel 18-20
A-1090 Vienna
AUSTRIA
Tel. +43 1 404 005464
Fax +43 1 404 004030
heinz.gisslinger@meduniwien.ac.at

Dr Lucy A. GODLEY
Department of Medicine
Section of Hematology/Oncology
University of Chicago Medicine
5841 South Maryland Avenue, MC 2115
Chicago IL 60637
USA
Tel. +1 773 702 4140
Fax +1 773 702 9268
lgodley@medicine.bsd.uchicago.edu

Dr Peter L. GREENBERG
Hematology Division
Stanford University Cancer Center
875 Blake Wilbur Drive, Room 2335
Stanford CA 94305-5821
USA
Tel. +1 650 725 8355
Fax +1 650 723 1269
peterg@stanford.edu

Dr Karen L. GROGG
Mayo Medical Laboratories
Department of Laboratory Medicine and
Pathology, Mayo Clinic
200 First Street South-west
Rochester MN 55905
USA
Tel. +1 507 538 1180
Fax +1 507 284 1599
grogg.karen@mayo.edu

Dr Margarita GUENOVA
Laboratory of Haematopathology & Immuno-
logy, National Specialized Hospital for Active
Treatment of Haematological Diseases
6 Plovdivsko Pole Street
1756 Sofia
BULGARIA
Tel. +359 88 8248 324
Fax +359 2 870 7316
margenova@mail.bg

Dr Julien HAROCHE
Internal Medicine
Pitié-Salpêtrière Hospital
47-83, Boulevard de l'Hôpital
75013 Paris
FRANCE
Tel. +33 1 42 17 80 37
Fax +33 1 42 16 58 04
julien.haroche@aphp.fr

Dr Nancy Lee HARRIS
Pathology Department
Massachusetts General Hospital
55 Fruit Street, Warren 2
Boston MA 02114
USA
Tel. +1 617 724 1458
Fax +1 617 726 5626
nlharris@partners.org

Dr Robert Paul HASSERJIAN #
Pathology Department
Massachusetts General Hospital
55 Fruit Street, Warren 219
Boston MA 02114-2698
USA
Tel. +1 617 724 1445
Fax +1 617 726 7474
rhasserjian@partners.org

Dr Eva HELLSTRÖM-LINDBERG #
Division of Hematology, Dep. of Medicine
Karolinska Univ. Hospital, Huddinge
Karolinska Institutet
SE-141 86 Stockholm
SWEDEN
Tel. +46 8 585 860 36
Fax +46 8 585 836 05
eva.hellstrom-lindberg@ki.se

Dr Hans-Peter HORNY
Institute of Pathology
Ludwig Maximilians University
Thalkirchner Strasse 36
D-80337 Munich
GERMANY
Tel. +49 89 2180 73698
Fax +49 1 2180 73604
hans-peter.horny@med.uni-muenchen.de

Dr Giorgio G. INGHIRAMI #
Department of Pathology and Laboratory
Medicine, Weill Cornell Medical College
NewYork-Presbyterian Hospital, Cornell
Campus
525 East 68th Street, F709
New York NY 10065
USA
Tel. +1 212 746 5616
ggi9001@med.cornell.edu

Dr Peter G. ISAACSON
Department of Histopathology
UCL Medical School
University Street
London WC1E 6JJ
UNITED KINGDOM
Tel. +44 20 7679 6045
Fax +44 20 7387 3674
p.isaacson@ucl.ac.uk

Dr Elaine S. JAFFE #
Laboratory of Pathology
Center for Cancer Research, NCI, NIH
10 Center Drive, MSC-1500
Building 10, Room 3S 235
Bethesda MD 20892-1500
USA
Tel. +1 301 480 8040
Fax +1 301 480 8089
ejaffe@mail.nih.gov

Dr Ronald JAFFE #
Department of Pathology
Children's Hospital of Pittsburgh of UPMC
4404 Penn Avenue
Pittsburgh PA 15224
USA
Tel. +1 412 692 5657
Fax +1 412 692 6550
ronald.jaffe@chp.edu

Dr Daniel M. JONES #
Department of Pathology
Nichols Institute
14225 Newbrook Drive
Chantilly VA 20153
USA
Tel. +1 703 802 7257
Fax +1 703 802 7113
dan.jones@questdiagnostics.com
dajones@mdanderson.org

Dr Marshall E. KADIN #
Department of Dermatology and Skin Surgery
Roger Williams Medical Center
Boston University School of Medicine
50 Maude Street
Providence RI 02908
USA
Tel. +1 401 456 2521
Fax +1 401 456 6449
mkadin@chartercare.org; mkadin@rwmc.org

Dr Hiroshi KIMURA
Department of Virology
Nagoya University
Graduate School of Medicine
65 Tsurumai-cho, Showa-ku
Nagoya 466-8550
JAPAN
Tel. +81 52 744 2207
Fax +81 52 744 2452
hkimura@med.nagoya-u.ac.jp

Dr Marsha C. KINNEY #
Department of Pathology
University of Texas Health Science Center
7703 Floyd Curl Drive
San Antonio TX 78229-3900
USA
Tel. +1 210 567 4098
Fax +1 210 567 0409
kinneym@uthscsa.edu

Dr Philip M. KLUIN
Department of Pathology and Medical Biology
University Medical Center Groningen
University of Groningen
Hanzeplein 1, Groningen Postbus 30001
9713 GZ Groningen
THE NETHERLANDS
Tel. +31 50 361 1766; +31 50 361 0020
Fax +31 50 361 9107
p.m.kluin@umcg.nl

Dr Young-Hyeh KO
Department of Pathology
Samsung Medical Center
SKKU School of Medicine
50 Irwon-dong, Gangnam-gu
135-710 Seoul
REPUBLIC OF KOREA
Tel. +82 2 3410 2762
Fax +82 2 3410 0025
yhko310@skku.edu

Dr Alla M. KOVRIGINA #
Department of Pathology
National Research Center for Hematology
Ministry of Healthcare of Russian Federation
Novy Zykovskij proezd 4, Moscow
125167, RUSSIAN FEDERATION
Tel. +7 495 612 62 12
Fax +7 495 612 49 60
kovrigina.alla@gmail.com

Dr Laszlo KRENACS
Laboratory of Tumor Pathology
and Molecular Diagnostics
Jobb fasor 23B
Szeged, 6726
HUNGARY
Tel. +36 62 550 545
Fax +36 62 550 545
krenacsl@vipmail.hu; t-sejt@invitel.hu

Dr W. Michael KUEHL
Genetics Branch
Center for Cancer Research, NCI, NIH
Bethesda Naval Hospital
Building 37, Room 6002C
Bethesda MD 20892-4265
USA
Tel. +1 301 435 5421
Fax +1 301 496 0047
kuehlw@helix.nih.gov

Dr Hans Michael KVASNICKA
Senckenberg Institute of Pathology
Goethe University Frankfurt
Theodor-Stern-Kai 7
60590 Frankfurt am Main
GERMANY
Tel. +49 221 478 6369
Fax +49 221 478 6360
hans-michael.kvasnicka@kgu.de

Dr Robert A. KYLE #
Departments of Medicine and Laboratory
Medicine and Pathology
Mayo Clinic
200 First Street South-west
Rochester MN 55905
USA
Tel. +1 507 284 3039
Fax +1 507 266 9277
kyle.robert@mayo.edu

Dr Laurence LAMANT-ROCHAIX
Service Anatomie Pathologique
Institut Univ. du Cancer de Toulouse Oncopole
1, Avenue Irène Joliot-Curie
31059 Toulouse Cedex 9
FRANCE
Tel. +33 5 31 15 61 97
Fax +33 5 31 15 65 94
laurence.lamant@inserm.fr
lamant.l@chutoulouse.fr

Dr Richard A. LARSON
Department of Medicine
University of Chicago
Cancer Research Center
5841 South Maryland Avenue
MC2115 Chicago IL 60637
USA
Tel. +1 773 702 6783
Fax +1 773 702 3002
rlarson@medicine.bsd.uchicago.edu

Dr Michelle M. LE BEAU
Cancer Cytogenetics Laboratory
University of Chicago
Comprehensive Cancer Center
5841 South Maryland Avenue
MC1140 Chicago IL 60637
USA
Tel. +1 773 702 0795
Fax +1 773 702 9311
mlebeau@bsd.uchicago.edu

Dr Lorenzo LEONCINI
Dept. of Human Pathology and Oncology
University of Siena
Nuovo Policlinico Le Scotte
Via delle Scotte 6
53100 Siena
ITALY
Tel. +39 0577 233237
Fax +39 0577 233235
leoncinil@unisi.it

Dr Ross LEVINE
Human Oncology and Pathogenesis Program
Memorial Sloan Kettering Cancer Center
1275 York Avenue, Box 20
New York NY 10021
USA
Tel. +1 646 888 2796
leviner@mskcc.org

Dr Alan F. LIST #
Department of Malignant Hematology and
Administration, H. Lee Moffitt Cancer
Center & Research Institute
12902 Magnolia Drive, Mail Stop SRB-CEO
Tampa FL 33612-9497
USA
Tel. +1 813 745 6086
Fax +1 813 745 3090
alan.list@moffitt.org

Dr Kenneth A. MacLENNAN
Section of Pathology and Tumour Histology
University of Leeds
Leeds LS9 7TF
UNITED KINGDOM
Tel. +44 113 206 8919
Fax +44 113 392 6483
kenneth.maclennan@leedsth.nhs.uk

Dr William R. MACON [#]
Department of Laboratory
Medicine and Pathology
Mayo Clinic
200 First Street South-west
Rochester MN 55905
USA
Tel. +1 507 284 1198
Fax +1 507 284 5115
macon.william@mayo.edu

Dr Luca MALCOVATI
Department of Molecular Medicine
University of Pavia
Fondazione IRCCS Policlinico San Matteo
Piazzale Golgi 2
27100 Pavia
ITALY
Tel. +39 382 503 062
Fax +39 382 502 250
luca.malcovati@unipv.it

Dr Estella MATUTES
Haematopathology Unit
University Hospital Clínic de Barcelona
IDIBAPS, C/ Villarroel 170
08036 Barcelona
SPAIN
Tel. +34 66 310 9312
Fax +34 93 227 5572
estella.matutes.juan@gmail.com

Dr Robert W. McKENNA
Department of Laboratory
Medicine and Pathology
University of Minnesota
420 Delaware Street South-east
MMC 609 Minneapolis MN 55455
USA
Tel. +1 612 624 2637
Fax: +1 612 624 6662
mcken138@umn.edu

Dr Junia V. MELO
Professor of Haematology
University of Adelaide
Adelaide, SA 5000
AUSTRALIA
junia.melo@adelaide.edu.au

Dr Dean D. METCALFE
Laboratory of Allergic Diseases
NIAID, National Institutes of Health
10 Center Drive, MSC-1881
Building 10, Room 11C205/207
Bethesda MD 20892-1881
USA
Tel. +1 301 496 2165
Fax +1 301 480 8384
dmetcalfe@niaid.nih.gov

Dr Manuela MOLLEJO
Department of Pathology
Hospital Virgen de la Salud
Avenida de Barber 30
45004 Toledo
SPAIN
Tel. +34 925 269 245
Fax +34 925 253 613
mmollejov@sescam.jccm.es

Dr Peter MÖLLER
Department of Pathology
University of Ulm
Oberer Eselsberg M23
Albert-Einstein-Allee 11
89081 Ulm
GERMANY
Tel. +49 731 5005 6320
Fax +49 731 5005 6384
peter.moeller@uniklinik-ulm.de

Dr Emili MONTSERRAT
Department of Haematology
University Hospital Clínic de Barcelona
IDIBAPS, C/ Villarroel 170
08036 Barcelona
SPAIN
Tel. +34 93 227 5475
Fax +34 93 227 9811
emontse@clinic.ub.es

Dr William G. MORICE
Department of Pathology
and Laboratory Medicine
Mayo Clinic
200 First Street South-west, Hilton Building
Rochester MN 55905
USA
Tel. +1 507 284 2396
Fax +1 507 284 5115
morice.william@mayo.edu

Dr Hans Konrad MÜLLER-HERMELINK
Institute of Pathology
University of Würzburg
Josef-Schneider-Strasse 2
97080 Würzburg
GERMANY
Tel. +49 931 318 3751
Fax +49 431 597 2007
konrad.mh@mail.uni-wuerzburg.de

Dr Shigeo NAKAMURA
Department of Pathology and
Laboratory Medicine
Nagoya University Hospital
65 Tsurumai-cho, Showa-ku
Nagoya 466-8560
JAPAN
Tel. +81 52 744 2896
Fax +81 52 744 2897
snakamur@med.nagoya-u.ac.jp

Dr Bharat N. NATHWANI
Director of Pathology Consultation Services
City of Hope National Medical Center
1500 East Duarte Road, Room 2287B
Duarte CA 91010
USA
Tel. +1 626 359 8111 ext. 64101
Fax +1 626 218 9020
bharat.nathwani@gmail.com

Dr Charlotte M. NIEMEYER [#]
Department of Pediatrics and
Adolescent Medicine
University of Freiburg
Mathildenstrasse 1
79106 Freiburg im Breisgau
GERMANY
Tel. +49 761 270 45060
Fax +49 761 270 45180
charlotte.niemeyer@uniklinik-freiburg.de

Dr Koichi OHSHIMA
Department of Pathology
Kurume University School of Medicine
67 Asahi-machi
Kurume, Fukuoka 830-0011
JAPAN
Tel. +81 942 31 7547
Fax +81 942 31 0342
ohshima_kouichi@med.kurume-u.ac.jp

Dr Mihaela ONCIU
Oncometrix Laboratory
Poplar Healthcare
3495 Hacks Cross Road
Memphis TN 38120
USA
Tel. +1 901 435 2131
Fax +1 901 271 2648
m.onciu@oncometrix.com

Dr Attilio ORAZI [#]
Department of Pathology and
Laboratory Medicine
Weill Cornell Medical College
525 East 68th Street
New York NY 10021
USA
Tel. +1 212 746 2442
Fax +1 212 746 8173
ato9002@med.cornell.edu

Dr German OTT
Department of Clinical Pathology
Robert Bosch Hospital
Auerbachstrasse 110
70376 Stuttgart
GERMANY
Tel. +49 711 8101 3394
Fax +49 711 8101 3619
german.ott@rbk.de

Dr Marco PAULLI
Pathology Unit, Department of Molecular
Medicine, University of Pavia
Fondazione IRCCS Policlinico San Matteo
Via Forlanini 14
27100 Pavia
ITALY
Tel. +39 38 250 1241; +39 38 250 2953
Fax +39 38 252 5866
m.paulli@smatteo.pv.it

Dr LoAnn C. PETERSON
Department of Pathology
Northwestern University
Feinberg School of Medicine
251 East Huron Street
Chicago IL 60611
USA
loannc@northwestern.edu

Dr Tony PETRELLA
University of Montréal
Hôpital Maisonneuve-Rosemont
5415 Bd de l'Assomption
Montréal (QC) H1T2M4
CANADA
Tel. +1 514 377 4412
Fax +1 514 252 3538
tony.petrella@umontreal.ca

Dr Stefano A. PILERI (1)
Department of Experimental, Diagnostic and
Specialty Medicine
University of Bologna School of Medicine
St. Orsola Hospital, Building 8
Via Giuseppe Massarenti 9
40138 Bologna
ITALY
Tel. +39 051 636 3044
stefano.pileri@unibo.it

Dr Stefano A. PILERI (2)
European Institute of Oncology
Via Giuseppe Ripamonti 435
20141 Milano
ITALY
Tel: +39 02 574 89521
stefano.pileri@ieo.it

Dr Miguel A. PIRIS [#]
Department of Pathology
Fundación Jiménez Díaz
Av Reyes Católicos, 2
28040 Madrid
SPAIN
Tel. +34 91 550 4804
Fax +34 94 220 2492
miguel.piris@quironsalud.es

Dr Stefania PITTALUGA
Laboratory of Pathology
Center for Cancer Research, NCI, NIH
10 Center Drive, MSC-1500
Building 10, Room 2S 235
Bethesda MD 20892-1500
USA
Tel. +1 301 480 8465
Fax +1 301 480 8089
stefpitt@mail.nih.gov

Dr Maurilio PONZONI
Unit of Lymphoid Malignancies
San Raffaele Scientific Institute
Via Olgettina 60
20132 Milan
ITALY
Tel. +39 2 2643 2544
Fax +39 2 2643 2409
ponzoni.maurilio@hsr.it

Dr Sibrand POPPEMA
Board of the University of Groningen
University of Groningen
PO Box 72
9700 AB Groningen
THE NETHERLANDS
Tel. +31 50 363 52 82
Fax +31 50 363 48 47
s.poppema@rug.nl; i.h.j.bolwijn@rug.nl

Dr Anna PORWIT [#]
Lund University
Faculty of Medicine,
Department of Clinical Sciences
Division of Oncology and Pathology
Sölvegatan 25
SE-22185 Lund
SWEDEN
Tel. +46 46 17 48 60
anna.porwit@skane.se

Dr Leticia QUINTANILLA-MARTINEZ
Institute of Pathology, UKT
Eberhard Karls Universität Tübingen
Liebermeisterstrasse 8
72076 Tübingen
GERMANY
Tel. +49 707 1298 2266
Fax +49 707 1292 258
leticia.quintanilla-fend@med.uni-tuebingen.de

Dr Jerald P. RADICH [#]
Clinical Research Division
Fred Hutchinson Cancer Research Center
1100 Fairview Avenue North,
Box 19024, #D4-100
Seattle WA 98109-1024
USA
Tel. +1 206 667 4118
Fax +1 206 667 2917
jradich@fhcrc.org

Dr Andreas ROSENWALD
Institute of Pathology
University of Würzburg
Josef-Schneider-Strasse 2
97080 Würzburg
GERMANY
Tel. +49 931 31 81199
Fax +49 931 31 81224
rosenwald@mail.uni-wuerzburg.de

Dr Davide ROSSI
Department of Translational Medicine
Amedeo Avogadro Univ. of Eastern Piedmont
Via Paolo Solaroli 17
28100 Novara
ITALY
Tel. +39 321 660 698
Fax +39 321 320 421
rossidav@med.unipmn.it; davide.rossi@med.
unipmn.it

Dr Jonathan SAID
Department of Pathology and
Laboratory Medicine
Center for the Health Sciences, 13-222 UCLA
10833 Le Conte Avenue
Los Angeles CA 90095-1732
USA
Tel. +1 310 825 1149
Fax +1 310 825 5674
jsaid@mednet.ucla.edu

Dr Itziar SALAVERRIA
Molecular Pathology Laboratory
University Hospital Clínic de Barcelona
IDIBAPS, C/ Rosselló 153, Second floor
08036 Barcelona
SPAIN
Tel. +34 93 227 5400 ext. 4582
Fax +34 93 312 9407
isalaver@clinic.ub.es

Dr Christian A. SANDER
Department of Dermatology
Asklepios Klinik St. Georg
Lohmühlenstrasse 5
20099 Hamburg
GERMANY
Tel. +49 40 18 18 85 2220
Fax +49 40 18 18 85 2462
c.sander@asklepios.com

Dr Masao SETO
Department of Pathology
Kurume University School of Medicine
67 Asahi-machi
Kurume, Fukuoka 830-0011
JAPAN
Tel. +81 942 31 7547
Fax +81 842 31 0342
masaoseto@air.ocn.ne.jp; seto_masao@
kurume-u.ac.jp

Dr Reiner SIEBERT [#]
Institute of Human Genetics
University Hospital of Ulm
Albert-Einstein-Allee 11
D-89081 Ulm
GERMANY
Tel. +49 731 500 654 00
Fax +49 731 500 654 02
reiner.siebert@uni-ulm.de

Dr Bruce R. SMOLLER
Department of Pathology
College of Medicine
University of Arkansas for Medical Sciences
4301 West Markham Street
Little Rock AR 72205
USA
Tel. +1 501 686 5170
Fax +1 501 296 1184
smollerbrucer@uams.edu

Dr Ivy SNG
Department of Pathology
Singapore General Hospital
20 College Road, Academia
Level 10, Diagnostics Tower
Singapore 169856
SINGAPORE
Tel. +65 6321 4926
Fax +65 6227 6562
ivy.sng.t.y@sgh.com.sg

Dr Aliyah R. SOHANI
Pathology Department
Massachusetts General Hospital
55 Fruit Street
Boston MA 02114
USA
Tel. +1 617 726 3187
Fax +1 617 726 7474
arsohani@partners.org

Dr Dominic SPAGNOLO
PathWest Laboratory Medicine WA
Locked Bag 2009
Nedlands WA 6909
AUSTRALIA
Tel. +61 8 9346 2953
Fax +61 8 9346 4122
dominic.spagnolo@health.wa.gov.au

Dr Harald STEIN [#]
Pathodiagnostik Berlin
Komturstrasse 58-62
12099 Berlin
GERMANY
Tel. +49 30 236 084 210
Fax +49 30 236 084 219
+49 30 236 084 218
h.stein@pathodiagnostik.de

Dr Christer SUNDSTRÖM
Department of Pathology
Uppsala University Hospital
SE-751 85 Uppsala
SWEDEN
Tel. +46 18 611 3806
Fax +46 18 611 2665
christer.sundstrom@akademiska.se

Dr Steven H. SWERDLOW [#]
Division of Hematopathology
UPMC Presbyterian
200 Lothrop Street, Room G-335
Pittsburgh PA 15213-2582
USA
Tel. +1 412 647 5191
Fax +1 412 647 4008
swerdlowsh@upmc.edu

Dr Soo Yong TAN
Department of Pathology
Histopathology Laboratory
Singapore General Hospital
20 College Road
Singapore 169856
SINGAPORE
Tel. +65 9793 4357
drtansy@gmail.com

Dr Ayalew TEFFERI
Division of Hematology
Mayo Clinic
200 First Street South-west
Rochester MN 55905
USA
Tel. +1 507 284 3159
Fax +1 507 266 4972
tefferi.ayalew@mayo.edu

Dr Catherine THIEBLEMONT
Unit of Onco-Haematology
Saint-Louis Hospital
1 Avenue Claude Vellefaux
75010 Paris
FRANCE
Tel. +33 1 42 49 92 36
Fax +33 1 42 49 96 41
catherine.thieblemont@sls.aphp.fr

Dr Jürgen THIELE [#]
Institute for Pathology
University of Cologne
Kerpener Strasse 62
50924 Cologne
GERMANY
Tel. +49 511 544 8948
Fax +49 511 544 8493
j.thiele@uni-koeln.de

Dr Peter VALENT
Medical University of Vienna
Waehringer Guertel 18-20
A-1090 Vienna
AUSTRIA
Tel. +43 1 404 006085
Fax +43 1 404 004030
peter.valent@meduniwien.ac.at

Dr J. Han VAN KRIEKEN
Department of Pathology
Radboud University Nijmegen Medical Centre
PO Box 9101
6500 HB Nijmegen
THE NETHERLANDS
Tel. +31 24 361 4352
Fax +31 24 354 0520
han.vankrieken@radboudumc.nl

Dr James W. VARDIMAN [#]
Department of Pathology
University of Chicago Medical Center
5841 South Maryland Avenue
MC008, Room TW-055
Chicago IL 60637-1470
USA
Tel. +1 773 702 6196
Fax +1 773 702 1200
james.vardiman@uchospitals.edu

Dr Béatrice VERGIER
Service de Pathologie (Sud),
Hôpital Haut-Lévêque
CHU de Bordeaux, Avenue de Magellan
33604 Pessac
FRANCE
Tel. +33 5 57 65 60 26
Fax +33 5 57 65 63 72
beatrice.vergier@chu-bordeaux.fr

Dr Neus VILLAMOR
Haematopathology Unit
University Hospital Clínic de Barcelona
IDIBAPS, C/ Villarroel 170
08036 Barcelona
SPAIN
Tel. +34 93 227 5572
Fax +34 93 227 5572
villamor@clinic.ub.es; villamor@clinic.cat

Dr Steven A. WEBBER
Department of Pediatrics
Vanderbilt University School of Medicine
2200 Children's Way, Suite 2407
Nashville TN 37232-9900
USA
Tel. +1 615 322 3377
Fax +1 615 936 3330
steve.a.webber@vanderbilt.edu

Dr Dennis D. WEISENBURGER
Department of Pathology
City of Hope National Medical Center
1500 East Duarte Road
Duarte CA 91010-3600
USA
Tel. +1 626 256 4673 ext. 63584
Fax +1 626 301 8842
dweisenburger@coh.org

Dr Lawrence M. WEISS
Clarient Pathology Services Inc.
31 Columbia
Aliso Viejo CA 92656
USA
Tel. +1 626 227 6438
weiss11111@gmail.com

Dr Rein WILLEMZE
Department of Dermatology
Leiden University Medical Center
PO Box 9600, B1-Q-93
2300 RC Leiden
THE NETHERLANDS
Tel. +31 71 526 2421
Fax +31 71 524 8106
rein.willemze@planet.nl

Dr Wyndham H. WILSON
Lymphoma Therapeutics Section
Center for Cancer Research, NCI, NIH
9000 Rockville Pike, Metabolism Branch,
Building 10, Room 4N115
Bethesda MD 20892
USA
Tel. +1 301 435 2415, Fax +1 301 402 0172
wilsonw@mail.nih.gov

Dr Sean J. WHITTAKER [#]
Skin Cancer Unit, Division of Genetics &
Molecular Medicine, KCL, St John's Institute
of Dermatology, St Thomas' Hospital
Westminster Bridge Road
London SE1 7EH
UNITED KINGDOM
Tel. +44 20 7188 8076
Fax +44 20 7188 8050
sean.whittaker@kcl.ac.uk

Dr Tadashi YOSHINO
Dep. of Pathology Okayama Univ. Graduate
School of Medicine
2-5-1 Shikata-cho
Okayama 700-8558
JAPAN
Tel. +81 86 235 7149
Fax +81 86 235 7156
yoshino@md.okayama-u.ac.jp

Declaration of interests

Dr Akin reports receiving personal consulting fees from Novartis.

Dr Arber reports having received personal consulting fees from United States Diagnostic Standards.

Dr Baccarani reports receiving personal consulting and speaking fees from Ariad, Bristol-Myers Squibb, Novartis, and Pfizer.

Dr Béné reports having received travel and lodging support from Celgene, Beckman Coulter, Mundipharma, Roche and Chugai. She participated in COST EuGESMA, which covered travel and lodging expenses. She has received personal consulting fees from Beckman Coulter, and as head of the Harmonemia project also received travel and lodging support from Beckman Coulter.

Dr Bennett reports receiving personal consulting fees from Celgene and providing unremunerated consulting services to GlaxoSmithKline, Onconova Therapeutics, and Amgen.

Dr Birgegård reports that the Department of Medical Sciences at Uppsala University has received research funding from Shire. He also reports having received speaking fees from Shire and Renapharma AB, and consulting fees from Shire.

Dr Borowitz reports receiving research support from Bristol-Myers Squibb, Amgen, and MedImmune, and having received research support from Beckman Coulter. He reports receiving non-financial research support from Becton, Dickinson and Company.

Dr Brousse reports having received personal speaking fees from Roche, Kephren, and Acuitude.

Dr Chadburn reports receiving personal consulting fees from Clarient.

Dr Wing Chung Chan reports owning intellectual property rights in a patent (held by the United States National Cancer Institute) on the classification of B-cell lymphoma using gene expression signatures.

Dr Cook reports having received personal consulting fees from Medical Marketing Economics.

Dr de Jong reports receiving personal consulting fees from Millennium Pharmaceuticals and Celgene.

Dr Dogan reports receiving personal consulting fees from Janssen Pharmaceuticals.

Dr Escribano reports receiving travel support from Thermo Fisher Scientific Brazil.

Dr Falini reports having applied for a patent on the clinical use of nucleophosmin protein (NPM1) mutants.

Dr Feldman reports owning intellectual property rights in United States patents (held by Mayo Clinic) on reducing IRF4, DUSP22, or FLJ43663 polypeptide expression and on detecting $TBL1XR1$ and $TP63$ translocations.

Dr Fend reports having received travel support from Roche and Janssen Pharmaceuticals.

Dr Gascoyne reports receiving personal speaking fees and research support from Seattle Genetics. He reports receiving personal consulting fees from Celgene, Seattle Genetics, Genentech, Roche, and Janssen Pharmaceuticals.

Dr Gatterman reports receiving personal consulting fees and research support from Novartis and Celgene. He reports receiving personal speaking fees and travel support from Novartis.

Dr Germing reports that the MDS Registry, through the University of Düsseldorf, has received funding from Novartis, Celgene, Chugai, Amgen, and Johnson & Johnson. He reports receiving personal speaking fees from Celgene and Johnson & Johnson.

Dr Ghia reports receiving personal consulting fees from Gilead Sciences, Pharmacyclics, Merck, MedImmune, Roche, and AbbVie. He reports receiving personal speaking fees from Gilead Sciences and research support from Roche and GlaxoSmithKline.

Dr Hasserjian reports having received personal consulting fees from Sanofi and Incyte.

Dr Hellström-Lindberg reports receiving unrestricted research support from Celgene.

Dr Inghirami reports having received personal consulting fees from Menarini Diagnostics, Celgene, and Seattle Genetics.

Dr Elaine S. Jaffe reports receiving personal speaking fees from the French and Australasian Divisions of the International Academy of Pathology.

Dr Ronald Jaffe reports receiving personal consulting fees from GlaxoSmithKline.

Dr Jones reports that he is a director and shareholder at Quest Diagnostics.

Dr Kadin reports receiving personal consulting fees from Allergan.

Dr Kinney reports that the University of Texas Health Science Center at San Antonio has received fees from Seattle Genetics for her consulting services.

Dr Kovrigina reports receiving travel support and personal consulting fees from Novartis.

Dr Kyle reports being on monitoring committees or boards for Celgene, Novartis, Merck, Bristol-Myers Squibb, Aeterna Zentaris (Keryx), Onyx Pharmaceuticals (Amgen), and Pharmacyclics. He reports receiving personal consulting fees from Binding Site.

Dr List reports receiving personal consulting fees from Cell Therapeutics and Celgene. He reports having received research support from Celgene.

Dr Macon reports receiving personal consulting fees from Seattle Genetics.

Dr Niemeyer reports that the University of Freiburg receives fees from Celgene for her consulting services.

Dr Orazi reports receiving personal consulting fees from Incyte and speaking fees from Incyte and Novartis. He reports that the Department of Pathology and Laboratory Medicine at Weill Cornell Medical College has a contract with GlaxoSmithKline to review histology slides from patients with chronic idiopathic thrombocytopenic purpura who have received long-term recombinant thrombopoietin therapy.

Dr Piris reports receiving personal speaking fees from Takeda.

Dr Porwit reports receiving meeting travel support from Beckman Coulter and personal speaking fees from Novartis.

Dr Radich reports receiving honoraria from Novartis, Bristol-Myers Squibb, Ariad, and Pfizer. He reports that the Fred Hutchinson Cancer Research Center receives non-financial research support from Novartis.

Dr Siebert reports receiving non-financial research support from Abbott.

Dr Stein reports receiving technical research support from HistoGene.

Dr Swerdlow reports having received personal consulting fees from Centocor R&D, Travel Destinations Management Group, and Johnson & Johnson.

Dr Thiele reports having received personal consulting fees from Sanofi, Incyte and Novartis.

Dr Vardiman reports that his department at the University of Chicago has received fees from Celgene for his consulting services.

Dr Whittaker reports that his research unit at St John's Institute of Dermatology receives fees from Actelion, Yaupon Therapeutics, and ProStrakan for his consulting services. He reports that his unit has also received fees for his consulting services from Johnson & Johnson.

Clinical Advisory Committee (Leukaemias)

Dr Cem Akin
Allergy and Immunology
Brigham and Women's Hospital
Chestnut Hill, MA 02467, USA

Dr Robert J. Arceci
Phoenix Children's Hospital
College of Medicine
University of Arizona
Phoenix, AZ 85004, USA

Dr Michele Baccarani
Policlinico S. Orsola
University of Bologna
40138 Bologna, Italy

Dr Tiziano Barbui
Research Foundation
Ospedale Papa Giovanni XXIII
24127 Bergamo, Italy

Dr Giovanni Barosi
Fondazione IRCCS
Policlinico San Matteo
27100 Pavia, Italy

Dr John M. Bennett
University of Rochester
Medical Center
Rochester, NY 14642, USA

Dr Clara D. Bloomfield #
James Cancer Hospital
and Solove Research Institute
Ohio State University
Columbus, OH 43210, USA

Dr Alan K. Burnett
Cardiff University School
of Medicine
Cardiff CF14 FXN, UK

Dr William Carroll
NYU Cancer Institute
New York, NY 10016-6402,
USA

Dr Mario Cazzola #
Policlinico San Matteo
University of Pavia
27100 Pavia, Italy

Dr Hartmut Döhner
Internal Medicine
University of Ulm
89081 Ulm, Germany

Dr James R. Downing
St. Jude Children's Research
Hospital
Memphis, TN 38105, USA

Dr Elihu H. Estey
University of Washington
School of Medicine
Seattle Cancer Care Alliance
Seattle, WA 98109, USA

Dr Brunangelo Falini
University of Perugia
Polo di Monteluce
06123 Perugia, Italy

Dr Pierre Fenaux
Hôpital Saint-Louis
Université Paris 7
75475 Paris, France

Dr Robin Foà
Division of Hematology
Sapienza University of Rome
00161 Rome, Italy

Dr Ulrich Germing
Klinik für Hämatologie, Onkologie
und Klinische Immunologie
Heinrich Heine University
40225 Düsseldorf, Germany

Dr Heinz Gisslinger
Medical University of Vienna
1090 Vienna
Austria

Dr Jason Gotlib
Stanford University
Cancer Center
Stanford, CA 94305-5821, USA

Dr Peter L. Greenberg
Stanford University
Cancer Center
Stanford CA 94305-5821, USA

Dr David Grimwade
Guy's Hospital
London SW15 2RG, UK

Dr Rüdiger Hehlmann
Medical Faculty Mannheim
University of Heidelberg
68169 Mannheim, Germany

Dr Eva Hellström-Lindberg
Department of Medicine,
Karolinska Institutet
SE-171 77 Stockholm, Sweden

Dr Richard A. Larson
Department of Medicine
Hematology/Oncology
University of Chicago
Chicago, IL 60637, USA

Dr Ross Levine
Memorial Sloan Kettering
Cancer Center
New York, NY 10021, USA

Dr Alan F. List
Hematology/Oncology
Moffitt Cancer Center
Tampa, FL 33612, USA

Dr Luca Malcovati
Dept of Molecular Medicine
Policlinico San Matteo
27100 Pavia, Italy

Dr Tomoki Naoe
Graduate School of Medicine
Nagoya University
Nagoya 466-8550, Japan

Dr Charlotte M. Niemeyer
Department of Pediatrics and
Adolescent Medicine
University of Freiburg
79106 Freiburg, Germany

Dr Jerald P. Radich
Fred Hutchinson Cancer
Research Center
Seattle, WA 98109, USA

Dr Martin S. Tallman
Memorial Sloan Kettering
Cancer Center
New York, NY 10065, USA

Dr Ayalew Tefferi
Mayo Clinic
Rochester, MN 55905, USA

Dr Hwei-Fang Tien
National Taiwan University
Hospital
Taipei, Taiwan, China

A meeting with members of the Clinical Advisory Committees took place at the Gleacher Center, University of Chicago, 31 March to 1 April, 2014.
Co-chair

Clinical Advisory Committee (Lymphomas)

Dr Ranjana Advani #
Stanford University
Stanford, CA 94305-5821, USA

Dr Kenneth C. Anderson
Harvard Medical School
Dana-Farber Cancer Institute
Boston, MA 02115-6013, USA

Dr Wing Y. Au
Queen Mary Hospital
University of Hong Kong
Hong Kong SAR, China

Dr Peter Leif Bergsagel
Department of Medicine
Mayo Clinic
Scottsdale, AZ 85259, USA

Dr Joseph Connors
BC Cancer Agency
Vancouver Centre
Vancouver, BC V5Z 4E6, Canada

Dr Francesco d'Amore
Dept of Hematology
Aarhus University Hospital
Aarhus, Denmark

Dr Martin Dreyling
University Hospital
Ludwig Maximilian University
81377 Munich, Germany

Dr Arnold S. Freedman
Harvard Medical School
Dana-Farber Cancer Institute
Boston, MA 02115-6013, USA

Dr Jonathan Friedberg
James P. Wilmot Cancer Institute
University of Rochester
Rochester, NY 14642, USA

Dr Paolo Ghia
Università Vita-Salute
San Raffaele
20132 Milan, Italy

Dr Michele Ghielmini #
Oncology Institute of Southern
Switzerland
6500 Bellinzona, Switzerland

Dr John Gribben
London School of Medicine
London, E1 4NS
UK

Dr Anton Hagenbeek
Department of Haematology
Academic Medical Center
1105 AZ Amsterdam,
The Netherlands

Dr Peter Johnson
Southampton General Hospital
School of Medicine
Southampton S016 6YD, UK

Dr Brad S. Kahl
University of Wisconsin
UW Carbone Cancer Center
Madison, WI 53705-2275, USA

Dr Eva Kimby
Karolinska Institutet
Huddinge University Hospital
14186 Huddinge, Sweden

Dr Ann S. LaCasce
Harvard Medical School
Dana-Farber Cancer Institute
Boston, MA 02115-6013, USA

Dr John P. Leonard
New York-Presbyterian Hospital
Weill Cornell Medical Center
New York, NY 10803, USA

Dr Michael Link
Stanford University School
of Medicine
Palo Alto, CA 94304-1812, USA

Dr Armando López-Guillermo
Hospital Clinic
University of Barcelona
08036 Barcelona, Spain

Dr Michael Pfreundschuh
Department of Medicine I
Saarland University
D-66421 Homburg, Germany

Dr Steven Rosen
Robert H. Lurie
Comprehensive Cancer Center
Northwestern University
Chicago, IL 60611-3008, USA

Dr Gilles Andre Salles #
Hématologie
Centre Hospitalier Lyon-Sud
69495 Pierre-Bénite, France

Dr Kensei Tobinai
National Cancer Center Hospital
Tokyo 104-0045, Japan

Dr Steven P. Treon
Harvard Medical School
Dana-Farber Cancer Institute
Boston, MA 02115, USA

Dr Julie M. Vose
Oncology/Hematology
Nebraska Medical Center
Omaha, NE 681980-7680, USA

Dr Rein Willemze
Department of Dermatology
Leiden University Medical Center
2300 RC Leiden
The Netherlands

Dr Wyndham H. Wilson
Lymphoid Malignancy Branch
National Cancer Institute,
Bethesda, MD 20892, USA

Dr Anas Younes
Memorial Sloan Kettering
Cancer Center
New York, NY 10021, USA

Dr Andrew Zelenetz #
Memorial Sloan Kettering Cancer
Center
New York, NY 10065, USA

Dr Pier-Luigi Zinzani
Institute of Hematology Oncology
University of Bologna
40138 Bologna, Italy

Dr Emanuele Zucca
Oncology Insitute of Southern
Switzerland
6500 Bellinzona, Switzerland

Co-chair

IARC/WHO Committee for the International Classification of Diseases for Oncology (ICD-O)

Dr Daniel A. ARBER
Department of Pathology
University of Chicago
5841 S. Maryland Avenue,
S327, MC 3083
Chicago IL 60637
USA
Tel. +1 773 702 0647
Fax +1 773 834 5414
darber@uchicago.edu

Dr Freddie BRAY
Section of Cancer Surveillance
International Agency for Research on Cancer
150 Cours Albert Thomas
69372 Lyon
FRANCE
Tel. +33 4 72 73 84 53
Fax +33 4 72 73 86 96
brayf@iarc.fr

Mrs April FRITZ
A. Fritz and Associates, LLC
21361 Crestview Road
Reno NV 89521
USA
Tel. +1 775 636 7243
Fax +1 888 891 3012
april@afritz.org

Dr Robert JAKOB
Data Standards and Informatics
World Health Organization (WHO)
20 Avenue Appia
1211 Geneva 27
SWITZERLAND
Tel. +41 22 791 58 77
Fax +41 22 791 48 94
jakobr@who.int

Dr Paul KLEIHUES
Faculty of Medicine
University of Zurich
Pestalozzistrasse 5
8032 Zurich
SWITZERLAND
Tel. +41 44 362 21 10
Fax +41 44 251 06 65
kleihues@pathol.uzh.ch

Dr Hiroko OHGAKI
Section of Molecular Pathology
International Agency for Research on Cancer
150 Cours Albert Thomas
69372 Lyon
FRANCE
Tel. +33 4 72 73 85 34
Fax +33 4 72 73 86 98
ohgakih@iarc.fr

Dr Marion PIÑEROS
Section of Cancer Surveillance
International Agency for Research on Cancer
150 Cours Albert Thomas
69372 Lyon
FRANCE
Tel. +33 4 72 73 84 18
Fax +33 4 72 73 86 96
pinerosm@iarc.fr

Dr Brian ROUS
National Cancer Registration Service
Eastern Office
Victoria House, Capital Park
CB21 5XB, Fulbourn, Cambridge
UNITED KINGDOM
Tel. +44 1 223 213 625
Fax +44 1 223 213 571
brian.rous@phe.gov.uk

Dr Leslie H. SOBIN
Frederick National Laboratory for
Cancer Research - Cancer Human Biobank
National Cancer Institute
6110 Executive Blvd, Suite 250
Rockville MD 20852
USA
Tel. +1 301 443 7947
Fax +1 301 402 9325
leslie.sobin@nih.gov

Dr Steven H. SWERDLOW
Division of Hematopathology
UPMC Presbyterian
200 Lothrop Street, Room G-335
Pittsburgh PA 15213
USA
Tel. +1 412 647 5191
Fax +1 412 647 4008
swerdlowsh@upmc.edu

Sources of figures and tables

Sources of figures

1.01	Vardiman J.W.
1.02	Vardiman J.W.
1.03 A,B	Vardiman J.W.
1.04	Goasguen J. CHU, Université de Rennes, France
1.05	Porwit A.
1.06	Levine RL, Pardanani A, Tefferi A, Gilliland DG (2007). Role of JAK2 in the pathogenesis and therapy of myeloproliferative disorders. Nat Rev Cancer 7:673–83. Reprinted by permission from Macmillan Publishers Ltd. Copyright 2007.
2.01 A–C	Vardiman J.W.
2.02 A–D	Vardiman J.W.
2.03 A,B,D	Thiele J.
2.03 C	Vardiman J.W.
2.04 A,B	Vardiman J.W.
2.04 C	Thiele J.
2.05–2.07	Vardiman J.W.
2.08 A,B	Le Beau M.M.
2.09	Melo J.V.
2.10 A,B	Melo J.V.
2.11	Ann Hematol. CML--Where do we stand in 2015? 2015;94 Suppl 2:S103-5. Hehlmann R. With permission of Springer.
2.12 A,C,D	Vardiman J.W.
2.12 B	Reprinted with permission From: Anastasi J, Vardiman JW (2001). Chronic Myelogenous Leukemia and the Chronic Myeloproliferative Diseases. In: Neoplastic Hematopathology. 2nd Edition. Knowles DM (ed). Lippincott, Williams Wilkins. Philadelphia, USA. ©LWW
2.13 A,B	Thiele J.
2.14 A–D	Thiele J.
2.15	Vardiman J.W.
2.16 A	Vardiman J.W.
2.16 B–D	Thiele J.
2.17	Vardiman J.W.
2.18	Kvasnicka H.M.
2.19 A–C	Thiele J.
2.20 A–D	Thiele J.
2.21 A,B	Vardiman J.W.
2.22 A,B	Thiele J.
2.23 A	Vardiman J.W.
2.23 B–D	Thiele J.
2.24 A–C	Vardiman J.W.
2.25 A–D	Thiele J.
2.26 A,B	Kvasnicka H.M.
2.27 A,B	Vardiman J.W.
2.28	Vardiman J.W.
2.29	Vardiman J.W.
2.30 A,B	Kvasnicka H.M.
2.31	Kvasnicka H.M.
3.01 A,B	Medenica M. University of Chicago, USA (deceased)
3.01 C–3.03	Longley J.B. Department of Dermatology, University of Wisconsin School of Medicine and Public Health, Madison, WI, USA
3.04 A,B	Vardiman J.W.
3.05	Brunning R.D.
3.06 A	Jaffe E.S.
3.06 B	Vardiman J.W.
3.07–3.10	Vardiman J.W.
3.11 A,B	Horny H.-P.
4.01	Bain B.J.
4.02	Bain B.J.
4.03 A–C	Bain B.J.
4.04 A–C	Vardiman J.W.
4.05	Horny H.-P.
5.01 A,B	Vardiman J.W.
5.01 C	Orazi A.
5.02	Vardiman J.W.
5.03 A–C	Vardiman J.W.
5.03 D	Orazi A.
5.04 A–C	Vardiman J.W.
5.05 A,B	Vardiman J.W.
5.06–5.07	Orazi A.
5.08 A–C	Vardiman J.W.
5.09 A,B	Vardiman J.W.
5.10	Baumann I.
5.11 A,B	Vardiman J.W.
5.12	Niemeyer C.M.
5.13 A,B	Vardiman J.W.
5.13 C,D	Husain A. Department of Pathology, University of Chicago Medical Center, Chicago, IL USA
5.14 A–D	Vardiman J.W.
5.15 A–C	Bueso-Ramos C.
6.01–6.06	Brunning R.D.
6.07 A,B	Orazi A.
6.08–6.11	Brunning R.D.
6.12 A	Orazi A.
6.12 B	Thiele J.
6.13–6.15	Brunning R.D.
6.16 A	Brunning R.D.
6.16 B,C	Hasserjian R.P.
6.17	Hasserjian R.P.
6.18–6.20	Brunning R.D.
6.21 A	Brunning R.D.
6.21 B	Hasserjian R.P.
6.22–6.25	Baumann I.
7.01 A,B	Peterson L.C.
7.02 A–C	Vardiman J.W.
8.01	Arber D.A.
8.02	Brunning R.D.
8.03	Flandrin G. Laboratoire Central d'Hématopathologie Hôpital Necker Paris, France
8.04 A,B	Hirsch B. Dept. of Laboratory Medicine and Pathology, University of Minnesota Medical School, Minneapolis, MN, USA
8.05 A	Flandrin G. Laboratoire Central d'Hématopathologie Hôpital Necker, Paris, France
8.05 B	Brunning R.D.
8.06	Brunning R.D.
8.07	Falini B.
8.08 A,B	Hirsch B. Dept. of Laboratory Medicine and Pathology, University of Minnesota Medical School, Minneapolis, MN, USA
8.09 A,B	Brunning R.D.
8.10 A,B	Brunning R.D.
8.11	Vardiman J.W.
8.12	Arber D.A.
8.13 A–C	Brunning R.D.
8.14 A–D	Falini B.
8.15 A–C	Falini B.
8.16	Republished with permission of the American Society of Hematology, from: Mrózek K, Marcucci G, Paschka P, Whitman SP, Bloomfield CD. Clinical relevance of mutations and gene-expression changes in adult acute myeloid leukemia with normal cytogenetics: are we ready for a prognostically prioritized molecular classification? Blood. 2007; 109:431–48, and Döhner K, Schlenk RF, Habdank M, Scholl C, Rücker FG, Corbacioglu A, Bullinger L, Fröhling S, Döhner H. Mutant nucleophosmin (NPM1) predicts favorable prognosis in younger adults with acute myeloid leukemia and normal cytogenetics: interaction with other gene mutations. Blood. 2005;106:3740–6. Permission conveyed through Copyright Clearance

8.17   Center, Inc.
       From: Falini B, Mecucci C,
       Tiacci E, Alcalay M, Rosati R,
       Pasqualucci L, La Starza R,
       Diverio D, Colombo E,
       Santucci A, Bigerna B,
       Pacini R, Pucciarini A,
       Liso A, Vignetti M, Fazi P,
       Meani N, Pettirossi V,
       Saglio G, Mandelli F,
       Lo-Coco F, Pelicci PG,
       Martelli MF (2005). GIMEMA
       Acute Leukemia Working
       Party. Cytoplasmic nucleo-
       phosmin in acute myelo-
       genous leukemia with a
       normal karyotype.
       N Engl J Med. 352:254–66.
       Copyright Massachusetts
       Medical Society. Reprinted
       with permission from Massa-
       chusetts Medical Society

8.18   From: Schlenk RF, Döhner
       K, Krauter J, Fröhling S,
       Corbacioglu A, Bullinger
       L, Habdank M, Späth D,
       Morgan M, Benner A,
       Schlegelberger B, Heil G,
       Ganser A, Döhner H (2008).
       German-Austrian Acute Mye-
       loid Leukemia Study Group.
       Mutations and treatment
       outcome in cytogenetically
       normal acute myeloid
       leukemia. N Engl J Med.
       358:1909–18. Copyright
       ©2008 Massachusetts Medi-
       cal Society. Reprinted with
       permission from Massachu-
       setts Medical Society.

8.19   Republished with permission
       from American Society of
       Hematology.
       From: Taskesen E,
       Bullinger L, Corbacioglu A,
       Sanders MA, Erpelinck CA,
       Wouters BJ, van der Poel-
       van de Luytgaarde SC,
       Damm F, Krauter J,
       Ganser A, Schlenk RF,
       Löwenberg B, Delwel R,
       Döhner H, Valk PJ, Döhner
       K (2011). Prognostic impact,
       concurrent genetic muta-
       tions, and gene expression
       features of AML with CEBPA
       mutations in a cohort of 1182
       cytogenetically normal AML
       patients: further evidence
       for CEBPA double mutant
       AML as a distinctive disease
       entity. Blood. 117:2469–75.
       Permission conveyed
       through Copyright Clearance
       Center, Inc.
8.20 A,B   Arber D.A.
8.21   Reprinted with permission.
       From: Grimwade D,
       Walker H, Oliver F,
       Wheatley K, Harrison C,
       Harrison G, Rees J, Hann I,
       Stevens R, Burnett A,
       Goldstone A (1998).

         The importance of diagnostic
         cytogenetics on outcome
         in AML: analysis of 1,612
         patients entered into the
         MRC AML 10 trial. The Medi-
         cal Research Council Adult
         and Children's Leukaemia
         Working Parties.
         Blood 92:2322–33.
8.22   Vardiman J.W.
8.23 A–C Vardiman J.W.
8.24 A   Flandrin G.
         Laboratoire Central
         d'Hématopathologie
         Hôpital Necker,
         Paris, France
8.24 B   Brunning R.D.
8.25 A   Arber D.A.
8.25 B   Flandrin G.
         Laboratoire Central
         d'Hématopathologie
         Hôpital Necker,
         Paris, France
8.26   Brunning R.D.
8.27 A–C Brunning R.D.
8.28 A–C Flandrin G.
         Laboratoire Central
         d'Hématopathologie
         Hôpital Necker,
         Paris, France
8.29   Orazi A.
8.30 A,B Brunning R.D.
8.31 A,B Brunning R.D.
8.32   Brunning R.D.
8.33 A,B Falini B.
8.34 A,B Flandrin G.
         Laboratoire Central
         d'Hématopathologie
         Hôpital Necker,
         Paris, France
8.35   Orazi A.
8.36 A,B Brunning R.D.
8.37–8.38 A Flandrin G.
         Laboratoire Central
         d'Hématopathologie
         Hôpital Necker,
         Paris, France
8.38 B   Brunning R.D.
8.39 A   Brunning R.D.
8.39 B–D Orazi A.
8.40   Pileri S.A.
8.41   Pileri S.A.
8.42   Pileri S.A.
8.43   Baumann I.
8.44 A,B Baumann I.
8.44 C   Brunning R.D.
8.45   Baumann I.

9.01–9.04 Facchetti F.

10.01   Borowitz M.J.
10.02   Matutes E.
10.03–10.06 Borowitz M.J.

11.01   Adapted with permission
         of the American Society of
         Hematology, from Patho-
         biology of peripheral
         T-cell lymphomas. Jaffe ES.
         Hematology Am Soc

           Hematol Educ Program.
           2006:317–22; permission
           conveyed through Copyright
           Clearance Center Inc.
11.02   Stein H.
11.03   Campo E.
11.04   Campo E.
11.05   Jaffe E.S.
11.06   Jaffe E.S.
11.07   Vose J.M.
         Oncology/Hematology
         Nebraska Medical Center
         Omaha NE, USA
11.08   Jaffe E.S.

12.01 A,B Brunning R.D.
12.02 A,B Brunning R.D.
12.03 A,B Jaffe E.S.
12.04–12.06 Brunning R.D.
12.07–12.09 Carroll A.J.
         Department of Genetics,
         University of Alabama School
         of Medicine,
         Birmingham, AL, USA
12.10   Hasserjian R.P.
12.11 A,B Brunning R.D.
12.12 A,B Nathwani B.N.
12.13   Chan J.K.C.
12.14   Jaffe E.S.

13.01 A–C Rozman M.
         Hospital Clinic Barcelona,
         Barcelona, Spain
13.02 A,B Müller-Hermelink H.K.
13.03 A,B Müller-Hermelink H.K.
13.04 A–C Campo E.
13.05   Villamor N.
13.06   Campo E.
13.07   Campo E.
13.08 A–E Swerdlow S.H.
13.09   Reprinted with permission
         from: Rawstron AC,
         Shanafelt T, Lanasa MC,
         Landgren O, Hanson C,
         Orfao A, Hillmen P, Ghia P
         (2010). Different biology and
         clinical outcome according
         to the absolute numbers of
         clonal B-cells in monoclonal
         B-cell lymphocytosis (MBL).
         Cytometry B Clin Cytom. 78
         Suppl 1:19–23.
13.10   Matutes E.
13.11   Jaffe E.S.
13.12   Jaffe E.S.
13.13–13.17 Isaacson P.G.
13.18   Harris N.L.
13.19–13.21 Foucar K.
13.22 A,B Foucar K.
13.22 C,D Falini B.
13.23 A–C Piris M.A.
13.24 A–D Piris M.A.
13.25 A   Matutes E.
13.25 B   Piris M.A.
13.26 A,B Swerdlow S.H.
13.26 C   Pileri S.A
13.27 A–C Swerdlow S.H.
13.28 A,B Swerdlow S.H.
13.29   Sohani A.R.
13.30   Cook J.R.
13.31   From: Munshi NC,

Digumarthy S, Rahemtullah A (2008). Case records of the Massachusetts General Hospital. Case 13-2008. A 46-year-old man with rheumatoid arthritis and lymphadenopathy. N Engl J Med. 358:1838–48. ©2008 Massachusetts Medical Society. Reprinted with permission.

13.32 Grogan T.M. University of Arizona College of Medicine, Tucson, AZ, USA

13.33 A,B Cook J.R.

13.34 Cook J.R.

13.35 – 13.36 From: Munshi NC, Digumarthy S, Rahemtullah A (2008). Case records of the Massachusetts General Hospital. Case 13-2008. A 46-year-old man with rheumatoid arthritis and lymphadenopathy. N Engl J Med. 358:1838–48. ©2008 Massachusetts Medical Society. Reprinted with permission.

13.37 A,B Isaacson P.G.

13.38 A Jaffe E.S.

13.38 B– Grogan T.M.

13.39 A University of Arizona College of Medicine, Tucson, AZ, USA

13.39 B Jaffe E.S.

13.40 A,B McKenna R.W.

13.41 A,B Grogan T.M. University of Arizona College of Medicine, Tucson, AZ, USA

13.42 Wians F.H. Department of Pathology Texas Tech University El Paso, TX, USA

13.43 Grogan T.M. University of Arizona College of Medicine, Tucson, AZ, USA

13.44 A McKenna R.W.

13.44 B – 13.46 Grogan T.M. University of Arizona College of Medicine, Tucson, AZ, USA

13.47 McKenna R.W.

13.48 A–D Fonseca R., Multiple Myeloma Lab. Mayo Clinic, Phoenix AZ, USA

13.49 A–D Roschke A., Gabrea A., Kuehl M.W. Genetics Branch, Center for Cancer Research, National Cancer Institute, NIH, Bethesda, MD, USA

13.50 – 13.56 Grogan T.M. University of Arizona College of Medicine, Tucson, AZ, USA

13.57 – 13.63 Isaacson P.G.

13.64 Cook J.R.

13.65 A,B Isaacson P.G.

13.66 A Campo E. & Swerdlow S.H.

13.66 B–E Campo E. & Jaffe E.S.

13.67 A,B Jaffe E.S.

13.68 Jaffe E.S.

13.69 Jaffe E.S.

13.70 A Nathwani B.N.

13.70 B–E Jaffe E.S.

13.71 A–C Jaffe E.S.

13.72 Nathwani B.N.

13.73 A–C Nathwani B.N.

13.74 A,B de Leval L.

13.75 A–D Jaffe E.S.

13.76 A,B de Leval L.

13.77 Jaffe E.S.

13.78 A Nathwani B.N.

13.78 B Jaffe E.S.

13.79 A–D Jaffe E.S.

13.80 A C de Leval L.

13.81 Adapted with permission from: Takata K, Tanino M, Ennishi D, Tari A, Sato Y, Okada H, Maeda Y, Goto N, Araki H, Harada M, Ando M, Iwamuro M, Tanimoto M, Yamamoto K, Gascoyne RD, Yoshino T. Duodenal follicular lymphoma: comprehensive gene expression analysis with insights into pathogenesis. Cancer Sci. 2014;105:608–15.

13.82 A–C Yoshino T.

13.83 A–E Jaffe E.S.

13.83 F Yoshino T.

13.84 A–F Jaffe E.S.

13.85 Pittaluga S.

13.86 Jaffe E.S.

13.87 A–C Pittaluga S.

13.87 D Jaffe E.S.

13.88 Pittaluga S.

13.89 – 13.92 A Willemze R.

13.92 B Vergier B.

13.92 C–E Willemze R.

13.93 A,B Harris N.L.

13.94 A–C Campo E.

13.95 A–C Swerdlow S.H.

13.96 Swerdlow S.H.

13.97 Republished with permission of J Clin Invest. From: Jares P, Colomer D, Campo E (2012). Molecular pathogenesis of mantle cell lymphoma. J Clin Invest. 122:3416–23. Permission conveyed through Copyright Clearance Center, Inc.

13.98 – 13.100 Swerdlow S.H.

13.101 Jaffe E.S.

13.102 A,B Jaffe E.S.

13.103 A Harris N.L.

13.103 B Warnke R.A. Department of Pathology Stanford University School of Medicine, Stanford, CA, USA

13.104 Gascoyne R.D.

13.105 Gascoyne R.D.

13.106 From: Scott DW, Mottok A, Ennishi D, Wright GW, Farinha P, Ben-Neriah S, et al. (2015). Prognostic Significance of Diffuse Large B-Cell Lymphoma Cell of Origin Determined by Digital Gene Expression in Formalin-Fixed Paraffin-Embedded Tissue Biopsies. J Clin Oncol. 33:2848–56. Reprinted with permission. ©2015 by American Society of Clinical Oncology. All rights reserved.

13.107 From: Nowakowski GS, LaPlant B, Macon WR, Reeder CB, Foran JM, Nelson GD, Thompson CA, Rivera CE, Inwards DJ, Micallef IN, Johnston PB, Porrata LF, Ansell SM, Gascoyne RD, Habermann TM, Witzig TE (2015). Lenalidomide combined with R-CHOP overcomes negative prognostic impact of non-germinal center B-cell phenotype in newly diagnosed diffuse large B-Cell lymphoma: a phase II study. J Clin Oncol. 33:251–7. Reprinted with permission. © 2015 American Society of Clinical Oncology. All rights reserved.

13.108 A–C Gascoyne R.D.

13.109 A,B De Wolf-Peeters C. Department of Pathology, University Hospitals K.U. Leuven, Leuven, Belgium

13.110 A,B Graus F. Hospital Clínic, University of Barcelona, Barcelona, Spain.

13.111 A,B van Baarlen J. Laboratorium Pathologie Oost-Nederland (LabPON), Hengelo, The Netherlands

13.112 A–C Kluin P.

13.113 Deckert M.

13.114 Willemze R.

13.115 A,B Willemze R.

13.116 A–C Willemze R.

13.117 A–C Nakamura S. & Murase T. Liaison Medical Marunouchi Nagoya, Japan

13.118 A–C Jaffe E.S.

13.119 A–C Nakamura S. & Murase T. Liaison Medical Marunouchi Nagoya, Japan

13.120 Jaffe E.S.

13.121 A–C Jaffe E.S.

13.122 A–D Jaffe E.S.

13.123 – 13.124 Aozasa K.

13.125 Reprinted with permission. From: Nishiu M, Tomita Y, Nakatsuka S, Takakuwa T, Iizuka N, Hoshida Y, Ikeda J, Iuchi K, Yanagawa R, Nakamura Y, Aozasa K (2004). Distinct pattern of gene expression in pyothorax-associated lymphoma (PAL), a lymphoma developing in long-standing inflammation. Cancer Sci. 95:828–34.

13.126 A–C Aozasa K.

13.127 A–C	Chan J.K.C.
13.128–13.131	Jaffe E.S.
13.132	Harris N.L.
13.133 A,B	Diebold J.
	Department of Anatomic Pathology and Cytology, Hotel-Dieu, University Denis Diderot, Paris, France
13.133 C	Harris N.L.
13.133 D	Banks P.M.
	Ventana Medical Systems, Tucson, AZ, USA
13.134–13.135	Diebold J.
	Department of Anatomic Pathology and Cytology, Hotel-Dieu, University Denis Diderot, Paris, France
13.136 A,B	Gaulard P.
13.137 A,B	Reprinted with permission from: Matsue K, Hayama BY, Iwama K, Koyama T, Fujiwara H, Yamakura M, Takeuchi M, O'uchi T (2011). High frequency of neuro-lymphomatosis as a relapse disease of intravascular large B-cell lymphoma. Cancer. 117:4512–21.
13.138–13.139	Nakamura S. & Murase T. Liaison Medical Marunouchi Nagoya, Japan
13.139 D	Diebold J.
	Department of Anatomic Pathology and Cytology, Hotel-Dieu, University Denis Diderot, Paris, France
13.140 A,B	Nakamura S.
13.140 C	Diebold J.
	Department of Anatomic Pathology and Cytology, Hotel-Dieu, University Denis Diderot, Paris, France
13.141 A,B	Delsol G.
	Centre Hospitalier Universitaire (CHU).
	Centre de Recherche en Cancerologie de Toulouse-Purpan, Toulouse, France
13.142 A–C	Diebold J.
	Department of Anatomic Pathology and Cytology, Hotel-Dieu, University Denis Diderot, Paris, France
13.143 A,B	Stein H.
13.144 A,B	Stein H.
13.144 C	Harris N.L.
13.145	Said J.
13.146	Said J.
13.147 A,B	Said J.
13.148–13.151	Isaacson P.G.
13.152 A–D	Said J.
13.153 A–C	Said J.
13.154–13.157	Jaffe E.S.
13.158 A	Pileri S.A.
13.158 B	Leoncini L.
13.158 C,D	Kluin P.M.
13.159 A,B	Kluin P.M.
13.159 C	Permission granted. From: Haralambieva E, Schuuring E, Rosati S, van Noesel C, Jansen P, Appel I, Guikema J, Wabinga H, Bleggi-Torres LF, Lam K, van den Berg E, Mellink C, van Zelderen-Bhola S, Kluin P (2004). Interphase fluorescence in situ hybridization for detection of 8q24/MYC breakpoints on routine histologic sections: validation in Burkitt lymphomas from three geographic regions. Genes Chromosomes Cancer. 40:10–8.
13.160	Adapted from: Campo E (2012). New pathogenic mechanisms in Burkitt lymphoma. Nat Genet. 44:1288–9. Copyright permission from Macmillan Publishers Ltd
13.161	Klapper W. Department of Pathology and Lymph Node Registry, Kiel University Hospital, Kiel, Germany
13.162	Salaverria I.
13.163–13.175	Kluin P.M.
13.176–13.179	Jaffe E.S.
13.180 A,B	Pack S. Laboratory of Pathology National Cancer Institute, Bethesda, MD, USA
14.01	Matutes E.
14.02 A,B	Müller-Hermelink H.K.
14.03 A,B	Müller-Hermelink H.K.
14.04	Müller-Hermelink H.K.
14.05	Chan J.K.C.
14.06 A,B	Chan W.C.
14.07 A	Morice W.G.
14.07 B,C	Osuji N. Croydon University Hospital, Croydon, UK
14.08	Reprinted with permission from: Jerez A, Clemente MJ, Makishima H, et al. (2012). STAT3 mutations unify the pathogenesis of chronic lymphoproliferative disorders of NK cells and T-cell large granular lymphocyte leukemia. Blood. 120:3048–57.
14.09	Morice W.G.
14.10 A–C	Villamor N.
14.10 D	Morice W.G
14.11–14.15	Chan J.K.C.
14.16 A–D	Ko Y.-H.
14.17–14.18	Quintanilla-Martinez L.
14.19 A–C	Jaffe E.S.
14.20 A–C	Jaffe E.S.
14.21 A,B	Quintanilla-Martinez L.
14.22 A–D	Jaffe E.S.
14.23 A–C	Quintanilla-Martinez L.
14.24 A–C	Ko Y.-H.
14.25 A–C	Quintanilla-Martinez L.
14.26 A–D	Quintanilla-Martinez L.
14.27	Jaffe E.S.
14.28 A–C	Jaffe E.S.
14.29–14.31	Quintanilla-Martinez L.
14.32 A–C	Ohshima K.
14.33	Ohshima K.
14.34	Jaffe E.S.
14.35	Ohshima K.
14.36 A,B	Kikuchi M. Pathology Department, School of Medicine, Kyushu University, Fukuoka city, Japan (deceased)
14.37	Ohshima K.
14.38 A	Ohshima K.
14.38 B	Kikuchi M. Pathology Department, School of Medicine, Kyushu University, Fukuoka city, Japan (deceased)
14.38 C	Jaffe E.S.
14.39 A,B	Ohshima K.
14.40	Jaffe E.S.
14.41	Jaffe E.S.
14.42	Ohshima K.
14.43	Jaffe E.S.
14.44 A,B	Kikuchi M. Pathology Department, School of Medicine, Kyushu University, Fukuoka city, Japan (deceased)
14.45	With permission from: Katsuya H, Ishitsuka K, Utsunomiya A, Hanada S, Eto T, Moriuchi Y, Saburi Y, Miyahara M, Sueoka E, Uike N, Yoshida S, Yamashita K, Tsukasaki K, Suzushima H, Ohno Y, Matsuoka H, Jo T, Amano M, Hino R, Shimokawa M, Kawai K, Suzumiya J, Tamura K. (2015). ATL-Prognostic Index Project. Treatment and survival among 1594 patients with ATL. Blood. 126:2570–7.
14.46 A,B	Chan J.K.C.
14.47	Chan J.K.C.
14.48	Jaffe E.S.
14.49 A–D	Chan J.K.C.
14.50–14.54	Chan J.K.C.
14.55	Harris N.L.
14.56	Bhagat G.
14.57	Wright D.H. University of Southampton, UK
14.58 A,B	Isaacson P.G.
14.58 C	Wright D.H. University of Southampton, UK
14.59 A–D	Isaacson P.G.
14.60	Isaacson P.G.
14.61 A,B	Bhagat G.
14.62–14.66	Jaffe E.S.
14.67	Tan S.Y.
14.68	Jaffe E.S.
14.69	Reprinted with permission from: Perry AM, Warnke RA, Hu Q, et al. (2013) Indolent T-cell lymphoproliferative disease of the gastrointestinal tract. Blood. 122:3599–606
14.70–14.74	Jaffe E.S.
14.75 A	Gaulard P.
14.75 B–D	Jaffe E.S.
14.76	Cerroni L.
14.77 A,B	Jaffe E.S.

14.78   Cerroni L.
14.79–14.81 Jaffe E.S.
14.82–14.89 Cerroni L.
14.90   Jaffe E.S.
14.91–14.97 Cerroni L.
14.98–14.100 Ralfkiaer E.
             Department of Pathology,
             Rigshospitalet,
             Copenhagen, Denmark
14.101–14.106 Willemze R.
14.107   Kadin M.E.
14.108 A–C   Kadin M.E.
14.109–14.114 Willemze R.
14.115   Jaffe E.S.
14.116 A–D   Toro J.R.
             Dermatology Branch,
             National Cancer Institute,
             NIH
             Bethesda, MD, USA
14.117   Jaffe E.S.
14.118 A–D   Jaffe E.S.
14.119   Jaffe E.S.
14.120   Willemze R.
14.121   Jaffe E.S.
14.122   Jaffe E.S.
14.123   Petrella T.
14.124 A   Carpentier O.
             Service de Dermatologie,
             Hôpital Claude Huriez,
             CHRU De Lille,
             Lille, France
14.124 B   Petrella T.
14.124 C   Dalle S.
             Université Claude Bernard,
             Lyon, France
14.125–14.130 Petrella T.
14.131 A,B   Willemze R.
14.132 A–C   Willemze R.
14.133 A–C   Ralfkiaer E.
             Department of Pathology,
             Rigshospitalet,
             Copenhagen, Denmark
14.134 A,B   Ralfkiaer E.
             Department of Pathology,
             Rigshospitalet,
             Copenhagen, Denmark
14.134 C,D   Jaffe E.S.
14.135–14.140 Pileri S.A.
14.141   Chan J.K.C.
14.142   Chan J.K.C.
14.143   Reprinted with permission
             from: Iqbal J, Wright G,
             Wang C, Rosenwald A,
             Gascoyne RD,
             Weisenburger DD, et al.
             (2014). Gene expres-
             sion signatures delineate
             biological and prognostic
             subgroups in peripheral
             T-cell lymphoma. Blood.
             123:2915–23.
14.144   Pileri S.A.
14.145   Pileri S.A.
14.146   de Leval L.
14.147 A–C   Dogan A.
14.148 A   Dogan A.
14.148 B   Jaffe E.S.
14.149–14.158 Dogan A.
14.159–14.161 Delsol G.
             Centre Hospitalier
             Universitaire (CHU).
             Centre de Recherche en
             Cancerologie de Toulouse-

14.162 A   Purpan,
             Toulouse, France
             Ralfkiaer E.
             Department of Pathology,
             Rigshospitalet,
             Copenhagen, Denmark
14.162 B   Delsol G.
             Centre Hospitalier
             Universitaire (CHU)
             Centre de Recherche en
             Cancerologie de Toulouse-
             Purpan,
             Toulouse, France
14.163–14.167 Delsol G.
             Centre Hospitalier
             Universitaire (CHU)
             Centre de Recherche en
             Cancerologie de Toulouse-
             Purpan,
             Toulouse, France
14.168 A,B   Chan J.K.C.
14.169   From: Lamant L, McCarthy K,
             d'Amore E, Klapper W,
             Nakagawa A, Fraga M,
             Maldyk J, Simonitsch-
             Klupp I, Oschlies I, Delsol G,
             Mauguen A, Brugières L,
             Le Deley MC (2011).
             Prognostic impact of
             morphologic and phenotypic
             features of childhood ALK-
             positive anaplastic large-cell
             lymphoma: results of the
             ALCL99 study. J Clin Oncol
             29:4669–76.
             Reprinted with permission.
             © 2011 American Society of
             Clinical Oncology. All rights
             reserved.
14.170   Delsol G.
             Centre Hospitalier
             Universitaire (CHU).
             Centre de Recherche en
             Cancerologie de Toulouse-
             Purpan,
             Toulouse, France
14.171–14.172 Mason D.Y.
             Haematology Department,
             John Radcliffe Hospital,
             University of Oxford, UK
             (deceased)
14.173 A,B   Feldman A.L.
14.174 A–D   Mason D.Y.
             Haematology Department,
             John Radcliffe Hospital,
             University of Oxford, UK
             (deceased)
14.175–14.176 Jaffe E.S.

15.01   Jaffe E.S.
15.02–15.04 Stein H.
15.05   Jaffe E.S.
15.06–15.14 Stein H.
15.15 A,B   Stein H.
15.16   Stein H.
15.17   Reproduced with permission
             from: Fan Z, Natkunam Y,
             Bair E, Tibshirani R,
             Warnke RA (2003). Charac-
             terization of variant patterns
             of nodular lymphocyte pre-
             dominant hodgkin lymphoma

             with immunohistologic and
             clinical correlation. Am J
             Surg Pathol. 27:1346–56.
15.18–15.20 Stein H.
15.21–15.29 Jaffe E.S.
15.30 A,B   Stein H.
15.31   Jaffe E.S.
15.32   Jaffe E.S.
15.33   Stein H.
15.34–15.39 Jaffe E.S.
15.40   Stein H.
15.41 A,B   From: Shimabukuro-
             Vornhagen A, Haverkamp H,
             Engert A, Balleisen L,
             Majunke P, Heil G, Eich HT,
             Stein H, Diehl V, Josting A
             (2005). Lymphocyte-rich
             classical Hodgkin's lym-
             phoma: clinical presentation
             and treatment outcome in
             100 patients treated within
             German Hodgkin's Study
             Group trials. J Clin Oncol.
             23:5739–45. Reprinted with
             permission. © 2005 American
             Society of Clinical Oncology.
             All rights reserved.
15.42 A,B   Stein H.
15.43 A   Jaffe E.S.
15.43 B   Stein H.
15.44   Stein H.
15.45 A–C   Stein H.
15.46–15.47 Jaffe E.S.

16.01   Pittaluga S.
16.02–16.04 Jaffe E.S.
16.05 A,C   Harris N.L.
16.05 B   Jaffe E.S.
16.06–16.08 Jaffe E.S.
16.09 A   Said J.
16.09 B,C   Raphaël M.
             Université Paris-Sud,
             INSERM U802,
             Le Kremlin-Bicêtre,
             Paris, France
16.09 D   Jaffe E.S.
16.10   Said J.
16.11   Jaffe E.S.
16.12 A   Jaffe E.S.
16.12 B,C   Raphaël M.
             Université Paris-Sud,
             INSERM U802,
             Le Kremlin-Bicêtre,
             Paris, France
16.13 A,B   Said J.
16.14 A–E   Harris N.L.
16.15 A   Webber S.A.
16.15 B,C   Swerdlow S.H.
16.16 A,B   Swerdlow S.H. &
             Nelson B.P.
             Feinberg School of Medicine,
             Northwestern University,
             Chicago, IL, USA
16.17 A–C   Swerdlow S.H.
16.18 A–C   Swerdlow S.H.
16.19 A–C   Harris N.L.
16.19 D   Swerdlow S.H.
16.20   Swerdlow S.H.
16.21 A,B   Harris N.L.
16.22 A–C   Swerdlow S.H.
16.23 A,B   Harris N.L.
16.24   Harris N.L.

17.01	Pileri S.A.
17.02–17.03	Grogan T.M. University of Arizona College of Medicine, Tucson, AZ, USA
17.04 A,B	Weiss L.M.
17.04 C	Grogan T.M. University of Arizona College of Medicine, Tucson, AZ, USA
17.05 A,B	Jaffe E.S.
17.06	Weiss L.M.
17.07 A–C	Weiss L.M.
17.08 A,B	Weiss L.M.
17.09 A	Grogan T.M. University of Arizona College of Medicine, Tucson, AZ, USA
17.09 B	Weiss L.M.
17.10 A–D	Falini B.
17.11 A–D	Jaffe E.S.
17.12 A,B	Jaffe E.S.
17.13 A,B	Weiss L.M.
17.14 A	Weiss L.M.
17.14 B	Spagnolo D.
17.15	Jaffe E.S.
17.16–17.17	Grogan T.M. University of Arizona College of Medicine, Tucson, AZ, USA
17.18–17.19	Weiss L.M.
17.20–17.23	Chan J.K.C.
17.24 A–C	Weiss L.M.
17.25	Weiss L.M.
17.26–17.31	Chan J.K.C.
17.32	O'Malley D.P. Clarient/NeoGenomics Aliso Viejo, CA, USA
17.33 A,B	Jaffe E.S.
17.34 A	From: Case records of the Massachusetts General Hospital. Weekly clinico-pathological exercises. Case 9-2000. A 41-year-old man with multiple bony lesions and adjacent soft-tissue masses. N Engl J Med. 342:875–83. © 2000 Massachusetts Medical Society. Reprinted with permission from Massachusetts Medical Society, Boston, USA
17.34 B	From: Mills JA, Gonzalez RG, Jaffe R. Case records of the Massachusetts General Hospital. Case 25-2008. A 43-year-old man with fatigue and lesions in the pituitary and cerebellum. N Engl J Med. 359:736–47. © 2008 Massachusetts Medical Society. Reprinted with permission.
17.35–17.36	Charlotte F. Service d'Anatomie Pathologique Hôpital Pitié-Salpêtrière, APHP-UPMC Paris, France
17.37	Jaffe E.S.
17.38	Jaffe E.S.

Sources of tables

2.04	Adapted from Thiele J, Kvasnicka HM. (2009) The 2008 WHO diagnostic criteria for polycythemia vera, essential thrombocythemia, and primary myelofibrosis. Curr Hematol Malig Rep.4:33-40. With permission of Springer.
2.05	Reprinted by permission from Macmillan Publishers Ltd: Leukemia. Barosi G, Mesa RA, Thiele J, Cervantes F, Campbell PJ, Verstovsek S, et al. Proposed criteria for the diagnosis of post-polycythemia vera and post-essential thrombocythemia myelofibrosis: a consensus statement from the International Working Group for Myelofibrosis Research and Treatment. Leukemia. 2008;22:437-8. Copyright 2008.
2.09	Thiele J, Kvasnicka HM, Facchetti F, Franco V, van der Walt J, Orazi A. (2005) European consensus on grading bone marrow fibrosis and assessment of cellularity. Haematologica. 90:1128–32. Obtained from the Haematologica Journal website http://www.haematologica.org
2.13	Reprinted by permission from Macmillan Publishers Ltd: Leukemia. Barosi G, Mesa RA, Thiele J, Cervantes F, Campbell PJ, Verstovsek S, et al. Proposed criteria for the diagnosis of post-polycythemia vera and post-essential thrombocythemia myelofibrosis: a consensus statement from the International Working Group for Myelofibrosis Research and Treatment. Leukemia. 2008; 22:437–8. Copyright 2008.
4.03	Reprinted from Immunol Allergy Clin North Am. 27. Bain BJ, Fletcher SH. Chronic eosinophilic leukemias and the myeloproliferative variant of the hypereosinophilic syndrome. 377-88. Copyright 2007. With permission from Elsevier.
4.05	Reprinted from Immunol Allergy Clin North Am. 27. Bain BJ, Fletcher SH. Chronic eosinophilic leukemias and the myeloproliferative variant

	of the hypereosinophilic syndrome. 377-88. Copyright 2007. With permission from Elsevier. {131} Macdonald D, Reiter A, Cross NC. (2002) The 8p11 myeloproliferative syndrome: a distinct clinical entity caused by constitutive activation of FGFR1. Acta Haematol. 107:101–7. With kind permission from S. Karger AG, Basel. {1354}
5.03	Reprinted with permission From: Locatelli F, Niemeyer CM. (2015) How I treat juvenile myelomonocytic leukemia. Blood. 125:1083–90.
6.05	Reprinted with permission From: Schanz J, Tüchler H, Solé F, Mallo M, Luño E, Cervera J, et al. (2012) New comprehensive cytogenetic scoring system for primary myelodysplastic syndromes (MDS) and oligoblastic acute myeloid leukemia after MDS derived from an international database merge. J Clin Oncol. 30:820–9.
6.06	With permission from Greenberg PL, Tuechler H, Schanz J, Sanz G, Garcia-Manero G, Solé F, et al. (2012) Revised international prognostic scoring system for myelodysplastic syndromes. Blood. 120:2454–65.
7.02	Reprinted from Churpek JE, Lorenz R, Nedumgottil S, Onel K, Olopade OI, Sorrell A, et al. (2013) Proposal for the clinical detection and management of patients and their family members with familial myelodysplastic syndrome/acute leukemia predisposition syndromes. Leuk Lymphoma. 54:28–35.
8.01	Hirsch B. Dept. of Laboratory Medicine and Pathology University of Minnesota Medical School Minneapolis, MN, USA, Susana Raimondi Cytogenetics Laboratory Department of Pathology St. Jude Children's Research Hospital Memphis, TN, USA, Soheil Meschinchi Hutchinson Cancer Research Center University of Washington School of Medicine Seattle, WA, USA, Nyla Heerema Department of Pathology The Ohio State University Columbus, OH, USA, Carroll

A.J. Department of Genetics, University of Alabama School of Medicine, Birmingham, AL, USA And Reprinted with permission from: Arber DA, Orazi A, Hasserjian R, et al. (2016) The 2016 revision to the World Health Organization classification of myeloid neoplasms and acute leukemia. Blood. 127(20):2391-405.

8.02 Mrózek K Department of Internal Medicine Comprehensive Cancer Center The Ohio State University Columbus, OH, USA And Reprinted with permission from: Arber DA, Orazi A, Hasserjian R, et al. (2016) The 2016 revision to the World Health Organization classification of myeloid neoplasms and acute leukemia. Blood. 127(20):2391-405.

13.01 Modified with permission from Kröber A, Seiler T, Benner A, Bullinger L, Brückle E, Lichter P, et al. V(H) mutation status, CD38 expression level, genomic aberrations, and survival in chronic lymphocytic leukemia. Blood. (2002) 15;100(4):1410–6.

13.03 Adapted from Lancet Oncol. 15(12). Rajkumar SV, Dimopoulos MA, Palumbo A, Blade J, Merlini G, Mateos MV, et al. International Myeloma Working Group updated criteria for the diagnosis of multiple myeloma. :e538-48. Copyright 2014. With permission from Elsevier.

13.05 Reprinted from Lancet Oncol. 15(12). Rajkumar SV, Dimopoulos MA, Palumbo A, Blade J, Merlini G, Mateos MV, et al. International Myeloma Working Group updated criteria for the diagnosis of multiple myeloma. e538–48. Copyright 2014. With permission from Elsevier.

13.06 Reprinted from Lancet Haematol. 1(1). Kyle RA, Larson DR, Therneau TM, Dispenzieri A, Melton LJ 3rd, Benson JT, et al. Clinical course of light-chain smouldering multiple myeloma (idiopathic Bence Jones proteinuria): a retrospective cohort study. e28–e36. Copyright 2014. With permission from Elsevier.

13.07 Adapted from Lancet Oncol. 15(12). Rajkumar SV, Dimopoulos MA, Palumbo A, Blade J, Merlini G, Mateos MV, et al. International Myeloma Working Group updated criteria for the diagnosis of multiple myeloma. :e538-48. Copyright 2014. With permission from Elsevier.

13.08 Adapted by permission from Macmillan Publishers Ltd: Leukemia. Fonseca R, Bergsagel PL, Drach J, Shaughnessy J, Gutierrez N, Stewart AK, et al. International Myeloma Working Group molecular classification of multiple myeloma: spotlight review. 23:2210-21. Copyright 2009.

13.09 Adapted by permission from Macmillan Publishers Ltd: Leukemia. Fonseca R, Bergsagel PL, Drach J, Shaughnessy J, Gutierrez N, Stewart AK, et al. International Myeloma Working Group molecular classification of multiple myeloma: spotlight review. 23:2210-21. Copyright 2009.

13.10 With permission from Kuehl WM, Bergsagel PL. (2012) Molecular pathogenesis of multiple myeloma and its premalignant precursor. J Clin Invest. 122:3456–63.

13.11 Greipp PR, San Miguel J, Durie BG, Crowley JJ, Barlogie B, Bladé J, et al. International staging system for multiple myeloma. J Clin Oncol. 2005. 20;23(15):3412–20. Reprinted with permission. © 2005 American Society of Clinical Oncology. All rights reserved.

13.12 Chesi M, Bergsagel PL. (2013) Molecular pathogenesis of multiple myeloma: basic and clinical updates. Int J Hematol. 97:313-23. Figure 3 is reused by the courtesy of the International Journal of Hematology.

13.13 Reprinted from Lancet Oncol. 15(12). Rajkumar SV, Dimopoulos MA, Palumbo A, Blade J, Merlini G, Mateos MV, et al. International Myeloma Working Group updated criteria for the diagnosis of multiple myeloma. :e538-48. Copyright 2014. With permission from Elsevier.

13.15 Reprinted from Blood Rev. 21(6), Dispenzieri A. POEMS syndrome. Pages No. 285–99. Copyright 2007, with permission from Elsevier

13.19 Reprinted with permission from Jegalian AG, Eberle FC, Pack SD, Mirvis M, Raffeld M, Pittaluga S, et al. (2011) Follicular lymphoma in situ: clinical implications and comparisons with partial involvement by follicular lymphoma. Blood. 118:2976-84.

14.03 Modified with permission from Shimoyama M. Diagnostic criteria and classification of clinical subtypes of adult T-cell leukaemia-lymphoma. A report from the Lymphoma Study Group (1984–87). Br J Haematol. 1991 Nov;79(3):428–37.

14.06 Reprinted with permission from Olsen E, Vonderheid E, Pimpinelli N, Willemze R, Kim Y, Knobler R, et al. (2007) Revisions to the staging and classification of mycosis fungoides and Sezary syndrome: a proposal of the International Society for Cutaneous Lymphomas (ISCL) and the cutaneous lymphoma task force of the European Organization of Research and Treatment of Cancer (EORTC). Blood. 110:1713–22.

Sources of figures on front cover

Top left	Grogan T.M. (Fig. 13.39A)
Top centre	Matsue K. et al.(Fig. 13.137A)
Top right	Jaffe E.S. (Fig. 13.129B)
Middle left	Brunning R.D. (Fig. 8.26)
Middle centre	Diebold J. (Fig. 13.142A)
Middle right	Jaffe E.S. (Fig. 15.05)
Bottom left	Roschke A., Gabrea A., Kuehl M.W. (Fig. 13.49B)
Bottom centre	Borowitz M.J. (Fig. 10.06F)
Bottom right	Pack S. (Fig. 13.180B)

References

1. A clinical evaluation of the International Lymphoma Study Group classification of non-Hodgkin's lymphoma; the Non-Hodgkin's Lymphoma Classification Project (1997). Blood. 89:3909–18. PMID:9166827

2. A predictive model for aggressive non-Hodgkin's lymphoma; the International Non-Hodgkin's Lymphoma Prognostic Factors Project (1993). N Engl J Med. 329:987–94. PMID:8141877

3. Aalbers AM, van den Heuvel-Eibrink MM, Baumann I, et al. (2015). Bone marrow immunophenotyping by flow cytometry in refractory cytopenia of childhood. Haematologica. 100:315–23. PMID:25425683

4. Aalbers AM, van den Heuvel-Eibrink MM, de Haas V, et al. (2013). Applicability of a reproducible flow cytometry scoring system in the diagnosis of refractory cytopenia of childhood. Leukemia. 27:1923–5. PMID:234930265

5. Aalbers AM, van der Velden VH, Yoshimi A, et al. (2014). The clinical relevance of minor paroxysmal nocturnal hemoglobinuria clones in refractory cytopenia of childhood: a prospective study by EWOG-MDS. Leukemia. 28:189–92. PMID:23807769

6. Aarts WM, Willemze R, Bende RJ, et al. (1998). VH gene analysis of primary cutaneous B-cell lymphomas: evidence for ongoing somatic hypermutation and isotype switching. Blood. 92:3857–64. PMID:9808579

7. Abadie V, Jabri B (2014). IL-15: a central regulator of celiac disease immunopathology. Immunol Rev. 260:221–34. PMID:24942692

7A. Abate F, da Silva-Almeida AC, Zairis S, et al. (2017). Activating mutations and translocations in the guanine exchange factor VAV1 in peripheral T-cell lymphomas. Proc Natl Acad Sci U S A. 114:764–9. PMID:28062691

8. Abate F, Ambrosio MR, Mundo L, et al. (2015). Distinct viral and mutational spectrum of endemic Burkitt lymphoma. PLoS Pathog. 11:e1005158. PMID:26468873

8A. Abruzzo LV, Jaffe ES, Cotelingam JD, et al. (1992). T-cell lymphoblastic lymphoma with eosinophilia associated with subsequent myeloid malignancy. Am J Surg Pathol. 16:236–45. PMID:1599015

8B. Abruzzo LV, Schmidt K, Weiss LM, et al. (1993). B-cell lymphoma after angioimmunoblastic lymphadenopathy: a case with oligoclonal gene rearrangements associated with Epstein-Barr virus. Blood. 82:241–6. PMID:8391875

9. Abdel-Wahab O, Levine RL (2013). Mutations in epigenetic modifiers in the pathogenesis and therapy of acute myeloid leukemia. Blood. 121:3563–72. PMID:23640996

10. Abdul-Wahab A, Tang SY, Robson A, et al. (2014). Chromosomal anomalies in primary cutaneous follicle center cell lymphoma do not portend a poor prognosis. J Am Acad Dermatol. 70:1010–20. PMID:24679486

11. Abdulkarim K, Ridell B, Johansson P, et al. (2011). The impact of peripheral blood values and bone marrow findings on prognosis for patients with essential thrombocythemia and polycythemia vera. Eur J Haematol. 86:148–55. PMID:21059102

12. Abramov D, Oschlies I, Zimmermann M, et al. (2013). Expression of CD8 is associated with non-common type morphology and outcome in pediatric anaplastic lymphoma kinase-positive anaplastic large cell lymphoma. Haematologica. 98:1547–53. PMID:23716548

13. Abramson JS (2006). T-cell/histiocyte-rich B-cell lymphoma: biology, diagnosis, and management. Oncologist. 11:384–92. PMID:16614234

14. Abrey LE, DeAngelis LM, Yahalom J (1998). Long-term survival in primary CNS lymphoma. J Clin Oncol. 16:859–63. PMID:9508166

15. Abruzzo LV, Jaffe ES, Cotelingam JD, et al. (1992). T-cell lymphoblastic lymphoma with eosinophilia associated with subsequent myeloid malignancy. Am J Surg Pathol. 16:236–45. PMID:1599015

16. Abruzzo LV, Rosales CM, Medeiros LJ, et al. (2002). Epstein-Barr virus-positive B-cell lymphoproliferative disorders arising in immunodeficient patients previously treated with fludarabine for low-grade B-cell neoplasms. Am J Surg Pathol. 26:630–6. PMID:11979093

17. Abstracts of CHEST 2013. October 26-31, 2013. Chicago, Illinois, USA (2013). Chest 144:2A–1029A. PMID:24153593

18. Achten R, Verhoef G, Vanuytsel L, et al. (2002). Histiocyte-rich, T-cell-rich B-cell lymphoma: a distinct diffuse large B-cell lymphoma subtype showing characteristic morphologic and immunophenotypic features. Histopathology. 40:31–45. PMID:11903596

19. Achten R, Verhoef G, Vanuytsel L, et al. (2002). T-cell/histiocyte-rich large B-cell lymphoma: a distinct clinicopathologic entity. J Clin Oncol. 20:1269–77. PMID:11870169

20. Adam P, Czapiewski P, Colak S, et al. (2014). Prevalence of Achromobacter xylosoxidans in pulmonary mucosa-associated lymphoid tissue lymphoma in different regions of Europe. Br J Haematol. 164:804–10. PMID:24372375

21. Adam P, Katzenberger T, Eifert M, et al. (2005). Presence of preserved reactive germinal centers in follicular lymphoma is a strong histopathologic indicator of limited disease stage. Am J Surg Pathol. 29:1661–4. PMID:16327439

22. Adam P, Katzenberger T, Seeberger H, et al. (2003). A case of a diffuse large B-cell lymphoma of plasmablastic type associated with the t(2;5)(p23;q35) chromosome translocation. Am J Surg Pathol. 27:1473–6. PMID:14576483

22A. Adam P, Schiefer A, et al. (2012) Incidence of preclinical manifestations of mantle cell lymphoma and mantle cell lymphoma in situ in reactive lymphoid tissues. Mod Pathol. 25:1629–36. PMID:22790016

23. Adams H, Campidelli C, Dirnhofer S, et al. (2009). Clinical, phenotypic and genetic similarities and disparities between post-transplant and classical Hodgkin lymphomas with respect to therapeutic targets. Expert Opin Ther Targets. 13:1137–45. PMID:19705967

24. Adams HJ, Kwee TC, de Keizer B, et al. (2014). FDG PET/CT for the detection of bone marrow involvement in diffuse large B-cell lymphoma: systematic review and meta-analysis. Eur J Nucl Med Mol Imaging. 41:565–74. PMID:24281821

25. Adélaïde J, Pérot C, Gelsi-Boyer V, et al. (2006). A t(8;9) translocation with PCM1-JAK2 fusion in a patient with T-cell lymphoma. Leukemia. 20:536–7. PMID:16424865

26. Affer M, Chesi M, Chen WD, et al. (2014). Promiscuous MYC locus rearrangements hijack enhancers but mostly super-enhancers to dysregulate MYC expression in multiple myeloma. Leukemia. 28:1725–35. PMID:24518206

27. Agar NS, Wedgeworth E, Crichton S, et al. (2010). Survival outcomes and prognostic factors in mycosis fungoides/Sézary syndrome: validation of the revised International Society for Cutaneous Lymphomas/European Organisation for Research and Treatment of Cancer staging proposal. J Clin Oncol. 28:4730–9. PMID:20855822

28. Agathangelidis A, Darzentas N, Hadzidimitriou A, et al. (2012). Stereotyped B-cell receptors in one-third of chronic lymphocytic leukemia: a molecular classification with implications for targeted therapies. Blood. 119:4467–75. PMID:22415752

29. Aggarwal N, Pongpruttipan T, Patel S, et al. (2015). Expression of S100 protein in CD4-positive T-cell lymphomas is often associated with T-cell prolymphocytic leukemia. Am J Surg Pathol. 39:1679–87. PMID:26379148

30. Agnarsson BA, Vonderheid EC, Kadin ME (1990). Cutaneous T cell lymphoma with suppressor/cytotoxic (CD8) phenotype: identification of rapidly progressive and chronic subtypes. J Am Acad Dermatol. 22:569–77. PMID:2138636

31. Agnelli L, Mereu E, Pellegrino E, et al. (2012). Identification of a 3-gene model as a powerful diagnostic tool for the recognition of ALK-negative anaplastic large-cell lymphoma. Blood. 120:1274–81. PMID:22740451

32. Agnello V, Chung RT, Kaplan LM (1992). A role for hepatitis C virus infection in type II cryoglobulinemia. N Engl J Med. 327:1490–5. PMID:1383822

33. Agopian J, Navarro JM, Gac AC, et al. (2009). Agricultural pesticide exposure and the molecular connection to lymphomagenesis. J Exp Med. 206:1473–83. PMID:19506050

34. Agostinelli C, Hartmann S, Klapper W, et al. (2011). Peripheral T cell lymphomas with follicular T helper phenotype: a new basket or a distinct entity? Revising Karl Lennert's personal archive. Histopathology. 59:679–91. PMID:22014049

35. Agostinelli C, Paterson JC, Gupta R, et al. (2012). Detection of LIM domain only 2 (LMO2) in normal human tissues and haematopoietic and non-haematopoietic tumours using a newly developed rabbit monoclonal antibody. Histopathology. 61:33–46. PMID:22394247

36. Aguilar C, Beltran B, Quiñones P, et al. (2015). Large B-cell lymphoma arising in cardiac myxoma or intracardiac fibrinous mass: a localized lymphoma usually associated with Epstein-Barr virus? Cardiovasc Pathol. 24:60–4. PMID:25307939

37. Aguilera NS, Tomaszewski MM, Moad JC, et al. (2001). Cutaneous follicle center lymphoma: a clinicopathologic study of 19 cases. Mod Pathol. 14:828–35. PMID:11557777

38. Agur A, Amir G, Paltiel O, et al. (2015). CD68 staining correlates with the size of residual mass but not with survival in classical Hodgkin lymphoma. Leuk Lymphoma. 56:1315–9. PMID:25204373

39. Ait-Tahar K, Damm-Welk C, Burkhardt B, et al. (2010). Correlation of the autoantibody response to the ALK oncoantigen in pediatric anaplastic lymphoma kinase-positive anaplastic large cell lymphoma with tumor dissemination and relapse risk. Blood. 115:3314–9. PMID:20185586

40. Akasaka T, Ueda C, Kurata M, et al. (2000). Nonimmunoglobulin (non-Ig)/BCL6 gene fusion in diffuse large B-cell lymphoma results in worse prognosis than Ig/BCL6. Blood. 96:2907–9. PMID:11023530

41. Akhter A, Mahe E, Street L, et al. (2015). CD10-positive mantle cell lymphoma: biologically distinct entity or an aberrant immunophenotype? Insight, through gene expression profile in a unique case series. J Clin Pathol. 68:844–8. PMID:26124315

42. Akin C, Fumo G, Yavuz AS, et al. (2004). A novel form of mastocytosis associated with a transmembrane c-kit mutation and response to imatinib. Blood. 103:3222–5. PMID:15070706

43. Akin C, Valent P, Metcalfe DD (2010). Mast cell activation syndrome: Proposed diagnostic criteria. J Allergy Clin Immunol. 126:1099–104.e4. PMID:21035176

44. Akyurek N, Uner A, Benekli M, et al. (2012). Prognostic significance of MYC, BCL2, and BCL6 rearrangements in patients with diffuse large B-cell lymphoma treated with cyclophosphamide, doxorubicin, vincristine, and prednisone plus rituximab. Cancer. 118:4173–83. PMID:22213394

45. Al Daama SA, Housawi YH, Dridi W, et al. (2013). A missense mutation in ANKRD26 segregates with thrombocytopenia. Blood. 122:461–2. PMID:23869080

46. Al-Hamadani M, Habermann TM, Cerhan JR, et al. (2015). Non-Hodgkin lymphoma subtype distribution, geodemographic patterns, and survival in the US: A longitudinal analysis of the National Cancer Data Base from 1998 to 2011. Am J Hematol. 90:790–5. PMID:26096944

47. Al-Mansour Z, Nelson BP, Evens AM (2013). Post-transplant lymphoproliferative disease (PTLD): risk factors, diagnosis, and current treatment strategies. Curr Hematol Malig Rep. 8:173–83. PMID:23737188

48. Al-Saleem T, Al-Mondhiry H (2005). Immunoproliferative small intestinal disease (IPSID): a model for mature B-cell neoplasms. Blood. 105:2274–80. PMID:15542584

49. Al-Toma A, Goerres MS, Meijer JW, et al. (2006). Human leukocyte antigen-DQ2 homozygosity and the development of refractory celiac disease and enteropathy-associated T-cell lymphoma. Clin Gastroenterol Hepatol. 4:315–9. PMID:16527694

50. Al-Toma A, Verbeek WH, Hadithi M, et al. (2007). Survival in refractory coeliac disease and enteropathy-associated T-cell lymphoma: retrospective evaluation of single-centre experience. Gut. 56:1373–8. PMID:17470479

50A. Alachkar H, Santhanam R, Maharry K, et al. (2014). SPARC promotes leukemic cell growth and predicts acute myeloid leukemia outcome. J Clin Invest. 124:1512–24. PMID:24590286

51. Aladily TN, Medeiros LJ, Amin MB, et al. (2012). Anaplastic large cell lymphoma associated with breast implants: a report of 13 cases. Am J Surg Pathol. 36:1000–8. PMID:22613996

52. Alapat D, Coviello-Malle J, Owens R, et al. (2012). Diagnostic usefulness and prognostic

impact of CD200 expression in lymphoid malignancies and plasma cell myeloma. Am J Clin Pathol. 137:93–100. PMID:22180482
53. Alayed K, Patel KP, Konoplev S, et al. (2013). TET2 mutations, myelodysplastic features, and a distinct immunoprofile characterize blastic plasmacytoid dendritic cell neoplasm in the bone marrow. Am J Hematol. 88:1055–61. PMID:23940084
54. Alcalay M, Tiacci E, Bergomas R, et al. (2005). Acute myeloid leukemia bearing cytoplasmic nucleophosmin (NPMc+ AML) shows a distinct gene expression profile characterized by up-regulation of genes involved in stem-cell maintenance. Blood. 106:899–902. PMID:15831697
55. Alcindor T, Bridges KR (2002). Sideroblastic anaemias. Br J Haematol. 116:733–43. PMID:11886376
56. Alencar AJ, Malumbres R, Kozloski GA, et al. (2011). MicroRNAs are independent predictors of outcome in diffuse large B-cell lymphoma patients treated with R-CHOP. Clin Cancer Res. 17:4125–35. PMID:21525173
57. Alexander A, Anicito I, Buxbaum J (1988). Gamma heavy chain disease in man. Genomic sequence reveals two noncontiguous deletions in a single gene. J Clin Invest. 82:1244–52. PMID:3139711
58. Alexander S, Kraveka JM, Weitzman S, et al. (2014). Advanced stage anaplastic large cell lymphoma in children and adolescents: results of ANHL0131, a randomized phase III trial of APO versus a modified regimen with vinblastine: a report from the children's oncology group. Pediatr Blood Cancer. 61:2236–42. PMID:25156886
59. Alexanian S, Said J, Lones M, et al. (2013). KSHV/HHV8-negative effusion-based lymphoma, a distinct entity associated with fluid overload states. Am J Surg Pathol. 37:241–9. PMID:23282971
60. Alexiev BA, Wang W, Ning Y, et al. (2007). Myeloid sarcomas: a histologic, immunohistochemical, and cytogenetic study. Diagn Pathol. 2:42. PMID:17974004
61. Alexiou C, Kau RJ, Dietzfelbinger H, et al. (1999). Extramedullary plasmacytoma: tumor occurrence and therapeutic concepts. Cancer. 85:2305–14. PMID:10357398
62. Algara P, Mateo MS, Sanchez-Beato M, et al. (2002). Analysis of the IgV(H) somatic mutations in splenic marginal zone lymphoma defines a group of unmutated cases with frequent 7q deletion and adverse clinical course. Blood. 99:1299–304. PMID:11830479
63. Alhan C, Westers TM, Cremers EM, et al. (2014). High flow cytometric scores identify adverse prognostic subgroups within the revised international prognostic scoring system for myelodysplastic syndromes. Br J Haematol. 167:100–9. PMID:24976502
64. Alhan C, Westers TM, van der Helm LH, et al. (2014). Absence of aberrant myeloid progenitors by flow cytometry is associated with favorable response to azacitidine in higher risk myelodysplastic syndromes. Cytometry B Clin Cytom. 86:207–15. PMID:24474614
65. Ali S, Olszewski AJ (2014). Disparate survival and risk of secondary non-Hodgkin lymphoma in histologic subtypes of Hodgkin lymphoma: a population-based study. Leuk Lymphoma. 55:1570–7. PMID:24067135
66. Alimena G, Breccia M, Latagliata R, et al. (2006). Sudden blast crisis in patients with Philadelphia chromosome-positive chronic myeloid leukemia who achieved complete cytogenetic remission after imatinib therapy. Cancer. 107:1008–13. PMID:16878324
67. Alizadeh AA, Eisen MB, Davis RE, et al. (2000). Distinct types of diffuse large B-cell lymphoma identified by gene expression profiling. Nature. 403:503–11. PMID:10676951
68. Alizadeh AA, Gentles AJ, Alencar AJ, et al. (2011). Prediction of survival in diffuse large B-cell lymphoma based on the expression of 2 genes reflecting tumor and microenvironment. Blood. 118:1350–8. PMID:21670469
69. Allan JM, Wild CP, Rollinson S, et al. (2001). Polymorphism in glutathione S-transferase P1 is associated with susceptibility to chemotherapy-induced leukemia. Proc Natl Acad Sci U S A. 98:11592–7. PMID:11553769
70. Allemani C, Sant M, De Angelis R, et al. (2006). Hodgkin disease survival in Europe and the U.S.: prognostic significance of morphologic groups. Cancer. 107:352–60. PMID:16770772
71. Allen CE, Parsons DW (2015). Biological and clinical significance of somatic mutations in Langerhans cell histiocytosis and related histiocytic neoplastic disorders. Hematology Am Soc Hematol Educ Program. 2015:559–64. PMID:26637772
72. Allen U, Preiksaitis J; AST Infectious Diseases Community of Practice (2009). Epstein-barr virus and posttransplant lymphoproliferative disorder in solid organ transplant recipients. Am J Transplant. 9 Suppl 4:S87–96. PMID:20070701
73. Almeida J, Orfao A, Ocqueteau M, et al. (1999). High-sensitive immunophenotyping and DNA ploidy studies for the investigation of minimal residual disease in multiple myeloma. Br J Haematol. 107:121–31. PMID:10520032
74. Alobaid A, Torlakovic E, Kongkham P (2015). Primary Central Nervous System Immunomodulatory Therapy-Induced Lymphoproliferative Disorder in a Patient with Ulcerative Colitis: A Case Report and Review of the Literature. World Neurosurg. 84:2074.e15–9. PMID:26171889
75. Alonsozana EL, Stamberg J, Kumar D, et al. (1997). Isochromosome 7q: the primary cytogenetic abnormality in hepatosplenic gammadelta T cell lymphoma. Leukemia. 11:1367–72. PMID:9264394
76. Alsabeh R, Brynes RK, Slovak ML, et al. (1997). Acute myeloid leukemia with t(6;9) (p23;q34): association with myelodysplasia, basophilia, and initial CD34 negative immunophenotype. Am J Clin Pathol. 107:430–7. PMID:9124211
77. Alsabeh R, Medeiros LJ, Glackin C, et al. (1997). Transformation of follicular lymphoma into CD30-large cell lymphoma with anaplastic cytologic features. Am J Surg Pathol. 21:528–36. PMID:9158676
78. Alter BP, Caruso JP, Drachtman RA, et al. (2000). Fanconi anemia: myelodysplasia as a predictor of outcome. Cancer Genet Cytogenet. 117:125–31. PMID:10704682
79. Alter BP, Scalise A, McCombs J, et al. (1993). Clonal chromosomal abnormalities in Fanconi's anaemia: what do they really mean? Br J Haematol. 85:627–30. PMID:8136289
80. Altieri A, Bermejo JL, Hemminki K (2005). Familial aggregation of lymphoplasmacytic lymphoma with non-Hodgkin lymphoma and other neoplasms. Leukemia. 19:2342–3. PMID:16224483
81. Altura RA, Head DR, Wang WC (2000). Long-term survival of infants with idiopathic myelofibrosis. Br J Haematol. 109:459–62. PMID:10848842
82. Alvarez-Larrán A, Angona A, Ancochea A, et al. (2016). Masked polycythaemia vera: presenting features, response to treatment and clinical outcomes. Eur J Haematol. 96:83–9. PMID:25810304
83. Álvarez-Twose I, Jara-Acevedo M, Morgado JM, et al. (2015). Clinical, immunophenotypic, and molecular characteristics of well-differentiated systemic mastocytosis. J Allergy Clin Immunol. 137:168–78.e1 PMID:26100086
84. Amato T, Abate F, Piccaluga P, et al. (2016). Clonality Analysis of Immunoglobulin Gene Rearrangement by Next-Generation Sequencing in Endemic Burkitt Lymphoma Suggests Antigen Drive Activation of BCR as Opposed to Sporadic Burkitt Lymphoma. Am J Clin Pathol. 145:116–27. PMID:26712879
85. Ambrosio MR, Navari M, Di Lisio L, et al. (2014). The Epstein Barr-encoded BART-6-3p microRNA affects regulation of cell growth and immuno response in Burkitt lymphoma. Infect Agent Cancer. 9:12. PMID:24731550
86. Ambrosio MR, Piccaluga PP, Ponzoni M, et al. (2012). The alteration of lipid metabolism in Burkitt lymphoma identifies a novel marker: adipophilin. PLoS One. 7:e44315. PMID:22952953
87. Ameis A, Ko HS, Pruzanski W (1976). M components-a review of 1242 cases. Can Med Assoc J. 114:889–92, 895. PMID:817789
88. Amenomori T, Tomonaga M, Yoshida Y, et al. (1986). Cytogenetic evidence for partially committed myeloid progenitor cell origin of chronic myelomonocytic leukaemia and juvenile chronic myeloid leukaemia: both granulocyte-macrophage precursors and erythroid precursors carry identical marker chromosome. Br J Haematol. 64:539–46. PMID:2947609
89. Amin HM, Yang Y, Shen Y, et al. (2005). Having a higher blast percentage in circulation than bone marrow: clinical implications in myelodysplastic syndrome and acute lymphoid and myeloid leukemias. Leukemia. 19:1567–72. PMID:16049515
90. Amiot A, Allez M, Treton X, et al. (2012). High frequency of fatal haemophagocytic lymphohistiocytosis syndrome in enteropathy-associated T cell lymphoma. Dig Liver Dis. 44:343–9. PMID:22100722
91. Anagnostopoulos I, Hansmann ML, Franssila K, et al. (2000). European Task Force on Lymphoma project on lymphocyte predominance Hodgkin disease: histologic and immunohistologic analysis of submitted cases reveals 2 types of Hodgkin disease with a nodular growth pattern and abundant lymphocytes. Blood. 96:1889–99. PMID:10961891
92. Anagnostopoulos I, Hummel M, Finn T, et al. (1992). Heterogeneous Epstein-Barr virus infection patterns in peripheral T-cell lymphoma of angioimmunoblastic lymphadenopathy type. Blood. 80:1804–12. PMID:1327284
93. Anastasi J, Vardiman JW (2001). Chronic myelogenous leukemia and the chronic myeloproliferative diseases. In: Knowles DM, editor. Neoplastic hematopathology. 2nd ed. Philadelphia: Lippincott Williams & Wilkins.
94. Andersen MK, Larson RA, Mauritzson N, et al. (2002). Balanced chromosome abnormalities inv(16) and t(15;17) in therapy-related myelodysplastic syndromes and acute leukemia: report from an international workshop. Genes Chromosomes Cancer. 33:395–400. PMID:11921273
95. Anderson JR, Armitage JO, Weisenburger DD (1998). Epidemiology of the non-Hodgkin's lymphomas: distributions of the major subtypes differ by geographic locations. Non-Hodgkin's Lymphoma Classification Project. Ann Oncol. 9:717–20. PMID:9739436
96. Anderson K, Arvidsson I, Jacobsson B, et al. (2002). Fluorescence in situ hybridization for the study of cell lineage involvement in myelodysplastic syndromes with chromosome 5 anomalies. Cancer Genet Cytogenet. 136:101–7. PMID:12237232
97. Anderson KC, Carrasco RD (2011). Pathogenesis of myeloma. Annu Rev Pathol. 6:249–74. PMID:21261519
98. Anderson T, Bender RA, Fisher RI, et al. (1977). Combination chemotherapy in non-Hodgkin's lymphoma: results of long-term followup. Cancer Treat Rep. 61:1057–66. PMID:71205
99. Andersson AK, Ma J, Wang J, et al. (2015). The landscape of somatic mutations in infant MLL-rearranged acute lymphoblastic leukemias. Nat Genet. 47:330–7. PMID:25730765
100. Ando M, Sato Y, Takata K, et al. (2013). A20 (TNFAIP3) deletion in Epstein-Barr virus-associated lymphoproliferative disorders/lymphomas. PLoS One. 8:e56741. PMID:23418597
101. Andréasson B, Swolin B, Kutti J (2002). Patients with idiopathic myelofibrosis show increased CD34+ cell concentrations in peripheral blood compared to patients with polycythaemia vera and essential thrombocythaemia. Eur J Haematol. 68:189–93. PMID:12071933
102. Andrieux JL, Demory JL (2005). Karyotype and molecular cytogenetic studies in polycythemia vera. Curr Hematol Rep. 4:224–9. PMID:15865876
103. Andriko JA, Swerdlow SH, Aguilera NI, et al. (2001). Is lymphoplasmacytic lymphoma/immunocytoma a distinct entity? A clinicopathologic study of 20 cases. Am J Surg Pathol. 25:742–51. PMID:11395551
104. Andriko JW, Kaldjian EP, Tsokos M, et al. (1998). Reticulum cell neoplasms of lymph nodes: a clinicopathologic study of 11 cases with recognition of a new subtype derived from fibroblastic reticular cells. Am J Surg Pathol. 22:1048–58. PMID:9737236
105. Angelini DF, Ottone T, Guerrera G, et al. (2015). A Leukemia-Associated CD34/CD123/CD25/CD99+ Immunophenotype Identifies FLT3-Mutated Clones in Acute Myeloid Leukemia. Clin Cancer Res. 21:3977–85. PMID:25957287
106. Angelopoulou MK, Kalpadakis C, Pangalis GA, et al. (2014). Nodal marginal zone lymphoma. Leuk Lymphoma. 55:1240–50. PMID:24004184
107. Angelot-Delettre F, Biichle S, Ferrand C, et al. (2012). Intracytoplasmic detection of TCL1–but not ILT7-by flow cytometry is useful for blastic plasmacytoid dendritic cell leukemia diagnosis. Cytometry A. 81:718–24. PMID:22674796
108. Angelot-Delettre F, Roggy A, Frankel AE, et al. (2015). In vivo and in vitro sensitivity of blastic plasmacytoid dendritic cell neoplasm to SL-401, an interleukin-3 receptor targeted biologic agent. Haematologica. 100:223–30. PMID:25381130
109. Annunziata CM, Davis RE, Demchenko Y, et al. (2007). Frequent engagement of the classical and alternative NF-kappaB pathways by diverse genetic abnormalities in multiple myeloma. Cancer Cell. 12:115–30. PMID:17692804
110. Ansari MQ, Dawson DB, Nador R, et al. (1996). Primary body cavity-based AIDS-related lymphomas. Am J Clin Pathol. 105:221–9. PMID:8607449
111. Ansari-Lari MA, Yang CF, Tinawi-Aljundi R, et al. (2004). FLT3 mutations in myeloid sarcoma. Br J Haematol. 126:785–91. PMID:15352981
112. Ansell SM, Armitage JO (2012). Positron emission tomographic scans in lymphoma: convention and controversy. Mayo Clin Proc. 87:571–80. PMID:22677077
113. Ansell SM, Lesokhin AM, Borrello I, et al. (2015). PD-1 blockade with nivolumab in relapsed or refractory Hodgkin's lymphoma. N Engl J Med. 372:311–9. PMID:25482239
114. Antony-Debré I, Steidl U (2015). Functionally relevant RNA helicase mutations in familial and sporadic myeloid malignancies. Cancer Cell. 27:609–11. PMID:25965566
115. Aoki T, Izutsu K, Suzuki R, et al. (2014). Prognostic significance of pleural or pericardial effusion and the implication of optimal treatment in primary mediastinal large B-cell lymphoma: a multicenter retrospective study in Japan.

Haematologica. 99:1817–25. PMID:25216682
116. Aoki Y, Yarchoan R, Braun J, et al. (2000). Viral and cellular cytokines in AIDS-related malignant lymphomatous effusions. Blood. 96:1599–601. PMID:10942415
117. Aozasa K (1990). Hashimoto's thyroiditis as a risk factor of thyroid lymphoma. Acta Pathol Jpn. 40:459–68. PMID:2220394
118. Aozasa K (2006). Pyothorax-associated lymphoma. J Clin Exp Hematop. 46:5–10. PMID:17058803
119. Aozasa K, Ohsawa M, Iuchi K, et al. (1991). Prognostic factors for pleural lymphoma patients. Jpn J Clin Oncol. 21:417–21. PMID:1805046
120. Aozasa K, Ohsawa M, Iuchi K, et al. (1993). Artificial pneumothorax as a risk factor for development of pleural lymphoma. Jpn J Cancer Res. 84:55–7. PMID:8449828
121. Aozasa K, Takakuwa T, Nakatsuka S (2005). Pyothorax-associated lymphoma: a lymphoma developing in chronic inflammation. Adv Anat Pathol. 12:324–31. PMID:16330929
122. Apperley JF (2007). Part I: mechanisms of resistance to imatinib in chronic myeloid leukaemia. Lancet Oncol. 8:1018–29. PMID:17976612
123. Apperley JF, Gardembas M, Melo JV, et al. (2002). Response to imatinib mesylate in patients with chronic myeloproliferative diseases with rearrangements of the platelet-derived growth factor receptor beta. N Engl J Med. 347:481–7. PMID:12181402
124. Arai A, Imadome K, Watanabe Y, et al. (2011). Clinical features of adult-onset chronic active Epstein-Barr virus infection: a retrospective analysis. Int J Hematol. 93:602–9. PMID:21491104
125. Araujo I, Bittencourt AL, Barbosa HS, et al. (2006). The high frequency of EBV infection in pediatric Hodgkin lymphoma is related to the classical type in Bahia, Brazil. Virchows Arch. 449:315–9. PMID:16896892
126. Arber DA, Carter NH, Ikle D, et al. (2003). Value of combined morphologic, cytochemical, and immunophenotypic features in predicting recurrent cytogenetic abnormalities in acute myeloid leukemia. Hum Pathol. 34:479–83. PMID:12792922
127. Arber DA, Chang KL, Lyda MH, et al. (2003). Detection of NPM/MLF1 fusion in t(3;5)-positive acute myeloid leukemia and myelodysplasia. Hum Pathol. 34:809–13. PMID:14506644
128. Arber DA, George TI (2005). Bone marrow biopsy involvement by non-Hodgkin's lymphoma: frequency of lymphoma types, patterns, blood involvement, and discordance with other sites in 450 specimens. Am J Surg Pathol. 29:1549–57. PMID:16327427
129. Arber DA, Kamel OW, van de Rijn M, et al. (1995). Frequent presence of the Epstein-Barr virus in inflammatory pseudotumor. Hum Pathol. 26:1093–8. PMID:7557942
129A. Arber DA, Orazi A, Hasserjian R, et al. (2016). The 2016 revision to the World Health Organization classification of myeloid neoplasms and acute leukemia. Blood. 127:2391–405. PMID:27069254
130. Arber DA, Slovak ML, Popplewell L, et al. (2002). Therapy-related acute myeloid leukemia/myelodysplasia with balanced 21q22 translocations. Am J Clin Pathol. 117:306–13. PMID:11863228
131. Arber DA, Snyder DS, Fine M, et al. (2001). Myeloperoxidase immunoreactivity in adult acute lymphoblastic leukemia. Am J Clin Pathol. 116:25–33. PMID:11447748
132. Arber DA, Stein AS, Carter NH, et al. (2003). Prognostic impact of acute myeloid leukemia classification. Importance of detection of recurring cytogenetic abnormalities and multilineage dysplasia on survival. Am J Clin Pathol. 119:672–80. PMID:12760285
133. Arber DA, Weiss LM, Albújar PF, et al. (1993). Nasal lymphomas in Peru. High incidence of T-cell immunophenotype and Epstein-Barr virus infection. Am J Surg Pathol. 17:392–9. PMID:8388175
134. Arber DA, Weiss LM, Chang KL (1998). Detection of Epstein-Barr Virus in inflammatory pseudotumor. Semin Diagn Pathol. 15:155–60. PMID:9606806
135. Arcaini L, Lazzarino M, Colombo N, et al. (2006). Splenic marginal zone lymphoma: a prognostic model for clinical use. Blood. 107:4643–9. PMID:16493005
136. Arcaini L, Lucioni M, Boveri E, et al. (2009). Nodal marginal zone lymphoma: current knowledge and future directions of an heterogeneous disease. Eur J Haematol. 83:165–74. PMID:19548917
137. Arcaini L, Paulli M, Burcheri S, et al. (2007). Primary nodal marginal zone B-cell lymphoma: clinical features and prognostic assessment of a rare disease. Br J Haematol. 136:301–4. PMID:17233821
138. Arcaini L, Zibellini S, Boveri E, et al. (2012). The BRAF V600E mutation in hairy cell leukemia and other mature B-cell neoplasms. Blood. 119:188–91. PMID:22072557
139. Argatoff LH, Connors JM, Klasa RJ, et al. (1997). Mantle cell lymphoma: a clinicopathologic study of 80 cases. Blood. 89:2067–78. PMID:9058729
140. Arguelles-Grande C, Brar P, Green PH, et al. (2013). Immunohistochemical and T-cell receptor gene rearrangement analyses as predictors of morbidity and mortality in refractory celiac disease. J Clin Gastroenterol. 47:593–601. PMID:23470642
141. Aricò M, Danesino C (2001). Langerhans' cell histiocytosis: is there a role for genetics? Haematologica. 86:1009–14. PMID:11602405
142. Aricò M, Girschikofsky M, Généreau T, et al. (2003). Langerhans cell histiocytosis in adults. Report from the International Registry of the Histiocyte Society. Eur J Cancer. 39:2341–8. PMID:14556926
143. Aricò M, Haupt R, Russotto VS, et al. (2001). Langerhans cell histiocytosis in two generations: a new family and review of the literature. Med Pediatr Oncol. 36:314–6. PMID:11452942
144. Aricò M, Mussolin L, Carraro E, et al. (2015). Non-Hodgkin lymphoma in children with an associated inherited condition: A retrospective analysis of the Associazione Italiana Ematologia Oncologia Pediatrica (AIEOP). Pediatr Blood Cancer. 62:1782–9. PMID:26011068
145. Aricò M, Nichols K, Whitlock JA, et al. (1999). Familial clustering of Langerhans cell histiocytosis. Br J Haematol. 107:883–8. PMID:10606898
146. Aricò M, Valsecchi MG, Camitta B, et al. (2000). Outcome of treatment in children with Philadelphia chromosome-positive acute lymphoblastic leukemia. N Engl J Med. 342:998–1006. PMID:10749961
147. Armes JE, Angus P, Southey MC, et al. (1994). Lymphoproliferative disease of donor origin arising in patients after orthotopic liver transplantation. Cancer. 74:2436–41. PMID:7922997
148. Armitage JO, Weisenburger DD (1998). New approach to classifying non-Hodgkin's lymphomas: clinical features of the major histologic subtypes. Non-Hodgkin's Lymphoma Classification Project. J Clin Oncol. 16:2780–95. PMID:9704731
149. Armstrong SA, Kung AL, Mabon ME, et al. (2003). Inhibition of FLT3 in MLL. Validation of a therapeutic target identified by gene expression based classification. Cancer Cell. 3:173–83. PMID:12620411
149A. Arnaud L, Gorochov G, Charlotte F, et al. (2011). Systemic perturbation of cytokine and chemokine networks in Erdheim-Chester disease: a single-center series of 37 patients. Blood. 117:2783–90. PMID:21205927
149B. Arnaud L, Hervier B, Néel A, et al. (2011). CNS involvement and treatment with interferon-α are independent prognostic factors in Erdheim-Chester disease: a multicenter survival analysis of 53 patients. Blood. 117:2778–82. PMID:21239701
149C. Arnaud L, Malek Z, Archambaud F, et al. (2009). 18F-fluorodeoxyglucose-positron emission tomography scanning is more useful in followup than in the initial assessment of patients with Erdheim-Chester disease. Arthritis Rheum. 60:3128–38. PMID:19790052
150. Arnulf B, Copie-Bergman C, Delfau-Larue MH, et al. (1998). Nonhepatosplenic gammadelta T-cell lymphoma: a subset of cytotoxic lymphomas with mucosal or skin localization. Blood. 91:1723–31. PMID:9473239
151. Arons E, Sorbara L, Raffeld M, et al. (2006). Characterization of T-cell repertoire in hairy cell leukemia patients before and after recombinant immunotoxin BL22 therapy. Cancer Immunol Immunother. 55:1100–10. PMID:16311729
152. Arons E, Sunshine J, Suntum T, et al. (2006). Somatic hypermutation and VH gene usage in hairy cell leukaemia. Br J Haematol. 133:504–12. PMID:16681637
153. Arons E, Suntum T, Stetler-Stevenson M, et al. (2009). VH4-34+ hairy cell leukemia, a new variant with poor prognosis despite standard therapy. Blood. 114:4687–95. PMID:19745070
154. Arribas AJ, Campos-Martín Y, Gómez-Abad C, et al. (2012). Nodal marginal zone lymphoma: gene expression and miRNA profiling identify diagnostic markers and potential therapeutic targets. Blood. 119:e9–21. PMID:22110251
155. Arulogun SO, Prince HM, Ng J, et al. (2008). Long-term outcomes of patients with advanced-stage cutaneous T-cell lymphoma and large cell transformation. Blood. 112:3082–7. PMID:18647960
156. Arvanitakis L, Geras-Raaka E, Varma A, et al. (1997). Human herpesvirus KSHV encodes a constitutively active G-protein-coupled receptor linked to cell proliferation. Nature. 385:347–50. PMID:9002520
157. Arvanitakis L, Mesri EA, Nador RG, et al. (1996). Establishment and characterization of a primary effusion (body cavity-based) lymphoma cell line (BC-3) harboring kaposi's sarcoma-associated herpesvirus (KSHV/HHV-8) in the absence of Epstein-Barr virus. Blood. 88:2648–54. PMID:8839859
158. Arvey A, Ojesina AI, Pedamallu CS, et al. (2015). The tumor virus landscape of AIDS-related lymphomas. Blood. 125:e14–22. PMID:25827832
159. Arzoo KK, Bu X, Espina BM, et al. (2004). T-cell lymphoma in HIV-infected patients. J Acquir Immune Defic Syndr. 36:1020–7. PMID:15247554
160. Asada H (2007). Hypersensitivity to mosquito bites: a unique pathogenic mechanism linking Epstein-Barr virus infection, allergy and oncogenesis. J Dermatol Sci. 45:153–60. PMID:17169531
161. Asada H, Miyagawa S, Sumikawa Y, et al. (2003). CD4+ T-lymphocyte-induced Epstein-Barr virus reactivation in a patient with severe hypersensitivity to mosquito bites and Epstein-Barr virus-infected NK cell lymphocytosis. Arch Dermatol. 139:1601–7. PMID:14676078
162. Asada H, Saito-Katsuragi M, Niizeki H, et al. (2005). Mosquito salivary gland extracts induce EBV-infected NK cell oncogenesis via CD4 T cells in patients with hypersensitivity to mosquito bites. J Invest Dermatol. 125:956–61. PMID:16297196
163. Asano N, Kinoshita T, Tamaru J, et al. (2011). Cytotoxic molecule-positive classical Hodgkin's lymphoma: a clinicopathological comparison with cytotoxic molecule-positive peripheral T-cell lymphoma of not otherwise specified type. Haematologica. 96:1636–43. PMID:21859738
164. Asano N, Suzuki R, Kagami Y, et al. (2005). Clinicopathologic and prognostic significance of cytotoxic molecule expression in nodal peripheral T-cell lymphoma, unspecified. Am J Surg Pathol. 29:1284–93. PMID:16160469
165. Asano N, Yamamoto K, Tamaru J, et al. (2009). Age-related Epstein-Barr virus (EBV)-associated B-cell lymphoproliferative disorders: comparison with EBV-positive classic Hodgkin lymphoma in elderly patients. Blood. 113:2629–36. PMID:19075188
166. Ascani S, Piccioli M, Poggi S, et al. (1997). Pyothorax-associated lymphoma: description of the first two cases detected in Italy. Ann Oncol. 8:1133–8. PMID:9426333
167. Aschebrook-Kilfoy B, Cocco P, La Vecchia C, et al. (2014). Medical history, lifestyle, family history, and occupational risk factors for mycosis fungoides and Sézary syndrome: the InterLymph Non-Hodgkin Lymphoma Subtypes Project. J Natl Cancer Inst Monogr. 2014:98–105. PMID:25174030
168. Ascoli V, Lo Coco F, Artini M, et al. (1998). Extranodal lymphomas associated with hepatitis C virus infection. Am J Clin Pathol. 109:600–9. PMID:9576580
169. Ashton-Key M, Diss TC, Pan L, et al. (1997). Molecular analysis of T-cell clonality in ulcerative jejunitis and enteropathy-associated T-cell lymphoma. Am J Pathol. 151:493–8. PMID:9250161
170. Ashton-Key M, Thorpe PA, Allen JP, et al. (1995). Follicular Hodgkin's disease. Am J Surg Pathol. 19:1294–9. PMID:7573692
171. Askling J, Linet M, Gridley G, et al. (2002). Cancer incidence in a population-based cohort of individuals hospitalized with celiac disease or dermatitis herpetiformis. Gastroenterology. 123:1428–35. PMID:12404215
172. Asou H, Said JW, Yang R, et al. (1998). Mechanisms of growth control of Kaposi's sarcoma-associated herpes virus-associated primary effusion lymphoma cells. Blood. 91:2475–81. PMID:9516148
173. Assaf C, Gellrich S, Whittaker S, et al. (2007). CD56-positive haematological neoplasms of the skin: a multicentre study of the Cutaneous Lymphoma Project Group of the European Organisation for Research and Treatment of Cancer. J Clin Pathol. 60:981–9. PMID:17018683
174. Atayar C, Kok K, Kluiver J, et al. (2006). BCL6 alternative breakpoint region break and homozygous deletion of 17q24 in the nodular lymphocyte predominance type of Hodgkin's lymphoma-derived cell line DEV. Hum Pathol. 37:675–83. PMID:16733207
175. Atayar C, Poppema S, Visser L, et al. (2006). Cytokine gene expression profile distinguishes CD4+/CD57+ T cells of the nodular lymphocyte predominance type of Hodgkin's lymphoma from their tonsillar counterparts. J Pathol. 208:423–30. PMID:16353293
176. Attarbaschi A, Beishuizen A, Mann G, et al. (2013). Children and adolescents with follicular lymphoma have an excellent prognosis with either limited chemotherapy or with a "Watch and wait" strategy after complete resection. Ann Hematol. 92:1537–41. PMID:23665980
177. Attygalle A, Al-Jehani R, Diss TC, et al.

(2002). Neoplastic T cells in angioimmunoblastic T-cell lymphoma express CD10. Blood. 99:627–33. PMID:11781247
178. Attygalle AD, Cabeçadas J, Gaulard P, et al. (2014). Peripheral T-cell and NK-cell lymphomas and their mimics; taking a step forward - report on the lymphoma workshop of the XVIth meeting of the European Association for Haematopathology and the Society for Hematopathology. Histopathology. 64:171–99. PMID:24128129
179. Attygalle AD, Chuang SS, Diss TC, et al. (2007). Distinguishing angioimmunoblastic T-cell lymphoma from peripheral T-cell lymphoma, unspecified, using morphology, immunophenotype and molecular genetics. Histopathology. 50:498–508. PMID:17448026
180. Attygalle AD, Diss TC, Munson P, et al. (2004). CD10 expression in extranodal dissemination of angioimmunoblastic T-cell lymphoma. Am J Surg Pathol. 28:54–61. PMID:14707864
181. Attygalle AD, Feldman AL, Dogan A (2013). ITK/SYK translocation in angioimmunoblastic T-cell lymphoma. Am J Surg Pathol. 37:1456–7. PMID:24076779
182. Attygalle AD, Kyriakou C, Dupuis J, et al. (2007). Histologic evolution of angioimmunoblastic T-cell lymphoma in consecutive biopsies: clinical correlation and insights into natural history and disease progression. Am J Surg Pathol. 31:1077–88. PMID:17592275
183. Attygalle AD, Liu H, Shirali S, et al. (2004). Atypical marginal zone hyperplasia of mucosa-associated lymphoid tissue: a reactive condition of childhood showing immunoglobulin lambda light-chain restriction. Blood. 104:3343–8. PMID:15256428
184. Au WY, Gascoyne RD, Gallagher RE, et al. (2004). Hodgkin's lymphoma in Chinese migrants to British Columbia: a 25-year survey. Ann Oncol. 15:626–30. PMID:15033671
185. Au WY, Horsman DE, Gascoyne RD, et al. (2004). The spectrum of lymphoma with 8q24 aberrations: a clinical, pathological and cytogenetic study of 87 consecutive cases. Leuk Lymphoma. 45:519–28. PMID:15160914
186. Au WY, Lam CC, Lie AK, et al. (2003). T-cell large granular lymphocyte leukemia of donor origin after allogeneic bone marrow transplantation. Am J Clin Pathol. 120:626–30. PMID:14560574
187. Au WY, Ma SY, Chim CS, et al. (2005). Clinicopathologic features and treatment outcome of mature T-cell and natural killer-cell lymphomas diagnosed according to the World Health Organization classification scheme: a single center experience of 10 years. Ann Oncol. 16:206–14. PMID:15668271
188. Au WY, Pang A, Choy C, et al. (2004). Quantification of circulating Epstein-Barr virus (EBV) DNA in the diagnosis and monitoring of natural killer cell and EBV-positive lymphomas in immunocompetent patients. Blood. 104:243–9. PMID:15031209
189. Au WY, Weisenburger DD, Intragumtornchai T, et al. (2009). Clinical differences between nasal and extranasal natural killer/T-cell lymphoma: a study of 136 cases from the International Peripheral T-Cell Lymphoma Project. Blood. 113:3931–7. PMID:19029440
190. Aucouturier P, Khamlichi AA, Touchard G, et al. (1993). Brief report: heavy-chain deposition disease. N Engl J Med. 329:1389–93. PMID:8413435
191. Audouin J, Diebold J, Pallesen G (1992). Frequent expression of Epstein-Barr virus latent membrane protein-1 in tumour cells of Hodgkin's disease in HIV-positive patients. J Pathol. 167:381–4. PMID:1328576
192. Auewarakul CU, Leecharendkeat A, Thongnoppakhun W, et al. (2006). Mutations of AML1 in non-M0 acute myeloid leukemia: six novel mutations and a high incidence of cooperative events in a South-east Asian population. Haematologica. 91:675–8. PMID:16627249
193. Aukema SM, Kreuz M, Kohler CW, et al. (2014). Biological characterization of adult MYC-translocation-positive mature B-cell lymphomas other than molecular Burkitt lymphoma. Haematologica. 99:726–35. PMID:24179151
194. Aukema SM, Siebert R, Schuuring E, et al. (2011). Double-hit B-cell lymphomas. Blood. 117:2319–31. PMID:21119107
195. Aukema SM, Theil L, Rohde M, et al. (2015). Sequential karyotyping in Burkitt lymphoma reveals a linear clonal evolution with increase in karyotype complexity and a high frequency of recurrent secondary aberrations. Br J Haematol. 170:814–25. PMID:26104998
196. Aul C, Bowen DT, Yoshida Y (1998). Pathogenesis, etiology and epidemiology of myelodysplastic syndromes. Haematologica. 83:71–86. PMID:9542325
197. Aul C, Gattermann N, Germing U, et al. (1997). Fatal hyperleukocytic syndrome in a patient with chronic myelomonocytic leukemia. Leuk Res. 21:249–53. PMID:9111170
198. Aul C, Gattermann N, Heyll A, et al. (1992). Primary myelodysplastic syndromes: analysis of prognostic factors in 235 patients and proposals for an improved scoring system. Leukemia. 6:52–9. PMID:1736014
199. Aul C, Gattermann N, Schneider W (1992). Age-related incidence and other epidemiological aspects of myelodysplastic syndromes. Br J Haematol. 82:358–67. PMID:1419819
200. Avet-Loiseau H, Attal M, Moreau P, et al. (2007). Genetic abnormalities and survival in multiple myeloma: the experience of the Intergroupe Francophone du Myélome. Blood. 109:3489–95. PMID:17209057
201. Avet-Loiseau H, Daviet A, Brigaudeau C, et al. (2001). Cytogenetic, interphase, and multicolor fluorescence in situ hybridization analyses in primary plasma cell leukemia: a study of 40 patients at diagnosis, on behalf of the Intergroupe Francophone du Myélome and the Groupe Français de Cytogénétique Hématologique. Blood. 97:822–5. PMID:11157506
202. Avet-Loiseau H, Facon T, Grosbois B, et al. (2002). Oncogenesis of multiple myeloma: 14q32 and 13q chromosomal abnormalities are not randomly distributed, but correlate with natural history, immunological features, and clinical presentation. Blood. 99:2185–91. PMID:11877296
203. Ayton PM, Cleary ML (2001). Molecular mechanisms of leukemogenesis mediated by MLL fusion proteins. Oncogene. 20:5695–707. PMID:11607819
204. Azambuja D, Natkunam Y, Biasoli I, et al. (2012). Lack of association of tumor-associated macrophages with clinical outcome in patients with classical Hodgkin's lymphoma. Ann Oncol. 23:736–42. PMID:21602260
205. Stewart BW, Wild CP, editors (2014). World Cancer Report 2014. Lyon: IARC.
206. Babushok DV, Bessler M (2015). Genetic predisposition syndromes: when should they be considered in the work-up of MDS? Best Pract Res Clin Haematol. 28:55–68. PMID:25659730
207. Baccarani M, Deininger MW, Rosti G, et al. (2013). European LeukemiaNet recommendations for the management of chronic myeloid leukemia: 2013. Blood. 122:872–84. PMID:23803709
208. Bacher U, Haferlach C, Alpermann T, et al. (2013). Patients with therapy-related myelodysplastic syndromes and acute myeloid leukemia share genetic features but can be separated by blast counts and cytogenetic risk profiles into prognostically relevant subgroups. Leuk Lymphoma. 54:639–42. PMID:22853779
209. Bacher U, Haferlach T, Kern W, et al. (2007). A comparative study of molecular mutations in 381 patients with myelodysplastic syndrome and in 4130 patients with acute myeloid leukemia. Haematologica. 92:744–52. PMID:17550846
210. Bacher U, Kern W, Alpermann T, et al. (2011). Prognosis in patients with MDS or AML and bone marrow blasts between 10% and 30% is not associated with blast counts but depends on cytogenetic and molecular genetic characteristics. Leukemia. 25:1361–4. PMID:21494258
211. Bacher U, Schnittger S, Macijewski K, et al. (2012). Multilineage dysplasia does not influence prognosis in CEBPA-mutated AML, supporting the WHO proposal to classify these patients as a unique entity. Blood. 119:4719–22. PMID:22442349
212. Bachy E, Salles G (2015). Treatment approach to newly diagnosed diffuse large B-cell lymphoma. Semin Hematol. 52:107–18. PMID:25805590
213. Bacon CM, Paterson JC, Liu H, et al. (2008). Peripheral T-cell lymphoma with a follicular growth pattern: derivation from follicular helper T cells and relationship to angioimmunoblastic T-cell lymphoma. Br J Haematol. 143:439–41. PMID:18729855
214. Bacon CM, Ye H, Diss TC, et al. (2007). Primary follicular lymphoma of the testis and epididymis in adults. Am J Surg Pathol. 31:1050–8. PMID:17592272
215. Badalian-Very G, Vergilio JA, Degar BA, et al. (2010). Recurrent BRAF mutations in Langerhans cell histiocytosis. Blood. 116:1919–23. PMID:20519626
216. Baddoura FK, Hanson C, Chan WC (1992). Plasmacytoid monocyte proliferation associated with myeloproliferative disorders. Cancer. 69:1457–67. PMID:1540883
217. Bader-Meunier B, Tchernia G, Miélot F, et al. (1997). Occurrence of myeloproliferative disorder in patients with Noonan syndrome. J Pediatr. 130:885–9. PMID:9202609
218. Bae E, Park CJ, Cho YU, et al. (2013). Differential diagnosis of myelofibrosis based on WHO 2008 criteria: acute panmyelosis with myelofibrosis, acute megakaryoblastic leukemia with myelofibrosis, primary myelofibrosis and myelodysplastic syndrome with myelofibrosis. Int J Lab Hematol. 35:629–36. PMID:23693053
219. Baecklund E, Smedby KE, Sutton LA, et al. (2014). Lymphoma development in patients with autoimmune and inflammatory disorders–what are the driving forces? Semin Cancer Biol. 24:61–70. PMID:24333759
220. Baecklund E, Sundström C, Ekbom A, et al. (2003). Lymphoma subtypes in patients with rheumatoid arthritis: increased proportion of diffuse large B cell lymphoma. Arthritis Rheum. 48:1543–50. PMID:12794821
221. Baer MR, Stewart CC, Lawrence D, et al. (1997). Expression of the neural cell adhesion molecule CD56 is associated with short remission duration and survival in acute myeloid leukemia with t(8;21)(q22;q22). Blood. 90:1643–8. PMID:9269784
222. Bagby GC, Meyers G (2007). Bone marrow failure as a risk factor for clonal evolution: prospects for leukemia prevention. Hematology Am Soc Hematol Educ Program. 40–6. PMID:18024607
223. Bagdi E, Diss TC, Munson P, et al. (1999). Mucosal intra-epithelial lymphocytes in enteropathy-associated T-cell lymphoma, ulcerative jejunitis, and refractory celiac disease constitute a neoplastic population. Blood. 94:260–4. PMID:10381521
224. Bahler DW, Aguilera NS, Chen CC, et al. (2000). Histological and immunoglobulin VH gene analysis of interfollicular small lymphocytic lymphoma provides evidence for two types. Am J Pathol. 157:1063–70. PMID:11021809
225. Bain B (2006). Ringed sideroblasts with thrombocytosis: an uncommon mixed myelodysplastic/myeloproliferative disease in older adults. Br J Haematol. 134:340, author reply 340–1. PMID:16787502
226. Bain BJ (1996). Eosinophilic leukaemias and the idiopathic hypereosinophilic syndrome. Br J Haematol. 95:2–9. PMID:8857931
227. Bain BJ (1999). The relationship between the myelodysplastic syndromes and the myeloproliferative disorders. Leuk Lymphoma. 34:443–9. PMID:10492067
228. Bain BJ (2004). Relationship between idiopathic hypereosinophilic syndrome, eosinophilic leukemia, and systemic mastocytosis. Am J Hematol. 77:82–5. PMID:15307112
229. Bain BJ (2015). Blood cells: a practical guide. 5th ed. Oxford: Wiley-Blackwell.
230. Bain BJ, Ahmad S (2014). Should myeloid and lymphoid neoplasms with PCM1-JAK2 and other rearrangements of JAK2 be recognized as specific entities? Br J Haematol. 166:809–17. PMID:24913195
231. Bain BJ, Ahmad S (2015). Chronic neutrophilic leukaemia and plasma cell-related neutrophilic leukaemoid reactions. Br J Haematol. 171:400–10. PMID:26218186
232. Bain BJ, Chakravorty S, Ancliff P (2015). Congenital acute megakaryoblastic leukemia. Am J Hematol. 90:963. PMID:26148249
233. Bain BJ, Fletcher SH (2007). Chronic eosinophilic leukemias and the myeloproliferative variant of the hypereosinophilic syndrome. Immunol Allergy Clin North Am. 27:377–88. PMID:17868855
234. Bains A, Luthra R, Medeiros LJ, et al. (2011). FLT3 and NPM1 mutations in myelodysplastic syndromes: Frequency and potential value for predicting progression to acute myeloid leukemia. Am J Clin Pathol. 135:62–9. PMID:21173125
235. Bairey O, Goldschmidt N, Ruchlemer R, et al. (2012). Insect-bite-like reaction in patients with chronic lymphocytic leukemia: a study from the Israeli Chronic Lymphocytic Leukemia Study Group. Eur J Haematol. 89:491–6. PMID:23033927
236. Bakker NA, van Imhoff GW, Verschuuren EA, et al. (2005). Early onset post-transplant lymphoproliferative disease is associated with allograft localization. Clin Transplant. 19:327–34. PMID:15877793
237. Bakkus MH, Heirman C, Van Riet I, et al. (1992). Evidence that multiple myeloma Ig heavy chain VDJ genes contain somatic mutations but show no intraclonal variation. Blood. 80:2326–35. PMID:1421403
238. Bakst RL, Tallman MS, Douer D, et al. (2011). How I treat extramedullary acute myeloid leukemia. Blood. 118:3785–93. PMID:21795742
238A. Balagué O, Martínez A, Colomo L, et al. (2007). Epstein-Barr virus negative clonal plasma cell proliferations and lymphomas in peripheral T-cell lymphomas: a phenomenon with distinctive clinicopathologic features. Am J Surg Pathol. 31:1310–22. PMID:17721185
239. Baldini L, Goldaniga M, Guffanti A, et al. (2005). Immunoglobulin M monoclonal gammopathies of undetermined significance and indolent Waldenstrom's macroglobulinemia recognize the same determinants of evolution into symptomatic lymphoid disorders: proposal for a common prognostic scoring system. J Clin Oncol. 23:4662–8. PMID:16034042
239A. Baldus CD, Tanner SM, Ruppert AS, et al. (2003). BAALC expression predicts clinical outcome of de novo acute myeloid leukemia patients with normal cytogenetics: a

Cancer and Leukemia Group B Study. Blood. 102:1613–8. PMID:12750167
239B. Baldus CD, Thiede C, Soucek S, et al. (2006). BAALC expression and FLT3 internal tandem duplication mutations in acute myeloid leukemia patients with normal cytogenetics: prognostic implications. J Clin Oncol. 24:790–7. PMID:16418499
239C. Balgobind BV, Raimondi SC, Harbott J, et al. (2009). Novel prognostic subgroups in childhood 11q23/MLL-rearranged acute myeloid leukemia: results of an international retrospective study. Blood. 114:2489–96. PMID:19528532
240. Baliakas P, Agathangelidis A, Hadzidimitriou A, et al. (2015). Not all IGHV3-21 chronic lymphocytic leukemias are equal: prognostic considerations. Blood. 125:856–9. PMID:25634617
241. Baliakas P, Hadzidimitriou A, Sutton LA, et al. (2015). Recurrent mutations refine prognosis in chronic lymphocytic leukemia. Leukemia. 29:329–36. PMID:24943832
242. Ballard HS, Hamilton LM, Marcus AJ, et al. (1970). A new variant of heavy-chain disease (mu-chain disease). N Engl J Med. 282:1060–2. PMID:5438427
243. Ballester B, Ramuz O, Gisselbrecht C, et al. (2006). Gene expression profiling identifies molecular subgroups among nodal peripheral T-cell lymphomas. Oncogene. 25:1560–70. PMID:16288225
244. Banchereau J, Briere F, Caux C, et al. (2000). Immunobiology of dendritic cells. Annu Rev Immunol. 18:767–811. PMID:10837075
245. Banks PM, Chan J, Cleary ML, et al. (1992). Mantle cell lymphoma. A proposal for unification of morphologic, immunologic, and molecular data. Am J Surg Pathol. 16:637–40. PMID:1530105
246. Barber NA, Loberiza FR Jr, Perry AM, et al. (2013). Does functional imaging distinguish nodular lymphocyte-predominant hodgkin lymphoma from T-cell/histiocyte-rich large B-cell lymphoma? Clin Lymphoma Myeloma Leuk. 13:392–7. PMID:23773450
247. Barbui T, Carobbio A, Rumi E, et al. (2014). In contemporary patients with polycythemia vera, rates of thrombosis and risk factors delineate a new clinical epidemiology. Blood. 124:3021–3. PMID:25377561
248. Barbui T, Thiele J, Carobbio A, et al. (2014). Masked polycythemia vera diagnosed according to WHO and BCSH classification. Am J Hematol. 89:199–202. PMID:24166817
249. Barbui T, Thiele J, Carobbio A, et al. (2014). Discriminating between essential thrombocythemia and masked polycythemia vera in JAK2 mutated patients. Am J Hematol. 89:588–90. PMID:24535932
250. Barbui T, Thiele J, Carobbio A, et al. (2015). The rate of transformation from JAK2-mutated ET to PV is influenced by an accurate WHO-defined clinico-morphological diagnosis. Leukemia. 29:992–3. PMID:25425199
251. Barbui T, Thiele J, Gisslinger H, et al. (2014). Masked polycythemia vera (mPV): results of an international study. Am J Hematol. 89:52–4. PMID:23996471
252. Barbui T, Thiele J, Kvasnicka HM, et al. (2014). Essential thrombocythemia with high hemoglobin levels according to the revised WHO classification. Leukemia. 28:2092–4. PMID:24888272
253. Barbui T, Thiele J, Passamonti F, et al. (2012). Initial bone marrow reticulin fibrosis in polycythemia vera exerts an impact on clinical outcome. Blood. 119:2239–41. PMID:22246040
254. Barbui T, Thiele J, Passamonti F, et al. (2011). Survival and disease progression in essential thrombocythemia are significantly influenced by accurate morphologic diagnosis: an international study. J Clin Oncol. 29:3179–84. PMID:21747083
255. Barbui T, Thiele J, Vannucchi AM, et al. (2013). Problems and pitfalls regarding WHO-defined diagnosis of early/prefibrotic primary myelofibrosis versus essential thrombocythemia. Leukemia. 27:1953–8. PMID:23467025
256. Barbui T, Thiele J, Vannucchi AM, et al. (2014). Rethinking the diagnostic criteria of polycythemia vera. Leukemia. 28:1191–5. PMID:24352199
257. Barbui T, Thiele J, Vannucchi AM, et al. (2015). Myeloproliferative neoplasms: Morphology and clinical practice. Am J Hematol. 91:430–3 PMID:26718907
258. Barbui T, Thiele J, Vannucchi AM, et al. (2015). Rationale for revision and proposed changes of the WHO diagnostic criteria for polycythemia vera, essential thrombocythemia and primary myelofibrosis. Blood Cancer J. 5:e337. PMID:26832847
258A. Bardet V, Costa LD, Elie C, et al. (2006). Nucleophosmin status may influence the therapeutic decision in de novo acute myeloid leukemia with normal karyotype. Leukemia. 20:1644–6. PMID:16791266
259. Bardet V, Wagner-Ballon O, Guy J, et al. (2015). Multicentric study underlining the interest of adding CD5, CD7 and CD56 expression assessment to the flow cytometric Ogata score in myelodysplastic syndromes and myelodysplastic/myeloproliferative neoplasms. Haematologica. 100:472–8. PMID:25637056
260. Bareau B, Rey J, Hamidou M, et al. (2010). Analysis of a French cohort of patients with large granular lymphocyte leukemia: a report on 229 cases. Haematologica. 95:1534–41. PMID:20378561
261. Barlow JL, Drynan LF, Hewett DR, et al. (2010). A p53-dependent mechanism underlies macrocytic anemia in a mouse model of human 5q- syndrome. Nat Med. 16:59–66. PMID:19966810
262. Baró C, Salido M, Domingo A, et al. (2006). Translocation t(9;14)(p13;q32) in cases of splenic marginal zone lymphoma. Haematologica. 91:1289–91. PMID:16956840
263. Barosi G (2014). Essential thrombocythemia vs. early/prefibrotic myelofibrosis: why does it matter. Best Pract Res Clin Haematol. 27:129–40. PMID:25189724
264. Barosi G, Hoffman R (2005). Idiopathic myelofibrosis. Semin Hematol. 42:248–58. PMID:16210038
265. Barosi G, Mesa RA, Thiele J, et al. (2008). Proposed criteria for the diagnosis of post-polycythemia vera and post-essential thrombocythemia myelofibrosis: a consensus statement from the International Working Group for Myelofibrosis Research and Treatment. Leukemia. 22:437–8. PMID:17728787
266. Barosi G, Rosti V, Bonetti E, et al. (2012). Evidence that prefibrotic myelofibrosis is aligned along a clinical and biological continuum featuring primary myelofibrosis. PLoS One. 7:e35631. PMID:22536419
267. Barosi G, Rosti V, Massa M, et al. (2004). Spleen neoangiogenesis in patients with myelofibrosis with myeloid metaplasia. Br J Haematol. 124:618–25. PMID:14871248
268. Barosi G, Viarengo G, Pecci A, et al. (2001). Diagnostic and clinical relevance of the number of circulating CD34(+) cells in myelofibrosis with myeloid metaplasia. Blood. 98:3249–55. PMID:11719361
269. Barrans S, Crouch S, Smith A, et al. (2010). Rearrangement of MYC is associated with poor prognosis in patients with diffuse large B-cell lymphoma treated in the era of rituximab. J Clin Oncol. 28:3360–5. PMID:20498406
270. Barrans SL, Evans PA, O'Connor SJ, et al. (2003). The t(14;18) is associated with germinal center-derived diffuse large B-cell lymphoma and is a strong predictor of outcome. Clin Cancer Res. 9:2133–9. PMID:12796378
271. Barrans SL, Fenton JA, Banham A, et al. (2004). Strong expression of FOXP1 identifies a distinct subset of diffuse large B-cell lymphoma (DLBCL) patients with poor outcome. Blood. 104:2933–5. PMID:15238418
272. Barrans SL, O'Connor SJ, Evans PA, et al. (2002). Rearrangement of the BCL6 locus at 3q27 is an independent poor prognostic factor in nodal diffuse large B-cell lymphoma. Br J Haematol. 117:322–32. PMID:11972514
273. Barrington SF, Mikhaeel NG, Kostakoglu L, et al. (2014). Role of imaging in the staging and response assessment of lymphoma: consensus of the International Conference on Malignant Lymphomas Imaging Working Group. J Clin Oncol. 32:3048–58. PMID:25113771
274. Barrionuevo C, Anderson VM, Zevallos-Giampietri E, et al. (2002). Hydroa-like cutaneous T-cell lymphoma: a clinicopathologic and molecular genetic study of 16 pediatric cases from Peru. Appl Immunohistochem Mol Morphol. 10:7–14. PMID:11893040
275. Barrionuevo C, Zaharia M, Martinez MT, et al. (2007). Extranodal NK/T-cell lymphoma, nasal type: study of clinicopathologic and prognosis factors in a series of 78 cases from Peru. Appl Immunohistochem Mol Morphol. 15:38–44. PMID:17536305
276. Barros MH, Hassan R, Niedobitek G (2011). Disease patterns in pediatric classical Hodgkin lymphoma: a report from a developing area in Brazil. Hematol Oncol. 29:190–5. PMID:21374695
277. Barry TS, Jaffe ES, Sorbara L, et al. (2003). Peripheral T-cell lymphomas expressing CD30 and CD15. Am J Surg Pathol. 27:1513–22. PMID:14657710
278. Barta SK, Samuel MS, Xue X, et al. (2015). Changes in the influence of lymphoma- and HIV-specific factors on outcomes in AIDS-related non-Hodgkin lymphoma. Ann Oncol. 26:958–66. PMID:25632071
279. Barth TF, Leithäuser F, Joos S, et al. (2002). Mediastinal (thymic) large B-cell lymphoma: where do we stand? Lancet Oncol. 3:229–34. PMID:12067685
280. Barth TF, Müller S, Pawlita M, et al. (2004). Homogeneous immunophenotype and paucity of secondary genomic aberrations are distinctive features of endemic but not of sporadic Burkitt's lymphoma and diffuse large B-cell lymphoma with MYC rearrangement. J Pathol. 203:940–5. PMID:15258997
281. Bartl R, Frisch B, Fateh-Moghadam A, et al. (1987). Histologic classification and staging of multiple myeloma. A retrospective and prospective study of 674 cases. Am J Clin Pathol. 87:342–55. PMID:3825999
282. Bartram CR, de Klein A, Hagemeijer A, et al. (1983). Translocation of c-ab1 oncogene correlates with the presence of a Philadelphia chromosome in chronic myelocytic leukaemia. Nature. 306:277–80. PMID:6580527
283. Baruchel A, Cayuela JM, Ballerini P, et al. (1997). The majority of myeloid-antigen-positive (My+) childhood B-cell precursor acute lymphoblastic leukaemias express TEL-AML1 fusion transcripts. Br J Haematol. 99:101–6. PMID:9359509
284. Baseggio L, Berger F, Morel D, et al. (2006). Identification of circulating CD10 positive T cells in angioimmunoblastic T-cell lymphoma. Leukemia. 20:296–303. PMID:16341050
285. Baseggio L, Traverse-Glehen A, Petinataud F, et al. (2010). CD5 expression identifies a subset of splenic marginal zone lymphomas with higher lymphocytosis: a clinico-pathological, cytogenetic and molecular study of 24 cases. Haematologica. 95:604–12. PMID:20015887
286. Bassig BA, Cerhan JR, Au WY, et al. (2015). Genetic susceptibility to diffuse large B-cell lymphoma in a pooled study of three Eastern Asian populations. Eur J Haematol. 95:442–8. PMID:25611436
287. Basso K, Liso A, Tiacci E, et al. (2004). Gene expression profiling of hairy cell leukemia reveals a phenotype related to memory B cells with altered expression of chemokine and adhesion receptors. J Exp Med. 199:59–68. PMID:14707115
288. Bastard C, Deweindt C, Kerckaert JP, et al. (1994). LAZ3 rearrangements in non-Hodgkin's lymphoma: correlation with histology, immunophenotype, karyotype, and clinical outcome in 217 patients. Blood. 83:2423–7. PMID:8167331
289. Bataille R, Boccadoro M, Klein B, et al. (1992). C-reactive protein and beta-2 microglobulin produce a simple and powerful myeloma staging system. Blood. 80:733–7. PMID:1638024
290. Bataille R, Durie BG, Grenier J, et al. (1986). Prognostic factors and staging in multiple myeloma: a reappraisal. J Clin Oncol. 4:80–7. PMID:3510284
291. Bataille R, Jégo G, Robillard N, et al. (2006). The phenotype of normal, reactive and malignant plasma cells. Identification of "many and multiple myelomas" and of new targets for myeloma therapy. Haematologica. 91:1234–40. PMID:16956823
292. Bataille R, Pellat-Deceunynck C, Robillard N, et al. (2008). CD117 (c-kit) is aberrantly expressed in a subset of MGUS and multiple myeloma with unexpectedly good prognosis. Leuk Res. 32:379–82. PMID:17767956
293. Batchelor T, Loeffler JS (2006). Primary CNS lymphoma. J Clin Oncol. 24:1281–8. PMID:16525183
294. Batista DA, Vonderheid EC, Hawkins A, et al. (2006). Multicolor fluorescence in situ hybridization (SKY) in mycosis fungoides and Sézary syndrome: search for recurrent chromosome abnormalities. Genes Chromosomes Cancer. 45:383–91. PMID:16382449
295. Baudon JJ (2012). [A possible link between late milk production and reduced breast feeding duration]. Soins Pediatr Pueric. (269):10. PMID:23297587
296. Baumann I, Führer M, Behrendt S, et al. (2012). Morphological differentiation of severe aplastic anaemia from hypocellular refractory cytopenia of childhood: reproducibility of histopathological diagnostic criteria. Histopathology. 61:10–7. PMID:22458667
297. Baumgärtner AK, Zettl A, Chott A, et al. (2003). High frequency of genetic aberrations in enteropathy-type T-cell lymphoma. Lab Invest. 83:1509–16. PMID:14563952
298. Baxter EJ, Hochhaus A, Bolufer P, et al. (2002). The t(4;22)(q12;q11) in atypical chronic myeloid leukaemia fuses BCR to PDGFRA. Hum Mol Genet. 11:1391–7. PMID:12023981
299. Baxter EJ, Scott LM, Campbell PJ, et al. (2005). Acquired mutation of the tyrosine kinase JAK2 in human myeloproliferative disorders. Lancet. 365:1054–61. PMID:15781101
300. Bayerl MG, Rakozy CK, Mohamed AN, et al. (2002). Blastic natural killer cell lymphoma/leukemia: a report of seven cases. Am J Clin Pathol. 117:41–50. PMID:11789729
301. Bayle C, Charpentier A, Duchayne E, et al. (1999). Leukaemic presentation of small cell variant anaplastic large cell lymphoma: report of four cases. Br J Haematol. 104:680–8. PMID:10192426
302. Beà S, Ribas M, Hernández JM, et al. (1999). Increased number of chromosomal imbalances and high-level DNA amplifications

in mantle cell lymphoma are associated with blastoid variants. Blood. 93:4365–74. PMID:10361135

303. Beà S, Salaverria I, Armengol L, et al. (2009). Uniparental disomies, homozygous deletions, amplifications, and target genes in mantle cell lymphoma revealed by integrative high-resolution whole-genome profiling. Blood. 113:3059–69. PMID:18984860

304. Beà S, Tort F, Pinyol M, et al. (2001). BMI-1 gene amplification and overexpression in hematological malignancies occur mainly in mantle cell lymphomas. Cancer Res. 61:2409–12. PMID:11289106

305. Beà S, Valdés-Mas R, Navarro A, et al. (2013). Landscape of somatic mutations and clonal evolution in mantle cell lymphoma. Proc Natl Acad Sci U S A. 110:18250–5. PMID:24145436

306. Bea S, Zettl A, Wright G, et al. (2005). Diffuse large B-cell lymphoma subgroups have distinct genetic profiles that influence tumor biology and improve gene-expression-based survival prediction. Blood. 106:3183–90. PMID:16046532

307. Bearman RM, Pangalis GA, Rappaport H (1979). Acute ("malignant") myelosclerosis. Cancer. 43:279–93. PMID:367569

308. Beaty MW, Kumar S, Sorbara L, et al. (1999). A biophenotypic human herpesvirus 8–associated primary bowel lymphoma. Am J Surg Pathol. 23:992–4. PMID:10435572

309. Beaty MW, Toro J, Sorbara L, et al. (2001). Cutaneous lymphomatoid granulomatosis: correlation of clinical and biologic features. Am J Surg Pathol. 25:1111–20. PMID:11688570

310. Becker H, Marcucci G, Maharry K, et al. (2010). Favorable prognostic impact of NPM1 mutations in older patients with cytogenetically normal de novo acute myeloid leukemia and associated gene- and microRNA-expression signatures: a Cancer and Leukemia Group B study. J Clin Oncol. 28:596–604. PMID:20026798

311. Bejar R (2014). Clinical and genetic predictors of prognosis in myelodysplastic syndromes. Haematologica. 99:956–64. PMID:24881041

312. Bejar R, Stevenson K, Abdel-Wahab O, et al. (2011). Clinical effect of point mutations in myelodysplastic syndromes. N Engl J Med. 364:2496–506. PMID:21714648

313. Bejar R, Stevenson KE, Caughey B, et al. (2014). Somatic mutations predict poor outcome in patients with myelodysplastic syndrome after hematopoietic stem-cell transplantation. J Clin Oncol. 32:2691–8. PMID:25092778

314. Bekkenk MW, Geelen FA, van Voorst Vader PC, et al. (2000). Primary and secondary cutaneous CD30(+) lymphoproliferative disorders: a report from the Dutch Cutaneous Lymphoma Group on the long-term follow-up data of 219 patients and guidelines for diagnosis and treatment. Blood. 95:3653–61. PMID:10845893

315. Bekkenk MW, Jansen PM, Meijer CJ, et al. (2004). CD56+ hematological neoplasms presenting in the skin: a retrospective analysis of 23 new cases and 130 cases from the literature. Ann Oncol. 15:1097–108. PMID:15205205

316. Bekkenk MW, Kluin PM, Jansen PM, et al. (2001). Lymphomatoid papulosis with a natural killer-cell phenotype. Br J Dermatol. 145:318–22. PMID:11531801

317. Bekkenk MW, Vermeer MH, Jansen PM, et al. (2003). Peripheral T-cell lymphomas unspecified presenting in the skin: analysis of prognostic factors in a group of 82 patients. Blood. 102:2213–9. PMID:12750155

318. Bélec L, Mohamed AS, Authier FJ, et al. (1999). Human herpesvirus 8 infection in patients with POEMS syndrome-associated multicentric Castleman's disease. Blood. 93:3643–53. PMID:10339470

319. Belhadj K, Reyes F, Farcet JP, et al. (2003). Hepatosplenic gammadelta T-cell lymphoma is a rare clinicopathologic entity with poor outcome: report on a series of 21 patients. Blood. 102:4261–9. PMID:12907441

320. Beljaards RC, Meijer CJ, Van der Putte SC, et al. (1994). Primary cutaneous T-cell lymphoma: clinicopathological features and prognostic parameters of 35 cases other than mycosis fungoides and CD30-positive large cell lymphoma. J Pathol. 172:53–60. PMID:7931828

321. Bell A, Rickinson AB (2003). Epstein-Barr virus, the TCL-1 oncogene and Burkitt's lymphoma. Trends Microbiol. 11:495–7. PMID:14607063

322. Bellanger D, Jacquemin V, Chopin M, et al. (2014). Recurrent JAK1 and JAK3 somatic mutations in T-cell prolymphocytic leukemia. Leukemia. 28:417–9. PMID:24048415

323. Beltraminelli H, Leinweber B, Kerl H, et al. (2009). Primary cutaneous CD4+ small-/medium-sized pleomorphic T-cell lymphoma: a cutaneous nodular proliferation of pleomorphic T lymphocytes of undetermined significance? A study of 136 cases. Am J Dermatopathol. 31:317–22. PMID:19461234

324. Beltraminelli H, Müllegger R, Cerroni L (2010). Indolent CD8+ lymphoid proliferation of the ear: a phenotypic variant of the small-medium pleomorphic cutaneous T-cell lymphoma? J Cutan Pathol. 37:81–4. PMID:19602068

325. Beltran BE, Castillo JJ, Morales D, et al. (2011). EBV-positive diffuse large B-cell lymphoma of the elderly: a case series from Peru. Am J Hematol. 86:663–7. PMID:21761432

326. Beltran BE, Morales D, Quiñones P, et al. (2011). EBV-positive diffuse large b-cell lymphoma in young immunocompetent individuals. Clin Lymphoma Myeloma Leuk. 11:512–6. PMID:21889434

327. Ben-Ezra J, Bailey A, Azumi N, et al. (1991). Malignant histiocytosis X. A distinct clinicopathologic entity. Cancer. 68:1050–60. PMID:1913475

328. Bende RJ, Smit LA, Bossenbroek JG, et al. (2003). Primary follicular lymphoma of the small intestine: alpha4beta7 expression and immunoglobulin configuration suggest an origin from local antigen-experienced B cells. Am J Pathol. 162:105–13. PMID:12507894

329. Bendriss-Vermare N, Chaperot L, Peoc'h M, et al. (2004). In situ leukemic plasmacytoid dendritic cells pattern of chemokine receptors expression and in vitro migratory response. Leukemia. 18:1491–8. PMID:15284853

330. Béné MC, Bernier M, Casasnovas RO, et al. (2001). Acute myeloid leukaemia M0: haematological, immunophenotypic and cytogenetic characteristics and their prognostic significance: an analysis in 241 patients. Br J Haematol. 113:737–45. PMID:11380465

331. Bene MC, Bernier M, Casasnovas RO, et al. (1998). The reliability and specificity of c-kit for the diagnosis of acute myeloid leukemias and undifferentiated leukemias. Blood. 92:596–9. PMID:9657760

332. Bene MC, Castoldi G, Knapp W, et al. (1995). Proposals for the immunological classification of acute leukemias. Leukemia. 9:1783–6. PMID:7564526

333. Bénet C, Gomez A, Aguilar C, et al. (2011). Histologic and immunohistologic characterization of skin localization of myeloid disorders: a study of 173 cases. Am J Clin Pathol. 135:278–90. PMID:21228369

334. Benharroch D, Levy A, Gopas J, et al. (2008). Lymphocyte-depleted classic Hodgkin lymphoma-a neglected entity? Virchows Arch. 453:611–6. PMID:18958495

335. Benharroch D, Meguerian-Bedoyan Z, Lamant L, et al. (1998). ALK-positive lymphoma: a single disease with a broad spectrum of morphology. Blood. 91:2076–84. PMID:9490693

336. Benner MF, Jansen PM, Meijer CJ, et al. (2009). Diagnostic and prognostic evaluation of phenotypic markers TRAF1, MUM1, BCL2 and CD15 in cutaneous CD30-positive lymphoproliferative disorders. Br J Dermatol. 161:121–7. PMID:19416236

337. Benner MF, Jansen PM, Vermeer MH, et al. (2012). Prognostic factors in transformed mycosis fungoides: a retrospective analysis of 100 cases. Blood. 119:1643–9. PMID:22160616

338. Benner MF, Willemze R (2009). Applicability and prognostic value of the new TNM classification system in 135 patients with primary cutaneous anaplastic large cell lymphoma. Arch Dermatol. 145:1399–404. PMID:20026848

338A. Bennett JM, Catovsky D, Daniel MT, et al. (1976). Proposals for the classification of the acute leukaemias. French-American-British (FAB) co-operative group. Br J Haematol. 33:451–8. PMID:188440

339. Bennett JM, Catovsky D, Daniel MT, et al. (1994). The chronic myeloid leukaemias: guidelines for distinguishing chronic granulocytic, atypical chronic myeloid, and chronic myelomonocytic leukaemia. Br J Haematol. 87:746–54. PMID:7986717

340. Bennett JM, Catovsky D, Daniel MT, et al. (1982). Proposals for the classification of the myelodysplastic syndromes. Br J Haematol. 51:189–99. PMID:6952920

341. Bennett JM, Catovsky D, Daniel MT, et al. (1989). Proposals for the classification of chronic (mature) B and T lymphoid leukaemias. J Clin Pathol. 42:567–84. PMID:2738163

342. Bennett JM, Orazi A (2009). Diagnostic criteria to distinguish hypocellular acute myeloid leukemia from hypocellular myelodysplastic syndromes and aplastic anemia: recommendations for a standardized approach. Haematologica. 94:264–8. PMID:19144661

343. Benton EC, Crichton S, Talpur R, et al. (2013). A cutaneous lymphoma international prognostic index (CLIPi) for mycosis fungoides and Sezary syndrome. Eur J Cancer. 49:2859–68. PMID:23735705

344. Bentz M, Barth TF, Brüderlein S, et al. (2001). Gain of chromosome arm 9p is characteristic of primary mediastinal B-cell lymphoma (MBL): comprehensive molecular cytogenetic analysis and presentation of a novel MBL cell line. Genes Chromosomes Cancer. 30:393–401. PMID:11241792

345. Beral V, Peterman T, Berkelman R, et al. (1991). AIDS-associated non-Hodgkin lymphoma. Lancet. 337:805–9. PMID:1672911

345A. Beran M, Luthra R, Kantarjian H, et al. (2004). FLT3 mutation and response to intensive chemotherapy in young adult and elderly patients with normal karyotype. Leuk Res. 28:547–50. PMID:15120929

346. Berger F, Felman P, Sonet A, et al. (1994). Nonfollicular small B-cell lymphomas: a heterogeneous group of patients with distinct clinical features and outcome. Blood. 83:2829–35. PMID:8180379

347. Berger F, Felman P, Thieblemont C, et al. (2000). Non-MALT marginal zone B-cell lymphomas: a description of clinical presentation and outcome in 124 patients. Blood. 95:1950–6. PMID:10706860

348. Berglund M, Thunberg U, Amini RM, et al. (2005). Evaluation of immunophenotype in diffuse large B-cell lymphoma and its impact on prognosis. Mod Pathol. 18:1113–20. PMID:15920553

349. Bergmann AK, Schneppenheim S, Seifert M, et al. (2014). Recurrent mutation of JAK3 in T-cell prolymphocytic leukemia. Genes Chromosomes Cancer. 53:309–16. PMID:24446122

350. Bergsagel PL, Kuehl WM (2001). Chromosome translocations in multiple myeloma. Oncogene. 20:5611–22. PMID:11607813

351. Bergsagel PL, Kuehl WM, Zhan F, et al. (2005). Cyclin D dysregulation: an early and unifying pathogenic event in multiple myeloma. Blood. 106:296–303. PMID:15755896

352. Berman EL, Zauber NP, Rickert RR, et al. (1998). Enteropathy-associated T cell lymphoma with brain involvement. J Clin Gastroenterol. 26:337–41. PMID:9649024

353. Bermudez G, González de Villambrosía S, Martínez-López A, et al. (2016). Incidental and Isolated Follicular Lymphoma In Situ and Mantle Cell Lymphoma In Situ Lack Clinical Significance. Am J Surg Pathol. PMID:26945339

354. Bernard A, Murphy SB, Melvin S, et al. (1982). Non-T, non-B lymphomas are rare in childhood and associated with cutaneous tumor. Blood. 59:549–54. PMID:6977384

355. Berndt SI, Skibola CF, Joseph V, et al. (2013). Genome-wide association study identifies multiple risk loci for chronic lymphocytic leukemia. Nat Genet. 45:868–76. PMID:23770605

356. Bernengo MG, Novelli M, Quaglino P, et al. (2001). The relevance of the CD4+ CD26- subset in the identification of circulating Sézary cells. Br J Dermatol. 144:125–35. PMID:11167693

357. Bernstein J, Dastugue N, Haas OA, et al. (2000). Nineteen cases of the t(1;22)(p13;q13) acute megakaryblastic leukaemia of infants/children and a review of 39 cases: report from a t(1;22) study group. Leukemia. 14:216–8. PMID:10637500

358. Berti E, Alessi E, Caputo R, et al. (1988). Reticulohistiocytoma of the dorsum. J Am Acad Dermatol. 19:259–72. PMID:3049688

359. Berti E, Cerri A, Cavicchini S, et al. (1991). Primary cutaneous gamma/delta T-cell lymphoma presenting as disseminated pagetoid reticulosis. J Invest Dermatol. 96:718–23. PMID:1827136

360. Berti E, Gianotti R, Alessi E (1988). Unusual cutaneous histiocytosis expressing an intermediate immunophenotype between Langerhans' cells and dermal macrophages. Arch Dermatol. 124:1250–3. PMID:3401031

361. Berti E, Tomasini D, Vermeer MH, et al. (1999). Primary cutaneous CD8-positive epidermotropic cytotoxic T cell lymphomas. A distinct clinicopathological entity with an aggressive clinical behavior. Am J Pathol. 155:483–92. PMID:10433941

362. Bertrand P, Bastard C, Maingonnat C, et al. (2007). Mapping of MYC breakpoints in 8q24 rearrangements involving non-immunoglobulin partners in B-cell lymphomas. Leukemia. 21:515–23. PMID:17230227

363. Besson C, Goubar A, Gabarre J, et al. (2001). Changes in AIDS-related lymphoma since the era of highly active antiretroviral therapy. Blood. 98:2339–44. PMID:11588028

364. Bethel KJ, Sharpe RW (2003). Pathology of hairy-cell leukaemia. Best Pract Res Clin Haematol. 16:15–31. PMID:12670462

364A. Beverloo HB, Panagopoulos I, Isaksson M, et al. (2001). Fusion of the homeobox gene HLXB9 and the ETV6 gene in infant acute myeloid leukemias with the t(7;12)(q36;p13). Cancer Res. 61:5374–7. PMID:11454678

365. Beylot-Barry M, Vergier B, Masquelier B, et al. (1999). The Spectrum of Cutaneous Lymphomas in HIV infection: a study of 21 cases. Am J Surg Pathol. 23:1208–16. PMID:10524521

366. Bhargava P, Rushin JM, Rusnock EJ, et al. (2007). Pulmonary light chain deposition disease: report of five cases and review of

the literature. Am J Surg Pathol. 31:267–76. PMID:17255772
366A. Bhavsar T, Lee JC, Perner Y, et al. (2017). KSHV-associated and EBV-associated Germinotropic Lymphoproliferative Disorder: New Findings and Review of the Literature. Am J Surg Pathol. 41:795-800.
367. Bhatia S (2013). Therapy-related myelodysplasia and acute myeloid leukemia. Semin Oncol. 40:666–75. PMID:24331189
368. Bhatt VR, Akhtari M, Bociek RG, et al. (2014). Allogeneic stem cell transplantation for Philadelphia chromosome-positive acute myeloid leukemia. J Natl Compr Canc Netw. 12:963–8. PMID:24994916
369. Bhatta S, Kut V, Petronic-Rosic V, et al. (2010). Therapy-related myeloid sarcoma with an NPM1 mutation. Leuk Lymphoma. 51:2130–1. PMID:20858094
370. Bianchi G, Anderson KC, Harris NL, et al. (2014). The heavy chain diseases: clinical and pathologic features. Oncology (Williston Park). 28:45–53. PMID:24683718
371. Bieliauskas S, Tubbs RR, Bacon CM, et al. (2012). Gamma heavy-chain disease: defining the spectrum of associated lymphoproliferative disorders through analysis of 13 cases. Am J Surg Pathol. 36:534–43. PMID:22301495
372. Bienz M, Ludwig M, Leibundgut EO, et al. (2005). Risk assessment in patients with acute myeloid leukemia and a normal karyotype. Clin Cancer Res. 11:1416–24. PMID:15746041
373. Biggar RJ, Chaturvedi AK, Goedert JJ, et al. (2007). AIDS-related cancer and severity of immunosuppression in persons with AIDS. J Natl Cancer Inst. 99:962–72. PMID:17565153
374. Biggar RJ, Jaffe ES, Goedert JJ, et al. (2006). Hodgkin lymphoma and immunodeficiency in persons with HIV/AIDS. Blood. 108:3786–91. PMID:16917006
375. Bigley V, Collin M (2011). Dendritic cell, monocyte, B and NK lymphoid deficiency defines the lost lineages of a new GATA-2 dependent myelodysplastic syndrome. Haematologica. 96:1081–3. PMID:21810969
376. Bigoni R, Cuneo A, Milani R, et al. (2001). Multilineage involvement in the 5q- syndrome: a fluorescent in situ hybridization study on bone marrow smears. Haematologica. 86:375–81. PMID:11325642
377. Bigouret V, Hoffmann T, Arlettaz L, et al. (2003). Monoclonal T-cell expansions in asymptomatic individuals and in patients with large granular leukemia consist of cytotoxic effector T cells expressing the activating CD94:NKG-2C/E and NKD2D killer cell receptors. Blood. 101:3198–204. PMID:12480700
378. Bikos V, Darzentas N, Hadzidimitriou A, et al. (2012). Over 30% of patients with splenic marginal zone lymphoma express the same immunoglobulin heavy variable gene: ontogenetic implications. Leukemia. 26:1638–46. PMID:22222599
379. Billecke L, Murga Penas EM, May AM, et al. (2013). Cytogenetics of extramedullary manifestations in multiple myeloma. Br J Haematol. 161:87–94. PMID:23368088
380. Bilsing A (1978). The effect of optical and acoustical stimuli on heart rate of guinea-pigs under various acoustical conditions. Act Nerv Super (Praha). 20:1–2. PMID:636748
381. Bindels EM, Havermans M, Lugthart S, et al. (2012). EVI1 is critical for the pathogenesis of a subset of MLL-AF9-rearranged AMLs. Blood. 119:5838–49. PMID:22553314
382. Binet JL, Auquier A, Dighiero G, et al. (1981). A new prognostic classification of chronic lymphocytic leukemia derived from a multivariate survival analysis. Cancer. 48:198–206. PMID:7237385
383. Binet JL, Caligaris-Cappio F, Catovsky D, et al. (2006). Perspectives on the use of new diagnostic tools in the treatment of chronic lymphocytic leukemia. Blood. 107:859–61. PMID:16223776
384. Bink K, Haralambieva E, Kremer M, et al. (2008). Primary extramedullary plasmacytoma: similarities with and differences from multiple myeloma revealed by interphase cytogenetics. Haematologica. 93:623–6. PMID:18326524
385. Birkeland SA, Hamilton-Dutoit S (2003). Is posttransplant lymphoproliferative disorder (PTLD) caused by any specific immunosuppressive drug or by the transplantation per se? Transplantation. 76:984–8. PMID:14508366
386. Bitter MA, Neilly ME, Le Beau MM, et al. (1985). Rearrangements of chromosome 3 involving bands 3q21 and 3q26 are associated with normal or elevated platelet counts in acute nonlymphocytic leukemia. Blood. 66:1362–70. PMID:4063525
387. Bizzozero OJ Jr, Johnson KG, Ciocco A (1966). Radiation-related leukemia in Hiroshima and Nagasaki, 1946-1964. I. Distribution, incidence and appearance time. N Engl J Med. 274:1095–101. PMID:5932020
388. Björkholm M, Derolf AR, Hultcrantz M, et al. (2011). Treatment-related risk factors for transformation to acute myeloid leukemia and myelodysplastic syndromes in myeloproliferative neoplasms. J Clin Oncol. 29:2410–5. PMID:21537037
389. Björkholm M, Hultcrantz M, Derolf ÅR (2014). Leukemic transformation in myeloproliferative neoplasms: therapy-related or unrelated? Best Pract Res Clin Haematol. 27:141–53. PMID:25189725
390. Bladé J, Kyle RA, Greipp PR (1996). Multiple myeloma in patients younger than 30 years. Report of 10 cases and review of the literature. Arch Intern Med. 156:1463–8. PMID:8678716
391. Blombery P, Kothari J, Yong K, et al. (2014). Plasma cell neoplasm associated chronic neutrophilic leukemia with membrane proximal and truncating CSF3R mutations. Leuk Lymphoma. 55:1661–2. PMID:24033109
391A. Blombery P, Thompson ER, Jones K, et al. (2016). Whole exome sequencing reveals activating JAK1 and STAT3 mutations in breast implant-associated anaplastic large cell lymphoma. Haematologica 101:e387–390. PMID:27198716
392. Bloomfield CD, Archer KJ, Mrózek K, et al. (2002). 11q23 balanced chromosome aberrations in treatment-related myelodysplastic syndromes and acute leukemia: report from an international workshop. Genes Chromosomes Cancer. 33:362–78. PMID:11921271
393. Bloomfield CD, Lawrence D, Byrd JC, et al. (1998). Frequency of prolonged remission duration after high-dose cytarabine intensification in acute myeloid leukemia varies by cytogenetic subtype. Cancer Res. 58:4173–9. PMID:9751631
394. Bob R, Falini B, Marafioti T, et al. (2013). Nodal reactive and neoplastic proliferation of monocytoid and marginal zone B cells: an immunoarchitectural and molecular study highlighting the relevance of IRTA1 and T-bet as positive markers. Histopathology. 63:482–98. PMID:23855758
395. Boccara O, Blanche S, de Prost Y, et al. (2012). Cutaneous hematologic disorders in children. Pediatr Blood Cancer. 58:226–32. PMID:21445946
396. Bochtler T, Hegenbart U, Cremer FW, et al. (2008). Evaluation of the cytogenetic aberration pattern in amyloid light chain amyloidosis as compared with monoclonal gammopathy of undetermined significance reveals common pathways of karyotypic instability. Blood. 111:4700–5. PMID:18305218
396A. Boddicker RL, Razidlo GL, Dasari S, et al. (2016). Integrated mate-pair and RNA sequencing identifies novel, targetable gene fusions in peripheral T-cell lymphoma. Blood. 128:1234–45. PMID:27297792
397. Boer JM, Koenders JE, van der Holt B, et al. (2015). Expression profiling of adult acute lymphoblastic leukemia identifies a BCR-ABL1-like subgroup characterized by high non-response and relapse rates. Haematologica. 100:e261–4. PMID:25769542
398. Boer JM, Marchante JR, Evans WE, et al. (2015). BCR-ABL1-like cases in pediatric acute lymphoblastic leukemia: a comparison between DCOG/Erasmus MC and COG/St. Jude signatures. Haematologica. 100:e354–7. PMID:26045294
399. Boerkamp KM, van Steenbeek FG, Penning LC, et al. (2014). The two main forms of histiocytic sarcoma in the predisposed Flatcoated retriever dog display variation in gene expression. PLoS One. 9:e98258. PMID:24886914
400. Bogusz AM, Seegmiller AC, Garcia R, et al. (2009). Plasmablastic lymphomas with MYC/IgH rearrangement: report of three cases and review of the literature. Am J Clin Pathol. 132:597–605. PMID:19762538
401. Bohn OL, Ruiz-Argüelles G, Navarro L, et al. (2007). Cutaneous Langerhans cell sarcoma: a case report and review of the literature. Int J Hematol. 85:116–20. PMID:17321988
402. Boi M, Rinaldi A, Kwee I, et al. (2013). PRDM1/BLIMP1 is commonly inactivated in anaplastic large T-cell lymphoma. Blood. 122:2683–93. PMID:24004669
403. Boi M, Zucca E, Inghirami G, et al. (2015). Advances in understanding the pathogenesis of systemic anaplastic large cell lymphomas. Br J Haematol. 168:771–83. PMID:25559471
404. Boiocchi L, Espinal-Witter R, Geyer JT, et al. (2013). Development of monocytosis in patients with primary myelofibrosis indicates an accelerated phase of the disease. Mod Pathol. 26:204–12. PMID:23018876
405. Boiocchi L, Gianelli U, Iurlo A, et al. (2015). Neutrophilic leukocytosis in advanced stage polycythemia vera: hematopathologic features and prognostic implications. Mod Pathol. 28:1448–57. PMID:26336886
406. Boiocchi L, Lonardi S, Vermi W, et al. (2013). BDCA-2 (CD303): a highly specific marker for normal and neoplastic plasmacytoid dendritic cells. Blood. 122:296–7. PMID:23847189
407. Boiocchi L, Mathew S, Gianelli U, et al. (2013). Morphologic and cytogenetic differences between post-polycythemic myelofibrosis and primary myelofibrosis in fibrotic stage. Mod Pathol. 26:1577–85. PMID:23787440
408. Boissel N, Auclerc MF, Lhéritier V, et al. (2003). Should adolescents with acute lymphoblastic leukemia be treated as old children or young adults? Comparison of the French FRALLE-93 and LALA-94 trials. J Clin Oncol. 21:774–80. PMID:12610173
408A. Boissel N, Leroy H, Brethon B, et al. (2006). Incidence and prognostic impact of c-Kit, FLT3, and Ras gene mutations in core binding factor acute myeloid leukemia (CBF-AML). Leukemia. 20:965–70. PMID:16598313
408B. Boissel N, Nibourel O, Renneville A, et al. (2010). Prognostic impact of isocitrate dehydrogenase enzyme isoforms 1 and 2 mutations in acute myeloid leukemia: a study by the Acute Leukemia French Association group. J Clin Oncol. 28:3717–23. PMID:20625116
408C. Boissel N, Renneville A, Biggio V, et al. (2005). Prevalence, clinical profile, and prognosis of NPM mutations in AML with normal karyotype. Blood. 106:3618–20. PMID:16046528
409. Boissinot M, Garand R, Hamidou M, et al. (2006). The JAK2-V617F mutation and essential thrombocythemia features in a subset of patients with refractory anemia with ring sideroblasts (RARS). Blood. 108:1781–2. PMID:16926301
410. Boll M, Parkins E, O'Connor SJ, et al. (2010). Extramedullary plasmacytoma are characterized by a 'myeloma-like' immunophenotype and genotype and occult bone marrow involvement. Br J Haematol. 151:525–7. PMID:20880115
411. Bonato M, Pittaluga S, Tierens A, et al. (1998). Lymph node histology in typical and atypical chronic lymphocytic leukemia. Am J Surg Pathol. 22:49–56. PMID:9422315
412. Bonetti F, Knowles DM 2nd, Chilosi M, et al. (1985). A distinctive cutaneous malignant neoplasm expressing the Langerhans cell phenotype. Synchronous occurrence with B-chronic lymphocytic leukemia. Cancer. 55:2417–25. PMID:3886125
413. Bonzheim I, Geissinger E, Roth S, et al. (2004). Anaplastic large cell lymphomas lack the expression of T-cell receptor molecules or molecules of proximal T-cell receptor signaling. Blood. 104:3358–60. PMID:15297316
414. Bonzheim I, Salaverria I, Haake A, et al. (2011). A unique case of follicular lymphoma provides insights to the clonal evolution from follicular lymphoma in situ to manifest follicular lymphoma. Blood. 118:3442–4. PMID:21940830
415. Booman M, Douwes J, Glas AM, et al. (2006). Mechanisms and effects of loss of human leukocyte antigen class II expression in immune-privileged site-associated B-cell lymphoma. Clin Cancer Res. 12:2698–705. PMID:16675561
416. Booman M, Douwes J, Legdeur MC, et al. (2007). From brain to testis: immune escape and clonal selection in a B cell lymphoma with selective outgrowth in two immune sanctuaries [correction of sanctuariesy]. [correction of sanctuariesy]. Haematologica. 92:e69–71. PMID:17650453
417. Borenstein J, Pezzella F, Gatter KC (2007). Plasmablastic lymphomas may occur as post-transplant lymphoproliferative disorders. Histopathology. 51:774–7. PMID:17944927
418. Boroumand N, Ly TL, Sonstein J, et al. (2012). Microscopic diffuse large B-cell lymphoma (DLBCL) occurring in pseudocysts: do these tumors belong to the category of DLBCL associated with chronic inflammation? Am J Surg Pathol. 36:1074–80. PMID:22472958
419. Borowitz MJ, Croker BP, Metzgar RS (1983). Lymphoblastic lymphoma with the phenotype of common acute lymphoblastic leukemia. Am J Clin Pathol. 79:387–91. PMID:6338702
420. Borowitz MJ, Hunger SP, Carroll AJ, et al. (1993). Predictability of the t(1;19)(q23;p13) from surface antigen phenotype: implications for screening cases of childhood acute lymphoblastic leukemia for molecular analysis: a Pediatric Oncology Group study. Blood. 82:1086–91. PMID:8353275
421. Borowitz MJ, Rubnitz J, Nash M, et al. (1998). Surface antigen phenotype can predict TEL-AML1 rearrangement in childhood B-precursor ALL: a Pediatric Oncology Group study. Leukemia. 12:1764–70. PMID:9823952
422. Bosch F, Campo E, Jares P, et al. (1995). Increased expression of the PRAD-1/CCND1 gene in hairy cell leukaemia. Br J Haematol. 91:1025–30. PMID:8547115
423. Bosch F, López-Guillermo A, Campo E, et al. (1998). Mantle cell lymphoma: presenting features, response to therapy, and prognostic factors. Cancer. 82:567–75. PMID:9452276
424. Bosga-Bouwer AG, van den Berg A, Haralambieva E, et al. (2006). Molecular, cytogenetic, and immunophenotypic characterization of follicular lymphoma grade 3B; a

separate entity or part of the spectrum of diffuse large B-cell lymphoma or follicular lymphoma? Hum Pathol. 37:528–33. PMID:16647949

425. Boshoff C, Weiss RA (2001). Epidemiology and pathogenesis of Kaposi's sarcoma-associated herpesvirus. Philos Trans R Soc Lond B Biol Sci. 356:517–34. PMID:11313009

426. Bosisio F, Boi S, Caputo V, et al. (2015). Lobular panniculitic infiltrates with overlapping histopathologic features of lupus panniculitis (lupus profundus) and subcutaneous T-cell lymphoma: a conceptual and practical dilemma. Am J Surg Pathol. 39:206–11. PMID:25118815

427. Bossard C, Dobay MP, Parrens M, et al. (2014). Immunohistochemistry as a valuable tool to assess CD30 expression in peripheral T-cell lymphomas: high correlation with mRNA levels. Blood. 124:2983–6. PMID:25224410

428. Bouabdallah R, Mounier N, Guettier C, et al. (2003). T-cell/histiocyte-rich large B-cell lymphomas and classical diffuse large B-cell lymphomas have similar outcome after chemotherapy: a matched-control analysis. J Clin Oncol. 21:1271–7. PMID:12663714

429. Bouchekioua A, Scourzic L, de Wever O, et al. (2014). JAK3 deregulation by activating mutations confers invasive growth advantage in extranodal nasal-type natural killer cell lymphoma. Leukemia. 28:338–48. PMID:23689514

429A. Boudová L, Torlakovic E, Delabie J, et al. (2003). Nodular lymphocyte-predominant Hodgkin lymphoma with nodules resembling T-cell/histiocyte-rich B-cell lymphoma: differential diagnosis between nodular lymphocyte-predominant Hodgkin lymphoma and T-cell/histiocyte-rich B-cell lymphoma. Blood. 102:3753–8. PMID:12881319

430. Boué F, Gabarre J, Gisselbrecht C, et al. (2006). Phase II trial of CHOP plus rituximab in patients with HIV-associated non-Hodgkin's lymphoma. J Clin Oncol. 24:4123–8. PMID:16896005

431. Boulanger E, Hermine O, Fermand JP, et al. (2004). Human herpesvirus 8 (HHV-8)-associated peritoneal primary effusion lymphoma (PEL) in two HIV-negative elderly patients. Am J Hematol. 76:88–91. PMID:15114607

432. Boulland ML, Wechsler J, Bagot M, et al. (2000). Primary CD30-positive cutaneous T-cell lymphomas and lymphomatoid papulosis frequently express cytotoxic proteins. Histopathology. 36:136–44. PMID:10672058

433. Boultwood J, Fidler C, Strickson AJ, et al. (2002). Narrowing and genomic annotation of the commonly deleted region of the 5q- syndrome. Blood. 99:4638–41. PMID:12036901

434. Boultwood J, Lewis S, Wainscoat JS (1994). The 5q-syndrome. Blood. 84:3253–60. PMID:7949083

435. Bourquin JP, Subramanian A, Langebrake C, et al. (2006). Identification of distinct molecular phenotypes in acute megakaryoblastic leukemia by gene expression profiling. Proc Natl Acad Sci U S A. 103:3339–44. PMID:16492768

436. Bousquet M, Quelen C, De Mas V, et al. (2005). The t(8;9)(p22;p24) translocation in atypical chronic myeloid leukaemia yields a new PCM1-JAK2 fusion gene. Oncogene. 24:7248–52. PMID:16091753

437. Boveri E, Arcaini L, Merli M, et al. (2009). Bone marrow histology in marginal zone B-cell lymphomas: correlation with clinical parameters and flow cytometry in 120 patients. Ann Oncol. 20:129–36. PMID:18718888

438. Boveri E, Passamonti F, Rumi E, et al. (2008). Bone marrow microvessel density in chronic myeloproliferative disorders: a study of 115 patients with clinicopathological and molecular correlations. Br J Haematol. 140:162–8. PMID:18028479

439. Bowen D, Culligan D, Jowitt S, et al. (2003). Guidelines for the diagnosis and therapy of adult myelodysplastic syndromes. Br J Haematol. 120:187–200. PMID:12542475

439A. Bowen D, Groves MJ, Burnett AK, et al. (2009). TP53 gene mutation is frequent in patients with acute myeloid leukemia and complex karyotype, and is associated with very poor prognosis. Leukemia. 23:203–6. PMID:18596741

440. Bower M, Pria AD, Coyle C, et al. (2014). Diagnostic criteria schemes for multicentric Castleman disease in 75 cases. J Acquir Immune Defic Syndr. 65:e80–2. PMID:24442228

440A. Boyer DF, McKelvie PA, de Leval L, et al. (2017). Fibrin-associated EBV-positive large B-cell lymphoma: An indolent neoplasm with features distinct from diffuse large B-cell lymphoma associated with chronic inflammation. Am J Surg Pathol. 41:299-312. PMID:28195879

441. Boztug H, Schumich A, Pötschger U, et al. (2013). Blast cell deficiency of CD11a as a marker of acute megakaryoblastic leukemia and transient myeloproliferative disease in children with and without Down syndrome. Cytometry B Clin Cytom. 84:370–8. PMID:23450818

442. Bracci PM, Benavente Y, Turner JJ, et al. (2014). Medical history, lifestyle, family history, and occupational risk factors for marginal zone lymphoma: the InterLymph Non-Hodgkin Lymphoma Subtypes Project. J Natl Cancer Inst Monogr. 2014:52–65. PMID:25174026

443. Braggio E, Dogan A, Keats JJ, et al. (2012). Genomic analysis of marginal zone and lymphoplasmacytic lymphomas identified common and disease-specific abnormalities. Mod Pathol. 25:651–60. PMID:22301699

444. Braggio E, Fonseca R (2013). Genomic abnormalities of Waldenström macroglobulinemia and related low-grade B-cell lymphomas. Clin Lymphoma Myeloma Leuk. 13:198–201. PMID:23477936

445. Brar P, Lee S, Lewis S, et al. (2007). Budesonide in the treatment of refractory celiac disease. Am J Gastroenterol. 102:2265–9. PMID:17581265

446. Braun T, de Botton S, Taksin AL, et al. (2011). Characteristics and outcome of myelodysplastic syndromes (MDS) with isolated 20q deletion: a report on 62 cases. Leuk Res. 35:863–7. PMID:21396711

447. Breccia M, Biondo F, Latagliata R, et al. (2006). Identification of risk factors in atypical chronic myeloid leukemia. Haematologica. 91:1566–8. PMID:17043019

448. Breccia M, Carmosino I, Biondo F, et al. (2006). Usefulness and prognostic impact on survival of WHO reclassification in FAB low risk myelodysplastic syndromes. Leuk Res. 30:178–82. PMID:16102825

449. Breccia M, Finsinger P, Loglisci G, et al. (2012). Prognostic features of patients with myelodysplastic syndromes aged < 50 years: update of a single-institution experience. Leuk Lymphoma. 53:2439–43. PMID:22647078

450. Breccia M, Latagliata R, Cannella L, et al. (2010). Refractory cytopenia with unilineage dysplasia: analysis of prognostic factors and survival in 126 patients. Leuk Lymphoma. 51:783–8. PMID:20302387

451. Breccia M, Loglisci G, Loglisci MG, et al. (2013). FLT3-ITD confers poor prognosis in patients with acute promyelocytic leukemia treated with AIDA protocols: long-term follow-up analysis. Haematologica. 98:e161–3. PMID:24323990

452. Breccia M, Mandelli F, Petti MC, et al. (2004). Clinico-pathological characteristics of myeloid sarcoma at diagnosis and during follow-up: report of 12 cases from a single institution. Leuk Res. 28:1165–9. PMID:15380340

453. Brecher M, Banks PM (1990). Hodgkin's disease variant of Richter's syndrome. Report of eight cases. Am J Clin Pathol. 93:333–9. PMID:1689938

454. Breen KA, Grimwade D, Hunt BJ (2012). The pathogenesis and management of the coagulopathy of acute promyelocytic leukaemia. Br J Haematol. 156:24–36. PMID:22050876

455. Brenner I, Roth S, Puppe B, et al. (2013). Primary cutaneous marginal zone lymphomas with plasmacytic differentiation show frequent IgG4 expression. Mod Pathol. 26:1568–76. PMID:23765244

456. Brink DS (2006). Transient leukemia (transient myeloproliferative disorder, transient abnormal myelopoiesis) of Down syndrome. Adv Anat Pathol. 13:256–62. PMID:16998319

457. Brito-Babapulle V, Catovsky D (1991). Inversions and tandem translocations involving chromosome 14q11 and 14q32 in T-prolymphocytic leukemia and T-cell leukemias in patients with ataxia telangiectasia. Cancer Genet Cytogenet. 55:1–9. PMID:1913594

458. Brito-Babapulle V, Hamoudi R, Matutes E, et al. (2000). p53 allele deletion and protein accumulation occurs in the absence of p53 gene mutation in T-prolymphocytic leukemia and Sezary syndrome. Br J Haematol. 110:180–7. PMID:10930996

459. Brito-Babapulle V, Pittman S, Melo JV, et al. (1987). Cytogenetic studies on prolymphocytic leukemia. 1. B-cell prolymphocytic leukemia. Hematol Pathol. 1:27–33. PMID:3509770

460. Brizard A, Huret JL, Lamotte F, et al. (1989). Three cases of myelodysplastic-myeloproliferative disorder with abnormal chromatin clumping in granulocytes. Br J Haematol. 72:294–5. PMID:2757974

461. Brody GS, Deapen D, Taylor CR, et al. (2015). Anaplastic large cell lymphoma occurring in women with breast implants: analysis of 173 cases. Plast Reconstr Surg. 135:695–705. PMID:25490535

462. Broséus J, Alpermann T, Wulfert M, et al. (2013). Age, JAK2(V617F) and SF3B1 mutations are the main predicting factors for survival in refractory anaemia with ring sideroblasts and marked thrombocytosis. Leukemia. 27:1826–31. PMID:23594705

463. Broseus J, Florensa L, Zipperer E, et al. (2012). Clinical features and course of refractory anemia with ring sideroblasts associated with marked thrombocytosis. Haematologica. 97:1036–41. PMID:22532522

464. Brouet JC, Sasportes M, Flandrin G, et al. (1975). Chronic lymphocytic leukaemia of T-cell origin. Immunological and clinical evaluation in eleven patients. Lancet. 2:890–3. PMID:53372

465. Brousset P, Rochaix P, Chittal S, et al. (1993). High incidence of Epstein-Barr virus detection in Hodgkin's disease and absence of detection in anaplastic large-cell lymphoma in children. Histopathology. 23:189–91. PMID:8406393

466. Brousset P, Schlaifer D, Meggetto F, et al. (1994). Persistence of the same viral strain in early and late relapses of Epstein-Barr virus-associated Hodgkin's disease. Blood. 84:2447–51. PMID:7919364

467. Brown L, Cheng JT, Chen Q, et al. (1990). Site-specific recombination of the tal-1 gene is a common occurrence in human T cell leukemia. EMBO J. 9:3343–51. PMID:2209547

468. Brown LM, Linet MS, Greenberg RS, et al. (1999). Multiple myeloma and family history of cancer among blacks and whites in the U.S. Cancer. 85:2385–90. PMID:10357409

469. Brown NA, Furtado LV, Betz BL, et al. (2014). High prevalence of somatic MAP2K1 mutations in BRAF V600E-negative

Langerhans cell histiocytosis. Blood. 124:1655–8. PMID:24982505

470. Brown P, McIntyre E, Rau R, et al. (2007). The incidence and clinical significance of nucleophosmin mutations in childhood AML. Blood. 110:979–85. PMID:17440048

471. Brown SL, Greene MH, Gershon SK, et al. (2002). Tumor necrosis factor antagonist therapy and lymphoma development: twenty-six cases reported to the Food and Drug Administration. Arthritis Rheum. 46:3151–8. PMID:12483718

472. Browne P, Petrosyan K, Hernandez A, et al. (2003). The B-cell transcription factors BSAP, Oct-2, and BOB.1 and the pan-B-cell markers CD20, CD22, and CD79a are useful in the differential diagnosis of classic Hodgkin lymphoma. Am J Clin Pathol. 120:767–77. PMID:14608905

473. Broyl A, Hose D, Lokhorst H, et al. (2010). Gene expression profiling for molecular classification of multiple myeloma in newly diagnosed patients. Blood. 116:2543–53. PMID:20574050

474. Brudno J, Tadmor T, Pittaluga S, et al. (2016). Discordant bone marrow involvement in non-Hodgkin lymphoma. Blood. 127:965–70. PMID:26679865

475. Brugières L, Deley MC, Pacquement H, et al. (1998). CD30(+) anaplastic large-cell lymphoma in children: analysis of 82 patients enrolled in two consecutive studies of the French Society of Pediatric Oncology. Blood. 92:3591–8. PMID:9808552

476. Brugnoni D, Airó P, Rossi G, et al. (1996). A case of hypereosinophilic syndrome is associated with the expansion of a CD3-CD4+ T-cell population able to secrete large amounts of interleukin-5. Blood. 87:1416–22. PMID:8608231

477. Brune V, Tiacci E, Pfeil I, et al. (2008). Origin and pathogenesis of nodular lymphocyte-predominant Hodgkin lymphoma as revealed by global gene expression analysis. J Exp Med. 205:2251–68. PMID:18794340

478. Brunn A, Nagel I, Montesinos-Rongen M, et al. (2013). Frequent triple-hit expression of MYC, BCL2, and BCL6 in primary lymphoma of the central nervous system and absence of a favorable MYC(low)BCL2 (low) subgroup may underlie the inferior prognosis as compared to systemic diffuse large B cell lymphomas. Acta Neuropathol. 126:603–5. PMID:24061549

479. Brunner P, Rufle A, Dirnhofer S, et al. (2014). Follicular lymphoma transformation into histiocytic sarcoma: indications for a common neoplastic progenitor. Leukemia. 28:1937–40. PMID:24850291

480. Brunning RD, McKenna RW (1994). Plasma cell dyscrasias and related disorders. In: AFIP atlas of tumor pathology, 3rd series. Washington (DC): ARP Press; pp. 323–67.

481. Brunning RD, McKenna RW (1994). Tumors of the bone marrow. In: AFIP atlas of tumor pathology, 3rd series. Washington (DC): ARP Press.

482. Bruno A, Boisselier B, Labreche K, et al. (2014). Mutational analysis of primary central nervous system lymphoma. Oncotarget. 5:5065–75. PMID:24970810

483. Bryce AH, Ketterling RP, Gertz MA, et al. (2008). A novel report of cig-FISH and cytogenetics in POEMS syndrome. Am J Hematol. 83:840–1. PMID:18839437

484. Bryce AH, Ketterling RP, Gertz MA, et al. (2009). Translocation t(11;14) and survival of patients with light chain (AL) amyloidosis. Haematologica. 94:380–6. PMID:19211640

485. Brück W, Brunn A, Klapper W, et al. (2013). [Differential diagnosis of lymphoid infiltrates in the central nervous system: experience of the Network Lymphomas and Lymphomatoid Lesions in the Nervous System]. Pathologe.

34:186–97. PMID:23471726
486. Bräuninger A, Hansmann ML, Strickler JG, et al. (1999). Identification of common germinal-center B-cell precursors in two patients with both Hodgkin's disease and non-Hodgkin's lymphoma. N Engl J Med. 340:1239–47. PMID:10210707
487. Bräuninger A, Küppers R, Spieker T, et al. (1999). Molecular analysis of single B cells from T-cell-rich B-cell lymphoma shows the derivation of the tumor cells from mutating germinal center B cells and exemplifies means by which immunoglobulin genes are modified in germinal center B cells. Blood. 93:2679–87. PMID:10194448
488. Bräuninger A, Wacker HH, Rajewsky K, et al. (2003). Typing the histogenetic origin of the tumor cells of lymphocyte-rich classical Hodgkin's lymphoma in relation to tumor cells of classical and lymphocyte-predominance Hodgkin's lymphoma. Cancer Res. 63:1644–51. PMID:12670918
489. Bubolz AM, Weissinger SE, Stenzinger A, et al. (2014). Potential clinical implications of BRAF mutations in histiocytic proliferations. Oncotarget. 5:4060–70. PMID:24938183
490. Buesche G, Hehlmann R, Hecker H, et al. (2003). Marrow fibrosis, indicator of therapy failure in chronic myeloid leukemia - prospective long-term results from a randomized-controlled trial. Leukemia. 17:2444–53. PMID:14562117
491. Buesche G, Teoman H, Wilczak W, et al. (2008). Marrow fibrosis predicts early fatal marrow failure in patients with myelodysplastic syndromes. Leukemia. 22:313–22. PMID:18033321
492. Buettner M, Greiner A, Avramidou A, et al. (2005). Evidence of abortive plasma cell differentiation in Hodgkin and Reed-Sternberg cells of classical Hodgkin lymphoma. Hematol Oncol. 23:127–32. PMID:16342298
493. Bug S, Dürig J, Oyen F, et al. (2009). Recurrent loss, but lack of mutations, of the SMARCB1 tumor suppressor gene in T-cell prolymphocytic leukemia with TCL1A-TCRAD juxtaposition. Cancer Genet Cytogenet. 192:44–7. PMID:19480937
494. Buhr T, Büsche G, Choritz H, et al. (2003). Evolution of myelofibrosis in chronic idiopathic myelofibrosis as evidenced in sequential bone marrow biopsy specimens. Am J Clin Pathol. 119:152–8. PMID:12520711
495. Buhr T, Choritz H, Georgii A (1992). The impact of megakaryocyte proliferation of the evolution of myelofibrosis. Histological follow-up study in 186 patients with chronic myeloid leukaemia. Virchows Arch A Pathol Anat Histopathol. 420:473–8. PMID:1609507
496. Buhr T, Georgii A, Choritz H (1993). Myelofibrosis in chronic myeloproliferative disorders. Incidence among subtypes according to the Hannover Classification. Pathol Res Pract. 189:121–32. PMID:8321741
497. Bunda S, Qin K, Kommaraju K, et al. (2015). Juvenile myelomonocytic leukaemia-associated mutation in Cbl promotes resistance to apoptosis via the Lyn-PI3K/AKT pathway. Oncogene. 34:789–97. PMID:24469048
498. Bunn B, van Heerden W (2015). EBV-positive mucocutaneous ulcer of the oral cavity associated with HIV/AIDS. Oral Surg Oral Med Oral Pathol Oral Radiol. 120:725–32. PMID:26254983
499. Bunn PA Jr, Schechter GP, Jaffe E, et al. (1983). Clinical course of retrovirus-associated adult T-cell lymphoma in the United States. N Engl J Med. 309:257–64. PMID:6602943
500. Burg G, Kempf W, Kazakov DV, et al. (2003). Pyogenic lymphoma of the skin: a peculiar variant of primary cutaneous neutrophil-rich CD30+ anaplastic large-cell lymphoma. Clinicopathological study of four cases and review of the literature. Br J Dermatol. 148:580–6. PMID:12653754
501. Burke AP, Andriko JA, Virmani R (2000). Anaplastic large cell lymphoma (CD 30+), T-phenotype, in the heart of an HIV-positive man. Cardiovasc Pathol. 9:49–52. PMID:10739907
502. Burke JS (1999). Are there site-specific differences among the MALT lymphomas–morphologic, clinical? Am J Clin Pathol. 111:S133–43. PMID:9894478
503. Burkitt D (1958). A sarcoma involving the jaws in African children. Br J Surg. 46:218–23. PMID:13628987
504. Burmester GR, Panaccione R, Gordon KB, et al. (2013). Adalimumab: long-term safety in 23 458 patients from global clinical trials in rheumatoid arthritis, juvenile idiopathic arthritis, ankylosing spondylitis, psoriatic arthritis, psoriasis and Crohn's disease. Ann Rheum Dis. 72:517–24. PMID:22562972
505. Burnett AK, Russell NH, Hills RK, et al. (2015). Arsenic trioxide and all-trans retinoic acid treatment for acute promyelocytic leukaemia in all risk groups (AML17): results of a randomised, controlled, phase 3 trial. Lancet Oncol. 16:1295–305. PMID:26384238
506. Busfield SJ, Biondo M, Wong M, et al. (2014). Targeting of acute myeloid leukemia in vitro and in vivo with an anti-CD123 mAb engineered for optimal ADCC. Leukemia. 28:2213–21. PMID:24705479
507. Busque L, Gilliland DG, Prchal JT, et al. (1995). Clonality in juvenile chronic myelogenous leukemia. Blood. 85:21–30. PMID:7803795
508. Butcher EC (1990). Warner-Lambert/Parke-Davis Award lecture. Cellular and molecular mechanisms that direct leukocyte traffic. Am J Pathol. 136:3–11. PMID:2404417
509. Buxbaum J (1992). Mechanisms of disease: monoclonal immunoglobulin deposition. Amyloidosis, light chain deposition disease, and light and heavy chain deposition disease. Hematol Oncol Clin North Am. 6:323–46. PMID:1582976
510. Buxbaum J, Gallo G (1999). Nonamyloidotic monoclonal immunoglobulin deposition disease. Light-chain, heavy-chain, and light- and heavy-chain deposition diseases. Hematol Oncol Clin North Am. 13:1235–48. PMID:10626147
511. Byrd JC, Mrózek K, Dodge RK, et al. (2002). Pretreatment cytogenetic abnormalities are predictive of induction success, cumulative incidence of relapse, and overall survival in adult patients with de novo acute myeloid leukemia: results from Cancer and Leukemia Group B (CALGB 8461). Blood. 100:4325–36. PMID:12393746
512. Byun YJ, Park BB, Lee ES, et al. (2014). A case of chronic myeloid leukemia with features of essential thrombocythemia in peripheral blood and bone marrow. Blood Res. 49:127–9. PMID:25025015
513. Bödör C, Grossmann V, Popov N, et al. (2013). EZH2 mutations are frequent and represent an early event in follicular lymphoma. Blood. 122:3165–8. PMID:24052547
514. Bödör C, Renneville A, Smith M, et al. (2012). Germ-line GATA2 p.THR354MET mutation in familial myelodysplastic syndrome with acquired monosomy 7 and ASXL1 mutation demonstrating rapid onset and poor survival. Haematologica. 97:890–4. PMID:22271902
515. Böhm J, Schaefer HE (2002). Chronic neutrophilic leukaemia: 14 new cases of an uncommon myeloproliferative disease. J Clin Pathol. 55:862–4. PMID:12401827
516. Bönig H, Göbel U, Nürnberger W (2002). Bilateral exopthalmus due to retro-orbital chloromas in a boy with t(8;21)-positive acute myeloblastic acute leukemia. Pediatr Hematol Oncol. 19:597–600. PMID:12487837
517. Cabagnols X, Favale F, Pasquier F, et al. (2016). Presence of atypical thrombopoietin receptor (MPL) mutations in triple-negative essential thrombocythemia patients. Blood. 127:333–42. PMID:26450985
518. Cabrera ME, Eizuru Y, Itoh T, et al. (2007). Nasal natural killer/T-cell lymphoma and its association with type "i"/XhoI loss strain Epstein-Barr virus in Chile. J Clin Pathol. 60:656–60. PMID:16775124
519. Cady FM, O'Neill BP, Law ME, et al. (2008). Del(6)(q22) and BCL6 rearrangements in primary CNS lymphoma are indicators of an aggressive clinical course. J Clin Oncol. 26:4814–9. PMID:18645192
520. Cai W, He X, Chen S, et al. (2015). [Clinical and laboratory characteristics of 12 Ph/BCR-ABL positive acute myeloid leukemia patients]. Zhonghua Xue Ye Xue Za Zhi. 36:398–402. PMID:26031527
521. Caillard S, Dharnidharka V, Agodoa L, et al. (2005). Posttransplant lymphoproliferative disorders after renal transplantation in the United States in era of modern immunosuppression. Transplantation. 80:1233–43. PMID:16314791
522. Caillard S, Lelong C, Pessione F, et al. (2006). Post-transplant lymphoproliferative disorders occurring after renal transplantation in adults: report of 230 cases from the French Registry. Am J Transplant. 6:2735–42. PMID:17049061
523. Cairns RA, Iqbal J, Lemonnier F, et al. (2012). IDH2 mutations are frequent in angioimmunoblastic T-cell lymphoma. Blood. 119:1901–3. PMID:22215888
523A. Cairoli R, Beghini A, Grillo G, et al. (2006). Prognostic impact of c-KIT mutations in core binding factor leukemias: an Italian retrospective study. Blood. 107:3463–8. PMID:16384925
524. Calaminici M, Piper K, Lee AM, et al. (2004). CD23 expression in mediastinal large B-cell lymphomas. Histopathology. 45:619–24. PMID:15569053
525. Calderón-Cabrera C, Montero I, Morales RM, et al. (2013). Differential cytogenetic profile in advanced chronic myeloid leukemia with sequential lymphoblastic and myeloblastic blast crisis. Leuk Res Rep. 2:79–81. PMID:24371788
526. Caldwell GG, Kelley DB, Heath CW Jr, et al. (1984). Polycythemia vera among participants of a nuclear weapons test. JAMA. 252:662–4. PMID:6737671
526A. Caligiuri MA, Strout MP, Lawrence D, et al. (1998). Rearrangement of ALL1 (MLL) in acute myeloid leukemia with normal cytogenetics. Cancer Res. 58:55–9. PMID:9426057
527. Callan MF (2004). Epstein-Barr virus, arthritis, and the development of lymphoma in arthritis patients. Curr Opin Rheumatol. 16:399–405. PMID:15201603
528. Callen JP (2007). Complications and adverse reactions in the use of newer biologic agents. Semin Cutan Med Surg. 26:6–14. PMID:17349557
529. Callens C, Chevret S, Cayuela JM, et al. (2005). Prognostic implication of FLT3 and Ras gene mutations in patients with acute promyelocytic leukemia (APL): a retrospective study from the European APL Group. Leukemia. 19:1153–60. PMID:15889156
530. Calvo KR, Price S, Braylan RC, et al. (2015). JMML and RALD (Ras-associated autoimmune leukoproliferative disorder): common genetic etiology yet clinically distinct entities. Blood. 125:2753–8. PMID:25691160
531. Calvo KR, Vinh DC, Maric I, et al. (2011). Myelodysplasia in autosomal dominant and sporadic monocytopenia immunodeficiency syndrome: diagnostic features and clinical implications. Haematologica. 96:1221–5. PMID:21508125
532. Camacho E, Hernández L, Hernández S, et al. (2002). ATM gene inactivation in mantle cell lymphoma mainly occurs by truncating mutations and missense mutations involving the phosphatidylinositol-3 kinase domain and is associated with increasing numbers of chromosomal imbalances. Blood. 99:238–44. PMID:11756177
533. Camacho FI, Algara P, Mollejo M, et al. (2003). Nodal marginal zone lymphoma: a heterogeneous tumor: a comprehensive analysis of a series of 27 cases. Am J Surg Pathol. 27:762–71. PMID:12766579
534. Camacho FI, Algara P, Rodríguez A, et al. (2003). Molecular heterogeneity in MCL defined by the use of specific VH genes and the frequency of somatic mutations. Blood. 101:4042–6. PMID:12511405
535. Camacho FI, García JF, Cigudosa JC, et al. (2004). Aberrant Bcl6 protein expression in mantle cell lymphoma. Am J Surg Pathol. 28:1051–6. PMID:15252312
536. Camilleri-Broët S, Davi F, Feuillard J, et al. (1997). AIDS-related primary brain lymphomas: histopathologic and immunohistochemical study of 51 cases. Hum Pathol. 28:367–74. PMID:9042803
537. Campana D, Coustan-Smith E (2004). Minimal residual disease studies by flow cytometry in acute leukemia. Acta Haematol. 112:8–15. PMID:15178999
538. Campbell J, Seymour JF, Matthews J, et al. (2006). The prognostic impact of bone marrow involvement in patients with diffuse large cell lymphoma varies according to the degree of infiltration and presence of discordant marrow involvement. Eur J Haematol. 76:473–80. PMID:16529599
539. Campbell JJ, Clark RA, Watanabe R, et al. (2010). Sezary syndrome and mycosis fungoides arise from distinct T-cell subsets: a biologic rationale for their distinct clinical behaviors. Blood. 116:767–71. PMID:20484084
540. Campbell PJ, Scott LM, Buck G, et al. (2005). Definition of subtypes of essential thrombocythaemia and relation to polycythaemia vera based on JAK2 V617F mutation status: a prospective study. Lancet. 366:1945–53. PMID:16325696
540A. Campo E (2012). New pathogenic mechanisms in Burkitt lymphoma. Nat Genet. 44:1288-9. PMID:23192177
541. Campo E (2015). MYC in DLBCL: partners matter. Blood. 126:2439–40. PMID:26612895
542. Campo E, Miquel R, Krenacs L, et al. (1999). Primary nodal marginal zone lymphomas of splenic and MALT type. Am J Surg Pathol. 23:59–68. PMID:9888704
543. Campo E, Raffeld M, Jaffe ES (1999). Mantle-cell lymphoma. Semin Hematol. 36:115–27. PMID:10319380
544. Campo E, Rule S (2015). Mantle cell lymphoma: evolving management strategies. Blood. 125:48–55. PMID:25499451
544A. Campochiaro C, Tomelleri A, Cavalli G, et al. (2015). Erdheim-Chester disease. Eur J Intern Med. 26:223–9. PMID:25865950
545. Cancer Genome Atlas Research Network (2013). Genomic and epigenomic landscapes of adult de novo acute myeloid leukemia. N Engl J Med. 368:2059–74. PMID:23634996
546. Canioni D, Arnulf B, Asso-Bonnet M, et al. (2001). Nasal natural killer lymphoma associated with Epstein-Barr virus in a patient infected with human immunodeficiency virus. Arch Pathol Lab Med. 125:660–2. PMID:11300939
547. Canioni D, Jabado N, MacIntyre E, et al. (2001). Lymphoproliferative disorders in children with primary immunodeficiencies:

immunological status may be more predictive of the outcome than other criteria. Histopathology. 38:146–59. PMID:11207828
548. Cao Y, Hunter ZR, Liu X, et al. (2015). The WHIM-like CXCR4(S338X) somatic mutation activates AKT and ERK, and promotes resistance to ibrutinib and other agents used in the treatment of Waldenstrom's Macroglobulinemia. Leukemia. 29:169–76. PMID:24912431
549. Cao Y, Hunter ZR, Liu X, et al. (2015). CXCR4 WHIM-like frameshift and nonsense mutations promote ibrutinib resistance but do not supplant MYD88(L265P) -directed survival signalling in Waldenström macroglobulinaemia cells. Br J Haematol. 168:701–7. PMID:25371371
550. Capello D, Rossi D, Gaidano G (2005). Post-transplant lymphoproliferative disorders: molecular basis of disease histogenesis and pathogenesis. Hematol Oncol. 23:61–7. PMID:16216037
551. Caponetti GC, Dave BJ, Perry AM, et al. (2015). Isolated MYC cytogenetic abnormalities in diffuse large B-cell lymphoma do not predict an adverse clinical outcome. Leuk Lymphoma. 56:3082–9. PMID:25827211
552. Caprini E, Cristofoletti C, Arcelli D, et al. (2009). Identification of key regions and genes important in the pathogenesis of sezary syndrome by combining genomic and expression microarrays. Cancer Res. 69:8438–46. PMID:19843862
553. Carbone A (1997). The Spectrum of AIDS-Related Lymphoproliferative Disorders. Adv Clin Path. 1:13–9. PMID:10352465
554. Carbone A (2002). AIDS-related non-Hodgkin's lymphomas: from pathology and molecular pathogenesis to treatment. Hum Pathol. 33:392–404. PMID:12055673
555. Carbone A (2003). Emerging pathways in the development of AIDS-related lymphomas. Lancet Oncol. 4:22–9. PMID:12517536
556. Carbone A, De Paoli P, Gloghini A, et al. (2015). KSHV-associated multicentric Castleman disease: A tangle of different entities requiring multitarget treatment strategies. Int J Cancer. 137:251–61. PMID:24771491
557. Carbone A, Gloghini A (2005). AIDS-related lymphomas: from pathogenesis to pathology. Br J Haematol. 130:662–70. PMID:16115121
558. Carbone A, Gloghini A, Vaccher E, et al. (2005). KSHV/HHV-8 associated lymph node based lymphomas in HIV seronegative subjects. Report of two cases with anaplastic large cell morphology and plasmablastic immunophenotype. J Clin Pathol. 58:1039–45. PMID:16189148
559. Carbone PP, Kaplan HS, Musshoff K, et al. (1971). Report of the Committee on Hodgkin's Disease Staging Classification. Cancer Res. 31:1860–1. PMID:5121694
560. Carbonell F, Swansbury J, Min T, et al. (1996). Cytogenetic findings in acute biphenotypic leukaemia. Leukemia. 10:1283–7. PMID:8709632
561. Carbonnel F, d'Almagne H, Lavergne A, et al. (1999). The clinicopathological features of extensive small intestinal CD4 T cell infiltration. Gut. 45:662–7. PMID:10517900
562. Carbonnel F, Grollet-Bioul L, Brouet JC, et al. (1998). Are complicated forms of celiac disease cryptic T-cell lymphomas? Blood. 92:3879–86. PMID:9808581
563. Carbonnel F, Lavergne A, Messing B, et al. (1994). Extensive small intestinal T-cell lymphoma of low-grade malignancy associated with a new chromosomal translocation. Cancer. 73:1286–91. PMID:8313332
564. Carde P, Hagenbeek A, Hayat M, et al. (1993). Clinical staging versus laparotomy and combined modality with MOPP versus ABVD in early-stage Hodgkin's disease: the H6 twin randomized trials from the European Organization for Research and Treatment of Cancer Lymphoma Cooperative Group. J Clin Oncol. 11:2258–72. PMID:7693881
564A. Care RS, Valk PJ, Goodeve AC, et al. (2003). Incidence and prognosis of c-KIT and FLT3 mutations in core binding factor (CBF) acute myeloid leukaemias. Br J Haematol. 121:775–7. PMID:12780793
565. Carney JP, Maser RS, Olivares H, et al. (1998). The hMre11/hRad50 protein complex and Nijmegen breakage syndrome: linkage of double-strand break repair to the cellular DNA damage response. Cell. 93:477–86. PMID:9590181
566. Carobbio A, Thiele J, Passamonti F, et al. (2011). Risk factors for arterial and venous thrombosis in WHO-defined essential thrombocythemia: an international study of 891 patients. Blood. 117:5857–9. PMID:21490340
567. Carroll A, Civin C, Schneider N, et al. (1991). The t(1;22) (p13;q13) is nonrandom and restricted to infants with acute megakaryoblastic leukemia: a Pediatric Oncology Group Study. Blood. 78:748–52. PMID:1859887
568. Carson KR, Bartlett NL, McDonald JR, et al. (2012). Increased body mass index is associated with improved survival in United States veterans with diffuse large B-cell lymphoma. J Clin Oncol. 30:3217–22. PMID:22649138
569. Carter MC, Clayton ST, Komarow HD, et al. (2015). Assessment of clinical findings, tryptase levels, and bone marrow histopathology in the management of pediatric mastocytosis. J Allergy Clin Immunol. 136:1673–79.e1–3. PMID:26044856
570. Carter MC, Metcalfe DD, Komarow HD (2014). Mastocytosis. Immunol Allergy Clin North Am. 34:181–96. PMID:24262698
571. Carvajal-Cuenca A, Sua LF, Silva NM, et al. (2012). In situ mantle cell lymphoma: clinical implications of an incidental finding with indolent clinical behavior. Haematologica. 97:270–8. PMID:22058203
572. Cassidy JF, Clinton C, Breen W, et al. (1993). Novel electrochemical device for the detection of cholesterol or glucose. Analyst. 118:415–8. PMID:8388178
573. Castagnetti F, Gugliotta G, Breccia M, et al. (2015). Long-term outcome of chronic myeloid leukemia patients treated frontline with imatinib. Leukemia. 29:1823–31. PMID:26088952
574. Castaigne S, Chomienne C, Daniel MT, et al. (1990). All-trans retinoic acid as a differentiation therapy for acute promyelocytic leukemia. I. Clinical results. Blood. 76:1704–9. PMID:2224119
575. Castellano-Sanchez AA, Li S, Qian J, et al. (2004). Primary central nervous system post-transplant lymphoproliferative disorders. Am J Clin Pathol. 121:246–53. PMID:14983939
576. Castells M, Metcalfe DD, Escribano L (2011). Diagnosis and treatment of cutaneous mastocytosis in children: practical recommendations. Am J Clin Dermatol. 12:259–70. PMID:21668033
577. Castillo J, Pantanowitz L, Dezube BJ (2008). HIV-associated plasmablastic lymphoma: lessons learned from 112 published cases. Am J Hematol. 83:804–9. PMID:18756521
578. Castillo JJ, Bibas M, Miranda RN (2015). The biology and treatment of plasmablastic lymphoma. Blood. 125:2323–30. PMID:25636338
579. Castillo JJ, Olszewski AJ, Kanan S, et al. (2015). Overall survival and competing risks of death in patients with Waldenström macroglobulinaemia: an analysis of the Surveillance, Epidemiology and End Results database. Br J Haematol. 169:81–9. PMID:25521528
580. Castor A, Nilsson L, Astrand-Grundström I, et al. (2005). Distinct patterns of hematopoietic stem cell involvement in acute lymphoblastic leukemia. Nat Med. 11:630–7. PMID:15908956
581. Castro-Malaspina H, Schaison G, Passe S, et al. (1984). Subacute and chronic myelomonocytic leukemia in children (juvenile CML). Clinical and hematologic observations, and identification of prognostic factors. Cancer. 54:675–86. PMID:6589029
582. Casulo C, Schöder H, Feeney J, et al. (2013). 18F-fluorodeoxyglucose positron emission tomography in the staging and prognosis of T cell lymphoma. Leuk Lymphoma. 54:2163–7. PMID:23369041
583. Catassi C, Bearzi I, Holmes GK (2005). Association of celiac disease and intestinal lymphomas and other cancers. Gastroenterology. 128:S79–86. PMID:15825131
584. Cattoretti G, Chang CC, Cechova K, et al. (1995). BCL-6 protein is expressed in germinal-center B cells. Blood. 86:45–53. PMID:7795255
585. Cattoretti G, Villa A, Vezzoni P, et al. (1990). Malignant histiocytosis. A phenotypic and genotypic investigation. Am J Pathol. 136:1009–19. PMID:2349962
586. Cawley JC (2006). The pathophysiology of the hairy cell. Hematol Oncol Clin North Am. 20:1011–21. PMID:16990104
587. Caye A, Strullu M, Guidez F, et al. (2015). Juvenile myelomonocytic leukemia displays mutations in components of the RAS pathway and the PRC2 network. Nat Genet. 47:1334–40. PMID:26457648
588. Cazals-Hatem D, André M, Mounier N, et al. (2001). Pathologic and clinical features of 77 Hodgkin's lymphoma patients treated in a lymphoma protocol (LNH87): a GELA study. Am J Surg Pathol. 25:297–306. PMID:11224599
589. Cazals-Hatem D, Lepage E, Brice P, et al. (1996). Primary mediastinal large B-cell lymphoma. A clinicopathologic study of 141 cases compared with 916 nonmediastinal large B-cell lymphomas, a GELA ("Groupe d'Etude des Lymphomes de l'Adulte") study. Am J Surg Pathol. 20:877–88. PMID:8669537
590. Cazzaniga G, Dell'Oro MG, Mecucci C, et al. (2005). Nucleophosmin mutations in childhood acute myelogenous leukemia with normal karyotype. Blood. 106:1419–22. PMID:15870172
591. Cazzola M, Invernizzi R, Bergamaschi G, et al. (2003). Mitochondrial ferritin expression in erythroid cells from patients with sideroblastic anemia. Blood. 101:1996–2000. PMID:12406866
592. Cazzola M, Malcovati L (2005). Myelodysplastic syndromes–coping with ineffective hematopoiesis. N Engl J Med. 352:536–8. PMID:15703418
593. Cazzola M, Rossi M, Malcovati L, et al. (2013). Biologic and clinical significance of somatic mutations of SF3B1 in myeloid and lymphoid neoplasms. Blood. 121:260–9. PMID:23160465
594. Ceesay MM, Lea NC, Ingram W, et al. (2006). The JAK2 V617F mutation is rare in RARS but common in RARS-T. Leukemia. 20:2060–1. PMID:16932338
595. Cehreli C, Undar B, Akkoc N, et al. (1994). Coexistence of chronic neutrophilic leukemia with light chain myeloma. Acta Haematol. 91:32–4. PMID:8171934
596. Cejkova P, Zettl A, Baumgärtner AK, et al. (2005). Amplification of NOTCH1 and ABL1 gene loci is a frequent aberration in enteropathy-type T-cell lymphoma. Virchows Arch. 446:416–20. PMID:15756589
597. Cella M, Facchetti F, Lanzavecchia A, et al. (2000). Plasmacytoid dendritic cells activated by influenza virus and CD40L drive a potent TH1 polarization. Nat Immunol. 1:305–10. PMID:11017101
598. Cella M, Jarrossay D, Facchetti F, et al. (1999). Plasmacytoid monocytes migrate to inflamed lymph nodes and produce large amounts of type I interferon. Nat Med. 5:919–23. PMID:10426316
599. Cellier C, Delabesse E, Helmer C, et al. (2000). Refractory sprue, coeliac disease, and enteropathy-associated T-cell lymphoma. Lancet. 356:203–8. PMID:10963198
600. Cencini E, Fabbri A, Rigacci L, et al. (2017). Evaluation of the prognostic role of tumour-associated macrophages in newly diagnosed classical Hodgkin lymphoma and correlation with early FDG-PET assessment. Hematol Oncol. 35:69–78. PMID:26251194
601. Cerf-Bensussan N, Brousse N, Cellier C (2002). From hyperplasia to T cell lymphoma. Gut. 51:304–5. PMID:12171943
602. Cerhan JR, Berndt SI, Vijai J, et al. (2014). Genome-wide association study identifies multiple susceptibility loci for diffuse large B cell lymphoma. Nat Genet. 46:1233–8. PMID:25261932
603. Cerhan JR, Slager SL (2015). Familial predisposition and genetic risk factors for lymphoma. Blood. 126:2265–73. PMID:26405224
604. Cerhan JR, Wang S, Maurer MJ, et al. (2007). Prognostic significance of host immune gene polymorphisms in follicular lymphoma survival. Blood. 109:5439–46. PMID:17327408
605. Ceriani L, Martelli M, Zinzani PL, et al. (2015). Utility of baseline 18FDG-PET/CT functional parameters in defining prognosis of primary mediastinal (thymic) large B-cell lymphoma. Blood. 126:950–6. PMID:26089397
605A. Cerroni L (2014). Skin lymphoma. The illustrated guide. 4th ed. Oxford: Wiley-Blackwell.
605B. Ceribelli M, Hou ZE, Kelly PN et al. (2016). A Druggable TCF4- and BRD4-dependent transcriptional network sustains malignancy in blastic plasmacytoid dendritic cell neoplasm. Cancer Cell. 14;30:764-778. PMID:27846392
606. Cerroni L, Arzberger E, Pütz B, et al. (2000). Primary cutaneous follicle center cell lymphoma with follicular growth pattern. Blood. 95:3922–8. PMID:10845929
607. Cerroni L, El-Shabrawi-Caelen L, Fink-Puches R, et al. (2000). Cutaneous spindle-cell B-cell lymphoma: a morphologic variant of cutaneous large B-cell lymphoma. Am J Dermatopathol. 22:299–304. PMID:10949453
608. Cerroni L, Fink-Puches R, Bäck B, et al. (2002). Follicular mucinosis: a critical reappraisal of clinicopathologic features and association with mycosis fungoides and Sézary syndrome. Arch Dermatol. 138:182–9. PMID:11843637
609. Cerroni L, Rieger E, Hödl S, et al. (1992). Clinicopathologic and immunologic features associated with transformation of mycosis fungoides to large-cell lymphoma. Am J Surg Pathol. 16:543–52. PMID:1599034
610. Cerroni L, Volkenandt M, Rieger E, et al. (1994). bcl-2 protein expression and correlation with the interchromosomal 14;18 translocation in cutaneous lymphomas and pseudolymphomas. J Invest Dermatol. 102:231–5. PMID:8106752
611. Cerroni L, Zöchling N, Pütz B, et al. (1997). Infection by Borrelia burgdorferi and cutaneous B-cell lymphoma. J Cutan Pathol. 24:457–61. PMID:9331890
612. Cervantes F, Alvarez-Larrán A, Talarn C, et al. (2002). Myelofibrosis with myeloid metaplasia following essential thrombocythaemia: actuarial probability, presenting characteristics and evolution in a series of 195 patients. Br J Haematol. 118:786–90. PMID:12181046
613. Cervantes F, Barosi G (2005). Myelofibrosis with myeloid metaplasia: diagnosis,

prognostic factors, and staging. Semin Oncol. 32:395–402. PMID:16202685
614. Cervantes F, Barosi G, Demory JL, et al. (1998). Myelofibrosis with myeloid metaplasia in young individuals: disease characteristics, prognostic factors and identification of risk groups. Br J Haematol. 102:684–90. PMID:9722294
615. Cervantes F, Dupriez B, Passamonti F, et al. (2012). Improving survival trends in primary myelofibrosis: an international study. J Clin Oncol. 30:2981–7. PMID:22826273
616. Cervantes F, Dupriez B, Pereira A, et al. (2009). New prognostic scoring system for primary myelofibrosis based on a study of the International Working Group for Myelofibrosis Research and Treatment. Blood. 113:2895–901. PMID:18988864
617. Cervantes F, Ribera JM, Sanchez-Bisono J, et al. (1984). Myeloproliferative disease in two young siblings. Cancer. 54:899–902. PMID:6744217
618. Cervantes F, Urbano-Ispizua A, Villamor N, et al. (1993). Ph-positive chronic myeloid leukemia mimicking essential thrombocythemia and terminating into megakaryoblastic blast crisis: report of two cases with molecular studies. Leukemia. 7:327–30. PMID:8426485
619. Cervantes F, Villamor N, Esteve J, et al. (1998). 'Lymphoid' blast crisis of chronic myeloid leukaemia is associated with distinct clinicohaematological features. Br J Haematol. 100:123–8. PMID:9450800
620. Cervera N, Itzykson R, Coppin E, et al. (2014). Gene mutations differently impact the prognosis of the myelodysplastic and myeloproliferative classes of chronic myelomonocytic leukemia. Am J Hematol. 89:604–9. PMID:24595958
621. Cesana C, Barbarano L, Miqueleiz S, et al. (2005). Clinical characteristics and outcome of immunoglobulin M-related disorders. Clin Lymphoma. 5:261–4. PMID:15794861
622. Cesarman E, Chadburn A, Liu YF, et al. (1998). BCL-6 gene mutations in posttransplantation lymphoproliferative disorders predict response to therapy and clinical outcome. Blood. 92:2294–302. PMID:9746767
623. Cesarman E, Chang Y, Moore PS, et al. (1995). Kaposi's sarcoma-associated herpesvirus-like DNA sequences in AIDS-related body-cavity-based lymphomas. N Engl J Med. 332:1186–91. PMID:7700311
624. Cessna MH, Hartung L, Tripp S, et al. (2005). Hairy cell leukemia variant: fact or fiction. Am J Clin Pathol. 123:132–8. PMID:15762289
625. Cetinözman F, Jansen PM, Vermeer MH, et al. (2012). Differential expression of programmed death-1 (PD-1) in Sézary syndrome and mycosis fungoides. Arch Dermatol. 148:1379–85. PMID:23247480
626. Cetinözman F, Jansen PM, Willemze R (2012). Expression of programmed death-1 in primary cutaneous CD4-positive small/medium-sized pleomorphic T-cell lymphoma, cutaneous pseudo-T-cell lymphoma, and other types of cutaneous T-cell lymphoma. Am J Surg Pathol. 36:109–16. PMID:21989349
627. Chacón JI, Mollejo M, Muñoz E, et al. (2002). Splenic marginal zone lymphoma: clinical characteristics and prognostic factors in a series of 60 patients. Blood. 100:1648–54. PMID:12176884
628. Chadburn A, Cesarman E, Liu YF, et al. (1995). Molecular genetic analysis demonstrates that multiple posttransplantation lymphoproliferative disorders occurring in one anatomic site in a single patient represent distinct primary lymphoid neoplasms. Cancer. 75:2747–56. PMID:7743481
629. Chadburn A, Chen JM, Hsu DT, et al. (1998). The morphologic and molecular genetic categories of posttransplantation lymphoproliferative disorders are clinically relevant. Cancer. 82:1978–87. PMID:9587133
630. Chadburn A, Chiu A, Lee JY, et al. (2009). Immunophenotypic analysis of AIDS-related diffuse large B-cell lymphoma and clinical implications in patients from AIDS Malignancies Consortium clinical trials 010 and 034. J Clin Oncol. 27:5039–48. PMID:19752343
631. Chadburn A, Hyjek E, Mathew S, et al. (2004). KSHV-positive solid lymphomas represent an extra-cavitary variant of primary effusion lymphoma. Am J Surg Pathol. 28:1401–16. PMID:15489644
632. Chadburn A, Suciu-Foca N, Cesarman E, et al. (1995). Post-transplantation lymphoproliferative disorders arising in solid organ transplant recipients are usually of recipient origin. Am J Pathol. 147:1862–70. PMID:7495309
633. Chaganti RS, Ladanyi M, Samaniego F, et al. (1989). Leukemic differentiation of a mediastinal germ cell tumor. Genes Chromosomes Cancer. 1:83–7. PMID:2562115
634. Chakraborty R, Hampton OA, Shen X, et al. (2014). Mutually exclusive recurrent somatic mutations in MAP2K1 and BRAF support a central role for ERK activation in LCH pathogenesis. Blood. 124:3007–15. PMID:25202140
635. Challa-Malladi M, Lieu YK, Califano O, et al. (2011). Combined genetic inactivation of β2-Microglobulin and CD58 reveals frequent escape from immune recognition in diffuse large B cell lymphoma. Cancer Cell. 20:728–40. PMID:22137796
636. Challagundla P, Medeiros LJ, Kanagal-Shamanna R, et al. (2014). Differential expression of CD200 in B-cell neoplasms by flow cytometry can assist in diagnosis, subclassification, and bone marrow staging. Am J Clin Pathol. 142:837–44. PMID:25389338
637. Chalmers ZR, Ali SM, Ohgami RS, et al. (2015). Comprehensive genomic profiling identifies a novel TNKS2-PDGFRA fusion that defines a myeloid neoplasm with eosinophilia that responded dramatically to imatinib therapy. Blood Cancer J. 5:e278. PMID:25658984
638. Chan AC, Chan KW, Chan JK, et al. (2001). Development of follicular dendritic cell sarcoma in hyaline-vascular Castleman's disease of the nasopharynx: tracing its evolution by sequential biopsies. Histopathology. 38:510–8. PMID:11422494
639. Chan AC, Serrano-Olmo J, Erlandson RA, et al. (2000). Cytokeratin-positive malignant tumors with reticulum cell morphology: a subtype of fibroblastic reticulum cell neoplasm? Am J Surg Pathol. 24:107–16. PMID:10632494
640. Chan JK (1998). Natural killer cell neoplasms. Anat Pathol. 3:77–145. PMID:10389582
641. Chan JK (2003). Splenic involvement by peripheral T-cell and NK-cell neoplasms. Semin Diagn Pathol. 20:105–20. PMID:12945934
642. Chan JKC (1997). Proliferative lesions of follicular dendritic cells: an overview, including a detailed account of follicular dendritic cell sarcoma, a neoplasm with many faces and uncommon etiologic associations. Adv Anat Pathol. 4:387–411.
643. Chan JK, Buchanan R, Fletcher CD (1990). Sarcomatoid variant of anaplastic large-cell Ki-1 lymphoma. Am J Surg Pathol. 14:983–8. PMID:2206085
644. Chan JK, Chan AC, Cheuk W, et al. (2011). Type II enteropathy-associated T-cell lymphoma: a distinct aggressive lymphoma with frequent γδ T-cell receptor expression. Am J Surg Pathol. 35:1557–69. PMID:21921780
645. Chan JK, Fletcher CD, Nayler SJ, et al. (1997). Follicular dendritic cell sarcoma. Clinicopathologic analysis of 17 cases suggesting a malignant potential higher than currently recognized. Cancer. 79:294–313. PMID:9010103
646. Chan JK, Lamant L, Algar E, et al. (2008). ALK+ histiocytosis: a novel type of systemic histiocytic proliferative disorder of early infancy. Blood. 112:2965–8. PMID:18660380
647. Chan JK, Sin VC, Wong KF, et al. (1997). Nonnasal lymphoma expressing the natural killer cell marker CD56: a clinicopathologic study of 49 cases of an uncommon aggressive neoplasm. Blood. 89:4501–13. PMID:9192774
648. Chan JK, Tsang WY, Ng CS (1996). Clarification of CD3 immunoreactivity in nasal T/natural killer cell lymphomas: the neoplastic cells are often CD3 epsilon+. Blood. 87:839–41. PMID:8555511
649. Chan JK, Yip TT, Tsang WY, et al. (1994). Detection of Epstein-Barr viral RNA in malignant lymphomas of the upper aerodigestive tract. Am J Surg Pathol. 18:938–46. PMID:8067515
650. Chan WC, Link S, Mawle A, et al. (1986). Heterogeneity of large granular lymphocyte proliferations: delineation of two major subtypes. Blood. 68:1142–53. PMID:3490288
651. Chan WC, Zaatari G (1986). Lymph node interdigitating reticulum cell sarcoma. Am J Clin Pathol. 85:739–44. PMID:2939710
651A. Chandran R, Gardiner SK, Simon M, et al. (2012). Survival trends in mantle cell lymphoma in the United States over 16 years 1992-2007. Leuk Lymphoma. 53:1488–93. PMID:22242824
652. Chang HW, Leong KH, Koh DR, et al. (1999). Clonality of isolated eosinophils in the hypereosinophilic syndrome. Blood. 93:1651–7. PMID:10029594
653. Chang KC, Khen NT, Jones D, et al. (2005). Epstein-Barr virus is associated with all histological subtypes of Hodgkin lymphoma in Vietnamese children with special emphasis on the entity of lymphocyte predominance subtype. Hum Pathol. 36:747–55. PMID:16084943
654. Chang SE, Cho S, Choi JC, et al. (2001). Clinicohistopathologic comparison of adult type and juvenile type xanthogranulomas in Korea. J Dermatol. 28:413–8. PMID:11560157
655. Chang SE, Yoon GS, Huh J, et al. (2002). Comparison of primary and secondary cutaneous CD56+ NK/T cell lymphomas. Appl Immunohistochem Mol Morphol. 10:163–70. PMID:12051636
656. Chang ST, Lu CL, Chuang SS (2007). CD52 expression in non-mycotic T- and NK/T-cell lymphomas. Leuk Lymphoma. 48:117–21. PMID:17325855
657. Chanudet E, Ye H, Ferry J, et al. (2009). A20 deletion is associated with copy number gain at the TNFA/B/C locus and occurs preferentially in translocation-negative MALT lymphoma of the ocular adnexa and salivary glands. J Pathol. 217:420–30. PMID:19006194
658. Chanudet E, Zhou Y, Bacon CM, et al. (2006). Chlamydia psittaci is variably associated with ocular adnexal MALT lymphoma in different geographical regions. J Pathol. 209:344–51. PMID:16583361
659. Chao C, Silverberg MJ, Martínez-Maza O, et al. (2012). Epstein-Barr virus infection and expression of B-cell oncogenic markers in HIV-related diffuse large B-cell Lymphoma. Clin Cancer Res. 18:4702–12. PMID:22711707
660. Chao C, Silverberg MJ, Xu L, et al. (2015). A comparative study of molecular characteristics of diffuse large B-cell lymphoma from patients with and without human immunodeficiency virus infection. Clin Cancer Res. 21:1429–37. PMID:25589617
661. Chao C, Xu L, Silverberg MJ, et al. (2015). Stromal immune infiltration in HIV-related diffuse large B-cell lymphoma is associated with HIV disease history and patient survival. AIDS. 29:1943–51. PMID:26355571
662. Chao MW, Gibbs P, Wirth A, et al. (2005). Radiotherapy in the management of solitary extramedullary plasmacytoma. Intern Med J. 35:211–5. PMID:15836498
663. Chaperot L, Bendriss N, Manches O, et al. (2001). Identification of a leukemic counterpart of the plasmacytoid dendritic cells. Blood. 97:3210–7. PMID:11342451
664. Chaperot L, Perrot I, Jacob MC, et al. (2004). Leukemic plasmacytoid dendritic cells share phenotypic and functional features with their normal counterparts. Eur J Immunol. 34:418–26. PMID:14768046
665. Chapuy B, Roemer MG, Stewart C, et al. (2016). Targetable genetic features of primary testicular and primary central nervous system lymphomas. Blood. 127:869–81. PMID:26702065
666. Chawla SS, Kumar SK, Dispenzieri A, et al. (2015). Clinical course and prognosis of non-secretory multiple myeloma. Eur J Haematol. 95:57–64. PMID:25382589
667. Cheah CY, George A, Giné E, et al. (2013). Central nervous system involvement in mantle cell lymphoma: clinical features, prognostic factors and outcomes from the European Mantle Cell Lymphoma Network. Ann Oncol. 24:2119–23. PMID:23616279
668. Chen BJ, Chapuy B, Ouyang J, et al. (2013). PD-L1 expression is characteristic of a subset of aggressive B-cell lymphomas and virus-associated malignancies. Clin Cancer Res. 19:3462–73. PMID:23674495
669. Chen CY, Chou WC, Tsay W, et al. (2013). Hierarchical cluster analysis of immunophenotype classify AML patients with NPM1 gene mutation into two groups with distinct prognosis. BMC Cancer. 13:107. PMID:23496932
670. Chen D, Gao Y, Nicholas J (2014). Human herpesvirus 8 interleukin-6 contributes to primary effusion lymphoma cell viability via suppression of proapoptotic cathepsin D, a cointeraction partner of vitamin K epoxide reductase complex subunit 1 variant 2. J Virol. 88:1025–38. PMID:24198402
671. Chen D, Hoyer JD, Ketterling RP, et al. (2009). Dysgranulopoiesis is an independent adverse prognostic factor in chronic myeloid disorders with an isolated interstitial deletion of chromosome 5q. Leukemia. 23:796–800. PMID:18946493
672. Chen G, Yim AP, Ma L, et al. (2011). Primary pulmonary large B-cell lymphoma–mediastinal type? Histopathology. 58:324–6. PMID:21323958
673. Chen J, Deangelo DJ, Kutok JL, et al. (2004). PKC412 inhibits the zinc finger 198-fibroblast growth factor receptor 1 fusion tyrosine kinase and is active in treatment of stem cell myeloproliferative disorder. Proc Natl Acad Sci U S A. 101:14479–84. PMID:15448205
674. Chen JS, Coustan-Smith E, Suzuki T, et al. (2001). Identification of novel markers for monitoring minimal residual disease in acute lymphoblastic leukemia. Blood. 97:2115–20. PMID:11264179
675. Chen JS, Tzeng CC, Tsao CJ, et al. (1997). Clonal karyotype abnormalities in EBV-associated hemophagocytic syndrome. Haematologica. 82:572–6. PMID:9407723
676. Chen LT, Lin JT, Shyu RY, et al. (2001). Prospective study of Helicobacter pylori eradication therapy in stage I(E) high-grade mucosa-associated lymphoid tissue lymphoma of the stomach. J Clin Oncol. 19:4245–51. PMID:11709568
677. Chen MH, Atenafu E, Craddock KJ, et al. (2013). CD11b expression correlates with monosomal karyotype and predicts an extremely poor prognosis in cytogenetically unfavorable acute myeloid leukemia. Leuk Res. 37:122–8. PMID:23092917

678. Chen W, Jaffe R, Zhang L, et al. (2013). Langerhans Cell Sarcoma Arising from Chronic Lymphocytic Lymphoma/Small Lymphocytic Leukemia: Lineage Analysis and BRAF V600E Mutation Study. N Am J Med Sci. 5:386–91. PMID:23923114

679. Chen W, Kesler MV, Karandikar NJ, et al. (2006). Flow cytometric features of angioimmunoblastic T-cell lymphoma. Cytometry B Clin Cytom. 70:142–8. PMID:16572417

680. Chen W, Lau SK, Fong D, et al. (2009). High frequency of clonal immunoglobulin receptor gene rearrangements in sporadic histiocytic/dendritic cell sarcomas. Am J Surg Pathol. 33:863–73. PMID:19145200

681. Chen W, Wang J, Wang E, et al. (2010). Detection of clonal lymphoid receptor gene rearrangements in langerhans cell histiocytosis. Am J Surg Pathol. 34:1049–57. PMID:20551822

682. Chen X, Rutledge JC, Wu D, et al. (2013). Chronic myelogenous leukemia presenting in blast phase with nodal, bilineal myeloid sarcoma and T-lymphoblastic lymphoma in a child. Pediatr Dev Pathol. 16:91–6. PMID:23171293

683. Chen Y, Shi H, Li H, et al. (2016). Clinicopathological features of inflammatory pseudotumor-like follicular dendritic cell tumor of the abdomen. Histopathology. 68:858–65. PMID:26332157

684. Chen YC, Chou JM, Ketterling RP, et al. (2003). Histologic and immunohistochemical study of bone marrow monocytic nodules in 21 cases with myelodysplasia. Am J Clin Pathol. 120:874–81. PMID:14671976

685. Chen YH, Tallman MS, Goolsby C, et al. (2006). Immunophenotypic variations in hairy cell leukemia. Am J Clin Pathol. 125:251–9. PMID:16393677

686. Chen YW, Guo T, Shen L, et al. (2015). Receptor-type tyrosine-protein phosphatase κ directly targets STAT3 activation for tumor suppression in nasal NK/T-cell lymphoma. Blood. 125:1589–600. PMID:25612622

687. Chen YW, Hu XT, Liang AC, et al. (2006). High BCL6 expression predicts better prognosis, independent of BCL6 translocation status, translocation partner, or BCL6-deregulating mutations, in gastric lymphoma. Blood. 108:2373–83. PMID:16772602

688. Chene A, Donati D, Orem J, et al. (2009). Endemic Burkitt's lymphoma as a polymicrobial disease: new insights on the interaction between Plasmodium falciparum and Epstein-Barr virus. Semin Cancer Biol. 19:411–20. PMID:19897039

689. Chereda B, Melo JV (2015). Natural course and biology of CML. Ann Hematol. 94 Suppl 2:S107–21. PMID:25814077

690. Chesi M, Bergsagel PL (2013). Molecular pathogenesis of multiple myeloma: basic and clinical updates. Int J Hematol. 97:313–23. PMID:23456262

691. Cheson BD, Fisher RI, Barrington SF, et al. (2014). Recommendations for initial evaluation, staging, and response assessment of Hodgkin and non-Hodgkin lymphoma: the Lugano classification. J Clin Oncol. 32:3059–68. PMID:25113753

692. Cheson BD, Pfistner B, Juweid ME, et al. (2007). Revised response criteria for malignant lymphoma. J Clin Oncol. 25:579–86. PMID:17242396

693. Chester W (1930). Über Lipoidgranulomatose. Virchows Arch Pathol Anat Physiol Klin Med. 279:561–602.

694. Chetty R, Biddolph S, Gatter K (1997). An immunohistochemical analysis of Reed-Sternberg-like cells in posttransplantation lymphoproliferative disorders: the possible pathogenetic relationship to Reed-Sternberg cells in Hodgkin's disease and Reed-Sternberg-like cells in non-Hodgkin's lymphomas and reactive conditions. Hum Pathol. 28:493–8. PMID:9104951

695. Chetty R, Pulford K, Jones M, et al. (1995). SCL/Tal-1 expression in T-acute lymphoblastic leukemia: an immunohistochemical and genotypic study. Hum Pathol. 26:994–8. PMID:7672800

696. Cheuk W, Chan AC, Chan JK, et al. (2005). Metallic implant-associated lymphoma: a distinct subgroup of large B-cell lymphoma related to pyothorax-associated lymphoma? Am J Surg Pathol. 29:832–6. PMID:15897752

697. Cheuk W, Chan JK, Shek TW, et al. (2001). Inflammatory pseudotumor-like follicular dendritic cell tumor: a distinctive low-grade malignant intra-abdominal neoplasm with consistent Epstein-Barr virus association. Am J Surg Pathol. 25:721–31. PMID:11395549

698. Cheuk W, Hill RW, Bacchi C, et al. (2000). Hypocellular anaplastic large cell lymphoma mimicking inflammatory lesions of lymph nodes. Am J Surg Pathol. 24:1537–43. PMID:11075856

699. Cheuk W, Walford N, Lou J, et al. (2001). Primary histiocytic lymphoma of the central nervous system: a neoplasm frequently overshadowed by a prominent inflammatory component. Am J Surg Pathol. 25:1372–9. PMID:11684953

700. Cheuk W, Wong KO, Wong CS, et al. (2004). Consistent immunostaining for cyclin D1 can be achieved on a routine basis using a newly available rabbit monoclonal antibody. Am J Surg Pathol. 28:801–7. PMID:15166673

701. Cheung KJ, Horsman DE, Gascoyne RD (2009). The significance of TP53 in lymphoid malignancies: mutation prevalence, regulation, prognostic impact and potential as a therapeutic target. Br J Haematol. 146:257–69. PMID:19500100

702. Cheung KJ, Johnson NA, Affleck JG, et al. (2010). Acquired TNFRSF14 mutations in follicular lymphoma are associated with worse prognosis. Cancer Res. 70:9166–74. PMID:20884631

703. Cheung MC, Bailey D, Pennell N, et al. (2009). In situ localization of follicular lymphoma: evidence for subclinical systemic disease with detection of an identical BCL-2/IGH fusion gene in blood and lymph node. Leukemia. 23:1176–9. PMID:19212334

704. Cheung MM, Chan JK, Lau WH, et al. (1998). Primary non-Hodgkin's lymphoma of the nose and nasopharynx: clinical features, tumor immunophenotype, and treatment outcome in 113 patients. J Clin Oncol. 16:70–7. PMID:9440725

705. Cheung MM, Chan JK, Lau WH, et al. (2002). Early stage nasal NK/T-cell lymphoma: clinical outcome, prognostic factors, and the effect of treatment modality. Int J Radiat Oncol Biol Phys. 54:182–90. PMID:12182990

706. Chevallier P, Mohty M, Lioure B, et al. (2008). Allogeneic hematopoietic stem-cell transplantation for myeloid sarcoma: a retrospective study from the SFGM-TC. J Clin Oncol. 26:4940–3. PMID:18606981

707. Chi Y, Lindgren V, Quigley S, et al. (2008). Acute myelogenous leukemia with t(6;9)(p23;q34) and marrow basophilia: an overview. Arch Pathol Lab Med. 132:1835–7. PMID:18976025

708. Chiang AK, Wong KY, Liang AC, et al. (1999). Comparative analysis of Epstein-Barr virus gene polymorphisms in nasal T/NK-cell lymphomas and normal nasal tissues: implications on virus strain selection in malignancy. Int J Cancer. 80:356–64. PMID:9935174

709. Chiarle R, Gong JZ, Guasparri I, et al. (2003). NPM-ALK transgenic mice spontaneously develop T-cell lymphomas and plasma cell tumors. Blood. 101:1919–27. PMID:12424201

710. Chiarle R, Simmons WJ, Cai H, et al. (2005). Stat3 is required for ALK-mediated lymphomagenesis and provides a possible therapeutic target. Nat Med. 11:623–9. PMID:15895073

711. Chiecchio L, Dagrada GP, Ibrahim AH, et al. (2009). Timing of acquisition of deletion 13 in plasma cell dyscrasias is dependent on genetic context. Haematologica. 94:1708–13. PMID:19996118

712. Chigrinova E, Rinaldi A, Kwee I, et al. (2013). Two main genetic pathways lead to the transformation of chronic lymphocytic leukemia to Richter syndrome. Blood. 122:2673–82. PMID:24004666

713. Chikatsu N, Kojima H, Suzukawa K, et al. (2003). ALK+, CD30-, CD20- large B-cell lymphoma containing anaplastic lymphoma kinase (ALK) fused to clathrin heavy chain gene (CLTC). Mod Pathol. 16:828–32. PMID:12920229

714. Chikwava K, Jaffe R (2004). Langerin (CD207) staining in normal pediatric tissues, reactive lymph nodes, and childhood histiocytic disorders. Pediatr Dev Pathol. 7:607–14. PMID:15630529

715. Child FJ, Russell-Jones R, Woolford AJ, et al. (2001). Absence of the t(14;18) chromosomal translocation in primary cutaneous B-cell lymphoma. Br J Dermatol. 144:735–44. PMID:11298531

716. Chilosi M, Pizzolo G, Caligaris-Cappio F, et al. (1985). Immunohistochemical demonstration of follicular dendritic cells in bone marrow involvement of B-cell chronic lymphocytic leukemia. Cancer. 56:328–32. PMID:3891066

717. Chim CS, Kwong YL, Lie AK, et al. (2005). Long-term outcome of 231 patients with essential thrombocythemia: prognostic factors for thrombosis, bleeding, myelofibrosis, and leukemia. Arch Intern Med. 165:2651–8. PMID:16344424

718. Chim CS, Ma ES, Loong F, et al. (2005). Diagnostic cues for natural killer cell lymphoma: primary nodal presentation and the role of in situ hybridisation for Epstein-Barr virus encoded early small RNA in detecting occult bone marrow involvement. J Clin Pathol. 58:443–5. PMID:15790718

719. Chim CS, Ma SY, Au WY, et al. (2004). Primary nasal natural killer cell lymphoma: long-term treatment outcome and relationship with the International Prognostic Index. Blood. 103:216–21. PMID:12933580

720. Chinnock R, Webber SA, Dipchand AI, et al. (2012). A 16-year multi-institutional study of the role of age and EBV status on PTLD incidence among pediatric heart transplant recipients. Am J Transplant. 12:3061–8. PMID:23072522

721. Chiorazzi N, Rai KR, Ferrarini M (2005). Chronic lymphocytic leukemia. N Engl J Med. 352:804–15. PMID:15728813

722. Chisholm KM, Bangs CD, Bacchi CE, et al. (2015). Expression profiles of MYC protein and MYC gene rearrangement in lymphomas. Am J Surg Pathol. 39:294–303. PMID:25581730

723. Chittal SM, Alard C, Rossi JF, et al. (1990). Further phenotypic evidence that nodular, lymphocyte-predominant Hodgkin's disease is a large B-cell lymphoma in evolution. Am J Surg Pathol. 14:1024–35. PMID:2240355

724. Chittal SM, Caverivière P, Schwarting R, et al. (1988). Monoclonal antibodies in the diagnosis of Hodgkin's disease. The search for a rational panel. Am J Surg Pathol. 12:9–21. PMID:2827535

725. Chiu A, Frizzera G, Mathew S, et al. (2009). Diffuse blastoid B-cell lymphoma: a histologically aggressive variant of t(14;18)-negative follicular lymphoma. Mod Pathol. 22:1507–17. PMID:19633642

726. Chmielecki J, Peifer M, Viale A, et al. (2012). Systematic screen for tyrosine kinase rearrangements identifies a novel C6orf204-PDGFRB fusion in a patient with recurrent T-ALL and an associated myeloproliferative neoplasm. Genes Chromosomes Cancer. 51:54–65. PMID:21938754

727. Chng WJ, Schop RF, Price-Troska T, et al. (2006). Gene-expression profiling of Waldenstrom macroglobulinemia reveals a phenotype more similar to chronic lymphocytic leukemia than multiple myeloma. Blood. 108:2755–63. PMID:16804116

728. Chng WJ, Van Wier SA, Ahmann GJ, et al. (2005). A validated FISH trisomy index demonstrates the hyperdiploid and nonhyperdiploid dichotomy in MGUS. Blood. 106:2156–61. PMID:15920009

729. Chng WJ, Winkler JM, Greipp PR, et al. (2006). Ploidy status rarely changes in myeloma patients at disease progression. Leuk Res. 30:266–71. PMID:16111750

730. Cho JH, Kim HS, Ko YH, et al. (2006). Epstein-Barr virus infected natural killer cell lymphoma in a patient with hypersensitivity to mosquito bite. J Infect. 52:e173–6. PMID:16246422

731. Cho KH, Kim CW, Heo DS, et al. (2001). Epstein-Barr virus-associated peripheral T-cell lymphoma in adults with hydroa vacciniforme-like lesions. Clin Exp Dermatol. 26:242–7. PMID:11422165

732. Cho KH, Lee SH, Kim CW, et al. (2004). Epstein-Barr virus-associated lymphoproliferative lesions presenting as a hydroa vacciniforme-like eruption: an analysis of six cases. Br J Dermatol. 151:372–80. PMID:15327544

733. Choe JY, Go H, Jeon YK, et al. (2013). Inflammatory pseudotumor-like follicular dendritic cell sarcoma of the spleen: a report of six cases with increased IgG4-positive plasma cells. Pathol Int. 63:245–51. PMID:23714251

734. Choe JY, Yun JY, Na HY, et al. (2016). MYC overexpression correlates with MYC amplification or translocation, and is associated with poor prognosis in mantle cell lymphoma. Histopathology. 68:442–9. PMID:26100211

735. Choi IK, Kim BS, Lee KA, et al. (2004). Efficacy of imatinib mesylate (STI571) in chronic neutrophilic leukemia with t(15;19): case report. Am J Hematol. 77:366–9. PMID:15551277

736. Choi J, Goh G, Walradt T, et al. (2015). Genomic landscape of cutaneous T cell lymphoma. Nat Genet. 47:1011–9. PMID:26192916

737. Choi PC, To KF, Lai FM, et al. (2000). Follicular dendritic cell sarcoma of the neck: report of two cases complicated by pulmonary metastases. Cancer. 89:664–72. PMID:10931467

738. Choi WW, Weisenburger DD, Greiner TC, et al. (2009). A new immunostain algorithm classifies diffuse large B-cell lymphoma into molecular subtypes with high accuracy. Clin Cancer Res. 15:5494–502. PMID:19706817

739. Choi Y, Lee JH, Kim SD, et al. (2013). Prognostic implications of CD14 positivity in acute myeloid leukemia arising from myelodysplastic syndrome. Int J Hematol. 97:246–55. PMID:23371544

740. Choi YL, Park JH, Namkung JH, et al. (2009). Extranodal NK/T-cell lymphoma with cutaneous involvement: 'nasal' vs. 'nasal-type' subgroups–a retrospective study of 18 patients. Br J Dermatol. 160:333–7. PMID:19014396

741. Choquet S, Leblond V, Herbrecht R, et al. (2006). Efficacy and safety of rituximab in B-cell post-transplantation lymphoproliferative disorders: results of a prospective multicenter phase 2 study. Blood. 107:3053–7. PMID:16254143

742. Choquet S, Trappe R, Leblond V, et al. (2007). CHOP-21 for the treatment of post-transplant lymphoproliferative disorders

(PTLD) following solid organ transplantation. Haematologica. 92:273–4. PMID:17296588

743. Chott A, Dragosics B, Radaszkiewicz T (1992). Peripheral T-cell lymphomas of the intestine. Am J Pathol. 141:1361–71. PMID:1466400

744. Chott A, Gisslinger H, Thiele J, et al. (1990). Interferon-alpha-induced morphological changes of megakaryocytes: a histomorphometrical study on bone marrow biopsies in chronic myeloproliferative disorders with excessive thrombocytosis. Br J Haematol. 74:10–6. PMID:2310690

745. Chott A, Guenther P, Huebner A, et al. (2003). Morphologic and immunophenotypic properties of neoplastic cells in a case of mast cell sarcoma. Am J Surg Pathol. 27:1013–9. PMID:12826896

746. Chott A, Haedicke W, Mosberger I, et al. (1998). Most CD56+ intestinal lymphomas are CD8+CD5-T-cell lymphomas of monomorphic small to medium size histology. Am J Pathol. 153:1483–90. PMID:9811340

747. Chott A, Vesely M, Simonitsch I, et al. (1999). Classification of intestinal T-cell neoplasms and their differential diagnosis. Am J Clin Pathol. 111:S68–74. PMID:9894471

748. Chott A, Vonderheid EC, Olbricht S, et al. (1996). The dominant T cell clone is present in multiple regressing skin lesions and associated T cell lymphomas of patients with lymphomatoid papulosis. J Invest Dermatol. 106:696–700. PMID:8618007

748 A. Chou WC, Huang HH, Hou HA, et al. (2010). Distinct clinical and biological features of de novo acute myeloid leukemia with additional sex comb-like 1 (ASXL1) mutations. Blood. 116:4086–94. PMID:20693432

749. Chou WC, Tang JL, Lin LI, et al. (2006). Nucleophosmin mutations in de novo acute myeloid leukemia: the age-dependent incidences and the stability during disease evolution. Cancer Res. 66:3310–6. PMID:16540685

750. Christian B, Zhao W, Hamadani M, et al. (2010). Mantle cell lymphoma 12 years after allogeneic bone marrow transplantation occurring simultaneously in recipient and donor. J Clin Oncol. 28:e629–32. PMID:20733121

751. Christiansen DH, Andersen MK, Pedersen-Bjergaard J (2004). Mutations of AML1 are common in therapy-related myelodysplasia following therapy with alkylating agents and are significantly associated with deletion or loss of chromosome arm 7q and with subsequent leukemic transformation. Blood. 104:1474–81. PMID:15142876

752. Christie LJ, Evans AT, Bray SE, et al. (2006). Lesions resembling Langerhans cell histiocytosis in association with other lymphoproliferative disorders: a reactive or neoplastic phenomenon? Hum Pathol. 37:32–9. PMID:16360413

753. Chu LC, Eberhart CG, Grossman SA, et al. (2006). Epigenetic silencing of multiple genes in primary CNS lymphoma. Int J Cancer. 119:2487–91. PMID:16858686

754. Chuang WY, Chang H, Shih LY, et al. (2015). CD5 positivity is an independent adverse prognostic factor in elderly patients with diffuse large B cell lymphoma. Virchows Arch. 467:571–82. PMID:26369546

755. Chung SS, Kim E, Park JH, et al. (2014). Hematopoietic stem cell origin of BRAFV600E mutations in hairy cell leukemia. Sci Transl Med. 6:238ra71. PMID:24871132

756. Churpek JE, Larson RA (2013). The evolving challenge of therapy-related myeloid neoplasms. Best Pract Res Clin Haematol. 26:309–17. PMID:24507808

757. Churpek JE, Lorenz R, Nedumgottil S, et al. (2013). Proposal for the clinical detection and management of patients and their

family members with familial myelodysplastic syndrome/acute leukemia predisposition syndromes. Leuk Lymphoma. 54:28–35. PMID:22691122

758. Churpek JE, Marquez R, Neistadt B, et al. (2016). Inherited mutations in cancer susceptibility genes are common among survivors of breast cancer who develop therapy-related leukemia. Cancer. 122:304–11. PMID:26641009

759. Chusid MJ, Dale DC, West BC, et al. (1975). The hypereosinophilic syndrome: analysis of fourteen cases with review of the literature. Medicine (Baltimore). 54:1–27. PMID:1090795

760. Ciccone M, Agostinelli C, Rigolin GM, et al. (2012). Proliferation centers in chronic lymphocytic leukemia: correlation with cytogenetic and clinicobiological features in consecutive patients analyzed on tissue microarrays. Leukemia. 26:499–508. PMID:21941366

761. Claessens YE, Bouscary D, Dupont JM, et al. (2002). In vitro proliferation and differentiation of erythroid progenitors from patients with myelodysplastic syndromes: evidence for Fas-dependent apoptosis. Blood. 99:1594–601. PMID:11861273

762. Clarke CA, Glaser SL, Keegan TH, et al. (2005). Neighborhood socioeconomic status and Hodgkin's lymphoma incidence in California. Cancer Epidemiol Biomarkers Prev. 14:1441–7. PMID:15941953

763. Clarke CA, Morton LM, Lynch C, et al. (2013). Risk of lymphoma subtypes after solid organ transplantation in the United States. Br J Cancer. 109:280–8. PMID:23756857

764. Clarke M, Gaynon P, Hann I, et al. (2003). CNS-directed therapy for childhood acute lymphoblastic leukemia: Childhood ALL Collaborative Group overview of 43 randomized trials. J Clin Oncol. 21:1798–809. PMID:12721257

765. Cleary ML, Meeker TC, Levy S, et al. (1986). Clustering of extensive somatic mutations in the variable region of an immunoglobulin heavy chain gene from a human B cell lymphoma. Cell. 44:97–106. PMID:3079673

766. Cleary ML, Nalesnik MA, Shearer WT, et al. (1988). Clonal analysis of transplant-associated lymphoproliferations based on the structure of the genomic termini of the Epstein-Barr virus. Blood. 72:349–52. PMID:2839256

767. Cleary ML, Warnke R, Sklar J (1984). Monoclonality of lymphoproliferative lesions in cardiac-transplant recipients. Clonal analysis based on immunoglobulin-gene rearrangements. N Engl J Med. 310:477–82. PMID:6363929

768. Clemente MJ, Przychodzen B, Jerez A, et al. (2013). Deep sequencing of the T-cell receptor repertoire in CD8+ T-large granular lymphocyte leukemia identifies signature landscapes. Blood. 122:4077–85. PMID:24149287

769. Cleven AH, Nardi V, Ok CY, et al. (2015). High p53 protein expression in therapy-related myeloid neoplasms is associated with adverse karyotype and poor outcome. Mod Pathol. 28:552–63. PMID:25412846

770. Clifford GM, Polesel J, Rickenbach M, et al. (2005). Cancer risk in the Swiss HIV Cohort Study: associations with immunodeficiency, smoking, and highly active antiretroviral therapy. J Natl Cancer Inst. 97:425–32. PMID:15770006

771. Clipson A, Wang M, de Leval L, et al. (2015). KLF2 mutation is the most frequent somatic change in splenic marginal zone lymphoma and identifies a subset with distinct genotype. Leukemia. 29:1177–85. PMID:25428260

772. Cobaleda C, Busslinger M (2008). Developmental plasticity of lymphocytes. Curr Opin Immunol. 20:139–48. PMID:18472258

773. Cobaleda C, Gutiérrez-Cianca N, Pérez-Losada J, et al. (2000). A primitive

hematopoietic cell is the target for the leukemic transformation in human philadelphia-positive acute lymphoblastic leukemia. Blood. 95:1007–13. PMID:10648416

774. Cobbers JM, Wolter M, Reifenberger J, et al. (1998). Frequent inactivation of CDKN2A and rare mutation of TP53 in PCNSL. Brain Pathol. 8:263–76. PMID:9546285

775. Cobo F, Hernández S, Hernández L, et al. (1999). Expression of potentially oncogenic HHV-8 genes in an EBV-negative primary effusion lymphoma occurring in an HIV-seronegative patient. J Pathol. 189:288–93. PMID:10547588

776. Cocco P, t'Mannetje A, Fadda D, et al. (2010). Occupational exposure to solvents and risk of lymphoma subtypes: results from the Epilymph case-control study. Occup Environ Med. 67:341–7. PMID:20447988

776A. Coenen EA, Zwaan CM, Reinhardt D, et al. (2013). Pediatric acute myeloid leukemia with t(8;16)(p11;p13), a distinct clinical and biological entity: a collaborative study by the International-Berlin-Frankfurt-Munster AML-study group. Blood. 122:2704–13. PMID:23974201

777. Cogle CR, Craig BM, Rollison DE, et al. (2011). Incidence of the myelodysplastic syndromes using a novel claims-based algorithm: high number of uncaptured cases by cancer registries. Blood. 117:7121–5. PMID:21531980

778. Cohen JB, Geyer SM, Lozanski G, et al. (2014). Complete response to induction therapy in patients with Myc-positive and double-hit non-Hodgkin lymphoma is associated with prolonged progression-free survival. Cancer. 120:1677–85. PMID:24578014

779. Cohen JI, Jaffe ES, Dale JK, et al. (2011). Characterization and treatment of chronic active Epstein-Barr virus disease: a 28-year experience in the United States. Blood. 117:5835–49. PMID:21454450

780. Cohen JI, Kimura H, Nakamura S, et al. (2009). Epstein-Barr virus-associated lymphoproliferative disease in non-immunocompromised hosts: a status report and summary of an international meeting, 8-9 September 2008. Ann Oncol. 20:1472–82. PMID:19515747

781. Cohen M, Narbaitz M, Metrebian F, et al. (2014). Epstein-Barr virus-positive diffuse large B-cell lymphoma association is not only restricted to elderly patients. Int J Cancer. 135:2816–24. PMID:24789501

782. Colby TV, Hoppe RT, Warnke RA (1982). Hodgkin's disease: a clinicopathologic study of 659 cases. Cancer. 49:1848–58. PMID:7074584

783. Coles FB, Cartun RW, Pastuszak WT (1988). Hodgkin's disease, lymphocyte-predominant type: immunoreactivity with B-cell antibodies. Mod Pathol. 1:274–8. PMID:3266337

784. Collin M, Dickinson R, Bigley V (2015). Haematopoietic and immune defects associated with GATA2 mutation. Br J Haematol. 169:173–87. PMID:25707267

785. Colomo L, Loong F, Rives S, et al. (2004). Diffuse large B-cell lymphomas with plasmablastic differentiation represent a heterogeneous group of disease entities. Am J Surg Pathol. 28:736–47. PMID:15166665

786. Colomo L, López-Guillermo A, Perales M, et al. (2003). Clinical impact of the differentiation profile assessed by immunophenotyping in patients with diffuse large B-cell lymphoma. Blood. 101:78–84. PMID:12393466

787. Colt JS, Davis S, Severson RK, et al. (2006). Residential insecticide use and risk of non-Hodgkin's lymphoma. Cancer Epidemiol Biomarkers Prev. 15:251–7. PMID:16492912

788. Comenzo RL, Zhou P, Fleisher M, et al. (2006). Seeking confidence in the diagnosis of systemic AL (Ig light-chain) amyloidosis:

patients can have both monoclonal gammopathies and hereditary amyloid proteins. Blood. 107:3489–91. PMID:16439680

789. Cong P, Raffeld M, Teruya-Feldstein J, et al. (2002). In situ localization of follicular lymphoma: description and analysis by laser capture microdissection. Blood. 99:3376–82. PMID:11964306

790. Connors JM (2005). State-of-the-art therapeutics: Hodgkin's lymphoma. J Clin Oncol. 23:6400–8. PMID:16155026

791. Connors JM (2015). Risk assessment in the management of newly diagnosed classical Hodgkin lymphoma. Blood. 125:1693–702. PMID:25575542

792. Cook JR, Aguilera NI, Reshmi S, et al. (2005). Deletion 6q is not a characteristic marker of nodal lymphoplasmacytic lymphoma. Cancer Genet Cytogenet. 162:85–8. PMID:16157207

793. Cook JR, Aguilera NI, Reshmi-Skarja S, et al. (2004). Lack of PAX5 rearrangements in lymphoplasmacytic lymphomas: reassessing the reported association with t(9;14). Hum Pathol. 35:447–54. PMID:15116325

794. Cook JR, Goldman B, Tubbs RR, et al. (2014). Clinical significance of MYC expression and/or "high-grade" morphology in non-Burkitt, diffuse aggressive B-cell lymphomas: a SWOG S9704 correlative study. Am J Surg Pathol. 38:494–501. PMID:24625415

795. Cook JR, Hsi ED, Worley S, et al. (2006). Immunohistochemical analysis identifies two cyclin D1+ subsets of plasma cell myeloma, each associated with favorable survival. Am J Clin Pathol. 125:615–24. PMID:16627271

796. Cook LB, Melamed A, Niederer H, et al. (2014). The role of HTLV-1 clonality, proviral structure, and genomic integration site in adult T-cell leukemia/lymphoma. Blood. 123:3925–31. PMID:24735963

797. Cooke CB, Krenacs L, Stetler-Stevenson M, et al. (1996). Hepatosplenic T-cell lymphoma: a distinct clinicopathologic entity of cytotoxic gamma delta T-cell origin. Blood. 88:4265–74. PMID:8943863

798. Cools J, DeAngelo DJ, Gotlib J, et al. (2003). A tyrosine kinase created by fusion of the PDGFRA and FIP1L1 genes as a therapeutic target of imatinib in idiopathic hypereosinophilic syndrome. N Engl J Med. 348:1201–14. PMID:12660384

799. Cools J, Mentens N, Odero MD, et al. (2002). Evidence for position effects as a variant ETV6-mediated leukemogenic mechanism in myeloid leukemias with a t(4;12)(q11-q12;p13) or t(5;12)(q31;p13). Blood. 99:1776–84. PMID:11861295

800. Cools J, Stover EH, Boulton CL, et al. (2003). PKC412 overcomes resistance to imatinib in a murine model of FIP1L1-PDGFRα-induced myeloproliferative disease. Cancer Cell. 3:459–69. PMID:12781364

801. Cools J, Wlodarska I, Somers R, et al. (2002). Identification of novel fusion partners of ALK, the anaplastic lymphoma kinase, in anaplastic large-cell lymphoma and inflammatory myofibroblastic tumor. Genes Chromosomes Cancer. 34:354–62. PMID:12112524

802. Copie-Bergman C, Cuillière-Dartigues P, Baia M, et al. (2015). MYC-IG rearrangements are negative predictors of survival in DLBCL patients treated with immunochemotherapy: a GELA/LYSA study. Blood. 126:2466–74. PMID:26373676

803. Copie-Bergman C, Gaulard P, Maouche-Chrétien L, et al. (1999). The MAL gene is expressed in primary mediastinal large B-cell lymphoma. Blood. 94:3567–75. PMID:10552968

804. Copie-Bergman C, Niedobitek G, Mangham DC, et al. (1997). Epstein-Barr virus

in B-cell lymphomas associated with chronic suppurative inflammation. J Pathol. 183:287–92. PMID:9422983
805. Copie-Bergman C, Plonquet A, Alonso MA, et al. (2002). MAL expression in lymphoid cells: further evidence for MAL as a distinct molecular marker of primary mediastinal large B-cell lymphomas. Mod Pathol. 15:1172–80. PMID:12429796
806. Copie-Bergman C, Wotherspoon AC, Norton AJ, et al. (1998). True histiocytic lymphoma: a morphologic, immunohistochemical, and molecular genetic study of 13 cases. Am J Surg Pathol. 22:1386–92. PMID:9808131
807. Corazzelli G, Capobianco G, Russo F, et al. (2005). Pentostatin (2'-deoxycoformycin) for the treatment of hepatosplenic gammadelta T-cell lymphomas. Haematologica. 90:ECR14. PMID:15753055
808. Corbin AS, Agarwal A, Loriaux M, et al. (2011). Human chronic myeloid leukemia stem cells are insensitive to imatinib despite inhibition of BCR-ABL activity. J Clin Invest. 121:396–409. PMID:21157039
809. Corces-Zimmerman MR, Hong WJ, Weissman IL, et al. (2014). Preleukemic mutations in human acute myeloid leukemia affect epigenetic regulators and persist in remission. Proc Natl Acad Sci U S A. 111:2548–53. PMID:24550281
810. Corcoran MM, Mould SJ, Orchard JA, et al. (1999). Dysregulation of cyclin dependent kinase 6 expression in splenic marginal zone lymphoma through chromosome 7q translocations. Oncogene. 18:6271–7. PMID:10597225
811. Cordeddu V, Yin JC, Gunnarsson C, et al. (2015). Activating Mutations Affecting the Dbl Homology Domain of SOS2 Cause Noonan Syndrome. Hum Mutat. 36:1080–7. PMID:26173643
812. Corey SJ, Locker J, Oliveri DR, et al. (1994). A non-classical translocation involving 17q12 (retinoic acid receptor alpha) in acute promyelocytic leukemia (APML) with atypical features. Leukemia. 8:1350–3. PMID:8057672
813. Coriu D, Weaver K, Schell M, et al. (2004). A molecular basis for nonsecretory myeloma. Blood. 104:829–31. PMID:15090444
814. Corrao G, Corazza GR, Bagnardi V, et al. (2001). Mortality in patients with coeliac disease and their relatives: a cohort study. Lancet. 358:356–61. PMID:11502314
815. Corso A, Lazzarino M, Morra E, et al. (1995). Chronic myelogenous leukemia and exposure to ionizing radiation–a retrospective study of 443 patients. Ann Hematol. 70:79–82. PMID:7880928
816. Cortes J (2003). CMML: a biologically distinct myeloproliferative disease. Curr Hematol Rep. 2:202–8. PMID:12901341
817. Cortes JE, Talpaz M, O'Brien S, et al. (2006). Staging of chronic myeloid leukemia in the imatinib era: an evaluation of the World Health Organization proposal. Cancer. 106:1306–15. PMID:16463391
818. Costa D, Queralt R, Aymerich M, et al. (2003). High levels of chromosomal imbalances in typical and small-cell variants of T-cell prolymphocytic leukemia. Cancer Genet Cytogenet. 147:36–43. PMID:14580769
819. Costes-Martineau V, Delfour C, Obled S, et al. (2002). Anaplastic lymphoma kinase (ALK) protein expressing lymphoma after liver transplantation: case report and literature review. J Clin Pathol. 55:868–71. PMID:12401829
820. Cota C, Vale E, Viana I, et al. (2010). Cutaneous manifestations of blastic plasmacytoid dendritic cell neoplasm-morphologic and phenotypic variability in a series of 33 patients. Am J Surg Pathol. 34:75–87. PMID:19956058
821. Coté TR, Manns A, Hardy CR, et al. (1996). Epidemiology of brain lymphoma among people with or without acquired immunodeficiency syndrome. J Natl Cancer Inst. 88:675–9. PMID:8627644
822. Cotta CV, Bueso-Ramos CE (2007). New insights into the pathobiology and treatment of chronic myelogenous leukemia. Ann Diagn Pathol. 11:68–78. PMID:17240312
823. Cottone M, Termini A, Oliva L, et al. (1999). Mortality and causes of death in celiac disease in a Mediterranean area. Dig Dis Sci. 44:2538–41. PMID:10630509
824. Coupland SE, Charlotte F, Mansour G, et al. (2005). HHV-8-associated T-cell lymphoma in a lymph node with concurrent peritoneal effusion in an HIV-positive man. Am J Surg Pathol. 29:647–52. PMID:15832089
825. Courts C, Montesinos-Rongen M, Brunn A, et al. (2008). Recurrent inactivation of the PRDM1 gene in primary central nervous system lymphoma. J Neuropathol Exp Neurol. 67:720–7. PMID:18596541
826. Courville EL, Sohani AR, Hasserjian RP, et al. (2014). Diverse clinicopathologic features in human herpesvirus 8-associated lymphomas lead to diagnostic problems. Am J Clin Pathol. 142:816–29. PMID:25389336
827. Courville EL, Wu Y, Kourda J, et al. (2013). Clinicopathologic analysis of acute myeloid leukemia arising from chronic myelomonocytic leukemia. Mod Pathol. 26:751–61. PMID:23307061
828. Coustan-Smith E, Mullighan CG, Onciu M, et al. (2009). Early T-cell precursor leukaemia: a subtype of very high-risk acute lymphoblastic leukaemia. Lancet Oncol. 10:147–56. PMID:19147408
829. Coustan-Smith E, Sancho J, Hancock ML, et al. (2000). Clinical importance of minimal residual disease in childhood acute lymphoblastic leukemia. Blood. 96:2691–6. PMID:11023499
830. Coutinho R, Clear AJ, Owen A, et al. (2013). Poor concordance among nine immunohistochemistry classifiers of cell-of-origin for diffuse large B-cell lymphoma: implications for therapeutic strategies. Clin Cancer Res. 19:6686–95. PMID:24122791
831. Cox MC, Nofroni I, Ruco L, et al. (2008). Low absolute lymphocyte count is a poor prognostic factor in diffuse-large-B-cell-lymphoma. Leuk Lymphoma. 49:1745–51. PMID:18798109
832. Craig FE, Johnson LR, Harvey SA, et al. (2007). Gene expression profiling of Epstein-Barr virus-positive and -negative monomorphic B-cell posttransplant lymphoproliferative disorders. Diagn Mol Pathol. 16:158–68. PMID:17721324
833. Cramer P, Hallek M (2011). Prognostic factors in chronic lymphocytic leukemia-what do we need to know? Nat Rev Clin Oncol. 8:38–47. PMID:20956983
834. Crane GM, Ambinder RF, Shirley CM, et al. (2014). HHV-8-positive and EBV-positive intravascular lymphoma: an unusual presentation of extracavitary primary effusion lymphoma. Am J Surg Pathol. 38:426–32. PMID:24525514
835. Crescenzi B, La Starza R, Nozzoli C, et al. (2007). Molecular cytogenetic findings in a four-way t(1;12;5;12)(p36;p13;q33;q24) underlying the ETV6-PDGFRB fusion gene in chronic myelomonocytic leukemia. Cancer Genet Cytogenet. 176:67–71. PMID:17574967
836. Crescenzo R, Abate F, Lasorsa E, et al. (2015). Convergent mutations and kinase fusions lead to oncogenic STAT3 activation in anaplastic large cell lymphoma. Cancer Cell. 27:516–32. PMID:25873174
837. Creutzig U, Harbott J, Sperling C, et al. (1995). Clinical significance of surface antigen expression in children with acute myeloid leukemia: results of study AML-BFM-87. Blood. 86:3097–108. PMID:7579404
838. Criel A, Michaux L, De Wolf-Peeters C (1999). The concept of typical and atypical chronic lymphocytic leukaemia. Leuk Lymphoma. 33:33–45. PMID:10194119
839. Criscione VD, Weinstock MA (2007). Incidence of cutaneous T-cell lymphoma in the United States, 1973-2002. Arch Dermatol. 143:854–9. PMID:17638728
840. Crusoe EdeQ, da Silva AM, Agareno J, et al. (2015). Multiple myeloma: a rare case in an 8-year-old child. Clin Lymphoma Myeloma Leuk. 15:e31–3. PMID:25441111
841. Cuadra-Garcia I, Proulx GM, Wu CL, et al. (1999). Sinonasal lymphoma: a clinicopathologic analysis of 58 cases from the Massachusetts General Hospital. Am J Surg Pathol. 23:1356–69. PMID:10555004
842. Cuadros M, Dave SS, Jaffe ES, et al. (2007). Identification of a proliferation signature related to survival in nodal peripheral T-cell lymphomas. J Clin Oncol. 25:3321–9. PMID:17577022
843. Cuccuini W, Briere J, Mounier N, et al. (2012). MYC+ diffuse large B-cell lymphoma is not salvaged by classical R-ICE or R-DHAP followed by BEAM plus autologous stem cell transplantation. Blood. 119:4619–24. PMID:22408263
844. Cudennec CA, Johnson GR (1981). Presence of multipotential hemopoietic cells in teratocarcinoma cultures. J Embryol Exp Morphol. 61:51–9. PMID:7264551
845. Cui R, Gale RP, Xu Z, et al. (2012). Clinical importance of SF3B1 mutations in Chinese with myelodysplastic syndromes with ring sideroblasts. Leuk Res. 36:1428–33. PMID:22921018
846. Cui Y, Li B, Gale RP, et al. (2014). CSF3R, SETBP1 and CALR mutations in chronic neutrophilic leukemia. J Hematol Oncol. 7:77. PMID:25316523
847. Cuneo A, Bigoni R, Rigolin GM, et al. (1999). Cytogenetic profile of lymphoma of follicle mantle lineage: correlation with clinicobiologic features. Blood. 93:1372–80. PMID:9949181
848. Cunningham D, Hawkes EA, Jack A, et al. (2013). Rituximab plus cyclophosphamide, doxorubicin, vincristine, and prednisolone in patients with newly diagnosed diffuse large B-cell non-Hodgkin lymphoma: a phase 3 comparison of dose intensification with 14-day versus 21-day cycles. Lancet. 381:1817–26. PMID:23615461
848A. Curiel-Olmo S, Mondéjar R, Almaraz CA, et al. (2017). Splenic diffuse red pulp small B-cell lymphoma displays increased expression of cyclin D3 and recurrent CCND3 mutations. Blood. 129:1042-5. PMID:28069605
849. Curtis CE, Grand FH, Musto P, et al. (2007). Two novel imatinib-responsive PDGFRA fusion genes in chronic eosinophilic leukaemia. Br J Haematol. 138:77–81. PMID:17555450
850. Curtis CE, Grand FH, Waghorn K, et al. (2007). A novel ETV6-PDGFRB fusion transcript missed by standard screening in a patient with an imatinib responsive chronic myeloproliferative disease. Leukemia. 21:1839–41. PMID:17508004
851. Curtis RE, Travis LB, Rowlings PA, et al. (1999). Risk of lymphoproliferative disorders after bone marrow transplantation: a multi-institutional study. Blood. 94:2208–16. PMID:10498590
852. Czader M, Orazi A (2009). Therapy-related myeloid neoplasms. Am J Clin Pathol. 132:410–25. PMID:19687318
853. Czader M, Orazi A (2015). Acute Myeloid Leukemia and Other Types of Disease Progression in Myeloproliferative Neoplasms. Am J Clin Pathol. 144:188–206. PMID:26185305
854. Czuchlewski DR, Peterson LC (2016). Myeloid Neoplasms with Germline Predisposition: A New Provisional Entity Within the World Health Organization Classification. Surg Pathol Clin. 9:165–76. PMID:26940275
855. d'Amore F, Relander T, Lauritzsen GF, et al. (2012). Up-front autologous stem-cell transplantation in peripheral T-cell lymphoma: NLG-T-01. J Clin Oncol. 30:3093–9. PMID:22851556
856. D'Souza A, Lacy M, Gertz M, et al. (2012). Long-term outcomes after autologous stem cell transplantation for patients with POEMS syndrome (osteosclerotic myeloma): a single-center experience. Blood. 120:56–62. PMID:22611150
857. Dacic S, Trusky C, Bakker A, et al. (2003). Genotypic analysis of pulmonary Langerhans cell histiocytosis. Hum Pathol. 34:1345–9. PMID:14691922
858. Dalal BI, Horsman DE, Bruyère H, et al. (2007). Imatinib mesylate responsiveness in aggressive systemic mastocytosis: novel association with a platelet derived growth factor receptor beta mutation. Am J Hematol. 82:77–9. PMID:17133421
859. Dalia S, Jaglal M, Chervenick P, et al. (2014). Clinicopathologic characteristics and outcomes of histiocytic and dendritic cell neoplasms: the moffitt cancer center experience over the last twenty five years. Cancers (Basel). 6:2275–95. PMID:25405526
860. Dalia S, Shao H, Sagatys E, et al. (2014). Dendritic cell and histiocytic neoplasms: biology, diagnosis, and treatment. Cancer Control. 21:290–300. PMID:25310210
861. Dalle S, Beylot-Barry M, Bagot M, et al. (2010). Blastic plasmacytoid dendritic cell neoplasm: is transplantation the treatment of choice? Br J Dermatol. 162:74–9. PMID:19689477
862. Dallenbach FE, Stein H (1989). Expression of T-cell-receptor beta chain in Reed-Sternberg cells. Lancet. 2:828–30. PMID:2477655
863. Damle RN, Wasil T, Fais F, et al. (1999). Ig V gene mutation status and CD38 expression as novel prognostic indicators in chronic lymphocytic leukemia. Blood. 94:1840–7. PMID:10477712
864. Damm F, Kosmider O, Gelsi-Boyer V, et al. (2012). Mutations affecting mRNA splicing define distinct clinical phenotypes and correlate with patient outcome in myelodysplastic syndromes. Blood. 119:3211–8. PMID:22343920
864A. Damm F, Markus B, Thol F, et al. (2014). TET2 mutations in cytogenetically normal acute myeloid leukemia: clinical implications and evolutionary patterns. Genes Chromosomes Cancer. 53:824–32. PMID:24898826
865. Damm-Welk C, Mussolin L, Zimmermann M, et al. (2014). Early assessment of minimal residual disease identifies patients at very high relapse risk in NPM-ALK-positive anaplastic large-cell lymphoma. Blood. 123:334–7. PMID:24297868
866. Dang H, Chen Y, Kamel-Reid S, et al. (2013). CD34 expression predicts an adverse outcome in patients with NPM1-positive acute myeloid leukemia. Hum Pathol. 44:2038–46. PMID:23701943
867. Dao LN, Hanson CA, Dispenzieri A, et al. (2011). Bone marrow histopathology in POEMS syndrome: a distinctive combination of plasma cell, lymphoid, and myeloid findings in 87 patients. Blood. 117:6438–44. PMID:21385854
868. Darenkov IA, Marcarelli MA, Basadonna GP, et al. (1997). Reduced incidence of Epstein-Barr virus-associated posttransplant lymphoproliferative disorder using preemptive antiviral therapy. Transplantation. 64:848–52. PMID:9326409
869. Dargent JL, Delannoy A, Pieron P, et al. (2011). Cutaneous accumulation of plasmacytoid dendritic cells associated with acute myeloid leukemia: a rare condition distinct from

blastic plasmacytoid dendritic cell neoplasm. J Cutan Pathol. 38:893–8. PMID:21883371
870. Dargent JL, Henne S, Pranger D, et al. (2016). Tumor-forming plasmacytoid dendritic cells associated with myeloid neoplasms. Report of a peculiar case with histopathologic features masquerading as lupus erythematosus. J Cutan Pathol. 43:280–6 PMID:26449631
871. Dash A, Gilliland DG (2001). Molecular genetics of acute myeloid leukaemia. Best Pract Res Clin Haematol. 14:49–64. PMID:11355923
872. Dastugue N, Duchayne E, Kuhlein E, et al. (1997). Acute basophilic leukaemia and translocation t(X;6)(p11;q23). Br J Haematol. 98:170–6. PMID:9233581
873. Dastugue N, Lafage-Pochitaloff M, Pagès MP, et al. (2002). Cytogenetic profile of childhood and adult megakaryoblastic leukemia (M7): a study of the Groupe Français de Cytogénétique Hématologique (GFCH). Blood. 100:618–26. PMID:12091356
874. Daum S, Cellier C, Mulder CJ (2005). Refractory coeliac disease. Best Pract Res Clin Gastroenterol. 19:413–24. PMID:15925846
875. Daum S, Ipczynski R, Schumann M, et al. (2009). High rates of complications and substantial mortality in both types of refractory sprue. Eur J Gastroenterol Hepatol. 21:66–70. PMID:19011576
876. Daum S, Ullrich R, Heise W, et al. (2003). Intestinal non-Hodgkin's lymphoma: a multicenter prospective clinical study from the German Study Group on Intestinal non-Hodgkin's Lymphoma. J Clin Oncol. 21:2740–6. PMID:12860953
877. Dave SS, Fu K, Wright GW, et al. (2006). Molecular diagnosis of Burkitt's lymphoma. N Engl J Med. 354:2431–42. PMID:16760443
878. Dave SS, Wright G, Tan B, et al. (2004). Prediction of survival in follicular lymphoma based on molecular features of tumor-infiltrating immune cells. N Engl J Med. 351:2159–69. PMID:15548776
879. Daver N, Kantarjian H, Marcucci G, et al. (2015). Clinical characteristics and outcomes in patients with acute promyelocytic leukaemia and hyperleucocytosis. Br J Haematol. 168:646–53. PMID:25312977
880. Daver N, Strati P, Jabbour E, et al. (2013). FLT3 mutations in myelodysplastic syndrome and chronic myelomonocytic leukemia. Am J Hematol. 88:56–9. PMID:23115106
881. Davi F, Delecluse HJ, Guiet P, et al. (1998). Burkitt-like lymphomas in AIDS patients: characterization within a series of 103 human immunodeficiency virus-associated non-Hodgkin's lymphomas. J Clin Oncol. 16:3788–95. PMID:9850023
882. David JA, Huang JZ (2016). Diagnostic Utility of Flow Cytometry Analysis of Reactive T Cells in Nodular Lymphocyte-Predominant Hodgkin Lymphoma. Am J Clin Pathol. 145:107–15. PMID:26712878
883. David M, Cross NC, Burgstaller S, et al. (2007). Durable responses to imatinib in patients with PDGFRB fusion gene-positive and BCR-ABL-negative chronic myeloproliferative disorders. Blood. 109:61–4. PMID:16960151
884. Davies AJ, Rosenwald A, Wright G, et al. (2007). Transformation of follicular lymphoma to diffuse large B-cell lymphoma proceeds by distinct oncogenic mechanisms. Br J Haematol. 136:286–93. PMID:17278262
885. Davis KL, Marina N, Arber DA, et al. (2013). Pediatric acute myeloid leukemia as classified using 2008 WHO criteria: a single-center experience. Am J Clin Pathol. 139:818–25. PMID:23690127
886. Davis RE, Ngo VN, Lenz G, et al. (2010). Chronic active B-cell-receptor signalling in diffuse large B-cell lymphoma. Nature. 463:88–92. PMID:20054396
887. Davis TH, Morton CC, Miller-Cassman R, et al. (1992). Hodgkin's disease, lymphomatoid papulosis, and cutaneous T-cell lymphoma derived from a common T-cell clone. N Engl J Med. 326:1115–22. PMID:1532439
888. de Baaij LR, Berkhof J, van de Water JM, et al. (2015). A New and Validated Clinical Prognostic Model (EPI) for Enteropathy-Associated T-cell Lymphoma. Clin Cancer Res. 21:3013–9. PMID:25779949
889. de Boer CJ, van Krieken JH, Kluin-Nelemans HC, et al. (1995). Cyclin D1 messenger RNA overexpression as a marker for mantle cell lymphoma. Oncogene. 10:1833–40. PMID:7753558
890. De Brabander M, Schaper W (1971). Quantitative histology of the canine coronary collateral circulation in localized myocardial ischemia. Life Sci I. 10:857–68. PMID:4935723
891. de Bruin PC, Beljaards RC, van Heerde P, et al. (1993). Differences in clinical behaviour and immunophenotype between primary cutaneous and primary nodal anaplastic large cell lymphoma of T-cell or null cell phenotype. Histopathology. 23:127–35. PMID:8406384
892. de Coninck EC, Kim YH, Varghese A, et al. (2001). Clinical characteristics and outcome of patients with extracutaneous mycosis fungoides. J Clin Oncol. 19:779–84. PMID:11157031
893. De Filippi P, Badulli C, Cuccia M, et al. (2006). Specific polymorphisms of cytokine genes are associated with different risks to develop single-system or multi-system childhood Langerhans cell histiocytosis. Br J Haematol. 132:784–7. PMID:16487180
894. De J, Zanjani R, Hibbard M, et al. (2007). Immunophenotypic profile predictive of KIT activating mutations in AML1-ETO leukemia. Am J Clin Pathol. 128:550–7. PMID:17875504
895. de Jong D, Vasmel WL, de Boer JP, et al. (2008). Anaplastic large-cell lymphoma in women with breast implants. JAMA. 300:2030–5. PMID:18984890
896. De Jong D, Voetdijk BM, Beverstock GC, et al. (1988). Activation of the c-myc oncogene in a precursor-B-cell blast crisis of follicular lymphoma, presenting as composite lymphoma. N Engl J Med. 318:1373–8. PMID:3285208
897. De Keersmaecker K, Marynen P, Cools J (2005). Genetic insights in the pathogenesis of T-cell acute lymphoblastic leukemia. Haematologica. 90:1116–27. PMID:16079112
898. de Leval L, Bonnet C, Copie-Bergman C, et al. (2012). Diffuse large B-cell lymphoma of Waldeyer's ring has distinct clinicopathologic features: a GELA study. Ann Oncol. 23:3143–51. PMID:22700993
899. de Leval L, Ferry JA, Falini B, et al. (2001). Expression of bcl-6 and CD10 in primary mediastinal large B-cell lymphoma: evidence for derivation from germinal center B cells? Am J Surg Pathol. 25:1277–82. PMID:11688462
900. de Leval L, Gaulard P (2014). Cellular origin of T-cell lymphomas. Blood. 123:2909–10. PMID:24810625
901. de Leval L, Gisselbrecht C, Gaulard P (2010). Advances in the understanding and management of angioimmunoblastic T-cell lymphoma. Br J Haematol. 148:673–89. PMID:19961485
902. de Leval L, Harris NL (2003). Variability in immunophenotype in diffuse large B-cell lymphoma and its clinical relevance. Histopathology. 43:509–28. PMID:14636252
903. de Leval L, Harris NL, Longtine J, et al. (2001). Cutaneous b-cell lymphomas of follicular and marginal zone types: use of Bcl-6, CD10, Bcl-2, and CD21 in differential diagnosis and classification. Am J Surg Pathol. 25:732–41. PMID:11395550
904. de Leval L, Parrens M, Le Bras F, et al. (2015). Angioimmunoblastic T-cell lymphoma is the most common T-cell lymphoma in two distinct French information data sets. Haematologica. 100:e361–4. PMID:26045291
905. de Leval L, Rickman DS, Thielen C, et al. (2007). The gene expression profile of nodal peripheral T-cell lymphoma demonstrates a molecular link between angioimmunoblastic T-cell lymphoma (AITL) and follicular helper T (TFH) cells. Blood. 109:4952–63. PMID:17284527
906. de Leval L, Savilo E, Longtine J, et al. (2001). Peripheral T-cell lymphoma with follicular involvement and a CD4+/bcl-6+ phenotype. Am J Surg Pathol. 25:395–400. PMID:11224611
907. De Paepe P, Baens M, van Krieken H, et al. (2003). ALK activation by the CLTC-ALK fusion is a recurrent event in large B-cell lymphoma. Blood. 102:2638–41. PMID:12750159
908. De Re V, De Vita S, Marzotto A, et al. (2000). Sequence analysis of the immunoglobulin antigen receptor of hepatitis C virus-associated non-Hodgkin lymphomas suggests that the malignant cells are derived from the rheumatoid factor-producing cells that occur mainly in type II cryoglobulinemia. Blood. 96:3578–84. PMID:11071657
908A. de Rooij JD, Hollink IH, Arentsen-Peters ST, et al. (2013). NUP98/JARID1A is a novel recurrent abnormality in pediatric acute megakaryoblastic leukemia with a distinct HOX gene expression pattern. Leukemia. 27:2280–8. PMID:23531517
909. de Sanjose S, Benavente Y, Vajdic CM, et al. (2008). Hepatitis C and non-Hodgkin lymphoma among 4784 cases and 6269 controls from the International Lymphoma Epidemiology Consortium. Clin Gastroenterol Hepatol. 6:451–8. PMID:18387498
910. de Souza A, el-Azhary RA, Camilleri MJ, et al. (2012). In search of prognostic indicators for lymphomatoid papulosis: a retrospective study of 123 patients. J Am Acad Dermatol. 66:928–37. PMID:21982062
911. de Thé H, Chomienne C, Lanotte M, et al. (1990). The t(15;17) translocation of acute promyelocytic leukaemia fuses the retinoic acid receptor alpha gene to a novel transcribed locus. Nature. 347:558–61. PMID:2170850
912. De Vita S, Sacco C, Sansonno D, et al. (1997). Characterization of overt B-cell lymphomas in patients with hepatitis C virus infection. Blood. 90:776–82. PMID:9226178
913. De Wolf-Peeters C, Achten R (2000). Anaplastic large cell lymphoma: what's in a name? J Clin Pathol. 53:407–8. PMID:10911796
914. De Zen L, Orfao A, Cazzaniga G, et al. (2000). Quantitative multiparametric immunophenotyping in acute lymphoblastic leukemia: correlation with specific genotype. I. ETV6/AML1 ALLs identification. Leukemia. 14:1225–31. PMID:10914546
915. de-Thé G, Geser A, Day NE, et al. (1978). Epidemiological evidence for causal relationship between Epstein-Barr virus and Burkitt's lymphoma from Ugandan prospective study. Nature. 274:756–61. PMID:210392
916. Dearden CE (2006). T-cell prolymphocytic leukemia. Med Oncol. 23:17–22. PMID:16645226
917. Dearden CE, Matutes E, Cazin B, et al. (2001). High remission rate in T-cell prolymphocytic leukemia with CAMPATH-1H. Blood. 98:1721–6. PMID:11535503
918. Deckert M, Brunn A, Montesinos-Rongen M, et al. (2014). Primary lymphoma of the central nervous system–a diagnostic challenge. Hematol Oncol. 32:57–67. PMID:23949943
919. Deckert M, Engert A, Brück W, et al. (2011). Modern concepts in the biology, diagnosis, differential diagnosis and treatment of primary central nervous system lymphoma. Leukemia. 25:1797–807. PMID:21818113
920. DeCoteau JF, Butmarc JR, Kinney MC, et al. (1996). The t(2;5) chromosomal translocation is not a common feature of primary cutaneous CD30+ lymphoproliferative disorders: comparison with anaplastic large-cell lymphoma of nodal origin. Blood. 87:3437–41. PMID:8605362
921. Dedic K (2003). Hairy cell leukemia: an autopsy study. Acta Medica (Hradec Kralove). 46:175–7. PMID:14965169
922. Deepak P, Sifuentes H, Sherid M, et al. (2013). T-cell non-Hodgkin's lymphomas reported to the FDA AERS with tumor necrosis factor-alpha (TNF-α) inhibitors: results of the REFURBISH study. Am J Gastroenterol. 108:99–105. PMID:23032984
923. Deffis-Court M, Alvarado-Ibarra M, Ruiz-Argüelles GJ, et al. (2014). Diagnosing and treating mixed phenotype acute leukemia: a multicenter 10-year experience in México. Ann Hematol. 93:595–601. PMID:24146232
925. Dehner LP (2003). Juvenile xanthogranulomas in the first two decades of life: a clinicopathologic study of 174 cases with cutaneous and extracutaneous manifestations. Am J Surg Pathol. 27:579–93. PMID:12717244
926. Dekmezian R, Kantarjian HM, Keating MJ, et al. (1987). The relevance of reticulin stain-measured fibrosis at diagnosis in chronic myelogenous leukemia. Cancer. 59:1739–43. PMID:2435399
927. Del Giudice I, Davis Z, Matutes E, et al. (2006). IgVH genes mutation and usage, ZAP-70 and CD38 expression provide new insights on B-cell prolymphocytic leukemia (B-PLL). Leukemia. 20:1231–7. PMID:16642047
928. Del Giudice I, Messina M, Chiaretti S, et al. (2012). Behind the scenes of non-nodal MCL: downmodulation of genes involved in actin cytoskeleton organization, cell projection, cell adhesion, tumour invasion, TP53 pathway and mutated status of immunoglobulin heavy chain genes. Br J Haematol. 156:601–11. PMID:22150124
929. Del Giudice I, Osuji N, Dexter T, et al. (2009). B-cell prolymphocytic leukemia and chronic lymphocytic leukemia have distinctive gene expression signatures. Leukemia. 23:2160–7. PMID:19641528
930. del Rey M, Benito R, Fontanillo C, et al. (2015). Deregulation of genes related to iron and mitochondrial metabolism in refractory anemia with ring sideroblasts. PLoS One. 10:e0126555. PMID:25955609
931. Delabesse E, Bernard M, Meyer V, et al. (1998). TAL1 expression does not occur in the majority of T-ALL blasts. Br J Haematol. 102:449–57. PMID:9695959
932. Delabie J, Holte H, Vose JM, et al. (2011). Enteropathy-associated T-cell lymphoma: clinical and histological findings from the international peripheral T-cell lymphoma project. Blood. 118:148–55. PMID:21566094
933. Delas A, Sophie D, Brousset P, et al. (2013). Unusual concomitant rearrangements of Cyclin D1 and MYC genes in blastoid variant of mantle cell lymphoma: Case report and review of literature. Pathol Res Pract. 209:115–9. PMID:23313364
934. Delauche-Cavallier MC, Laredo JD, Wybier M, et al. (1988). Solitary plasmacytoma of the spine. Long-term clinical course. Cancer. 61:1707–14. PMID:3349431
935. Delaunay J, Vey N, Leblanc T, et al. (2003). Prognosis of inv(16)/t(16;16) acute myeloid leukemia (AML): a survey of 110 cases from the French AML Intergroup. Blood. 102:462–9. PMID:12649129
936. Delecluse HJ, Anagnostopoulos I, Dallenbach F, et al. (1997). Plasmablastic lymphomas of the oral cavity: a new entity associated with

the human immunodeficiency virus infection. Blood. 89:1413–20. PMID:9028965
937. Deleeuw RJ, Zettl A, Klinker E, et al. (2007). Whole-genome analysis and HLA genotyping of enteropathy-type T-cell lymphoma reveals 2 distinct lymphoma subtypes. Gastroenterology. 132:1902–11. PMID:17484883
938. Delfau-Larue MH, de Leval L, Joly B, et al. (2012). Targeting intratumoral B cells with rituximab in addition to CHOP in angioimmunoblastic T-cell lymphoma. A clinicobiological study of the GELA. Haematologica. 97:1594–602. PMID:22371178
939. Delfau-Larue MH, Klapper W, Berger F, et al. (2015). High-dose cytarabine does not overcome the adverse prognostic value of CDKN2A and TP53 deletions in mantle cell lymphoma. Blood. 126:604–11. PMID:26022239
940. Delgado J, Salaverria I, Baumann T, et al. (2014). Genomic complexity and IGHV mutational status are key predictors of outcome of chronic lymphocytic leukemia patients with TP53 disruption. Haematologica. 99:e231–4. PMID:24997154
941. Della Porta MG, Malcovati L (2011). Myelodysplastic syndromes with bone marrow fibrosis. Haematologica. 96:180–3. PMID:21282718
942. Della Porta MG, Malcovati L, Boveri E, et al. (2009). Clinical relevance of bone marrow fibrosis and CD34-positive cell clusters in primary myelodysplastic syndromes. J Clin Oncol. 27:754–62. PMID:19103730
943. Della Porta MG, Malcovati L, Galli A, et al. (2005). Mitochondrial ferritin expression and clonality of hematopoiesis in patients with refractory anemia with ringed sideroblasts. Blood. 106:3444.
944. Della Porta MG, Malcovati L, Invernizzi R, et al. (2006). Flow cytometry evaluation of erythroid dysplasia in patients with myelodysplastic syndrome. Leukemia. 20:549–55. PMID:16498394
945. Della Porta MG, Picone C, Pascutto C, et al. (2012). Multicenter validation of a reproducible flow cytometric score for the diagnosis of low-grade myelodysplastic syndromes: results of a European LeukemiaNET study. Haematologica. 97:1209–17. PMID:22315489
946. Della Porta MG, Picone C, Tenore A, et al. (2014). Prognostic significance of reproducible immunophenotypic markers of marrow dysplasia. Haematologica. 99:e8–10. PMID:24425693
947. Della Porta MG, Travaglino E, Boveri E, et al. (2015). Minimal morphological criteria for defining bone marrow dysplasia: a basis for clinical implementation of WHO classification of myelodysplastic syndromes. Leukemia. 29:66–75. PMID:24935723
948. Della Porta MG, Tuechler H, Malcovati L, et al. (2015). Validation of WHO classification-based Prognostic Scoring System (WPSS) for myelodysplastic syndromes and comparison with the revised International Prognostic Scoring System (IPSS-R). A study of the International Working Group for Prognosis in Myelodysplasia (IWG-PM). Leukemia. 29:1502–13. PMID:25721895
949. Delsol G, Al Saati T, Gatter KC, et al. (1988). Coexpression of epithelial membrane antigen (EMA), Ki-1, and interleukin-2 receptor by anaplastic large cell lymphomas. Diagnostic value in so-called malignant histiocytosis. Am J Pathol. 130:59–70. PMID:2827494
950. Delsol G, Brousset P, Chittal S, et al. (1992). Correlation of the expression of Epstein-Barr virus latent membrane protein and in situ hybridization with biotinylated BamHI-W probes in Hodgkin's disease. Am J Pathol. 140:247–53. PMID:1310829
951. Delsol G, Lamant L, Mariamé B, et al. (1997). A new subtype of large B-cell lymphoma expressing the ALK kinase and lacking the 2; 5 translocation. Blood. 89:1483–90. PMID:9057627
952. deMent SH (1990). Association between mediastinal germ cell tumors and hematologic malignancies: an update. Hum Pathol. 21:699–703. PMID:2163361
953. Demirkesen C, Tüzüner N, Esen T, et al. (2011). The expression of IgM is helpful in the differentiation of primary cutaneous diffuse large B cell lymphoma and follicle center lymphoma. Leuk Res. 35:1269–72. PMID:21700336
954. Deng L, Xu-Monette ZY, Loghavi S, et al. (2016). Primary testicular diffuse large B-cell lymphoma displays distinct clinical and biological features for treatment failure in rituximab era: a report from the International PTL Consortium. Leukemia. 30:361–72. PMID:26308769
955. DePond W, Said JW, Tasaka T, et al. (1997). Kaposi's sarcoma-associated herpesvirus and human herpesvirus 8 (KSHV/HHV8)-associated lymphoma of the bowel. Report of two cases in HIV-positive men with secondary effusion lymphomas. Am J Surg Pathol. 21:719–24. PMID:9199651
956. Dereure O, Cheval J, Du Thanh A, et al. (2013). No evidence for viral sequences in mycosis fungoides and Sézary syndrome skin lesions: a high-throughput sequencing approach. J Invest Dermatol. 133:853–5. PMID:23096719
957. Derringer GA, Thompson LD, Frommelt RA, et al. (2000). Malignant lymphoma of the thyroid gland: a clinicopathologic study of 108 cases. Am J Surg Pathol. 24:623–39. PMID:10800981
958. Desai M, Liu S, Parker S (2015). Clinical characteristics, prognostic factors, and survival of 393 patients with mycosis fungoides and Sézary syndrome in the southeastern United States: a single-institution cohort. J Am Acad Dermatol. 72:276–85. PMID:25458019
959. Desar IM, Keuter M, Raemaekers JM, et al. (2006). Extranodal marginal zone (MALT) lymphoma in common variable immunodeficiency. Neth J Med. 64:136–40. PMID:16702611
960. Deschler B, Lübbert M (2006). Acute myeloid leukemia: epidemiology and etiology. Cancer. 107:2099–107. PMID:17019734
961. Despouy G, Joiner M, Le Toriellec E, et al. (2007). The TCL1 oncoprotein inhibits activation-induced cell death by impairing PKCtheta and ERK pathways. Blood. 110:4406–16. PMID:17846228
962. Determann O, Hoster E, Ott G, et al. (2008). Ki-67 predicts outcome in advanced-stage mantle cell lymphoma patients treated with anti-CD20 immunochemotherapy: results from randomized trials of the European MCL Network and the German Low Grade Lymphoma Study Group. Blood. 111:2385–7. PMID:18077791
963. Devillier R, Gelsi-Boyer V, Brecqueville M, et al. (2012). Acute myeloid leukemia with myelodysplasia-related changes are characterized by a specific molecular pattern with high frequency of ASXL1 mutations. Am J Hematol. 87:659–62. PMID:22535592
964. Devillier R, Mansat-De Mas V, Gelsi-Boyer V, et al. (2015). Role of ASXL1 and TP53 mutations in the molecular classification and prognosis of acute myeloid leukemias with myelodysplasia-related changes. Oncotarget. 6:8388–96. PMID:25860933
965. DeVita VT Jr, Simon RM, Hubbard SM, et al. (1980). Curability of advanced Hodgkin's disease with chemotherapy. Long-term follow-up of MOPP-treated patients at the National Cancer Institute. Ann Intern Med. 92:587–95. PMID:6892984
966. Dharnidharka VR, Tejani AH, Ho PL, et al. (2002). Post-transplant lymphoproliferative disorder in the United States: young Caucasian males are at highest risk. Am J Transplant. 2:993–8. PMID:12482154
967. Dhodapkar MV, Li CY, Lust JA, et al. (1994). Clinical spectrum of clonal proliferations of T-large granular lymphocytes: a T-cell clonopathy of undetermined significance? Blood. 84:1620–7. PMID:8068951
968. Dhodapkar MV, Merlini G, Solomon A (1997). Biology and therapy of immunoglobulin deposition diseases. Hematol Oncol Clin North Am. 11:89–110. PMID:9081206
969. Dhodapkar MV, Sexton R, Waheed S, et al. (2014). Clinical, genomic, and imaging predictors of myeloma progression from asymptomatic monoclonal gammopathies (SWOG S0120). Blood. 123:78–85. PMID:24144643
970. Di Donato C, Croci G, Lazzari S, et al. (1986). Chronic neutrophilic leukemia: description of a new case with karyotypic abnormalities. Am J Clin Pathol. 85:369–71. PMID:3463191
971. Di Napoli A, Giubettini M, Duranti E, et al. (2011). Iatrogenic EBV-positive lymphoproliferative disorder with features of EBV+ mucocutaneous ulcer: evidence for concomitant TCRγ/IGH rearrangements in the Hodgkin-like neoplastic cells. Virchows Arch. 458:631–6. PMID:21399965
972. Diab A, Zickl L, Abdel-Wahab O, et al. (2013). Acute myeloid leukemia with translocation t(8;16) presents with features which mimic acute promyelocytic leukemia and is associated with poor prognosis. Leuk Res. 37:32–6. PMID:23102703
973. Diamandidou E, Colome M, Fayad L, et al. (1999). Prognostic factor analysis in mycosis fungoides/Sézary syndrome. J Am Acad Dermatol. 40:914–24. PMID:10365922
974. Diamond C, Taylor TH, Im T, et al. (2006). Presentation and outcomes of systemic non-Hodgkin's lymphoma: a comparison between patients with acquired immunodeficiency syndrome (AIDS) treated with highly active antiretroviral therapy and patients without AIDS. Leuk Lymphoma. 47:1822–9. PMID:17064995
974A. Diamond EL, Dagna L, Hyman DM, et al. (2014). Consensus guidelines for the diagnosis and clinical management of Erdheim-Chester disease. Blood. 124:483–92. PMID:24850756
974B. Díaz-Beyá M, Brunet S, Nomdedéu J, et al. (2015). The expression level of BAALC-associated microRNA miR-3151 is an independent prognostic factor in younger patients with cytogenetic intermediate-risk acute myeloid leukemia. Blood Cancer J. 5:e352. PMID:26430723
975. Díaz-Beyá M, Rozman M, Pratcorona M, et al. (2010). The prognostic value of multilineage dysplasia in de novo acute myeloid leukemia patients with intermediate-risk cytogenetics is dependent on NPM1 mutational status. Blood. 116:6147–8. PMID:21183700
976. Dicker F, Haferlach C, Kern W, et al. (2007). Trisomy 13 is strongly associated with AML1/RUNX1 mutations and increased FLT3 expression in acute myeloid leukemia. Blood. 110:1308–16. PMID:17485549
977. Dickinson RE, Griffin H, Bigley V, et al. (2011). Exome sequencing identifies GATA-2 mutation as the cause of dendritic cell, monocyte, B and NK lymphoid deficiency. Blood. 118:2656–8. PMID:21765025
978. Dickinson RE, Milne P, Jardine L, et al. (2014). The evolution of cellular deficiency in GATA2 mutation. Blood. 123:863–74. PMID:24345756
979. Diehl V, Engert A, Re D (2007). New strategies for the treatment of advanced-stage Hodgkin's lymphoma. Hematol Oncol Clin North Am. 21:897–914. PMID:17908627
980. Diehl V, Sextro M, Franklin J, et al. (1999). Clinical presentation, course, and prognostic factors in lymphocyte-predominant Hodgkin's disease and lymphocyte-rich classical Hodgkin's disease: report from the European Task Force on Lymphoma Project on Lymphocyte-Predominant Hodgkin's Disease. J Clin Oncol. 17:776–83. PMID:10071266
981. Dierickx D, Tousseyn T, Sagaert X, et al. (2013). Single-center analysis of biopsy-confirmed posttransplant lymphoproliferative disorder: incidence, clinicopathological characteristics and prognostic factors. Leuk Lymphoma. 54:2433–40. PMID:23442063
982. Dierlamm J, Baens M, Wlodarska I, et al. (1999). The apoptosis inhibitor gene API2 and a novel 18q gene, MLT, are recurrently rearranged in the t(11;18)(q21;q21) associated with mucosa-associated lymphoid tissue lymphomas. Blood. 93:3601–9. PMID:10339464
983. Dierlamm J, Wlodarska I, Michaux L, et al. (2000). Genetic abnormalities in marginal zone B-cell lymphoma. Hematol Oncol. 18:1–13. PMID:10797525
984. Dietrich S, Andrulis M, Hegenbart U, et al. (2011). Blastic plasmacytoid dendritic cell neoplasia (BPDC) in elderly patients: results of a treatment algorithm employing allogeneic stem cell transplantation with moderately reduced conditioning intensity. Biol Blood Marrow Transplant. 17:1250–4. PMID:21215813
985. DiGiuseppe JA, Louie DC, Williams JE, et al. (1997). Blastic natural killer cell leukemia/lymphoma: a clinicopathologic study. Am J Surg Pathol. 21:1223–30. PMID:9331296
986. Dijkman R, Tensen CP, Jordanova ES, et al. (2006). Array-based comparative genomic hybridization analysis reveals recurrent chromosomal alterations and prognostic parameters in primary cutaneous large B-cell lymphoma. J Clin Oncol. 24:296–305. PMID:16330669
987. Dijkman R, van Doorn R, Szuhai K, et al. (2007). Gene-expression profiling and array-based CGH classify CD4+CD56+ hematodermic neoplasm and cutaneous myelomonocytic leukemia as distinct disease entities. Blood. 109:1720–7. PMID:17068154
988. Dimopoulos M, Terpos E, Comenzo RL, et al. (2009). International myeloma working group consensus statement and guidelines regarding the current role of imaging techniques in the diagnosis and monitoring of multiple Myeloma. Leukemia. 23:1545–56. PMID:19421229
989. Dimopoulos MA, Hamilos G (2002). Solitary bone plasmacytoma and extramedullary plasmacytoma. Curr Treat Options Oncol. 3:255–9. PMID:12057071
990. Dimopoulos MA, Kiamouris C, Moulopoulos LA (1999). Solitary plasmacytoma of bone and extramedullary plasmacytoma. Hematol Oncol Clin North Am. 13:1249–57. PMID:10626148
991. Dimopoulos MA, Kyle RA, Anagnostopoulos A, et al. (2005). Diagnosis and management of Waldenstrom's macroglobulinemia. J Clin Oncol. 23:1564–77. PMID:15735132
992. Dimopoulos MA, Moulopoulos LA, Maniatis A, et al. (2000). Solitary plasmacytoma of bone and asymptomatic multiple myeloma. Blood. 96:2037–44. PMID:10979944
993. Dimopoulos MA, Palumbo A, Delasalle KB, et al. (1994). Primary plasma cell leukaemia. Br J Haematol. 88:754–9. PMID:7819100
994. DiNardo CD, Daver N, Jain N, et al. (2014). Myelodysplastic/myeloproliferative neoplasms, unclassifiable (MDS/MPN, U): natural history and clinical outcome by treatment strategy. Leukemia. 28:958–61. PMID:24492324
995. Dinçol G, Nalçaci M, Doğan O, et al. (2002). Coexistence of chronic neutrophilic leukemia with multiple myeloma. Leuk Lymphoma. 43:649–51. PMID:12002774
996. Dingli D, Grand FH, Mahaffey V, et al. (2005). Der(6)t(1;6)(q21-23;p21.3): a specific

cytogenetic abnormality in myelofibrosis with myeloid metaplasia. Br J Haematol. 130:229–32. PMID:16029451
997. Dingli D, Kyle RA, Rajkumar SV, et al. (2006). Immunoglobulin free light chains and solitary plasmacytoma of bone. Blood. 108:1979–83. PMID:16741249
998. Dingli D, Mesa RA, Tefferi A (2004). Myelofibrosis with myeloid metaplasia: new developments in pathogenesis and treatment. Intern Med. 43:540–7. PMID:15335177
999. Dinmohamed AG, van Norden Y, Visser O, et al. (2015). The use of medical claims to assess incidence, diagnostic procedures and initial treatment of myelodysplastic syndromes and chronic myelomonocytic leukemia in the Netherlands. Leuk Res. 39:177–82. PMID:25533930
1000. Dirnhofer S, Angeles-Angeles A, Ortiz-Hidalgo C, et al. (1999). High prevalence of a 30-base pair deletion in the Epstein-Barr virus (EBV) latent membrane protein 1 gene and of strain type B EBV in Mexican classical Hodgkin's disease and reactive lymphoid tissue. Hum Pathol. 30:781–7. PMID:10414496
1001. Dispenzieri A (2007). POEMS syndrome. Blood Rev. 21:285–99. PMID:17850941
1002. Dispenzieri A (2008). Castleman disease. Cancer Treat Res. 142:293–330. PMID:18283792
1003. Dispenzieri A (2014). POEMS syndrome: 2014 update on diagnosis, risk-stratification, and management. Am J Hematol. 89:214–23. PMID:24532337
1004. Dispenzieri A, Katzmann JA, Kyle RA, et al. (2010). Prevalence and risk of progression of light-chain monoclonal gammopathy of undetermined significance: a retrospective population-based cohort study. Lancet. 375:1721–8. PMID:20472173
1005. Dispenzieri A, Kyle RA, Katzmann JA, et al. (2008). Immunoglobulin free light chain ratio is an independent risk factor for progression of smoldering (asymptomatic) multiple myeloma. Blood. 111:785–9. PMID:17942755
1006. Dispenzieri A, Kyle RA, Lacy MQ, et al. (2003). POEMS syndrome: definitions and long-term outcome. Blood. 101:2496–506. PMID:12456500
1007. Dispenzieri A, Stewart AK, Chanan-Khan A, et al. (2013). Smoldering multiple myeloma requiring treatment: time for a new definition? Blood. 122:4172–81. PMID:24144641
1008. Dittmer DP (2014). Not like a wrecking ball: EBV fine-tunes MYC lymphomagenesis. Blood. 123:460–1. PMID:24458272
1009. Dixon N, Kishnani PS, Zimmerman S (2006). Clinical manifestations of hematologic and oncologic disorders in patients with Down syndrome. Am J Med Genet C Semin Med Genet. 142C:149–57. PMID:17048354
1010. Djokic M, Le Beau MM, Swinnen LJ, et al. (2006). Post-transplant lymphoproliferative disorder subtypes correlate with different recurring chromosomal abnormalities. Genes Chromosomes Cancer. 45:313–8. PMID:16283619
1010A. Dobay MP, Lemonnier F, Missiaglia E, et al. (2017). Integrative clinicopathological and molecular analyses of angioimmunoblastic T-cell lymphoma and other nodal lymphomas of follicular helper T-cell origin. Haematologica 102:e148-e151. PMID:28082343.
1011. Dobo I, Boiret N, Lippert E, et al. (2004). A standardized endogenous megakaryocytic erythroid colony assay for the diagnosis of essential thrombocythemia. Haematologica. 89:1207–12. PMID:15477205
1012. Doeden K, Molina-Kirsch H, Perez E, et al. (2008). Hydroa-like lymphoma with CD56 expression. J Cutan Pathol. 35:488–94. PMID:17976208
1013. Dogan A, Attygalle AD, Kyriakou C (2003). Angioimmunoblastic T-cell lymphoma. Br J Haematol. 121:681–91. PMID:12780782
1014. Dogan A, Burke JS, Goteri G, et al. (2003). Micronodular T-cell/histiocyte-rich large B-cell lymphoma of the spleen: histology, immunophenotype, and differential diagnosis. Am J Surg Pathol. 27:903–11. PMID:12826882
1015. Dogan A, Du MQ, Aiello A, et al. (1998). Follicular lymphomas contain a clonally linked but phenotypically distinct neoplastic B-cell population in the interfollicular zone. Blood. 91:4708–14. PMID:9616169
1016. Doglioni C, Wotherspoon AC, Moschini A, et al. (1992). High incidence of primary gastric lymphoma in northeastern Italy. Lancet. 339:834–5. PMID:1347858
1017. Dojcinov SD, Venkataraman G, Pittaluga S, et al. (2011). Age-related EBV-associated lymphoproliferative disorders in the Western population: a spectrum of reactive lymphoid hyperplasia and lymphoma. Blood. 117:4726–35. PMID:21385849
1018. Dojcinov SD, Venkataraman G, Raffeld M, et al. (2010). EBV positive mucocutaneous ulcer–a study of 26 cases associated with various sources of immunosuppression. Am J Surg Pathol. 34:405–17. PMID:20154586
1019. Dolatshad H, Pellagatti A, Fernandez-Mercado M, et al. (2015). Disruption of SF3B1 results in deregulated expression and splicing of key genes and pathways in myelodysplastic syndrome hematopoietic stem and progenitor cells. Leukemia. 29:1092–103. PMID:25428262
1020. Dominguez-Sola D, Victora GD, Ying CY, et al. (2012). The proto-oncogene MYC is required for selection in the germinal center and cyclic reentry. Nat Immunol. 13:1083–91. PMID:23001145
1021. Donadieu J, Chalard F, Jeziorski E (2012). Medical management of langerhans cell histiocytosis from diagnosis to treatment. Expert Opin Pharmacother. 13:1309–22. PMID:22578036
1022. Donadini MP, Dentali F, Ageno W (2012). Splanchnic vein thrombosis: new risk factors and management. Thromb Res. 129 Suppl 1:S93–6. PMID:22682143
1023. Dong HY, Scadden DT, de Leval L, et al. (2005). Plasmablastic lymphoma in HIV-positive patients: an aggressive Epstein-Barr virus-associated extramedullary plasmacytic neoplasm. Am J Surg Pathol. 29:1633–41. PMID:16327436
1024. Dong HY, Weisberger J, Liu Z, et al. (2009). Immunophenotypic analysis of CD103+ B-lymphoproliferative disorders: hairy cell leukemia and its mimics. Am J Clin Pathol. 131:586–95. PMID:19289595
1025. Dores GM, Matsuno RK, Weisenburger DD, et al. (2008). Hairy cell leukaemia: a heterogeneous disease? Br J Haematol. 142:45–51. PMID:18477040
1026. Dorfman DM, Brown JA, Shahsafaei A, et al. (2006). Programmed death-1 (PD-1) is a marker of germinal center-associated T cells and angioimmunoblastic T-cell lymphoma. Am J Surg Pathol. 30:802–10. PMID:16819321
1027. Dorfman DM, Shahsafaei A (2010). CD200 (OX-2 membrane glycoprotein) expression in b cell-derived neoplasms. Am J Clin Pathol. 134:726–33. PMID:20959655
1028. Dorfman DM, Shahsafaei A (2011). CD200 (OX-2 membrane glycoprotein) is expressed by follicular T helper cells and in angioimmunoblastic T-cell lymphoma. Am J Surg Pathol. 35:76–83. PMID:21164290
1029. Dossier A, Meignin V, Fieschi C, et al. (2013). Human herpesvirus 8-related Castleman disease in the absence of HIV infection. Clin Infect Dis. 56:833–42. PMID:23223599
1030. Dotti G, Fiocchi R, Motta T, et al. (1999). Primary effusion lymphoma after heart transplantation: a new entity associated with human herpesvirus-8. Leukemia. 13:664–70. PMID:10374868
1031. Doubrovina E, Oflaz-Sozmen B, Prockop SE, et al. (2012). Adoptive immunotherapy with unselected or EBV-specific T cells for biopsy-proven EBV+ lymphomas after allogeneic hematopoietic cell transplantation. Blood. 119:2644–56. PMID:22138512
1032. Downing JR (1999). The AML1-ETO chimaeric transcription factor in acute myeloid leukaemia: biology and clinical significance. Br J Haematol. 106:296–308. PMID:10460585
1033. Doyle LA, Sepehr GJ, Hamilton MJ, et al. (2014). A clinicopathologic study of 24 cases of systemic mastocytosis involving the gastrointestinal tract and assessment of mucosal mast cell density in irritable bowel syndrome and asymptomatic patients. Am J Surg Pathol. 38:832–43. PMID:24618605
1034. Doyle TJ, Venkatachalam KK, Maeda K, et al. (1983). Hodgkin's disease in renal transplant recipients. Cancer. 51:245–7. PMID:6185199
1035. Drake MT, Maurer MJ, Link BK, et al. (2010). Vitamin D insufficiency and prognosis in non-Hodgkin's lymphoma. J Clin Oncol. 28:4191–8. PMID:20713849
1036. Drayson M, Tang LX, Drew R, et al. (2001). Serum free light-chain measurements for identifying and monitoring patients with nonsecretory multiple myeloma. Blood. 97:2900–2. PMID:11313287
1037. Dreyling M; European Mantle Cell Lymphoma Network (2014). Mantle cell lymphoma: biology, clinical presentation, and therapeutic approaches. Am Soc Clin Oncol Educ Book. 191–8. PMID:24857076
1038. Dreyling M, Ferrero S, Vogt N, et al. (2014). New paradigms in mantle cell lymphoma: is it time to risk-stratify treatment based on the proliferative signature? Clin Cancer Res. 20:5194–206. PMID:25320369
1039. Driessen EM, van Roon EH, Spijkers-Hagelstein JA, et al. (2013). Frequencies and prognostic impact of RAS mutations in MLL-rearranged acute lymphoblastic leukemia in infants. Haematologica. 98:937–44. PMID:23403319
1040. Druker BJ, Guilhot F, O'Brien SG, et al. (2006). Five-year follow-up of patients receiving imatinib for chronic myeloid leukemia. N Engl J Med. 355:2408–17. PMID:17151364
1041. Druker BJ, Talpaz M, Resta DJ, et al. (2001). Efficacy and safety of a specific inhibitor of the BCR-ABL tyrosine kinase in chronic myeloid leukemia. N Engl J Med. 344:1031–7. PMID:11287972
1042. Druker BJ, Tamura S, Buchdunger E, et al. (1996). Effects of a selective inhibitor of the Abl tyrosine kinase on the growth of Bcr-Abl positive cells. Nat Med. 2:561–6. PMID:8616716
1043. Du M, Diss TC, Xu C, et al. (1996). Ongoing mutation in MALT lymphoma immunoglobulin gene suggests that antigen stimulation plays a role in the clonal expansion. Leukemia. 10:1190–7. PMID:8684001
1044. Du MQ (2007). MALT lymphoma: recent advances in aetiology and molecular genetics. J Clin Exp Hematop. 47:31–42. PMID:18040143
1045. Du MQ (2011). MALT lymphoma: many roads lead to nuclear factor-κb activation. Histopathology. 58:26–38. PMID:21261681
1046. Du MQ, Bacon CM, Isaacson PG (2007). Kaposi sarcoma-associated herpesvirus/human herpesvirus 8 and lymphoproliferative disorders. J Clin Pathol. 60:1350–7. PMID:18042691
1047. Du MQ, Diss TC, Liu H, et al. (2002). KSHV- and EBV-associated germinotropic lymphoproliferative disorder. Blood. 100:3415–8. PMID:12384445
1048. Du MQ, Liu H, Diss TC, et al. (2001). Kaposi sarcoma-associated herpesvirus infects monotypic (IgM lambda) but polyclonal naive B cells in Castleman disease and associated lymphoproliferative disorders. Blood. 97:2130–6. PMID:11264181
1049. Dubois S, Viailly PJ, Mareschal S, et al. (2016). Next-generation sequencing in diffuse large B-cell lymphoma highlights molecular divergence and therapeutic opportunities: a LYSA study. Clin Cancer Res. 22:2919–28. PMID:26819451
1050. Duchayne E, Fenneteau O, Pages MP, et al. (2003). Acute megakaryoblastic leukaemia: a national clinical and biological study of 53 adult and childhood cases by the Groupe Français d'Hématologie Cellulaire (GFHC). Leuk Lymphoma. 44:49–58. PMID:12691142
1051. Duckworth CB, Zhang L, Li S (2014). Systemic mastocytosis with associated myeloproliferative neoplasm with t(8;19)(p12;q13.1) and abnormality of FGFR1: report of a unique case. Int J Clin Exp Pathol. 7:801–7. PMID:24551307
1052. Dufour A, Schneider F, Metzeler KH, et al. (2010). Acute myeloid leukemia with biallelic CEBPA gene mutations and normal karyotype represents a distinct genetic entity associated with a favorable clinical outcome. J Clin Oncol. 28:570–7. PMID:20038735
1053. Dul JL, Argon Y (1990). A single amino acid substitution in the variable region of the light chain specifically blocks immunoglobulin secretion. Proc Natl Acad Sci U S A. 87:8135–9. PMID:2122454
1054. Dulai PS, Thompson KD, Blunt HB, et al. (2014). Risks of serious infection or lymphoma with anti-tumor necrosis factor therapy for pediatric inflammatory bowel disease: a systematic review. Clin Gastroenterol Hepatol. 12:1443–51, quiz e88–9. PMID:24462626
1055. Dunleavy K (2014). Double-hit lymphomas: current paradigms and novel treatment approaches. Hematology Am Soc Hematol Educ Program. 2014:107–12. PMID:25696842
1056. Dunleavy K, Little RF, Pittaluga S, et al. (2010). The role of tumor histogenesis, FDG-PET, and short-course EPOCH with dose-dense rituximab (SC-EPOCH-RR) in HIV-associated diffuse large B-cell lymphoma. Blood. 115:3017–24. PMID:20130244
1057. Dunleavy K, Pittaluga S, Czuczman MS, et al. (2009). Differential efficacy of bortezomib plus chemotherapy within molecular subtypes of diffuse large B-cell lymphoma. Blood. 113:6069–76. PMID:19380866
1058. Dunleavy K, Pittaluga S, Maeda LS, et al. (2013). Dose-adjusted EPOCH-rituximab therapy in primary mediastinal B-cell lymphoma. N Engl J Med. 368:1408–16. PMID:23574119
1059. Dunleavy K, Steidl C (2015). Emerging biological insights and novel treatment strategies in primary mediastinal large B-cell lymphoma. Semin Hematol. 52:119–25. PMID:25805591
1060. Dunleavy K, Wilson WH (2015). Primary mediastinal B-cell lymphoma and mediastinal gray zone lymphoma: do they require a unique therapeutic approach? Blood. 125:33–9. PMID:25499450
1061. Dunleavy K, Wilson WH, Jaffe ES (2007). Angioimmunoblastic T cell lymphoma: pathobiological insights and clinical implications. Curr Opin Hematol. 14:348–53. PMID:17534160
1062. Dunphy CH, Gardner LJ, Grosso LE, et al. (2002). Flow cytometric immunophenotyping in posttransplant lymphoproliferative disorders. Am J Clin Pathol. 117:24–8. PMID:11789726
1063. Dunphy CH, Orton SO, Mantell J (2004).

Relative contributions of enzyme cytochemistry and flow cytometric immunophenotyping to the evaluation of acute myeloid leukemias with a monocytic component and of flow cytometric immunophenotyping to the evaluation of absolute monocytoses. Am J Clin Pathol. 122:865–74. PMID:15539379

1064. Dupin N, Diss TL, Kellam P, et al. (2000). HHV-8 is associated with a plasmablastic variant of Castleman disease that is linked to HHV-8-positive plasmablastic lymphoma. Blood. 95:1406–12. PMID:10666218

1065. Dupin N, Fisher C, Kellam P, et al. (1999). Distribution of human herpesvirus-8 latently infected cells in Kaposi's sarcoma, multicentric Castleman's disease, and primary effusion lymphoma. Proc Natl Acad Sci U S A. 96:4546–51. PMID:10200299

1066. Duplantier JE, Seyama K, Day NK, et al. (2001). Immunologic reconstitution following bone marrow transplantation for X-linked hyper IgM syndrome. Clin Immunol. 98:313–8. PMID:11237554

1067. Dupuis J, Boye K, Martin N, et al. (2006). Expression of CXCL13 by neoplastic cells in angioimmunoblastic T-cell lymphoma (AITL): a new diagnostic marker providing evidence that AITL derives from follicular helper T cells. Am J Surg Pathol. 30:490–4. PMID:16625095

1068. Dupuis J, Emile JF, Mounier N, et al. (2006). Prognostic significance of Epstein-Barr virus in nodal peripheral T-cell lymphoma, unspecified: A Groupe d'Etude des Lymphomes de l'Adulte (GELA) study. Blood. 108:4163–9. PMID:16902151

1069. Durot E, Patey M, Luquet I, et al. (2013). An aggressive B-cell lymphoma with rearrangements of MYC and CCND1 genes: a rare subtype of double-hit lymphoma. Leuk Lymphoma. 54:649–52. PMID:22784333

1070. Dyck PJ, Engelstad J, Dispenzieri A (2006). Vascular endothelial growth factor and POEMS. Neurology. 66:10–2. PMID:16401837

1071. Dyhdalo KS, Lanigan C, Tubbs RR, et al. (2013). Immunoarchitectural patterns of germinal center antigens including LMO2 assist in the differential diagnosis of marginal zone lymphoma vs follicular lymphoma. Am J Clin Pathol. 140:149–54. PMID:23897248

1072. Dühren-von Minden M, Übelhart R, Schneider D, et al. (2012). Chronic lymphocytic leukaemia is driven by antigen-independent cell-autonomous signalling. Nature. 489:309–12. PMID:22885698

1073. Döhner H, Stilgenbauer S, Benner A, et al. (2000). Genomic aberrations and survival in chronic lymphocytic leukemia. N Engl J Med. 343:1910–6. PMID:11136261

1074. Döhner H, Weisdorf DJ, Bloomfield CD (2015). Acute Myeloid Leukemia. N Engl J Med. 373:1136–52. PMID:26376137

1075. Döhner K, Schlenk RF, Habdank M, et al. (2005). Mutant nucleophosmin (NPM1) predicts favorable prognosis in younger adults with acute myeloid leukemia and normal cytogenetics: interaction with other gene mutations. Blood. 106:3740–6. PMID:16051734

1075A. Döhner K, Tobis K, Ulrich R, et al. (2002). Prognostic significance of partial tandem duplications of the MLL gene in adult patients 16 to 60 years old with acute myeloid leukemia and normal cytogenetics: a study of the Acute Myeloid Leukemia Study Group Ulm. J Clin Oncol. 20:3254–61. PMID:12149299

1076. Dölken G, Dölken L, Hirt C, et al. (2008). Age-dependent prevalence and frequency of circulating t(14;18)-positive cells in the peripheral blood of healthy individuals. J Natl Cancer Inst Monogr. (39):44–7. PMID:18648002

1077. Eberle FC, Salaverria I, Steidl C, et al. (2011). Gray zone lymphoma: chromosomal aberrations with immunophenotypic and clinical correlations. Mod Pathol. 24:1586–97. PMID:21822207

1078. Eberle FC, Song JY, Xi L, et al. (2012). Nodal involvement by cutaneous CD30-positive T-cell lymphoma mimicking classical Hodgkin lymphoma. Am J Surg Pathol. 36:716–25. PMID:22367293

1078A. Ebert BL, Pretz J, Bosco J, et al. (2008). Identification of RPS14 as a 5q-syndrome gene by RNA interference screen. Nature. 17:451(7176):335-9. PMID: 18202658

1079. Edelmann J, Holzmann K, Miller F, et al. (2012). High-resolution genomic profiling of chronic lymphocytic leukemia reveals new recurrent genomic alterations. Blood. 120:4783–94. PMID:23047824

1080. Edinger JT, Kant JA, Swerdlow SH (2010). Cutaneous marginal zone lymphomas have distinctive features and include 2 subsets. Am J Surg Pathol. 34:1830–41. PMID:21107089

1081. Egan LJ, Walsh SV, Stevens FM, et al. (1995). Celiac-associated lymphoma. A single institution experience of 30 cases in the combination chemotherapy era. J Clin Gastroenterol. 21:123–9. PMID:8583077

1082. Egawa N, Fukayama M, Kawaguchi K, et al. (1995). Relapsing oral and colonic ulcers with monoclonal T-cell infiltration. A low grade mucosal T-lymphoproliferative disease of the digestive tract. Cancer. 75:1728–33. PMID:8826934

1083. Ehlers A, Oker E, Bentink S, et al. (2008). Histone acetylation and DNA demethylation of B cells result in a Hodgkin-like phenotype. Leukemia. 22:835–41. PMID:18256685

1084. Ehrentraut S, Nagel S, Scherr ME, et al. (2013). t(8;9)(p22;p24)/PCM1-JAK2 activates SOCS2 and SOCS3 via STAT5. PLoS One. 8:e53767. PMID:23372669

1085. Eisele L, Dürig J, Hüttmann A, et al. (2012). Prevalence and progression of monoclonal gammopathy of undetermined significance and light-chain MGUS in Germany. Ann Hematol. 91:243–8. PMID:21789623

1085A. Eisfeld AK, Marcucci G, Maharry K, et al. (2012). miR-3151 interplays with its host gene BAALC and independently affects outcome of patients with cytogenetically normal acute myeloid leukemia. Blood. 120:249–58. PMID:22529287

1086. Ejerblad E, Kvasnicka HM, Thiele J, et al. (2013). Diagnosis according to World Health Organization determines the long-term prognosis in patients with myeloproliferative neoplasms treated with anagrelide: results of a prospective long-term follow-up. Hematology. 18:8–13. PMID:22990042

1087. El Rassi F, Bergsagel JD, Arellano M, et al. (2015). Predicting early blast transformation in chronic-phase chronic myeloid leukemia: is immunophenotyping the missing link? Cancer. 121:872–5. PMID:25387987

1088. El Shabrawi-Caelen L, Kerl H, Cerroni L (2004). Lymphomatoid papulosis: reappraisal of clinicopathologic presentation and classification into subtypes A, B, and C. Arch Dermatol. 140:441–7. PMID:15096372

1089. Elenitoba-Johnson KS, Gascoyne RD, Lim MS, et al. (1998). Homozygous deletions at chromosome 9p21 involving p16 and p15 are associated with histologic progression in follicle center lymphoma. Blood. 91:4677–85. PMID:9616165

1090. Elenitoba-Johnson KS, Jaffe ES (1997). Lymphoproliferative disorders associated with congenital immunodeficiencies. Semin Diagn Pathol. 14:35–47. PMID:9044508

1091. Elenitoba-Johnson KS, Zarate-Osorno A, Meneses A, et al. (1998). Cytotoxic granular protein expression, Epstein-Barr virus strain type, and latent membrane protein-1 oncogene deletions in nasal T-lymphocyte/natural killer cell lymphomas from Mexico. Mod Pathol. 11:754–61. PMID:9720504

1092. Elgui de Oliveira D, Bacchi MM, Abreu ES, et al. (2002). Hodgkin disease in adult and juvenile groups from two different geographic regions in Brazil: characterization of clinicopathologic aspects and relationship with Epstein-Barr virus infection. Am J Clin Pathol. 118:25–30. PMID:12109852

1093. Elling C, Erben P, Walz C, et al. (2011). Novel imatinib-sensitive PDGFRA-activating point mutations in hypereosinophilic syndrome induce growth factor independence and leukemia-like disease. Blood. 117:2935–43. PMID:21224473

1094. Elliott MA, Hanson CA, Dewald GW, et al. (2005). WHO-defined chronic neutrophilic leukemia: a long-term analysis of 12 cases and a critical review of the literature. Leukemia. 19:313–7. PMID:15549147

1095. Elliott MA, Pardanani A, Hanson CA, et al. (2015). ASXL1 mutations are frequent and prognostically detrimental in CSF3R-mutated chronic neutrophilic leukemia. Am J Hematol. 90:653–6. PMID:25850813

1096. Elliott MA, Tefferi A (2005). Thrombosis and haemorrhage in polycythaemia vera and essential thrombocythaemia. Br J Haematol. 128:275–90. PMID:15667529

1096A. Elliott MA, Tefferi A (2016). Chronic neutrophilic leukemia 2016: Update on diagnosis, molecular genetics, prognosis, and management. Am J Haematol. 91:341-349. PMID:26700908

1097. Elliott MA, Verstovsek S, Dingli D, et al. (2007). Monocytosis is an adverse prognostic factor for survival in younger patients with primary myelofibrosis. Leuk Res. 31:1503–9. PMID:17397921

1098. Ellis JT, Peterson P, Geller SA, et al. (1986). Studies of the bone marrow in polycythemia vera and the evolution of myelofibrosis and second hematologic malignancies. Semin Hematol. 23:144–55. PMID:3704666

1099. Elstrom RL, Andreadis C, Aqui NA, et al. (2006). Treatment of PTLD with rituximab or chemotherapy. Am J Transplant. 6:569–76. PMID:16468968

1100. Emanuel PD, Bates LJ, Castleberry RP, et al. (1991). Selective hypersensitivity to granulocyte-macrophage colony-stimulating factor by juvenile chronic myeloid leukemia hematopoietic progenitors. Blood. 77:925–9. PMID:1704804

1101. Emile JF, Abla O, Fraitag S, et al. (2016). Revised classification of histiocytoses and neoplasms of the macrophage-dendritic cell lineages. Blood. 127:2672–81. PMID:26966089

1102. Emile JF, Charlotte F, Amoura Z, et al. (2013). BRAF mutations in Erdheim-Chester disease. J Clin Oncol. 31:398. PMID:23248255

1103. Enblom A, Lindskog E, Hasselbalch H, et al. (2015). High rate of abnormal blood values and vascular complications before diagnosis of myeloproliferative neoplasms. Eur J Intern Med. 26:344–7. PMID:25863408

1104. Endly DC, Weenig RH, Peters MS, et al. (2013). Indolent course of cutaneous gamma-delta T-cell lymphoma. J Cutan Pathol. 40:896–902. PMID:23379625

1105. Engelhard M, Brittinger G, Huhn D, et al. (1997). Subclassification of diffuse large B-cell lymphomas according to the Kiel classification: distinction of centroblastic and immunoblastic lymphomas is a significant prognostic risk factor. Blood. 89:2291–7. PMID:9116271

1106. Engels EA, Pfeiffer RM, Fraumeni JF Jr, et al. (2011). Spectrum of cancer risk among US solid organ transplant recipients. JAMA. 306:1891–901. PMID:22045767

1107. Engels EA, Pfeiffer RM, Goedert JJ, et al. (2006). Trends in cancer risk among people with AIDS in the United States 1980-2002. AIDS. 20:1645–54. PMID:16868446

1108. Engels EA, Pittaluga S, Whitby D, et al. (2003). Immunoblastic lymphoma in persons with AIDS-associated Kaposi's sarcoma: a role for Kaposi's sarcoma-associated herpesvirus. Mod Pathol. 16:424–9. PMID:12748248

1109. Engert A, Ballova V, Haverkamp H, et al. (2005). Hodgkin's lymphoma in elderly patients: a comprehensive retrospective analysis from the German Hodgkin's Study Group. J Clin Oncol. 23:5052–60. PMID:15955904

1110. Ennishi D, Takeuchi K, Yokoyama M, et al. (2008). CD5 expression is potentially predictive of poor outcome among biomarkers in patients with diffuse large B-cell lymphoma receiving rituximab plus CHOP therapy. Ann Oncol. 19:1921–6. PMID:18573805

1111. Ensor HM, Schwab C, Russell LJ, et al. (2011). Demographic, clinical, and outcome features of children with acute lymphoblastic leukemia and CRLF2 deregulation: results from the MRC ALL97 clinical trial. Blood. 117:2129–36. PMID:21106984

1112. Epling-Burnette PK, Liu JH, Catlett-Falcone R, et al. (2001). Inhibition of STAT3 signaling leads to apoptosis of leukemic large granular lymphocytes and decreased Mcl-1 expression. J Clin Invest. 107:351–62. PMID:11160159

1113. Epling-Burnette PK, Painter JS, Chaurasia P, et al. (2004). Dysregulated NK receptor expression in patients with lymphoproliferative disease of granular lymphocytes. Blood. 103:3431–9. PMID:14726391

1114. Escribano L, Orfao A, Díaz-Agustin B, et al. (1998). Indolent systemic mast cell disease in adults: immunophenotypic characterization of bone marrow mast cells and its diagnostic implications. Blood. 91:2731–6. PMID:9531582

1115. Espinet B, Ferrer A, Bellosillo B, et al. (2014). Distinction between asymptomatic monoclonal B-cell lymphocytosis with cyclin D1 overexpression and mantle cell lymphoma: from molecular profiling to flow cytometry. Clin Cancer Res. 20:1007–19. PMID:24352646

1116. Estey E, Garcia-Manero G, Ferrajoli A, et al. (2006). Use of all-trans retinoic acid plus arsenic trioxide as an alternative to chemotherapy in untreated acute promyelocytic leukemia. Blood. 107:3469–73. PMID:16373661

1116A. Ettersperger J, Montcuquet N, Malamut G, et al. (2016). Interleukin-15-dependent T-cell-like innate intraepithelial lymphocytes develop in the intestine and transform into lymphomas in celiac disease. Immunity. 45:610-25. PMID:27612641

1117. Evans PA, Pott Ch, Groenen PJ, et al. (2007). Significantly improved PCR-based clonality testing in B-cell malignancies by use of multiple immunoglobulin gene targets. Report of the BIOMED-2 Concerted Action BHM4-CT98-3936. Leukemia. 21:207–14. PMID:17170731

1118. Eve HE, Furtado MV, Hamon MD, et al. (2009). Time to treatment does not influence overall survival in newly diagnosed mantle-cell lymphoma. J Clin Oncol. 27:e189–90, author reply e191. PMID:19805667

1119. Evens AM, Choquet S, Kroll-Desrosiers AR, et al. (2013). Primary CNS posttransplant lymphoproliferative disease (PTLD): an international report of 84 cases in the modern era. Am J Transplant. 13:1512–22. PMID:23721553

1120. Evens AM, David KA, Helenowski I, et al. (2010). Multicenter analysis of 80 solid organ transplantation recipients with post-transplantation lymphoproliferative disease: outcomes and prognostic factors in the modern era. J Clin

Oncol. 28:1038–46. PMID:20085936
1121. Evens AM, Kanakry JA, Sehn LH, et al. (2015). Gray zone lymphoma with features intermediate between classical Hodgkin lymphoma and diffuse large B-cell lymphoma: characteristics, outcomes, and prognostication among a large multicenter cohort. Am J Hematol. 90:778–83. PMID:26044261
1122. Evens AM, Roy R, Sterrenberg D, et al. (2010). Post-transplantation lymphoproliferative disorders: diagnosis, prognosis, and current approaches to therapy. Curr Oncol Rep. 12:383–94. PMID:20963522
1123. Exner M, Thalhammer R, Kapiotis S, et al. (2000). The "typical" immunophenotype of acute promyelocytic leukemia (APL-M3): does it prove true for the M3-variant? Cytometry. 42:106–9. PMID:10797447
1124. Fabarius A, Leitner A, Hochhaus A, et al. (2011). Impact of additional cytogenetic aberrations at diagnosis on prognosis of CML: long-term observation of 1151 patients from the randomized CML Study IV. Blood. 118:6760–8. PMID:22039253
1125. Fabbri G, Khiabanian H, Holmes AB, et al. (2013). Genetic lesions associated with chronic lymphocytic leukemia transformation to Richter syndrome. J Exp Med. 210:2273–88. PMID:24127483
1126. Facchetti F, Cigognetti M, Fisogni S, et al. (2016). Neoplasms derived from plasmacytoid dendritic cells. Mod Pathol. 29:98–111. PMID:26743477
1127. Facchetti F, De Wolf-Peeters C, Kennes C, et al. (1990). Leukemia-associated lymph node infiltrates of plasmacytoid monocytes (so-called plasmacytoid T-cells). Evidence for two distinct histological and immunophenotypical patterns. Am J Surg Pathol. 14:101–12. PMID:2301697
1128. Facchetti F, Pileri SA, Agostinelli C, et al. (2009). Cytoplasmic nucleophosmin is not detected in blastic plasmacytoid dendritic cell neoplasm. Haematologica. 94:285–8. PMID:19066330
1129. Facchetti F, Vermi W, Mason D, et al. (2003). The plasmacytoid monocyte/interferon producing cells. Virchows Arch. 443:703–17. PMID:14586652
1130. Facchetti F, Vermi W, Santoro A, et al. (2003). Neoplasms derived from plasmacytoid monocytes/interferon-producing cells: variability of CD56 and granzyme B expression. Am J Surg Pathol. 27:1489–92, author reply 1492–3. PMID:14576486
1131. Faderl S, Talpaz M, Estrov Z, et al. (1999). The biology of chronic myeloid leukemia. N Engl J Med. 341:164–72. PMID:10403855
1132. Faguet GB, Barton BP, Smith LL, et al. (1977). Gamma heavy chain disease: clinical aspects and characterization of a deleted, noncovalently linked gamma1 heavy chain dimer (BAZ). Blood. 49:495–505. PMID:402960
1132A. Fajgenbaum DC, Uldrick TS, Bagg A, et al. (2017). International, evidence-based consensus diagnostic criteria for HHV-8-negative/idiopathic multicentric Castleman disease. Blood. 129:1646-57. PMID:28087540
1133. Fajgenbaum DC, van Rhee F, Nabel CS (2014). HHV-8-negative, idiopathic multicentric Castleman disease: novel insights into biology, pathogenesis, and therapy. Blood. 123:2924–33. PMID:24622327
1134. Falchi L, Keating MJ, Marom EM, et al. (2014). Correlation between FDG/PET, histology, characteristics, and survival in 332 patients with chronic lymphoid leukemia. Blood. 123:2783–90. PMID:24615780
1135. Falchook GS, Vega F, Dang NH, et al. (2009). Hepatosplenic gamma-delta T-cell lymphoma: clinicopathological features and treatment. Ann Oncol. 20:1080–5. PMID:19237479
1136. Falini B (2001). Anaplastic large cell lymphoma: pathological, molecular and clinical features. Br J Haematol. 114:741–60. PMID:11564061
1137. Falini B, Agostinelli C, Bigerna B, et al. (2012). IRTA1 is selectively expressed in nodal and extranodal marginal zone lymphomas. Histopathology. 61:930–41. PMID:22716304
1138. Falini B, Bigerna B, Fizzotti M, et al. (1998). ALK expression defines a distinct group of T/null lymphomas ("ALK lymphomas") with a wide morphological spectrum. Am J Pathol. 153:875–86. PMID:9736036
1139. Falini B, Bigerna B, Pasqualucci L, et al. (1996). Distinctive expression pattern of the BCL-6 protein in nodular lymphocyte predominance Hodgkin's disease. Blood. 87:465–71. PMID:8555467
1140. Falini B, Bolli N, Liso A, et al. (2009). Altered nucleophosmin transport in acute myeloid leukaemia with mutated NPM1: molecular basis and clinical implications. Leukemia. 23:1731–43. PMID:19516275
1141. Falini B, Fizzotti M, Pucciarini A, et al. (2000). A monoclonal antibody (MUM1p) detects expression of the MUM1/IRF4 protein in a subset of germinal center B cells, plasma cells, and activated T cells. Blood. 95:2084–92. PMID:10706878
1142. Falini B, Flenghi L, Fagioli M, et al. (1997). Immunocytochemical diagnosis of acute promyelocytic leukemia (M3) with the monoclonal antibody PG-M3 (anti-PML). Blood. 90:4046–53. PMID:9354674
1143. Falini B, Flenghi L, Pileri S, et al. (1993). PG-M1: a new monoclonal antibody directed against a fixative-resistant epitope on the macrophage-restricted form of the CD68 molecule. Am J Pathol. 142:1359–72. PMID:7684194
1144. Falini B, Lenze D, Hasserjian R, et al. (2007). Cytoplasmic mutated nucleophosmin (NPM) defines the molecular status of a significant fraction of myeloid sarcomas. Leukemia. 21:1566–70. PMID:17443224
1145. Falini B, Macijewski K, Weiss T, et al. (2010). Multilineage dysplasia has no impact on biologic, clinicopathologic, and prognostic features of AML with mutated nucleophosmin (NPM1). Blood. 115:3776–86. PMID:20203266
1146. Falini B, Martelli MP, Bolli N, et al. (2006). Immunohistochemistry predicts nucleophosmin (NPM) mutations in acute myeloid leukemia. Blood. 108:1999–2005. PMID:16720834
1147. Falini B, Mason DY (2002). Proteins encoded by genes involved in chromosomal alterations in lymphoma and leukemia: clinical value of their detection by immunocytochemistry. Blood. 99:409–26. PMID:11781220
1148. Falini B, Mecucci C, Saglio G, et al. (2008). NPM1 mutations and cytoplasmic nucleophosmin are mutually exclusive of recurrent genetic abnormalities: a comparative analysis of 2562 patients with acute myeloid leukemia. Haematologica. 93:439–42. PMID:18268276
1149. Falini B, Mecucci C, Tiacci E, et al. (2005). Cytoplasmic nucleophosmin in acute myelogenous leukemia with a normal karyotype. N Engl J Med. 352:254–66. PMID:15659725
1150. Falini B, Nicoletti I, Martelli MF, et al. (2007). Acute myeloid leukemia carrying cytoplasmic/mutated nucleophosmin (NPMc+ AML): biologic and clinical features. Blood. 109:874–85. PMID:17008539
1151. Falini B, Pileri S, Zinzani PL, et al. (1999). ALK+ lymphoma: clinico-pathological findings and outcome. Blood. 93:2697–706. PMID:10194450
1152. Falini B, Pulford K, Pucciarini A, et al. (1999). Lymphomas expressing ALK fusion protein(s) other than NPM-ALK. Blood. 94:3509–15. PMID:10552961
1153. Falini B, Tiacci E, Liso A, et al. (2004). Simple diagnostic assay for hairy cell leukaemia by immunocytochemical detection of annexin A1 (ANXA1). Lancet. 363:1869–70. PMID:15183626
1154. Falini B, Tiacci E, Pucciarini A, et al. (2003). Expression of the IRTA1 receptor identifies intraepithelial and subepithelial marginal zone B cells of the mucosa-associated lymphoid tissue (MALT). Blood. 102:3684–92. PMID:12881317
1155. Fallah M, Liu X, Ji J, et al. (2014). Autoimmune diseases associated with non-Hodgkin lymphoma: a nationwide cohort study. Ann Oncol. 25:2025–30. PMID:25081899
1156. Fallah M, Liu X, Ji J, et al. (2014). Hodgkin lymphoma after autoimmune diseases by age at diagnosis and histological subtype. Ann Oncol. 25:1397–404. PMID:24718892
1157. Fan L, Miao Y, Wu YJ, et al. (2015). Expression patterns of CD200 and CD148 in leukemic B-cell chronic lymphoproliferative disorders and their potential value in differential diagnosis. Leuk Lymphoma. 56:3329–35. PMID:25791119
1158. Fan PC, Chang HN (1995). Hypersensitivity to mosquito bite: a case report. Gaoxiong Yi Xue Ke Xue Za Zhi. 11:420–4. PMID:7650782
1159. Fan Z, Natkunam Y, Bair E, et al. (2003). Characterization of variant patterns of nodular lymphocyte predominant hodgkin lymphoma with immunohistologic and clinical correlation. Am J Surg Pathol. 27:1346–56. PMID:14508396
1160. Fanale MA, Horwitz SM, Forero-Torres A, et al. (2014). Brentuximab vedotin in the frontline treatment of patients with CD30+ peripheral T-cell lymphomas: results of a phase I study. J Clin Oncol. 32:3137–43. PMID:25135998
1161. Farag SS, Ruppert AS, Mrózek K, et al. (2004). Prognostic significance of additional cytogenetic abnormalities in newly diagnosed patients with Philadelphia chromosome-positive chronic myelogenous leukemia treated with interferon-alpha: a Cancer and Leukemia Group B study. Int J Oncol. 25:143–51. PMID:15201999
1162. Farstad IN, Johansen FE, Vlatkovic L, et al. (2002). Heterogeneity of intraepithelial lymphocytes in refractory sprue: potential implications of CD30 expression. Gut. 51:372–8. PMID:12171959
1163. Fasan A, Kern W, Grossmann V, et al. (2013). STAT3 mutations are highly specific for large granular lymphocytic leukemia. Leukemia. 27:1598–600. PMID:23207521
1165. Favara BE, Feller AC, Pauli M, et al. (1997). Contemporary classification of histiocytic disorders. Med Pediatr Oncol. 29:157–66. PMID:9212839
1166. Favara BE, Jaffe R, Egeler RM (2002). Macrophage activation and hemophagocytic syndrome in langerhans cell histiocytosis: report of 30 cases. Pediatr Dev Pathol. 5:130–40. PMID:11910507
1167. Fazi C, Scarfò L, Pecciarini L, et al. (2011). General population low-count CLL-like MBL persists over time without clinical progression, although carrying the same cytogenetic abnormalities of CLL. Blood. 118:6618–25. PMID:21876118
1168. Federico M, Bellei M, Marcheselli L, et al. (2009). Follicular lymphoma international prognostic index 2: a new prognostic index for follicular lymphoma developed by the international follicular lymphoma prognostic factor project. J Clin Oncol. 27:4555–62. PMID:19652063
1169. Federico M, Rudiger T, Bellei M, et al. (2013). Clinicopathologic characteristics of angioimmunoblastic T-cell lymphoma: analysis of the international peripheral T-cell lymphoma project. J Clin Oncol. 31:240–6. PMID:22869878
1170. Federmann B, Abele M, Rosero Cuesta DS, et al. (2014). The detection of SRSF2 mutations in routinely processed bone marrow biopsies is useful in the diagnosis of chronic myelomonocytic leukemia. Hum Pathol. 45:2471–9. PMID:25305095
1171. Fei XH, Wu SL, Sun RJ, et al. (2012). [Clinical analysis of 12 cases of acute myeloid leukemia with Ph chromosome and BCR-ABL positive]. Zhongguo Shi Yan Xue Ye Xue Za Zhi. 20:545–8. PMID:22739152
1172. Feldman AL, Arber DA, Pittaluga S, et al. (2008). Clonally related follicular lymphomas and histiocytic/dendritic cell sarcomas: evidence for transdifferentiation of the follicular lymphoma clone. Blood. 111:5433–9. PMID:18272816
1173. Feldman AL, Berthold F, Arceci RJ, et al. (2005). Clonal relationship between precursor T-lymphoblastic leukaemia/lymphoma and Langerhans-cell histiocytosis. Lancet Oncol. 6:435–7. PMID:15925822
1174. Feldman AL, Dogan A, Smith DI, et al. (2011). Discovery of recurrent t(6;7)(p25.3;q32.3) translocations in ALK-negative anaplastic large cell lymphomas by massively parallel genomic sequencing. Blood. 117:915–9. PMID:21030553
1175. Feldman AL, Law ME, Inwards DJ, et al. (2010). PAX5-positive T-cell anaplastic large cell lymphomas associated with extra copies of the PAX5 gene locus. Mod Pathol. 23:593–602. PMID:20118907
1176. Feldman AL, Minniti C, Santi M, et al. (2004). Histiocytic sarcoma after acute lymphoblastic leukaemia: a common clonal origin. Lancet Oncol. 5:248–50. PMID:15050956
1177. Feldman AL, Vasmatzis G, Asmann YW, et al. (2013). Novel TRAF1-ALK fusion identified by deep RNA sequencing of anaplastic large cell lymphoma. Genes Chromosomes Cancer. 52:1097–102. PMID:23999969
1177A. Felix CA, Lange BJ (1999). Leukemia in infants. Oncologist. 4:225–40. PMID:10394590
1178. Felman P, Bryon PA, Gentilhomme O, et al. (1988). The syndrome of abnormal chromatin clumping in leucocytes: a myelodysplastic disorder with proliferative features? Br J Haematol. 70:49–54. PMID:3179227
1179. Feltkamp CA, van Heerde P, Feltkamp-Vroom TM, et al. (1981). A malignant tumor arising from interdigitating cells; light microscopical, ultrastructural, immuno-and enzyme-histochemical characteristics. Virchows Arch A Pathol Anat Histol. 393:183–92. PMID:6270876
1180. Fenaux P, Beuscart R, Lai JL, et al. (1988). Prognostic factors in adult chronic myelomonocytic leukemia: an analysis of 107 cases. J Clin Oncol. 6:1417–24. PMID:3166485
1181. Fenaux P, Jouet JP, Zandecki M, et al. (1987). Chronic and subacute myelomonocytic leukaemia in the adult: a report of 60 cases with special reference to prognostic factors. Br J Haematol. 65:101–6. PMID:3468995
1182. Fenaux P, Morel P, Lai JL (1996). Cytogenetics of myelodysplastic syndromes. Semin Hematol. 33:127–38. PMID:8722683
1183. Fenaux P, Mufti GJ, Hellstrom-Lindberg E, et al. (2009). Efficacy of azacitidine compared with that of conventional care regimens in the treatment of higher-risk myelodysplastic syndromes: a randomised, open-label, phase III study. Lancet Oncol. 10:223–32. PMID:19230772
1184. Fend F, Horn T, Koch I, et al. (2008). Atypical chronic myeloid leukemia as defined in the WHO classification is a JAK2 V617F negative neoplasm. Leuk Res. 32:1931–5. PMID:18555525

1185. Fernández de Larrea C, Kyle RA, Durie BG, et al. (2013). Plasma cell leukemia: consensus statement on diagnostic requirements, response criteria and treatment recommendations by the International Myeloma Working Group. Leukemia. 27:780–91. PMID:23288300
1186. Fernàndez V, Hartmann E, Ott G, et al. (2005). Pathogenesis of mantle-cell lymphoma: all oncogenic roads lead to dysregulation of cell cycle and DNA damage response pathways. J Clin Oncol. 23:6364–9. PMID:16155021
1187. Fernàndez V, Salamero O, Espinet B, et al. (2010). Genomic and gene expression profiling defines indolent forms of mantle cell lymphoma. Cancer Res. 70:1408–18. PMID:20124476
1188. Ferrando AA (2013). SOX11 is a mantle cell lymphoma oncogene. Blood. 121:2169–70. PMID:23520328
1189. Ferrando AA, Neuberg DS, Staunton J, et al. (2002). Gene expression signatures define novel oncogenic pathways in T cell acute lymphoblastic leukemia. Cancer Cell. 1:75–87. PMID:12086890
1190. Ferreira JM, Klumb CE, de Souza Reis R, et al. (2012). Lymphoma subtype incidence rates in children and adolescents: first report from Brazil. Cancer Epidemiol. 36:e221–6. PMID:22552334
1191. Ferreiro JF, Morscio J, Dierickx D, et al. (2015). Post-transplant molecularly defined Burkitt lymphomas are frequently MYC-negative and characterized by the 11q-gain/loss pattern. Haematologica. 100:e275–9. PMID:25795716
1192. Ferrer A, Salaverria I, Bosch F, et al. (2007). Leukemic involvement is a common feature in mantle cell lymphoma. Cancer. 109:2473–80. PMID:17477385
1193. Ferreri AJ, Campo E, Seymour JF, et al. (2004). Intravascular lymphoma: clinical presentation, natural history, management and prognostic factors in a series of 38 cases, with special emphasis on the 'cutaneous variant'. Br J Haematol. 127:173–83. PMID:15461623
1194. Ferreri AJ, Dell'Oro S, Capello D, et al. (2004). Aberrant methylation in the promoter region of the reduced folate carrier gene is a potential mechanism of resistance to methotrexate in primary central nervous system lymphomas. Br J Haematol. 126:657–64. PMID:15327516
1195. Ferreri AJ, Dognini GP, Bairey O, et al. (2008). The addition of rituximab to anthracycline-based chemotherapy significantly improves outcome in 'Western' patients with intravascular large B-cell lymphoma. Br J Haematol. 143:253–7. PMID:18699850
1196. Ferreri AJ, Dognini GP, Campo E, et al. (2007). Variations in clinical presentation, frequency of hemophagocytosis and clinical behavior of intravascular lymphoma diagnosed in different geographical regions. Haematologica. 92:486–92. PMID:17488659
1197. Ferreri AJ, Dognini GP, Govi S, et al. (2008). Can rituximab change the usually dismal prognosis of patients with intravascular large B-cell lymphoma? J Clin Oncol. 26:5134–6, author reply 5136–7. PMID:18838697
1198. Ferreri AJ, Ernberg I, Copie-Bergman C (2009). Infectious agents and lymphoma development: molecular and clinical aspects. J Intern Med. 265:421–38. PMID:19298458
1199. Ferreri AJ, Govi S, Ponzoni M (2013). Marginal zone lymphomas and infectious agents. Semin Cancer Biol. 23:431–40. PMID:24090976
1200. Ferreri AJ, Govi S, Raderer M, et al. (2012). Helicobacter pylori eradication as exclusive treatment for limited-stage gastric diffuse large B-cell lymphoma: results of a multicenter phase 2 trial. Blood. 120:3858–60. PMID:23118214
1201. Ferreri AJ, Ponzoni M, Guidoboni M, et al. (2006). Bacteria-eradicating therapy with doxycycline in ocular adnexal MALT lymphoma: a multicenter prospective trial. J Natl Cancer Inst. 98:1375–82. PMID:17018784
1202. Ferringer T, Banks PM, Metcalf JS (2006). Langerhans cell sarcoma. Am J Dermatopathol. 28:36–9. PMID:16456323
1203. Ferry JA, Fung CY, Zukerberg L, et al. (2007). Lymphoma of the ocular adnexa: A study of 353 cases. Am J Surg Pathol. 31:170–84. PMID:17255761
1204. Ferry JA, Harris NL, Picker LJ, et al. (1988). Intravascular lymphomatosis (malignant angioendotheliomatosis). A B-cell neoplasm expressing surface homing receptors. Mod Pathol. 1:444–52. PMID:3065781
1205. Ferry JA, Jacobson JO, Conti D, et al. (1989). Lymphoproliferative disorders and hematologic malignancies following organ transplantation. Mod Pathol. 2:583–92. PMID:2587566
1206. Ferry JA, Sohani AR, Longtine JA, et al. (2009). HHV8-positive, EBV-positive Hodgkin lymphoma-like large B-cell lymphoma and HHV8-positive intravascular large B-cell lymphoma. Mod Pathol. 22:618–26. PMID:19287457
1207. Ferry JA, Zukerberg LR, Harris NL (1992). Florid progressive transformation of germinal centers. A syndrome affecting young men, without early progression to nodular lymphocyte predominance Hodgkin's disease. Am J Surg Pathol. 16:252–8. PMID:1599017
1208. Feuerhake F, Kutok JL, Monti S, et al. (2005). NFkappaB activity, function, and target-gene signatures in primary mediastinal large B-cell lymphoma and diffuse large B-cell lymphoma subtypes. Blood. 106:1392–9. PMID:15870177
1209. Feuillard J, Jacob MC, Valensi F, et al. (2002). Clinical and biologic features of CD4(+) CD56(+) malignancies. Blood. 99:1556–63. PMID:11861268
1210. Fialkow PJ, Jacobson RJ, Papayannopoulou T (1977). Chronic myelocytic leukemia: clonal origin in a stem cell common to the granulocyte, erythrocyte, platelet and monocyte/macrophage. Am J Med. 63:125–30. PMID:267431
1211. Fianchi L, Pagano L, Piciocchi A, et al. (2015). Characteristics and outcome of therapy-related myeloid neoplasms: Report from the Italian network on secondary leukemias. Am J Hematol. 90:E80–5. PMID:25653205
1212. Fiedler W, Weh HJ, Zeller W, et al. (1991). Translocation (14; 18) and (8; 22) in three patients with acute leukemia/lymphoma following centrocytic/centroblastic non-Hodgkin's lymphoma. Ann Hematol. 63:282–7. PMID:1958753
1213. Fierro MT, Comessatti A, Quaglino P, et al. (2006). Expression pattern of chemokine receptors and chemokine release in inflammatory erythroderma and Sézary syndrome. Dermatology. 213:284–92. PMID:17135733
1214. Finalet Ferreiro J, Rouhigharabaei L, Urbankova H, et al. (2014). Integrative genomic and transcriptomic analysis identified candidate genes implicated in the pathogenesis of hepatosplenic T-cell lymphoma. PLoS One. 9:e102977. PMID:25057852
1215. Finazzi G, Carobbio A, Thiele J, et al. (2012). Incidence and risk factors for bleeding in 1104 patients with essential thrombocythemia or prefibrotic myelofibrosis diagnosed according to the 2008 WHO criteria. Leukemia. 26:716–9. PMID:21926959
1216. Finazzi G, Caruso V, Marchioli R, et al. (2005). Acute leukemia in polycythemia vera: an analysis of 1638 patients enrolled in a prospective observational study. Blood. 105:2664–70. PMID:15585653
1217. Finazzi G, Harrison C (2005). Essential thrombocythemia. Semin Hematol. 42:230–8. PMID:16210036
1218. Fink-Puches R, Chott A, Ardigó M, et al. (2004). The spectrum of cutaneous lymphomas in patients less than 20 years of age. Pediatr Dermatol. 21:525–33. PMID:15461755
1219. Finn LS, Viswanatha DS, Belasco JB, et al. (1999). Primary follicular lymphoma of the testis in childhood. Cancer. 85:1626–35. PMID:10193956
1220. Fioretos T, Strömbeck B, Sandberg T, et al. (1999). Isochromosome 17q in blast crisis of chronic myeloid leukemia and in other hematologic malignancies is the result of clustered breakpoints in 17p11 and is not associated with coding TP53 mutations. Blood. 94:225–32. PMID:10381517
1221. Fish K, Chen J, Longnecker R (2014). Epstein-Barr virus latent membrane protein 2A enhances MYC-driven cell cycle progression in a mouse model of B lymphoma. Blood. 123:530–40. PMID:24174629
1222. Flaig MJ, Cerroni L, Schuhmann K, et al. (2001). Follicular mycosis fungoides. A histopathologic analysis of nine cases. J Cutan Pathol. 28:525–30. PMID:11737522
1223. Flann S, Orchard GE, Wain EM, et al. (2006). Three cases of lymphomatoid papulosis with a CD56+ immunophenotype. J Am Acad Dermatol. 55:903–6. PMID:17052504
1224. Flatley E, Chen AI, Zhao X, et al. (2014). Aberrations of MYC are a common event in B-cell prolymphocytic leukemia. Am J Clin Pathol. 142:347–54. PMID:25125625
1225. Flavell KJ, Murray PG (2000). Hodgkin's disease and the Epstein-Barr virus. Mol Pathol. 53:262–9. PMID:11091850
1226. Fletcher S, Abdalla S, Edwards M, et al. (2007). Case 32. Eosinophilia: reactive or neoplastic? Leuk Lymphoma. 48:174–6. PMID:17325861
1227. Florena AM, Tripodo C, Iannitto E, et al. (2004). Value of bone marrow biopsy in the diagnosis of essential thrombocythemia. Haematologica. 89:911–9. PMID:15339673
1228. Fonatsch C, Gudat H, Lengfelder E, et al. (1994). Correlation of cytogenetic findings with clinical features in 18 patients with inv(3)(q21q26) or t(3;3)(q21;q26). Leukemia. 8:1318–26. PMID:8057667
1229. Fong CT, Brodeur GM (1987). Down's syndrome and leukemia: epidemiology, genetics, cytogenetics and mechanisms of leukemogenesis. Cancer Genet Cytogenet. 28:55–76. PMID:2955886
1230. Fonseca R, Bailey RJ, Ahmann GJ, et al. (2002). Genomic abnormalities in monoclonal gammopathy of undetermined significance. Blood. 100:1417–24. PMID:12149226
1231. Fonseca R, Barlogie B, Bataille R, et al. (2004). Genetics and cytogenetics of multiple myeloma: a workshop report. Cancer Res. 64:1546–58. PMID:14989251
1232. Fonseca R, Bergsagel PL, Drach J, et al. (2009). International Myeloma Working Group molecular classification of multiple myeloma: spotlight review. Leukemia. 23:2210–21. PMID:19798094
1233. Font P, Loscertales J, Soto C, et al. (2015). Interobserver variance in myelodysplastic syndromes with less than 5 % bone marrow blasts: unilineage vs. multilineage dysplasia and reproducibility of the threshold of 2 % blasts. Ann Hematol. 94:565–73. PMID:25387664
1234. Ford AM, Fasching K, Panzer-Grümayer ER, et al. (2001). Origins of "late" relapse in childhood acute lymphoblastic leukemia with TEL-AML1 fusion genes. Blood. 98:558–64. PMID:11468150
1235. Ford AM, Pombo-de-Oliveira MS, McCarthy KP, et al. (1997). Monoclonal origin of concordant T-cell malignancy in identical twins. Blood. 89:281–5. PMID:8978302
1236. Forestier E, Heim S, Blennow E, et al. (2003). Cytogenetic abnormalities in childhood acute myeloid leukaemia: a Nordic series comprising all children enrolled in the NOPHO-93-AML trial between 1993 and 2001. Br J Haematol. 121:566–77. PMID:12752097
1237. Foss HD, Anagnostopoulos I, Araujo I, et al. (1996). Anaplastic large-cell lymphomas of T-cell and null-cell phenotype express cytotoxic molecules. Blood. 88:4005–11. PMID:8916967
1238. Foss HD, Reusch R, Demel G, et al. (1999). Frequent expression of the B-cell-specific activator protein in Reed-Sternberg cells of classical Hodgkin's disease provides further evidence for its B-cell origin. Blood. 94:3108–13. PMID:10556196
1239. Fraga M, Brousset P, Schlaifer D, et al. (1995). Bone marrow involvement in anaplastic large cell lymphoma. Immunohistochemical detection of minimal disease and its prognostic significance. Am J Clin Pathol. 103:82–9. PMID:7817951
1240. Fraga M, Sánchez-Verde L, Forteza J, et al. (2002). T-cell/histiocyte-rich large B-cell lymphoma is a disseminated aggressive neoplasm: differential diagnosis from Hodgkin's lymphoma. Histopathology. 41:216–29. PMID:12207783
1241. Franchini G (1995). Molecular mechanisms of human T-cell leukemia/lymphotropic virus type I infection. Blood. 86:3619–39. PMID:7579327
1242. Franco V, Florena AM, Campesi G (1996). Intrasinusoidal bone marrow infiltration: a possible hallmark of splenic lymphoma. Histopathology. 29:571–5. PMID:8971565
1243. Frangione B, Franklin EC (1973). Heavy chain diseases: clinical features and molecular significance of the disordered immunoglobulin structure. Semin Hematol. 10:53–64. PMID:4567166
1244. Frangione B, Franklin EC, Prelli F (1976). Mu heavy-chain disease–a defect in immunoglobulin assembly. Structural studies of the kappa chain. Scand J Immunol. 5:623–7. PMID:824712
1245. Frank D, Cesarman E, Liu YF, et al. (1995). Posttransplantation lymphoproliferative disorders frequently contain type A and not type B Epstein-Barr virus. Blood. 85:1396–403. PMID:7858270
1246. Franke S, Wlodarska I, Maes B, et al. (2002). Comparative genomic hybridization pattern distinguishes T-cell/histiocyte-rich B-cell lymphoma from nodular lymphocyte predominance Hodgkin's lymphoma. Am J Pathol. 161:1861–7. PMID:12414532
1247. Franke S, Wlodarska I, Maes B, et al. (2001). Lymphocyte predominance Hodgkin disease is characterized by recurrent genomic imbalances. Blood. 97:1845–53. PMID:11238128
1248. Frankel AE, Woo JH, Ahn C, et al. (2014). Activity of SL-401, a targeted therapy directed to interleukin-3 receptor, in blastic plasmacytoid dendritic cell neoplasm patients. Blood. 124:385–92. PMID:24859366
1249. Franklin EC, Kyle R, Seligmann M, et al. (1979). Correlation of protein structure and immunoglobulin gene organization in the light of two new deleted heavy chain disease proteins. Mol Immunol. 16:919–21. PMID:118919
1250. Fraser CR, Wang W, Gomez M, et al. (2009). Transformation of chronic lymphocytic leukemia/small lymphocytic lymphoma to interdigitating dendritic cell sarcoma: evidence for

transdifferentiation of the lymphoma clone. Am J Clin Pathol. 132:928–39. PMID:19926586
1251. Freedman A (2014). Follicular lymphoma: 2014 update on diagnosis and management. Am J Hematol. 89:429–36. PMID:24687887
1252. Freedman A (2015). Follicular lymphoma: 2015 update on diagnosis and management. Am J Hematol. 90:1171–8. PMID:26769125
1253. French LE, Alcindor T, Shapiro M, et al. (2002). Identification of amplified clonal T cell populations in the blood of patients with chronic graft-versus-host disease: positive correlation with response to photopheresis. Bone Marrow Transplant. 30:509–15. PMID:12379890
1254. Fresquet V, Robles EF, Parker A, et al. (2012). High-throughput sequencing analysis of the chromosome 7q32 deletion reveals IRF5 as a potential tumour suppressor in splenic marginal-zone lymphoma. Br J Haematol. 158:712–26. PMID:22816737
1255. Freud AG, Caligiuri MA (2006). Human natural killer cell development. Immunol Rev. 214:56–72. PMID:17100876
1256. Freyer DR, Kennedy R, Bostrom BC, et al. (1996). Juvenile xanthogranuloma: forms of systemic disease and their clinical implications. J Pediatr. 129:227–37. PMID:8765620
1257. Fritschi L, Benke G, Hughes AM, et al. (2005). Occupational exposure to pesticides and risk of non-Hodgkin's lymphoma. Am J Epidemiol. 162:849–57. PMID:16177143
1257A. Fritz A, Percy C, Jack A, et al. (2013) International Classification of Diseases for Oncology. 3rd ed. First revision.
Geneva: WHO Press.
1258. Frizzera G, Hanto DW, Gajl-Peczalska KJ, et al. (1981). Polymorphic diffuse B-cell hyperplasias and lymphomas in renal transplant recipients. Cancer Res. 41:4262–79. PMID:7030473
1259. Froberg MK, Brunning RD, Dorion P, et al. (1998). Demonstration of clonality in neutrophils using FISH in a case of chronic neutrophilic leukemia. Leukemia. 12:623–6. PMID:9557623
1259A. Fröhling S, Schlenk RF, Breitruck J, et al. (2002). Prognostic significance of activating FLT3 mutations in younger adults (16 to 60 years) with acute myeloid leukemia and normal cytogenetics: a study of the AML Study Group Ulm. Blood. 100:4372–80. PMID:12393388
1260. Fröhling S, Schlenk RF, Stolze I, et al. (2004). CEBPA mutations in younger adults with acute myeloid leukemia and normal cytogenetics: prognostic relevance and analysis of cooperating mutations. J Clin Oncol. 22:624–33. PMID:14726504
1261. Fu B, Jaso JM, Sargent RL, et al. (2014). Bone marrow fibrosis in patients with primary myelodysplastic syndromes has prognostic value using current therapies and new risk stratification systems. Mod Pathol. 27:681–9. PMID:24186132
1262. Fu K, Weisenburger DD, Greiner TC, et al. (2005). Cyclin D1-negative mantle cell lymphoma: a clinicopathologic study based on gene expression profiling. Blood. 106:4315–21. PMID:16123218
1263. Fujimoto M, Haga H, Okamoto M, et al. (2008). EBV-associated diffuse large B-cell lymphoma arising in the chest wall with surgical mesh implant. Pathol Int. 58:668–71. PMID:18801089
1264. Fukayama M, Ibuka T, Hayashi Y, et al. (1993). Epstein-Barr virus in pyothorax-associated pleural lymphoma. Am J Pathol. 143:1044–9. PMID:8214001
1265. Funch DP, Walker AM, Schneider G, et al. (2005). Ganciclovir and acyclovir reduce the risk of post-transplant lymphoproliferative disorder in renal transplant recipients. Am J Transplant. 5:2894–900. PMID:16303002
1266. Funkhouser AW, Katzman PJ, Sickel JZ, et al. (1998). CD30-positive anaplastic large cell lymphoma (ALCL) of T-cell lineage in a 14-month-old infant with perinatally acquired HIV-1 infection. J Pediatr Hematol Oncol. 20:556–9. PMID:9856678
1267. Gachard N, Parrens M, Soubeyran I, et al. (2013). IGHV gene features and MYD88 L265P mutation separate the three marginal zone lymphoma entities and Waldenström macroglobulinemia/lymphoplasmacytic lymphomas. Leukemia. 27:183–9. PMID:22944768
1268. Gadner H, Grois N, Arico M, et al. (2001). A randomized trial of treatment for multisystem Langerhans' cell histiocytosis. J Pediatr. 138:728–34. PMID:11343051
1269. Gaertner EM, Tsokos M, Derringer GA, et al. (2001). Interdigitating dendritic cell sarcoma. A report of four cases and review of the literature. Am J Clin Pathol. 115:589–97. PMID:11293908
1270. Gahn B, Haase D, Unterhalt M, et al. (1996). De novo AML with dysplastic hematopoiesis: cytogenetic and prognostic significance. Leukemia. 10:946–51. PMID:8667650
1271. Gaidano G, Capello D, Cilia AM, et al. (1999). Genetic characterization of HHV-8/KSHV-positive primary effusion lymphoma reveals frequent mutations of BCL6: implications for disease pathogenesis and histogenesis. Genes Chromosomes Cancer. 24:16–23. PMID:9892104
1272. Gaidano G, Carbone A, Pastore C, et al. (1997). Frequent mutation of the 5' noncoding region of the BCL-6 gene in acquired immunodeficiency syndrome-related non-Hodgkin's lymphomas. Blood. 89:3755–62. PMID:9160681
1273. Gaidano G, Cerri M, Capello D, et al. (2002). Molecular histogenesis of plasmablastic lymphoma of the oral cavity. Br J Haematol. 119:622–8. PMID:12437635
1274. Gaidzik VI, Bullinger L, Schlenk RF, et al. (2011). RUNX1 mutations in acute myeloid leukemia: results from a comprehensive genetic and clinical analysis from the AML study group. J Clin Oncol. 29:1364–72. PMID:21343560
1274A. Gaidzik VI, Paschka P, Späth D, et al. (2012). TET2 mutations in acute myeloid leukemia (AML): results from a comprehensive genetic and clinical analysis of the AML study group. J Clin Oncol. 30:1350–7. PMID:22430270
1274B. Gaidzik VI, Schlenk RF, Moschny S, et al. (2009). Prognostic impact of WT1 mutations in cytogenetically normal acute myeloid leukemia: a study of the German-Austrian AML Study Group. Blood. 113:4505–11. PMID:19221039
1274C. Gaidzik VI, Schlenk RF, Paschka P, et al. (2013). Clinical impact of DNMT3A mutations in younger adult patients with acute myeloid leukemia: results of the AML Study Group (AMLSG). Blood. 121:4769–77. PMID:23632886
1275. Gajendra S, Sachdev R, Dorwal P, et al. (2014). Mixed-phenotypic acute leukemia: cytochemically myeloid and phenotypically early T-cell precursor acute lymphoblastic leukemia. Blood Res. 49:196–8. PMID:25325041
1276. Gale J, Simmonds PD, Mead GM, et al. (2000). Enteropathy-type intestinal T-cell lymphoma: clinical features and treatment of 31 patients in a single center. J Clin Oncol. 18:795–803. PMID:10673521
1277. Gale KB, Ford AM, Repp R, et al. (1997). Backtracking leukemia to birth: identification of clonotypic gene fusion sequences in neonatal blood spots. Proc Natl Acad Sci U S A. 94:13950–4. PMID:9391133
1278. Gale RE, Green C, Allen C, et al. (2008). The impact of FLT3 internal tandem duplication mutant level, number, size, and interaction with NPM1 mutations in a large cohort of young adult patients with acute myeloid leukemia. Blood. 111:2776–84. PMID:17957027
1279. Galieni P, Cavo M, Pulsoni A, et al. (2000). Clinical outcome of extramedullary plasmacytoma. Haematologica. 85:47–51. PMID:10629591
1280. Gallagher CJ, Gregory WM, Jones AE, et al. (1986). Follicular lymphoma: prognostic factors for response and survival. J Clin Oncol. 4:1470–80. PMID:3531422
1281. Gallamini A, Hutchings M, Rigacci L, et al. (2007). Early interim 2-[18F]fluoro-2-deoxy-D-glucose positron emission tomography is prognostically superior to international prognostic score in advanced-stage Hodgkin's lymphoma: a report from a joint Italian-Danish study. J Clin Oncol. 25:3746–52. PMID:17646666
1282. Gallamini A, Stelitano C, Calvi R, et al. (2004). Peripheral T-cell lymphoma unspecified (PTCL-U): a new prognostic model from a retrospective multicentric clinical study. Blood. 103:2474–9. PMID:14645001
1283. Gallo G, Goñi F, Boctor F, et al. (1996). Light chain cardiomyopathy. Structural analysis of the light chain tissue deposits. Am J Pathol. 148:1397–406. PMID:8623912
1284. Galton DA, Goldman JM, Wiltshaw E, et al. (1974). Prolymphocytic leukaemia. Br J Haematol. 27:7–23. PMID:4137136
1285. Gambacorti-Passerini C, Messa C, Pogliani EM (2011). Crizotinib in anaplastic large-cell lymphoma. N Engl J Med. 364:775–6. PMID:21345110
1286. Gambacorti-Passerini CB, Donadoni C, Parmiani A, et al. (2015). Recurrent ETNK1 mutations in atypical chronic myeloid leukemia. Blood. 125:499–503. PMID:25343957
1287. Gamis AS, Woods WG, Alonzo TA, et al. (2003). Increased age at diagnosis has a significantly negative effect on outcome in children with Down syndrome and acute myeloid leukemia: a report from the Children's Cancer Group Study 2891. J Clin Oncol. 21:3415–22. PMID:12885836
1288. Ganapathi KA, Pittaluga S, Odejide OO, et al. (2014). Early lymphoid lesions: conceptual, diagnostic and clinical challenges. Haematologica. 99:1421–32. PMID:25176983
1289. Ganapathi KA, Townsley DM, Hsu AP, et al. (2015). GATA2 deficiency-associated bone marrow disorder differs from idiopathic aplastic anemia. Blood. 125:56–70. PMID:25359990
1290. Gangat N, Caramazza D, Vaidya R, et al. (2011). DIPSS plus: a refined Dynamic International Prognostic Scoring System for primary myelofibrosis that incorporates prognostic information from karyotype, platelet count, and transfusion status. J Clin Oncol. 29:392–7. PMID:21149668
1291. Ganly P, Walker LC, Morris CM (2004). Familial mutations of the transcription factor RUNX1 (AML1, CBFA2) predispose to acute myeloid leukemia. Leuk Lymphoma. 45:1–10. PMID:15061191
1292. Gao J, Chen YH, Peterson LC (2015). GATA family transcriptional factors: emerging suspects in hematologic disorders. Exp Hematol Oncol. 4:28. PMID:26445707
1293. Gao J, Gentzler RD, Timms AE, et al. (2014). Heritable GATA2 mutations associated with familial AML-MDS: a case report and review of literature. J Hematol Oncol. 7:36. PMID:24754962
1294. Gao J, Peterson L, Nelson B, et al. (2009). Immunophenotypic variations in mantle cell lymphoma. Am J Clin Pathol. 132:699–706. PMID:19846810
1295. Gao Y, Kristinsson SY, Goldin LR, et al. (2009). Increased risk for non-Hodgkin lymphoma in individuals with celiac disease and a potential familial association. Gastroenterology. 136:91–8. PMID:18950631
1296. Garand R, Goasguen J, Brizard A, et al. (1998). Indolent course as a relatively frequent presentation in T-prolymphocytic leukaemia. Groupe Français d'Hématologie Cellulaire. Br J Haematol. 103:488–94. PMID:9827924
1297. García JF, Mollejo M, Fraga M, et al. (2005). Large B-cell lymphoma with Hodgkin's features. Histopathology. 47:101–10. PMID:15982329
1298. Garcia-Herrera A, Colomo L, Camós M, et al. (2008). Primary cutaneous small/medium CD4+ T-cell lymphomas: a heterogeneous group of tumors with different clinicopathologic features and outcome. J Clin Oncol. 26:3364–71. PMID:18541895
1299. Garcia-Herrera A, Song JY, Chuang SS, et al. (2011). Nonhepatosplenic γδ T-cell lymphomas represent a spectrum of aggressive cytotoxic T-cell lymphomas with a mainly extranodal presentation. Am J Surg Pathol. 35:1214–25. PMID:21753698
1300. García-Sanz R, Orfão A, González M, et al. (1999). Primary plasma cell leukemia: clinical, immunophenotypic, DNA ploidy, and cytogenetic characteristics. Blood. 93:1032–7. PMID:9920853
1301. Gardner RV, Velez MC, Ode DL, et al. (2004). Gamma/delta T-cell lymphoma as a recurrent complication after transplantation. Leuk Lymphoma. 45:2355–9. PMID:15512831
1302. Garnache Ottou F, Chandesris MO, Lhermitte L, et al. (2014). Peripheral blood 8 colour flow cytometry monitoring of hairy cell leukaemia allows detection of high-risk patients. Br J Haematol. 166:50–9. PMID:24661013
1303. Garnache-Ottou F, Feuillard J, Ferrand C, et al. (2009). Extended diagnostic criteria for plasmacytoid dendritic cell leukaemia. Br J Haematol. 145:624–36. PMID:19388928
1304. Garzon R, Garofalo M, Martelli MP, et al. (2008). Distinctive microRNA signature of acute myeloid leukemia bearing cytoplasmic mutated nucleophosmin. Proc Natl Acad Sci U S A. 105:3945–50. PMID:18308931
1305. Gascoyne RD, Adomat SA, Krajewski S, et al. (1997). Prognostic significance of Bcl-2 protein expression and Bcl-2 gene rearrangement in diffuse aggressive non-Hodgkin's lymphoma. Blood. 90:244–51. PMID:9207459
1306. Gascoyne RD, Aoun P, Wu D, et al. (1999). Prognostic significance of anaplastic lymphoma kinase (ALK) protein expression in adults with anaplastic large cell lymphoma. Blood. 93:3913–21. PMID:10339500
1307. Gascoyne RD, Lamant L, Martin-Subero JI, et al. (2003). ALK-positive diffuse large B-cell lymphoma is associated with Clathrin-ALK rearrangements: report of 6 cases. Blood. 102:2568–73. PMID:12763927
1308. Gatalica Z, Bilalovic N, Palazzo JP, et al. (2015). Disseminated histiocytoses biomarkers beyond BRAFV600E: frequent expression of PD-L1. Oncotarget. 6:19819–25. PMID:26110571
1309. Gattermann N, Aul C, Schneider W (1990). Two types of acquired idiopathic sideroblastic anaemia (AISA). Br J Haematol. 74:45–52. PMID:2310696
1310. Gattermann N, Billiet J, Kronenwett R, et al. (2007). High frequency of the JAK2 V617F mutation in patients with thrombocytosis (platelet count>600x109/L) and ringed sideroblasts more than 15% considered as MDS/MPD, unclassifiable. Blood. 109:1334–5. PMID:17244688
1310A. Gaulard P, Bourquelot P, Kanavaros P, et al. (1990). Expression of the alpha/beta and gamma/delta T-cell receptors in 57 cases of peripheral T-cell lymphomas. Identification of a subset of gamma/delta T-cell lymphomas. Am J

Pathol. 137:617–28. PMID:1698028
1311. Gauwerky CE, Hoxie J, Nowell PC, et al. (1988). Pre-B-cell leukemia with a t(8; 14) and a t(14; 18) translocation is preceded by follicular lymphoma. Oncogene. 2:431–5. PMID:3131717
1312. Gavrilescu LC, Cross NCP, Van Etten RA (2008). Distinct leukemogenic activity and imatinib responsiveness of a BCR-PDGFR alpha fusion tyrosine kinase. Blood. 108:Abstract 3634.
1313. Gebauer N, Bernard V, Feller AC, et al. (2013). ID3 mutations are recurrent events in double-hit B-cell lymphomas. Anticancer Res. 33:4771–8. PMID:24222112
1314. Gebauer N, Bernard V, Gebauer W, et al. (2015). TP53 mutations are frequent events in double-hit B-cell lymphomas with MYC and BCL2 but not MYC and BCL6 translocations. Leuk Lymphoma. 56:179–85. PMID:24679006
1315. Gebauer N, Bernard V, Thorns C, et al. (2015). Oncogenic MYD88 mutations are rare events in double-hit B-cell lymphomas. Acta Haematol. 133:113–5. PMID:25247317
1316. Gebauer N, Gebauer J, Hardel TT, et al. (2015). Prevalence of targetable oncogenic mutations and genomic alterations in Epstein-Barr virus-associated diffuse large B-cell lymphoma of the elderly. Leuk Lymphoma. 56:1100–6. PMID:25030036
1317. Gebauer N, Nissen EJ, Driesch Pv, et al. (2014). Intravascular natural killer cell lymphoma mimicking mycosis fungoides: a case report and review of the literature. Am J Dermatopathol. 36:e100–4. PMID:24803068
1318. Geelen FA, Vermeer MH, Meijer CJ, et al. (1998). bcl-2 protein expression in primary cutaneous large B-cell lymphoma is site-related. J Clin Oncol. 16:2080–5. PMID:9626207
1319. Geisler CH, Kolstad A, Laurell A, et al. (2010). The Mantle Cell Lymphoma International Prognostic Index (MIPI) is superior to the International Prognostic Index (IPI) in predicting survival following intensive first-line immunochemotherapy and autologous stem cell transplantation (ASCT). Blood. 115:1530–3. PMID:20032504
1320. Geissinger E, Bonzheim I, Krenács L, et al. (2006). Nodal peripheral T-cell lymphomas correspond to distinct mature T-cell populations. J Pathol. 210:172–80. PMID:16924587
1321. Geissinger E, Odenwald T, Lee SS, et al. (2004). Nodal peripheral T-cell lymphomas and, in particular, their lymphoepithelioid (Lennert's) variant are often derived from CD8(+) cytotoxic T-cells. Virchows Arch. 445:334–43. PMID:15480768
1322. Geissinger E, Sadler P, Roth S, et al. (2010). Disturbed expression of the T-cell receptor/CD3 complex and associated signaling molecules in CD30+ T-cell lymphoproliferations. Haematologica. 95:1697–704. PMID:20511667
1323. Geissmann F, Dieu-Nosjean MC, Dezutter C, et al. (2002). Accumulation of immature Langerhans cells in human lymph nodes draining chronically inflamed skin. J Exp Med. 196:417–30. PMID:12186835
1324. Geissmann F, Ruskoné-Fourmestraux A, Hermine O, et al. (1998). Homing receptor alpha4beta7 integrin expression predicts digestive tract involvement in mantle cell lymphoma. Am J Pathol. 153:1701–5. PMID:9846960
1325. Gellrich S, Rutz S, Golembowski S, et al. (2001). Primary cutaneous follicle center cell lymphomas and large B cell lymphomas of the leg descend from germinal center cells. A single cell polymerase chain reaction analysis. J Invest Dermatol. 117:1512–20. PMID:11886516
1326. Genovese G, Kähler AK, Handsaker RE, et al. (2014). Clonal hematopoiesis and blood-cancer risk inferred from blood DNA sequence. N Engl J Med. 371:2477–87. PMID:25426838
1327. Gentile TC, Uner AH, Hutchison RE, et al. (1994). CD3+, CD56+ aggressive variant of large granular lymphocyte leukemia. Blood. 84:2315–21. PMID:7522625
1327A. Gentry M, Bodo J, Durkin L, et al. (2017). Performance of a commercially available MAL antibody in the diagnosis of primary mediastinal large B-Cell lymphoma. Am J Surg Pathol. 41:189-94. PMID:27879516
1328. George TI, Wrede JE, Bangs CD, et al. (2005). Low-grade B-Cell lymphomas with plasmacytic differentiation lack PAX5 gene rearrangements. J Mol Diagn. 7:346–51. PMID:16049306
1329. Georgii A, Buesche G, Kreft A (1998). The histopathology of chronic myeloproliferative diseases. Baillieres Clin Haematol. 11:721–49. PMID:10640214
1330. Georgii A, Vykoupil KF, Buhr T, et al. (1990). Chronic myeloproliferative disorders in bone marrow biopsies. Pathol Res Pract. 186:3–27. PMID:2179909
1330A. Gerard-Marchant R, Hamlin I, Lennert K, et al. (1974). Classification of non-Hodgkin's lymphoma. Lancet. 2:406–8.
1331. Géraud C, Goerdt S, Klemke CD (2011). Primary cutaneous CD8+ small/medium-sized pleomorphic T-cell lymphoma, ear-type: a unique cutaneous T-cell lymphoma with a favourable prognosis. Br J Dermatol. 164:456–8. PMID:20969565
1332. Gerdes J, Van Baarlen J, Pileri S, et al. (1987). Tumor cell growth fraction in Hodgkin's disease. Am J Pathol. 128:390–3. PMID:3307442
1333. Germing U, Gattermann N, Aivado M, et al. (2000). Two types of acquired idiopathic sideroblastic anaemia (AISA): a time-tested distinction. Br J Haematol. 108:724–8. PMID:10792275
1334. Germing U, Gattermann N, Minning H, et al. (1998). Problems in the classification of CMML–dysplastic versus proliferative type. Leuk Res. 22:871–8. PMID:9766745
1335. Germing U, Gattermann N, Strupp C, et al. (2000). Validation of the WHO proposals for a new classification of primary myelodysplastic syndromes: a retrospective analysis of 1600 patients. Leuk Res. 24:983–92. PMID:11077111
1336. Germing U, Kündgen A, Gattermann N (2004). Risk assessment in chronic myelomonocytic leukemia (CMML). Leuk Lymphoma. 45:1311–8. PMID:15359628
1337. Germing U, Lauseker M, Hildebrandt B, et al. (2012). Survival, prognostic factors and rates of leukemic transformation in 381 untreated patients with MDS and del(5q): a multicenter study. Leukemia. 26:1286–92. PMID:22289990
1338. Germing U, Strupp C, Giagounidis A, et al. (2012). Evaluation of dysplasia through detailed cytomorphology in 3156 patients from the Düsseldorf Registry on myelodysplastic syndromes. Leuk Res. 36:727–34. PMID:22421409
1339. Germing U, Strupp C, Knipp S, et al. (2007). Chronic myelomonocytic leukemia in the light of the WHO proposals. Haematologica. 92:974–7. PMID:17606449
1340. Germing U, Strupp C, Kuendgen A, et al. (2006). Refractory anaemia with excess of blasts (RAEB): analysis of reclassification according to the WHO proposals. Br J Haematol. 132:162–7. PMID:16398650
1341. Germing U, Strupp C, Kuendgen A, et al. (2006). Prospective validation of the WHO proposals for the classification of myelodysplastic syndromes. Haematologica. 91:1596–604. PMID:17145595
1342. Germing U, Strupp C, Kündgen A, et al. (2004). No increase in age-specific incidence of myelodysplastic syndromes. Haematologica. 89:905–10. PMID:15339672
1343. Gerr H, Zimmermann M, Schrappe M, et al. (2010). Acute leukaemias of ambiguous lineage in children: characterization, prognosis and therapy recommendations. Br J Haematol. 149:84–92. PMID:20085575
1344. Gerstung M, Pellagatti A, Malcovati L, et al. (2015). Combining gene mutation with gene expression data improves outcome prediction in myelodysplastic syndromes. Nat Commun. 6:5901. PMID:25574665
1345. Gertz MA (2013). Immunoglobulin light chain amyloidosis: 2013 update on diagnosis, prognosis, and treatment. Am J Hematol. 88:416–25. PMID:23605846
1346. Gertz MA, Kyle RA (2003). Amyloidosis with IgM monoclonal gammopathies. Semin Oncol. 30:325–8. PMID:12720162
1347. Gertz MA, Kyle RA, Noel P (1993). Primary systemic amyloidosis: a rare complication of immunoglobulin M monoclonal gammopathies and Waldenström's macroglobulinemia. J Clin Oncol. 11:914–20. PMID:8487054
1348. Gesk S, Gascoyne RD, Schnitzer B, et al. (2005). ALK-positive diffuse large B-cell lymphoma with ALK-Clathrin fusion belongs to the spectrum of pediatric lymphomas. Leukemia. 19:1839–40. PMID:16107887
1349. Geyer JT, Subramaniyam S, Jiang Y, et al. (2015). Lymphoblastic transformation of follicular lymphoma: a clinicopathologic and molecular analysis of 7 patients. Hum Pathol. 46:260–71. PMID:25529125
1350. Geyer JT, Verma S, Mathew S, et al. (2013). Bone marrow morphology predicts additional chromosomal abnormalities in patients with myelodysplastic syndrome with del(5q). Hum Pathol. 44:346–56. PMID:22995330
1351. Ghesquieres H, Slager SL, Jardin F, et al. (2015). Genome-Wide Association Study of Event-Free Survival in Diffuse Large B-Cell Lymphoma Treated With Immunochemotherapy. J Clin Oncol. 33:3930–7. PMID:26460308
1352. Ghez D, Lepelletier Y, Lambert S, et al. (2006). Neuropilin-1 is involved in human T-cell lymphotropic virus type 1 entry. J Virol. 80:6844–54. PMID:16809290
1353. Ghia P, Prato G, Scielzo C, et al. (2004). Monoclonal CD5+ and CD5- B-lymphocyte expansions are frequent in the peripheral blood of the elderly. Blood. 103:2337–42. PMID:14630808
1354. Ghigna MR, Reineke T, Rincé P, et al. (2013). Epstein-Barr virus infection and altered control of apoptotic pathways in posttransplant lymphoproliferative disorders. Pathobiology. 80:53–9. PMID:22868923
1355. Ghobrial IM, Habermann TM, Macon WR, et al. (2005). Differences between early and late posttransplant lymphoproliferative disorders in solid organ transplant patients: are they two different diseases? Transplantation. 79:244–7. PMID:15665775
1356. Ghobrial IM, Habermann TM, Maurer MJ, et al. (2005). Prognostic analysis for survival in adult solid organ transplant recipients with post-transplantation lymphoproliferative disorders. J Clin Oncol. 23:7574–82. PMID:16186599
1357. Ghosh SK, Wood C, Boise LH, et al. (2003). Potentiation of TRAIL-induced apoptosis in primary effusion lymphoma through azidothymidine-mediated inhibition of NF-kappa B. Blood. 101:2321–7. PMID:12406882
1358. Giagounidis AA, Germing U, Haase S, et al. (2004). Clinical, morphological, cytogenetic, and prognostic features of patients with myelodysplastic syndromes and del(5q) including band q31. Leukemia. 18:113–9. PMID:14586479
1359. Giagounidis AA, Germing U, Strupp C, et al. (2005). Prognosis of patients with del(5q) MDS and complex karyotype and the possible role of lenalidomide in this patient subgroup. Ann Hematol. 84:569–71. PMID:15891887
1360. Giagounidis AA, Hildebrandt B, Heinsch M, et al. (2001). Acute basophilic leukemia. Eur J Haematol. 67:72–6. PMID:11722593
1361. Gianelli U, Bossi A, Cortinovis I, et al. (2014). Reproducibility of the WHO histological criteria for the diagnosis of Philadelphia chromosome-negative myeloproliferative neoplasms. Mod Pathol. 27:814–22. PMID:24201120
1361A. Gianelli U, Cattaneo D, Bossi A, et al. (2017). The myeloproliferative neoplasms, unclassifiable: clinical and pathological considerations. Mod Pathol. 30:169-179. PMID:27739437
1362. Gianelli U, Iurlo A, Cattaneo D, et al. (2015). Discrepancies between bone marrow histopathology and clinical phenotype in BCR-ABL1-negative myeloproliferative neoplasms associated with splanchnic vein thrombosis. Leuk Res. 39:525–9. PMID:25840747
1363. Gianelli U, Iurlo A, Cattaneo D, et al. (2014). Cooperation between pathologists and clinicians allows a better diagnosis of Philadelphia chromosome-negative myeloproliferative neoplasms. Expert Rev Hematol. 7:255–64. PMID:24524231
1364. Gianelli U, Iurlo A, Vener C, et al. (2008). The significance of bone marrow biopsy and JAK2V617F mutation in the differential diagnosis between the "early" prepolycythemic phase of polycythemia vera and essential thrombocythemia. Am J Clin Pathol. 130:336–42. PMID:18701405
1365. Gianelli U, Vener C, Bossi A, et al. (2012). The European Consensus on grading of bone marrow fibrosis allows a better prognostication of patients with primary myelofibrosis. Mod Pathol. 25:1193–202. PMID:22627739
1366. Gianelli U, Vener C, Raviele PR, et al. (2006). Essential thrombocythemia or chronic idiopathic myelofibrosis? A single-center study based on hematopoietic bone marrow histology. Leuk Lymphoma. 47:1774–81. PMID:17064987
1367. Gibson SE, Hsi ED (2009). Epstein-Barr virus-positive B-cell lymphoma of the elderly at a United States tertiary medical center: an uncommon aggressive lymphoma with a nongerminal center B-cell phenotype. Hum Pathol. 40:653–61. PMID:19144386
1368. Gibson SE, Swerdlow SH, Craig FE, et al. (2011). EBV-positive extranodal marginal zone lymphoma of mucosa-associated lymphoid tissue in the posttransplant setting: a distinct type of posttransplant lymphoproliferative disorder? Am J Surg Pathol. 35:807–15. PMID:21552113
1369. Gibson SE, Swerdlow SH, Ferry JA, et al. (2011). Reassessment of small lymphocytic lymphoma in the era of monoclonal B-cell lymphocytosis. Haematologica. 96:1144–52. PMID:21546505
1370. Gibson TM, Morton LM, Shiels MS, et al. (2014). Risk of non-Hodgkin lymphoma subtypes in HIV-infected people during the HAART era: a population-based study. AIDS. 28:2313–8. PMID:25111081
1371. Gilmour KC, Cranston T, Jones A, et al. (2000). Diagnosis of X-linked lymphoproliferative disease by analysis of SLAM-associated protein expression. Eur J Immunol. 30:1691–7. PMID:10898506
1372. Gilmour KC, Gaspar HB (2003). Pathogenesis and diagnosis of X-linked lymphoproliferative disease. Expert Rev Mol Diagn. 3:549–61. PMID:14510176
1373. Giné E, Martinez A, Villamor N, et al. (2010). Expanded and highly active proliferation centers identify a histological subtype of chronic lymphocytic leukemia ("accelerated" chronic lymphocytic leukemia) with aggressive

clinical behavior. Haematologica. 95:1526–33. PMID:20421272
1374. Giona F, Putti MC, Micalizzi C, et al. (2015). Long-term results of high-dose imatinib in children and adolescents with chronic myeloid leukaemia in chronic phase: the Italian experience. Br J Haematol. 170:398–407. PMID:25891192
1375. Giona F, Teofili L, Moleti ML, et al. (2012). Thrombocythemia and polycythemia in patients younger than 20 years at diagnosis: clinical and biologic features, treatment, and long-term outcome. Blood. 119:2219–27. PMID:22262773
1376. Girard T, Luquet-Besson I, Baran-Marszak F, et al. (2005). HIV+ MALT lymphoma remission induced by highly active antiretroviral therapy alone. Eur J Haematol. 74:70–2. PMID:15613110
1377. Girodon F, Dutrillaux F, Broséus J, et al. (2010). Leukocytosis is associated with poor survival but not with increased risk of thrombosis in essential thrombocythemia: a population-based study of 311 patients. Leukemia. 24:900–3. PMID:20130601
1378. Gisslinger H (2006). Update on diagnosis and management of essential thrombocythemia. Semin Thromb Hemost. 32:430–6. PMID:16810619
1379. Gisslinger H, Gotic M, Holowiecki J, et al. (2013). Anagrelide compared with hydroxyurea in WHO-classified essential thrombocythemia: the ANAHYDRET Study, a randomized controlled trial. Blood. 121:1720–8. PMID:23315161
1380. Gisslinger H, Jeryczynski G, Gisslinger B, et al. (2016). Clinical impact of bone marrow morphology for the diagnosis of essential thrombocythemia: comparison between the BCSH and the WHO criteria. Leukemia. 30:1126–32 PMID:26710883
1381. Giulino-Roth L, Wang K, MacDonald TY, et al. (2012). Targeted genomic sequencing of pediatric Burkitt lymphoma identifies recurrent alterations in antiapoptotic and chromatin-remodeling genes. Blood. 120:5181–4. PMID:23091298
1382. Glas AM, Knoops L, Delahaye L, et al. (2007). Gene-expression and immunohistochemical study of specific T-cell subsets and accessory cell types in the transformation and prognosis of follicular lymphoma. J Clin Oncol. 25:390–8. PMID:17200149
1383. Glaser SL, Keegan TH, Clarke CA, et al. (2005). Exposure to childhood infections and risk of Epstein-Barr virus–defined Hodgkin's lymphoma in women. Int J Cancer. 115:599–605. PMID:15700307
1384. Glaser SL, Lin RJ, Stewart SL, et al. (1997). Epstein-Barr virus-associated Hodgkin's disease: epidemiologic characteristics in international data. Int J Cancer. 70:375–82. PMID:9033642
1385. Gloghini A, Volpi CC, Caccia D, et al. (2014). Primary effusion lymphoma: secretome analysis reveals novel candidate biomarkers with potential pathogenetic significance. Am J Pathol. 184:618–30. PMID:24521760
1386. Go H, Jeon YK, Huh J, et al. (2014). Frequent detection of BRAF(V600E) mutations in histiocytic and dendritic cell neoplasms. Histopathology. 65:261–72. PMID:24720374
1387. Goasguen JE, Bennett JM, Bain BJ, et al. (2014). Proposal for refining the definition of dysgranulopoiesis in acute myeloid leukemia and myelodysplastic syndromes. Leuk Res. 38:447–53. PMID:24439566
1388. Goasguen JE, Bennett JM, Bain BJ, et al. (2016). Quality control initiative on the evaluation of the dysmegakaryopoiesis in myeloid neoplasms: Difficulties in the assessment of dysplasia. Leuk Res. 45:75–81. PMID:27107657
1389. Gobbi C, Buess M, Probst A, et al. (2003). Enteropathy-associated T-cell lymphoma with initial manifestation in the CNS. Neurology. 60:1718–9. PMID:12771280
1390. Godley LA (2014). Inherited predisposition to acute myeloid leukemia. Semin Hematol. 51:306–21. PMID:25311743
1391. Goedert JJ, Bower M (2012). Impact of highly effective antiretroviral therapy on the risk for Hodgkin lymphoma among people with human immunodeficiency virus infection. Curr Opin Oncol. 24:531–6. PMID:22729154
1392. Goemans BF, Zwaan CM, Miller M, et al. (2005). Mutations in KIT and RAS are frequent events in pediatric core-binding factor acute myeloid leukemia. Leukemia. 19:1536–42. PMID:16015387
1393. Goldberg JM, Silverman LB, Levy DE, et al. (2003). Childhood T-cell acute lymphoblastic leukemia: the Dana-Farber Cancer Institute acute lymphoblastic leukemia consortium experience. J Clin Oncol. 21:3616–22. PMID:14512392
1394. Goldberg SL, Chen E, Corral M, et al. (2010). Incidence and clinical complications of myelodysplastic syndromes among United States Medicare beneficiaries. J Clin Oncol. 28:2847–52. PMID:20421543
1395. Goldgeier MH, Nordlund JJ, Lucky AW, et al. (1982). Hydroa vacciniforme: diagnosis and therapy. Arch Dermatol. 118:588–91. PMID:7103528
1396. Goldin LR, Pfeiffer RM, Li X, et al. (2004). Familial risk of lymphoproliferative tumors in families of patients with chronic lymphocytic leukemia: results from the Swedish Family-Cancer Database. Blood. 104:1850–4. PMID:15161669
1397. Golomb HM, Rowley JD, Vardiman JW, et al. (1980). "Microgranular" acute promyelocytic leukemia: a distinct clinical, ultrastructural, and cytogenetic entity. Blood. 55:253–9. PMID:6928105
1398. Golub TR, Barker GF, Lovett M, et al. (1994). Fusion of PDGF receptor beta to a novel ets-like gene, tel, in chronic myelomonocytic leukemia with t(5;12) chromosomal translocation. Cell. 77:307–16. PMID:8168137
1399. Gong S, Auer I, Duggal R, et al. (2015). Epstein-Barr virus-associated inflammatory pseudotumor presenting as a colonic mass. Hum Pathol. 46:1956–61. PMID:26477709
1400. Gonsalves WI, Rajkumar SV, Go RS, et al. (2014). Trends in survival of patients with primary plasma cell leukemia: a population-based analysis. Blood. 124:907–12. PMID:24957143
1401. Gonzalez CL, Medeiros LJ, Braziel RM, et al. (1991). T-cell lymphoma involving subcutaneous tissue. A clinicopathologic entity commonly associated with hemophagocytic syndrome. Am J Surg Pathol. 15:17–27. PMID:1985499
1402. Gonzalez CL, Medeiros LJ, Jaffe ES (1991). Composite lymphoma. A clinicopathologic analysis of nine patients with Hodgkin's disease and B-cell non-Hodgkin's lymphoma. Am J Clin Pathol. 96:81–9. PMID:2069139
1403. Gonzalez-Aguilar A, Idbaih A, Boisselier B, et al. (2012). Recurrent mutations of MYD88 and TBL1XR1 in primary central nervous system lymphomas. Clin Cancer Res. 18:5203–11. PMID:22837180
1404. González-Barca E, Domingo-Domenech E, Capote FJ, et al. (2007). Prospective phase II trial of extended treatment with rituximab in patients with B-cell post-transplant lymphoproliferative disease. Haematologica. 92:1489–94. PMID:18024397
1404A. Gonzalez-Farre B, Martinez D, Lopez-Guerra M, et al. (2017). HHV8-related lymphoid proliferations: a broad spectrum of lesions from reactive lymphoid hyperplasia to overt lymphoma. Mod Pathol. 30:745–60. PMID:28084335
1405. Gonzalez-Farre B, Rovira J, Martinez D, et al. (2014). In vivo intratumoral Epstein-Barr virus replication is associated with XBP1 activation and early-onset post-transplant lymphoproliferative disorders with prognostic implications. Mod Pathol. 27:1599–611. PMID:24762547
1406. Goodlad JR (2001). Spindle-cell B-cell lymphoma presenting in the skin. Br J Dermatol. 145:313–7. PMID:11531800
1407. Goodlad JR, Batstone PJ, Hamilton D, et al. (2003). Follicular lymphoma with marginal zone differentiation: cytogenetic findings in support of a high-risk variant of follicular lymphoma. Histopathology. 42:292–8. PMID:12605649
1408. Goodlad JR, Krajewski AS, Batstone PJ, et al. (2002). Primary cutaneous follicular lymphoma: a clinicopathologic and molecular study of 16 cases in support of a distinct entity. Am J Surg Pathol. 26:733–41. PMID:12023577
1409. Goodlad JR, Krajewski AS, Batstone PJ, et al. (2003). Primary cutaneous diffuse large B-cell lymphoma: prognostic significance of clinicopathological subtypes. Am J Surg Pathol. 27:1538–45. PMID:14657713
1410. Gopcsa L, Banyai A, Jakab K, et al. (2005). Extensive flow cytometric characterization of plasmacytoid dendritic cell leukemia cells. Eur J Haematol. 75:346–51. PMID:16146542
1411. Gordeuk VR, Stockton DW, Prchal JT (2005). Congenital polycythemias/erythrocytoses. Haematologica. 90:109–16. PMID:15642677
1412. Gordon S (2007). The macrophage: past, present and future. Eur J Immunol. 37 Suppl 1:S9–17. PMID:17972350
1413. Gordon S, Taylor PR (2005). Monocyte and macrophage heterogeneity. Nat Rev Immunol. 5:953–64. PMID:16322748
1414. Gotlib J, Maxson JE, George TI, et al. (2013). The new genetics of chronic neutrophilic leukemia and atypical CML: implications for diagnosis and treatment. Blood. 122:1707–11. PMID:23896413
1415. Gould VE, Warren WH, Faber LP, et al. (1990). Malignant cells of epithelial phenotype limited to thoracic lymph nodes. Eur J Cancer. 26:1121–6. PMID:2149993
1416. Goy A, Kalayoglu Besisik S, Drach J, et al. (2015). Longer-term follow-up and outcome by tumour cell proliferation rate (Ki-67) in patients with relapsed/refractory mantle cell lymphoma treated with lenalidomide on MCL-001(EMERGE) pivotal trial. Br J Haematol. 170:496–503. PMID:25921098
1417. Goyal RK, McEvoy L, Wilson DB (1996). Hodgkin disease after renal transplantation in childhood. J Pediatr Hematol Oncol. 18:392–5. PMID:8888750
1418. Gradowski JF, Jaffe ES, Warnke RA, et al. (2010). Follicular lymphomas with plasmacytic differentiation include two subtypes. Mod Pathol. 23:71–9. PMID:19838161
1419. Gradowski JF, Sargent RL, Craig FE, et al. (2012). Chronic lymphocytic leukemia/small lymphocytic lymphoma with cyclin D1 positive proliferation centers do not have CCND1 translocations or gains and lack SOX11 expression. Am J Clin Pathol. 138:132–9. PMID:22706868
1420. Granfeldt Østgård LS, Medeiros BC, Sengeløv H, et al. (2015). Epidemiology and Clinical Significance of Secondary and Therapy-Related Acute Myeloid Leukemia: A National Population-Based Cohort Study. J Clin Oncol. 33:3641–9. PMID:26304885
1421. Grange F, Bekkenk MW, Wechsler J, et al. (2001). Prognostic factors in primary cutaneous large B-cell lymphomas: a European multicenter study. J Clin Oncol. 19:3602–10. PMID:11504742
1422. Grange F, Beylot-Barry M, Courville P, et al. (2007). Primary cutaneous diffuse large B-cell lymphoma, leg type: clinicopathologic features and prognostic analysis in 60 cases. Arch Dermatol. 143:1144–50. PMID:17875875
1423. Grange F, Joly P, Barbe C, et al. (2014). Improvement of survival in patients with primary cutaneous diffuse large B-cell lymphoma, leg type, in France. JAMA Dermatol. 150:535–41. PMID:24647650
1424. Grange F, Petrella T, Beylot-Barry M, et al. (2004). Bcl-2 protein expression is the strongest independent prognostic factor of survival in primary cutaneous large B-cell lymphomas. Blood. 103:3662–8. PMID:14726400
1425. Grasso JA, Myers TJ, Hines JD, et al. (1980). Energy-dispersive X-ray analysis of the mitochondria of sideroblastic anaemia. Br J Haematol. 46:57–72. PMID:6932957
1426. Graux C, Cools J, Michaux L, et al. (2006). Cytogenetics and molecular genetics of T-cell acute lymphoblastic leukemia: from thymocyte to lymphoblast. Leukemia. 20:1496–510. PMID:16826225
1427. Gravel S, Delsol G, Al Saati T (1998). Single-cell analysis of the t(14;18)(q32;q21) chromosomal translocation in Hodgkin's disease demonstrates the absence of this translocation in neoplastic Hodgkin and Reed-Sternberg cells. Blood. 91:2866–74. PMID:9531597
1428. Greaves MF (2004). Biological models for leukaemia and lymphoma. IARC Sci Publ. (157):351–72. PMID:15055306
1429. Green CL, Koo KK, Hills RK, et al. (2010). Prognostic significance of CEBPA mutations in a large cohort of younger adult patients with acute myeloid leukemia: impact of double CEBPA mutations and the interaction with FLT3 and NPM1 mutations. J Clin Oncol. 28:2739–47. PMID:20439648
1430. Green CL, Tawana K, Hills RK, et al. (2013). GATA2 mutations in sporadic and familial acute myeloid leukaemia patients with CEBPA mutations. Br J Haematol. 161:701–5. PMID:23560626
1431. Green M, Kaufmann M, Wilson J, et al. (1997). Comparison of intravenous ganciclovir followed by oral acyclovir with intravenous ganciclovir alone for prevention of cytomegalovirus and Epstein-Barr virus disease after liver transplantation in children. Clin Infect Dis. 25:1344–9. PMID:9431375
1432. Green MR, Alizadeh AA (2014). Common progenitor cells in mature B-cell malignancies: implications for therapy. Curr Opin Hematol. 21:333–40. PMID:24811163
1433. Green MR, Aya-Bonilla C, Gandhi MK, et al. (2011). Integrative genomic profiling reveals conserved genetic mechanisms for tumorigenesis in common entities of non-Hodgkin's lymphoma. Genes Chromosomes Cancer. 50:313–26. PMID:21305641
1434. Green MR, Gentles AJ, Nair RV, et al. (2013). Hierarchy in somatic mutations arising during genomic evolution and progression of follicular lymphoma. Blood. 121:1604–11. PMID:23297126
1435. Green MR, Kihira S, Liu CL, et al. (2015). Mutations in early follicular lymphoma progenitors are associated with suppressed antigen presentation. Proc Natl Acad Sci U S A. 112:E1116–25. PMID:25713363
1436. Green MR, Monti S, Rodig SJ, et al. (2010). Integrative analysis reveals selective 9p24.1 amplification, increased PD-1 ligand expression, and further induction via JAK2 in nodular sclerosing Hodgkin lymphoma and primary mediastinal large B-cell lymphoma. Blood. 116:3268–77. PMID:20628145
1437. Green PH, Cellier C (2007). Celiac disease. N Engl J Med. 357:1731–43. PMID:17960014

1438. Green PH, Fleischauer AT, Bhagat G, et al. (2003). Risk of malignancy in patients with celiac disease. Am J Med. 115:191–5. PMID:12935825

1439. Green TM, Nielsen O, de Stricker K, et al. (2012). High levels of nuclear MYC protein predict the presence of MYC rearrangement in diffuse large B-cell lymphoma. Am J Surg Pathol. 36:612–9. PMID:22314191

1440. Green TM, Young KH, Visco C, et al. (2012). Immunohistochemical double-hit score is a strong predictor of outcome in patients with diffuse large B-cell lymphoma treated with rituximab plus cyclophosphamide, doxorubicin, vincristine, and prednisone. J Clin Oncol. 30:3460–7. PMID:22665537

1441. Greenberg AJ, Rajkumar SV, Vachon CM (2012). Familial monoclonal gammopathy of undetermined significance and multiple myeloma: epidemiology, risk factors, and biological characteristics. Blood. 119:5359–66. PMID:22354002

1442. Greenberg P, Cox C, LeBeau MM, et al. (1997). International scoring system for evaluating prognosis in myelodysplastic syndromes. Blood. 89:2079–88. PMID:9058730

1442A. Greenberg P, Cox C, LeBeau MM, et al. (1998). Erratum. Blood 91:1100

1443. Greenberg PL, Stone RM, Bejar R, et al. (2015). Myelodysplastic syndromes, version 2.2015. J Natl Compr Canc Netw. 13:261–72. PMID:25736003

1444. Greenberg PL, Tuechler H, Schanz J, et al. (2012). Revised international prognostic scoring system for myelodysplastic syndromes. Blood. 120:2454–65. PMID:22740453

1444A. Greenberg PL, Tuechler H, Schanz J, et al. (2016). Cytopenia levels for aiding establishment of the diagnosis of myelodysplastic syndromes. Blood. 128:2096–7. PMID:27535995

1445. Greenberg PL, Young NS, Gattermann N (2002). Myelodysplastic syndromes. Hematology Am Soc Hematol Educ Program. 136–61. PMID:12446422

1446. Greenblatt D, Ally M, Child F, et al. (2013). Indolent CD8(+) lymphoid proliferation of acral sites: a clinicopathologic study of six patients with some atypical features. J Cutan Pathol. 40:248–58. PMID:23189944

1447. Greene ME, Mundschau G, Wechsler J, et al. (2003). Mutations in GATA1 in both transient myeloproliferative disorder and acute megakaryoblastic leukemia of Down syndrome. Blood Cells Mol Dis. 31:351–6. PMID:14636651

1448. Greer JP, Macon WR, Lamar RE, et al. (1995). T-cell-rich B-cell lymphomas: diagnosis and response to therapy of 44 patients. J Clin Oncol. 13:1742–50. PMID:7602364

1449. Gregg XT, Reddy V, Prchal JT (2002). Copper deficiency masquerading as myelodysplastic syndrome. Blood. 100:1493–5. PMID:12149237

1450. Greif PA, Dufour A, Konstandin NP, et al. (2012). GATA2 zinc finger 1 mutations associated with biallelic CEBPA mutations define a unique genetic entity of acute myeloid leukemia. Blood. 120:395–403. PMID:22649106

1451. Greiner A, Tobollik S, Buettner M, et al. (2005). Differential expression of activation-induced cytidine deaminase (AID) in nodular lymphocyte-predominant and classical Hodgkin lymphoma. J Pathol. 205:541–7. PMID:15732141

1452. Greiner TC, Gascoyne RD, Anderson ME, et al. (1996). Nodular lymphocyte-predominant Hodgkin's disease associated with large-cell lymphoma: analysis of Ig gene rearrangements by V-J polymerase chain reaction. Blood. 88:657–66. PMID:8695813

1453. Greiner TC, Moynihan MJ, Chan WC, et al. (1996). p53 mutations in mantle cell lymphoma are associated with variant cytology and predict a poor prognosis. Blood. 87:4302–10. PMID:8639789

1454. Greipp PR, Leong T, Bennett JM, et al. (1998). Plasmablastic morphology–an independent prognostic factor with clinical and laboratory correlates: Eastern Cooperative Oncology Group (ECOG) myeloma trial E9486 report by the ECOG Myeloma Laboratory Group. Blood. 91:2501–7. PMID:9516151

1455. Greipp PR, Lust JA, O'Fallon WM, et al. (1993). Plasma cell labeling index and beta 2-microglobulin predict survival independent of thymidine kinase and C-reactive protein in multiple myeloma. Blood. 81:3382–7. PMID:8507875

1456. Greipp PR, San Miguel J, Durie BG, et al. (2005). International staging system for multiple myeloma. J Clin Oncol. 23:3412–20. PMID:15809451

1457. Greisman HA, Lu Z, Tsai AG, et al. (2012). IgH partner breakpoint sequences provide evidence that AID initiates t(11;14) and t(8;14) chromosomal breaks in mantle cell and Burkitt lymphomas. Blood. 120:2864–7. PMID:22915650

1458. Grever MR (2010). How I treat hairy cell leukemia. Blood. 115:21–8. PMID:19843881

1459. Griffin CA, Hawkins AL, Dvorak C, et al. (1999). Recurrent involvement of 2p23 in inflammatory myofibroblastic tumors. Cancer Res. 59:2776–80. PMID:10383129

1460. Griffin GK, Sholl LM, Lindeman NI, et al. (2016). Targeted genomic sequencing of follicular dendritic cell sarcoma reveals recurrent alterations in NF-κB regulatory genes. Mod Pathol. 29:67–74. PMID:26564005

1461. Griffin JH, Leung J, Bruner RJ, et al. (2003). Discovery of a fusion kinase in EOL-1 cells and idiopathic hypereosinophilic syndrome. Proc Natl Acad Sci U S A. 100:7830–5. PMID:12808148

1462. Grigg AP, Gascoyne RD, Phillips GL, et al. (1993). Clinical, haematological and cytogenetic features in 24 patients with structural rearrangements of the Q arm of chromosome 3. Br J Haematol. 83:158–65. PMID:8435325

1463. Grimaldi JC, Meeker TC (1989). The t(5;14) chromosomal translocation in a case of acute lymphocytic leukemia joins the interleukin-3 gene to the immunoglobulin heavy chain gene. Blood. 73:2081–5. PMID:2499362

1464. Grimwade D, Hills RK, Moorman AV, et al. (2010). Refinement of cytogenetic classification in acute myeloid leukemia: determination of prognostic significance of rare recurring chromosomal abnormalities among 5876 younger adult patients treated in the United Kingdom Medical Research Council trials. Blood. 116:354–65. PMID:20385793

1465. Grimwade D, Mrózek K (2011). Diagnostic and prognostic value of cytogenetics in acute myeloid leukemia. Hematol Oncol Clin North Am. 25:1135–61, vii. [vii.] PMID:22093581

1466. Grimwade D, Walker H, Oliver F, et al. (1998). The importance of diagnostic cytogenetics on outcome in AML: analysis of 1,612 patients entered into the MRC AML 10 trial. Blood. 92:2322–33. PMID:9746770

1467. Gritti C, Dastot H, Soulier J, et al. (1998). Transgenic mice for MTCP1 develop T-cell prolymphocytic leukemia. Blood. 92:368–73. PMID:9657733

1468. Grogan TM, Lippman SM, Spier CM, et al. (1988). Independent prognostic significance of a nuclear proliferation antigen in diffuse large cell lymphomas as determined by the monoclonal antibody Ki-67. Blood. 71:1157–60. PMID:3281723

1469. Grogg KL, Attygalle AD, Macon WR, et al. (2006). Expression of CXCL13, a chemokine highly upregulated in germinal center T-helper cells, distinguishes angioimmunoblastic T-cell lymphoma from peripheral T-cell lymphoma, unspecified. Mod Pathol. 19:1101–7. PMID:16680156

1470. Grogg KL, Attygalle AD, Macon WR, et al. (2005). Angioimmunoblastic T-cell lymphoma: a neoplasm of germinal-center T-helper cells? Blood. 106:1501–2. PMID:16079436

1471. Grogg KL, Jung S, Erickson LA, et al. (2008). Primary cutaneous CD4-positive small/medium-sized pleomorphic T-cell lymphoma: a clonal T-cell lymphoproliferative disorder with indolent behavior. Mod Pathol. 21:708–15. PMID:18311111

1472. Grogg KL, Lae ME, Kurtin PJ, et al. (2004). Clusterin expression distinguishes follicular dendritic cell tumors from other dendritic cell neoplasms: report of a novel follicular dendritic cell marker and clinicopathologic data on 12 additional follicular dendritic cell tumors and 6 additional interdigitating dendritic cell tumors. Am J Surg Pathol. 28:988–98. PMID:15252304

1473. Grogg KL, Macon WR, Kurtin PJ, et al. (2005). A survey of clusterin and fascin expression in sarcomas and spindle cell neoplasms: strong clusterin immunostaining is highly specific for follicular dendritic cell tumor. Mod Pathol. 18:260–6. PMID:15467709

1474. Gross TG, Bucuvalas JC, Park JR, et al. (2005). Low-dose chemotherapy for Epstein-Barr virus-positive post-transplantation lymphoproliferative disease in children after solid organ transplantation. J Clin Oncol. 23:6481–8. PMID:16170157

1475. Grossmann V, Bacher U, Haferlach C, et al. (2013). Acute erythroid leukemia (AEL) can be separated into distinct prognostic subsets based on cytogenetic and molecular genetic characteristics. Leukemia. 27:1940–3. PMID:23648669

1476. Grouard G, Rissoan MC, Filgueira L, et al. (1997). The enigmatic plasmacytoid T cells develop into dendritic cells with interleukin (IL)-3 and CD40-ligand. J Exp Med. 185:1101–11. PMID:9091583

1477. Groves FD, Linet MS, Travis LB, et al. (2000). Cancer surveillance series: non-Hodgkin's lymphoma incidence by histologic subtype in the United States from 1978 through 1995. J Natl Cancer Inst. 92:1240–51. PMID:10922409

1477A. Gruber TA, Larson Gedman A, Zhang J, et al. (2012). An Inv(16)(p13.3q24.3)-encoded CBFA2T3-GLIS2 fusion protein defines an aggressive subtype of pediatric acute megakaryoblastic leukemia. Cancer Cell. 22:683–97. PMID:23153540

1478. Grulich AE, Vajdic CM, Cozen W (2007). Altered immunity as a risk factor for non-Hodgkin lymphoma. Cancer Epidemiol Biomarkers Prev. 16:405–8. PMID:17337643

1479. Gruver AM, Huba MA, Dogan A, et al. (2012). Fibrin-associated large B-cell lymphoma: part of the spectrum of cardiac lymphomas. Am J Surg Pathol. 36:1527–37. PMID:22982895

1479A. Gröschel S, Lugthart S, Schlenk RF, et al. (2010). High EVI1 expression predicts outcome in younger adult patients with acute myeloid leukemia and is associated with distinct cytogenetic abnormalities. J Clin Oncol. 28:2101–7. PMID:20308656

1480. Gröschel S, Sanders MA, Hoogenboezem R, et al. (2014). A single oncogenic enhancer rearrangement causes concomitant EVI1 and GATA2 deregulation in leukemia. Cell. 157:369–81. PMID:24703711

1481. Gröschel S, Sanders MA, Hoogenboezem R, et al. (2015). Mutational spectrum of myeloid malignancies with inv(3)/t(3;3) reveals a predominant involvement of RAS/RTK signaling pathways. Blood. 125:133–9. PMID:25381062

1482. Gröschel S, Schlenk RF, Engelmann J, et al. (2013). Deregulated expression of EVI1 defines a poor prognostic subset of MLL-rearranged acute myeloid leukemias: a study of the German-Austrian Acute Myeloid Leukemia Study Group and the Dutch-Belgian-Swiss HOVON/SAKK Cooperative Group. J Clin Oncol. 31:95–103. PMID:23008312

1483. Grønbaek K, Straten PT, Ralfkiaer E, et al. (1998). Somatic Fas mutations in non-Hodgkin's lymphoma: association with extranodal disease and autoimmunity. Blood. 92:3018–24. PMID:9787134

1484. Gualco G, Domeny-Duarte P, Chioato L, et al. (2011). Clinicopathologic and molecular features of 122 Brazilian cases of nodal and extranodal NK/T-cell lymphoma, nasal type, with EBV subtyping analysis. Am J Surg Pathol. 35:1195–203. PMID:21716086

1485. Guenova E, Schanz S, Hoetzenecker W, et al. (2014). Systemic corticosteroids for subcutaneous panniculitis-like T-cell lymphoma. Br J Dermatol. 171:891–4. PMID:24725144

1486. Guglielmelli P, Lasho TL, Rotunno G, et al. (2014). The number of prognostically detrimental mutations and prognosis in primary myelofibrosis: an international study of 797 patients. Leukemia. 28:1804–10. PMID:24549259

1487. Guidelines Working Group of UK Myeloma Forum; British Commitee for Standards in Haematology, British Society for Haematology (2004). Guidelines on the diagnosis and management of AL amyloidosis. Br J Haematol. 125:681–700. PMID:15180858

1488. Guillaume T, Beguin Y, Tabrizi R, et al. (2015). Allogeneic hematopoietic stem cell transplantation for T-prolymphocytic leukemia: a report from the French society for stem cell transplantation (SFGM-TC). Eur J Haematol. 94:265–9. PMID:25130897

1489. Guillem VM, Collado M, Terol MJ, et al. (2007). Role of MTHFR (677, 1298) haplotype in the risk of developing secondary leukemia after treatment of breast cancer and hematological malignancies. Leukemia. 21:1413–22. PMID:17476281

1490. Guinee D Jr, Jaffe E, Kingma D, et al. (1994). Pulmonary lymphomatoid granulomatosis. Evidence for a proliferation of Epstein-Barr virus infected B-lymphocytes with a prominent T-cell component and vasculitis. Am J Surg Pathol. 18:753–64. PMID:8037289

1491. Guinee DG Jr, Perkins SL, Travis WD, et al. (1998). Proliferation and cellular phenotype in lymphomatoid granulomatosis: implications of a higher proliferation index in B cells. Am J Surg Pathol. 22:1093–100. PMID:9737242

1492. Guitart J (2000). HIV-1 and an HTLV-II-associated cutaneous T-cell lymphoma. N Engl J Med. 343:303–4. PMID:10928885

1493. Guitart J, Weisenburger DD, Subtil A, et al. (2012). Cutaneous γδ T-cell lymphomas: a spectrum of presentations with overlap with other cytotoxic lymphomas. Am J Surg Pathol. 36:1656–65. PMID:23073324

1494. Gulia A, Saggini A, Wiesner T, et al. (2011). Clinicopathologic features of early lesions of primary cutaneous follicle center lymphoma, diffuse type: implications for early diagnosis and treatment. J Am Acad Dermatol. 65:991–1000. PMID:21704419

1495. Gunawardana J, Chan FC, Telenius A, et al. (2014). Recurrent somatic mutations of PTPN1 in primary mediastinal B cell lymphoma and Hodgkin lymphoma. Nat Genet. 46:329–35. PMID:24531327

1496. Gunsilius E, Duba HC, Petzer AL, et al. (2000). Evidence from a leukaemia model for maintenance of vascular endothelium by bone-marrow-derived endothelial cells. Lancet. 355:1688–91. PMID:10905245

1497. Guo RJ, Bahmanyar M, Minden MD, et

al. (2016). CD33, not early precursor T-cell phenotype, is associated with adverse outcome in adult T-cell acute lymphoblastic leukaemia. Br J Haematol. 172:823–5. PMID:26123477

1498. Gupta G, Man I, Kemmett D (2000). Hydroa vacciniforme: A clinical and follow-up study of 17 cases. J Am Acad Dermatol. 42:208–13. PMID:10642674

1499. Gupta R, Abdalla SH, Bain BJ (1999). Thrombocytosis with sideroblastic erythropoiesis: a mixed myeloproliferative myelodysplastic syndrome. Leuk Lymphoma. 34:615–9. PMID:10492088

1500. Gupta R, Soupir CP, Johari V, et al. (2007). Myelodysplastic syndrome with isolated deletion of chromosome 20q: an indolent disease with minimal morphological dysplasia and frequent thrombocytopenic presentation. Br J Haematol. 139:265–8. PMID:17764468

1501. Gurney JG, Smith MA, Bunin GR (1995). CNS and miscellaneous intracranial and intraspinal neoplasms. In: Ries LAG, Smith MA, Gurney JG, et al., editors. Cancer incidence and survival among children and adolescents. United States SEER Program 1975-1995. NIH Pub no. 99-4649. Bethesda: National Cancer Institute.

1502. Gutiérrez NC, Ocio EM, de Las Rivas J, et al. (2007). Gene expression profiling of B lymphocytes and plasma cells from Waldenström's macroglobulinemia: comparison with expression patterns of the same cell counterparts from chronic lymphocytic leukemia, multiple myeloma and normal individuals. Leukemia. 21:541–9. PMID:17252022

1503. Gyan E, Dreyfus F, Fenaux P (2015). Refractory thrombocytopenia and neutropenia: a diagnostic challenge. Mediterr J Hematol Infect Dis. 7:e2015018. PMID:25745545

1504. Göhring G, Michalova K, Beverloo HB, et al. (2010). Complex karyotype newly defined: the strongest prognostic factor in advanced childhood myelodysplastic syndrome. Blood. 116:3766–9. PMID:20802024

1505. Ha SY, Sung J, Ju H, et al. (2013). Epstein-Barr virus-positive nodal peripheral T cell lymphomas: clinicopathologic and gene expression profiling study. Pathol Res Pract. 209:448–54. PMID:23735590

1506. Hadfield KA, Swalla BJ, Jeffery WR (1995). Multiple origins of anural development in ascidians inferred from rDNA sequences. J Mol Evol. 40:413–27. PMID:7646666

1507. Hadithi M, Mallant M, Oudejans J, et al. (2006). 18F-FDG PET versus CT for the detection of enteropathy-associated T-cell lymphoma in refractory celiac disease. J Nucl Med. 47:1622–7. PMID:17015897

1508. Hadzić N, Pagliuca A, Rela M, et al. (2000). Correction of the hyper-IgM syndrome after liver and bone marrow transplantation. N Engl J Med. 342:320–4. PMID:10655530

1509. Hadzidimitriou A, Agathangelidis A, Darzentas N, et al. (2011). Is there a role for antigen selection in mantle cell lymphoma? Immunogenetic support from a series of 807 cases. Blood. 118:3088–95. PMID:21791422

1510. Haferlach C, Dicker F, Schnittger S, et al. (2007). Comprehensive genetic characterization of CLL: a study on 506 cases analysed with chromosome banding analysis, interphase FISH, IgV(H) status and immunophenotyping. Leukemia. 21:2442–51. PMID:17805327

1511. Haferlach C, Mecucci C, Schnittger S, et al. (2009). AML with mutated NPM1 carrying a normal or aberrant karyotype show overlapping biologic, pathologic, immunophenotypic, and prognostic features. Blood. 114:3024–32. PMID:19429869

1512. Haferlach T, Kohlmann A, Klein HU, et al. (2009). AML with translocation t(8;16)(p11;p13) demonstrates unique cytomorphological,

cytogenetic, molecular and prognostic features. Leukemia. 23:934–43. PMID:19194466

1513. Haferlach T, Nagata Y, Grossmann V, et al. (2014). Landscape of genetic lesions in 944 patients with myelodysplastic syndromes. Leukemia. 28:241–7. PMID:24220272

1514. Haferlach T, Schoch C, Löffler H, et al. (2003). Morphologic dysplasia in de novo acute myeloid leukemia (AML) is related to unfavorable cytogenetics but has no independent prognostic relevance under the conditions of intensive induction therapy: results of a multiparameter analysis from the German AML Cooperative Group studies. J Clin Oncol. 21:256–65. PMID:12525517

1515. Hagen JW, Magro CM (2014). Indolent CD8+ lymphoid proliferation of the face with eyelid involvement. Am J Dermatopathol. 36:137–41. PMID:24556898

1516. Haghighi B, Smoller BR, LeBoit PE, et al. (2000). Pagetoid reticulosis (Woringer-Kolopp disease): an immunophenotypic, molecular, and clinicopathologic study. Mod Pathol. 13:502–10. PMID:10824921

1517. Hahm C, Huh HJ, Mun YC, et al. (2015). Genomic aberrations of myeloproliferative and myelodysplastic/myeloproliferative neoplasms in chronic phase and during disease progression. Int J Lab Hematol. 37:181–9. PMID:24845343

1518. Hahn CN, Chong CE, Carmichael CL, et al. (2011). Heritable GATA2 mutations associated with familial myelodysplastic syndrome and acute myeloid leukemia. Nat Genet. 43:1012–7. PMID:21892162

1519. Hahtola S, Tuomela S, Elo L, et al. (2006). Th1 response and cytotoxicity genes are down-regulated in cutaneous T-cell lymphoma. Clin Cancer Res. 12:4812–21. PMID:16914566

1520. Hall J, Foucar K (2010). Diagnosing myelodysplastic/myeloproliferative neoplasms: laboratory testing strategies to exclude other disorders. Int J Lab Hematol. 32:559–71. PMID:20670271

1521. Hallböök H, Gustafsson G, Smedmyr B, et al. (2006). Treatment outcome in young adults and children >10 years of age with acute lymphoblastic leukemia in Sweden: a comparison between a pediatric protocol and an adult protocol. Cancer. 107:1551–61. PMID:16955505

1522. Hallek M, Bergsagel PL, Anderson KC (1998). Multiple myeloma: increasing evidence for a multistep transformation process. Blood. 91:3–21. PMID:9414264

1523. Hallek M, Cheson BD, Catovsky D, et al. (2008). Guidelines for the diagnosis and treatment of chronic lymphocytic leukemia: a report from the International Workshop on Chronic Lymphocytic Leukemia updating the National Cancer Institute-Working Group 1996 guidelines. Blood. 111:5446–56. PMID:18216293

1524. Hallermann C, Kaune KM, Gesk S, et al. (2004). Molecular cytogenetic analysis of chromosomal breakpoints in the IGH, MYC, BCL6, and MALT1 gene loci in primary cutaneous B-cell lymphomas. J Invest Dermatol. 123:213–9. PMID:15191563

1525. Hallermann C, Kaune KM, Siebert R, et al. (2004). Chromosomal aberration patterns differ in subtypes of primary cutaneous B cell lymphomas. J Invest Dermatol. 122:1495–502. PMID:15175042

1526. Hamadeh F, MacNamara S, Bacon CM, et al. (2014). Gamma heavy chain disease lacks the MYD88 L265P mutation associated with lymphoplasmacytic lymphoma. Haematologica. 99:e154–5. PMID:24859878

1527. Hamadeh F, MacNamara SP, Aguilera NS, et al. (2015). MYD88 L265P mutation analysis helps define nodal lymphoplasmacytic

lymphoma. Mod Pathol. 28:564–74. PMID:25216226

1528. Hamblin TJ, Davis Z, Gardiner A, et al. (1999). Unmutated Ig V(H) genes are associated with a more aggressive form of chronic lymphocytic leukemia. Blood. 94:1848–54. PMID:10477713

1529. Hamilton A, Helgason GV, Schemionek M, et al. (2012). Chronic myeloid leukemia stem cells are not dependent on Bcr-Abl kinase activity for their survival. Blood. 119:1501–10. PMID:22184410

1530. Hamilton SN, Wai ES, Tan K, et al. (2013). Treatment and outcomes in patients with primary cutaneous B-cell lymphoma: the BC Cancer Agency experience. Int J Radiat Oncol Biol Phys. 87:719–25. PMID:24001373

1531. Hamilton-Dutoit SJ, Raphael M, Audouin J, et al. (1993). In situ demonstration of Epstein-Barr virus small RNAs (EBER 1) in acquired immunodeficiency syndrome-related lymphomas: correlation with tumor morphology and primary site. Blood. 82:619–24. PMID:8392401

1532. Hammer RD, Glick AD, Greer JP, et al. (1996). Splenic marginal zone lymphoma. A distinct B-cell neoplasm. Am J Surg Pathol. 20:613–26. PMID:8619426

1533. Han JY, Theil KS (2006). The Philadelphia chromosome as a secondary abnormality in inv(3)(q21q26) acute myeloid leukemia at diagnosis: confirmation of p190 BCR-ABL mRNA by real-time quantitative polymerase chain reaction. Cancer Genet Cytogenet. 165:70–4. PMID:16490599

1534. Han X, Bueso-Ramos CE (2007). Precursor T-cell acute lymphoblastic leukemia/lymphoblastic lymphoma and acute biphenotypic leukemias. Am J Clin Pathol. 127:528–44. PMID:17369128

1535. Hanfstein B, Müller MC, Hochhaus A (2015). Response-related predictors of survival in CML. Ann Hematol. 94 Suppl 2:S227–39. PMID:25814089

1536. Hanna J, Markoulaki S, Schorderet P, et al. (2008). Direct reprogramming of terminally differentiated mature B lymphocytes to pluripotency. Cell. 133:250–64. PMID:18423197

1537. Hans CP, Weisenburger DD, Greiner TC, et al. (2004). Confirmation of the molecular classification of diffuse large B-cell lymphoma by immunohistochemistry using a tissue microarray. Blood. 103:275–82. PMID:14504078

1538. Hansmann ML, Stein H, Fellbaum C, et al. (1989). Nodular paragranuloma can transform into high-grade malignant lymphoma of B type. Hum Pathol. 20:1169–75. PMID:2591946

1539. Hanson CA, Abaza M, Sheldon S, et al. (1993). Acute biphenotypic leukaemia: immunophenotypic and cytogenetic analysis. Br J Haematol. 84:49–60. PMID:7687860

1540. Hanson CA, Jaszcz W, Kersey JH, et al. (1989). True histiocytic lymphoma: histopathologic, immunophenotypic and genotypic analysis. Br J Haematol. 73:187–98. PMID:2684258

1541. Hanto DW, Gajl-Peczalska KJ, Frizzera G, et al. (1983). Epstein-Barr virus (EBV) induced polyclonal and monoclonal B-cell lymphoproliferative diseases occurring after renal transplantation. Clinical, pathologic, and virologic findings and implications for therapy. Ann Surg. 198:356–69. PMID:6311121

1542. Hao X, Wei X, Huang F, et al. (2015). The expression of CD30 based on immunohistochemistry predicts inferior outcome in patients with diffuse large B-cell lymphoma. PLoS One. 10:e0126615. PMID:25974110

1543. Hapgood G, Savage KJ (2015). The biology and management of systemic anaplastic large cell lymphoma. Blood. 126:17–25. PMID:25869285

1544. Haque AK, Myers JL, Hudnall SD, et al. (1998). Pulmonary lymphomatoid

granulomatosis in acquired immunodeficiency syndrome: lesions with Epstein-Barr virus infection. Mod Pathol. 11:347–56. PMID:9578085

1545. Haque T, McAulay KA, Kelly D, et al. (2010). Allogeneic T-cell therapy for Epstein-Barr virus-positive posttransplant lymphoproliferative disease: long-term follow-up. Transplantation. 90:93–4. PMID:20606564

1546. Harada H, Harada Y, Tanaka H, et al. (2003). Implications of somatic mutations in the AML1 gene in radiation-associated and therapy-related myelodysplastic syndrome/acute myeloid leukemia. Blood. 101:673–80. PMID:12393679

1547. Haralambieva E, Boerma EJ, van Imhoff GW, et al. (2005). Clinical, immunophenotypic, and genetic analysis of adult lymphomas with morphologic features of Burkitt lymphoma. Am J Surg Pathol. 29:1086–94. PMID:16006805

1548. Haralambieva E, Pulford KA, Lamant L, et al. (2000). Anaplastic large-cell lymphomas of B-cell phenotype are anaplastic lymphoma kinase (ALK) negative and belong to the spectrum of diffuse large B-cell lymphomas. Br J Haematol. 109:584–91. PMID:10886208

1549. Haralambieva E, Rosati S, van Noesel C, et al. (2004). Florid granulomatous reaction in Epstein-Barr virus-positive nonendemic Burkitt lymphomas: report of four cases. Am J Surg Pathol. 28:379–83. PMID:15104301

1550. Haralambieva E, Schuuring E, Rosati S, et al. (2004). Interphase fluorescence in situ hybridization for detection of 8q24/MYC breakpoints on routine histologic sections: validation in Burkitt lymphomas from three geographic regions. Genes Chromosomes Cancer. 40:10–8. PMID:15034863

1551. Harif M, Barsaoui S, Benchekroun S, et al. (2005). [Treatment of childhood cancer in Africa. Preliminary results of the French-African paediatric oncology group]. Arch Pediatr. 12:851–3. PMID:15904826

1552. Harney J, Pope A, Short SC (2004). Primary central nervous system lymphoma with testicular relapse. Clin Oncol (R Coll Radiol). 16:193–5. PMID:15191006

1552A. Haroche J, Abla O (2015). Uncommon histiocytic disorders: Rosai-Dorfman, juvenile xanthogranuloma, and Erdheim-Chester disease. Hematology Am Soc Hematol Educ Program. 2015:571–8. PMID:26637774

1553. Haroche J, Charlotte F, Arnaud L, et al. (2012). High prevalence of BRAF V600E mutations in Erdheim-Chester disease but not in other non-Langerhans cell histiocytoses. Blood. 120:2700–3. PMID:22879539

1553A. Haroche J, Cohen-Aubart F, Emile JF, et al. (2015). Reproducible and sustained efficacy of targeted therapy with vemurafenib in patients with BRAF(V600E)-mutated Erdheim-Chester disease. J Clin Oncol. 33:411–8. PMID:25422482

1554. Harris MB, Shuster JJ, Carroll A, et al. (1992). Trisomy of leukemic cell chromosomes 4 and 10 identifies children with B-progenitor cell acute lymphoblastic leukemia with a very low risk of treatment failure: a Pediatric Oncology Group study. Blood. 79:3316–24. PMID:1596572

1555. Harris NL, Demirjian Z (1991). Plasmacytoid T-zone cell proliferation in a patient with chronic myelomonocytic leukemia. Histologic and immunohistologic characterization. Am J Surg Pathol. 15:87–95. PMID:1845925

1556. Harris NL, Jaffe ES, Diebold J, et al. (1999). World Health Organization classification of neoplastic diseases of the hematopoietic and lymphoid tissues: report of the Clinical Advisory Committee meeting-Airlie House, Virginia, November 1997. J Clin Oncol. 17:3835–49. PMID:10577857

1557. Harris NL, Jaffe ES, Stein H, et al. (1994).

A revised European-American classification of lymphoid neoplasms: a proposal from the International Lymphoma Study Group. Blood. 84:1361–92. PMID:8068936
1558. Harris NL, Nadler LM, Bhan AK (1984). Immunohistologic characterization of two malignant lymphomas of germinal center type (centroblastic/centrocytic and centrocytic) with monoclonal antibodies. Follicular and diffuse lymphomas of small-cleaved-cell type are related but distinct entities. Am J Pathol. 117:262–72. PMID:6437232
1559. Harrison CJ, Hills RK, Moorman AV, et al. (2010). Cytogenetics of childhood acute myeloid leukemia: United Kingdom Medical Research Council Treatment trials AML 10 and 12. J Clin Oncol. 28:2674–81. PMID:20439644
1560. Harrison CJ, Moorman AV, Broadfield ZJ, et al. (2004). Three distinct subgroups of hypodiploidy in acute lymphoblastic leukaemia. Br J Haematol. 125:552–9. PMID:15147369
1561. Harrison CJ, Moorman AV, Schwab C, et al. (2014). An international study of intrachromosomal amplification of chromosome 21 (iAMP21): cytogenetic characterization and outcome. Leukemia. 28:1015–21. PMID:24166298
1562. Harrison CN, Bareford D, Butt N, et al. (2010). Guideline for investigation and management of adults and children presenting with a thrombocytosis. Br J Haematol. 149:352–75. PMID:20331456
1563. Harrison CN, Green AR (2003). Essential thrombocythemia. Hematol Oncol Clin North Am. 17:1175–90, vii. [vii.] PMID:14560781
1563A. Harrison CN, Vannucchi AM, Kiladjian JJ, et al. (2016). Long-term findings from Comfort-II, a phase 3 study of ruxolitinib vs best available therapy for myelofibrosis. Leukemia. 30:1701–7. PMID:27211272
1564. Hart DN, Baker BW, Inglis MJ, et al. (1992). Epstein-Barr viral DNA in acute large granular lymphocyte (natural killer) leukemic cells. Blood. 79:2116–23. PMID:1314113
1565. Hart M, Thakral B, Yohe S, et al. (2014). EBV-positive mucocutaneous ulcer in organ transplant recipients: a localized indolent posttransplant lymphoproliferative disorder. Am J Surg Pathol. 38:1522–9. PMID:25007145
1566. Hartge P, Colt JS, Severson RK, et al. (2005). Residential herbicide use and risk of non-Hodgkin lymphoma. Cancer Epidemiol Biomarkers Prev. 14:934–7. PMID:15824166
1567. Hartmann K, Escribano L, Grattan C, et al. (2016). Cutaneous manifestations in patients with mastocytosis: Consensus report of the European Competence Network on Mastocytosis; the American Academy of Allergy, Asthma & Immunology; and the European Academy of Allergology and Clinical Immunology. J Allergy Clin Immunol. 137:35–45 PMID:26476479
1568. Hartmann K, Henz BM (2002). Cutaneous mastocytosis – clinical heterogeneity. Int Arch Allergy Immunol. 127:143–6. PMID:11919426
1569. Hartmann S, Agostinelli C, Klapper W, et al. (2011). Revising the historical collection of epithelioid cell-rich lymphomas of the Kiel Lymph Node Registry: what is Lennert's lymphoma nowadays? Histopathology. 59:1173–82. PMID:22175897
1569A. Hartmann S, Döring C, Agostinelli C, et al. (2016) miRNA expression profiling divides follicular dendritic cell sarcomas into two groups, related to fibroblasts and myopericytomas or Castleman's disease. Eur J Cancer. 64:159–66. PMID:27423414
1570. Hartmann S, Döring C, Jakobus C, et al. (2013). Nodular lymphocyte predominant hodgkin lymphoma and T cell/histiocyte rich large B cell lymphoma–endpoints of a spectrum of one disease? PLoS One. 8:e78812. PMID:24244368
1571. Hartmann S, Döring C, Vucic E, et al. (2015). Array comparative genomic hybridization reveals similarities between nodular lymphocyte predominant Hodgkin lymphoma and T cell/histiocyte rich large B cell lymphoma. Br J Haematol. 169:415–22. PMID:25644177
1572. Hartmann S, Eichenauer DA, Plütschow A, et al. (2013). The prognostic impact of variant histology in nodular lymphocyte-predominant Hodgkin lymphoma: a report from the German Hodgkin Study Group (GHSG). Blood. 122:4246–52, quiz 4292. PMID:24100447
1573. Hartmann S, Gesk S, Scholtysik R, et al. (2010). High resolution SNP array genomic profiling of peripheral T cell lymphomas, not otherwise specified, identifies a subgroup with chromosomal aberrations affecting the REL locus. Br J Haematol. 148:402–12. PMID:19863542
1574. Hartmann S, Jakobus C, Rengstl B, et al. (2013). Spindle-shaped CD163+ rosetting macrophages replace CD4+ T-cells in HIV-related classical Hodgkin lymphoma. Mod Pathol. 26:648–57. PMID:23307058
1575. Hartmann S, Schuhmacher B, Rausch T, et al. (2016). Highly recurrent mutations of SGK1, DUSP2 and JUNB in nodular lymphocyte predominant Hodgkin lymphoma. Leukemia. 30:844–53 PMID:26658840
1576. Hartmann S, Tousseyn T, Döring C, et al. (2013). Macrophages in T cell/histiocyte rich large B cell lymphoma strongly express metal-binding proteins and show a bi-activated phenotype. Int J Cancer. 133:2609–18. PMID:23686423
1577. Harvey RC, Mullighan CG, Chen IM, et al. (2010). Rearrangement of CRLF2 is associated with mutation of JAK kinases, alteration of IKZF1, Hispanic/Latino ethnicity, and a poor outcome in pediatric B-progenitor acute lymphoblastic leukemia. Blood. 115:5312–21. PMID:20139093
1578. Hasegawa D, Bugarin C, Giordan M, et al. (2013). Validation of flow cytometric phospho-STAT5 as a diagnostic tool for juvenile myelomonocytic leukemia. Blood Cancer J. 3:e160. PMID:24241400
1579. Hasegawa D, Chen X, Hirabayashi S, et al. (2014). Clinical characteristics and treatment outcome in 65 cases with refractory cytopenia of childhood defined according to the WHO 2008 classification. Br J Haematol. 166:758–66. PMID:24894311
1580. Hasegawa D, Manabe A, Yagasaki H, et al. (2009). Treatment of children with refractory anemia: the Japanese Childhood MDS Study Group trial (MDS99). Pediatr Blood Cancer. 53:1011–5. PMID:19499580
1581. Hasenclever D, Diehl V (1998). A prognostic score for advanced Hodgkin's disease. International Prognostic Factors Project on Advanced Hodgkin's Disease. N Engl J Med. 339:1506–14. PMID:9819449
1582. Hasford J, Baccarani M, Hoffmann V, et al. (2011). Predicting complete cytogenetic response and subsequent progression-free survival in 2060 patients with CML on imatinib treatment: the EUTOS score. Blood. 118:686–92. PMID:21536864
1583. Hashimoto A, Chiba N, Tsuno H, et al. (2015). Incidence of malignancy and the risk of lymphoma in Japanese patients with rheumatoid arthritis compared to the general population. J Rheumatol. 42:564–71. PMID:25593236
1584. Hashimoto M, Yamashita Y, Mori N (2002). Immunohistochemical detection of CD79a expression in precursor T cell lymphoblastic lymphoma/leukaemias. J Pathol. 197:341–7. PMID:12115880
1585. Hasle H (1994). Myelodysplastic syndromes in childhood–classification, epidemiology, and treatment. Leuk Lymphoma. 13:11–26. PMID:8025513
1586. Hasle H, Niemeyer CM (2011). Advances in the prognostication and management of advanced MDS in children. Br J Haematol. 154:185–95. PMID:21554264
1587. Hasle H, Niemeyer CM, Chessells JM, et al. (2003). A pediatric approach to the WHO classification of myelodysplastic and myeloproliferative diseases. Leukemia. 17:277–82. PMID:12592323
1588. Hasle H, Olesen G, Kerndrup G, et al. (1996). Chronic neutrophil leukaemia in adolescence and young adulthood. Br J Haematol. 94:628–30. PMID:8826884
1589. Hasselblom S, Ridell B, Sigurdardottir M, et al. (2008). Low rather than high Ki-67 protein expression is an adverse prognostic factor in diffuse large B-cell lymphoma. Leuk Lymphoma. 49:1501–9. PMID:18766962
1590. Hasserjian RP, Campigotto F, Klepeis V, et al. (2014). De novo acute myeloid leukemia with 20-29% blasts is less aggressive than acute myeloid leukemia with ≥30% blasts in older adults: a Bone Marrow Pathology Group study. Am J Hematol. 89:E193–9. PMID:25042343
1591. Hasserjian RP, Harris NL (2007). NK-cell lymphomas and leukemias: a spectrum of tumors with variable manifestations and immunophenotype. Am J Clin Pathol. 127:860–8. PMID:17509983
1592. Hasserjian RP, Zuo Z, Garcia C, et al. (2010). Acute erythroid leukemia: a reassessment using criteria refined in the 2008 WHO classification. Blood. 115:1985–92. PMID:20040759
1593. Hayday A, Theodoridis E, Ramsburg E, et al. (2001). Intraepithelial lymphocytes: exploring the Third Way in immunology. Nat Immunol. 2:997–1003. PMID:11685222
1594. Hayman SR, Bailey RJ, Jalal SM, et al. (2001). Translocations involving the immunoglobulin heavy-chain locus are possible early genetic events in patients with primary systemic amyloidosis. Blood. 98:2266–8. PMID:11568015
1595. Head DR (1996). Revised classification of acute myeloid leukemia. Leukemia. 10:1826–31. PMID:8892688
1596. Hebert J, Cayuela JM, Berkeley J, et al. (1994). Candidate tumor-suppressor genes MTS1 (p16INK4A) and MTS2 (p15INK4B) display frequent homozygous deletions in primary cells from T- but not from B-cell lineage acute lymphoblastic leukemias. Blood. 84:4038–44. PMID:7994022
1597. Heerema NA, Carroll AJ, Devidas M, et al. (2013). Intrachromosomal amplification of chromosome 21 is associated with inferior outcomes in children with acute lymphoblastic leukemia treated in contemporary standard-risk children's oncology group studies: a report from the children's oncology group. J Clin Oncol. 31:3397–402. PMID:23940221
1598. Heerema NA, Raimondi SC, Anderson JR, et al. (2007). Specific extra chromosomes occur in a modal number dependent pattern in pediatric acute lymphoblastic leukemia. Genes Chromosomes Cancer. 46:684–93. PMID:17431878
1599. Heesch S, Neumann M, Schwartz S, et al. (2013). Acute leukemias of ambiguous lineage in adults: molecular and clinical characterization. Ann Hematol. 92:747–58. PMID:23412561
1600. Hegewisch S, Mainzer K, Braumann D (1987). IgE myelomatosis. Presentation of a new case and summary of literature. Blut. 55:55–60. PMID:3607296
1601. Hehlmann R (2012). How I treat CML blast crisis. Blood. 120:737–47. PMID:22653972
1602. Hehlmann R (2015). CML–Where do we stand in 2015? Ann Hematol. 94 Suppl 2:S103–5. PMID:25814076
1603. Heiligenberg W (1990). Electrosensory systems in fish. Synapse. 6:196–206. PMID:2237781
1604. Heinicke T, Hütten H, Kalinski T, et al. (2015). Sustained remission of blastic plasmacytoid dendritic cell neoplasm after unrelated allogeneic stem cell transplantation–a single center experience. Ann Hematol. 94:283–7. PMID:25138222
1605. Helbig G, Kyrcz-Krzemien S (2013). Myeloid neoplasms with eosinophilia and FIP1L1-PDGFRA fusion gene: another point of view. Leuk Lymphoma. 54:897–8. PMID:23025324
1606. Helbig G, Soja A, Bartkowska-Chrobok A, et al. (2012). Chronic eosinophilic leukemia-not otherwise specified has a poor prognosis with unresponsiveness to conventional treatment and high risk of acute transformation. Am J Hematol. 87:643–5. PMID:22473587
1607. Helbig G, Wieczorkiewicz A, Dziaczkowska-Suszek J, et al. (2009). T-cell abnormalities are present at high frequencies in patients with hypereosinophilic syndrome. Haematologica. 94:1236–41. PMID:19734416
1608. Heller KN, Teruya-Feldstein J, La Quaglia MP, et al. (2004). Primary follicular lymphoma of the testis: excellent outcome following surgical resection without adjuvant chemotherapy. J Pediatr Hematol Oncol. 26:104–7. PMID:14767197
1609. Henderson R, Spence L (2006). Down syndrome with myelodysplasia of megakaryoblastic lineage. Clin Lab Sci. 19:161–4. PMID:16910232
1610. Henopp T, Quintanilla-Martínez L, Fend F, et al. (2011). Prevalence of follicular lymphoma in situ in consecutively analysed reactive lymph nodes. Histopathology. 59:139–42. PMID:21771030
1611. Henter JI, Horne A, Aricó M, et al. (2007). HLH-2004: Diagnostic and therapeutic guidelines for hemophagocytic lymphohistiocytosis. Pediatr Blood Cancer. 48:124–31. PMID:16937360
1612. Herbst H, Dallenbach F, Hummel M, et al. (1991). Epstein-Barr virus latent membrane protein expression in Hodgkin and Reed-Sternberg cells. Proc Natl Acad Sci U S A. 88:4766–70. PMID:1647016
1613. Herbst H, Foss HD, Samol J, et al. (1996). Frequent expression of interleukin-10 by Epstein-Barr virus-harboring tumor cells of Hodgkin's disease. Blood. 87:2918–29. PMID:8639912
1614. Herbst H, Niedobitek G, Kneba M, et al. (1990). High incidence of Epstein-Barr virus genomes in Hodgkin's disease. Am J Pathol. 137:13–8. PMID:2164775
1615. Herling M, Jones D (2007). CD4+/CD56+ hematodermic tumor: the features of an evolving entity and its relationship to dendritic cells. Am J Clin Pathol. 127:687–700. PMID:17439829
1616. Herling M, Khoury JD, Washington LT, et al. (2004). A systematic approach to diagnosis of mature T-cell leukemias reveals heterogeneity among WHO categories. Blood. 104:328–35. PMID:15044256
1617. Herling M, Patel KA, Teitell MA, et al. (2008). High TCL1 expression and intact T-cell receptor signaling define a hyperproliferative subset of T-cell prolymphocytic leukemia. Blood. 111:328–37. PMID:17890451
1618. Herling M, Teitell MA, Shen RR, et al. (2003). TCL1 expression in plasmacytoid dendritic cells (DC2s) and the related CD4+ CD56+ blastic tumors of skin. Blood. 101:5007–9. PMID:12576313
1619. Hermine O, Haioun C, Lepage E, et al. (1996). Prognostic significance of bcl-2 protein expression in aggressive non-Hodgkin's

lymphoma. Groupe d'Etude des Lymphomes de l'Adulte (GELA). Blood. 87:265–72. PMID:8547651
1620. Hermine O, Lefrère F, Bronowicki JP, et al. (2002). Regression of splenic lymphoma with villous lymphocytes after treatment of hepatitis C virus infection. N Engl J Med. 347:89–94. PMID:12110736
1620A. Hermkens MC, van den Heuvel-Eibrink MM, Arentsen-Peters ST, et al. (2013). The clinical relevance of BAALC and ERG expression levels in pediatric AML. Leukemia. 27:735–7. PMID:22895118
1621. Hernández JM, del Cañizo MC, Cuneo A, et al. (2000). Clinical, hematological and cytogenetic characteristics of atypical chronic myeloid leukemia. Ann Oncol. 11:441–4. PMID:10847463
1622. Hernández L, Beà S, Pinyol M, et al. (2005). CDK4 and MDM2 gene alterations mainly occur in highly proliferative and aggressive mantle cell lymphomas with wild-type INK4a/ARF locus. Cancer Res. 65:2199–206. PMID:15781632
1623. Hernández L, Pinyol M, Hernández S, et al. (1999). TRK-fused gene (TFG) is a new partner of ALK in anaplastic large cell lymphoma producing two structurally different TFG-ALK translocations. Blood. 94:3265–8. PMID:10556217
1624. Herndier BG, Sanchez HC, Chang KL, et al. (1993). High prevalence of Epstein-Barr virus in the Reed-Sternberg cells of HIV-associated Hodgkin's disease. Am J Pathol. 142:1073–9. PMID:8386441
1625. Herreman A, Dierickx D, Morscio J, et al. (2013). Clinicopathological characteristics of posttransplant lymphoproliferative disorders of T-cell origin: single-center series of nine cases and meta-analysis of 147 reported cases. Leuk Lymphoma. 54:2190–9. PMID:23402267
1626. Herrinton LJ, Liu L, Weng X, et al. (2011). Role of thiopurine and anti-TNF therapy in lymphoma in inflammatory bowel disease. Am J Gastroenterol. 106:2146–53. PMID:22031357
1627. Herzenberg AM, Lien J, Magil AB (1996). Monoclonal heavy chain (immunoglobulin G3) deposition disease: report of a case. Am J Kidney Dis. 28:128–31. PMID:8712207
1628. Heslop HE (2005). Biology and treatment of Epstein-Barr virus-associated non-Hodgkin lymphomas. Hematology Am Soc Hematol Educ Program. 260–6. PMID:16304390
1629. Heslop HE, Slobod KS, Pule MA, et al. (2010). Long-term outcome of EBV-specific T-cell infusions to prevent or treat EBV-related lymphoproliferative disease in transplant recipients. Blood. 115:925–35. PMID:19880495
1630. Hess JL, Bodis S, Pinkus G, et al. (1994). Histopathologic grading of nodular sclerosis Hodgkin's disease. Lack of prognostic significance in 254 surgically staged patients. Cancer. 74:708–14. PMID:8033052
1631. Hetet G, Dastot H, Baens M, et al. (2000). Recurrent molecular deletion of the 12p13 region, centromeric to ETV6/TEL, in T-cell prolymphocytic leukemia. Hematol J. 1:42–7. PMID:11920168
1631A. Heuser M, Beutel G, Krauter J, et al. (2006). High meningioma 1 (MN1) expression as a predictor for poor outcome in acute myeloid leukemia with normal cytogenetics. Blood. 108:3898–905. PMID:16912223
1632. Hiddemann W, Cheson BD (2014). How we manage follicular lymphoma. Leukemia. 28:1388–95. PMID:24577532
1633. Higgins JP, Warnke RA (1999). CD30 expression is common in mediastinal large B-cell lymphoma. Am J Clin Pathol. 112:241–7. PMID:10439805
1634. Hill BT, Tubbs RR, Smith MR (2015). Complete remission of CD30-positive diffuse large B-cell lymphoma in a patient with post-transplant lymphoproliferative disorder and end-stage renal disease treated with single-agent brentuximab vedotin. Leuk Lymphoma. 56:1552–3. PMID:24717110
1635. Hill QA, Rawstron AC, de Tute RM, et al. (2014). Outcome prediction in plasmacytoma of bone: a risk model utilizing bone marrow flow cytometry and light-chain analysis. Blood. 124:1296–9. PMID:24939658
1636. Hinds GA, Heald P (2009). Cutaneous T-cell lymphoma in skin of color. J Am Acad Dermatol. 60:359–75, quiz 376–8. PMID:19231637
1637. Hinz M, Lemke P, Anagnostopoulos I, et al. (2002). Nuclear factor kappaB-dependent gene expression profiling of Hodgkin's disease tumor cells, pathogenetic significance, and link to constitutive signal transducer and activator of transcription 5a activity. J Exp Med. 196:605–17. PMID:12208876
1638. Hinz M, Löser P, Mathas S, et al. (2001). Constitutive NF-kappaB maintains high expression of a characteristic gene network, including CD40, CD86, and a set of antiapoptotic genes in Hodgkin/Reed-Sternberg cells. Blood. 97:2798–807. PMID:11313274
1639. Hirai Y, Yamamoto T, Kimura H, et al. (2012). Hydroa vacciniforme is associated with increased numbers of Epstein-Barr virus-infected γδT cells. J Invest Dermatol. 132:1401–8. PMID:22297643
1640. Hirakawa K, Fuchigami T, Nakamura S, et al. (1996). Primary gastrointestinal T-cell lymphoma resembling multiple lymphomatous polyposis. Gastroenterology. 111:778–82. PMID:8780585
1641. Hirose Y, Masaki Y, Sugai S (2002). Leukemic transformation with trisomy 8 in essential thrombocythemia: a report of four cases. Eur J Haematol. 68:112–6. PMID:12061320
1641A. Hirsch BA, Alonzo TA, Gerbing RB, et al. (2013). Abnormalities of 12p are associated with high-risk acute myeloid leukemia: a Children's Oncology Group report [meeting abstract]. Blood. 122:612.
1642. Hishikawa N, Niwa H, Hara T, et al. (2011). An autopsy case of lymphomatosis cerebri showing pathological changes of intravascular large B-cell lymphoma in visceral organs. Neuropathology. 31:612–9. PMID:21382094
1643. Hishima T, Oyaizu N, Fujii T, et al. (2006). Decrease in Epstein-Barr virus-positive AIDS-related lymphoma in the era of highly active antiretroviral therapy. Microbes Infect. 8:1301–7. PMID:16697236
1643A. Histiocytosis syndromes in children; Writing Group of the Histiocyte Society (1987). Lancet. 1:208–9. PMID:2880029
1644. Hitzler JK, Cheung J, Li Y, et al. (2003). GATA1 mutations in transient leukemia and acute megakaryoblastic leukemia of Down syndrome. Blood. 101:4301–4. PMID:12586620
1645. Ho FC, Choy D, Loke SL, et al. (1990). Polymorphic reticulosis and conventional lymphomas of the nose and upper aerodigestive tract: a clinicopathologic study of 70 cases, and immunophenotypic studies of 16 cases. Hum Pathol. 21:1041–50. PMID:2210727
1646. Ho FC, Srivastava G, Loke SL, et al. (1990). Presence of Epstein-Barr virus DNA in nasal lymphomas of B and 'T' cell type. Hematol Oncol. 8:271–81. PMID:1979042
1646A. Ho PA, Zeng R, Alonzo TA, et al. (2010). Prevalence and prognostic implications of WT1 mutations in pediatric acute myeloid leukemia (AML): a report from the Children's Oncology Group. Blood. 116:702–10. PMID:20413658
1647. Hockley SL, Else M, Morilla A, et al. (2012). The prognostic impact of clinical and molecular features in hairy cell leukaemia variant and splenic marginal zone lymphoma. Br J Haematol. 158:347–54. PMID:22594855
1648. Hockley SL, Giannouli S, Morilla A, et al. (2010). Insight into the molecular pathogenesis of hairy cell leukaemia, hairy cell leukaemia variant and splenic marginal zone lymphoma, provided by the analysis of their IGH rearrangements and somatic hypermutation patterns. Br J Haematol. 148:666–9. PMID:19863540
1649. Hockley SL, Morgan GJ, Leone PE, et al. (2011). High-resolution genomic profiling in hairy cell leukemia-variant compared with typical hairy cell leukemia. Leukemia. 25:1189–92. PMID:21436839
1650. Hodges KB, Collins RD, Greer JP, et al. (1999). Transformation of the small cell variant Ki-1+ lymphoma to anaplastic large cell lymphoma: pathologic and clinical features. Am J Surg Pathol. 23:49–58. PMID:9888703
1651. Hodgkin (1832). On some morbid appearances of the absorbent glands and spleen. Med Chir Trans. 17:68–114.
1652. Hodgson K, Ferrer G, Montserrat E, et al. (2011). Chronic lymphocytic leukemia and autoimmunity: a systematic review. Haematologica. 96:752–61. PMID:21242190
1653. Hoefnagel JJ, Dijkman R, Basso K, et al. (2005). Distinct types of primary cutaneous large B-cell lymphoma identified by gene expression profiling. Blood. 105:3671–8. PMID:15308563
1654. Hoefnagel JJ, Vermeer MH, Jansen PM, et al. (2003). Bcl-2, Bcl-6 and CD10 expression in cutaneous B-cell lymphoma: further support for a follicle centre cell origin and differential diagnostic significance. Br J Dermatol. 149:1183–91. PMID:14674895
1655. Hoeller S, Tzankov A, Pileri SA, et al. (2010). Epstein-Barr virus-positive diffuse large B-cell lymphoma in elderly patients is rare in Western populations. Hum Pathol. 41:352–7. PMID:19913281
1656. Hoeller S, Walz C, Reiter A, et al. (2011). PCM1-JAK2-fusion: a potential treatment target in myelodysplastic-myeloproliferative and other hemato-lymphoid neoplasms. Expert Opin Ther Targets. 15:53–62. PMID:21091042
1657. Hoffmann C, Hentrich M, Gillor D, et al. (2015). Hodgkin lymphoma is as common as non-Hodgkin lymphoma in HIV-positive patients with sustained viral suppression and limited immune deficiency: a prospective cohort study. HIV Med. 16:261–4. PMID:25252101
1658. Hoffmann K, Dreger CK, Olins AL, et al. (2002). Mutations in the gene encoding the lamin B receptor produce an altered nuclear morphology in granulocytes (Pelger-Huët anomaly). Nat Genet. 31:410–4. PMID:12118250
1659. Hoffmann M, Kletter K, Becherer A, et al. (2003). 18F-fluorodeoxyglucose positron emission tomography (18F-FDG-PET) for staging and follow-up of marginal zone B-cell lymphoma. Oncology. 64:336–40. PMID:12759529
1660. Hoffmann M, Vogelsang H, Kletter K, et al. (2003). 18F-fluoro-deoxy-glucose positron emission tomography (18F-FDG-PET) for assessment of enteropathy-type T cell lymphoma. Gut. 52:347–51. PMID:12584214
1661. Hoffmann T, De Libero G, Colonna M, et al. (2000). Natural killer-type receptors for HLA class I antigens are clonally expressed in lymphoproliferative disorders of natural killer and T-cell type. Br J Haematol. 110:525–36. PMID:10997961
1662. Hoffmann VS, Baccarani M, Hasford J, et al. (2015). The EUTOS population-based registry: incidence and clinical characteristics of 2904 CML patients in 20 European Countries. Leukemia. 29:1336–43. PMID:25783795
1663. Hofscheier A, Ponciano A, Bonzheim I, et al. (2011). Geographic variation in the prevalence of Epstein-Barr virus-positive diffuse large B-cell lymphoma of the elderly: a comparative analysis of a Mexican and a German population. Mod Pathol. 24:1046–54. PMID:21499229
1664. Holland J, Trenkner DA, Wasserman TH, et al. (1992). Plasmacytoma. Treatment results and conversion to myeloma. Cancer. 69:1513–7. PMID:1540888
1665. Hollander P, Rostgaard K, Smedby KE, et al. (2015). Autoimmune and Atopic Disorders and Risk of Classical Hodgkin Lymphoma. Am J Epidemiol. 182:624–32. PMID:26346543
1666. Hollingsworth HC, Longo DL, Jaffe ES (1993). Small noncleaved cell lymphoma associated with florid epithelioid granulomatous response. A clinicopathologic study of seven patients. Am J Surg Pathol. 17:51–9. PMID:8447509
1667. Hollingsworth HC, Stetler-Stevenson M, Gagneten D, et al. (1994). Immunodeficiency-associated malignant lymphoma. Three cases showing genotypic evidence of both T- and B-cell lineages. Am J Surg Pathol. 18:1092–101. PMID:7943530
1668. Hollink IH, van den Heuvel-Eibrink MM, Arentsen-Peters ST, et al. (2011). Characterization of CEBPA mutations and promoter hypermethylation in pediatric acute myeloid leukemia. Haematologica. 96:384–92. PMID:21134981
1668A. Hollink IH, van den Heuvel-Eibrink MM, Arentsen-Peters ST, et al. (2011). NUP98/NSD1 characterizes a novel poor prognostic group in acute myeloid leukemia with a distinct HOX gene expression pattern. Blood. 118:3645–56. PMID:21813447
1668B. Hollink IH, van den Heuvel-Eibrink MM, Zimmermann M, et al. (2009). Clinical relevance of Wilms tumor 1 gene mutations in childhood acute myeloid leukemia. Blood. 113:5951–60. PMID:19171881
1669. Hollon JR, Cureton PA, Martin ML, et al. (2013). Trace gluten contamination may play a role in mucosal and clinical recovery in a subgroup of diet-adherent non-responsive celiac disease patients. BMC Gastroenterol. 13:40. PMID:23448408
1670. Hollowood K, Stamp G, Zouvani I, et al. (1995). Extranodal follicular dendritic cell sarcoma of the gastrointestinal tract. Morphologic, immunohistochemical and ultrastructural analysis of two cases. Am J Clin Pathol. 103:90–7. PMID:7817952
1671. Holm LE, Blomgren H, Löwhagen T (1985). Cancer risks in patients with chronic lymphocytic thyroiditis. N Engl J Med. 312:601–4. PMID:3838363
1672. Holmes GK, Prior P, Lane MR, et al. (1989). Malignancy in coeliac disease–effect of a gluten free diet. Gut. 30:333–8. PMID:2707633
1673. Hong F, Habermann TM, Gordon LI, et al. (2014). The role of body mass index in survival outcome for lymphoma patients: US intergroup experience. Ann Oncol. 25:669–74. PMID:24567515
1674. Hong JY, Ko YH, Kim SJ, et al. (2015). Epstein-Barr virus-positive diffuse large B-cell lymphoma of the elderly: a concise review and update. Curr Opin Oncol. 27:392–8. PMID:26258272
1675. Hong JY, Yoon DH, Suh C, et al. (2015). EBV-positive diffuse large B-cell lymphoma in young adults: is this a distinct disease entity? Ann Oncol. 26:548–55. PMID:25475080
1676. Hong M, Ko YH, Yoo KH, et al. (2013). EBV-Positive T/NK-Cell Lymphoproliferative Disease of Childhood. Korean J Pathol. 47:137–47. PMID:23667373
1677. Hong WJ, Gotlib J (2014). Hereditary erythrocytosis, thrombocytosis and neutrophilia. Best Pract Res Clin Haematol. 27:95–106. PMID:25189721
1678. Hongyo T, Hoshida Y, Nakatsuka S, et al.

(2005). p53, K-ras, c-kit and beta-catenin gene mutations in sinonasal NK/T-cell lymphoma in Korea and Japan. Oncol Rep. 13:265–71. PMID:15643509

1679. Hongyo T, Kurooka M, Taniguchi E, et al. (1998). Frequent p53 mutations at dipyrimidine sites in patients with pyothorax-associated lymphoma. Cancer Res. 58:1105–7. PMID:9515788

1680. Honig GR, Suarez CR, Vida LN, et al. (1998). Juvenile myelomonocytic leukemia (JMML) with the hematologic phenotype of severe beta thalassemia. Am J Hematol. 58:67–71. PMID:9590152

1681. Honma K, Tsuzuki S, Nakagawa M, et al. (2009). TNFAIP3/A20 functions as a novel tumor suppressor gene in several subtypes of non-Hodgkin lymphomas. Blood. 114:2467–75. PMID:19608751

1682. Honorat JF, Ragab A, Lamant L, et al. (2006). SHP1 tyrosine phosphatase negatively regulates NPM-ALK tyrosine kinase signaling. Blood. 107:4130–8. PMID:16469875

1683. Horenstein MG, Nador RG, Chadburn A, et al. (1997). Epstein-Barr virus latent gene expression in primary effusion lymphomas containing Kaposi's sarcoma-associated herpesvirus/human herpesvirus-8. Blood. 90:1186–91. PMID:9242551

1684. Horn H, Schmelter C, Leich E, et al. (2011). Follicular lymphoma grade 3B is a distinct neoplasm according to cytogenetic and immunohistochemical profiles. Haematologica. 96:1327–34. PMID:21659362

1685. Horn H, Staiger AM, Vöhringer M, et al. (2015). Diffuse large B-cell lymphomas of immunoblastic type are a major reservoir for MYC-IGH translocations. Am J Surg Pathol. 39:61–6. PMID:25229766

1686. Horn H, Ziepert M, Becher C, et al. (2013). MYC status in concert with BCL2 and BCL6 expression predicts outcome in diffuse large B-cell lymphoma. Blood. 121:2253–63. PMID:23335369

1687. Horna P, Zhang L, Sotomayor EM, et al. (2014). Diagnostic immunophenotype of acute promyelocytic leukemia before and early during therapy with all-trans retinoic acid. Am J Clin Pathol. 142:546–52. PMID:25239423

1688. Hornick JL, Jaffe ES, Fletcher CD (2004). Extranodal histiocytic sarcoma: clinicopathologic analysis of 14 cases of a rare epithelioid malignancy. Am J Surg Pathol. 28:1133–44. PMID:15316312

1689. Horning SJ, Rosenberg SA (1984). The natural history of initially untreated low-grade non-Hodgkin's lymphomas. N Engl J Med. 311:1471–5. PMID:6548796

1690. Horny HP, Kaiserling E, Campbell M, et al. (1989). Liver findings in generalized mastocytosis. A clinicopathologic study. Cancer. 63:532–8. PMID:2643456

1691. Horny HP, Kaiserling E, Handgretinger R, et al. (1995). Evidence for a lymphotropic nature of circulating plasmacytoid monocytes: findings from a case of CD56+ chronic myelomonocytic leukemia. Eur J Haematol. 54:209–16. PMID:7540556

1692. Horny HP, Kaiserling E, Parwaresch MR, et al. (1992). Lymph node findings in generalized mastocytosis. Histopathology. 21:439–46. PMID:1452127

1693. Horny HP, Parwaresch MR, Kaiserling E, et al. (1986). Mast cell sarcoma of the larynx. J Clin Pathol. 39:596–602. PMID:3088063

1694. Horny HP, Ruck M, Wehrmann M, et al. (1990). Blood findings in generalized mastocytosis: evidence of frequent simultaneous occurrence of myeloproliferative disorders. Br J Haematol. 76:186–93. PMID:2128807

1695. Horny HP, Ruck MT, Kaiserling E (1992). Spleen findings in generalized mastocytosis. A clinicopathologic study. Cancer. 70:459–68. PMID:1617595

1696. Horny HP, Sotlar K, Reiter A, et al. (2014). Myelomastocytic leukemia: histopathological features, diagnostic criteria and differential diagnosis. Expert Rev Hematol. 7:431–7. PMID:25025369

1697. Horny HP, Sotlar K, Sperr WR, et al. (2004). Systemic mastocytosis with associated clonal haematological non-mast cell lineage diseases: a histopathological challenge. J Clin Pathol. 57:604–8. PMID:15166264

1698. Horny HP, Valent P (2001). Diagnosis of mastocytosis: general histopathological aspects, morphological criteria, and immunohistochemical findings. Leuk Res. 25:543–51. PMID:11377679

1699. Horny HP, Valent P (2002). Histopathological and immunohistochemical aspects of mastocytosis. Int Arch Allergy Immunol. 127:115–7. PMID:11919419

1700. Horsman DE, Gascoyne RD, Coupland RW, et al. (1995). Comparison of cytogenetic analysis, southern analysis, and polymerase chain reaction for the detection of t(14; 18) in follicular lymphoma. Am J Clin Pathol. 103:472–8. PMID:7726146

1701. Horwitz SM, Advani RH, Bartlett NL, et al. (2014). Objective responses in relapsed T-cell lymphomas with single-agent brentuximab vedotin. Blood. 123:3095–100. PMID:24652992

1702. Hoshida Y, Li T, Dong Z, et al. (2001). Lymphoproliferative disorders in renal transplant patients in Japan. Int J Cancer. 91:869–75. PMID:11275994

1703. Hoshida Y, Xu JX, Fujita S, et al. (2007). Lymphoproliferative disorders in rheumatoid arthritis: clinicopathological analysis of 76 cases in relation to methotrexate medication. J Rheumatol. 34:322–31. PMID:17117491

1704. Hoster E, Dreyling M, Klapper W, et al. (2008). A new prognostic index (MIPI) for patients with advanced-stage mantle cell lymphoma. Blood. 111:558–65. PMID:17962512

1705. Hou HA, Lin LI, Chen CY, et al. (2009). Reply to 'Heterogeneity within AML with CEBPA mutations; only CEBPA double mutations, but not single CEBPA mutations are associated with favorable prognosis'. Br J Cancer. 101:738–40. PMID:19623175

1706. Howat AJ, McPhie JL, Smith DA, et al. (1995). Cavitation of mesenteric lymph nodes: a rare complication of coeliac disease, associated with a poor outcome. Histopathology. 27:349–54. PMID:8847065

1707. Howe RB, Porwit-MacDonald A, Wanat R, et al. (2004). The WHO classification of MDS does make a difference. Blood. 103:3265–70. PMID:14684416

1708. Howell WM, Leung ST, Jones DB, et al. (1995). HLA-DRB, -DQA, and -DQB polymorphism in celiac disease and enteropathy-associated T-cell lymphoma. Common features and additional risk factors for malignancy. Hum Immunol. 43:29–37. PMID:7558926

1709. Howlett C, Snedecor SJ, Landsburg DJ, et al. (2015). Front-line, dose-escalated immunochemotherapy is associated with a significant progression-free survival advantage in patients with double-hit lymphomas: a systematic review and meta-analysis. Br J Haematol. 170:504–14. PMID:25907897

1710. Hoyle CF, Sherrington P, Hayhoe FG (1988). Translocation (3;6)(q21;p21) in acute myeloid leukemia with abnormal thrombopoiesis and basophilia. Cancer Genet Cytogenet. 30:261–7. PMID:3422580

1711. Hoyle CF, Sherrington PD, Fischer P, et al. (1989). Basophils in acute myeloid leukaemia. J Clin Pathol. 42:785–92. PMID:2671051

1712. Hrusák O, Porwit-MacDonald A (2002). Antigen expression patterns reflecting genotype of acute leukemias. Leukemia. 16:1233–58. PMID:12094248

1713. Hsi AC, Robirds DH, Luo J, et al. (2014). T-cell prolymphocytic leukemia frequently shows cutaneous involvement and is associated with gains of MYC, loss of ATM, and TCL1A rearrangement. Am J Surg Pathol. 38:1468–83. PMID:25310835

1714. Hsiao SC, Cortada IR, Colomo L, et al. (2012). SOX11 is useful in differentiating cyclin D1-positive diffuse large B-cell lymphoma from mantle cell lymphoma. Histopathology. 61:685–93. PMID:22642745

1715. Hsu AP, Sampaio EP, Khan J, et al. (2011). Mutations in GATA2 are associated with the autosomal dominant and sporadic monocytopenia and mycobacterial infection (MonoMAC) syndrome. Blood. 118:2653–5. PMID:21670465

1716. Hsu SM, Jaffe ES (1984). Leu M1 and peanut agglutinin stain the neoplastic cells of Hodgkin's disease. Am J Clin Pathol. 82:29–32. PMID:6741873

1717. Hu S, Xu-Monette ZY, Balasubramanyam A, et al. (2013). CD30 expression defines a novel subgroup of diffuse large B-cell lymphoma with favorable prognosis and distinct gene expression signature: a report from the International DLBCL Rituximab-CHOP Consortium Program Study. Blood. 121:2715–24. PMID:23343832

1718. Hu S, Xu-Monette ZY, Tzankov A, et al. (2013). MYC/BCL2 protein coexpression contributes to the inferior survival of activated B-cell subtype of diffuse large B-cell lymphoma and demonstrates high-risk gene expression signatures: a report from The International DLBCL Rituximab-CHOP Consortium Program. Blood. 121:4021–31, quiz 4250. PMID:23449635

1719. Huang JZ, Sanger WG, Greiner TC, et al. (2002). The t(14;18) defines a unique subset of diffuse large B-cell lymphoma with a germinal center B-cell gene expression profile. Blood. 99:2285–90. PMID:11895757

1720. Huang KP, Weinstock MA, Clarke CA, et al. (2007). Second lymphomas and other malignant neoplasms in patients with mycosis fungoides and Sezary syndrome: evidence from population-based and clinical cohorts. Arch Dermatol. 143:45–50. PMID:17224541

1721. Huang Q, Chang KL, Gaal KK, et al. (2004). KSHV/HHV8-associated lymphoma simulating anaplastic large cell lymphoma. Am J Surg Pathol. 28:693–7. PMID:15105661

1722. Huang Q, Chang KL, Gaal KK, et al. (2005). An aggressive extranodal NK-cell lymphoma arising from indolent NK-cell lymphoproliferative disorder. Am J Surg Pathol. 29:1540–3. PMID:16224224

1722A. Huang SJ, Gillan TL, Gerrie AS, et al. (2016). Influence of clone and deletion size on outcome in chronic lymphocytic leukemia patients with an isolated deletion 13q in a population-based analysis in British Columbia, Canada. Genes Chromosomes Cancer. 55:16–24. PMID:26391112

1723. Huang TC, Ko BS, Tang JL, et al. (2008). Comparison of hypoplastic myelodysplastic syndrome (MDS) with normo-/hypercellular MDS by International Prognostic Scoring System, cytogenetic and genetic studies. Leukemia. 22:544–50. PMID:18094713

1724. Huang WT, Chang KC, Huang GC, et al. (2005). Bone marrow that is positive for Epstein-Barr virus encoded RNA-1 by in situ hybridization is related with a poor prognosis in patients with extranodal natural killer/T-cell lymphoma, nasal type. Haematologica. 90:1063–9. PMID:16079105

1725. Huang X, Cortes J, Kantarjian H (2012). Estimations of the increasing prevalence and plateau prevalence of chronic myeloid leukemia in the era of tyrosine kinase inhibitor therapy. Cancer. 118:3123–7. PMID:22294282

1726. Huang X, Kushekhar K, Nolte I, et al. (2012). HLA associations in classical Hodgkin lymphoma: EBV status matters. PLoS One. 7:e39986. PMID:22808081

1727. Huang Y, de Leval L, Gaulard P (2013). Molecular underpinning of extranodal NK/T-cell lymphoma. Best Pract Res Clin Haematol. 26:57–74. PMID:23768641

1728. Huang Y, de Reyniès A, de Leval L, et al. (2010). Gene expression profiling identifies emerging oncogenic pathways operating in extranodal NK/T-cell lymphoma, nasal type. Blood. 115:1226–37. PMID:19965620

1729. Huang Y, Moreau A, Dupuis J, et al. (2009). Peripheral T-cell lymphomas with a follicular growth pattern are derived from follicular helper T cells (TFH) and may show overlapping features with angioimmunoblastic T-cell lymphomas. Am J Surg Pathol. 33:682–90. PMID:19295409

1730. Huh YO, Schweighofer CD, Ketterling RP, et al. (2011). Chronic lymphocytic leukemia with t(14;19)(q32;q13) is characterized by atypical morphologic and immunophenotypic features and distinctive genetic features. Am J Clin Pathol. 135:686–96. PMID:21502423

1731. Hummel M, Anagnostopoulos I, Dallenbach F, et al. (1992). EBV infection patterns in Hodgkin's disease and normal lymphoid tissue: expression and cellular localization of EBV gene products. Br J Haematol. 82:689–94. PMID:1336392

1732. Hummel M, Bentink S, Berger H, et al. (2006). A biologic definition of Burkitt's lymphoma from transcriptional and genomic profiling. N Engl J Med. 354:2419–30. PMID:16760442

1733. Hummel M, Tamaru J, Kalvelage B, et al. (1994). Mantle cell (previously centrocytic) lymphomas express VH genes with no or very little somatic mutations like the physiologic cells of the follicle mantle. Blood. 84:403–7. PMID:8025269

1734. Hunger SP, Mullighan CG (2015). Redefining ALL classification: toward detecting high-risk ALL and implementing precision medicine. Blood. 125:3977–87. PMID:25999453

1735. Hunter ZR, Xu L, Yang G, et al. (2014). The genomic landscape of Waldenstrom macroglobulinemia is characterized by highly recurring MYD88 and WHIM-like CXCR4 mutations, and small somatic deletions associated with B-cell lymphomagenesis. Blood. 123:1637–46. PMID:24366360

1736. Huppmann AR, Nicolae A, Slack GW, et al. (2014). EBV may be expressed in the LP cells of nodular lymphocyte-predominant Hodgkin lymphoma (NLPHL) in both children and adults. Am J Surg Pathol. 38:316–24. PMID:24525501

1736A. Huppmann AR, Roullet MR, Raffeld M, et al. (2013). Angioimmunoblastic T-cell lymphoma partially obscured by an Epstein-Barr virus-negative clonal plasma cell proliferation. J Clin Oncol. 31:e28–30. PMID:23213091

1737. Huppmann AR, Xi L, Raffeld M, et al. (2013). Subcutaneous panniculitis-like T-cell lymphoma in the pediatric age group: a lymphoma of low malignant potential. Pediatr Blood Cancer. 60:1165–70. PMID:23382035

1738. Hurwitz CA, Raimondi SC, Head D, et al. (1992). Distinctive immunophenotypic features of t(8;21)(q22;q22) acute myeloblastic leukemia in children. Blood. 80:3182–8. PMID:1467524

1739. Husby G, Blichfeldt P, Brinch L, et al. (1998). Chronic arthritis and gamma heavy chain disease: coincidence or pathogenic link? Scand J Rheumatol. 27:257–64. PMID:9751465

1740. Hussein K, Bock O, Theophile K, et

al. (2008). Chronic myeloproliferative diseases with concurrent BCR-ABL junction and JAK2V617F mutation. Leukemia. 22:1059–62. PMID:17972958

1741. Hussell T, Isaacson PG, Crabtree JE, et al. (1993). The response of cells from low-grade B-cell gastric lymphomas of mucosa-associated lymphoid tissue to Helicobacter pylori. Lancet. 342:571–4. PMID:8102718

1742. Hussong JW, Perkins SL, Schnitzer B, et al. (1999). Extramedullary plasmacytoma. A form of marginal zone cell lymphoma? Am J Clin Pathol. 111:111–6. PMID:9894461

1743. Hutchings M, Loft A, Hansen M, et al. (2006). Position emission tomography with or without computed tomography in the primary staging of Hodgkin's lymphoma. Haematologica. 91:482–9. PMID:16585015

1744. Hutchings M, Loft A, Hansen M, et al. (2006). FDG-PET after two cycles of chemotherapy predicts treatment failure and progression-free survival in Hodgkin lymphoma. Blood. 107:52–9. PMID:16150944

1745. Hwang HS, Park CS, Yoon DH, et al. (2014). High concordance of gene expression profiling-correlated immunohistochemistry algorithms in diffuse large B-cell lymphoma, not otherwise specified. Am J Surg Pathol. 38:1046–57. PMID:24705314

1746. Hwang Y, Huh J, Mun Y, et al. (2011). Characteristics of myelodysplastic syndrome, unclassifiable by WHO classification 2008. Ann Hematol. 90:469–71. PMID:20567825

1747. Hüe S, Mention JJ, Monteiro RC, et al. (2004). A direct role for NKG2D/MICA interaction in villous atrophy during celiac disease. Immunity. 21:367–77. PMID:15357948

1748. Hyjek E, Vardiman JW (2011). Myelodysplastic/myeloproliferative neoplasms. Semin Diagn Pathol. 28:283–97. PMID:22195406

1749. Höglund M, Sandin F, Simonsson B (2015). Epidemiology of chronic myeloid leukaemia: an update. Ann Hematol. 94 Suppl 2:S241–7. PMID:25814090

1750. Höglund M, Sehn L, Connors JM, et al. (2004). Identification of cytogenetic subgroups and karyotypic pathways of clonal evolution in follicular lymphomas. Genes Chromosomes Cancer. 39:195–204. PMID:14732921

1751. Höpken UE, Foss HD, Meyer D, et al. (2002). Up-regulation of the chemokine receptor CCR7 in classical but not in lymphocyte-predominant Hodgkin disease correlates with distinct dissemination of neoplastic cells in lymphoid organs. Blood. 99:1109–16. PMID:11830455

1752. Ichikawa A, Arakawa F, Kiyasu J, et al. (2013). Methotrexate/iatrogenic lymphoproliferative disorders in rheumatoid arthritis: histology, Epstein-Barr virus, and clonality are important predictors of disease progression and regression. Eur J Haematol. 91:20–8. PMID:23560463

1753. Ichinohasama R, Miura I, Kobayashi N, et al. (1998). Herpes virus type 8-negative primary effusion lymphoma associated with PAX-5 gene rearrangement and hepatitis C virus: a case report and review of the literature. Am J Surg Pathol. 22:1528–37. PMID:9850179

1754. Ilowite NT, Fligner CL, Ochs HD, et al. (1986). Pulmonary angiitis with atypical lymphoreticular infiltrates in Wiskott-Aldrich syndrome: possible relationship of lymphomatoid granulomatosis and EBV infection. Clin Immunol Immunopathol. 41:479–84. PMID:3022973

1755. Ilus T, Kaukinen K, Virta LJ, et al. (2014). Refractory coeliac disease in a country with a high prevalence of clinically-diagnosed coeliac disease. Aliment Pharmacol Ther. 39:418–25. PMID:24387637

1756. Imamura N, Kusunoki Y, Kawa-Ha K, et al. (1990). Aggressive natural killer cell leukaemia/lymphoma: report of four cases and review of the literature. Possible existence of a new clinical entity originating from the third lineage of lymphoid cells. Br J Haematol. 75:49–59. PMID:2375924

1756A. Inaba H, Zhou Y, Abla O, et al. (2015). Heterogeneous cytogenetic subgroups and outcomes in childhood acute megakaryoblastic leukemia: a retrospective international study. Blood. 126:1575–84. PMID:26215111

1757. Inamdar KV, Medeiros LJ, Jorgensen JL, et al. (2008). Bone marrow involvement by marginal zone B-cell lymphomas of different types. Am J Clin Pathol. 129:714–22. PMID:18426730

1758. Inghirami G, Foitl DR, Sabichi A, et al. (1991). Autoantibody-associated cross-reactive idiotype-bearing human B lymphocytes: distribution and characterization, including Ig VH gene and CD5 antigen expression. Blood. 78:1503–15. PMID:1715792

1758A. Inghirami G, Chan WC, Pileri S (2015). Peripheral T-cell and NK cell lymphoproliferative disorders: cell of origin, clinical and pathological implications. Immunol Rev. 263:124-59. PMID: 25510275

1759. Ingram W, Lea NC, Cervera J, et al. (2006). The JAK2 V617F mutation identifies a subgroup of MDS patients with isolated deletion 5q and a proliferative bone marrow. Leukemia. 20:1319–21. PMID:16617322

1760. Inhorn RC, Aster JC, Roach SA, et al. (1995). A syndrome of lymphoblastic lymphoma, eosinophilia, and myeloid hyperplasia/malignancy associated with t(8;13)(p11;q11): description of a distinctive clinicopathologic entity. Blood. 85:1881–7. PMID:7661940

1761. Insuasti-Beltran G, Steidler NL, Kang H, et al. (2012). CD34+ megakaryocytes (≥30%) are associated with megaloblastic anaemia and non-acute myeloid neoplasia. Histopathology. 61:694–701. PMID:22651817

1762. International Myeloma Working Group (2003). Criteria for the classification of monoclonal gammopathies, multiple myeloma and related disorders: a report of the International Myeloma Working Group. Br J Haematol. 121:749–57. PMID:12780789

1763. Intlekofer AM, Younes A (2014). Precision therapy for lymphoma–current state and future directions. Nat Rev Clin Oncol. 11:585–96. PMID:25135367

1764. Inui Y, Matsuoka H, Yakushijin K, et al. (2015). Methotrexate-associated lymphoproliferative disorders: management by watchful waiting and observation of early lymphocyte recovery after methotrexate withdrawal. Leuk Lymphoma. 56:3045–51. PMID:25721751

1765. Inukai T, Kiyokawa N, Campana D, et al. (2012). Clinical significance of early T-cell precursor acute lymphoblastic leukaemia: results of the Tokyo Children's Cancer Study Group Study L99-15. Br J Haematol. 156:358–65. PMID:22128890

1766. Invernizzi R, Custodi P, de Fazio P, et al. (1990). The syndrome of abnormal chromatin clumping in leucocytes: clinical and biological study of a case. Haematologica. 75:532–6. PMID:2098294

1767. Inwald DP, Peters MJ, Walshe D, et al. (2000). Absence of platelet CD40L identifies patients with X-linked hyper IgM syndrome. Clin Exp Immunol. 120:499–502. PMID:10844529

1768. Iqbal J, Greiner TC, Patel K, et al. (2007). Distinctive patterns of BCL6 molecular alterations and their functional consequences in different subgroups of diffuse large B-cell lymphoma. Leukemia. 21:2332–43. PMID:17625604

1769. Iqbal J, Meyer PN, Smith LM, et al. (2011). BCL2 predicts survival in germinal center B-cell-like diffuse large B-cell lymphoma treated with CHOP-like therapy and rituximab.

Clin Cancer Res. 17:7785–95. PMID:21933893

1770. Iqbal J, Neppalli VT, Wright G, et al. (2006). BCL2 expression is a prognostic marker for the activated B-cell-like type of diffuse large B-cell lymphoma. J Clin Oncol. 24:961–8. PMID:16418494

1771. Iqbal J, Sanger WG, Horsman DE, et al. (2004). BCL2 translocation defines a unique tumor subset within the germinal center B-cell-like diffuse large B-cell lymphoma. Am J Pathol. 165:159–66. PMID:15215171

1772. Iqbal J, Shen Y, Huang X, et al. (2015). Global microRNA expression profiling uncovers molecular markers for classification and prognosis in aggressive B-cell lymphoma. Blood. 125:1137–45. PMID:25498913

1773. Iqbal J, Weisenburger DD, Chowdhury A, et al. (2011). Natural killer cell lymphoma shares strikingly similar molecular features with a group of non-hepatosplenic γδ T-cell lymphoma and is highly sensitive to a novel aurora kinase A inhibitor in vitro. Leukemia. 25:348–58. PMID:21052088

1774. Iqbal J, Weisenburger DD, Greiner TC, et al. (2010). Molecular signatures to improve diagnosis in peripheral T-cell lymphoma and prognostication in angioimmunoblastic T-cell lymphoma. Blood. 115:1026–36. PMID:19965671

1775. Iqbal J, Wright G, Wang C, et al. (2014). Gene expression signatures delineate biological and prognostic subgroups in peripheral T-cell lymphoma. Blood. 123:2915–23. PMID:24632715

1776. Iriyama N, Asou N, Miyazaki Y, et al. (2014). Normal karyotype acute myeloid leukemia with the CD7+ CD15+ CD34+ HLA-DR+ immunophenotype is a clinically distinct entity with a favorable outcome. Ann Hematol. 93:957–63. PMID:24441947

1777. Iriyama N, Hatta Y, Takeuchi J, et al. (2013). CD56 expression is an independent prognostic factor for relapse in acute myeloid leukemia with t(8;21). Leuk Res. 37:1021–6. PMID:23810283

1778. Irving JA, Mattman A, Lockitch G, et al. (2003). Element of caution: a case of reversible cytopenias associated with excessive zinc supplementation. CMAJ. 169:129–31. PMID:12874162

1779. Isaacson PG (1994). Gastrointestinal lymphoma. Hum Pathol. 25:1020–9. PMID:7927306

1780. Isaacson PG (1996). Malignant lymphomas with a follicular growth pattern. Histopathology. 28:487–95. PMID:8803592

1781. Isaacson PG, Dogan A, Price SK, et al. (1989). Immunoproliferative small-intestinal disease. An immunohistochemical study. Am J Surg Pathol. 13:1023–33. PMID:2512818

1782. Isaacson PG, Du MQ (2004). MALT lymphoma: from morphology to molecules. Nat Rev Cancer. 4:644–53. PMID:15286744

1783. Isaacson PG, Matutes E, Burke M, et al. (1994). The histopathology of splenic lymphoma with villous lymphocytes. Blood. 84:3828–34. PMID:7949139

1784. Isaacson PG, Spencer J (1987). Malignant lymphoma of mucosa-associated lymphoid tissue. Histopathology. 11:445–62. PMID:3497084

1785. Isaacson PG, Wotherspoon AC, Diss T, et al. (1991). Follicular colonization in B-cell lymphoma of mucosa-associated lymphoid tissue. Am J Surg Pathol. 15:819–28. PMID:1951841

1786. Ishida F (2015). [Recent progress of diagnosis and treatment in NK cell neoplasms]. Rinsho Ketsueki. 56:645–50. PMID:26256874

1787. Ishida M, Hodohara K, Yoshii M, et al. (2013). Methotrexate-related Epstein-Barr virus-associated lymphoproliferative disorder occurring in the gingiva of a patient with

rheumatoid arthritis. Int J Clin Exp Pathol. 6:2237–41. PMID:24133604

1788. Ishihara S, Ohshima K, Tokura Y, et al. (1997). Hypersensitivity to mosquito bites conceals clonal lymphoproliferation of Epstein-Barr viral DNA-positive natural killer cells. Jpn J Cancer Res. 88:82–7. PMID:9045900

1789. Ishihara S, Okada S, Wakiguchi H, et al. (1997). Clonal lymphoproliferation following chronic active Epstein-Barr virus infection and hypersensitivity to mosquito bites. Am J Hematol. 54:276–81. PMID:9092681

1790. Isimbaldi G, Bandiera L, d'Amore ES, et al. (2006). ALK-positive plasmablastic B-cell lymphoma with the clathrin-ALK gene rearrangement. Pediatr Blood Cancer. 46:390–1. PMID:16086416

1791. Isobe Y, Aritaka N, Sasaki M, et al. (2009). Spontaneous regression of natural killer cell lymphoma. J Clin Pathol. 62:647–50. PMID:19561234

1792. Isobe Y, Aritaka N, Setoguchi Y, et al. (2012). T/NK cell type chronic active Epstein-Barr virus disease in adults: an underlying condition for Epstein-Barr virus-associated T/NK-cell lymphoma. J Clin Pathol. 65:278–82. PMID:22247563

1793. Isohisa I, Shima K, Koyama T, et al. (1986). [Increased creatine phosphokinase (CPK) level and muscle symptoms during beta-blocker therapy]. Nihon Naika Gakkai Zasshi. 75:1400–4. PMID:2879876

1794. Isomoto H, Maeda T, Akashi T, et al. (2004). Multiple lymphomatous polyposis of the colon originating from T-cells: a case report. Dig Liver Dis. 36:218–21. PMID:15046193

1795. Itzykson R, Kosmider O, Renneville A, et al. (2013). Prognostic score including gene mutations in chronic myelomonocytic leukemia. J Clin Oncol. 31:2428–36. PMID:23690417

1796. Itzykson R, Thépot S, Quesnel B, et al. (2011). Prognostic factors for response and overall survival in 282 patients with higher-risk myelodysplastic syndromes treated with azacitidine. Blood. 117:403–11. PMID:20940414

1797. Iuchi K, Aozasa K, Yamamoto S, et al. (1989). Non-Hodgkin's lymphoma of the pleural cavity developing from long-standing pyothorax. Summary of clinical and pathological findings in thirty-seven cases. Jpn J Clin Oncol. 19:249–57. PMID:2681886

1798. Iurlo A, Cattaneo D, Boiocchi L, et al. (2015). Clinical and morphologic features in five post-polycythemic myelofibrosis patients treated with ruxolitinib. Ann Hematol. 94:1749–51. PMID:26082334

1799. Iurlo A, Gianelli U, Beghini A, et al. (2014). Identification of kit(M541L) somatic mutation in chronic eosinophilic leukemia, not otherwise specified and its implication in low-dose imatinib response. Oncotarget. 5:4665–70. PMID:25015329

1799A. Iurlo A, Gianelli U, Cattaneo D, et al. (2017). Impact of the 2016 revised WHO criteria for myeloproliferative neoplasms, unclassifiable: Comparison with the 2008 version. Am J Hematol. 92:E48–E51. PMID:28109016

1800. Iurlo A, Gianelli U, Rapezzi D, et al. (2014). Imatinib and ruxolitinib association: first experience in two patients. Haematologica. 99:e76–7. PMID:24633869

1801. Ivanovski M, Silvestri F, Pozzato G, et al. (1998). Somatic hypermutation, clonal diversity, and preferential expression of the VH 51p1/VL kv325 immunoglobulin gene combination in hepatitis C virus-associated immunocytomas. Blood. 91:2433–42. PMID:9516143

1802. Iwamuro M, Okada H, Kawano S, et al. (2015). A multicenter survey of enteroscopy for the diagnosis of intestinal follicular lymphoma. Oncol Lett. 10:131–6. PMID:26170988

1803. Iwasaki H, Akashi K (2007).

Myeloid lineage commitment from the hematopoietic stem cell. Immunity. 26:726–40. PMID:17582345
1804. Iwata S, Wada K, Tobita S, et al. (2010). Quantitative analysis of Epstein-Barr virus (EBV)-related gene expression in patients with chronic active EBV infection. J Gen Virol. 91:42–50. PMID:19793909
1805. Iwatsuki K, Ohtsuka M, Akiba H, et al. (1999). Atypical hydroa vacciniforme in childhood: from a smoldering stage to Epstein-Barr virus-associated lymphoid malignancy. J Am Acad Dermatol. 40:283–4. PMID:10025766
1806. Iwatsuki K, Satoh M, Yamamoto T, et al. (2006). Pathogenic link between hydroa vacciniforme and Epstein-Barr virus-associated hematologic disorders. Arch Dermatol. 142:587–95. PMID:16702496
1807. Iwatsuki K, Xu Z, Takata M, et al. (1999). The association of latent Epstein-Barr virus infection with hydroa vacciniforme. Br J Dermatol. 140:715–21. PMID:10233328
1808. Izumi M, Mochizuki M, Kuroda M, et al. (2002). Angiomyoid proliferative lesion: an unusual stroma-rich variant of Castleman's disease of hyaline-vascular type. Virchows Arch. 441:400–5. PMID:12404066
1809. Jabbour E, Kantarjian H (2014). Chronic myeloid leukemia: 2014 update on diagnosis, monitoring, and management. Am J Hematol. 89:547–56. PMID:24729196
1810. Jacknow G, Frizzera G, Gajl-Peczalska K, et al. (1985). Extramedullary presentation of the blast crisis of chronic myelogenous leukaemia. Br J Haematol. 61:225–36. PMID:3862425
1811. Jackson A, Scarffe JH (1990). Prognostic significance of osteopenia and immunoparesis at presentation in patients with solitary myeloma of bone. Eur J Cancer. 26:363–71. PMID:2141495
1812. Jacob MC, Chaperot L, Mossuz P, et al. (2003). CD4+ CD56+ lineage negative malignancies: a new entity developed from malignant early plasmacytoid dendritic cells. Haematologica. 88:941–55. PMID:12935983
1813. Jacoby MA, De Jesus Pizarro RE, Shao J, et al. (2014). The DNA double-strand break response is abnormal in myeloblasts from patients with therapy-related acute myeloid leukemia. Leukemia. 28:1242–51. PMID:24304937
1814. Jaffe ES (1995). Nasal and nasal-type T/NK cell lymphoma: a unique form of lymphoma associated with the Epstein-Barr virus. Histopathology. 27:581–3. PMID:8838342
1815. Jaffe ES (2001). Anaplastic large cell lymphoma: the shifting sands of diagnostic hematopathology. Mod Pathol. 14:219–28. PMID:11266530
1816. Jaffe ES (2006). Pathobiology of peripheral T-cell lymphomas. Hematology Am Soc Hematol Educ Program. 317–22. PMID:17124078
1817. Jaffe ES (2013). Follicular lymphomas: a tapestry of common and contrasting threads. Haematologica. 98:1163–5. PMID:23904232
1818. Jaffe ES, Blattner WA, Blayney DW, et al. (1984). The pathologic spectrum of adult T-cell leukemia/lymphoma in the United States. Human T-cell leukemia/lymphoma virus-associated lymphoid malignancies. Am J Surg Pathol. 8:263–75. PMID:6324600
1819. Jaffe ES, Chan JK, Su IJ, et al. (1996). Report of the Workshop on Nasal and Related Extranodal Angiocentric T/Natural Killer Cell Lymphomas. Definitions, differential diagnosis, and epidemiology. Am J Surg Pathol. 20:103–11. PMID:8540601
1820. Jaffe ES, Harris NL, Stein H, et al., editors. (2001). World Health Organization classification of tumours. Pathology and genetics of tumours of haematopoietic and lymphoid tissues. 3rd ed. Lyon: IARC Press.
1821. Jaffe ES, Krenacs L, Raffeld M (2003). Classification of cytotoxic T-cell and natural killer cell lymphomas. Semin Hematol. 40:175–84. PMID:12876666
1822. Jaffe ES, Puck JM, Jackson CE, et al. (1999). Increased risk for diverse lymphomas in autoimmune lymphoproliferative syndrome (ALPS), an inherited disorder due to defective lymphocyte apoptosis. Blood. 94:597a.
1823. Jaffe ES, Wilson WH (1997). Lymphomatoid granulomatosis: pathogenesis, pathology and clinical implications. Cancer Surv. 30:233–48. PMID:9547995
1824. Jaffe ES, Zarate-Osorno A, Kingma DW, et al. (1994). The interrelationship between Hodgkin's disease and non-Hodgkin's lymphomas. Ann Oncol. 5 Suppl 1:7–11. PMID:8172822
1825. Jaffe ES, Zarate-Osorno A, Medeiros LJ (1992). The interrelationship of Hodgkin's disease and non-Hodgkin's lymphomas–lessons learned from composite and sequential malignancies. Semin Diagn Pathol. 9:297–303. PMID:1480852
1826. Jaffe R (2004). Liver involvement in the histiocytic disorders of childhood. Pediatr Dev Pathol. 7:214–25. PMID:15022067
1827. Jaffe ES, Harris NL, Vardiman JW, et al., editors (2010). Hematopathology. 1st ed. St. Louis: Elsevier Saunders.
1828. Jahnke K, Thiel E, Martus P, et al. (2006). Relapse of primary central nervous system lymphoma: clinical features, outcome and prognostic factors. J Neurooncol. 80:159–65. PMID:16699873
1829. Jain N, Khoury JD, Pemmaraju N, et al. (2013). Imatinib therapy in a patient with suspected chronic neutrophilic leukemia and FIP1L1-PDGFRA rearrangement. Blood. 122:3387–8. PMID:24203930
1830. Jaiswal S, Fontanillas P, Flannick J, et al. (2014). Age-related clonal hematopoiesis associated with adverse outcomes. N Engl J Med. 371:2488–98. PMID:25426837
1831. James C, Ugo V, Le Couédic JP, et al. (2005). A unique clonal JAK2 mutation leading to constitutive signalling causes polycythaemia vera. Nature. 434:1144–8. PMID:15793561
1832. James E, Sokhn JG, Gibson JF, et al. (2015). CD4 + primary cutaneous small/medium-sized pleomorphic T-cell lymphoma: a retrospective case series and review of literature. Leuk Lymphoma. 56:951–7. PMID:24996443
1833. Jamieson C, Hasserjian R, Gotlib J, et al. (2015). Effect of treatment with a JAK2-selective inhibitor, fedratinib, on bone marrow fibrosis in patients with myelofibrosis. J Transl Med. 13:294. PMID:26357842
1834. Janka GE (2007). Hemophagocytic syndromes. Blood Rev. 21:245–53. PMID:17590250
1835. Janssen D, Fölster-Holst R, Harms D, et al. (2007). Clonality in juvenile xanthogranuloma. Am J Surg Pathol. 31:812–3. PMID:17460468
1836. Janssen D, Harms D (2005). Juvenile xanthogranuloma in childhood and adolescence: a clinicopathologic study of 129 patients from the kiel pediatric tumor registry. Am J Surg Pathol. 29:21–8. PMID:15613853
1837. Janssen JW, Ludwig WD, Sterry W, et al. (1993). SIL-TAL1 deletion in T-cell acute lymphoblastic leukemia. Leukemia. 7:1204–10. PMID:8350619
1838. Janz M, Hummel M, Truss M, et al. (2006). Classical Hodgkin lymphoma is characterized by high constitutive expression of activating transcription factor 3 (ATF3), which promotes viability of Hodgkin/Reed-Sternberg cells. Blood. 107:2536–9. PMID:16263788
1839. Jardin F, Jais JP, Molina TJ, et al. (2010). Diffuse large B-cell lymphomas with CDKN2A deletion have a distinct gene expression signature and a poor prognosis under R-CHOP treatment: a GELA study. Blood. 116:1092–104. PMID:20435884
1840. Jardin F, Ruminy P, Parmentier F, et al. (2011). TET2 and TP53 mutations are frequently observed in blastic plasmacytoid dendritic cell neoplasm. Br J Haematol. 153:413–6. PMID:21275969
1841. Jares P, Campo E, Pinyol M, et al. (1996). Expression of retinoblastoma gene product (pRb) in mantle cell lymphomas. Correlation with cyclin D1 (PRAD1/CCND1) mRNA levels and proliferative activity. Am J Pathol. 148:1591–600. PMID:8623927
1842. Jares P, Colomer D, Campo E (2007). Genetic and molecular pathogenesis of mantle cell lymphoma: perspectives for new targeted therapeutics. Nat Rev Cancer. 7:750–62. PMID:17891190
1843. Jares P, Colomer D, Campo E (2012). Molecular pathogenesis of mantle cell lymphoma. J Clin Invest. 122:3416–23. PMID:23023712
1844. Jasionowski TM, Hartung L, Greenwood JH, et al. (2003). Analysis of CD10+ hairy cell leukemia. Am J Clin Pathol. 120:228–35. PMID:12931553
1845. Jaso JM, Yin CC, Wang SA, et al. (2013). Clinicopathologic features of CD5-positive nodal marginal zone lymphoma. Am J Clin Pathol. 140:693–700. PMID:24124149
1846. Jaye DL, Geigerman CM, Herling M, et al. (2006). Expression of the plasmacytoid dendritic cell marker BDCA-2 supports a spectrum of maturation among CD4+ CD56+ hematodermic neoplasms. Mod Pathol. 19:1555–62. PMID:16998465
1847. Jegalian AG, Buxbaum NP, Facchetti F, et al. (2010). Blastic plasmacytoid dendritic cell neoplasm in children: diagnostic features and clinical implications. Haematologica. 95:1873–9. PMID:20663945
1848. Jegalian AG, Eberle FC, Pack SD, et al. (2011). Follicular lymphoma in situ: clinical implications and comparisons with partial involvement by follicular lymphoma. Blood. 118:2976–84. PMID:21768298
1849. Jegalian AG, Facchetti F, Jaffe ES (2009). Plasmacytoid dendritic cells: physiologic roles and pathologic states. Adv Anat Pathol. 16:392–404. PMID:19851130
1850. Jeha S, Pei D, Raimondi SC, et al. (2009). Increased risk for CNS relapse in pre-B cell leukemia with the t(1;19)/TCF3-PBX1. Leukemia. 23:1406–9. PMID:19282835
1851. Jemal A, Siegel R, Ward E, et al. (2007). Cancer statistics, 2007. CA Cancer J Clin. 57:43–66. PMID:17237035
1852. Jenkins RB, Tefferi A, Solberg LA Jr, et al. (1989). Acute leukemia with abnormal thrombopoiesis and inversions of chromosome 3. Cancer Genet Cytogenet. 39:167–79. PMID:2752370
1853. Jensen RT (2000). Gastrointestinal abnormalities and involvement in systemic mastocytosis. Hematol Oncol Clin North Am. 14:579–623. PMID:10909042
1854. Jerez A, Clemente MJ, Makishima H, et al. (2012). STAT3 mutations unify the pathogenesis of chronic lymphoproliferative disorders of NK cells and T-cell large granular lymphocyte leukemia. Blood. 120:3048–57. PMID:22859607
1855. Jerez A, Clemente MJ, Makishima H, et al. (2013). STAT3 mutations indicate the presence of subclinical T-cell clones in a subset of aplastic anemia and myelodysplastic syndrome patients. Blood. 122:2453–9. PMID:23926297
1856. Jevremovic D, Timm MM, Reichard KK, et al. (2014). Loss of blast heterogeneity in myelodysplastic syndrome and other chronic myeloid neoplasms. Am J Clin Pathol. 142:292–8. PMID:25125617
1857. Jhala DN, Medeiros LJ, Lopez-Terrada D, et al. (2000). Neutrophil-rich anaplastic large cell lymphoma of T-cell lineage. A report of two cases arising in HIV-positive patients. Am J Clin Pathol. 114:478–82. PMID:10989649
1858. Jhuang JY, Chang ST, Weng SF, et al. (2015). Extranodal natural killer/T-cell lymphoma, nasal type in Taiwan: a relatively higher frequency of T-cell lineage and poor survival for extranasal tumors. Hum Pathol. 46:313–21. PMID:25554090
1859. Jiang L, Gu ZH, Yan ZX, et al. (2015). Exome sequencing identifies somatic mutations of DDX3X in natural killer/T-cell lymphoma. Nat Genet. 47:1061–6. PMID:26192917
1860. Jiang L, Li P, Wang H, et al. (2014). Prognostic significance of Ki-67 antigen expression in extranodal natural killer/T-cell lymphoma, nasal type. Med Oncol. 31:218. PMID:25204411
1861. Jiménez C, Sebastián E, Chillón MC, et al. (2013). MYD88 L265P is a marker highly characteristic of, but not restricted to, Waldenström's macroglobulinemia. Leukemia. 27:1722–8. PMID:23446312
1862. Jimenez-Zepeda VH, Neme-Yunes Y, Braggio E (2011). Chromosome abnormalities defined by conventional cytogenetics in plasma cell leukemia: what have we learned about its biology? Eur J Haematol. 87:20–7. PMID:21692850
1863. Johan MF, Goodeve AC, Bowen DT, et al. (2005). JAK2 V617F Mutation is uncommon in chronic myelomonocytic leukaemia. Br J Haematol. 130:968. PMID:16156870
1864. Johansson P (2006). Epidemiology of the myeloproliferative disorders polycythemia vera and essential thrombocythemia. Semin Thromb Hemost. 32:171–3. PMID:16673273
1865. Johnson NA, Savage KJ, Ludkovski O, et al. (2009). Lymphomas with concurrent BCL2 and MYC translocations: the critical factors associated with survival. Blood. 114:2273–9. PMID:19597184
1866. Johnson NA, Slack GW, Savage KJ, et al. (2012). Concurrent expression of MYC and BCL2 in diffuse large B-cell lymphoma treated with rituximab plus cyclophosphamide, doxorubicin, vincristine, and prednisone. J Clin Oncol. 30:3452–9. PMID:22851565
1867. Johnson PC, McAulay KA, Montgomery D, et al. (2015). Modeling HLA associations with EBV-positive and -negative Hodgkin lymphoma suggests distinct mechanisms in disease pathogenesis. Int J Cancer. 137:1066–75. PMID:25648508
1868. Johnson RC, Savage NM, Chiang T, et al. (2013). Hidden mastocytosis in acute myeloid leukemia with t(8;21)(q22;q22). Am J Clin Pathol. 140:525–35. PMID:24045550
1869. Johnston EE, LeBlanc RE, Kim J, et al. (2015). Subcutaneous panniculitis-like T-cell lymphoma: Pediatric case series demonstrating heterogeneous presentation and option for watchful waiting. Pediatr Blood Cancer. 62:2025–8. PMID:26146844
1870. Johnston WT, Mutalima N, Sun D, et al. (2014). Relationship between Plasmodium falciparum malaria prevalence, genetic diversity and endemic Burkitt lymphoma in Malawi. Sci Rep. 4:3741. PMID:24434689
1871. Jones AM, Gaspar HB (2000). Immunogenetics: changing the face of immunodeficiency. J Clin Pathol. 53:60–5. PMID:10767859
1872. Jones AV, Kreil S, Zoi K, et al. (2005). Widespread occurrence of the JAK2 V617F mutation in chronic myeloproliferative disorders. Blood. 106:2162–8. PMID:15920007
1873. Jones CL, Wain EM, Chu CC, et al.

(2010). Downregulation of Fas gene expression in Sézary syndrome is associated with promoter hypermethylation. J Invest Dermatol. 130:1116–25. PMID:19759548

1874. Jones D, Amin M, Ordonez NG, et al. (2001). Reticulum cell sarcoma of lymph node with mixed dendritic and fibroblastic features. Mod Pathol. 14:1059–67. PMID:11598178

1875. Jones D, Ballestas ME, Kaye KM, et al. (1998). Primary-effusion lymphoma and Kaposi's sarcoma in a cardiac-transplant recipient. N Engl J Med. 339:444–9. PMID:9700178

1876. Jones D, O'Hara C, Kraus MD, et al. (2000). Expression pattern of T-cell-associated chemokine receptors and their chemokines correlates with specific subtypes of T-cell non-Hodgkin lymphoma. Blood. 96:685–90. PMID:10887135

1876A. Jones D, Yao H, Romans A, et al. (2010). Modeling interactions between leukemia-specific chromosomal changes, somatic mutations, and gene expression patterns during progression of core-binding factor leukemias. Genes Chromosomes Cancer. 49:182–91. PMID:19908318

1877. Jones JF, Shurin S, Abramowsky C, et al. (1988). T-cell lymphomas containing Epstein-Barr viral DNA in patients with chronic Epstein-Barr virus infections. N Engl J Med. 318:733–41. PMID:2831453

1878. Jonkman-Berk BM, van den Berg JM, Ten Berge IJ, et al. (2015). Primary immunodeficiencies in the Netherlands: national patient data demonstrate the increased risk of malignancy. Clin Immunol. 156:154–62. PMID:25451158

1879. Joos S, Granzow M, Holtgreve-Grez H, et al. (2003). Hodgkin's lymphoma cell lines are characterized by frequent aberrations on chromosomes 2p and 9p including REL and JAK2. Int J Cancer. 103:489–95. PMID:12478664

1880. Joos S, Küpper M, Ohl S, et al. (2000). Genomic imbalances including amplification of the tyrosine kinase gene JAK2 in CD30+ Hodgkin cells. Cancer Res. 60:549–52. PMID:10676635

1881. Joos S, Otaño-Joos MI, Ziegler S, et al. (1996). Primary mediastinal (thymic) B-cell lymphoma is characterized by gains of chromosomal material including 9p and amplification of the REL gene. Blood. 87:1571–8. PMID:8608249

1882. Jordan MB, Allen CE, Weitzman S, et al. (2011). How I treat hemophagocytic lymphohistiocytosis. Blood. 118:4041–52. PMID:21828139

1883. Jordanova ES, Riemersma SA, Philippo K, et al. (2002). Hemizygous deletions in the HLA region account for loss of heterozygosity in the majority of diffuse large B-cell lymphomas of the testis and the central nervous system. Genes Chromosomes Cancer. 35:38–48. PMID:12203788

1884. Jorgensen C, Legouffe MC, Perney P, et al. (1996). Sicca syndrome associated with hepatitis C virus infection. Arthritis Rheum. 39:1166–71. PMID:8670326

1885. Joslin JM, Fernald AA, Tennant TR, et al. (2007). Haploinsufficiency of EGR1, a candidate gene in the del(5q), leads to the development of myeloid disorders. Blood. 110:719–26. PMID:17420284

1886. Josting A, Wolf J, Diehl V (2000). Hodgkin disease: prognostic factors and treatment strategies. Curr Opin Oncol. 12:403–11. PMID:10975546

1887. Julia F, Dalle S, Duru G, et al. (2014). Blastic plasmacytoid dendritic cell neoplasms: clinico-immunohistochemical correlations in a series of 91 patients. Am J Surg Pathol. 38:673–80. PMID:24441662

1888. Julia F, Petrella T, Beylot-Barry M, et al. (2013). Blastic plasmacytoid dendritic cell neoplasm: clinical features in 90 patients. Br J Dermatol. 169:579–86. PMID:23646868

1889. Juncà J, Garcia-Caro M, Granada I, et al. (2014). Correlation of CD11b and CD56 expression in adult acute myeloid leukemia with cytogenetic risk groups and prognosis. Ann Hematol. 93:1483–9. PMID:24782118

1890. Juneja SK, Imbert M, Jouault H, et al. (1983). Haematological features of primary myelodysplastic syndromes (PMDS) at initial presentation: a study of 118 cases. J Clin Pathol. 36:1129–35. PMID:6619310

1891. Juneja SK, Imbert M, Sigaux F, et al. (1983). Prevalence and distribution of ringed sideroblasts in primary myelodysplastic syndromes. J Clin Pathol. 36:566–9. PMID:6841648

1892. Junker AK, Thomas EE, Radcliffe A, et al. (1991). Epstein-Barr virus shedding in breast milk. Am J Med Sci. 302:220–3. PMID:1656752

1893. Juweid ME, Stroobants S, Hoekstra OS, et al. (2007). Use of positron emission tomography for response assessment of lymphoma: consensus of the Imaging Subcommittee of International Harmonization Project in Lymphoma. J Clin Oncol. 25:571–8. PMID:17242397

1894. Jädersten M, Saft L, Smith A, et al. (2011). TP53 mutations in low-risk myelodysplastic syndromes with del(5q) predict disease progression. J Clin Oncol. 29:1971–9. PMID:21519010

1895. Järviluoma A, Koopal S, Räsänen S, et al. (2004). KSHV viral cyclin binds to p27KIP1 in primary effusion lymphomas. Blood. 104:3349–54. PMID:15271792

1896. Jöhrens K, Stein H, Anagnostopoulos I (2007). T-bet transcription factor detection facilitates the diagnosis of minimal hairy cell leukemia infiltrates in bone marrow trephines. Am J Surg Pathol. 31:1181–5. PMID:17667540

1897. Kadin ME, Agnarsson BA, Ellingsworth LR, et al. (1990). Immunohistochemical evidence of a role for transforming growth factor beta in the pathogenesis of nodular sclerosing Hodgkin's disease. Am J Pathol. 136:1209–14. PMID:2356855

1898. Kadin ME, Hughey LC, Wood GS (2014). Large-cell transformation of mycosis fungoides-differential diagnosis with implications for clinical management: a consensus statement of the US Cutaneous Lymphoma Consortium. J Am Acad Dermatol. 70:374–6. PMID:24438952

1899. Kadin ME, Liebowitz DN (1999). Cytokines and cytokine receptors in Hodgkin's disease. In: Mauch P, Armitage JO, Diehl V, editors. Hodgkin's disease. Philadelphia: Lippincott Williams & Wilkins; p. 139.

1900. Kadin ME, Pinkus JL, Pinkus GS, et al. (2008). Primary cutaneous ALCL with phosphorylated/activated cytoplasmic ALK and novel phenotype: EMA/MUC1+, cutaneous lymphocyte antigen negative. Am J Surg Pathol. 32:1421–6. PMID:18670345

1901. Kagami Y, Suzuki R, Taji H, et al. (1999). Nodal cytotoxic lymphoma spectrum: a clinicopathologic study of 66 patients. Am J Surg Pathol. 23:1184–200. PMID:10524519

1902. Kako S, Kanda Y, Sato T, et al. (2007). Early relapse of JAK2 V617F-positive chronic neutrophilic leukemia with central nervous system infiltration after unrelated bone marrow transplantation. Am J Hematol. 82:386–90. PMID:17109389

1903. Kaleem Z, White G (2001). Diagnostic criteria for minimally differentiated acute myeloid leukemia (AML-M0). Evaluation and a proposal. Am J Clin Pathol. 115:876–84. PMID:11392885

1904. Kalmanti L, Saussele S, Lauseker M, et al. (2015). Safety and efficacy of imatinib in CML over a period of 10 years: data from the randomized CML-study IV. Leukemia. 29:1123–32. PMID:25676422

1905. Kalpadakis C, Pangalis GA, Vassilakopoulos TP, et al. (2014). Clinical aspects of malt lymphomas. Curr Hematol Malig Rep. 9:262–72. PMID:25240474

1906. Kambham N, Markowitz GS, Appel GB, et al. (1999). Heavy chain deposition disease: the disease spectrum. Am J Kidney Dis. 33:954–62. PMID:10213655

1907. Kameda K, Shono T, Takagishi S, et al. (2015). Epstein-Barr virus-positive diffuse large B-cell primary central nervous system lymphoma associated with organized chronic subdural hematoma: a case report and review of the literature. Pathol Int. 65:138–43. PMID:25597523

1908. Kamel OW (2002). Iatrogenic lymphoproliferative disorders in non-transplantation settings. Recent Results Cancer Res. 159:19–26. PMID:11785840

1909. Kamel OW, Gocke CD, Kell DL, et al. (1995). True histiocytic lymphoma: a study of 12 cases based on current definition. Leuk Lymphoma. 18:81–6. PMID:8580833

1910. Kamel OW, van de Rijn M, Weiss LM, et al. (1993). Brief report: reversible lymphomas associated with Epstein-Barr virus occurring during methotrexate therapy for rheumatoid arthritis and dermatomyositis. N Engl J Med. 328:1317–21. PMID:8385742

1911. Kamel OW, Weiss LM, van de Rijn M, et al. (1996). Hodgkin's disease and lymphoproliferations resembling Hodgkin's disease in patients receiving long-term low-dose methotrexate therapy. Am J Surg Pathol. 20:1279–87. PMID:8827036

1912. Kanagal-Shamanna R, Bueso-Ramos CE, Barkoh B, et al. (2012). Myeloid neoplasms with isolated isochromosome 17q represent a clinicopathologic entity associated with myelodysplastic/myeloproliferative features, a high risk of leukemic transformation, and wild-type TP53. Cancer. 118:2879–88. PMID:22038701

1913. Kanagal-Shamanna R, Luthra R, Yin CC, et al. (2016). Myeloid neoplasms with isolated isochromosome 17q demonstrate a high frequency of mutations in SETBP1, SRSF2, ASXL1 and NRAS. Oncotarget. 7:14251–8. PMID:26883102

1914. Kanagal-Shamanna R, Medeiros LJ, Lu G, et al. (2012). High-grade B cell lymphoma, unclassifiable, with blastoid features: an unusual morphological subgroup associated frequently with BCL2 and/or MYC gene rearrangements and a poor prognosis. Histopathology. 61:945–54. PMID:22804688

1915. Kanavaros P, Gaulard P, Charlotte F, et al. (1995). Discordant expression of immunoglobulin and its associated molecule mb-1/CD79a is frequently found in mediastinal large B cell lymphomas. Am J Pathol. 146:735–41. PMID:7887454

1916. Kanavaros P, Lescs MC, Brière J, et al. (1993). Nasal T-cell lymphoma: a clinicopathologic entity associated with peculiar phenotype and with Epstein-Barr virus. Blood. 81:2688–95. PMID:8387835

1917. Kanazawa T, Hiramatsu Y, Iwata S, et al. (2014). Anti-CCR4 monoclonal antibody mogamulizumab for the treatment of EBV-associated T- and NK-cell lymphoproliferative diseases. Clin Cancer Res. 20:5075–84. PMID:25117294

1918. Kanegane H, Bhatia K, Gutierrez M, et al. (1998). A syndrome of peripheral blood T-cell infection with Epstein-Barr virus (EBV) followed by EBV-positive T-cell lymphoma. Blood. 91:2085–91. PMID:9490694

1919. Kanegane H, Nomura K, Miyawaki T, et al. (2002). Biological aspects of Epstein-Barr virus (EBV)-infected lymphocytes in chronic active EBV infection and associated malignancies. Crit Rev Oncol Hematol. 44:239–49. PMID:12467964

1920. Kanellis G, Garcia-Alonso L, Camacho FI, et al. (2011). Hairy cell leukemia, blastic type: description of spleen morphology and immunophenotype of a distinctive case. Leuk Lymphoma. 52:1589–92. PMID:21534875

1921. Kanellis G, Mollejo M, Montes-Moreno S, et al. (2010). Splenic diffuse red pulp small B-cell lymphoma: revision of a series of cases reveals characteristic clinico-pathological features. Haematologica. 95:1122–9. PMID:20220064

1922. Kanellis G, Roncador G, Arribas A, et al. (2009). Identification of MNDA as a new marker for nodal marginal zone lymphoma. Leukemia. 23:1847–57. PMID:19474799

1923. Kanezaki R, Toki T, Terui K, et al. (2010). Down syndrome and GATA1 mutations in transient abnormal myeloproliferative disorder: mutation classes correlate with progression to myeloid leukemia. Blood. 116:4631–8. PMID:20729467

1924. Kang WY, Shen KN, Duan MH, et al. (2013). 14q32 translocations and 13q14 deletions are common cytogenetic abnormalities in POEMS syndrome. Eur J Haematol. 91:490–6. PMID:23957213

1925. Kanno H, Naka N, Yasunaga Y, et al. (1997). Production of the immunosuppressive cytokine interleukin-10 by Epstein-Barr-virus-expressing pyothorax-associated lymphoma: possible role in the development of overt lymphoma in immunocompetent hosts. Am J Pathol. 150:349–57. PMID:9006350

1926. Kanno H, Nakatsuka S, Iuchi K, et al. (2000). Sequences of cytotoxic T-lymphocyte epitopes in the Epstein-Barr virus (EBV) nuclear antigen-3B gene in a Japanese population with or without EBV-positive lymphoid malignancies. Int J Cancer. 88:626–32. PMID:11058881

1927. Kanno H, Ohsawa M, Hashimoto M, et al. (1999). HLA-A alleles of patients with pyothorax-associated lymphoma: anti-Epstein-Barr virus (EBV) host immune responses during the development of EBV latent antigen-positive lymphomas. Int J Cancer. 82:630–4. PMID:10417757

1928. Kanno H, Yasunaga Y, Iuchi K, et al. (1996). Interleukin-6-mediated growth enhancement of cell lines derived from pyothorax-associated lymphoma. Lab Invest. 75:167–73. PMID:8765317

1929. Kano A, Rouse AR, Gmitro AF (2013). Ultrathin single-channel fiberscopes for biomedical imaging. J Biomed Opt. 18:16013. PMID:23334688

1930. Kant JA, Hubbard SM, Longo DL, et al. (1986). The pathologic and clinical heterogeneity of lymphocyte-depleted Hodgkin's disease. J Clin Oncol. 4:284–94. PMID:3754003

1931. Kantarjian H, O'Brien S, Cortes J, et al. (2003). Sudden onset of the blastic phase of chronic myelogenous leukemia: patterns and implications. Cancer. 98:81–5. PMID:12833459

1932. Kantarjian HM, Bueso-Ramos CE, Talpaz M, et al. (2005). The degree of bone marrow fibrosis in chronic myelogenous leukemia is not a prognostic factor with imatinib mesylate therapy. Leuk Lymphoma. 46:993–7. PMID:16019549

1933. Kanungo A, Medeiros LJ, Abruzzo LV, et al. (2006). Lymphoid neoplasms associated with concurrent t(14;18) and 8q24/c-MYC translocation generally have a poor prognosis. Mod Pathol. 19:25–33. PMID:16258503

1934. Kanzler H, Küppers R, Hansmann ML, et al. (1996). Hodgkin and Reed-Sternberg cells in Hodgkin's disease represent the outgrowth of a dominant tumor clone derived from (crippled)

germinal center B cells. J Exp Med. 184:1495–505. PMID:8879220
1935. Kapelushnik J, Ariad S, Benharroch D, et al. (2001). Post renal transplantation human herpesvirus 8-associated lymphoproliferative disorder and Kaposi's sarcoma. Br J Haematol. 113:425–8. PMID:11380409
1936. Kaplan MA, Ferry JA, Harris NL, et al. (1994). Clonal analysis of posttransplant lymphoproliferative disorders, using both episomal Epstein-Barr virus and immunoglobulin genes as markers. Am J Clin Pathol. 101:590–6. PMID:8178765
1937. Kapp U, Yeh WC, Patterson B, et al. (1999). Interleukin 13 is secreted by and stimulates the growth of Hodgkin and Reed-Sternberg cells. J Exp Med. 189:1939–46. PMID:10377189
1938. Karai LJ, Kadin ME, Hsi ED, et al. (2013). Chromosomal rearrangements of 6p25.3 define a new subtype of lymphomatoid papulosis. Am J Surg Pathol. 37:1173–81. PMID:23648461
1939. Karandikar NJ, Aquino DB, McKenna RW, et al. (2001). Transient myeloproliferative disorder and acute myeloid leukemia in Down syndrome. An immunophenotypic analysis. Am J Clin Pathol. 116:204–10. PMID:11488066
1940. Kardos G, Baumann I, Passmore SJ, et al. (2003). Refractory anemia in childhood: a retrospective analysis of 67 patients with particular reference to monosomy 7. Blood. 102:1997–2003. PMID:12763938
1941. Kari L, Loboda A, Nebozhyn M, et al. (2003). Classification and prediction of survival in patients with the leukemic phase of cutaneous T cell lymphoma. J Exp Med. 197:1477–88. PMID:12782714
1942. Karow A, Flotho C, Schneider M, et al. (2010). Mutations of the Shwachman-Bodian-Diamond syndrome gene in patients presenting with refractory cytopenia–do we have to screen? Haematologica. 95:689–90. PMID:19951977
1943. Karube K, Campo E (2015). MYC alterations in diffuse large B-cell lymphomas. Semin Hematol. 52:97–106. PMID:25805589
1944. Karube K, Guo Y, Suzumiya J, et al. (2007). CD10-MUM1+ follicular lymphoma lacks BCL2 gene translocation and shows characteristic biologic and clinical features. Blood. 109:3076–9. PMID:17138820
1945. Karube K, Martínez D, Royo C, et al. (2014). Recurrent mutations of NOTCH genes in follicular lymphoma identify a distinctive subset of tumours. J Pathol. 234:423–30. PMID:25141821
1946. Karube K, Nakagawa M, Tsuzuki S, et al. (2011). Identification of FOXO3 and PRDM1 as tumor-suppressor gene candidates in NK-cell neoplasms by genomic and functional analyses. Blood. 118:3195–204. PMID:21690554
1947. Karube K, Niino D, Kimura Y, et al. (2013). Classical Hodgkin lymphoma, lymphocyte depleted type: clinicopathological analysis and prognostic comparison with other types of classical Hodgkin lymphoma. Pathol Res Pract. 209:201–7. PMID:23478005
1948. Karube K, Ohshima K, Tsuchiya T, et al. (2004). Expression of FoxP3, a key molecule in CD4CD25 regulatory T cells, in adult T-cell leukaemia/lymphoma cells. Br J Haematol. 126:81–4. PMID:15198736
1949. Karube K, Scarfò L, Campo E, et al. (2014). Monoclonal B cell lymphocytosis and "in situ" lymphoma. Semin Cancer Biol. 24:3–14. PMID:23999128
1950. Karube K, Ying G, Tagawa H, et al. (2008). BCL6 gene amplification/3q27 gain is associated with unique clinicopathological characteristics among follicular lymphoma without BCL2 gene translocation. Mod Pathol. 21:973–8. PMID:18500267
1951. Karuturi M, Shah N, Frank D, et al. (2013). Plasmacytic post-transplant lymphoproliferative disorder: a case series of nine patients. Transpl Int. 26:616–22. PMID:23551167
1952. Kasahara Y, Yachie A, Takei K, et al. (2001). Differential cellular targets of Epstein-Barr virus (EBV) infection between acute EBV-associated hemophagocytic lymphohistiocytosis and chronic active EBV infection. Blood. 98:1882–8. PMID:11535525
1953. Kassan SS, Thomas TL, Moutsopoulos HM, et al. (1978). Increased risk of lymphoma in sicca syndrome. Ann Intern Med. 89:888–92. PMID:102228
1954. Katagiri Y, Mitsuhashi Y, Kondo S, et al. (2003). Hydroa vacciniforme-like eruptions in a patient with chronic active EB virus infection. J Dermatol. 30:400–4. PMID:12773806
1955. Katakai T, Hara T, Lee JH, et al. (2004). A novel reticular stromal structure in lymph node cortex: an immuno-platform for interactions among dendritic cells, T cells and B cells. Int Immunol. 16:1133–42. PMID:15237106
1956. Katano H, Ali MA, Patera AC, et al. (2004). Chronic active Epstein-Barr virus infection associated with mutations in perforin that impair its maturation. Blood. 103:1244–52. PMID:14576041
1957. Kataoka K, Nagata Y, Kitanaka A, et al. (2015). Integrated molecular analysis of adult T cell leukemia/lymphoma. Nat Genet. 47:1304–15. PMID:26437031
1958. Kato H, Karube K, Yamamoto K, et al. (2014). Gene expression profiling of Epstein-Barr virus-positive diffuse large B-cell lymphoma of the elderly reveals alterations of characteristic oncogenetic pathways. Cancer Sci. 105:537–44. PMID:24581222
1959. Kato I, Tajima K, Suchi T, et al. (1985). Chronic thyroiditis as a risk factor of B-cell lymphoma in the thyroid gland. Jpn J Cancer Res. 76:1085–90. PMID:3936828
1960. Kato K, Ohshima K, Ishihara S, et al. (1998). Elevated serum soluble Fas ligand in natural killer cell proliferative disorders. Br J Haematol. 103:1164–6. PMID:9886336
1961. Katsuya H, Ishitsuka K, Utsunomiya A, et al. (2015). Treatment and survival among 1594 patients with ATL. Blood. 126:2570–7. PMID:26361794
1962. Katzenberger T, Kalla J, Leich E, et al. (2009). A distinctive subtype of t(14;18)-negative nodal follicular non-Hodgkin lymphoma characterized by a predominantly diffuse growth pattern and deletions in the chromosomal region 1p36. Blood. 113:1053–61. PMID:18978208
1963. Katzenberger T, Ott G, Klein T, et al. (2004). Cytogenetic alterations affecting BCL6 are predominantly found in follicular lymphomas grade 3B with a diffuse large B-cell component. Am J Pathol. 165:481–90. PMID:15277222
1964. Katzenberger T, Petzoldt C, Höller S, et al. (2006). The Ki67 proliferation index is a quantitative indicator of clinical risk in mantle cell lymphoma. Blood. 107:3407. PMID:16597597
1965. Katzenstein AL, Carrington CB, Liebow AA (1979). Lymphomatoid granulomatosis: a clinicopathologic study of 152 cases. Cancer. 43:360–73. PMID:761171
1966. Katzenstein AL, Doxtader E, Narendra S (2010). Lymphomatoid granulomatosis: insights gained over 4 decades. Am J Surg Pathol. 34:e35–48. PMID:21107080
1967. Katzenstein AL, Peiper SC (1990). Detection of Epstein-Barr virus genomes in lymphomatoid granulomatosis: analysis of 29 cases by the polymerase chain reaction technique. Mod Pathol. 3:435–41. PMID:2170969
1968. Katzmann JA, Abraham RS, Dispenzieri A, et al. (2005). Diagnostic performance of quantitative kappa and lambda free light chain assays in clinical practice. Clin Chem. 51:878–81. PMID:15774572
1969. Katzmann JA, Clark RJ, Rajkumar VS, et al. (2003). Monoclonal free light chains in sera from healthy individuals: FLC MGUS. Clin Chem. 49:A24.
1970. Kaufmann H, Ackermann J, Baldia C, et al. (2004). Both IGH translocations and chromosome 13q deletions are early events in monoclonal gammopathy of undetermined significance and do not evolve during transition to multiple myeloma. Leukemia. 18:1879–82. PMID:15385925
1971. Kawa-Ha K, Ishihara S, Ninomiya T, et al. (1989). CD3-negative lymphoproliferative disease of granular lymphocytes containing Epstein-Barr viral DNA. J Clin Invest. 84:51–5. PMID:2544630
1972. Kawabe S, Ito Y, Gotoh K, et al. (2012). Application of flow cytometric in situ hybridization assay to Epstein-Barr virus-associated T/natural killer cell lymphoproliferative diseases. Cancer Sci. 103:1481–8. PMID:22497716
1973. Kawajiri C, Tanaka H, Hashimoto S, et al. (2014). Successful treatment of Philadelphia chromosome-positive mixed phenotype acute leukemia by appropriate alternation of second-generation tyrosine kinase inhibitors according to BCR-ABL1 mutation status. Int J Hematol. 99:513–8. PMID:24532437
1974. Kawamoto H (2006). A close developmental relationship between the lymphoid and myeloid lineages. Trends Immunol. 27:169–75. PMID:16515884
1975. Kawano S, Tatsumi E, Yoneda N, et al. (1995). Novel leukemic lymphoma with probable derivation from immature stage of natural killer (NK) lineage in an aged patient. Hematol Oncol. 13:1–11. PMID:7538482
1976. Kayser S, Döhner K, Krauter J, et al. (2011). The impact of therapy-related acute myeloid leukemia (AML) on outcome in 2853 adult patients with newly diagnosed AML. Blood. 117:2137–45. PMID:21127174
1977. Kazakov DV, Mentzel T, Burg G, et al. (2003). Blastic natural killer-cell lymphoma of the skin associated with myelodysplastic syndrome or myelogenous leukaemia: a coincidence or more? Br J Dermatol. 149:869–76. PMID:14616384
1978. Keating MJ, Cazin B, Coutré S, et al. (2002). Campath-1H treatment of T-cell prolymphocytic leukemia in patients for whom at least one prior chemotherapy regimen has failed. J Clin Oncol. 20:205–13. PMID:11773171
1979. Keats JJ, Chesi M, Egan JB, et al. (2012). Clonal competition with alternating dominance in multiple myeloma. Blood. 120:1067–76. PMID:22498740
1980. Keene P, Mendelow B, Pinto MR, et al. (1987). Abnormalities of chromosome 12p13 and malignant proliferation of eosinophils: a nonrandom association. Br J Haematol. 67:25–31. PMID:3478077
1981. Kelly A, Richards SJ, Sivakumaran M, et al. (1994). Clonality of CD3 negative large granular lymphocyte proliferations determined by PCR based X-inactivation studies. J Clin Pathol. 47:399–404. PMID:8027391
1982. Kelly GL, Stylianou J, Rasaiyaah J, et al. (2013). Different patterns of Epstein-Barr virus latency in endemic Burkitt lymphoma (BL) lead to distinct variants within the BL-associated gene expression signature. J Virol. 87:2882–94. PMID:23269792
1983. Kelly JJ Jr, Kyle RA, Miles JM, et al. (1983). Osteosclerotic myeloma and peripheral neuropathy. Neurology. 33:202–10. PMID:6296727
1984. Kelly LM, Gilliland DG (2002). Genetics of myeloid leukemias. Annu Rev Genomics Hum Genet. 3:179–98. PMID:12194988
1985. Kelsen J, Dige A, Schwindt H, et al. (2011). Infliximab induces clonal expansion of γδ-T cells in Crohn's disease: a predictor of lymphoma risk? PLoS One. 6:e17890. PMID:21483853
1986. Kempf W (2006). CD30+ lymphoproliferative disorders: histopathology, differential diagnosis, new variants, and simulators. J Cutan Pathol. 33 Suppl 1:58–70. PMID:16412214
1987. Kempf W, Kazakov DV, Baumgartner HP, et al. (2013). Follicular lymphomatoid papulosis revisited: a study of 11 cases, with new histopathological findings. J Am Acad Dermatol. 68:809–16. PMID:23375516
1988. Kempf W, Kazakov DV, Schärer L, et al. (2013). Angioinvasive lymphomatoid papulosis: a new variant simulating aggressive lymphomas. Am J Surg Pathol. 37:1–13. PMID:23026936
1989. Kempf W, Ostheeren-Michaelis S, Paulli M, et al. (2008). Granulomatous mycosis fungoides and granulomatous slack skin: a multicenter study of the Cutaneous Lymphoma Histopathology Task Force Group of the European Organization For Research and Treatment of Cancer (EORTC). Arch Dermatol. 144:1609–17. PMID:19075143
1990. Kendrick SL, Redd L, Muranyi A, et al. (2014). BCL2 antibodies targeted at different epitopes detect varying levels of protein expression and correlate with frequent gene amplification in diffuse large B-cell lymphoma. Hum Pathol. 45:2144–53. PMID:25090918
1991. Kennedy GA, Kay TD, Johnson DW, et al. (2002). Neutrophil dysplasia characterised by a pseudo-Pelger-Huet anomaly occurring with the use of mycophenolate mofetil and ganciclovir following renal transplantation: a report of five cases. Pathology. 34:263–6. PMID:12109788
1992. Kern W, Bacher U, Haferlach C, et al. (2012). Monoclonal B-cell lymphocytosis is closely related to chronic lymphocytic leukaemia and may be better classified as early-stage CLL. Br J Haematol. 157:86–96. PMID:22224978
1993. Kern W, Bacher U, Haferlach C, et al. (2011). Acute monoblastic/monocytic leukemia and chronic myelomonocytic leukemia share common immunophenotypic features but differ in the extent of aberrantly expressed antigens and amount of granulocytic cells. Leuk Lymphoma. 52:92–100. PMID:21219126
1994. Kern W, Haferlach C, Schnittger S, et al. (2010). Clinical utility of multiparameter flow cytometry in the diagnosis of 1013 patients with suspected myelodysplastic syndrome: correlation to cytomorphology, cytogenetics, and clinical data. Cancer. 116:4549–63. PMID:20572043
1995. Kern W, Haferlach T, Schnittger S, et al. (2004). Prognosis in therapy-related acute myeloid leukemia and impact of karyotype. J Clin Oncol. 22:2510–1. PMID:15197216
1996. Kern WF, Spier CM, Hanneman EH, et al. (1992). Neural cell adhesion molecule-positive peripheral T-cell lymphoma: a rare variant with a propensity for unusual sites of involvement. Blood. 79:2432–7. PMID:1373974
1997. Khalidi HS, Brynes RK, Medeiros LJ, et al. (1998). The immunophenotype of blast transformation of chronic myelogenous leukemia: a high frequency of mixed lineage phenotype in "lymphoid" blasts and A comparison of morphologic, immunophenotypic, and molecular findings. Mod Pathol. 11:1211–21. PMID:9872654
1998. Khalidi HS, Chang KL, Medeiros LJ, et al. (1999). Acute lymphoblastic leukemia. Survey of immunophenotype, French-American-British classification, frequency of myeloid antigen

expression, and karyotypic abnormalities in 210 pediatric and adult cases. Am J Clin Pathol. 111:467–76. PMID:10191766
1999. Khalil MO, Morton LM, Devesa SS, et al. (2014). Incidence of marginal zone lymphoma in the United States, 2001-2009 with a focus on primary anatomic site. Br J Haematol. 165:67–77. PMID:24417667
2000. Khan AB, Barrington SF, Mikhaeel NG, et al. (2013). PET-CT staging of DLBCL accurately identifies and provides new insight into the clinical significance of bone marrow involvement. Blood. 122:61–7. PMID:23660958
2001. Khong PL, Pang CB, Liang R, et al. (2008). Fluorine-18 fluorodeoxyglucose positron emission tomography in mature T-cell and natural killer cell malignancies. Ann Hematol. 87:613–21. PMID:18509641
2002. Khoury H, Dalal BI, Nevill TJ, et al. (2003). Acute myelogenous leukemia with t(8;21)–identification of a specific immunophenotype. Leuk Lymphoma. 44:1713–8. PMID:14692523
2003. Khoury JD, Jones D, Yared MA, et al. (2004). Bone marrow involvement in patients with nodular lymphocyte predominant Hodgkin lymphoma. Am J Surg Pathol. 28:489–95. PMID:15087668
2004. Khoury JD, Medeiros LJ, Manning JT, et al. (2002). CD56(+) TdT(+) blastic natural killer cell tumor of the skin: a primitive systemic malignancy related to myelomonocytic leukemia. Cancer. 94:2401–8. PMID:12015765
2005. Kiel MJ, Sahasrabuddhe AA, Rolland DC, et al. (2015). Genomic analyses reveal recurrent mutations in epigenetic modifiers and the JAK-STAT pathway in Sézary syndrome. Nat Commun. 6:8470. PMID:26415585
2006. Kiel MJ, Velusamy T, Betz BL, et al. (2012). Whole-genome sequencing identifies recurrent somatic NOTCH2 mutations in splenic marginal zone lymphoma. J Exp Med. 209:1553–65. PMID:22891276
2007. Kiel MJ, Velusamy T, Rolland D, et al. (2014). Integrated genomic sequencing reveals mutational landscape of T-cell prolymphocytic leukemia. Blood. 124:1460–72. PMID:24825865
2008. Kienle D, Kröber A, Katzenberger T, et al. (2003). VH mutation status and VDJ rearrangement structure in mantle cell lymphoma: correlation with genomic aberrations, clinical characteristics, and outcome. Blood. 102:3003–9. PMID:12842981
2009. Kikuchi A, Hasegawa D, Ohtsuka Y, et al. (2012). Outcome of children with refractory anaemia with excess of blast (RAEB) and RAEB in transformation (RAEB-T) in the Japanese MDS99 study. Br J Haematol. 158:657–61. PMID:22734597
2010. Kikuchi K, Miyazaki Y, Tanaka A, et al. (2010). Methotrexate-related Epstein-Barr Virus (EBV)-associated lymphoproliferative disorder–so-called "Hodgkin-like lesion"–of the oral cavity in a patient with rheumatoid arthritis. Head Neck Pathol. 4:305–11. PMID:20676828
2011. Kikuta H, Sakiyama Y, Matsumoto S, et al. (1993). Fatal Epstein-Barr virus-associated hemophagocytic syndrome. Blood. 82:3259–64. PMID:8241498
2012. Kiladjian JJ, Cervantes F, Leebeek FW, et al. (2008). The impact of JAK2 and MPL mutations on diagnosis and prognosis of splanchnic vein thrombosis: a report on 241 cases. Blood. 111:4922–9. PMID:18250227
2013. Killick S, Matutes E, Powles RL, et al. (1999). Outcome of biphenotypic acute leukemia. Haematologica. 84:699–706. PMID:10457405
2014. Kilpivaara O, Levine RL (2008). JAK2 and MPL mutations in myeloproliferative neoplasms: discovery and science. Leukemia. 22:1813–7. PMID:18754026
2015. Kim AS, Goldstein SC, Luger S, et al. (2008). Sudden extramedullary T-lymphoblastic blast crisis in chronic myelogenous leukemia: a nonrandom event associated with imatinib? Am J Clin Pathol. 129:639–48. PMID:18343792
2016. Kim BK, Surti U, Pandya A, et al. (2005). Clinicopathologic, immunophenotypic, and molecular cytogenetic fluorescence in situ hybridization analysis of primary and secondary cutaneous follicular lymphomas. Am J Surg Pathol. 29:69–82. PMID:15613857
2016A. Kim HJ, Ahn HK, Jung CW, et al. (2013). KIT D816 mutation associates with adverse outcomes in core binding factor acute myeloid leukemia, especially in the subgroup with RUNX1/RUNX1T1 rearrangement. Ann Hematol. 92:163–71. PMID:23053179
2017. Kim HK, Park CJ, Jang S, et al. (2014). Bone marrow involvement of Langerhans cell histiocytosis: immunohistochemical evaluation of bone marrow for CD1a, Langerin, and S100 expression. Histopathology. 65:742–8. PMID:25138018
2018. Kim SJ, Kim BS, Choi CW, et al. (2007). Ki-67 expression is predictive of prognosis in patients with stage I/II extranodal NK/T-cell lymphoma, nasal type. Ann Oncol. 18:1382–7. PMID:17693651
2019. Kim SY, Im K, Park SN, et al. (2015). CALR, JAK2, and MPL mutation profiles in patients with four different subtypes of myeloproliferative neoplasms: primary myelofibrosis, essential thrombocythemia, polycythemia vera, and myeloproliferative neoplasm, unclassifiable. Am J Clin Pathol. 143:635–44. PMID:25873496
2020. Kim WY, Kim H, Jeon YK, et al. (2010). Follicular dendritic cell sarcoma with immature T-cell proliferation. Hum Pathol. 41:129–33. PMID:19740517
2021. Kim WY, Nam SJ, Kim S, et al. (2015). Prognostic implications of CD30 expression in extranodal natural killer/T-cell lymphoma according to treatment modalities. Leuk Lymphoma. 56:1778–86. PMID:25288491
2022. Kim YM, Ramírez JA, Mick JE, et al. (2007). Molecular characterization of the Tax-containing HTLV-1 enhancer complex reveals a prominent role for CREB phosphorylation in Tax transactivation. J Biol Chem. 282:18750–7. PMID:17449469
2023. Kimura H (2006). Pathogenesis of chronic active Epstein-Barr virus infection: is this an infectious disease, lymphoproliferative disorder, or immunodeficiency? Rev Med Virol. 16:251–61. PMID:16791843
2024. Kimura H, Hoshino Y, Hara S, et al. (2005). Differences between T cell-type and natural killer cell-type chronic active Epstein-Barr virus infection. J Infect Dis. 191:531–9. PMID:15655776
2025. Kimura H, Hoshino Y, Kanegane H, et al. (2001). Clinical and virologic characteristics of chronic active Epstein-Barr virus infection. Blood. 98:280–6. PMID:11435294
2026. Kimura H, Ito Y, Kawabe S, et al. (2012). EBV-associated T/NK-cell lymphoproliferative diseases in nonimmunocompromised hosts: prospective analysis of 108 cases. Blood. 119:673–86. PMID:22096243
2027. Kimura H, Karube K, Ito Y, et al. (2014). Rare occurrence of JAK3 mutations in natural killer cell neoplasms in Japan. Leuk Lymphoma. 55:962–3. PMID:23808814
2028. Kimura H, Morishima T, Kanegane H, et al. (2003). Prognostic factors for chronic active Epstein-Barr virus infection. J Infect Dis. 187:527–33. PMID:12599068
2029. King RL, Dao LN, McPhail ED, et al. (2016). Morphologic Features of ALK-negative Anaplastic Large Cell Lymphomas With DUSP22 Rearrangements. Am J Surg Pathol. 40:36–43 PMID:26379151
2030. Kingma DW, Mueller BU, Frekko K, et al. (1999). Low-grade monoclonal Epstein-Barr virus-associated lymphoproliferative disorder of the brain presenting as human immunodeficiency virus-associated encephalopathy in a child with acquired immunodeficiency syndrome. Arch Pathol Lab Med. 123:83–7. PMID:9923843
2031. Kinney MC, Collins RD, Greer JP, et al. (1993). A small-cell-predominant variant of primary Ki-1 (CD30)+ T-cell lymphoma. Am J Surg Pathol. 17:859–68. PMID:8394652
2032. Kipps TJ (1989). The CD5 B cell. Adv Immunol. 47:117–85. PMID:2479233
2033. Kirwan M, Walne AJ, Plagnol V, et al. (2012). Exome sequencing identifies autosomal-dominant SRP72 mutations associated with familial aplasia and myelodysplasia. Am J Hum Genet. 90:888–92. PMID:22541560
2034. Kita K, Nakase K, Miwa H, et al. (1992). Phenotypical characteristics of acute myelocytic leukemia associated with the t(8;21)(q22;q22) chromosomal abnormality: frequent expression of immature B-cell antigen CD19 together with stem cell antigen CD34. Blood. 80:470–7. PMID:1378322
2035. Kitano K, Ichikawa N, Mahbub B, et al. (1996). Eosinophilia associated with proliferation of CD(3+)4-(8-) alpha beta+ T cells with chromosome 16 anomalies. Br J Haematol. 92:315–7. PMID:8602991
2036. Kiyasu J, Miyoshi H, Hirata A, et al. (2015). Expression of programmed cell death ligand 1 is associated with poor overall survival in patients with diffuse large B-cell lymphoma. Blood. 126:2193–201. PMID:26239088
2037. Klampfl T, Gisslinger H, Harutyunyan AS, et al. (2013). Somatic mutations of calreticulin in myeloproliferative neoplasms. N Engl J Med. 369:2379–90. PMID:24325356
2038. Klapper W, Szczepanowski M, Burkhardt B, et al. (2008). Molecular profiling of pediatric mature B-cell lymphoma treated in population-based prospective clinical trials. Blood. 112:1374–81. PMID:18509088
2039. Klco JM, Welch JS, Nguyen TT, et al. (2011). State of the art in myeloid sarcoma. Int J Lab Hematol. 33:555–65. PMID:21883967
2040. Klein U, Gloghini A, Gaidano G, et al. (2003). Gene expression profile analysis of AIDS-related primary effusion lymphoma (PEL) suggests a plasmablastic derivation and identifies PEL-specific transcripts. Blood. 101:4115–21. PMID:12531789
2041. Klemke CD, Mansmann U, Poenitz N, et al. (2005). Prognostic factors and prediction of prognosis by the CTCL Severity Index in mycosis fungoides and Sézary syndrome. Br J Dermatol. 153:118–24. PMID:16029336
2042. Klimm B, Franklin J, Stein H, et al. (2011). Lymphocyte-depleted classical Hodgkin's lymphoma: a comprehensive analysis from the German Hodgkin study group. J Clin Oncol. 29:3914–20. PMID:21911729
2043. Klion AD (2015). How I treat hypereosinophilic syndromes. Blood. 126:1069–77. PMID:25964669
2044. Klion AD, Noel P, Akin C, et al. (2003). Elevated serum tryptase levels identify a subset of patients with a myeloproliferative variant of idiopathic hypereosinophilic syndrome associated with tissue fibrosis, poor prognosis, and imatinib responsiveness. Blood. 101:4660–6. PMID:12676775
2045. Klion AD, Robyn J, Akin C, et al. (2004). Molecular remission and reversal of myelofibrosis in response to imatinib mesylate treatment in patients with the myeloproliferative variant of hypereosinophilic syndrome. Blood. 103:473–8. PMID:14504092
2046. Kluin PM, Langerak AW, Beverdam-Vincent J, et al. (2015). Paediatric nodal marginal zone B-cell lymphadenopathy of the neck: a Haemophilus influenzae-driven immune disorder? J Pathol. 236:302–14. PMID:25722108
2047. Kluk MJ, Ashworth T, Wang H, et al. (2013). Gauging NOTCH1 Activation in Cancer Using Immunohistochemistry. PLoS One. 8:e67306. PMID:23825651
2048. Kluk MJ, Chapuy B, Sinha P, et al. (2012). Immunohistochemical detection of MYC-driven diffuse large B-cell lymphomas. PLoS One. 7:e33813. PMID:22511926
2049. Kluk MJ, Ho C, Yu H, et al. (2016). MYC Immunohistochemistry to Identify MYC-Driven B-Cell Lymphomas in Clinical Practice. Am J Clin Pathol. 145:166–79. PMID:26834124
2050. Klymenko S, Trott K, Atkinson M, et al. (2005). Aml1 gene rearrangements and mutations in radiation-associated acute myeloid leukemia and myelodysplastic syndromes. J Radiat Res. 46:249–55. PMID:15988144
2051. Knight JS, Tsodikov A, Cibrik DM, et al. (2009). Lymphoma after solid organ transplantation: risk, response to therapy, and survival at a transplantation center. J Clin Oncol. 27:3354–62. PMID:19451438
2052. Knipp S, Strupp C, Gattermann N, et al. (2008). Presence of peripheral blasts in refractory anemia and refractory cytopenia with multilineage dysplasia predicts an unfavourable outcome. Leuk Res. 32:33–7. PMID:17412418
2053. Knowles DM, Cesarman E, Chadburn A, et al. (1995). Correlative morphologic and molecular genetic analysis demonstrates three distinct categories of posttransplantation lymphoproliferative disorders. Blood. 85:552–65. PMID:7812011
2054. Knowles DM, Inghirami G, Ubriaco A, et al. (1989). Molecular genetic analysis of three AIDS-associated neoplasms of uncertain lineage demonstrates their B-cell derivation and the possible pathogenetic role of the Epstein-Barr virus. Blood. 73:792–9. PMID:2537119
2055. Knuutila S, Alitalo R, Ruutu T (1993). Power of the MAC (morphology-antibody-chromosomes) method in distinguishing reactive and clonal cells: report of a patient with acute lymphatic leukemia, eosinophilia, and t(5;14). Genes Chromosomes Cancer. 8:219–23. PMID:7512364
2056. Ko YH, Karnan S, Kim KM, et al. (2010). Enteropathy-associated T-cell lymphoma–a clinicopathologic and array comparative genomic hybridization study. Hum Pathol. 41:1231–7. PMID:20399483
2057. Ko YH, Park S, Kim K, et al. (2008). Aggressive natural killer cell leukemia: is Epstein-Barr virus negativity an indicator of a favorable prognosis? Acta Haematol. 120:199–206. PMID:19153474
2058. Ko YH, Ree HJ, Kim WS, et al. (2000). Clinicopathologic and genotypic study of extranodal nasal-type natural killer/T-cell lymphoma and natural killer precursor lymphoma among Koreans. Cancer. 89:2106–16. PMID:11066052
2059. Kobayashi K, Mitsui K, Ichikawa H, et al. (2014). ATF7IP as a novel PDGFRB fusion partner in acute lymphoblastic leukaemia in children. Br J Haematol. 165:836–41. PMID:24628626
2060. Kobe C, Dietlein M, Franklin J, et al. (2008). Positron emission tomography has a high negative predictive value for progression or early relapse for patients with residual disease after first-line chemotherapy in advanced-stage Hodgkin lymphoma. Blood. 112:3989–94. PMID:18757777
2061. Kobrin C, Cha SC, Qin H, et al. (2006). Molecular analysis of light-chain switch and acute lymphoblastic leukemia transformation in

two follicular lymphomas: implications for lymphomagenesis. Leuk Lymphoma. 47:1523–34. PMID:16966263
2062. Kodama K, Massone C, Chott A, et al. (2005). Primary cutaneous large B-cell lymphomas: clinicopathologic features, classification, and prognostic factors in a large series of patients. Blood. 106:2491–7. PMID:15947086
2063. Koeffler HP, Levine AM, Sparkes M, et al. (1980). Chronic myelocytic leukemia: eosinophils involved in the malignant clone. Blood. 55:1063–5. PMID:6929713
2064. Koenig G, Stevens TM, Peker D (2015). Plasmablastic microlymphoma arising in human herpesvirus-8-associated multicentric Castleman disease in a human immunodeficiency virus-seronegative patient with clinical response to anti-interleukin-6 therapy. Histopathology. 67:930–2. PMID:25900626
2065. Koens L, Senff NJ, Vermeer MH, et al. (2014). Methotrexate-associated B-cell lymphoproliferative disorders presenting in the skin: A clinicopathologic and immunophenotypical study of 10 cases. Am J Surg Pathol. 38:999–1006. PMID:24805861
2066. Koens L, Vermeer MH, Willemze R, et al. (2010). IgM expression on paraffin sections distinguishes primary cutaneous large B-cell lymphoma, leg type from primary cutaneous follicle center lymphoma. Am J Surg Pathol. 34:1043–8. PMID:20551823
2067. Koens L, Zoutman WH, Ngarmlertsirichai P, et al. (2014). Nuclear factor-κB pathway-activating gene aberrancies in primary cutaneous large B-cell lymphoma, leg type. J Invest Dermatol. 134:290–2. PMID:23863863
2068. Koeppen H, Newell K, Baunoch DA, et al. (1998). Morphologic bone marrow changes in patients with posttransplantation lymphoproliferative disorders. Am J Surg Pathol. 22:208–14. PMID:9500222
2069. Koh YW, Hwang HS, Park CS, et al. (2015). Prognostic effect of Ki-67 expression in rituximab, cyclophosphamide, doxorubicin, vincristine and prednisone-treated diffuse large B-cell lymphoma is limited to non-germinal center B-cell-like subtype in late-elderly patients. Leuk Lymphoma. 56:2630–6. PMID:25573205
2070. Koita H, Suzumiya J, Ohshima K, et al. (1997). Lymphoblastic lymphoma expressing natural killer cell phenotype with involvement of the mediastinum and nasal cavity. Am J Surg Pathol. 21:242–8. PMID:9042293
2071. Koizumi K, Sawada K, Nishio M, et al. (1997). Effective high-dose chemotherapy followed by autologous peripheral blood stem cell transplantation in a patient with the aggressive form of cytophagic histiocytic panniculitis. Bone Marrow Transplant. 20:171–3. PMID:9244423
2072. Kojima K, Yasukawa M, Hara M, et al. (1999). Familial occurrence of chronic neutrophilic leukaemia. Br J Haematol. 105:428–30. PMID:10233414
2073. Kojima M, Nakamura S, Itoh H, et al. (1999). Mast cell sarcoma with tissue eosinophilia arising in the ascending colon. Mod Pathol. 12:739–43. PMID:10430280
2074. Kojima M, Nishikii H, Takizawa J, et al. (2013). MYC rearrangements are useful for predicting outcomes following rituximab and chemotherapy: multicenter analysis of Japanese patients with diffuse large B-cell lymphoma. Leuk Lymphoma. 54:2149–54. PMID:23363269
2075. Kolar GR, Mehta D, Pelayo R, et al. (2007). A novel human B cell subpopulation representing the initial germinal center population to express AID. Blood. 109:2545–52. PMID:17132718
2076. Kolde G, Bröcker EB (1986). Multiple skin tumors of indeterminate cells in an adult. J Am Acad Dermatol. 15:591–7. PMID:3095403
2077. Koldehoff M, Beelen DW, Trenschel R, et al. (2004). Outcome of hematopoietic stem cell transplantation in patients with atypical chronic myeloid leukemia. Bone Marrow Transplant. 34:1047–50. PMID:15516946
2078. Komatsu H, Yoshida K, Seto M, et al. (1993). Overexpression of PRAD1 in a mantle zone lymphoma patient with a t(11;22)(q13;q11) translocation. Br J Haematol. 85:427–9. PMID:8280621
2079. Kondo S, Tanimoto K, Yamada K, et al. (2013). Mature T/NK-cell lymphoproliferative disease and Epstein-Barr virus infection are more frequent in patients with rheumatoid arthritis treated with methotrexate. Virchows Arch. 462:399–407. PMID:23494713
2080. Kondratiev S, Duraisamy S, Unitt CL, et al. (2011). Aberrant expression of the dendritic cell marker TNFAIP2 by the malignant cells of Hodgkin lymphoma and primary mediastinal large B-cell lymphoma distinguishes these tumor types from morphologically and phenotypically similar lymphomas. Am J Surg Pathol. 35:1531–9. PMID:21921781
2081. Konoplev S, Lin P, Qiu X, et al. (2010). Clonal relationship of extranodal marginal zone lymphomas of mucosa-associated lymphoid tissue involving different sites. Am J Clin Pathol. 134:112–8. PMID:20551275
2082. Konoplev S, Yin CC, Kornblau SM, et al. (2013). Molecular characterization of de novo Philadelphia chromosome-positive acute myeloid leukemia. Leuk Lymphoma. 54:138–44. PMID:22691121
2083. Koo GC, Tan SY, Tang T, et al. (2012). Janus kinase 3-activating mutations identified in natural killer/T-cell lymphoma. Cancer Discov. 2:591–7. PMID:22705984
2084. Korfel A, Schlegel U (2013). Diagnosis and treatment of primary CNS lymphoma. Nat Rev Neurol. 9:317–27. PMID:23670107
2085. Korgavkar K, Xiong M, Weinstock M (2013). Changing incidence trends of cutaneous T-cell lymphoma. JAMA Dermatol. 149:1295–9. PMID:24005876
2086. Koskela HL, Eldfors S, Ellonen P, et al. (2012). Somatic STAT3 mutations in large granular lymphocytic leukemia. N Engl J Med. 366:1905–13. PMID:22591296
2087. Koss MN, Hochholzer L, Langloss JM, et al. (1986). Lymphomatoid granulomatosis: a clinicopathologic study of 42 patients. Pathology. 18:283–8. PMID:3785978
2088. Koster A, Tromp HA, Raemaekers JM, et al. (2007). The prognostic significance of the intra-follicular tumor cell proliferative rate in follicular lymphoma. Haematologica. 92:184–90. PMID:17296567
2089. Kosugi N, Ebihara Y, Nakahata T, et al. (2005). CD34+CD7+ leukemic progenitor cells may be involved in maintenance and clonal evolution of chronic myeloid leukemia. Clin Cancer Res. 11:505–11. PMID:15701834
2090. Kotecha N, Flores NJ, Irish JM, et al. (2008). Single-cell profiling identifies aberrant STAT5 activation in myeloid malignancies with specific clinical and biologic correlates. Cancer Cell. 14:335–43. PMID:18835035
2091. Kotlyar DS, Osterman MT, Diamond RH, et al. (2011). A systematic review of factors that contribute to hepatosplenic T-cell lymphoma in patients with inflammatory bowel disease. Clin Gastroenterol Hepatol. 9:36–41. e1. PMID:20888436
2092. Kouides PA, Bennett JM (1996). Morphology and classification of the myelodysplastic syndromes and their pathologic variants. Semin Hematol. 33:95–110. PMID:8722681
2093. Kovalchuk AL, Ansarah-Sobrinho C, Hakim O, et al. (2012). Mouse model of endemic Burkitt translocations reveals the long-range boundaries of Ig-mediated oncogene deregulation. Proc Natl Acad Sci U S A. 109:10972–7. PMID:22711821
2094. Kovalszki A, Weller PF (2014). Eosinophilia in mast cell disease. Immunol Allergy Clin North Am. 34:357–64. PMID:24745679
2095. Kowal-Vern A, Cotelingam J, Schumacher HR (1992). The prognostic significance of proerythroblasts in acute erythroleukemia. Am J Clin Pathol. 98:34–40. PMID:1615923
2096. Kozyra EJ, Hirabayashi S, Pastor Loyola VB, et al. (2015). Clonal mutational landscape of childhood myelodysplastic syndromes. Blood. 126:1662.
2097. Kraan W, Horlings HM, van Keimpema M, et al. (2013). High prevalence of oncogenic MYD88 and CD79B mutations in diffuse large B-cell lymphomas presenting at immune-privileged sites. Blood Cancer J. 3:e139. PMID:24013661
2098. Kraan W, van Keimpema M, Horlings HM, et al. (2014). High prevalence of oncogenic MYD88 and CD79B mutations in primary testicular diffuse large B-cell lymphoma. Leukemia. 28:719–20. PMID:24253023
2099. Kralovics R, Passamonti F, Buser AS, et al. (2005). A gain-of-function mutation of JAK2 in myeloproliferative disorders. N Engl J Med. 352:1779–90. PMID:15858187
2100. Kramer MH, Hermans J, Wijburg E, et al. (1998). Clinical relevance of BCL2, BCL6, and MYC rearrangements in diffuse large B-cell lymphoma. Blood. 92:3152–62. PMID:9787151
2101. Kramer MH, Raghoebier S, Beverstock GC, et al. (1991). De novo acute B-cell leukemia with translocation t(14;18): an entity with a poor prognosis. Leukemia. 5:473–8. PMID:1711639
2102. Kratz CP, Franke L, Peters H, et al. (2015). Cancer spectrum and frequency among children with Noonan, Costello, and cardio-facio-cutaneous syndromes. Br J Cancer. 112:1392–7. PMID:25742478
2103. Kratz CP, Niemeyer CM, Castleberry RP, et al. (2005). The mutational spectrum of PTPN11 in juvenile myelomonocytic leukemia and Noonan syndrome/myeloproliferative disease. Blood. 106:2183–5. PMID:15928039
2104. Kraus MD, Haley JC, Ruiz R, et al. (2001). "Juvenile" xanthogranuloma: an immunophenotypic study with a reappraisal of histogenesis. Am J Dermatopathol. 23:104–11. PMID:11285404
2104A. Krauter J, Wagner K, Schäfer I, et al. (2009). Prognostic factors in adult patients up to 60 years old with acute myeloid leukemia and translocations of chromosome band 11q23: individual patient data-based meta-analysis of the German Acute Myeloid Leukemia Intergroup. J Clin Oncol. 27:3000–6. PMID:19380453
2104B. Krauth MT, Alpermann T, Bacher U, et al. (2015). WT1 mutations are secondary events in AML, show varying frequencies and impact on prognosis between genetic subgroups. Leukemia. 29:660–7. PMID:25110071
2105. Kreft A, Büche G, Ghalibafian M, et al. (2005). The incidence of myelofibrosis in essential thrombocythaemia, polycythaemia vera and chronic idiopathic myelofibrosis: a retrospective evaluation of sequential bone marrow biopsies. Acta Haematol. 113:137–43. PMID:15802893
2106. Kreitman RJ, Wilson W, Calvo KR, et al. (2013). Cladribine with immediate rituximab for the treatment of patients with variant hairy cell leukemia. Clin Cancer Res. 19:6873–81. PMID:24277451
2107. Kremer M, Ott G, Nathrath M, et al. (2005). Primary extramedullary plasmacytoma and multiple myeloma: phenotypic differences revealed by immunohistochemical analysis. J Pathol. 205:92–101. PMID:15586381
2108. Krenacs L, Schaerli P, Kis G, et al. (2006). Phenotype of neoplastic cells in angioimmunoblastic T-cell lymphoma is consistent with activated follicular B helper T cells. Blood. 108:1110–1. PMID:16861359
2109. Krenacs L, Smyth MJ, Bagdi E, et al. (2003). The serine protease granzyme M is preferentially expressed in NK-cell, gamma delta T-cell, and intestinal T-cell lymphomas: evidence of origin from lymphocytes involved in innate immunity. Blood. 101:3590–3. PMID:12506019
2110. Krenács L, Tiszalvicz L, Krenács T, et al. (1993). Immunohistochemical detection of CD1A antigen in formalin-fixed and paraffin-embedded tissue sections with monoclonal antibody 010. J Pathol. 171:99–104. PMID:7506772
2111. Krenacs L, Wellmann A, Sorbara L, et al. (1997). Cytotoxic cell antigen expression in anaplastic large cell lymphomas of T- and null-cell type and Hodgkin's disease: evidence for distinct cellular origin. Blood. 89:980–9. PMID:9028330
2112. Kretzmer H, Bernhart SH, Wang W, et al. (2015). DNA methylome analysis in Burkitt and follicular lymphomas identifies differentially methylated regions linked to somatic mutation and transcriptional control. Nat Genet. 47:1316–25. PMID:26437030
2113. Kreutzman A, Juvonen V, Kairisto V, et al. (2010). Mono/oligoclonal T and NK cells are common in chronic myeloid leukemia patients at diagnosis and expand during dasatinib therapy. Blood. 116:772–82. PMID:20413659
2114. Kriangkum J, Taylor BJ, Treon SP, et al. (2004). Clonotypic IgM V/D/J sequence analysis in Waldenstrom macroglobulinemia suggests an unusual B-cell origin and an expansion of polyclonal B cells in peripheral blood. Blood. 104:2134–42. PMID:14764523
2115. Kridel R, Meissner B, Rogic S, et al. (2012). Whole transcriptome sequencing reveals recurrent NOTCH1 mutations in mantle cell lymphoma. Blood. 119:1963–71. PMID:22210878
2116. Krishnan B, Else M, Tjonnfjord GE, et al. (2010). Stem cell transplantation after alemtuzumab in T-cell prolymphocytic leukaemia results in longer survival than after alemtuzumab alone: a multicentre retrospective study. Br J Haematol. 149:907–10. PMID:20201944
2117. Krishnan B, Matutes E, Dearden C (2006). Prolymphocytic leukemias. Semin Oncol. 33:257–63. PMID:16616073
2118. Krishnan J, Wallberg K, Frizzera G (1994). T-cell-rich large B-cell lymphoma. A study of 30 cases, supporting its histologic heterogeneity and lack of clinical distinctiveness. Am J Surg Pathol. 18:455–65. PMID:8172320
2119. Kristinsson SY, Holmberg E, Blimark C (2013). Treatment for high-risk smoldering myeloma. N Engl J Med. 369:1762–3. PMID:24171527
2120. Krivtsov AV, Figueroa ME, Sinha AU, et al. (2013). Cell of origin determines clinically relevant subtypes of MLL-rearranged AML. Leukemia. 27:852–60. PMID:23235717
2120A. Kröber A, Seiler T, Benner A, et al. (2002). V(H) mutation status, CD38 expression level, genomic aberrations, and survival in chronic lymphocytic leukemia. Blood. 2002;100:1410–6. PMID:12149225
2121. Kroft SH, Domiati-Saad R, Finn WG, et al. (2000). Precursor B-lymphoblastic transformation of grade I follicle center lymphoma. Am J Clin Pathol. 113:411–8. PMID:10705823
2122. Krokowski M, Sotlar K, Krauth MT, et al. (2005). Delineation of patterns of bone marrow mast cell infiltration in systemic mastocytosis: value of CD25, correlation with subvariants of the disease, and separation from mast cell

hyperplasia. Am J Clin Pathol. 124:560–8. PMID:16146815
2123. Krysov S, Dias S, Paterson A, et al. (2012). Surface IgM stimulation induces MEK1/2-dependent MYC expression in chronic lymphocytic leukemia cells. Blood. 119:170–9. PMID:22086413
2124. Kröger N, Brand R, van Biezen A, et al. (2009). Risk factors for therapy-related myelodysplastic syndrome and acute myeloid leukemia treated with allogeneic stem cell transplantation. Haematologica. 94:542–9. PMID:19278968
2125. Kröger N, Thiele J, Zander A, et al. (2007). Rapid regression of bone marrow fibrosis after dose-reduced allogeneic stem cell transplantation in patients with primary myelofibrosis. Exp Hematol. 35:1719–22. PMID:17976523
2126. Krönke J, Bullinger L, Teleanu V, et al. (2013). Clonal evolution in relapsed NPM1-mutated acute myeloid leukemia. Blood. 122:100–8. PMID:23704090
2127. Kueck BD, Smith RE, Parkin J, et al. (1991). Eosinophilic leukemia: a myeloproliferative disorder distinct from the hypereosinophilic syndrome. Hematol Pathol. 5:195–205. PMID:1794968
2128. Kuehl WM, Bergsagel PL (2012). Molecular pathogenesis of multiple myeloma and its premalignant precursor. J Clin Invest. 122:3456–63. PMID:23023717
2129. Kuiper R, Broyl A, de Knegt Y, et al. (2012). A gene expression signature for high-risk multiple myeloma. Leukemia. 26:2406–13. PMID:22722715
2129A. Kulasekararaj AG, Smith AE, Mian SA et al. (2013). TP53 mutations in myelodysplastic syndrome are strongly correlated with aberrations of chromosome 5, and correlate with adverse prognosis. Br J Haematol. 160:660–72. PMID: 23297687.
2130. Kulis M, Heath S, Bibikova M, et al. (2012). Epigenomic analysis detects widespread gene-body DNA hypomethylation in chronic lymphocytic leukemia. Nat Genet. 44:1236–42. PMID:23064414
2131. Kumar S, Dispenzieri A, Lacy MQ, et al. (2012). Revised prognostic staging system for light chain amyloidosis incorporating cardiac biomarkers and serum free light chain measurements. J Clin Oncol. 30:989–95. PMID:22331953
2132. Kumar S, Fend F, Quintanilla-Martinez L, et al. (2000). Epstein-Barr virus-positive primary gastrointestinal Hodgkin's disease: association with inflammatory bowel disease and immunosuppression. Am J Surg Pathol. 24:66–73. PMID:10632489
2133. Kumar S, Krenacs L, Medeiros J, et al. (1998). Subcutaneous panniculitic T-cell lymphoma is a tumor of cytotoxic T lymphocytes. Hum Pathol. 29:397–403. PMID:9563791
2134. Kumar S, Krenacs L, Otsuki T, et al. (1996). bc1-1 rearrangement and cyclin D1 protein expression in multiple lymphomatous polyposis. Am J Clin Pathol. 105:737–43. PMID:8659449
2135. Kumar V, Matsuo K, Takahashi A, et al. (2011). Common variants on 14q32 and 13q12 are associated with DLBCL susceptibility. J Hum Genet. 56:436–9. PMID:21471979
2136. Kummer JA, Vermeer MH, Dukers D, et al. (1997). Most primary cutaneous CD30-positive lymphoproliferative disorders have a CD4-positive cytotoxic T-cell phenotype. J Invest Dermatol. 109:636–40. PMID:9347791
2137. Kuo SH, Cheng AL (2013). Helicobacter pylori and mucosa-associated lymphoid tissue: what's new. Hematology Am Soc Hematol Educ Program. 2013:109–17. PMID:24319171
2138. Kuo TT, Chen MJ, Kuo MC (2006). Cutaneous intravascular NK-cell lymphoma: report of a rare variant associated with Epstein-Barr virus. Am J Surg Pathol. 30:1197–201. PMID:16931967
2139. Kuo TT, Shih LY, Tsang NM (2004). Nasal NK/T cell lymphoma in Taiwan: a clinicopathologic study of 22 cases, with analysis of histologic subtypes, Epstein-Barr virus LMP-1 gene association, and treatment modalities. Int J Surg Pathol. 12:375–87. PMID:15494863
2140. Kuper-Hommel MJ, van Krieken JH (2012). Molecular pathogenesis and histologic and clinical features of extranodal marginal zone lymphomas of mucosa-associated lymphoid tissue type. Leuk Lymphoma. 53:1032–45. PMID:21988643
2141. Kurata M, Hasegawa M, Nakagawa Y, et al. (2006). Expression dynamics of drug resistance genes, multidrug resistance 1 (MDR1) and lung resistance protein (LRP) during the evolution of overt leukemia in myelodysplastic syndromes. Exp Mol Pathol. 81:249–54. PMID:16566920
2142. Kurtin PJ, Dewald GW, Shields DJ, et al. (1996). Hematologic disorders associated with deletions of chromosome 20q: a clinicopathologic study of 107 patients. Am J Clin Pathol. 106:680–8. PMID:8929482
2143. Kurzrock R, Bueso-Ramos CE, Kantarjian H, et al. (2001). BCR rearrangement-negative chronic myelogenous leukemia revisited. J Clin Oncol. 19:2915–26. PMID:11387365
2144. Kurzwelly D, Glas M, Roth P, et al. (2010). Primary CNS lymphoma in the elderly: temozolomide therapy and MGMT status. J Neurooncol. 97:389–92. PMID:19841864
2145. Kussick SJ, Kalnoski M, Braziel RM, et al. (2004). Prominent clonal B-cell populations identified by flow cytometry in histologically reactive lymphoid proliferations. Am J Clin Pathol. 121:464–72. PMID:15080297
2146. Kuter DJ, Bain B, Mufti G, et al. (2007). Bone marrow fibrosis: pathophysiology and clinical significance of increased bone marrow stromal fibres. Br J Haematol. 139:351–62. PMID:17910625
2147. Kvasnicka HM (2013). WHO classification of myeloproliferative neoplasms (MPN): A critical update. Curr Hematol Malig Rep. 8:333–41. PMID:24146204
2148. Kvasnicka HM, Beham-Schmid C, Bob R, et al. (2016). Problems and pitfalls in grading of bone marrow fibrosis, collagen deposition and osteosclerosis - a consensus-based study. Histopathology. 68:905–15 PMID:26402166
2149. Kvasnicka HM, Thiele J (2004). Bone marrow angiogenesis: methods of quantification and changes evolving in chronic myeloproliferative disorders. Histol Histopathol. 19:1245–60. PMID:15375769
2150. Kvasnicka HM, Thiele J (2006). The impact of clinicopathological studies on staging and survival in essential thrombocythemia, chronic idiopathic myelofibrosis, and polycythemia rubra vera. Semin Thromb Hemost. 32:362–71. PMID:16810612
2151. Kvasnicka HM, Thiele J (2007). Classification of Ph-negative chronic myeloproliferative disorders–morphology as the yardstick of classification. Pathobiology. 74:63–71. PMID:17587877
2152. Kvasnicka HM, Thiele J (2010). Prodromal myeloproliferative neoplasms: the 2008 WHO classification. Am J Hematol. 85:62–9. PMID:19844986
2153. Kwok M, Korde N, Landgren O (2012). Bortezomib to treat the TEMPI syndrome. N Engl J Med. 366:1843–5. PMID:22571216
2154. Kwong YL, Chan AC, Liang R, et al. (1997). CD56+ NK lymphomas: clinicopathological features and prognosis. Br J Haematol. 97:821–9. PMID:9217183
2155. Kwong YL, Chan AC, Liang RH (1997). Natural killer cell lymphoma/leukemia: pathology and treatment. Hematol Oncol. 15:71–9. PMID:9375032
2156. Kwong YL, Lam CC, Chan TM (2000). Post-transplantation lymphoproliferative disease of natural killer cell lineage: a clinicopathological and molecular analysis. Br J Haematol. 110:197–202. PMID:10930998
2157. Kwong YL, Wong KF, Chan LC, et al. (1995). Large granular lymphocyte leukemia. A study of nine cases in a Chinese population. Am J Clin Pathol. 103:76–81. PMID:7817949
2158. Küçük C, Hu X, Jiang B, et al. (2015). Global promoter methylation analysis reveals novel candidate tumor suppressor genes in natural killer cell lymphoma. Clin Cancer Res. 21:1699–711. PMID:25614448
2159. Küçük C, Iqbal J, Hu X, et al. (2011). PRDM1 is a tumor suppressor gene in natural killer cell malignancies. Proc Natl Acad Sci U S A. 108:20119–24. PMID:22143801
2160. Küçük C, Jiang B, Hu X, et al. (2015). Activating mutations of STAT5B and STAT3 in lymphomas derived from γδ-T or NK cells. Nat Commun. 6:6025. PMID:25586472
2161. Küker W, Nägele T, Korfel A, et al. (2005). Primary central nervous system lymphomas (PCNSL): MRI features at presentation in 100 patients. J Neurooncol. 72:169–77. PMID:15925998
2162. Kyle RA, Dispenzieri A, Kumar S, et al. (2011). IgM monoclonal gammopathy of undetermined significance (MGUS) and smoldering Waldenström's macroglobulinemia (SWM). Clin Lymphoma Myeloma Leuk. 11:74–6. PMID:21454195
2163. Kyle RA, Gertz MA (1995). Primary systemic amyloidosis: clinical and laboratory features in 474 cases. Semin Hematol. 32:45–59. PMID:7878478
2164. Kyle RA, Gertz MA, Witzig TE, et al. (2003). Review of 1027 patients with newly diagnosed multiple myeloma. Mayo Clin Proc. 78:21–33. PMID:12528874
2165. Kyle RA, Greipp PR (1980). Smoldering multiple myeloma. N Engl J Med. 302:1347–9. PMID:7374679
2166. Kyle RA, Greipp PR, O'Fallon WM (1986). Primary systemic amyloidosis: multivariate analysis for prognostic factors in 168 cases. Blood. 68:220–4. PMID:3719098
2167. Kyle RA, Larson DR, Therneau TM, et al. (2014). Clinical course of light-chain smouldering multiple myeloma (idiopathic Bence Jones proteinuria): a retrospective cohort study. Lancet Haematol. 1:e28–36. PMID:25530988
2168. Kyle RA, Linos A, Beard CM, et al. (1992). Incidence and natural history of primary systemic amyloidosis in Olmsted County, Minnesota, 1950 through 1989. Blood. 79:1817–22. PMID:1558973
2169. Kyle RA, Maldonado JE, Bayrd ED (1974). Plasma cell leukemia. Report on 17 cases. Arch Intern Med. 133:813–8. PMID:4821776
2170. Kyle RA, Rajkumar SV (2004). Multiple myeloma. N Engl J Med. 351:1860–73. PMID:15509819
2171. Kyle RA, Rajkumar SV (2006). Monoclonal gammopathy of undetermined significance. Br J Haematol. 134:573–89. PMID:16938117
2172. Kyle RA, Rajkumar SV (2007). Monoclonal gammopathy of undetermined significance and smouldering multiple myeloma: emphasis on risk factors for progression. Br J Haematol. 139:730–43. PMID:18021088
2173. Kyle RA, Rajkumar SV, Therneau TM, et al. (2005). Prognostic factors and predictors of outcome of immunoglobulin M monoclonal gammopathy of undetermined significance. Clin Lymphoma. 5:257–60. PMID:15794860
2174. Kyle RA, Remstein ED, Therneau TM, et al. (2007). Clinical course and prognosis of smoldering (asymptomatic) multiple myeloma. N Engl J Med. 356:2582–90. PMID:17582068
2175. Kyle RA, Therneau TM, Rajkumar SV, et al. (2006). Prevalence of monoclonal gammopathy of undetermined significance. N Engl J Med. 354:1362–9. PMID:16571879
2176. Kyle RA, Therneau TM, Rajkumar SV, et al. (2002). A long-term study of prognosis in monoclonal gammopathy of undetermined significance. N Engl J Med. 346:564–9. PMID:11856795
2177. Kyle RA, Therneau TM, Rajkumar SV, et al. (2003). Long-term follow-up of IgM monoclonal gammopathy of undetermined significance. Blood. 102:3759–64. PMID:12881316
2178. Küppers R, Klein U, Schwering I, et al. (2003). Identification of Hodgkin and Reed-Sternberg cell-specific genes by gene expression profiling. J Clin Invest. 111:529–37. PMID:12588891
2179. Königsberg R, Ackermann J, Kaufmann H, et al. (2000). Deletions of chromosome 13q in monoclonal gammopathy of undetermined significance. Leukemia. 14:1975–9. PMID:11069034
2180. Königsberg R, Zojer N, Ackermann J, et al. (2000). Predictive role of interphase cytogenetics for survival of patients with multiple myeloma. J Clin Oncol. 18:804–12. PMID:10673522
2180A. Küppers R (2012). New insights in the biology of Hodgkin lymphoma. Hematology Am Soc Hematol Educ Program. 2012:328-34. PMID:23233600
2181. Lachenal F, Berger F, Ghesquières H, et al. (2007). Angioimmunoblastic T-cell lymphoma: clinical and laboratory features at diagnosis in 77 patients. Medicine (Baltimore). 86:282–92. PMID:17873758
2182. Lachmann HJ, Booth DR, Booth SE, et al. (2002). Misdiagnosis of hereditary amyloidosis as AL (primary) amyloidosis. N Engl J Med. 346:1786–91. PMID:12050338
2183. Lae ME, Ahmed I, Macon WR (2002). Clusterin is widely expressed in systemic anaplastic large cell lymphoma but fails to differentiate primary from secondary cutaneous anaplastic large cell lymphoma. Am J Clin Pathol. 118:773–9. PMID:12428799
2184. Laginestra MA, Piccaluga PP, Fuligni F, et al. (2014). Pathogenetic and diagnostic significance of microRNA deregulation in peripheral T-cell lymphoma not otherwise specified. Blood Cancer J. 4:259. PMID:25382608
2184A. Laginestra MA, Tripodo C, Agostinelli C, et al. (2017). Distinctive histogenesis and immunological microenvironment based on transcriptional profiles of follicular dendritic cell sarcomas. Mol Cancer Res. 15:541–52. PMID: 28130401
2185. Laharanne E, Oumouhou N, Bonnet F, et al. (2010). Genome-wide analysis of cutaneous T-cell lymphomas identifies three clinically relevant classes. J Invest Dermatol. 130:1707–18. PMID:20130593
2186. Lahortiga I, Vázquez I, Agirre X, et al. (2004). Molecular heterogeneity in AML/MDS patients with 3q21q26 rearrangements. Genes Chromosomes Cancer. 40:179–89. PMID:15138998
2187. Lai JL, Preudhomme C, Zandecki M, et al. (1995). Myelodysplastic syndromes and acute myeloid leukemia with 17p deletion. An entity characterized by specific dysgranulopoïesis and a high incidence of P53 mutations. Leukemia. 9:370–81. PMID:7885035
2188. Laï JL, Zandecki M, Mary JY, et al. (1995). Improved cytogenetics in multiple myeloma: a study of 151 patients including 117 patients at diagnosis. Blood. 85:2490–7. PMID:7537117
2189. Lai R, Arber DA, Chang KL, et al. (1998). Frequency of bcl-2 expression in non-Hodgkin's

lymphoma: a study of 778 cases with comparison of marginal zone lymphoma and monocytoid B-cell hyperplasia. Mod Pathol. 11:864–9. PMID:9758366

2190. Lai R, Weiss LM, Chang KL, et al. (1999). Frequency of CD43 expression in non-Hodgkin lymphoma. A survey of 742 cases and further characterization of rare CD43+ follicular lymphomas. Am J Clin Pathol. 111:488–94. PMID:10191768

2191. Lai YY, Li Y, Shi Y, et al. (2012). [Characteristics of 11 patients with acute myeloid leukemia accompanied with karyotype aberration t(6;9)]. Zhongguo Shi Yan Xue Ye Xue Za Zhi. 20:1293–6. PMID:23257419

2192. Laimer D, Dolznig H, Kollmann K, et al. (2012). PDGFR blockade is a rational and effective therapy for NPM-ALK-driven lymphomas. Nat Med. 18:1699–704. PMID:23064464

2193. Laiosa CV, Stadtfeld M, Graf T (2006). Determinants of lymphoid-myeloid lineage diversification. Annu Rev Immunol. 24:705–38. PMID:16551264

2194. Lakey MA, Pardanani A, Hoyer JD, et al. (2010). Bone marrow morphologic features in polycythemia vera with JAK2 exon 12 mutations. Am J Clin Pathol. 133:942–8. PMID:20472853

2195. Lamant L, Dastugue N, Pulford K, et al. (1999). A new fusion gene TPM3-ALK in anaplastic large cell lymphoma created by a (1;2)(q25;p23) translocation. Blood. 93:3088–95. PMID:10216106

2196. Lamant L, de Reyniès A, Duplantier MM, et al. (2007). Gene-expression profiling of systemic anaplastic large-cell lymphoma reveals differences based on ALK status and two distinct morphologic ALK+ subtypes. Blood. 109:2156–64. PMID:17077326

2197. Lamant L, Gascoyne RD, Duplantier MM, et al. (2003). Non-muscle myosin heavy chain (MYH9): a new partner fused to ALK in anaplastic large cell lymphoma. Genes Chromosomes Cancer. 37:427–32. PMID:12800156

2198. Lamant L, McCarthy K, d'Amore E, et al. (2011). Prognostic impact of morphologic and phenotypic features of childhood ALK-positive anaplastic large-cell lymphoma: results of the ALCL99 study. J Clin Oncol. 29:4669–76. PMID:22084369

2199. Lamant L, Meggetto F, al Saati T, et al. (1996). High incidence of the t(2;5)(p23;q35) translocation in anaplastic large cell lymphoma and its lack of detection in Hodgkin's disease. Comparison of cytogenetic analysis, reverse transcriptase-polymerase chain reaction, and P-80 immunostaining. Blood. 87:284–91. PMID:8547653

2200. Lamant L, Pileri S, Sabattini E, et al. (2010). Cutaneous presentation of ALK-positive anaplastic large cell lymphoma following insect bites: evidence for an association in five cases. Haematologica. 95:449–55. PMID:19951975

2201. Lambertenghi-Deliliers G, Orazi A, Luksch R, et al. (1991). Myelodysplastic syndrome with increased marrow fibrosis: a distinct clinico-pathological entity. Br J Haematol. 78:161–6. PMID:1712222

2202. Lampert IA, Wotherspoon A, Van Noorden S, et al. (1999). High expression of CD23 in the proliferation centers of chronic lymphocytic leukemia in lymph nodes and spleen. Hum Pathol. 30:648–54. PMID:10374772

2203. Lamy T, Loughran TP Jr (1999). Current concepts: large granular lymphocyte leukemia. Blood Rev. 13:230–40. PMID:10741898

2204. Lamy T, Loughran TP Jr (2003). Clinical features of large granular lymphocyte leukemia. Semin Hematol. 40:185–95. PMID:12876667

2205. Lamy T, Loughran TP Jr (2011). How I treat LGL leukemia. Blood. 117:2764–74. PMID:21190991

2206. Lan Q, Zheng T, Chanock S, et al. (2007). Genetic variants in caspase genes and susceptibility to non-Hodgkin lymphoma. Carcinogenesis. 28:823–7. PMID:17071630

2207. Landau DA, Carter SL, Stojanov P, et al. (2013). Evolution and impact of subclonal mutations in chronic lymphocytic leukemia. Cell. 152:714–26. PMID:23415222

2208. Landau DA, Tausch E, Taylor-Weiner AN, et al. (2015). Mutations driving CLL and their evolution in progression and relapse. Nature. 526:525–30. PMID:26466571

2209. Landgren O, Goldin LR, Kristinsson SY, et al. (2008). Increased risks of polycythemia vera, essential thrombocythemia, and myelofibrosis among 24,577 first-degree relatives of 11,039 patients with myeloproliferative neoplasms in Sweden. Blood. 112:2199–204. PMID:18451307

2210. Landgren O, Graubard BI, Katzmann JA, et al. (2014). Racial disparities in the prevalence of monoclonal gammopathies: a population-based study of 12,482 persons from the National Health and Nutritional Examination Survey. Leukemia. 28:1537–42. PMID:24441287

2211. Landgren O, Gridley G, Turesson I, et al. (2006). Risk of monoclonal gammopathy of undetermined significance (MGUS) and subsequent multiple myeloma among African American and white veterans in the United States. Blood. 107:904–6. PMID:16210333

2212. Landgren O, Kristinsson SY, Goldin LR, et al. (2009). Risk of plasma cell and lymphoproliferative disorders among 14621 first-degree relatives of 4458 patients with monoclonal gammopathy of undetermined significance in Sweden. Blood. 114:791–5. PMID:19182202

2213. Landgren O, Kyle RA, Pfeiffer RM, et al. (2009). Monoclonal gammopathy of undetermined significance (MGUS) consistently precedes multiple myeloma: a prospective study. Blood. 113:5412–7. PMID:19179464

2214. Landgren O, Staudt L (2012). MYD88 L265P somatic mutation in IgM MGUS. N Engl J Med. 367:2255–6, author reply 2256–7. PMID:23215570

2215. Landgren O, Weiss BM (2009). Patterns of monoclonal gammopathy of undetermined significance and multiple myeloma in various ethnic/racial groups: support for genetic factors in pathogenesis. Leukemia. 23:1691–7. PMID:19587704

2216. Lange BJ, Kobrinsky N, Barnard DR, et al. (1998). Distinctive demography, biology, and outcome of acute myeloid leukemia and myelodysplastic syndrome in children with Down syndrome: Children's Cancer Group Studies 2861 and 2891. Blood. 91:608–15. PMID:9427716

2217. Langebrake C, Creutzig U, Reinhardt D (2005). Immunophenotype of Down syndrome acute myeloid leukemia and transient myeloproliferative disease differs significantly from other diseases with morphologically identical or similar blasts. Klin Padiatr. 217:126–34. PMID:15858703

2217A. Langer C, Marcucci G, Holland KB, et al. (2009). Prognostic importance of MN1 transcript levels, and biologic insights from MN1-associated gene and microRNA expression signatures in cytogenetically normal acute myeloid leukemia: a cancer and leukemia group B study. J Clin Oncol. 27:3198–204. PMID:19451432

2218. Lanoy E, Rosenberg PS, Fily F, et al. (2011). HIV-associated Hodgkin lymphoma during the first months on combination antiretroviral therapy. Blood. 118:44–9. PMID:21551234

2219. Lardelli P, Bookman MA, Sundeen J, et al. (1990). Lymphocytic lymphoma of intermediate differentiation. Morphologic and immunophenotypic spectrum and clinical correlations. Am J Surg Pathol. 14:752–63. PMID:2198813

2220. Largent J, Oefelein M, Kaplan HM, et al. (2012). Risk of lymphoma in women with breast implants: analysis of clinical studies. Eur J Cancer Prev. 21:274–80. PMID:22456426

2221. Larson RA (2009). Therapy-related myeloid neoplasms. Haematologica. 94:454–9. PMID:19336749

2222. Larson RA (2012). Cytogenetics, not just previous therapy, determines the course of therapy-related myeloid neoplasms. J Clin Oncol. 30:2300–2. PMID:22585693

2223. Larson RA, Le Beau MM (2011). Prognosis and therapy when acute promyelocytic leukemia and other "good risk" acute myeloid leukemias occur as a therapy-related myeloid neoplasm. Mediterr J Hematol Infect Dis. 3:e2011032. PMID:21869918

2224. Larson RA, Wang Y, Banerjee M, et al. (1999). Prevalence of the inactivating 609C–>T polymorphism in the NAD(P)H:quinone oxidoreductase (NQO1) gene in patients with primary and therapy-related myeloid leukemia. Blood. 94:803–7. PMID:10397748

2225. Larson RS, Scott MA, McCurley TL, et al. (1996). Microsatellite analysis of posttransplant lymphoproliferative disorders: determination of donor/recipient origin and identification of putative lymphomagenic mechanism. Cancer Res. 56:4378–81. PMID:8813129

2226. Lasho TL, Mims A, Elliott MA, et al. (2014). Chronic neutrophilic leukemia with concurrent CSF3R and SETBP1 mutations: single colony clonality studies, in vitro sensitivity to JAK inhibitors and lack of treatment response to ruxolitinib. Leukemia. 28:1363–5. PMID:24445868

2227. Laszewski MJ, Kemp JD, Goeken JA, et al. (1990). Clonal immunoglobulin gene rearrangement in nodular lymphoid hyperplasia of the gastrointestinal tract associated with common variable immunodeficiency. Am J Clin Pathol. 94:338–43. PMID:2204266

2228. Launay E, Pangault C, Bertrand P, et al. (2012). High rate of TNFRSF14 gene alterations related to 1p36 region in de novo follicular lymphoma and impact on prognosis. Leukemia. 26:559–62. PMID:21941365

2229. Laurent C, Delas A, Gaulard P, et al. (2016). Breast implant-associated anaplastic large cell lymphoma: two distinct clinicopathological variants with different outcomes. Ann Oncol. 27:306–14 PMID:26598546

2230. Laurent C, Do C, Gascoyne RD, et al. (2009). Anaplastic lymphoma kinase-positive diffuse large B-cell lymphoma: a rare clinicopathologic entity with poor prognosis. J Clin Oncol. 27:4211–6. PMID:19636007

2230A. Laurent C, Do C, Gourraud P.A, et al. (2015). Prevalence of common Non-Hodgkin lymphomas and subtypes of Hodgkin lymphoma by nodal site of involvement: a systematic retrospective review of 938 cases. Medicine (Baltimore) 94:e987. PMID:26107683.

2231. Laurent C, Fazilleau N, Brousset P (2010). A novel subset of T-helper cells: follicular T-helper cells and their markers. Haematologica. 95:356–8. PMID:20207841

2232. Laurini JA, Perry AM, Boilesen E, et al. (2012). Classification of non-Hodgkin lymphoma in Central and South America: a review of 1028 cases. Blood. 120:4795–801. PMID:23086753

2233. Lazzarino M, Orlandi E, Paulli M, et al. (1993). Primary mediastinal B-cell lymphoma with sclerosis: an aggressive tumor with distinctive clinical and pathologic features. J Clin Oncol. 11:2306–13. PMID:8246020

2234. Lazzarino M, Orlandi E, Paulli M, et al. (1997). Treatment outcome and prognostic factors for primary mediastinal (thymic) B-cell lymphoma: a multicenter study of 106 patients. J Clin Oncol. 15:1646–53. PMID:9193365

2235. Lazzeri D, Agostini T, Bocci G, et al. (2011). ALK-1-negative anaplastic large cell lymphoma associated with breast implants: a new clinical entity. Clin Breast Cancer. 11:283–96. PMID:21729665

2236. Le Beau MM (2001). Role of cytogenetics in the diagnosis and classification of hematopoietic neoplasms. In: Knowles D, editor. Neoplastic hematopathology. 2nd ed. Philadelphia: Lippincott Williams & Wilkins; pp. 319–418.

2237. Le Gouill S, Talmant P, Touzeau C, et al. (2007). The clinical presentation and prognosis of diffuse large B-cell lymphoma with t(14;18) and 8q24/c-MYC rearrangement. Haematologica. 92:1335–42. PMID:18024371

2238. Lebbe C, Porcher R, Marcelin AG, et al. (2013). Human herpesvirus 8 (HHV8) transmission and related morbidity in organ recipients. Am J Transplant. 13:207–13. PMID:23057808

2239. Leblond V, Davi F, Charlotte F, et al. (1998). Posttransplant lymphoproliferative disorders not associated with Epstein-Barr virus: a distinct entity? J Clin Oncol. 16:2052–9. PMID:9626203

2240. Leblond V, Dhedin N, Mamzer Bruneel MF, et al. (2001). Identification of prognostic factors in 61 patients with posttransplantation lymphoproliferative disorders. J Clin Oncol. 19:772–8. PMID:11157030

2241. LeBoit PE (1994). Granulomatous slack skin. Dermatol Clin. 12:375–89. PMID:8045049

2242. LeBoit PE, Burg G, Weedon D, et al., editors. (2005). World Health Organization classification of tumours. Pathology and genetics of skin tumours. 3rd ed. Lyon: IARC Press.

2243. LeBrun DP (2003). E2A basic helix-loop-helix transcription factors in human leukemia. Front Biosci. 8:s206–22. PMID:12700034

2244. LeBrun DP, Ngan BY, Weiss LM, et al. (1994). The bcl-2 oncogene in Hodgkin's disease arising in the setting of follicular non-Hodgkin's lymphoma. Blood. 83:223–30. PMID:8274737

2245. Lechapt-Zalcman E, Challine D, Delfau-Larue MH, et al. (2001). Association of primary pleural effusion lymphoma of T-cell origin and human herpesvirus 8 in a human immunodeficiency virus-seronegative man. Arch Pathol Lab Med. 125:1246–8. PMID:11520284

2246. Lechner MG, Megiel C, Church CH, et al. (2012). Survival signals and targets for therapy in breast implant-associated ALK–anaplastic large cell lymphoma. Clin Cancer Res. 18:4549–59. PMID:22791880

2247. Lecluse Y, Lebailly P, Roulland S, et al. (2009). t(11;14)-positive clones can persist over a long period of time in the peripheral blood of healthy individuals. Leukemia. 23:1190–3. PMID:19242498

2248. Lecuit M, Abachin E, Martin A, et al. (2004). Immunoproliferative small intestinal disease associated with Campylobacter jejuni. N Engl J Med. 350:239–48. PMID:14724303

2249. Lee AY, Connors JM, Klimo P, et al. (1997). Late relapse in patients with diffuse large-cell lymphoma treated with MACOP-B. J Clin Oncol. 15:1745–53. PMID:9164181

2250. Lee IJ, Kim SC, Kim HS, et al. (1999). Paraneoplastic pemphigus associated with follicular dendritic cell sarcoma arising from Castleman's tumor. J Am Acad Dermatol. 40:294–7. PMID:10025851

2251. Lee J, Suh C, Park YH, et al. (2006). Extranodal natural killer T-cell lymphoma, nasal-type: a prognostic model from a retrospective multicenter study. J Clin Oncol. 24:612–8. PMID:16380410

2252. Lee JT, Innes DJ Jr, Williams ME (1989). Sequential bcl-2 and c-myc oncogene

rearrangements associated with the clinical transformation of non-Hodgkin's lymphoma. J Clin Invest. 84:1454–9. PMID:2509518
2253. Lee SH, Erber WN, Porwit A, et al. (2008). ICSH guidelines for the standardization of bone marrow specimens and reports. Int J Lab Hematol. 30:349–64. PMID:18822060
2254. Lee SH, Kim JS, Kim J, et al. (2015). A highly recurrent novel missense mutation in CD28 among angioimmunoblastic T-cell lymphoma patients. Haematologica. 100:e505–7. PMID:26405154
2255. Lefèvre G, Copin MC, Staumont-Sallé D, et al. (2014). The lymphoid variant of hypereosinophilic syndrome: study of 21 patients with CD3-CD4+ aberrant T-cell phenotype. Medicine (Baltimore). 93:255–66. PMID:25398061
2256. Leffler DA, Dennis M, Hyett B, et al. (2007). Etiologies and predictors of diagnosis in nonresponsive celiac disease. Clin Gastroenterol Hepatol. 5:445–50. PMID:17382600
2257. Legrand O, Perrot JY, Simonin G, et al. (1998). Adult biphenotypic acute leukaemia: an entity with poor prognosis which is related to unfavourable cytogenetics and P-glycoprotein over-expression. Br J Haematol. 100:147–55. PMID:9450804
2258. Leich E, Hoster E, Wartenberg M, et al. (2016). Similar clinical features in follicular lymphomas with and without breaks in the BCL2 locus. Leukemia. 30:854–60 PMID:26621338
2259. Leich E, Salaverria I, Bea S, et al. (2009). Follicular lymphomas with and without translocation t(14;18) differ in gene expression profiles and genetic alterations. Blood. 114:826–34. PMID:19471018
2260. Leith CP, Kopecky KJ, Chen IM, et al. (1999). Frequency and clinical significance of the expression of the multidrug resistance proteins MDR1/P-glycoprotein, MRP1, and LRP in acute myeloid leukemia: a Southwest Oncology Group Study. Blood. 94:1086–99. PMID:10419902
2261. Leith CP, Kopecky KJ, Godwin J, et al. (1997). Acute myeloid leukemia in the elderly: assessment of multidrug resistance (MDR1) and cytogenetics distinguishes biologic subgroups with remarkably distinct responses to standard chemotherapy. A Southwest Oncology Group study. Blood. 89:3323–9. PMID:9129038
2262. Leithäuser F, Bäuerle M, Huynh MQ, et al. (2001). Isotype-switched immunoglobulin genes with a high load of somatic hypermutation and lack of ongoing mutational activity are prevalent in mediastinal B-cell lymphoma. Blood. 98:2762–70. PMID:11675349
2263. Leleu X, O'Connor K, Ho AW, et al. (2007). Hepatitis C viral infection is not associated with Waldenström's macroglobulinemia. Am J Hematol. 82:83–4. PMID:16955461
2264. Lemonnier F, Couronné L, Parrens M, et al. (2012). Recurrent TET2 mutations in peripheral T-cell lymphomas correlate with TFH-like features and adverse clinical parameters. Blood. 120:1466–9. PMID:22760778
2265. Lengfelder E, Hochhaus A, Kronawitter U, et al. (1998). Should a platelet limit of 600 x 10(9)/l be used as a diagnostic criterion in essential thrombocythaemia? An analysis of the natural course including early stages. Br J Haematol. 100:15–23. PMID:9450785
2266. Lenglet J, Traullé C, Mounier N, et al. (2014). Long-term follow-up analysis of 100 patients with splenic marginal zone lymphoma treated with splenectomy as first-line treatment. Leuk Lymphoma. 55:1854–60. PMID:24206091
2267. Lennert K, editor. (1978). Malignant lymphomas other than Hodgkin's disease. New York: Springer Verlag.
2268. Lennert K, Parwaresch MR (1979). Mast cells and mast cell neoplasia: a review. Histopathology. 3:349–65. PMID:114472
2269. Lennert K, Stein H, Kaiserling E (1975). Cytological and functional criteria for the classification of malignant lymphomata. Br J Cancer Suppl. 2:29–43. PMID:52366
2270. Lens D, De Schouwer PJ, Hamoudi RA, et al. (1997). p53 abnormalities in B-cell prolymphocytic leukemia. Blood. 89:2015–23. PMID:9058723
2271. Lenz G, Davis RE, Ngo VN, et al. (2008). Oncogenic CARD11 mutations in human diffuse large B cell lymphoma. Science. 319:1676–9. PMID:18323416
2272. Lenz G, Staudt LM (2010). Aggressive lymphomas. N Engl J Med. 362:1417–29. PMID:20393178
2273. Lenz G, Wright G, Dave SS, et al. (2008). Stromal gene signatures in large-B-cell lymphomas. N Engl J Med. 359:2313–23. PMID:19038878
2274. Lenz G, Wright GW, Emre NC, et al. (2008). Molecular subtypes of diffuse large B-cell lymphoma arise by distinct genetic pathways. Proc Natl Acad Sci U S A. 105:13520–5. PMID:18765795
2275. Lenze D, Leoncini L, Hummel M, et al. (2011). The different epidemiologic subtypes of Burkitt lymphoma share a homogenous micro RNA profile distinct from diffuse large B-cell lymphoma. Leukemia. 25:1869–76. PMID:21701491
2276. Leoncini L, Spina D, Nyong'o A, et al. (1996). Neoplastic cells of Hodgkin's disease show differences in EBV expression between Kenya and Italy. Int J Cancer. 65:781–4. PMID:8631592
2277. Leong CF, Kalaichelvi AV, Cheong SK, et al. (2004). Comparison of myeloperoxidase detection by flow cytometry using two different clones of monoclonal antibodies. Malays J Pathol. 26:111–6. PMID:16329563
2278. Leroux D, Mugneret F, Callanan M, et al. (2002). CD4(+), CD56(+) DC2 acute leukemia is characterized by recurrent clonal chromosomal changes affecting 6 major targets: a study of 21 cases by the Groupe Français de Cytogénétique Hématologique. Blood. 99:4154–9. PMID:12010820
2279. Leroy K, Haioun C, Lepage E, et al. (2002). p53 gene mutations are associated with poor survival in low and low-intermediate risk diffuse large B-cell lymphomas. Ann Oncol. 13:1108–15. PMID:12176791
2280. Leroy K, Pujals A, Pelletier L (2014). Targeting STAT6 in PMBL. Oncotarget. 5:7216. PMID:25277174
2281. Lessard M, Struski S, Leymarie V, et al. (2005). Cytogenetic study of 75 erythroleukemias. Cancer Genet Cytogenet. 163:113–22. PMID:16337853
2282. Leucci E, Cocco M, Onnis A, et al. (2008). MYC translocation-negative classical Burkitt lymphoma cases: an alternative pathogenetic mechanism involving miRNA deregulation. J Pathol. 216:440–50. PMID:18802929
2283. Leucci E, Onnis A, Cocco M, et al. (2010). B-cell differentiation in EBV-positive Burkitt lymphoma is impaired at posttranscriptional level by miRNA-altered expression. Int J Cancer. 126:1316–26. PMID:19530237
2284. Leulier F, Lemaitre B (2008). Toll-like receptors–taking an evolutionary approach. Nat Rev Genet. 9:165–78. PMID:18227810
2285. Levine AM (1993). AIDS-related malignancies: the emerging epidemic. J Natl Cancer Inst. 85:1382–97. PMID:8350362
2286. Levine EG, Arthur DC, Machnicki J, et al. (1989). Four new recurring translocations in non-Hodgkin lymphoma. Blood. 74:1796–800. PMID:2506953
2287. Levine PH, Manns A, Jaffe ES, et al. (1994). The effect of ethnic differences on the pattern of HTLV-I-associated T-cell leukemia/lymphoma (HATL) in the United States. Int J Cancer. 56:177–81. PMID:8314298
2288. Levine RL, Loriaux M, Huntly BJ, et al. (2005). The JAK2V617F activating mutation occurs in chronic myelomonocytic leukemia and acute myeloid leukemia, but not in acute lymphoblastic leukemia or chronic lymphocytic leukemia. Blood. 106:3377–9. PMID:16081687
2289. Levine RL, Pardanani A, Tefferi A, et al. (2007). Role of JAK2 in the pathogenesis and therapy of myeloproliferative disorders. Nat Rev Cancer. 7:673–83. PMID:17721432
2290. Levine RL, Wadleigh M, Cools J, et al. (2005). Activating mutation in the tyrosine kinase JAK2 in polycythemia vera, essential thrombocythemia, and myeloid metaplasia with myelofibrosis. Cancer Cell. 7:387–97. PMID:15837627
2291. Lewinsohn M, Brown AL, Weinel LM, et al. (2016). Novel germ line DDX41 mutations define families with a lower age of MDS/AML onset and lymphoid malignancies. Blood. 127:1017–23. PMID:26712909
2292. Lewis EB (1963). Leukemia, multiple myeloma and anaplastic anemia in American Radiologists. Science. 142:1492–4. PMID:14077037
2293. Lewis JT, Gaffney RL, Casey MB, et al. (2003). Inflammatory pseudotumor of the spleen associated with a clonal Epstein-Barr virus genome. Case report and review of the literature. Am J Clin Pathol. 120:56–61. PMID:12866373
2294. Lewis MJ, Oelbaum MH, Coleman M, et al. (1986). An association between chronic neutrophilic leukaemia and multiple myeloma with a study of cobalamin-binding proteins. Br J Haematol. 63:173–80. PMID:3458500
2295. Lewis RE, Cruse JM, Sanders CM, et al. (2007). Aberrant expression of T-cell markers in acute myeloid leukemia. Exp Mol Pathol. 83:462–3. PMID:17927977
2296. Li C, Inagaki H, Kuo TT, et al. (2003). Primary cutaneous marginal zone B-cell lymphoma: a molecular and clinicopathologic study of 24 asian cases. Am J Surg Pathol. 27:1061–9. PMID:12883238
2297. Li C, Tian Y, Wang J, et al. (2014). Abnormal immunophenotype provides a key diagnostic marker: a report of 29 cases of de novo aggressive natural killer cell leukemia. Transl Res. 163:565–77. PMID:24524877
2298. Li F, Zhai YP, Tang YM, et al. (2012). Identification of a novel partner gene, TPR, fused to FGFR1 in 8p11 myeloproliferative syndrome. Genes Chromosomes Cancer. 51:890–7. PMID:22619110
2299. Li J, Sze DM, Brown RD, et al. (2010). Clonal expansions of cytotoxic T cells exist in the blood of patients with Waldenstrom macroglobulinemia but exhibit anergic properties and are eliminated by nucleoside analogue therapy. Blood. 115:3580–8. PMID:20190191
2300. Li J, Zhou DB (2013). New advances in the diagnosis and treatment of POEMS syndrome. Br J Haematol. 161:303–15. PMID:23398538
2301. Li JY, Gaillard F, Moreau A, et al. (1999). Detection of translocation t(11;14)(q13;q32) in mantle cell lymphoma by fluorescence in situ hybridization. Am J Pathol. 154:1449–52. PMID:10329598
2302. Li JY, Guitart J, Pulitzer MP, et al. (2014). Multicenter case series of indolent small/medium-sized CD8+ lymphoid proliferations with predilection for the ear and face. Am J Dermatopathol. 36:402–8. PMID:24394306
2303. Li KD, Miles R, Tripp SR, et al. (2015). Clinicopathologic evaluation of MYC expression in primary mediastinal (thymic) large B-cell lymphoma. Am J Clin Pathol. 143:598–604. PMID:25780014
2304. Li S, Desai P, Lin P, et al. (2016). MYC/BCL6 double-hit lymphoma (DHL): a tumour associated with an aggressive clinical course and poor prognosis. Histopathology. 68:1090–8 PMID:26426741
2305. Li S, Feng X, Li T, et al. (2013). Extranodal NK/T-cell lymphoma, nasal type: a report of 73 cases at MD Anderson Cancer Center. Am J Surg Pathol. 37:14–23. PMID:23232851
2306. Li S, Lin P, Fayad LE, et al. (2012). B-cell lymphomas with MYC/8q24 rearrangements and IGH@BCL2/t(14;18)(q32;q21): an aggressive disease with heterogeneous histology, germinal center B-cell immunophenotype and poor outcome. Mod Pathol. 25:145–56. PMID:22002575
2307. Li S, Seegmiller AC, Lin P, et al. (2015). B-cell lymphomas with concurrent MYC and BCL2 abnormalities other than translocations behave similarly to MYC/BCL2 double-hit lymphomas. Mod Pathol. 28:208–17. PMID:25103070
2308. Li T, Medeiros LJ, Lin P, et al. (2010). Immunohistochemical profile and fluorescence in situ hybridization analysis of diffuse large B-cell lymphoma in northern China. Arch Pathol Lab Med. 134:759–65. PMID:20441508
2309. Li X, Li J, Du W, et al. (2011). Relevance of immunophenotypes to prognostic subgroups of age, WBC, platelet count, and cytogenetics in de novo acute myeloid leukemia. APMIS. 119:76–84. PMID:21143529
2310. Li XQ, Cheuk W, Lam PW, et al. (2014). Inflammatory pseudotumor-like follicular dendritic cell tumor of liver and spleen: granulomatous and eosinophil-rich variants mimicking inflammatory or infective lesions. Am J Surg Pathol. 38:646–53. PMID:24503752
2311. Li XQ, Zhou XY, Sheng WQ, et al. (2009). Indolent CD8+ lymphoid proliferation of the ear: a new entity and possible occurrence of signet ring cells. Histopathology. 55:468–70. PMID:19817899
2312. Li Y, Gordon MW, Xu-Monette ZY, et al. (2013). Single nucleotide variation in the TP53 3' untranslated region in diffuse large B-cell lymphoma treated with rituximab-CHOP: a report from the International DLBCL Rituximab-CHOP Consortium Program. Blood. 121:4529–40. PMID:23515929
2313. Li Y, Hu S, Zuo Z, et al. (2015). CD5-positive follicular lymphoma: clinicopathologic correlations and outcome in 88 cases. Mod Pathol. 28:787–98. PMID:25743023
2314. Li Y, Schwab C, Ryan SL, et al. (2014). Constitutional and somatic rearrangement of chromosome 21 in acute lymphoblastic leukaemia. Nature. 508:98–102. PMID:24670643
2315. Li ZM, Rinaldi A, Cavalli A, et al. (2012). MYD88 somatic mutations in MALT lymphomas. Br J Haematol. 158:662–4. PMID:22640364
2316. Liang JH, Lu TX, Tian T, et al. (2015). Epstein-Barr virus (EBV) DNA in whole blood as a superior prognostic and monitoring factor than EBV-encoded small RNA in situ hybridization in diffuse large B-cell lymphoma. Clin Microbiol Infect. 21:596–602. PMID:25743579
2317. Liang R, Todd D, Chan TK, et al. (1995). Treatment outcome and prognostic factors for primary nasal lymphoma. J Clin Oncol. 13:666–70. PMID:7884427
2318. Liang X, Branchford B, Greffe B, et al. (2013). Dual ALK and MYC rearrangements leading to an aggressive variant of anaplastic large cell lymphoma. J Pediatr Hematol Oncol. 35:e209–13. PMID:23619105
2319. Liang Y, Yang Z, Qin B, et al. (2014). Primary Sjogren's syndrome and malignancy risk: a systematic review and meta-analysis. Ann Rheum Dis. 73:1151–6. PMID:23687261
2320. Liau JY, Chuang SS, Chu CY, et al. (2013). The presence of clusters of

plasmacytoid dendritic cells is a helpful feature for differentiating lupus panniculitis from subcutaneous panniculitis-like T-cell lymphoma. Histopathology. 62:1057–66. PMID:23600665
2321. Licht JD (2001). AML1 and the AML1-ETO fusion protein in the pathogenesis of t(8;21) AML. Oncogene. 20:5660–79. PMID:11607817
2322. Lichtman MA, Segel GB (2005). Uncommon phenotypes of acute myelogenous leukemia: basophilic, mast cell, eosinophilic, and myeloid dendritic cell subtypes: a review. Blood Cells Mol Dis. 35:370–83. PMID:16203163
2323. Lieberz D, Sextro M, Paulus U, et al. (2000). How to restrict liver biopsy to high-risk patients in early-stage Hodgkin's disease. Ann Hematol. 79:73–8. PMID:10741918
2324. Liebross RH, Ha CS, Cox JD, et al. (1998). Solitary bone plasmacytoma: outcome and prognostic factors following radiotherapy. Int J Radiat Oncol Biol Phys. 41:1063–7. PMID:9719116
2326. Lierman E, Folens C, Stover EH, et al. (2006). Sorafenib is a potent inhibitor of FIP1L1-PDGFRalpha and the imatinib-resistant FIP1L1-PDGFRalpha T674I mutant. Blood. 108:1374–6. PMID:16645167
2327. Lightfoot J, Hitzler JK, Zipursky A, et al. (2004). Distinct gene signatures of transient and acute megakaryoblastic leukemia in Down syndrome. Leukemia. 18:1617–23. PMID:15343346
2328. Lim EL, Trinh DL, Scott DW, et al. (2015). Comprehensive miRNA sequence analysis reveals survival differences in diffuse large B-cell lymphoma patients. Genome Biol. 16:18. PMID:25723320
2329. Lim KH, Tefferi A, Lasho TL, et al. (2009). Systemic mastocytosis in 342 consecutive adults: survival studies and prognostic factors. Blood. 113:5727–36. PMID:19363219
2330. Lim MS, Beaty M, Sorbara L, et al. (2002). T-cell/histiocyte-rich large B-cell lymphoma: a heterogeneous entity with derivation from germinal center B cells. Am J Surg Pathol. 26:1458–66. PMID:12409722
2331. Lim MS, Straus SE, Dale JK, et al. (1998). Pathological findings in human autoimmune lymphoproliferative syndrome. Am J Pathol. 153:1541–50. PMID:9811346
2332. Lim ST, Karim R, Nathwani BN, et al. (2005). AIDS-related Burkitt's lymphoma versus diffuse large-cell lymphoma in the pre-highly active antiretroviral therapy (HAART) and HAART eras: significant differences in survival with standard chemotherapy. J Clin Oncol. 23:4430–8. PMID:15883411
2333. Lim ST, Karim R, Tulpule A, et al. (2005). Prognostic factors in HIV-related diffuse large-cell lymphoma: before versus after highly active antiretroviral therapy. J Clin Oncol. 23:8477–82. PMID:16230675
2334. Lim ZY, Killick S, Germing U, et al. (2007). Low IPSS score and bone marrow hypocellularity in MDS patients predict hematological responses to antithymocyte globulin. Leukemia. 21:1436–41. PMID:17507999
2335. Lima M, Almeida J, Dos Anjos Teixeira M, et al. (2003). TCRalphabeta+/CD4+ large granular lymphocytosis: a new clonal T-cell lymphoproliferative disorder. Am J Pathol. 163:763–71. PMID:12875995
2336. Lima M, Almeida J, Montero AG, et al. (2004). Clinicobiological, immunophenotypic, and molecular characteristics of monoclonal CD56-/+dim chronic natural killer cell large granular lymphocytosis. Am J Pathol. 165:1117–27. PMID:15466379
2337. Lin CC, Hou HA, Chou WC, et al. (2014). SF3B1 mutations in patients with myelodysplastic syndromes: the mutation is stable during disease evolution. Am J Hematol. 89:E109–15. PMID:24723457
2338. Lin CW, Liu TY, Chen SU, et al. (2005). CD94 1A transcripts characterize lymphoblastic lymphoma/leukemia of immature natural killer cell origin with distinct clinical features. Blood. 106:3567–74. PMID:16046525
2339. Lin CW, O'Brien S, Faber J, et al. (1999). De novo CD5+ Burkitt lymphoma/leukemia. Am J Clin Pathol. 112:828–35. PMID:10587706
2340. Lin J, Markowitz GS, Valeri AM, et al. (2001). Renal monoclonal immunoglobulin deposition disease: the disease spectrum. J Am Soc Nephrol. 12:1482–92. PMID:11423577
2341. Lin LI, Chen CY, Lin DT, et al. (2005). Characterization of CEBPA mutations in acute myeloid leukemia: most patients with CEBPA mutations have biallelic mutations and show a distinct immunophenotype of the leukemic cells. Clin Cancer Res. 11:1372–9. PMID:15746035
2342. Lin O, Frizzera G (1997). Angiomyoid and follicular dendritic cell proliferative lesions in Castleman's disease of hyaline-vascular type: a study of 10 cases. Am J Surg Pathol. 21:1295–306. PMID:9351567
2343. Lin P, Bueso-Ramos C, Wilson CS, et al. (2003). Waldenstrom macroglobulinemia involving extramedullary sites: morphologic and immunophenotypic findings in 44 patients. Am J Surg Pathol. 27:1104–13. PMID:12883242
2344. Lin P, Dickason TJ, Fayad LE, et al. (2012). Prognostic value of MYC rearrangement in cases of B-cell lymphoma, unclassifiable, with features intermediate between diffuse large B-cell lymphoma and Burkitt lymphoma. Cancer. 118:1566–73. PMID:21882178
2345. Lin P, Jones D, Dorfman DM, et al. (2000). Precursor B-cell lymphoblastic lymphoma: a predominantly extranodal tumor with low propensity for leukemic involvement. Am J Surg Pathol. 24:1480–90. PMID:11075849
2346. Lin P, Mansoor A, Bueso-Ramos C, et al. (2003). Diffuse large B-cell lymphoma occurring in patients with lymphoplasmacytic lymphoma/Waldenström macroglobulinemia. Clinicopathologic features of 12 cases. Am J Clin Pathol. 120:246–53. PMID:12931555
2347. Lin P, Molina TJ, Cook JR, et al. (2011). Lymphoplasmacytic lymphoma and other non-marginal zone lymphomas with plasmacytic differentiation. Am J Clin Pathol. 136:195–210. PMID:21757593
2348. Lin P, Owens R, Tricot G, et al. (2004). Flow cytometric immunophenotypic analysis of 306 cases of multiple myeloma. Am J Clin Pathol. 121:482–8. PMID:15080299
2348A. Lin Y, Liu e, Sun Q, et al. (2015). The prevalence of JAK2, MPL, and CALR mutations in Chinese patients with BCR-ABL1-negative myeloproliferative neoplasms. Am J Clin Pathol. 144:165–71. PMID:26071474
2349. Lindfors KK, Meyer JE, Dedrick CG, et al. (1985). Thymic cysts in mediastinal Hodgkin disease. Radiology. 156:37–41. PMID:4001419
2350. Lindsley RC, LaCasce AS (2012). Biology of double-hit B-cell lymphomas. Curr Opin Hematol. 19:299–304. PMID:22504522
2351. Lindsley RC, Mar BG, Mazzola E, et al. (2015). Acute myeloid leukemia ontogeny is defined by distinct somatic mutations. Blood. 125:1367–76. PMID:25550361
2352. Lindström MS, Wiman KG (2002). Role of genetic and epigenetic changes in Burkitt lymphoma. Semin Cancer Biol. 12:381–7. PMID:12191637
2353. Linet MS, Harlow SD, McLaughlin JK (1987). A case-control study of multiple myeloma in whites: chronic antigenic stimulation, occupation, and drug use. Cancer Res. 47:2978–81. PMID:3567914
2354. Linet MS, Vajdic CM, Morton LM, et al. (2014). Medical history, lifestyle, family history, and occupational risk factors for follicular lymphoma: the InterLymph Non-Hodgkin Lymphoma Subtypes Project. J Natl Cancer Inst Monogr. 2014:26–40. PMID:25174024
2355. Ling YH, Zhu CM, Wen SH, et al. (2015). Pseudoepitheliomatous hyperplasia mimicking invasive squamous cell carcinoma in extranodal natural killer/T-cell lymphoma: a report of 34 cases. Histopathology. 67:404–9. PMID:25619876
2356. Link DC, Schuettpelz LG, Shen D, et al. (2011). Identification of a novel TP53 cancer susceptibility mutation through whole-genome sequencing of a patient with therapy-related AML. JAMA. 305:1568–76. PMID:21505135
2357. Lipford EH Jr, Margolick JB, Longo DL, et al. (1988). Angiocentric immunoproliferative lesions: a clinicopathologic spectrum of post-thymic T-cell proliferations. Blood. 72:1674–81. PMID:3263153
2358. Lipworth L, Tarone RE, McLaughlin JK (2009). Breast implants and lymphoma risk: a review of the epidemiologic evidence through 2008. Plast Reconstr Surg. 123:790–3. PMID:19319041
2359. Liso A, Capello D, Marafioti T, et al. (2006). Aberrant somatic hypermutation in tumor cells of nodular-lymphocyte-predominant and classic Hodgkin lymphoma. Blood. 108:1013–20. PMID:16614247
2360. Liso A, Tiacci E, Binazzi R, et al. (2004). Haploidentical peripheral-blood stem-cell transplantation for ALK-positive anaplastic large-cell lymphoma. Lancet Oncol. 5:127–8. PMID:14761818
2361. List A, Dewald G, Bennett J, et al. (2006). Lenalidomide in the myelodysplastic syndrome with chromosome 5q deletion. N Engl J Med. 355:1456–65. PMID:17021321
2362. Lister TA, Crowther D, Sutcliffe SB, et al. (1989). Report of a committee convened to discuss the evaluation and staging of patients with Hodgkin's disease: Cotswolds meeting. J Clin Oncol. 7:1630–6. PMID:2809679
2363. Litz CE, Davies S, Brunning RD, et al. (1995). Acute leukemia and the transient myeloproliferative disorder associated with Down syndrome: morphologic, immunophenotypic and cytogenetic manifestations. Leukemia. 9:1432–9. PMID:7658708
2364. Liu C, Iqbal J, Teruya-Feldstein J, et al. (2013). MicroRNA expression profiling identifies molecular signatures associated with anaplastic large cell lymphoma. Blood. 122:2083–92. PMID:23801630
2365. Liu F, Asano N, Tatematsu A, et al. (2012). Plasmablastic lymphoma of the elderly: a clinicopathological comparison with age-related Epstein-Barr virus-associated B cell lymphoproliferative disorder. Histopathology. 61:1183–97. PMID:22958176
2366. Liu H, Ruskon-Fourmestraux A, Lavergne-Slove A, et al. (2001). Resistance of t(11;18) positive gastric mucosa-associated lymphoid tissue lymphoma to Helicobacter pylori eradication therapy. Lancet. 357:39–40. PMID:11197361
2367. Liu HL, Hoppe RT, Kohler S, et al. (2003). CD30+ cutaneous lymphoproliferative disorders: the Stanford experience in lymphomatoid papulosis and primary cutaneous anaplastic large cell lymphoma. J Am Acad Dermatol. 49:1049–58. PMID:14639383
2368. Liu JH, Wei S, Lamy T, et al. (2000). Chronic neutropenia mediated by fas ligand. Blood. 95:3219–22. PMID:10807792
2369. Liu Q, Salaverria I, Pittaluga S, et al. (2013). Follicular lymphomas in children and young adults: a comparison of the pediatric variant with usual follicular lymphoma. Am J Surg Pathol. 37:333–43. PMID:23108024
2370. Liu TX, Becker MW, Jelinek J, et al. (2007). Chromosome 5q deletion and epigenetic suppression of the gene encoding alpha-catenin (CTNNA1) in myeloid cell transformation. Nat Med. 13:78–83. PMID:17159988
2371. Liu W, Hasserjian RP, Hu Y, et al. (2011). Pure erythroid leukemia: a reassessment of the entity using the 2008 World Health Organization classification. Mod Pathol. 24:375–83. PMID:21102413
2372. Liu Y, Zhang W, An J, et al. (2014). Cutaneous intravascular natural killer-cell lymphoma: a case report and review of the literature. Am J Clin Pathol. 142:243–7. PMID:25015867
2373. Liu YJ (2005). IPC: professional type 1 interferon-producing cells and plasmacytoid dendritic cell precursors. Annu Rev Immunol. 23:275–306. PMID:15771572
2374. Liu YJ, Zhang J, Lane PJ, et al. (1991). Sites of specific B cell activation in primary and secondary responses to T cell-dependent and T cell-independent antigens. Eur J Immunol. 21:2951–62. PMID:1748148
2375. Liu YR, Zhu HH, Ruan GR, et al. (2013). NPM1-mutated acute myeloid leukemia of monocytic or myeloid origin exhibit distinct immunophenotypes. Leuk Res. 37:737–41. PMID:23601747
2376. Lo-Coco F, Avvisati G, Vignetti M, et al. (2013). Retinoic acid and arsenic trioxide for acute promyelocytic leukemia. N Engl J Med. 369:111–21. PMID:23841729
2377. Locatelli F, Niemeyer CM (2015). How I treat juvenile myelomonocytic leukemia. Blood. 125:1083–90. PMID:25564399
2378. Locker J, Nalesnik M (1989). Molecular genetic analysis of lymphoid tumors arising after organ transplantation. Am J Pathol. 135:977–87. PMID:2556930
2379. Loddenkemper C, Anagnostopoulos I, Hummel M, et al. (2004). Differential Emu enhancer activity and expression of BOB.1/OBF.1, Oct2, PU.1, and immunoglobulin in reactive B-cell populations, B-cell non-Hodgkin lymphomas, and Hodgkin lymphomas. J Pathol. 202:60–9. PMID:14694522
2380. Loghavi S, Zuo Z, Ravandi F, et al. (2014). Clinical features of de novo acute myeloid leukemia with concurrent DNMT3A, FLT3 and NPM1 mutations. J Hematol Oncol. 7:74. PMID:25281355
2381. Loh ML, Sakai DS, Flotho C, et al. (2009). Mutations in CBL occur frequently in juvenile myelomonocytic leukemia. Blood. 114:1859–63. PMID:19571318
2382. Loh ML, Vattikuti S, Schubbert S, et al. (2004). Mutations in PTPN11 implicate the SHP-2 phosphatase in leukemogenesis. Blood. 103:2325–31. PMID:14644997
2383. Lohr JG, Stojanov P, Carter SL, et al. (2014). Widespread genetic heterogeneity in multiple myeloma: implications for targeted therapy. Cancer Cell. 25:91–101. PMID:24434212
2384. Lohr JG, Stojanov P, Lawrence MS, et al. (2012). Discovery and prioritization of somatic mutations in diffuse large B-cell lymphoma (DLBCL) by whole-exome sequencing. Proc Natl Acad Sci U S A. 109:3879–84. PMID:22343534
2384A. Lones MA, Cairo MS, Perkins SL (2000). T-cell-rich large B-cell lymphoma in children and adolescents: a clinicopathologic report of six cases from the Children's Cancer Group Study CCG-5961. Cancer. 88:2378–86. PMID:10820362
2385. Lones MA, Mishalani S, Shintaku IP, et al. (1995). Changes in tonsils and adenoids in children with posttransplant lymphoproliferative disorder: report of three cases with early involvement of Waldeyer's ring. Hum Pathol. 26:525–30. PMID:7750936

2386. Lones MA, Raphael M, McCarthy K, et al. (2012). Primary follicular lymphoma of the testis in children and adolescents. J Pediatr Hematol Oncol. 34:68–71. PMID:22215099
2387. Loo EY, Medeiros LJ, Aladily TN, et al. (2013). Classical Hodgkin lymphoma arising in the setting of iatrogenic immunodeficiency: a clinicopathologic study of 10 cases. Am J Surg Pathol. 37:1290–7. PMID:23774171
2388. Loong F, Chan AC, Ho BC, et al. (2010). Diffuse large B-cell lymphoma associated with chronic inflammation as an incidental finding and new clinical scenarios. Mod Pathol. 23:493–501. PMID:20062008
2389. Lopez-Olivo MA, Tayar JH, Martinez-Lopez JA, et al. (2012). Risk of malignancies in patients with rheumatoid arthritis treated with biologic therapy: a meta-analysis. JAMA. 308:898–908. PMID:22948700
2389A. Lorenzi L, Döring C, Rausch T, et al. (2017). Identification of novel follicular dendritic cell sarcoma markers, FDCSP and SRGN, by whole transcriptome sequencing. Oncotarget. 8:16463–72. PMID:28145886
2390. Lorenzi L, Lonardi S, Petrilli G, et al. (2012). Folliculocentric B-cell-rich follicular dendritic cells sarcoma: a hitherto unreported morphological variant mimicking lymphoproliferative disorders. Hum Pathol. 43:209–15. PMID:21835430
2391. Lorenzi L, Tabellini G, Vermi W, et al. (2013). Occurrence of nodular lymphocyte-predominant hodgkin lymphoma in hermansky-pudlak type 2 syndrome is associated to natural killer and natural killer T cell defects. PLoS One. 8:e80131. PMID:24302998
2393. Lorsbach RB, Shay-Seymore D, Moore J, et al. (2002). Clinicopathologic analysis of follicular lymphoma occurring in children. Blood. 99:1959–64. PMID:11877266
2394. Lossos C, Bayraktar S, Weinzierl E, et al. (2014). LMO2 and BCL6 are associated with improved survival in primary central nervous system lymphoma. Br J Haematol. 165:640–8. PMID:24571259
2395. Lossos IS, Alizadeh AA, Diehn M, et al. (2002). Transformation of follicular lymphoma to diffuse large-cell lymphoma: alternative patterns with increased or decreased expression of c-myc and its regulated genes. Proc Natl Acad Sci U S A. 99:8886–91. PMID:12077300
2396. Lossos IS, Jones CD, Warnke R, et al. (2001). Expression of a single gene, BCL-6, strongly predicts survival in patients with diffuse large B-cell lymphoma. Blood. 98:945–51. PMID:11493437
2397. Lossos IS, Morgensztern D (2006). Prognostic biomarkers in diffuse large B-cell lymphoma. J Clin Oncol. 24:995–1007. PMID:16418498
2398. Loughran TP Jr, Zambello R, Ashley R, et al. (1993). Failure to detect Epstein-Barr virus DNA in peripheral blood mononuclear cells of most patients with large granular lymphocyte leukemia. Blood. 81:2723–7. PMID:8387836
2399. Louie DC, Offit K, Jaslow R, et al. (1995). p53 overexpression as a marker of poor prognosis in mantle cell lymphomas with t(11;14)(q13;q32). Blood. 86:2892–9. PMID:7579380
2400. Louissaint A Jr, Ackerman AM, Dias-Santagata D, et al. (2012). Pediatric-type nodal follicular lymphoma: an indolent clonal proliferation in children and adults with high proliferation index and no BCL2 rearrangement. Blood. 128:2395–404. PMID:22855608
2400A. Louissaint A Jr, Schafernak KT, Geyer JT, et al. (2016). Pediatric-type nodal follicular lymphoma: a biologically distinct lymphoma with frequent MAPK pathway mutations. Blood. 128:1093–100. PMID:27325104
2401. Love C, Sun Z, Jima D, et al. (2012). The genetic landscape of mutations in Burkitt lymphoma. Nat Genet. 44:1321–5. PMID:23143597
2402. Lu J, Ashwani N, Zhang M, et al. (2015). Children Diagnosed as Mixed-Phenotype Acute Leukemia Didn't Benefit from the CCLG-2008 Protocol, Retrospective Analysis from Single Center. Indian J Hematol Blood Transfus. 31:32–7. PMID:25548442
2403. Lu J, Meng H, Zhang A, et al. (2015). Phenotype and function of tissue-resident unconventional Foxp3-expressing CD4(+) regulatory T cells. Cell Immunol. 297:53–9. PMID:26142700
2404. Lu TX, Fan L, Wang L, et al. (2015). MYC or BCL2 copy number aberration is a strong predictor of outcome in patients with diffuse large B-cell lymphoma. Oncotarget. 6:18374–88. PMID:26158410
2405. Lu TX, Liang JH, Miao Y, et al. (2015). Epstein-Barr virus positive diffuse large B-cell lymphoma predict poor outcome, regardless of the age. Sci Rep. 5:12168. PMID:26202875
2406. Lucas PC, Kuffa P, Gu S, et al. (2007). A dual role for the API2 moiety in API2-MALT1-dependent NF-kappaB activation: heterotypic oligomerization and TRAF2 recruitment. Oncogene. 26:5643–54. PMID:17334391
2407. Luciano L, Catalano L, Sarrantonio C, et al. (1999). AlphaIFN-induced hematologic and cytogenetic remission in chronic eosinophilic leukemia with t(1;5). Haematologica. 84:651–3. PMID:10406909
2408. Lucio P, Gaipa G, van Lochem EG, et al. (2001). BIOMED-I concerted action report: flow cytometric immunophenotyping of precursor B-ALL with standardized triple-stainings. BIOMED-1 Concerted Action Investigation of Minimal Residual Disease in Acute Leukemia: International Standardization and Clinical Evaluation. Leukemia. 15:1185–92. PMID:11480560
2409. Lucioni M, Novara F, Fiandrino G, et al. (2011). Twenty-one cases of blastic plasmacytoid dendritic cell neoplasm: focus on biallelic locus 9p21.3 deletion. Blood. 118:4591–4. PMID:21900200
2410. Lugthart S, Gröschel S, Beverloo HB, et al. (2010). Clinical, molecular, and prognostic significance of WHO type inv(3)(q21q26.2)/t(3;3)(q21;q26.2) and various other 3q abnormalities in acute myeloid leukemia. J Clin Oncol. 28:3890–8. PMID:20660833
2411. Luk IS, Shek TW, Tang VW, et al. (1999). Interdigitating dendritic cell tumor of the testis: a novel testicular spindle cell neoplasm. Am J Surg Pathol. 23:1141–8. PMID:10478677
2412. Lukes RJ, Butler JJ (1966). The pathology and nomenclature of Hodgkin's disease. Cancer Res. 26:1063–83. PMID:5947336
2412A. Lukes RJ, Collins RD (1974). Immunologic characterization of human malignant lymphomas. Cancer. 34:1488–503. PMID:4608683
2413. Lukes RJ, Craver L, Hall T, et al. (1966). Report of the nomenclature committee. Cancer Res. 26:1311.
2414. Luminari S, Cesaretti M, Marcheselli L, et al. (2010). Decreasing incidence of gastric MALT lymphomas in the era of anti-Helicobacter pylori interventions: results from a population-based study on extranodal marginal zone lymphomas. Ann Oncol. 21:855–9. PMID:19850642
2415. Luna-Fineman S, Shannon KM, Atwater SK, et al. (1999). Myelodysplastic and myeloproliferative disorders of childhood: a study of 167 patients. Blood. 93:459–66. PMID:9885207
2416. Lundell R, Hartung L, Hill S, et al. (2005). T-cell large granular lymphocyte leukemias have multiple phenotypic abnormalities involving pan-T-cell antigens and receptors for MHC molecules. Am J Clin Pathol. 124:937–46. PMID:16416744
2417. Luppi M, Barozzi P, Santagostino G, et al. (2000). Molecular evidence of organ-related transmission of Kaposi sarcoma-associated herpesvirus or human herpesvirus-8 in transplant patients. Blood. 96:3279–81. PMID:11050015
2418. Luppi M, Marasca R, Morselli M, et al. (1994). Clonal nature of hypereosinophilic syndrome. Blood. 84:349–50. PMID:8018930
2419. Luskin MR, Huen AO, Brooks SA, et al. (2015). NPM1 mutation is associated with leukemia cutis in acute myeloid leukemia with monocytic features. Haematologica. 100:e412–4. PMID:26113416
2420. Ma M, Wang X, Tang J, et al. (2012). Early T-cell precursor leukemia: a subtype of high risk childhood acute lymphoblastic leukemia. Front Med. 6:416–20. PMID:23065427
2421. Ma X, Does M, Raza A, et al. (2007). Myelodysplastic syndromes: incidence and survival in the United States. Cancer. 109:1536–42. PMID:17345612
2422. Ma Z, Morris SW, Valentine V, et al. (2001). Fusion of two novel genes, RBM15 and MKL1, in the t(1;22)(p13;q13) of acute megakaryoblastic leukemia. Nat Genet. 28:220–1. PMID:11431691
2423. Maassen A, Strupp C, Giagounidis A, et al. (2013). Validation and proposals for a refinement of the WHO 2008 classification of myelodysplastic syndromes without excess of blasts. Leuk Res. 37:64–70. PMID:23122806
2424. Macdonald D, Reiter A, Cross NC (2002). The 8p11 myeloproliferative syndrome: a distinct clinical entity caused by constitutive activation of FGFR1. Acta Haematol. 107:101–7. PMID:11919391
2425. Macgrogan G, Vergier B, Dubus P, et al. (1996). CD30-positive cutaneous large cell lymphomas. A comparative study of clinicopathologic and molecular features of 16 cases. Am J Clin Pathol. 105:440–50. PMID:8604686
2426. Mackey AC, Green L, Liang LC, et al. (2007). Hepatosplenic T cell lymphoma associated with infliximab use in young patients treated for inflammatory bowel disease. J Pediatr Gastroenterol Nutr. 44:265–7. PMID:17255842
2427. MacLennan IC (1994). Germinal centers. Annu Rev Immunol. 12:117–39. PMID:8011279
2428. MacLennan IC, Liu YJ, Oldfield S, et al. (1990). The evolution of B-cell clones. Curr Top Microbiol Immunol. 159:37–63. PMID:2189692
2429. MacLennan KA, Bennett MH, Tu A, et al. (1989). Relationship of histopathologic features to survival and relapse in nodular sclerosing Hodgkin's disease. A study of 1659 patients. Cancer. 64:1686–93. PMID:2790683
2430. MacLennan KA, Bennett MH, Vaughan Hudson B, et al. (1992). Diagnosis and grading of nodular sclerosing Hodgkin's disease: a study of 2190 patients. Int Rev Exp Pathol. 33:27–51. PMID:1733871
2431. Macon WR, Levy NB, Kurtin PJ, et al. (2001). Hepatosplenic alphabeta T-cell lymphomas: a report of 14 cases and comparison with hepatosplenic gammadelta T-cell lymphomas. Am J Surg Pathol. 25:285–96. PMID:11224598
2432. Macon WR, Williams ME, Greer JP, et al. (1995). Paracortical nodular T-cell lymphoma. Identification of an unusual variant of peripheral T-cell lymphoma. Am J Surg Pathol. 19:297–303. PMID:7872427
2433. Madelung AB, Bondo H, Stamp I, et al. (2013). World Health Organization-defined classification of myeloproliferative neoplasms: morphological reproducibility and clinical correlations–the Danish experience. Am J Hematol. 88:1012–6. PMID:23897670
2434. Madelung AB, Bondo H, Stamp I, et al. (2015). WHO classification 2008 of myeloproliferative neoplasms: a workshop learning effect–the Danish experience. APMIS. 123:787–92. PMID:26200697
2435. Maecker B, Jack T, Zimmermann M, et al. (2007). CNS or bone marrow involvement as risk factors for poor survival in post-transplantation lymphoproliferative disorders in children after solid organ transplantation. J Clin Oncol. 25:4902–8. PMID:17971586
2436. Maeda K, Matsuda M, Suzuki H, et al. (2002). Immunohistochemical recognition of human follicular dendritic cells (FDCs) in routinely processed paraffin sections. J Histochem Cytochem. 50:1475–86. PMID:12417613
2437. Maeda T, Murata K, Fukushima T, et al. (2005). A novel plasmacytoid dendritic cell line, CAL-1, established from a patient with blastic natural killer cell lymphoma. Int J Hematol. 81:148–54. PMID:15765784
2437A. Maes B, Anastasopoulou A, Kluin-Nelemans JC, et al. (2001). Among diffuse large B-cell lymphomas, T-cell-rich/histiocyte-rich BCL and CD30+ anaplastic B-cell subtypes exhibit distinct clinical features. Ann Oncol. 12:853–8. PMID:11484964
2438. Magalhães IQ, Splendore A, Emerenciano M, et al. (2006). GATA1 mutations in acute leukemia in children with Down syndrome. Cancer Genet Cytogenet. 166:112–6. PMID:16631466
2439. Magaña M, Massone C, Magaña P, et al. (2016). Clinicopathologic Features of Hydroa Vacciniforme-Like Lymphoma: A Series of 9 Patients. Am J Dermatopathol. 38:20–5 PMID:26368647
2440. Magaña M, Sangüeza P, Gil-Beristain J, et al. (1998). Angiocentric cutaneous T-cell lymphoma of childhood (hydroa-like lymphoma): a distinctive type of cutaneous T-cell lymphoma. J Am Acad Dermatol. 38:574–9. PMID:9580256
2441. Magrath I (2012). Epidemiology: clues to the pathogenesis of Burkitt lymphoma. Br J Haematol. 156:744–56. PMID:22260300
2442. Magrath IT (1991). African Burkitt's lymphoma. History, biology, clinical features, and treatment. Am J Pediatr Hematol Oncol. 13:222–46. PMID:2069232
2443. Magrath IT, Janus C, Edwards BK, et al. (1984). An effective therapy for both undifferentiated (including Burkitt's) lymphomas and lymphoblastic lymphomas in children and young adults. Blood. 63:1102–11. PMID:6546890
2444. Magrath IT, Sariban E (1985). Clinical features of Burkitt's lymphoma in the USA. IARC Sci Publ. (60):119–27. PMID:2998986
2445. Magro CM, Crowson AN, Kovatich AJ, et al. (2001). Lupus profundus, indeterminate lymphocytic lobular panniculitis and subcutaneous T-cell lymphoma: a spectrum of subcuticular T-cell lymphoid dyscrasia. J Cutan Pathol. 28:235–47. PMID:11401667
2446. Mahmoud AZ, George TI, Czuchlewski DR, et al. (2015). Scoring of MYC protein expression in diffuse large B-cell lymphomas: concordance rate among hematopathologists. Mod Pathol. 28:545–51. PMID:25431238
2447. Maini MK, Gudgeon N, Wedderburn LR, et al. (2000). Clonal expansions in acute EBV infection are detectable in the CD8 and not the CD4 subset and persist with a variable CD45 phenotype. J Immunol. 165:5729–37. PMID:11067931
2448. Maitra A, McKenna RW, Weinberg AG, et al. (2001). Precursor B-cell lymphoblastic lymphoma. A study of nine cases lacking blood and bone marrow involvement and review of the literature. Am J Clin Pathol. 115:868–75. PMID:11392884
2449. Majlis A, Pugh WC, Rodriguez MA, et al. (1997). Mantle cell lymphoma: correlation of clinical outcome and biologic features with three histologic variants. J Clin Oncol. 15:1664–71. PMID:9193367
2450. Majumdar G, Grace RJ, Singh AK, et al. (1992). The value of the bone marrow plasma

cell cytoplasmic light chain ratio in differentiating between multiple myeloma and monoclonal gammopathy of undetermined significance. Leuk Lymphoma. 8:491–3. PMID:1297481

2451. Mak V, Ip D, Mang O, et al. (2014). Preservation of lower incidence of chronic lymphocytic leukemia in Chinese residents in British Columbia: a 26-year survey from 1983 to 2008. Leuk Lymphoma. 55:824–7. PMID:23909397

2452. Makishima H, Ito T, Momose K, et al. (2007). Chemokine system and tissue infiltration in aggressive NK-cell leukemia. Leuk Res. 31:1237–45. PMID:17123604

2453. Makishima H, Jankowska AM, McDevitt MA, et al. (2011). CBL, CBLB, TET2, ASXL1, and IDH1/2 mutations and additional chromosomal aberrations constitute molecular events in chronic myelogenous leukemia. Blood. 117:e198–206. PMID:21346257

2454. Malamut G, Afchain P, Verkarre V, et al. (2009). Presentation and long-term follow-up of refractory celiac disease: comparison of type I with type II. Gastroenterology. 136:81–90. PMID:19014942

2455. Malamut G, Cellier C (2013). Refractory coeliac disease. Curr Opin Oncol. 25:445–51. PMID:23942290

2456. Malamut G, Chandesris O, Verkarre V, et al. (2013). Enteropathy associated T cell lymphoma in celiac disease: a large retrospective study. Dig Liver Dis. 45:377–84. PMID:23313469

2457. Malamut G, El Machhour R, Montcuquet N, et al. (2010). IL-15 triggers an antiapoptotic pathway in human intraepithelial lymphocytes that is a potential new target in celiac disease-associated inflammation and lymphomagenesis. J Clin Invest. 120:2131–43. PMID:20440074

2458. Malamut G, Meresse B, Cellier C, et al. (2012). Refractory celiac disease: from bench to bedside. Semin Immunopathol. 34:601–13. PMID:22810901

2459. Malbrain ML, Van den Bergh H, Zachée P (1996). Further evidence for the clonal nature of the idiopathic hypereosinophilic syndrome: complete haematological and cytogenetic remission induced by interferon-alpha in a case with a unique chromosomal abnormality. Br J Haematol. 92:176–83. PMID:8562393

2460. Malcovati L, Cazzola M (2013). Refractory anemia with ring sideroblasts. Best Pract Res Clin Haematol. 26:377–85. PMID:24507814

2461. Malcovati L, Della Porta MG, Pietra D, et al. (2009). Molecular and clinical features of refractory anemia with ringed sideroblasts associated with marked thrombocytosis. Blood. 114:3538–45. PMID:19692701

2462. Malcovati L, Germing U, Kuendgen A, et al. (2007). Time-dependent prognostic scoring system for predicting survival and leukemic evolution in myelodysplastic syndromes. J Clin Oncol. 25:3503–10. PMID:17687155

2463. Malcovati L, Hellström-Lindberg E, Bowen D, et al. (2013). Diagnosis and treatment of primary myelodysplastic syndromes in adults: recommendations from the European LeukemiaNet. Blood. 122:2943–64. PMID:23980065

2464. Malcovati L, Karimi M, Papaemmanuil E, et al. (2015). SF3B1 mutation identifies a distinct subset of myelodysplastic syndrome with ring sideroblasts. Blood. 126:233–41. PMID:25957392

2465. Malcovati L, Papaemmanuil E, Ambaglio I, et al. (2014). Driver somatic mutations identify distinct disease entities within myeloid neoplasms with myelodysplasia. Blood. 124:1513–21. PMID:24970933

2466. Malcovati L, Papaemmanuil E, Bowen DT, et al. (2011). Clinical significance of SF3B1

mutations in myelodysplastic syndromes and myelodysplastic/myeloproliferative neoplasms. Blood. 118:6239–46. PMID:21998214

2467. Malcovati L, Porta MG, Pascutto C, et al. (2005). Prognostic factors and life expectancy in myelodysplastic syndromes classified according to WHO criteria: a basis for clinical decision making. J Clin Oncol. 23:7594–603. PMID:16186598

2468. Malecka A, Tierens A, Østlie I, et al. (2015). Primary diffuse large B-cell lymphoma associated with clonally-related monoclonal B lymphocytosis indicates a common precursor cell. Haematologica. 100:e415–8. PMID:26001788

2469. Malek SN (2013). The biology and clinical significance of acquired genomic copy number aberrations and recurrent gene mutations in chronic lymphocytic leukemia. Oncogene. 32:2805–17. PMID:23001040

2470. Maljaei SH, Brito-Babapulle V, Hiorns LR, et al. (1998). Abnormalities of chromosomes 8, 11, 14, and X in T-prolymphocytic leukemia studied by fluorescence in situ hybridization. Cancer Genet Cytogenet. 103:110–6. PMID:9614908

2471. Malkin D, Nichols KE, Zelley K, et al. (2014). Predisposition to pediatric and hematologic cancers: a moving target. Am Soc Clin Oncol Educ Book. e44–55. PMID:24857136

2472. Mallett RB, Matutes E, Catovsky D, et al. (1995). Cutaneous infiltration in T-cell prolymphocytic leukaemia. Br J Dermatol. 132:263–6. PMID:7888364

2473. Mallo M, Cervera J, Schanz J, et al. (2011). Impact of adjunct cytogenetic abnormalities for prognostic stratification in patients with myelodysplastic syndrome and deletion 5q. Leukemia. 25:110–20. PMID:20882045

2474. Mallo M, Del Rey M, Ibáñez M, et al. (2013). Response to lenalidomide in myelodysplastic syndromes with del(5q): influence of cytogenetics and mutations. Br J Haematol. 162:74–86. PMID:23614682

2475. Mallo M, Espinet B, Salido M, et al. (2007). Gain of multiple copies of the CBFB gene: a new genetic aberration in a case of granulocytic sarcoma. Cancer Genet Cytogenet. 179:62–5. PMID:17981216

2476. Malpas J, Bergsagel D, Kyle R, et al., editors. (2004). Myeloma: biology and management. 3rd ed. Philadelphia: Saumders.

2477. Malpeli G, Barbi S, Moore PS, et al. (2004). Primary mediastinal B-cell lymphoma: hypermutation of the BCL6 gene targets motifs different from those in diffuse large B-cell and follicular lymphomas. Haematologica. 89:1091–9. PMID:15377470

2478. Malyukova A, Dohda T, von der Lehr N, et al. (2007). The tumor suppressor gene hCDC4 is frequently mutated in human T-cell acute lymphoblastic leukemia with functional consequences for Notch signaling. Cancer Res. 67:5611–6. PMID:17575125

2479. Mamessier E, Broussais-Guillaumot F, Chetaille B, et al. (2014). Nature and importance of follicular lymphoma precursors. Haematologica. 99:802–10. PMID:24790058

2480. Mamessier E, Song JY, Eberle FC, et al. (2014). Early lesions of follicular lymphoma: a genetic perspective. Haematologica. 99:481–8. PMID:24162788

2481. Manabe A, Yoshimasu T, Ebihara Y, et al. (2004). Viral infections in juvenile myelomonocytic leukemia: prevalence and clinical implications. J Pediatr Hematol Oncol. 26:636–41. PMID:15454834

2482. Manaloor EJ, Neiman RS, Heilman DK, et al. (2000). Immunohistochemistry can be used to subtype acute myeloid leukemia in routinely processed bone marrow biopsy specimens. Comparison with flow cytometry. Am J

Clin Pathol. 113:814–22. PMID:10874882

2483. Manasanch EE, Kristinsson SY, Landgren O (2013). Etiology of Waldenström macroglobulinemia: genetic factors and immune-related conditions. Clin Lymphoma Myeloma Leuk. 13:194–7. PMID:23473950

2484. Mani H, Jaffe ES (2009). Hodgkin lymphoma: an update on its biology with new insights into classification. Clin Lymphoma Myeloma. 9:206–16. PMID:19525189

2485. Mann RB, Berard CW (1983). Criteria for the cytologic subclassification of follicular lymphomas: a proposed alternative method. Hematol Oncol. 1:187–92. PMID:6376315

2486. Mannucci S, Luzzi A, Carugi A, et al. (2012). EBV Reactivation and Chromosomal Polysomies: Euphorbia tirucalli as a Possible Cofactor in Endemic Burkitt Lymphoma. Adv Hematol. 2012:149780. PMID:22593768

2487. Manola KN (2013). Cytogenetic abnormalities in acute leukaemia of ambiguous lineage: an overview. Br J Haematol. 163:24–39. PMID:23888868

2488. Manso R, Rodríguez-Pinilla SM, González-Rincón J, et al. (2015). Recurrent presence of the PLCG1 S345F mutation in nodal peripheral T-cell lymphomas. Haematologica. 100:e25–7. PMID:25304611

2489. Mansoor A, Medeiros LJ, Weber DM, et al. (2001). Cytogenetic findings in lymphoplasmacytic lymphoma/Waldenström macroglobulinemia. Chromosomal abnormalities are associated with the polymorphous subtype and an aggressive clinical course. Am J Clin Pathol. 116:543–9. PMID:11601139

2489A. Mansoor A, Pittaluga S, Beck PL, et al. (2011). NK-cell enteropathy: a benign NK-cell lymphoproliferative disease mimicking intestinal lymphoma: clinicopathologic features and follow-up in a unique case series. Blood. 117:1447-52. PMID:20966166

2490. Mansour S, Connell V, Steward C, et al. (2011). Emberger syndrome-primary lymphedema with myelodysplasia: report of seven new cases. Am J Med Genet A. 152A:2287–96. PMID:20803646

2491. Mao X, Lillington DM, Czepulkowski B, et al. (2003). Molecular cytogenetic characterization of Sézary syndrome. Genes Chromosomes Cancer. 36:250–60. PMID:12557225

2492. Mao Z, Quintanilla-Martinez L, Raffeld M, et al. (2007). IgVH mutational status and clonality analysis of Richter's transformation: diffuse large B-cell lymphoma and Hodgkin lymphoma in association with B-cell chronic lymphocytic leukemia (B-CLL) represent 2 different pathways of disease evolution. Am J Surg Pathol. 31:1605–14. PMID:17895764

2493. Marafioti T, Hummel M, Anagnostopoulos I, et al. (1997). Origin of nodular lymphocyte-predominant Hodgkin's disease from a clonal expansion of highly mutated germinal-center B cells. N Engl J Med. 337:453–8. PMID:9250847

2494. Marafioti T, Hummel M, Anagnostopoulos I, et al. (1999). Classical Hodgkin's disease and follicular lymphoma originating from the same germinal center B cell. J Clin Oncol. 17:3804–9. PMID:10577852

2495. Marafioti T, Hummel M, Foss HD, et al. (2000). Hodgkin and reed-sternberg cells represent an expansion of a single clone originating from a germinal center B-cell with functional immunoglobulin gene rearrangements but defective immunoglobulin transcription. Blood. 95:1443–50. PMID:10666223

2496. Marafioti T, Paterson JC, Ballabio E, et al. (2010). The inducible T-cell co-stimulator molecule is expressed on subsets of T cells and is a new marker of lymphomas of T follicular helper cell-derivation. Haematologica. 95:432–9. PMID:20207847

2497. Marafioti T, Paterson JC, Ballabio E, et al. (2008). Novel markers of normal and neoplastic human plasmacytoid dendritic cells. Blood. 111:3778–92. PMID:18218851

2498. Marafioti T, Pozzobon M, Hansmann ML, et al. (2004). Expression of intracellular signaling molecules in classical and lymphocyte predominance Hodgkin disease. Blood. 103:188–93. PMID:12881301

2499. Marasca R, Vaccari P, Luppi M, et al. (2001). Immunoglobulin gene mutations and frequent use of VH1-69 and VH4-34 segments in hepatitis C virus-positive and hepatitis C virus-negative nodal marginal zone B-cell lymphoma. Am J Pathol. 159:253–61. PMID:11438472

2500. Marchioli R, Finazzi G, Landolfi R, et al. (2005). Vascular and neoplastic risk in a large cohort of patients with polycythemia vera. J Clin Oncol. 23:2224–32. PMID:15710945

2501. Marchioli R, Finazzi G, Specchia G, et al. (2013). Cardiovascular events and intensity of treatment in polycythemia vera. N Engl J Med. 368:22–33. PMID:23216616

2501A. Marcucci G, Baldus CD, Ruppert AS, et al. (2005). Overexpression of the ETS-related gene, ERG, predicts a worse outcome in acute myeloid leukemia with normal karyotype: a Cancer and Leukemia Group B study. J Clin Oncol. 23:9234–42. PMID:16275934

2501B. Marcucci G, Maharry KS, Metzeler KH, et al. (2013). Clinical role of microRNAs in cytogenetically normal acute myeloid leukemia: miR-155 upregulation independently identifies high-risk patients. J Clin Oncol. 31:2086–93. PMID:23650424

2501C. Marcucci G, Maharry K, Whitman SP, et al. (2007). High expression levels of the ETS-related gene, ERG, predict adverse outcome and improve molecular risk-based classification of cytogenetically normal acute myeloid leukemia: a Cancer and Leukemia Group B Study. J Clin Oncol. 25:3337–43. PMID:17577018

2501D. Marcucci G, Maharry K, Wu YZ, et al. (2010). IDH1 and IDH2 gene mutations identify novel molecular subsets within de novo cytogenetically normal acute myeloid leukemia: a Cancer and Leukemia Group B study. J Clin Oncol. 28:2348–55. PMID:20368543

2501E. Marcucci G, Metzeler KH, Schwind S, et al. (2012). Age-related prognostic impact of different types of DNMT3A mutations in adults with primary cytogenetically normal acute myeloid leukemia. J Clin Oncol. 30:742–50. PMID:22291079

2502. Marcucci G, Mrózek K, Ruppert AS, et al. (2005). Prognostic factors and outcome of core binding factor acute myeloid leukemia patients with t(8;21) differ from those of patients with inv(16): a Cancer and Leukemia Group B study. J Clin Oncol. 23:5705–17. PMID:16110030

2503. Marcus A, Sadimin E, Richardson M, et al. (2012). Fluorescence microscopy is superior to polarized microscopy for detecting amyloid deposits in Congo red-stained trephine bone marrow biopsy specimens. Am J Clin Pathol. 138:590–3. PMID:23010714

2504. Mareschal S, Dubois S, Viailly PJ, et al. (2016). Whole exome sequencing of relapsed/refractory patients expands the repertoire of somatic mutations in diffuse large B-cell lymphoma. Genes Chromosomes Cancer. 55:251–67. PMID:26608593

2505. Mareschal S, Ruminy P, Bagacean C, et al. (2015). Accurate classification of germinal center b-cell-like/activated b-cell-like diffuse large b-cell lymphoma using a simple and rapid reverse transcriptase-multiplex ligation-dependent probe amplification assay: A CALYM study. J Mol Diagn. [Epub ahead of print]. PMID:25891505

2506. Margolskee E, Jobanputra V, Lewis SK,

et al. (2013). Indolent small intestinal CD4+ T-cell lymphoma is a distinct entity with unique biologic and clinical features. PLoS One. 8:e68343. PMID:23861889
2507. Maria Murga Penas E, Schilling G, Behrmann P, et al. (2014). Comprehensive cytogenetic and molecular cytogenetic analysis of 44 Burkitt lymphoma cell lines: secondary chromosomal changes characterization, karyotypic evolution, and comparison with primary samples. Genes Chromosomes Cancer. 53:497–515. PMID:24590883
2508. Maric I, Robyn J, Metcalfe DD, et al. (2007). KIT D816V-associated systemic mastocytosis with eosinophilia and FIP1L1/PDGFRA-associated chronic eosinophilic leukemia are distinct entities. J Allergy Clin Immunol. 120:680–7. PMID:17628645
2509. Mariette X, Cazals-Hatem D, Warszawki J, et al. (2002). Lymphomas in rheumatoid arthritis patients treated with methotrexate: a 3-year prospective study in France. Blood. 99:3909–15. PMID:12010788
2510. Mariette X, Matucci-Cerinic M, Pavelka K, et al. (2011). Malignancies associated with tumour necrosis factor inhibitors in registries and prospective observational studies: a systematic review and meta-analysis. Ann Rheum Dis. 70:1895–904. PMID:21885875
2511. Marinier DE, Mesa H, Rawal A, et al. (2010). Refractory cytopenias with unilineage dysplasia: a retrospective analysis of refractory neutropenia and refractory thrombocytopenia. Leuk Lymphoma. 51:1923–6. PMID:20919862
2512. Mariño-Enríquez A, Dal Cin P (2013). ALK as a paradigm of oncogenic promiscuity: different mechanisms of activation and different fusion partners drive tumors of different lineages. Cancer Genet. 206:357–73. PMID:24091028
2513. Marlton P, Keating M, Kantarjian H, et al. (1995). Cytogenetic and clinical correlates in AML patients with abnormalities of chromosome 16. Leukemia. 9:965–71. PMID:7596186
2514. Martelli M, Ceriani L, Zucca E, et al. (2014). [18F]fluorodeoxyglucose positron emission tomography predicts survival after chemoimmunotherapy for primary mediastinal large B-cell lymphoma: results of the International Extranodal Lymphoma Study Group IELSG-26 Study. J Clin Oncol. 32:1769–75. PMID:24799481
2515. Martelli MP, Pettirossi V, Thiede C, et al. (2010). CD34+ cells from AML with mutated NPM1 harbor cytoplasmic mutated nucleophosmin and generate leukemia in immunocompromised mice. Blood. 116:3907–22. PMID:20634376
2516. Marti GE, Rawstron AC, Ghia P, et al. (2005). Diagnostic criteria for monoclonal B-cell lymphocytosis. Br J Haematol. 130:325–32. PMID:16042682
2517. Martiat P, Michaux JL, Rodhain J (1991). Philadelphia-negative (Ph-) chronic myeloid leukemia (CML): comparison with Ph+ CML and chronic myelomonocytic leukemia. The Groupe Français de Cytogénétique Hématologique. Blood. 78:205–11. PMID:2070054
2518. Martin A, Capron F, Liguory-Brunaud MD, et al. (1994). Epstein-Barr virus-associated primary malignant lymphomas of the pleural cavity occurring in longstanding pleural chronic inflammation. Hum Pathol. 25:1314–8. PMID:8001926
2519. Martin A, Flaman JM, Frebourg T, et al. (1998). Functional analysis of the p53 protein in AIDS-related non-Hodgkin's lymphomas and polymorphic lymphoproliferations. Br J Haematol. 101:311–7. PMID:9609527
2520. Martin AR, Weisenburger DD, Chan WC, et al. (1995). Prognostic value of cellular proliferation and histologic grade in follicular lymphoma. Blood. 85:3671–8. PMID:7780151
2521. Martin F, Taylor GP, Jacobson S (2014). Inflammatory manifestations of HTLV-1 and their therapeutic options. Expert Rev Clin Immunol. 10:1531–46. PMID:25340428
2522. Martin P, Chadburn A, Christos P, et al. (2009). Outcome of deferred initial therapy in mantle-cell lymphoma. J Clin Oncol. 27:1209–13. PMID:19188674
2523. Martin PL, Look AT, Schnell S, et al. (1996). Comparison of fluorescence in situ hybridization, cytogenetic analysis, and DNA index analysis to detect chromosomes 4 and 10 aneuploidy in pediatric acute lymphoblastic leukemia: a Pediatric Oncology Group study. J Pediatr Hematol Oncol. 18:113–21. PMID:8846121
2524. Martin-Guerrero I, Salaverria I, Burkhardt B, et al. (2013). Recurrent loss of heterozygosity in 1p36 associated with TNFRSF14 mutations in IRF4 translocation negative pediatric follicular lymphomas. Haematologica. 98:1237–41. PMID:23445872
2525. Martín-Martín L, López A, Vidriales B, et al. (2015). Classification and clinical behavior of blastic plasmacytoid dendritic cell neoplasms according to their maturation-associated immunophenotypic profile. Oncotarget. 6:19204–16. PMID:26056082
2526. Martín-Subero JI, Klapper W, Sotnikova A, et al. (2006). Chromosomal breakpoints affecting immunoglobulin loci are recurrent in Hodgkin and Reed-Sternberg cells of classical Hodgkin lymphoma. Cancer Res. 66:10332–8. PMID:17079453
2527. Martín-Subero JI, Odero MD, Hernandez R, et al. (2005). Amplification of IGH/MYC fusion in clinically aggressive IGH/BCL2-positive germinal center B-cell lymphomas. Genes Chromosomes Cancer. 43:414–23. PMID:15852472
2528. Martinelli S, Stellacci E, Pannone L, et al. (2015). Molecular Diversity and Associated Phenotypic Spectrum of Germline CBL Mutations. Hum Mutat. 36:787–96. PMID:25952305
2529. Martinez A, Pittaluga S, Villamor N, et al. (2004). Clonal T-cell populations and increased risk for cytotoxic T-cell lymphomas in B-CLL patients: clinicopathologic observations and molecular analysis. Am J Surg Pathol. 28:849–58. PMID:15223953
2530. Martinez D, Navarro A, Martinez-Trillos A, et al. (2016). NOTCH1, TP53, and MAP2K1 Mutations in Splenic Diffuse Red Pulp Small B-cell Lymphoma Are Associated With Progressive Disease. Am J Surg Pathol. 40:192–201. PMID:26426381
2531. Martinez D, Valera A, Perez NS, et al. (2013). Plasmablastic transformation of low-grade B-cell lymphomas: report on 6 cases. Am J Surg Pathol. 37:272–81. PMID:23282972
2532. Martínez N, Almaraz C, Vaqué JP, et al. (2014). Whole-exome sequencing in splenic marginal zone lymphoma reveals mutations in genes involved in marginal zone differentiation. Leukemia. 28:1334–40. PMID:24296945
2532A. Martinez-Climent JA, Vizcarra E, Benet I, et al. (1998). Cytogenetic response induced by interferon alpha in the myeloproliferative disorder with eosinophilia, T cell lymphoma and the chromosomal translocation t(8;13)(p11;q12) Leukemia. 12:999–1000. PMID:9639434
2533. Martinez-Escala ME, Sidiropoulos M, Deonizio J, et al. (2015). γδ T-cell-rich variants of pityriasis lichenoides and lymphomatoid papulosis: benign cutaneous disorders to be distinguished from aggressive cutaneous γδ T-cell lymphomas. Br J Dermatol. 172:372–9 PMID:25143223
2534. Martinez-Lopez A, Curiel-Olmo S, Mollejo M, et al. (2015). MYD88 (L265P) somatic mutation in marginal zone B-cell lymphoma. Am J Surg Pathol. 39:644–51. PMID:25723115
2535. Marzano AV, Ghislanzoni M, Gianelli U, et al. (2005). Fatal CD8+ epidermotropic cytotoxic primary cutaneous T-cell lymphoma with multiorgan involvement. Dermatology. 211:281–5. PMID:16205076
2536. Marzano AV, Vezzoli P, Mariotti F, et al. (2005). Paraneoplastic pemphigus associated with follicular dendritic cell sarcoma and Castleman disease. Br J Dermatol. 153:214–5. PMID:16029358
2537. Masai R, Wakui H, Togashi M, et al. (2009). Clinicopathological features and prognosis in immunoglobulin light and heavy chain deposition disease. Clin Nephrol. 71:9–20. PMID:19203545
2538. Maschek H, Georgii A, Kaloutsi V, et al. (1992). Myelofibrosis in primary myelodysplastic syndromes: a retrospective study of 352 patients. Eur J Haematol. 48:208–14. PMID:1592101
2538A. Masetti R, Pigazzi M, Togni M, et al. (2013). CBFA2T3-GLIS2 fusion transcript is a novel common feature in pediatric, cytogenetically normal AML, not restricted to FAB M7 subtype. Blood. 121:3469–72. PMID:23407549
2539. Masih AS, Weisenburger DD, Vose JM, et al. (1992). Histologic grade does not predict prognosis in optimally treated, advanced-stage nodular sclerosing Hodgkin's disease. Cancer. 69:228–32. PMID:1727667
2540. Masir N, Campbell LJ, Jones M, et al. (2010). Pseudonegative BCL2 protein expression in a t(14;18) translocation positive lymphoma cell line: a need for an alternative BCL2 antibody. Pathology. 42:212–6. PMID:20350212
2541. Mason DY, Bastard C, Rimokh R, et al. (1990). CD30-positive large cell lymphomas ('Ki-1 lymphoma') are associated with a chromosomal translocation involving 5q35. Br J Haematol. 74:161–8. PMID:2156548
2542. Mason DY, Pulford KA, Bischof D, et al. (1998). Nucleolar localization of the nucleophosmin-anaplastic lymphoma kinase is not required for malignant transformation. Cancer Res. 58:1057–62. PMID:9500471
2543. Masqué-Soler N, Szczepanowski M, Kohler CW, et al. (2015). Clinical and pathological features of Burkitt lymphoma showing expression of BCL2–an analysis including gene expression in formalin-fixed paraffin-embedded tissue. Br J Haematol. 171:501–8. PMID:26218299
2543A. Massaro F, Molica M, Breccia M. (2017). How ruxolitinib modified the outcome in myelofibrosis: focus on overall survival, allele burden reduction and fibrosis changes. Expert Rev Hematol. 10:155–9. PMID:27983880
2544. Massey GV, Zipursky A, Chang MN, et al. (2006). A prospective study of the natural history of transient leukemia (TL) in neonates with Down syndrome (DS): Children's Oncology Group (COG) study POG-9481. Blood. 107:4606–13. PMID:16469874
2545. Massone C, Cerroni L (2014). Phenotypic variability in primary cutaneous anaplastic large T-cell lymphoma: a study on 35 patients. Am J Dermatopathol. 36:153–7. PMID:24394302
2546. Massone C, Chott A, Metze D, et al. (2004). Subcutaneous, blastic natural killer (NK), NK/T-cell, and other cytotoxic lymphomas of the skin: a morphologic, immunophenotypic, and molecular study of 50 patients. Am J Surg Pathol. 28:719–35. PMID:15166664
2547. Massone C, Crisman G, Kerl H, et al. (2008). The prognosis of early mycosis fungoides is not influenced by phenotype and T-cell clonality. Br J Dermatol. 159:881–6. PMID:18644018
2548. Massone C, El-Shabrawi-Caelen L, Kerl H, et al. (2008). The morphologic spectrum of primary cutaneous anaplastic large T-cell lymphoma: a histopathologic study on 66 biopsy specimens from 47 patients with report of rare variants. J Cutan Pathol. 35:46–53. PMID:18095994
2549. Massone C, Kodama K, Kerl H, et al. (2005). Histopathologic features of early (patch) lesions of mycosis fungoides: a morphologic study on 745 biopsy specimens from 427 patients. Am J Surg Pathol. 29:550–60. PMID:15767812
2550. Massone C, Kodama K, Salmhofer W, et al. (2005). Lupus erythematosus panniculitis (lupus profundus): clinical, histopathological, and molecular analysis of nine cases. J Cutan Pathol. 32:396–404. PMID:15953372
2551. Massone C, Lozzi GP, Egberts F, et al. (2006). The protean spectrum of non-Hodgkin lymphomas with prominent involvement of subcutaneous fat. J Cutan Pathol. 33:418–25. PMID:16776717
2552. Masuko K, Kato S, Hagihara M, et al. (1996). Stable clonal expansion of T cells induced by bone marrow transplantation. Blood. 87:789–99. PMID:8555504
2553. Matano S, Nakamura S, Kobayashi K, et al. (1997). Deletion of the long arm of chromosome 20 in a patient with chronic neutrophilic leukemia: cytogenetic findings in chronic neutrophilic leukemia. Am J Hematol. 54:72–5. PMID:8980264
2554. Matarraz S, Almeida J, Flores-Montero J, et al. (2017). Introduction to the diagnosis and classification of monocytic-lineage leukemias by flow cytometry. Cytometry B Clin Cytom. 92:218–27. PMID:26282340
2555. Matarraz S, López A, Barrena S, et al. (2008). The immunophenotype of different immature, myeloid and B-cell lineage-committed CD34+ hematopoietic cells allows discrimination between normal/reactive and myelodysplastic syndrome precursors. Leukemia. 22:1175–83. PMID:18337765
2555A. Matarraz S, López A, Barrena S et al. (2010). Bone marrow cells from myelodysplastic syndromes show altered immunophenotypic profiles that may contribute to the diagnosis and prognostic stratification of the disease: a pilot study on a series of 56 patients. Cytometry B Clin Cytom. 78:154–68. PMID: 20198685.
2556. Matarraz S, Paiva B, Diez-Campelo M, et al. (2012). Myelodysplasia-associated immunophenotypic alterations of bone marrow cells in myeloma: are they present at diagnosis or are they induced by lenalidomide? Haematologica. 97:1608–11. PMID:22511492
2557. Mateo G, Montalbán MA, Vidriales MB, et al. (2008). Prognostic value of immunophenotyping in multiple myeloma: a study by the PETHEMA/GEM cooperative study groups on patients uniformly treated with high-dose therapy. J Clin Oncol. 26:2737–44. PMID:18443352
2558. Mateos MV, San Miguel JF (2013). How should we treat newly diagnosed multiple myeloma patients? Hematology Am Soc Hematol Educ Program. 2013:488–95. PMID:24319223
2559. Mathas S, Hinz M, Anagnostopoulos I, et al. (2002). Aberrantly expressed c-Jun and JunB are a hallmark of Hodgkin lymphoma cells, stimulate proliferation and synergize with NF-kappa B. EMBO J. 21:4104–13. PMID:12145210
2560. Mathas S, Janz M, Hummel F, et al. (2006). Intrinsic inhibition of transcription factor E2A by HLH proteins ABF-1 and Id2 mediates reprogramming of neoplastic B cells in Hodgkin lymphoma. Nat Immunol. 7:207–15. PMID:16369535
2561. Mathew P, Tefferi A, Dewald GW, et al. (1993). The 5q- syndrome: a single-institution study of 43 consecutive patients. Blood.

81:1040–5. PMID:8427985
2562. Mathews Griner LA, Guha R, Shinn P, et al. (2014). High-throughput combinatorial screening identifies drugs that cooperate with ibrutinib to kill activated B-cell-like diffuse large B-cell lymphoma cells. Proc Natl Acad Sci U S A. 111:2349–54. PMID:24469833
2563. Mathis S, Chapuis N, Debord C, et al. (2013). Flow cytometric detection of dyserythropoiesis: a sensitive and powerful diagnostic tool for myelodysplastic syndromes. Leukemia. 27:1981–7. PMID:23765225
2564. Mationg-Kalaw E, Tan LH, Tay K, et al. (2012). Does the proliferation fraction help identify mature B cell lymphomas with double- and triple-hit translocations? Histopathology. 61:1214–8. PMID:23171357
2565. Matolcsy A, Nádor RG, Cesarman E, et al. (1998). Immunoglobulin VH gene mutational analysis suggests that primary effusion lymphomas derive from different stages of B cell maturation. Am J Pathol. 153:1609–14. PMID:9811353
2566. Matsuda A, Germing U, Jinnai I, et al. (2010). Differences in the distribution of subtypes according to the WHO classification 2008 between Japanese and German patients with refractory anemia according to the FAB classification in myelodysplastic syndromes. Leuk Res. 34:974–80. PMID:20022110
2567. Matsuda A, Germing U, Jinnai I, et al. (2007). Improvement of criteria for refractory cytopenia with multilineage dysplasia according to the WHO classification based on prognostic significance of morphological features in patients with refractory anemia according to the FAB classification. Leukemia. 21:678–86. PMID:17268513
2568. Matsuda A, Jinnai I, Iwanaga M, et al. (2013). Correlation between dysplastic lineage and type of cytopenia in myelodysplastic syndromes patients with refractory anemia according to the FAB classification. Am J Clin Pathol. 140:253–7. PMID:23897263
2569. Matsue K, Asada N, Odawara J, et al. (2011). Random skin biopsy and bone marrow biopsy for diagnosis of intravascular large B cell lymphoma. Ann Hematol. 90:417–21. PMID:20957365
2570. Matsue K, Hayama BY, Iwama K, et al. (2011). High frequency of neurolymphomatosis as a relapse disease of intravascular large B-cell lymphoma. Cancer. 117:4512–21. PMID:21448935
2571. Matsushima AY, Strauchen JA, Lee G, et al. (1999). Posttransplantation plasmacytic proliferations related to Kaposi's sarcoma-associated herpesvirus. Am J Surg Pathol. 23:1393–400. PMID:10555008
2572. Matsushita K, Margulies I, Onda M, et al. (2008). Soluble CD22 as a tumor marker for hairy cell leukemia. Blood. 112:2272–7. PMID:18596230
2573. Matuchansky C, Colin R, Hemet J, et al. (1984). Cavitation of mesenteric lymph nodes, splenic atrophy, and a flat small intestinal mucosa. Report of six cases. Gastroenterology. 87:606–14. PMID:6745613
2574. Matutes E (2006). Immunophenotyping and differential diagnosis of hairy cell leukemia. Hematol Oncol Clin North Am. 20:1051–63. PMID:16990106
2575. Matutes E, Brito-Babapulle V, Swansbury J, et al. (1991). Clinical and laboratory features of 78 cases of T-prolymphocytic leukemia. Blood. 78:3269–74. PMID:1742486
2576. Matutes E, Crockard AD, O'Brien M, et al. (1983). Ultrastructural cytochemistry of chronic T-cell leukaemias. A study with four acid hydrolases. Histochem J. 15:895–909. PMID:6605330
2577. Matutes E, Garcia Talavera J, O'Brien M, et al. (1986). The morphological spectrum of T-prolymphocytic leukaemia. Br J Haematol. 64:111–24. PMID:3489482
2578. Matutes E, Morilla R, Farahat N, et al. (1997). Definition of acute biphenotypic leukemia. Haematologica. 82:64–6. PMID:9107085
2579. Matutes E, Morilla R, Owusu-Ankomah K, et al. (1994). The immunophenotype of splenic lymphoma with villous lymphocytes and its relevance to the differential diagnosis with other B-cell disorders. Blood. 83:1558–62. PMID:8123845
2580. Matutes E, Oscier D, Garcia-Marco J, et al. (1996). Trisomy 12 defines a group of CLL with atypical morphology: correlation between cytogenetic, clinical and laboratory features in 544 patients. Br J Haematol. 92:382–8. PMID:8603004
2581. Matutes E, Oscier D, Montalban C, et al. (2008). Splenic marginal zone lymphoma proposals for a revision of diagnostic, staging and therapeutic criteria. Leukemia. 22:487–95. PMID:18094718
2582. Matutes E, Owusu-Ankomah K, Morilla R, et al. (1994). The immunological profile of B-cell disorders and proposal of a scoring system for the diagnosis of CLL. Leukemia. 8:1640–5. PMID:7523797
2583. Matutes E, Pickl WF, Van't Veer M, et al. (2011). Mixed-phenotype acute leukemia: clinical and laboratory features and outcome in 100 patients defined according to the WHO 2008 classification. Blood. 117:3163–71. PMID:21228332
2584. Matutes E, Wotherspoon A, Catovsky D (2003). The variant form of hairy-cell leukaemia. Best Pract Res Clin Haematol. 16:41–56. PMID:12670464
2585. Matutes E, Wotherspoon AC, Parker NE, et al. (2001). Transformation of T-cell large granular lymphocyte leukaemia into a high-grade large T-cell lymphoma. Br J Haematol. 115:801–6. PMID:11843812
2586. Maurer MJ, Micallef IN, Cerhan JR, et al. (2011). Elevated serum free light chains are associated with event-free and overall survival in two independent cohorts of patients with diffuse large B-cell lymphoma. J Clin Oncol. 29:1620–6. PMID:21383282
2587. Mauritzson N, Albin M, Rylander L, et al. (2002). Pooled analysis of clinical and cytogenetic features in treatment-related and de novo adult acute myeloid leukemia and myelodysplastic syndromes based on a consecutive series of 761 patients analyzed 1976-1993 and on 5098 unselected cases reported in the literature 1974-2001. Leukemia. 16:2366–78. PMID:12454741
2588. Maxson JE, Gotlib J, Pollyea DA, et al. (2013). Oncogenic CSF3R mutations in chronic neutrophilic leukemia and atypical CML. N Engl J Med. 368:1781–90. PMID:23656643
2589. Mazzaro C, Franzin F, Tulissi P, et al. (1996). Regression of monoclonal B-cell expansion in patients affected by mixed cryoglobulinemia responsive to alpha-interferon therapy. Cancer. 77:2604–13. PMID:8640712
2590. Mbulaiteye SM, Anderson WF, Ferlay J, et al. (2012). Pediatric, elderly, and emerging adult-onset peaks in Burkitt's lymphoma incidence diagnosed in four continents, excluding Africa. Am J Hematol. 87:573–8. PMID:22488262
2591. Mc Lornan DP, Percy MJ, Jones AV, et al. (2005). Chronic neutrophilic leukemia with an associated V617F JAK2 tyrosine kinase mutation. Haematologica. 90:1696–7. PMID:16330446
2592. McAulay KA, Haque T, Crawford DH (2009). Tumour necrosis factor gene polymorphism: a predictive factor for the development of post-transplant lymphoproliferative disease. Br J Cancer. 101:1019–27. PMID:19738620
2593. McClain KL, Leach CT, Jenson HB, et al. (2000). Molecular and virologic characteristics of lymphoid malignancies in children with AIDS. J Acquir Immune Defic Syndr. 23:152–9. PMID:10737430
2594. McClure RF, Dewald GW, Hoyer JD, et al. (1999). Isolated isochromosome 17q: a distinct type of mixed myeloproliferative disorder/myelodysplastic syndrome with an aggressive clinical course. Br J Haematol. 106:445–54. PMID:10460605
2595. McDiarmid SV, Jordan S, Kim GS, et al. (1998). Prevention and preemptive therapy of postransplant lymphoproliferative disease in pediatric liver recipients. Transplantation. 66:1604–11. PMID:9884246
2596. McElwaine S, Mulligan C, Groet J, et al. (2004). Microarray transcript profiling distinguishes the transient from the acute type of megakaryoblastic leukaemia (M7) in Down's syndrome, revealing PRAME as a specific discriminating marker. Br J Haematol. 125:729–42. PMID:15180862
2597. McGinness JL, Spicknall KE, Mutasim DF (2012). Azathioprine-induced EBV-positive mucocutaneous ulcer. J Cutan Pathol. 39:377–81. PMID:22236092
2598. McGirt LY, Jia P, Baerenwald DA, et al. (2015). Whole-genome sequencing reveals oncogenic mutations in mycosis fungoides. Blood. 126:508–19. PMID:26082451
2599. McKenna RW, Parkin J, Kersey JH, et al. (1977). Chronic lymphoproliferative disorder with unusual clinical, morphologic, ultrastructural and membrane surface marker characteristics. Am J Med. 62:588–96. PMID:192076
2600. McKenna RW, Washington LT, Aquino DB, et al. (2001). Immunophenotypic analysis of hematogones (B-lymphocyte precursors) in 662 consecutive bone marrow specimens by 4-color flow cytometry. Blood. 98:2498–507. PMID:11588048
2600A. McKinney M, Moffitt AB, Gaulard P, et al. (2017). The Genetic Basis of Hepatosplenic T-cell Lymphoma. Cancer Discov. 7:369-79. PMID:28122867
2601. McManus DT, Catherwood MA, Carey PD, et al. (2004). ALK-positive diffuse large B-cell lymphoma of the stomach associated with a clathrin-ALK rearrangement. Hum Pathol. 35:1285–8. PMID:15492998
2602. McMullin MF, Bareford D, Campbell P, et al. (2005). Guidelines for the diagnosis, investigation and management of polycythaemia/erythrocytosis. Br J Haematol. 130:174–95. PMID:16029446
2603. McMullin MF, Reilly JT, Campbell P, et al. (2007). Amendment to the guideline for diagnosis and investigation of polycythaemia/erythrocytosis. Br J Haematol. 138:821–2. PMID:17672880
2604. McNiff JM, Cooper D, Howe G, et al. (1996). Lymphomatoid granulomatosis of the skin and lung. An angiocentric T-cell-rich B-cell lymphoproliferative disorder. Arch Dermatol. 132:1464–70. PMID:8961876
2605. McWeeney SK, Pemberton LC, Loriaux MM, et al. (2010). A gene expression signature of CD34+ cells to predict major cytogenetic response in chronic-phase chronic myeloid leukemia patients treated with imatinib. Blood. 115:315–25. PMID:19837975
2606. Medeiros BC, Kohrt HE, Arber DA, et al. (2010). Immunophenotypic features of acute myeloid leukemia with inv(3)(q21q26.2)/t(3;3)(q21;q26.2). Leuk Res. 34:594–7. PMID:19781775
2607. Medeiros LJ, Peiper SC, Elwood L, et al. (1991). Angiocentric immunoproliferative lesions: a molecular analysis of eight cases. Hum Pathol. 22:1150–7. PMID:1743700
2608. Meech SJ, McGavran L, Odom LF, et al. (2001). Unusual childhood extramedullary hematologic malignancy with natural killer cell properties that contains tropomyosin 4–anaplastic lymphoma kinase gene fusion. Blood. 98:1209–16. PMID:11493472
2609. Meeker TC, Hardy D, Willman C, et al. (1990). Activation of the interleukin-3 gene by chromosome translocation in acute lymphocytic leukemia with eosinophilia. Blood. 76:285–9. PMID:2114933
2610. Meggendorfer M, Bacher U, Alpermann T, et al. (2013). SETBP1 mutations occur in 9% of MDS/MPN and in 4% of MPN cases and are strongly associated with atypical CML, monosomy 7, isochromosome i(17)(q10), ASXL1 and CBL mutations. Leukemia. 27:1852–60. PMID:23628959
2611. Meggendorfer M, Roller A, Haferlach T, et al. (2012). SRSF2 mutations in 275 cases with chronic myelomonocytic leukemia (CMML). Blood. 120:3080–8. PMID:22919025
2612. Méhes G, Irsai G, Bedekovics J, et al. (2014). Activating BRAF V600E mutation in aggressive pediatric Langerhans cell histiocytosis: demonstration by allele-specific PCR/direct sequencing and immunohistochemistry. Am J Surg Pathol. 38:1644–8. PMID:25118810
2613. Mehta J, Wang H, Iqbal SU, et al. (2014). Epidemiology of myeloproliferative neoplasms in the United States. Leuk Lymphoma. 55:595–600. PMID:23768070
2614. Meijerink JP (2010). Genetic rearrangements in relation to immunophenotype and outcome in T-cell acute lymphoblastic leukaemia. Best Pract Res Clin Haematol. 23:307–18. PMID:21112032
2615. Meissner B, Kridel R, Lim RS, et al. (2013). The E3 ubiquitin ligase UBR5 is recurrently mutated in mantle cell lymphoma. Blood. 121:3161–4. PMID:23407552
2616. Mele A, Pulsoni A, Bianco E, et al. (2003). Hepatitis C virus and B-cell non-Hodgkin lymphomas: an Italian multicenter case-control study. Blood. 102:996–9. PMID:12714514
2617. Meléndez B, Díaz-Uriarte R, Cuadros M, et al. (2004). Gene expression analysis of chromosomal regions with gain or loss of genetic material detected by comparative genomic hybridization. Genes Chromosomes Cancer. 41:353–65. PMID:15382261
2618. Melnick A, Licht JD (1999). Deconstructing a disease: RARalpha, its fusion partners, and their roles in the pathogenesis of acute promyelocytic leukemia. Blood. 93:3167–215. PMID:10233871
2619. Melo JV (1996). The diversity of BCR-ABL fusion proteins and their relationship to leukemia phenotype. Blood. 88:2375–84. PMID:8839828
2620. Melo JV, Barnes DJ (2007). Chronic myeloid leukaemia as a model of disease evolution in human cancer. Nat Rev Cancer. 7:441–53. PMID:17522713
2621. Melo JV, Catovsky D, Galton DA (1986). The relationship between chronic lymphocytic leukaemia and prolymphocytic leukaemia. I. Clinical and laboratory features of 300 patients and characterization of an intermediate group. Br J Haematol. 63:377–87. PMID:3487341
2622. Melo JV, Hegde U, Parreira A, et al. (1987). Splenic B cell lymphoma with circulating villous lymphocytes: differential diagnosis of B cell leukaemias with large spleens. J Clin Pathol. 40:642–51. PMID:3497180
2623. Melo JV, Myint H, Galton DA, et al. (1994). P190BCR-ABL chronic myeloid leukaemia: the missing link with chronic myelomonocytic leukaemia? Leukemia. 8:208–11. PMID:8289491

2624. Melzner I, Bucur AJ, Brüderlein S, et al. (2005). Biallelic mutation of SOCS-1 impairs JAK2 degradation and sustains phospho-JAK2 action in the MedB-1 mediastinal lymphoma line. Blood. 105:2535–42. PMID:15572583
2625. Melzner I, Weniger MA, Menz CK, et al. (2006). Absence of the JAK2 V617F activating mutation in classical Hodgkin lymphoma and primary mediastinal B-cell lymphoma. Leukemia. 20:157–8. PMID:16331280
2626. Mendizabal AM, Garcia-Gonzalez P, Levine PH (2013). Regional variations in age at diagnosis and overall survival among patients with chronic myeloid leukemia from low and middle income countries. Cancer Epidemiol. 37:247–54. PMID:23411044
2627. Mendler JH, Maharry K, Radmacher MD, et al. (2012). RUNX1 mutations are associated with poor outcome in younger and older patients with cytogenetically normal acute myeloid leukemia and with distinct gene and MicroRNA expression signatures. J Clin Oncol. 30:3109–18. PMID:22753902
2628. Menestrina F, Chilosi M, Bonetti F, et al. (1986). Mediastinal large-cell lymphoma of B-type, with sclerosis: histopathological and immunohistochemical study of eight cases. Histopathology. 10:589–600. PMID:3525372
2629. Menezes J, Acquadro F, Wiseman M, et al. (2014). Exome sequencing reveals novel and recurrent mutations with clinical impact in blastic plasmacytoid dendritic cell neoplasm. Leukemia. 28:823–9. PMID:24072100
2630. Menezes J, Makishima H, Gomez I, et al. (2013). CSF3R T618I co-occurs with mutations of splicing and epigenetic genes and with a new PIM3 truncated fusion gene in chronic neutrophilic leukemia. Blood Cancer J. 3:e158. PMID:24212483
2631. Menke DM, Horny HP, Griesser H, et al. (2001). Primary lymph node plasmacytomas (plasmacytic lymphomas). Am J Clin Pathol. 115:119–26. PMID:11190797
2632. Menon MP, Nicolae A, Meeker H, et al. (2015). Primary CNS T-cell Lymphomas: A Clinical, Morphologic, Immunophenotypic, and Molecular Analysis. Am J Surg Pathol. 39:1719–29. PMID:26379152
2633. Menter T, Dirnhofer S, Tzankov A (2015). LEF1: a highly specific marker for the diagnosis of chronic lymphocytic B cell leukaemia/small lymphocytic B cell lymphoma. J Clin Pathol. 68:473–8. PMID:25713417
2634. Menter T, Gasser A, Juskevicius D, et al. (2015). Diagnostic Utility of the Germinal Center-associated Markers GCET1, HGAL, and LMO2 in Hematolymphoid Neoplasms. Appl Immunohistochem Mol Morphol. 23:491–8. PMID:25203428
2635. Mention JJ, Ben Ahmed M, Bègue B, et al. (2003). Interleukin 15: a key to disrupted intraepithelial lymphocyte homeostasis and lymphomagenesis in celiac disease. Gastroenterology. 125:730–45. PMID:12949719
2636. Mercer LK, Davies R, Galloway JB, et al. (2013). Risk of cancer in patients receiving non-biologic disease-modifying therapy for rheumatoid arthritis compared with the UK general population. Rheumatology (Oxford). 52:91–8. PMID:23238979
2637. Mercher T, Coniat MB, Monni R, et al. (2001). Involvement of a human gene related to the Drosophila spen gene in the recurrent t(1;22) translocation of acute megakaryocytic leukemia. Proc Natl Acad Sci U S A. 98:5776–9. PMID:11344311
2638. Mercieca J, Puga M, Matutes E, et al. (1994). Incidence and significance of abdominal lymphadenopathy in hairy cell leukaemia. Leuk Lymphoma. 14 Suppl 1:79–83. PMID:7820058
2639. Meresse B, Chen Z, Ciszewski C, et al. (2004). Coordinated induction by IL15 of a TCR-independent NKG2D signaling pathway converts CTL into lymphokine-activated killer cells in celiac disease. Immunity. 21:357–66. PMID:15357947
2640. Merlini G, Seldin DC, Gertz MA (2011). Amyloidosis: pathogenesis and new therapeutic options. J Clin Oncol. 29:1924–33. PMID:21483018
2641. Merlini G, Stone MJ (2006). Dangerous small B-cell clones. Blood. 108:2520–30. PMID:16794250
2642. Mesa RA, Hanson CA, Rajkumar SV, et al. (2000). Evaluation and clinical correlations of bone marrow angiogenesis in myelofibrosis with myeloid metaplasia. Blood. 96:3374–80. PMID:11071630
2643. Mesa RA, Kantarjian H, Tefferi A, et al. (2011). Evaluating the serial use of the Myelofibrosis Symptom Assessment Form for measuring symptomatic improvement: performance in 87 myelofibrosis patients on a JAK1 and JAK2 inhibitor (INCB018424) clinical trial. Cancer. 117:4869–77. PMID:21480207
2644. Metcalf RA, Bashey S, Wysong A, et al. (2013). Intravascular ALK-negative anaplastic large cell lymphoma with localized cutaneous involvement and an indolent clinical course: toward recognition of a distinct clinicopathologic entity. Am J Surg Pathol. 37:617–23. PMID:23480896
2645. Metcalf RA, Monabati A, Vyas M, et al. (2014). Myeloid cell nuclear differentiation antigen is expressed in a subset of marginal zone lymphomas and is useful in the differential diagnosis with follicular lymphoma. Hum Pathol. 45:1730–6. PMID:24925224
2646. Metcalfe DD (1991). Classification and diagnosis of mastocytosis: current status. J Invest Dermatol. 96:2S–4S. PMID:16799601
2647. Metcalfe DD (1991). The liver, spleen, and lymph nodes in mastocytosis. J Invest Dermatol. 96:45S–46S. PMID:16799608
2648. Metchnikoff E (1883). Untersuchungen uber die intracellulare Verdauung bei wirbellosen Thieren. Arb Zoologischen Inst Univ Wien. 5:141.
2648A. Metzeler KH, Becker H, Maharry K, et al. (2011). ASXL1 mutations identify a high-risk subgroup of older patients with primary cytogenetically normal AML within the ELN Favorable genetic category. Blood. 118:6920–9. PMID:22031865
2648B. Metzeler KH, Dufour A, Benthaus T, et al. (2009). ERG expression is an independent prognostic factor and allows refined risk stratification in cytogenetically normal acute myeloid leukemia: a comprehensive analysis of ERG, MN1, and BAALC transcript levels using oligonucleotide microarrays. J Clin Oncol. 27:5031–8. PMID:19752345
2648C. Metzeler KH, Maharry K, Radmacher MD, et al. (2011). TET2 mutations improve the new European LeukemiaNet risk classification of acute myeloid leukemia: a Cancer and Leukemia Group B study. J Clin Oncol. 29:1373–81. PMID:21343549
2649. Metzgeroth G, Schwaab J, Gosenca D, et al. (2013). Long-term follow-up of treatment with imatinib in eosinophilia-associated myeloid/lymphoid neoplasms with PDGFR rearrangements in blast phase. Leukemia. 27:2254–6. PMID:23615556
2650. Metzgeroth G, Walz C, Score J, et al. (2007). Recurrent finding of the FIP1L1-PDGFRA fusion gene in eosinophilia-associated acute myeloid leukemia and lymphoblastic T-cell lymphoma. Leukemia. 21:1183–8. PMID:17377585
2651. Meyer C, Hofmann J, Burmeister T, et al. (2013). The MLL recombinome of acute leukemias in 2013. Leukemia. 27:2165–76. PMID:23628958
2652. Meyer PN, Fu K, Greiner TC, et al. (2011). Immunohistochemical methods for predicting cell of origin and survival in patients with diffuse large B-cell lymphoma treated with rituximab. J Clin Oncol. 29:200–7. PMID:21135273
2653. Michaux JL, Martiat P (1993). Chronic myelomonocytic leukaemia (CMML)–a myelodysplastic or myeloproliferative syndrome? Leuk Lymphoma. 9:35–41. PMID:8477199
2654. Michels SD, McKenna RW, Arthur DC, et al. (1985). Therapy-related acute myeloid leukemia and myelodysplastic syndrome: a clinical and morphologic study of 65 cases. Blood. 65:1364–72. PMID:3857944
2655. Michor F (2007). Chronic myeloid leukemia blast crisis arises from progenitors. Stem Cells. 25:1114–8. PMID:17218393
2656. Micol JB, Abdel-Wahab O (2014). Collaborating constitutive and somatic genetic events in myeloid malignancies: ASXL1 mutations in patients with germline GATA2 mutations. Haematologica. 99:201–3. PMID:24497555
2657. Micol JB, Duployez N, Boissel N, et al. (2014). Frequent ASXL2 mutations in acute myeloid leukemia patients with t(8;21)/RUNX1-RUNX1T1 chromosomal translocations. Blood. 124:1445–9. PMID:24973361
2658. Miesner M, Haferlach C, Bacher U, et al. (2010). Multilineage dysplasia (MLD) in acute myeloid leukemia (AML) correlates with MDS-related cytogenetic abnormalities and a prior history of MDS or MDS/MPN but has no independent prognostic relevance: a comparison of 408 cases classified as "AML not otherwise specified" (AML-NOS) or "AML with myelodysplasia-related changes" (AML-MRC). Blood. 116:2742–51. PMID:20581309
2659. Miettinen M, Fletcher CD, Lasota J (1993). True histiocytic lymphoma of small intestine. Analysis of two S-100 protein-positive cases with features of interdigitating reticulum cell sarcoma. Am J Clin Pathol. 100:285–92. PMID:8379537
2660. Miettinen M, Franssila KO, Saxén E (1983). Hodgkin's disease, lymphocytic predominance nodular. Increased risk for subsequent non-Hodgkin's lymphomas. Cancer. 51:2293–300. PMID:6850508
2661. Mikhael JR, Dingli D, Roy V, et al. (2013). Management of newly diagnosed symptomatic multiple myeloma: updated Mayo Stratification of Myeloma and Risk-Adapted Therapy (mSMART) consensus guidelines 2013. Mayo Clin Proc. 88:360–76. PMID:23541011
2662. Miles DK, Freedman MH, Stephens K, et al. (1996). Patterns of hematopoietic lineage involvement in children with neurofibromatosis type 1 and malignant myeloid disorders. Blood. 88:4314–20. PMID:8943868
2663. Miller DV, Firchau DJ, McClure RF, et al. (2010). Epstein-Barr virus-associated diffuse large B-cell lymphoma arising on cardiac prostheses. Am J Surg Pathol. 34:377–84. PMID:20139760
2664. Miller TP, Grogan TM, Dahlberg S, et al. (1994). Prognostic significance of the Ki-67-associated proliferative antigen in aggressive non-Hodgkin's lymphomas: a prospective Southwest Oncology Group trial. Blood. 83:1460–6. PMID:8123837
2665. Millot F, Traore P, Guilhot J, et al. (2005). Clinical and biological features at diagnosis in 40 children with chronic myeloid leukemia. Pediatrics. 116:140–3. PMID:15995044
2665A. Mills JA, Gonzalez RG, Jaffe R (2008). Case records of the Massachusetts General Hospital. Case 25-2008. A 43-year-old man with fatigue and lesions in the pituitary and cerebellum. N Engl J Med. 359:736–47. PMID:18703477
2666. Milosevic Feenstra JD, Nivarthi H, Gisslinger H, et al. (2016). Whole-exome sequencing identifies novel MPL and JAK2 mutations in triple-negative myeloproliferative neoplasms. Blood. 127:325–32. PMID:26423830
2667. Minard-Colin V, Brugières L, Reiter A, et al. (2015). Non-Hodgkin Lymphoma in Children and Adolescents: Progress Through Effective Collaboration, Current Knowledge, and Challenges Ahead. J Clin Oncol. 33:2963–74. PMID:26304908
2668. Minkov M, Grois N, Heitger A, et al. (2002). Response to initial treatment of multisystem Langerhans cell histiocytosis: an important prognostic indicator. Med Pediatr Oncol. 39:581–5. PMID:12376981
2669. Minkov M, Prosch H, Steiner M, et al. (2005). Langerhans cell histiocytosis in neonates. Pediatr Blood Cancer. 45:802–7. PMID:15770639
2670. Minkov M, Pötschger U, Grois N, et al. (2007). Bone marrow assessment in Langerhans cell histiocytosis. Pediatr Blood Cancer. 49:694–8. PMID:17455318
2671. Miralles GD, O'Fallon JR, Talley NJ (1992). Plasma-cell dyscrasia with polyneuropathy. The spectrum of POEMS syndrome. N Engl J Med. 327:1919–23. PMID:1333569
2672. Miranda RN, Aladily TN, Prince HM, et al. (2014). Breast implant-associated anaplastic large-cell lymphoma: long-term follow-up of 60 patients. J Clin Oncol. 32:114–20. PMID:24323027
2673. Miranda RN, Loo E, Medeiros LJ (2013). Iatrogenic immunodeficiency-associated classical hodgkin lymphoma: clinicopathologic features of 54 cases reported in the literature. Am J Surg Pathol. 37:1895–7. PMID:24145656
2674. Mirza I, Macpherson N, Paproski S, et al. (2002). Primary cutaneous follicular lymphoma: an assessment of clinical, histopathologic, immunophenotypic, and molecular features. J Clin Oncol. 20:647–55. PMID:11821444
2675. Misdraji J, Fernandez del Castillo C, Ferry JA (1997). Follicle center lymphoma of the ampulla of Vater presenting with jaundice: report of a case. Am J Surg Pathol. 21:484–8. PMID:9130997
2676. Misdraji J, Harris NL, Hasserjian RP, et al. (2011). Primary follicular lymphoma of the gastrointestinal tract. Am J Surg Pathol. 35:1255–63. PMID:21836483
2677. Mitsiades CS, McMillin DW, Klippel S, et al. (2007). The role of the bone marrow microenvironment in the pathophysiology of myeloma and its significance in the development of more effective therapies. Hematol Oncol Clin North Am. 21:1007–34, vii–viii. [vii-viii.] PMID:17996586
2678. Mittal K, Neri A, Feiner H, et al. (1990). Lymphomatoid granulomatosis in the acquired immunodeficiency syndrome. Evidence of Epstein-Barr virus infection and B-cell clonal selection without myc rearrangement. Cancer. 65:1345–9. PMID:2155052
2679. Mitus AJ, Stein R, Rappeport JM, et al. (1989). Monoclonal and oligoclonal gammopathy after bone marrow transplantation. Blood. 74:2764–8. PMID:2819246
2680. Miwa H, Takakuwa T, Nakatsuka S, et al. (2002). DNA sequences of the immunoglobulin heavy chain variable region gene in pyothorax-associated lymphoma. Oncology. 62:241–50. PMID:12065872
2681. Miyazaki K, Yamaguchi M, Suzuki R, et al. (2011). CD5-positive diffuse large B-cell lymphoma: a retrospective study in 337 patients treated by chemotherapy with or without rituximab. Ann Oncol. 22:1601–7. PMID:21199885
2682. Miyazaki Y, Kuriyama K, Miyawaki S, et al. (2003). Cytogenetic heterogeneity of acute myeloid leukaemia (AML) with trilineage dysplasia: Japan Adult Leukaemia Study

Group-AML 92 study. Br J Haematol. 120:56–62. PMID:12492577
2683. Moccia AA, Donaldson J, Chhanabhai M, et al. (2012). International Prognostic Score in advanced-stage Hodgkin's lymphoma: altered utility in the modern era. J Clin Oncol. 30:3383–8. PMID:22869887
2684. Mohammadi F, Wolverson MK, Bastani B (2012). A new case of TEMPI syndrome. Clin Kidney J. 5:556–8. PMID:26069800
2685. Moldenhauer G, Popov SW, Wotschke B, et al. (2006). AID expression identifies interfollicular large B cells as putative precursors of mature B-cell malignancies. Blood. 107:2470–3. PMID:16269615
2686. Molina TJ, Canioni D, Copie-Bergman C, et al. (2014). Young patients with non-germinal center B-cell-like diffuse large B-cell lymphoma benefit from intensified chemotherapy with ACVBP plus rituximab compared with CHOP plus rituximab: analysis of data from the Groupe d'Etudes des Lymphomes de l'Adulte/lymphoma study association phase III trial LNH 03-2B. J Clin Oncol. 32:3996–4003. PMID:25385729
2687. Molina TJ, Lin P, Swerdlow SH, et al. (2011). Marginal zone lymphomas with plasmacytic differentiation and related disorders. Am J Clin Pathol. 136:211–25. PMID:21757594
2688. Mollejo M, Algara P, Mateo MS, et al. (2003). Large B-cell lymphoma presenting in the spleen: identification of different clinicopathologic conditions. Am J Surg Pathol. 27:895–902. PMID:12826881
2689. Mollejo M, Algara P, Mateo MS, et al. (2002). Splenic small B-cell lymphoma with predominant red pulp involvement: a diffuse variant of splenic marginal zone lymphoma? Histopathology. 40:22–30. PMID:11903595
2690. Mollejo M, Menárguez J, Guisado-Vasco P, et al. (2014). Hepatitis C virus-related lymphoproliferative disorders encompass a broader clinical and morphological spectrum than previously recognized: a clinicopathological study. Mod Pathol. 27:281–93. PMID:23929267
2691. Mollejo M, Menárguez J, Lloret E, et al. (1995). Splenic marginal zone lymphoma: a distinctive type of low-grade B-cell lymphoma. A clinicopathological study of 13 cases. Am J Surg Pathol. 19:1146–57. PMID:7573673
2692. Molyneux EM, Rochford R, Griffin B, et al. (2012). Burkitt's lymphoma. Lancet. 379:1234–44. PMID:22333947
2693. Momose S, Weißbach S, Pischimarov J, et al. (2015). The diagnostic gray zone between Burkitt lymphoma and diffuse large B-cell lymphoma is also a gray zone of the mutational spectrum. Leukemia. 29:1789–91. PMID:25673238
2694. Momota H, Narita Y, Maeshima AM, et al. (2010). Prognostic value of immunohistochemical profile and response to high-dose methotrexate therapy in primary CNS lymphoma. J Neurooncol. 98:341–8. PMID:20012911
2695. Monda L, Warnke R, Rosai J (1986). A primary lymph node malignancy with features suggestive of dendritic reticulum cell differentiation. A report of 4 cases. Am J Pathol. 122:562–72. PMID:2420185
2696. Montalbán C, Abraira V, Arcaini L, et al. (2012). Risk stratification for Splenic Marginal Zone Lymphoma based on haemoglobin concentration, platelet count, high lactate dehydrogenase level and extrahilar lymphadenopathy: development and validation on 593 cases. Br J Haematol. 159:164–71. PMID:22924582
2697. Montanari F, O'Connor OA, Savage DG, et al. (2010). Bone marrow involvement in patients with posttransplant lymphoproliferative disorders: incidence and prognostic factors. Hum Pathol. 41:1150–8. PMID:20381113
2698. Montes-Moreno S, Castro Y, Rodríguez-Pinilla SM, et al. (2010). Intrafollicular neoplasia/in situ follicular lymphoma: review of a series of 13 cases. Histopathology. 56:658–62. PMID:20459579
2699. Montes-Moreno S, Gonzalez-Medina AR, Rodriguez-Pinilla SM, et al. (2010). Aggressive large B-cell lymphoma with plasma cell differentiation: immunohistochemical characterization of plasmablastic lymphoma and diffuse large B-cell lymphoma with partial plasmablastic phenotype. Haematologica. 95:1342–9. PMID:20418245
2700. Montes-Moreno S, Montalbán C, Piris MA (2012). Large B-cell lymphomas with plasmablastic differentiation: a biological and therapeutic challenge. Leuk Lymphoma. 53:185–94. PMID:21812534
2701. Montes-Moreno S, Odqvist L, Diaz-Perez JA, et al. (2012). EBV-positive diffuse large B-cell lymphoma of the elderly is an aggressive post-germinal center B-cell neoplasm characterized by prominent nuclear factor-kB activation. Mod Pathol. 25:968–82. PMID:22538516
2702. Montes-Moreno S, Ramos-Medina R, Martínez-López A, et al. (2013). SPIB, a novel immunohistochemical marker for human blastic plasmacytoid dendritic cell neoplasms: characterization of its expression in major hematolymphoid neoplasms. Blood. 121:643–7. PMID:23165482
2703. Montes-Moreno S, Roncador G, Maestre L, et al. (2008). Gcet1 (centerin), a highly restricted marker for a subset of germinal center-derived lymphomas. Blood. 111:351–8. PMID:17898315
2704. Montesinos P, Rayón C, Vellenga E, et al. (2011). Clinical significance of CD56 expression in patients with acute promyelocytic leukemia treated with all-trans retinoic acid and anthracycline-based regimens. Blood. 117:1799–805. PMID:21148082
2705. Montesinos-Rongen M, Besleaga R, Heinsohn S, et al. (2004). Absence of simian virus 40 DNA sequences in primary central nervous system lymphoma in HIV-negative patients. Virchows Arch. 444:436–8. PMID:15042369
2706. Montesinos-Rongen M, Brunn A, Bentink S, et al. (2008). Gene expression profiling suggests primary central nervous system lymphomas to be derived from a late germinal center B cell. Leukemia. 22:400–5. PMID:17989719
2707. Montesinos-Rongen M, Godlewska E, Brunn A, et al. (2011). Activating L265P mutations of the MYD88 gene are common in primary central nervous system lymphoma. Acta Neuropathol. 122:791–2. PMID:22020631
2708. Montesinos-Rongen M, Hans VH, Eis-Hübinger AM, et al. (2001). Human herpes virus-8 is not associated with primary central nervous system lymphoma in HIV-negative patients. Acta Neuropathol. 102:489–95. PMID:11699563
2709. Montesinos-Rongen M, Küppers R, Schlüter D, et al. (1999). Primary central nervous system lymphomas are derived from germinal-center B cells and show a preferential usage of the V4-34 gene segment. Am J Pathol. 155:2077–86. PMID:10595937
2710. Montesinos-Rongen M, Purschke FG, Brunn A, et al. (2015). Primary Central Nervous System (CNS) Lymphoma B Cell Receptors Recognize CNS Proteins. J Immunol. 195:1312–9. PMID:26116512
2711. Montesinos-Rongen M, Roers A, Küppers R, et al. (1999). Mutation of the p53 gene is not a typical feature of Hodgkin and Reed-Sternberg cells in Hodgkin's disease. Blood. 94:1755–60. PMID:10477701
2712. Montesinos-Rongen M, Schmitz R, Brunn A, et al. (2010). Mutations of CARD11 but not TNFAIP3 may activate the NF-kappaB pathway in primary CNS lymphoma. Acta Neuropathol. 120:529–35. PMID:20544211
2713. Montesinos-Rongen M, Schmitz R, Courts C, et al. (2005). Absence of immunoglobulin class switch in primary lymphomas of the central nervous system. Am J Pathol. 166:1773–9. PMID:15920162
2714. Montesinos-Rongen M, Schäfer E, Siebert R, et al. (2012). Genes regulating the B cell receptor pathway are recurrently mutated in primary central nervous system lymphoma. Acta Neuropathol. 124:905–6. PMID:23138649
2715. Montesinos-Rongen M, Van Roost D, Schaller C, et al. (2004). Primary diffuse large B-cell lymphomas of the central nervous system are targeted by aberrant somatic hypermutation. Blood. 103:1869–75. PMID:14592832
2716. Montesinos-Rongen M, Zühlke-Jenisch R, Gesk S, et al. (2002). Interphase cytogenetic analysis of lymphoma-associated chromosomal breakpoints in primary diffuse large B-cell lymphomas of the central nervous system. J Neuropathol Exp Neurol. 61:926–33. PMID:12387458
2717. Monteverde A, Sabattini E, Poggi S, et al. (1995). Bone marrow findings further support the hypothesis that essential mixed cryoglobulinemia type II is characterized by a monoclonal B-cell proliferation. Leuk Lymphoma. 20:119–24. PMID:8750632
2718. Monti S, Chapuy B, Takeyama K, et al. (2012). Integrative analysis reveals an outcome-associated and targetable pattern of p53 and cell cycle deregulation in diffuse large B cell lymphoma. Cancer Cell. 22:359–72. PMID:22975378
2719. Monti S, Savage KJ, Kutok JL, et al. (2005). Molecular profiling of diffuse large B-cell lymphoma identifies robust subtypes including one characterized by host inflammatory response. Blood. 105:1851–61. PMID:15550490
2720. Montserrat E, Villamor N, Reverter JC, et al. (1996). Bone marrow assessment in B-cell chronic lymphocytic leukaemia: aspirate or biopsy? A comparative study in 258 patients. Br J Haematol. 93:111–6. PMID:8611442
2720A. Moore EM, Aggarwal N, Surti U, Swerdlow SH (2017). Further exploration of the complexities of large B-cell lymphomas with MYC abnormalities and the importance of a blastoid morphology. Am J Surg Pathol, in press. PMID:28614202
2721. Moran NR, Webster B, Lee KM, et al. (2015). Epstein Barr virus-positive mucocutaneous ulcer of the colon associated Hodgkin lymphoma in Crohn's disease. World J Gastroenterol. 21:6072–6. PMID:26019475
2722. Moreau EJ, Matutes E, A'Hern RP, et al. (1997). Improvement of the chronic lymphocytic leukemia scoring system with the monoclonal antibody SN8 (CD79b). Am J Clin Pathol. 108:378–82. PMID:9322589
2723. Moreau P, Attal M, Facon T (2015). Frontline therapy of multiple myeloma. Blood. 125:3076–84. PMID:25838345
2724. Moreau P, Robillard N, Avet-Loiseau H, et al. (2004). Patients with CD45 negative multiple myeloma receiving high-dose therapy have a shorter survival than those with CD45 positive multiple myeloma. Haematologica. 89:547–51. PMID:15136217
2725. Moreau P, Robillard N, Jégo G, et al. (2006). Lack of CD27 in myeloma delineates different presentation and outcome. Br J Haematol. 132:168–70. PMID:16398651
2726. Morel P, Duhamel A, Gobbi P, et al. (2009). International prognostic scoring system for Waldenstrom macroglobulinemia. Blood. 113:4163–70. PMID:19196866
2727. Morel P, Lepage E, Brice P, et al. (1992). Prognosis and treatment of lymphoblastic lymphoma in adults: a report on 80 patients. J Clin Oncol. 10:1078–85. PMID:1607914
2728. Morerio C, Acquila M, Rosanda C, et al. (2004). HCMOGT-1 is a novel fusion partner to PDGFRB in juvenile myelomonocytic leukemia with t(5;17)(q33;p11.2). Cancer Res. 64:2649–51. PMID:15087372
2729. Morgado JM, Perbellini O, Johnson RC, et al. (2013). CD30 expression by bone marrow mast cells from different diagnostic variants of systemic mastocytosis. Histopathology. 63:780–7. PMID:24111625
2730. Morgan EA, Yu H, Pinkus JL, et al. (2013). Immunohistochemical detection of hairy cell leukemia in paraffin sections using a highly effective CD103 rabbit monoclonal antibody. Am J Clin Pathol. 139:220–30. PMID:23355207
2731. Mori H, Colman SM, Xiao Z, et al. (2002). Chromosome translocations and covert leukemic clones are generated during normal fetal development. Proc Natl Acad Sci U S A. 99:8242–7. PMID:12048236
2732. Mori M, Kobayashi Y, Maeshima AM, et al. (2010). The indolent course and high incidence of t(14;18) in primary duodenal follicular lymphoma. Ann Oncol. 21:1500–5. PMID:20022910
2733. Mori N, Yamashita Y, Tsuzuki T, et al. (2000). Lymphomatous features of aggressive NK cell leukaemia/lymphoma with massive necrosis, haemophagocytosis and EB virus infection. Histopathology. 37:363–71. PMID:11012744
2734. Mori N, Yatabe Y, Narita M, et al. (1996). Pyothorax-associated lymphoma. An unusual case with biphenotypic character of T and B cells. Am J Surg Pathol. 20:760–6. PMID:8651357
2735. Morice WG (2007). The immunophenotypic attributes of NK cells and NK-cell lineage lymphoproliferative disorders. Am J Clin Pathol. 127:881–6. PMID:17509985
2736. Morice WG, Chen D, Kurtin PJ, et al. (2009). Novel immunophenotypic features of marrow lymphoplasmacytic lymphoma and correlation with Waldenström's macroglobulinemia. Mod Pathol. 22:807–16. PMID:19287458
2737. Morice WG, Hodnefield JM, Kurtin PJ, et al. (2004). An unusual case of leukemic mantle cell lymphoma with a blastoid component showing loss of CD5 and aberrant expression of CD10. Am J Clin Pathol. 122:122–7. PMID:15272540
2738. Morice WG, Jevremovic D, Hanson CA (2007). The expression of the novel cytotoxic protein granzyme M by large granular lymphocytic leukaemias of both T-cell and NK-cell lineage: an unexpected finding with implications regarding the pathobiology of these disorders. Br J Haematol. 137:237–9. PMID:17408463
2739. Morice WG, Jevremovic D, Olteanu H, et al. (2010). Chronic lymphoproliferative disorder of natural killer cells: a distinct entity with subtypes correlating with normal natural killer cell subsets. Leukemia. 24:881–4. PMID:20111066
2740. Morice WG, Kurtin PJ, Leibson PJ, et al. (2003). Demonstration of aberrant T-cell and natural killer-cell antigen expression in all cases of granular lymphocytic leukaemia. Br J Haematol. 120:1026–36. PMID:12648073
2741. Morice WG, Kurtin PJ, Tefferi A, et al. (2002). Distinct bone marrow findings in T-cell granular lymphocytic leukemia revealed by paraffin section immunoperoxidase stains for CD8, TIA-1, and granzyme B. Blood. 99:268–74. PMID:11756181
2742. Morice WG, Macon WR, Dogan A, et al. (2006). NK-cell-associated receptor expression in hepatosplenic T-cell lymphoma, insights into pathogenesis. Leukemia. 20:883–6. PMID:16525496
2743. Morice WG, Rodriguez FJ, Hoyer JD,

et al. (2005). Diffuse large B-cell lymphoma with distinctive patterns of splenic and bone marrow involvement: clinicopathologic features of two cases. Mod Pathol. 18:495–502. PMID:15492760

2744. Morin RD, Johnson NA, Severson TM, et al. (2010). Somatic mutations altering EZH2 (Tyr641) in follicular and diffuse large B-cell lymphomas of germinal-center origin. Nat Genet. 42:181–5. PMID:20081860

2745. Morin RD, Mendez-Lago M, Mungall AJ, et al. (2011). Frequent mutation of histone-modifying genes in non-Hodgkin lymphoma. Nature. 476:298–303. PMID:21796119

2746. Morishima S, Nakamura S, Yamamoto K, et al. (2015). Increased T-cell responses to Epstein-Barr virus with high viral load in patients with Epstein-Barr virus-positive diffuse large B-cell lymphoma. Leuk Lymphoma. 56:1072–8. PMID:24975317

2747. Morita K, Nakamine H, Nakai T, et al. (2015). A retrospective study of patients with follicular lymphoma (FL): identification of in situ FL or FL-like B cells of uncertain significance in lymph nodes resected at the time of previous surgery for carcinomas. J Clin Pathol. 68:541–6. PMID:25862812

2748. Moritake H, Shimonodan H, Marutsuka K, et al. (2011). C-MYC rearrangement may induce an aggressive phenotype in anaplastic lymphoma kinase positive anaplastic large cell lymphoma: Identification of a novel fusion gene ALO17/C-MYC. Am J Hematol. 86:75–8. PMID:21080342

2749. Moriwaki K, Manabe A, Taketani T, et al. (2014). Cytogenetics and clinical features of pediatric myelodysplastic syndrome in Japan. Int J Hematol. 100:478–84. PMID:25261124

2750. Moroch J, Copie-Bergman C, de Leval L, et al. (2012). Follicular peripheral T-cell lymphoma expands the spectrum of classical Hodgkin lymphoma mimics. Am J Surg Pathol. 36:1636–46. PMID:23073322

2751. Morra E, Cesana C, Klersy C, et al. (2004). Clinical characteristics and factors predicting evolution of asymptomatic IgM monoclonal gammopathies and IgM-related disorders. Leukemia. 18:1512–7. PMID:15322559

2752. Morra E, Cesana C, Klersy C, et al. (2003). Predictive variables for malignant transformation in 452 patients with asymptomatic IgM monoclonal gammopathy. Semin Oncol. 30:172–7. PMID:12720131

2753. Morris SW, Kirstein MN, Valentine MB, et al. (1994). Fusion of a kinase gene, ALK, to a nucleolar protein gene, NPM, in non-Hodgkin's lymphoma. Science. 263:1281–4. PMID:8122112

2754. Morscio J, Dierickx D, Ferreiro JF, et al. (2013). Gene expression profiling reveals clear differences between EBV-positive and EBV-negative posttransplant lymphoproliferative disorders. Am J Transplant. 13:1305–16. PMID:23489474

2755. Morscio J, Dierickx D, Nijs J, et al. (2014). Clinicopathologic comparison of plasmablastic lymphoma in HIV-positive, immunocompetent, and posttransplant patients: single-center series of 25 cases and meta-analysis of 277 reported cases. Am J Surg Pathol. 38:875–86. PMID:24832164

2756. Morscio J, Dierickx D, Tousseyn T (2013). Molecular pathogenesis of B-cell posttransplant lymphoproliferative disorder: what do we know so far? Clin Dev Immunol. 2013:150835. PMID:23690819

2757. Morton LM, Dores GM, Tucker MA, et al. (2013). Evolving risk of therapy-related acute myeloid leukemia following cancer chemotherapy among adults in the United States, 1975-2008. Blood. 121:2996–3004. PMID:23412096

2758. Morton LM, Sampson JN, Cerhan JR,

et al. (2014). Rationale and Design of the International Lymphoma Epidemiology Consortium (InterLymph) Non-Hodgkin Lymphoma Subtypes Project. J Natl Cancer Inst Monogr. 2014:1–14. PMID:25174022

2759. Morton LM, Wang SS, Devesa SS, et al. (2006). Lymphoma incidence patterns by WHO subtype in the United States, 1992-2001. Blood. 107:265–76. PMID:16150940

2760. Mossuz P, Girodon F, Donnard M, et al. (2004). Diagnostic value of serum erythropoietin level in patients with absolute erythrocytosis. Haematologica. 89:1194–8. PMID:15477203

2761. Mottok A, Gascoyne RD (2015). Bromodomain inhibition in diffuse large B-cell lymphoma–giving MYC a brake. Clin Cancer Res. 21:4–6. PMID:25165099

2762. Mottok A, Hansmann ML, Bräuninger A (2005). Activation induced cytidine deaminase expression in lymphocyte predominant Hodgkin lymphoma. J Clin Pathol. 58:1002–4. PMID:16126891

2763. Mottok A, Woolcock B, Chan FC, et al. (2015). Genomic Alterations in CIITA Are Frequent in Primary Mediastinal Large B Cell Lymphoma and Are Associated with Diminished MHC Class II Expression. Cell Rep. 13:1418–31. PMID:26549456

2764. Moulard O, Mehta J, Fryzek J, et al. (2014). Epidemiology of myelofibrosis, essential thrombocythemia, and polycythemia vera in the European Union. Eur J Haematol. 92:289–97. PMID:24372927

2765. Moulopoulos LA, Dimopoulos MA, Weber D, et al. (1993). Magnetic resonance imaging in the staging of solitary plasmacytoma of bone. J Clin Oncol. 11:1311–5. PMID:8315427

2766. Mounier N, Briere J, Gisselbrecht C, et al. (2003). Rituximab plus CHOP (R-CHOP) overcomes bcl-2–associated resistance to chemotherapy in elderly patients with diffuse large B-cell lymphoma (DLBCL). Blood. 101:4279–84. PMID:12576316

2767. Mourad N, Mounier N, Brière J, et al. (2008). Clinical, biologic, and pathologic features in 157 patients with angioimmunoblastic T-cell lymphoma treated within the Groupe d'Etude des Lymphomes de l'Adulte (GELA) trials. Blood. 111:4463–70. PMID:18292286

2768. Movassaghian M, Brunner AM, Blonquist TM, et al. (2015). Presentation and outcomes among patients with isolated myeloid sarcoma: a Surveillance, Epidemiology, and End Results database analysis. Leuk Lymphoma. 56:1698–703. PMID:25213180

2769. Mozos A, Royo C, Hartmann E, et al. (2009). SOX11 expression is highly specific for mantle cell lymphoma and identifies the cyclin D1-negative subtype. Haematologica. 94:1555–62. PMID:19880778

2770. Mrózek K, Bloomfield CD (2006). Chromosome aberrations, gene mutations and expression changes, and prognosis in adult acute myeloid leukemia. Hematology Am Soc Hematol Educ Program. 169–77. PMID:17124057

2771. Mrózek K, Harper DP, Aplan PD (2009). Cytogenetics and molecular genetics of acute lymphoblastic leukemia. Hematol Oncol Clin North Am. 23:991–1010, v. [v.] PMID:19825449

2772. Mrózek K, Heinonen K, de la Chapelle A, et al. (1997). Clinical significance of cytogenetics in acute myeloid leukemia. Semin Oncol. 24:17–31. PMID:9045301

2773. Mrózek K, Heinonen K, Lawrence D, et al. (1997). Adult patients with de novo acute myeloid leukemia and t(9; 11)(p22; q23) have a superior outcome to patients with other translocations involving band 11q23: a cancer and leukemia group b study. Blood. 90:4532–8. PMID:9373264

2774. Mrózek K, Marcucci G, Paschka P, et

al. (2007). Clinical relevance of mutations and gene-expression changes in adult acute myeloid leukemia with normal cytogenetics: are we ready for a prognostically prioritized molecular classification? Blood. 109:431–48. PMID:16960150

2775. Mrózek K, Prior TW, Edwards C, et al. (2001). Comparison of cytogenetic and molecular genetic detection of t(8;21) and inv(16) in a prospective series of adults with de novo acute myeloid leukemia: a Cancer and Leukemia Group B Study. J Clin Oncol. 19:2482–92. PMID:11331327

2776. Muehleck SD, McKenna RW, Arthur DC, et al. (1984). Transformation of chronic myelogenous leukemia: clinical, morphologic, and cytogenetic features. Am J Clin Pathol. 82:1–14. PMID:6588747

2777. Mueller NE, Grufferman S (1999). The epidemiology of Hodgkin's disease. In: Mauch PM, Armitage JO, Diehl V, editors. Hodgkin's disease. Philadelphia: Lippincott Williams & Wilkins; p. 61.

2778. Mufti GJ, Bennett JM, Goasguen J, et al. (2008). Diagnosis and classification of myelodysplastic syndrome: International Working Group on Morphology of myelodysplastic syndrome (IWGM-MDS) consensus proposals for the definition and enumeration of myeloblasts and ring sideroblasts. Haematologica. 93:1712–7. PMID:18838480

2779. Mughal TI, Cross NC, Padron E, et al. (2015). An International MDS/MPN Working Group's perspective and recommendations on molecular pathogenesis, diagnosis and clinical characterization of myelodysplastic/myeloproliferative neoplasms. Haematologica. 100:1117–30. PMID:26341525

2780. Mullaney BP, Ng VL, Herndier BG, et al. (2000). Comparative genomic analyses of primary effusion lymphoma. Arch Pathol Lab Med. 124:824–6. PMID:10835513

2781. Mulligan SP, Matutes E, Dearden C, et al. (1991). Splenic lymphoma with villous lymphocytes: natural history and response to therapy in 50 cases. Br J Haematol. 78:206–9. PMID:2064958

2782. Mullighan CG, Kennedy A, Zhou X, et al. (2007). Pediatric acute myeloid leukemia with NPM1 mutations is characterized by a gene expression profile with dysregulated HOX gene expression distinct from MLL-rearranged leukemias. Leukemia. 21:2000–9. PMID:17597811

2783. Muñoz L, Nomdedéu JF, Villamor N, et al. (2003). Acute myeloid leukemia with MLL rearrangements: clinicobiological features, prognostic impact and value of flow cytometry in the detection of residual leukemic cells. Leukemia. 17:76–82. PMID:12529663

2784. Muñoz-Mármol AM, Sanz C, Tapia G, et al. (2013). MYC status determination in aggressive B-cell lymphoma: the impact of FISH probe selection. Histopathology. 63:418–24. PMID:23795946

2785. Munshi NC, Digumarthy S, Rahemtullah A (2008). Case records of the Massachusetts General Hospital. Case 13-2008. A 46-year-old man with rheumatoid arthritis and lymphadenopathy. N Engl J Med. 358:1838–48. PMID:18434654

2786. Murakami I, Matsushita M, Iwasaki T, et al. (2014). High viral load of Merkel cell polyomavirus DNA sequences in Langerhans cell sarcoma tissues. Infect Agent Cancer. 9:15. PMID:24834110

2787. Murakami I, Matsushita M, Iwasaki T, et al. (2015). Interleukin-1 loop model for pathogenesis of Langerhans cell histiocytosis. Cell Commun Signal. 13:13. PMID:25889448

2788. Muramatsu H, Makishima H, Jankowska AM, et al. (2010). Mutations of an E3 ubiquitin ligase c-Cbl but not TET2 mutations are

pathogenic in juvenile myelomonocytic leukemia. Blood. 115:1969–75. PMID:20008299

2789. Murase T, Yamaguchi M, Suzuki R, et al. (2007). Intravascular large B-cell lymphoma (IVLBCL): a clinicopathologic study of 96 cases with special reference to the immunophenotypic heterogeneity of CD5. Blood. 109:478–85. PMID:16985183

2790. Muris JJ, Meijer CJ, Vos W, et al. (2006). Immunohistochemical profiling based on Bcl-2, CD10 and MUM1 expression improves risk stratification in patients with primary nodal diffuse large B cell lymphoma. J Pathol. 208:714–23. PMID:16400625

2791. Murphy S, Peterson P, Iland H, et al. (1997). Experience of the Polycythemia Vera Study Group with essential thrombocythemia: a final report on diagnostic criteria, survival, and leukemic transition by treatment. Semin Hematol. 34:29–39. PMID:9025160

2792. Murphy SB (1978). Childhood non-Hodgkin's lymphoma. N Engl J Med. 299:1446–8. PMID:362210

2793. Murphy SB, Hustu HO (1980). A randomized trial of combined modality therapy of childhood non-Hodgkin's lymphoma. Cancer. 45:630–7. PMID:6986967

2794. Murray A, Cuevas EC, Jones DB, et al. (1995). Study of the immunohistochemistry and T cell clonality of enteropathy-associated T cell lymphoma. Am J Pathol. 146:509–19. PMID:7856760

2795. Murray JM, Morgello S (2004). Polyomaviruses and primary central nervous system lymphomas. Neurology. 63:1299–301. PMID:15477558

2796. Mustjoki S, Ekblom M, Arstila TP, et al. (2009). Clonal expansion of T/NK-cells during tyrosine kinase inhibitor dasatinib therapy. Leukemia. 23:1398–405. PMID:19295545

2797. Müller C, Murawski N, Wiesen MH, et al. (2012). The role of sex and weight on rituximab clearance and serum elimination half-life in elderly patients with DLBCL. Blood. 119:3276–84. PMID:22337718

2798. Müschen M, Rajewsky K, Bräuninger A, et al. (2000). Rare occurrence of classical Hodgkin's disease as a T cell lymphoma. J Exp Med. 191:387–94. PMID:10637283

2799. Möller P, Lämmler B, Herrmann B, et al. (1986). The primary mediastinal clear cell lymphoma of B-cell type has variable defects in MHC antigen expression. Immunology. 59:411–7. PMID:3491784

2800. Möller P, Moldenhauer G, Momburg F, et al. (1987). Mediastinal lymphoma of clear cell type is a tumor corresponding to terminal steps of B cell differentiation. Blood. 69:1087–95. PMID:3103712

2801. Nacheva EP, Grace CD, Brazma D, et al. (2013). Does BCR/ABL1 positive acute myeloid leukaemia exist? Br J Haematol. 161:541–50. PMID:23521501

2802. Nachman JB, Heerema NA, Sather H, et al. (2007). Outcome of treatment in children with hypodiploid acute lymphoblastic leukemia. Blood. 110:1112–5. PMID:17473063

2803. Nador RG, Cesarman E, Chadburn A, et al. (1996). Primary effusion lymphoma: a distinct clinicopathologic entity associated with the Kaposi's sarcoma-associated herpes virus. Blood. 88:645–56. PMID:8695812

2804. Nador RG, Chadburn A, Gundappa G, et al. (2003). Human immunodeficiency virus (HIV)-associated polymorphic lymphoproliferative disorders. Am J Surg Pathol. 27:293–302. PMID:12604885

2805. Nagai K, Nakano N, Iwai T, et al. (2014). Pediatric subcutaneous panniculitis-like T-cell lymphoma with favorable result by immunosuppressive therapy: a report of two cases. Pediatr Hematol Oncol. 31:528–33. PMID:24684413

2806. Nair C, Chopra H, Shinde S, et al. (1995). Immunophenotype and ultrastructural studies in blast crisis of chronic myeloid leukemia. Leuk Lymphoma. 19:309–13. PMID:8535224
2807. Nairismägi ML, Tan J, Lim JQ, et al. (2016). JAK-STAT and G-protein-coupled receptor signaling pathways are frequently altered in epitheliotropic intestinal T-cell lymphoma. Leukemia. 30:1311–9. PMID:26854024
2808. Nakagawa M, Schmitz R, Xiao W, et al. (2014). Gain-of-function CCR4 mutations in adult T cell leukemia/lymphoma. J Exp Med. 211:2497–505. PMID:25488980
2809. Nakajima Y, Waku M, Kojima A, et al. (1996). [Prognosis of the surgical treatment for non-Hodgkin lymphoma originating from chronic tuberculous empyema–analysis of 11 cases with pleuropneumonectomy]. Nihon Kyobu Geka Gakkai Zasshi. 44:484–92. PMID:8666866
2810. Nakamichi N, Fukuhara S, Aozasa K, et al. (2008). NK-cell intravascular lymphomatosis–a mini-review. Eur J Haematol. 81:1–7. PMID:18462254
2811. Nakamura N, Ohshima K, Abe M, et al. (2007). Demonstration of chimeric DNA of bcl-2 and immunoglobulin heavy chain in follicular lymphoma and subsequent Hodgkin lymphoma from the same patient. J Clin Exp Hematop. 47:9–13. PMID:17510532
2812. Nakamura S, Hara K, Suchi T, et al. (1988). Interdigitating cell sarcoma. A morphologic, immunohistologic, and enzyme-histochemical study. Cancer. 61:562–8. PMID:3338024
2813. Nakamura S, Koshikawa T, Kitoh K, et al. (1994). Interdigitating cell sarcoma: a morphologic and immunologic study of lymph node lesions in four cases. Pathol Int. 44:374–86. PMID:8044307
2814. Nakamura S, Shiota M, Nakagawa A, et al. (1997). Anaplastic large cell lymphoma: a distinct molecular pathologic entity: a reappraisal with special reference to p80(NPM/ALK) expression. Am J Surg Pathol. 21:1420–32. PMID:9414185
2815. Nakase K, Sartor M, Bradstock (1998). Detection of myeloperoxidase by flow cytometry in acute leukemia. Cytometry. 34:198–202. PMID:9725460
2816. Nakashima MO, Durkin L, Bodo J, et al. (2014). Utility and diagnostic pitfalls of SOX11 monoclonal antibodies in mantle cell lymphoma and other lymphoproliferative disorders. Appl Immunohistochem Mol Morphol. 22:720–7. PMID:25229384
2817. Nakashima Y, Tagawa H, Suzuki R, et al. (2005). Genome-wide array-based comparative genomic hybridization of natural killer cell lymphoma/leukemia: different genomic alteration patterns of aggressive NK-cell leukemia and extranodal Nk/T-cell lymphoma, nasal type. Genes Chromosomes Cancer. 44:247–55. PMID:16049916
2818. Nakatsuka S, Yao M, Hoshida Y, et al. (2002). Pyothorax-associated lymphoma: a review of 106 cases. J Clin Oncol. 20:4255–60. PMID:12377970
2819. Nalesnik MA, Jaffe R, Starzl TE, et al. (1988). The pathology of posttransplant lymphoproliferative disorders occurring in the setting of cyclosporine A-prednisone immunosuppression. Am J Pathol. 133:173–92. PMID:2845789
2820. Nalesnik MA, Randhawa P, Demetris AJ, et al. (1993). Lymphoma resembling Hodgkin disease after posttransplant lymphoproliferative disorder in a liver transplant recipient. Cancer. 72:2568–73. PMID:8402478
2821. Nam-Cha SH, Montes-Moreno S, Salcedo MT, et al. (2009). Lymphocyte-rich classical Hodgkin's lymphoma: distinctive tumor and microenvironment markers. Mod Pathol. 22:1006–15. PMID:19465900
2822. Nam-Cha SH, Roncador G, Sanchez-Verde L, et al. (2008). PD-1, a follicular T-cell marker useful for recognizing nodular lymphocyte-predominant Hodgkin lymphoma. Am J Surg Pathol. 32:1252–7. PMID:18594468
2823. Nangalia J, Massie CE, Baxter EJ, et al. (2013). Somatic CALR mutations in myeloproliferative neoplasms with nonmutated JAK2. N Engl J Med. 369:2391–405. PMID:24325359
2824. Nardi V, Winkfield KM, Ok CY, et al. (2012). Acute myeloid leukemia and myelodysplastic syndromes after radiation therapy are similar to de novo disease and differ from other therapy-related myeloid neoplasms. J Clin Oncol. 30:2340–7. PMID:22585703
2825. Narducci MG, Scala E, Bresin A, et al. (2006). Skin homing of Sézary cells involves SDF-1-CXCR4 signaling and down-regulation of CD26/dipeptidylpeptidase IV. Blood. 107:1108–15. PMID:16204308
2826. Naresh KN, Ibrahim HA, Lazzi S, et al. (2011). Diagnosis of Burkitt lymphoma using an algorithmic approach–applicable in both resource-poor and resource-rich countries. Br J Haematol. 154:770–6. PMID:21718280
2827. Narimatsu H, Ota Y, Kami M, et al. (2007). Clinicopathological features of pyothorax-associated lymphoma; a retrospective survey involving 98 patients. Ann Oncol. 18:122–8. PMID:17043091
2828. Narita M, Watanabe N, Yamahira A, et al. (2009). A leukemic plasmacytoid dendritic cell line, PMDC05, with the ability to secrete IFN-alpha by stimulation via Toll-like receptors and present antigens to naïve T cells. Leuk Res. 33:1224–32. PMID:19443030
2829. Narumi H, Kojima K, Matsuo Y, et al. (2004). T-cell large granular lymphocytic leukemia occurring after autologous peripheral blood stem cell transplantation. Bone Marrow Transplant. 33:99–101. PMID:14704662
2830. Nascimento AF, Pinkus JL, Pinkus GS (2004). Clusterin, a marker for anaplastic large cell lymphoma immunohistochemical profile in hematopoietic and nonhematopoietic malignant neoplasms. Am J Clin Pathol. 121:709–17. PMID:15151211
2831. Nash R, McSweeney P, Zambello R, et al. (1993). Clonal studies of CD3- lymphoproliferative disease of granular lymphocytes. Blood. 81:2363–8. PMID:8097633
2832. Nash RA, Dansey R, Storek J, et al. (2003). Epstein-Barr virus-associated post-transplantation lymphoproliferative disorder after high-dose immunosuppressive therapy and autologous CD34-selected hematopoietic stem cell transplantation for severe autoimmune diseases. Biol Blood Marrow Transplant. 9:583–91. PMID:14506660
2832A. Nassif S, Ozdemirli M (2013). EBV-positive low-grade marginal zone lymphoma in the breast with massive amyloid deposition arising in a heart transplant patient: a report of an unusual case. Pediatr Transplant. 17:E141–5. PMID:23773403
2833. Nathwani BN, Anderson JR, Armitage JO, et al. (1999). Clinical significance of follicular lymphoma with monocytoid B cells. Non-Hodgkin's Lymphoma Classification Project. Hum Pathol. 30:263–8. PMID:10088543
2834. Nathwani BN, Anderson JR, Armitage JO, et al. (1999). Marginal zone B-cell lymphoma: A clinical comparison of nodal and mucosa-associated lymphoid tissue types. Non-Hodgkin's Lymphoma Classification Project. J Clin Oncol. 17:2486–92. PMID:10561313
2835. Nathwani BN, Metter GE, Miller TP, et al. (1986). What should be the morphologic criteria for the subdivision of follicular lymphomas? Blood. 68:837–45. PMID:3530348
2836. National Cancer Institute sponsored study of classifications of non-Hodgkin's lymphomas: summary and description of a working formulation for clinical usage; the Non-Hodgkin's Lymphoma Pathologic Classification Project (1982). Cancer. 49:2112–35. PMID:6896167
2837. National Research Council (US) Committee on a Framework for Developing a New Taxonomy of Disease (2011). Toward precision medicine: building a knowledge network for biomedical research and a new taxonomy of disease. Washington (DC): National Academies Press (US).
2838. Natkunam Y, Farinha P, Hsi ED, et al. (2008). LMO2 protein expression predicts survival in patients with diffuse large B-cell lymphoma treated with anthracycline-based chemotherapy with and without rituximab. J Clin Oncol. 26:447–54. PMID:18086797
2839. Natkunam Y, Warnke RA, Haghighi B, et al. (2000). Co-expression of CD56 and CD30 in lymphomas with primary presentation in the skin: clinicopathologic, immunohistochemical and molecular analyses of seven cases. J Cutan Pathol. 27:392–9. PMID:10955685
2840. Natkunam Y, Zhao S, Mason DY, et al. (2007). The oncoprotein LMO2 is expressed in normal germinal-center B cells and in human B-cell lymphomas. Blood. 109:1636–42. PMID:17038524
2841. Navarro A, Clot G, Royo C, et al. (2012). Molecular subsets of mantle cell lymphoma defined by the IGHV mutational status and SOX11 expression have distinct biologic and clinical features. Cancer Res. 72:5307–16. PMID:22915760
2842. Navarro JT, Ribera JM, Mate JL, et al. (2003). Hepatosplenic T-gammadelta lymphoma in a patient with Crohn's disease treated with azathioprine. Leuk Lymphoma. 44:531–3. PMID:12688327
2843. Navas IC, Ortiz-Romero PL, Villuendas R, et al. (2000). p16(INK4a) gene alterations are frequent in lesions of mycosis fungoides. Am J Pathol. 156:1565–72. PMID:10793068
2844. Navid F, Mosijczuk AD, Head DR, et al. (1999). Acute lymphoblastic leukemia with the (8;14)(q24;q32) translocation and FAB L3 morphology associated with a B-precursor immunophenotype: the Pediatric Oncology Group experience. Leukemia. 13:135–41. PMID:10049049
2845. Nedeljkovic M, He S, Szer J, et al. (2014). Chronic neutrophilia associated with myeloma: is it clonal? Leuk Lymphoma. 55:439–40. PMID:23713456
2846. Neiman RS, Barcos M, Berard C, et al. (1981). Granulocytic sarcoma: a clinicopathologic study of 61 biopsied cases. Cancer. 48:1426–37. PMID:7023656
2847. Nelson AA, Harrington AM, Kroft S, et al. (2016). Presentation and management of post-allogeneic transplantation EBV-positive mucocutaneous ulcer. Bone Marrow Transplant. 51:300–2. PMID:26457913
2848. Nelson BP, Nalesnik MA, Bahler DW, et al. (2000). Epstein-Barr virus-negative post-transplant lymphoproliferative disorders: a distinct entity? Am J Surg Pathol. 24:375–85. PMID:10716151
2849. Nelson BP, Wolniak KL, Evens A, et al. (2012). Early posttransplant lymphoproliferative disease: clinicopathologic features and correlation with mTOR signaling pathway activation. Am J Clin Pathol. 138:568–78. PMID:23010712
2850. Nelson BP, Wolniak KL, Evens A, et al. (2012). Early posttransplant lymphoproliferative disease: clinicopathologic features and correlation with mTOR signaling pathway activation. Am J Clin Pathol. 138:568–78. PMID:23010712
2851. Nelson DS, Quispel W, Badalian-Very G, et al. (2014). Somatic activating ARAF mutations in Langerhans cell histiocytosis. Blood. 123:3152–5. PMID:24652991
2852. Nelson DS, van Halteren A, Quispel WT, et al. (2015). MAP2K1 and MAP3K1 mutations in Langerhans cell histiocytosis. Genes Chromosomes Cancer. 54:361–8. PMID:25899310
2853. Neubauer A, Thiede C, Morgner A, et al. (1997). Cure of Helicobacter pylori infection and duration of remission of low-grade gastric mucosa-associated lymphoid tissue lymphoma. J Natl Cancer Inst. 89:1350–5. PMID:9308704
2854. Neukirchen J, Schoonen WM, Strupp C, et al. (2011). Incidence and prevalence of myelodysplastic syndromes: data from the Düsseldorf MDS-registry. Leuk Res. 35:1591–6. PMID:21708407
2855. Neumann M, Coskun E, Fransecky L, et al. (2013). FLT3 mutations in early T-cell precursor ALL characterize a stem cell like leukemia and imply the clinical use of tyrosine kinase inhibitors. PLoS One. 8:e53190. PMID:23359050
2856. Neumann M, Heesch S, Schlee C, et al. (2013). Whole-exome sequencing in adult ETP-ALL reveals a high rate of DNMT3A mutations. Blood. 121:4749–52. PMID:23603912
2857. Neuwirtová R, Mociková K, Musilová J, et al. (1996). Mixed myelodysplastic and myeloproliferative syndromes. Leuk Res. 20:717–26. PMID:8947580
2858. Ng CS, Lo ST, Chan JK, et al. (1997). CD56+ putative natural killer cell lymphomas: production of cytolytic effectors and related proteins mediating tumor cell apoptosis? Hum Pathol. 28:1276–82. PMID:9385933
2859. Ng SB, Lai KW, Murugaya S, et al. (2004). Nasal-type extranodal natural killer/T-cell lymphomas: a clinicopathologic and genotypic study of 42 cases in Singapore. Mod Pathol. 17:1097–107. PMID:15195107
2860. Ngo VN, Young RM, Schmitz R, et al. (2011). Oncogenically active MYD88 mutations in human lymphoma. Nature. 470:115–9. PMID:21179087
2861. Ngoma T, Adde M, Durosinmi M, et al. (2012). Treatment of Burkitt lymphoma in equatorial Africa using a simple three-drug combination followed by a salvage regimen for patients with persistent or recurrent disease. Br J Haematol. 158:749–62. PMID:22844968
2862. Nguyen DT, Diamond LW, Hansmann ML, et al. (1994). Follicular dendritic cell sarcoma: identification by monoclonal antibodies in paraffin sections. Appl Immunohistochem. 2:60–4.
2863. Ni H, Barosi G, Hoffman R (2006). Quantitative evaluation of bone marrow angiogenesis in idiopathic myelofibrosis. Am J Clin Pathol. 126:241–7. PMID:16891200
2864. Ni H, Barosi G, Rondelli D, et al. (2005). Studies of the site and distribution of CD34+ cells in idiopathic myelofibrosis. Am J Clin Pathol. 123:833–9. PMID:15899773
2865. Nichols CR, Roth BJ, Heerema N, et al. (1990). Hematologic neoplasia associated with primary mediastinal germ-cell tumors. N Engl J Med. 322:1425–9. PMID:2158625
2866. Nickels EM, Soodalter J, Churpek JE, et al. (2013). Recognizing familial myeloid leukemia in adults. Ther Adv Hematol. 4:254–69. PMID:23926458
2866A. Nicolae A, Ganapathi K, Pittaluga S, et al. (2015). Aggressive NK-cell leukemia/lymphoma, EBV-negative – a report of 5 cases [meeting abstract]. Lab Invest. 95:368A.
2867. Nicolae A, Pittaluga S, Abdullah S, et al. (2015). EBV-positive large B-cell lymphomas in young patients: a nodal lymphoma with evidence for a tolerogenic immune environment. Blood. 126:863–72. PMID:25999451
2868. Nicolae A, Pittaluga S, Venkataraman G, et al. (2013). Peripheral T-cell lymphomas of

follicular T-helper cell derivation with Hodgkin/Reed-Sternberg cells of B-cell lineage: both EBV-positive and EBV-negative variants exist. Am J Surg Pathol. 37:816–26. PMID:23598959
2869. Nicolae A, Xi L, Pittaluga S, et al. (2014). Frequent STAT5B mutations in γδ hepatosplenic T-cell lymphomas. Leukemia. 28:2244–8. PMID:24947020
2869A. Nicolae A, Xi L, Pham TH, et al. (2016). Mutations in the JAK/STAT and RAS signaling pathways are common in intestinal T-cell lymphomas. Leukemia 30:2245-47. PMID:27389054
2870. Nicolae-Cristea AR, Benner MF, Zoutman WH, et al. (2015). Diagnostic and prognostic significance of CDKN2A/CDKN2B deletions in patients with transformed mycosis fungoides and primary cutaneous CD30-positive lymphoproliferative disease. Br J Dermatol. 172:784–8. PMID:25308604
2870A. Niederwieser C, Kohlschmidt J, Volinia S, et al. (2015). Prognostic and biologic significance of DNMT3B expression in older patients with cytogenetically normal primary acute myeloid leukemia. Leukemia. 29:567–75. PMID:25204569
2871. Niemeyer CM (2014). RAS diseases in children. Haematologica. 99:1653–62. PMID:25420281
2872. Niemeyer CM, Arico M, Basso G, et al. (1997). Chronic myelomonocytic leukemia in childhood: a retrospective analysis of 110 cases. Blood. 89:3534–43. PMID:9160658
2873. Niemeyer CM, Baumann I (2011). Classification of childhood aplastic anemia and myelodysplastic syndrome. Hematology Am Soc Hematol Educ Program. 2011:84–9. PMID:22160017
2874. Niemeyer CM, Kang MW, Shin DH, et al. (2010). Germline CBL mutations cause developmental abnormalities and predispose to juvenile myelomonocytic leukemia. Nat Genet. 42:794–800. PMID:20694012
2875. Nieters A, Kallinowski B, Brennan P, et al. (2006). Hepatitis C and risk of lymphoma: results of the European multicenter case-control study EPILYMPH. Gastroenterology. 131:1879–86. PMID:17087949
2876. Nieto WG, Almeida J, Romero A, et al. (2009). Increased frequency (12%) of circulating chronic lymphocytic leukemia-like B-cell clones in healthy subjects using a highly sensitive multicolor flow cytometry approach. Blood. 114:33–7. PMID:19420353
2877. Nievergall E, Ramshaw HS, Yong AS, et al. (2014). Monoclonal antibody targeting of IL-3 receptor α with CSL362 effectively depletes CML progenitor and stem cells. Blood. 123:1218–28. PMID:24363400
2878. Niitsu N, Okamoto M, Miura I, et al. (2009). Clinical features and prognosis of de novo diffuse large B-cell lymphoma with t(14;18) and 8q24/c-MYC translocations. Leukemia. 23:777–83. PMID:19151788
2879. Niitsu N, Okamoto M, Tamaru JI, et al. (2010). Clinicopathologic characteristics and treatment outcome of the addition of rituximab to chemotherapy for CD5-positive in comparison with CD5-negative diffuse large B-cell lymphoma. Ann Oncol. 21:2069–74. PMID:20231297
2880. Nijmegen breakage syndrome; the International Nijmegen Breakage Syndrome Study Group (2000). Arch Dis Child. 82:400–6. PMID:10799436
2881. Nikpour M, Scharenberg C, Liu A, et al. (2013). The transporter ABCB7 is a mediator of the phenotype of acquired refractory anemia with ring sideroblasts. Leukemia. 27:889–96. PMID:23070040
2882. Nishiu M, Tomita Y, Nakatsuka S, et al. (2004). Distinct pattern of gene expression in pyothorax-associated lymphoma (PAL), a lymphoma developing in long-standing inflammation. Cancer Sci. 95:828–34. PMID:15504251
2883. Nitta Y, Iwatsuki K, Kimura H, et al. (2005). Fatal natural killer cell lymphoma arising in a patient with a crop of Epstein-Barr virus-associated disorders. Eur J Dermatol. 15:503–6. PMID:16280311
2884. Nizze H, Cogliatti SB, von Schilling C, et al. (1991). Monocytoid B-cell lymphoma: morphological variants and relationship to low-grade B-cell lymphoma of the mucosa-associated lymphoid tissue. Histopathology. 18:403–14. PMID:1885166
2885. Nodit L, Bahler DW, Jacobs SA, et al. (2003). Indolent mantle cell lymphoma with nodal involvement and mutated immunoglobulin heavy chain genes. Hum Pathol. 34:1030–4. PMID:14608537
2886. Noel P, Kyle RA (1987). Plasma cell leukemia: an evaluation of response to therapy. Am J Med. 83:1062–8. PMID:3503574
2887. Noetzli L, Lo RW, Lee-Sherick AB, et al. (2015). Germline mutations in ETV6 are associated with thrombocytopenia, red cell macrocytosis and predisposition to lymphoblastic leukemia. Nat Genet. 47:535–8. PMID:25807284
2888. Nogová L, Reineke T, Brillant C, et al. (2008). Lymphocyte-predominant and classical Hodgkin's lymphoma: a comprehensive analysis from the German Hodgkin Study Group. J Clin Oncol. 26:434–9. PMID:18086799
2889. Nomdedéu J, Bussaglia E, Villamor N, et al. (2011). Immunophenotype of acute myeloid leukemia with NPM mutations: prognostic impact of the leukemic compartment size. Leuk Res. 35:163–8. PMID:20542566
2889A. Nomdedéu J, Hoyos M, Carricondo M, et al. (2012). Adverse impact of IDH1 and IDH2 mutations in primary AML: experience of the Spanish CETLAM group. Leuk Res. 36:990–7. PMID:22520341
2890. Nomdedéu JF, Mateu R, Altès A, et al. (1999). Enhanced myeloid specificity of CD117 compared with CD13 and CD33. Leuk Res. 23:341–7. PMID:10229319
2891. Nonami A, Yokoyama T, Takeshita M, et al. (2004). Human herpes virus 8-negative primary effusion lymphoma (PEL) in a patient after repeated chylous ascites and chylothorax. Intern Med. 43:236–42. PMID:15098608
2892. Nordström L, Sernbo S, Eden P, et al. (2014). SOX11 and TP53 add prognostic information to MIPI in a homogenously treated cohort of mantle cell lymphoma–a Nordic Lymphoma Group study. Br J Haematol. 166:98–108. PMID:24684350
2893. Noris P, Favier R, Alessi MC, et al. (2013). ANKRD26-related thrombocytopenia and myeloid malignancies. Blood. 122:1987–9. PMID:24030261
2894. Noris P, Perrotta S, Seri M, et al. (2011). Mutations in ANKRD26 are responsible for a frequent form of inherited thrombocytopenia: analysis of 78 patients from 21 families. Blood. 117:6673–80. PMID:21467542
2895. Norton A, Fisher C, Liu H, et al. (2007). Analysis of JAK3, JAK2, and C-MPL mutations in transient myeloproliferative disorder and myeloid leukemia of Down syndrome blasts in children with Down syndrome. Blood. 110:1077–9. PMID:17644747
2896. Norton AJ, Matthews J, Pappa V, et al. (1995). Mantle cell lymphoma: natural history defined in a serially biopsied population over a 20-year period. Ann Oncol. 6:249–56. PMID:7612490
2896A. Nosaka K, Miyamoto T, Sakai T, et al. (2002). Mechanism of hypercalcemia in adult T-cell leukemia: overexpression of receptor activator of nuclear factor kappaB ligand on adult T-cell leukemia cells. Blood. 99:634-40. PMID:11781248
2897. Notarangelo L, Casanova JL, Conley ME, et al. (2006). Primary immunodeficiency diseases: an update from the International Union of Immunological Societies Primary Immunodeficiency Diseases Classification Committee Meeting in Budapest, 2005. J Allergy Clin Immunol. 117:883–96. PMID:16680902
2898. Novak U, Rinaldi A, Kwee I, et al. (2009). The NF-kappaB negative regulator TNFAIP3 (A20) is inactivated by somatic mutations and genomic deletions in marginal zone lymphomas. Blood. 113:4918–21. PMID:19258598
2899. Novakovic BJ, Novakovic S, Frkovic-Grazio S (2006). A single-center report on clinical features and treatment response in patients with intestinal T cell non-Hodgkin's lymphomas. Oncol Rep. 16:191–5. PMID:16786145
2900. Novella E, D'Emilio A, Bernardi M, et al. (2009). Atypical myeloproliferative disorder presenting FIP1L1-PDGFRA rearrangement. Haematologica. 94 Suppl. 4:200.
2901. Nowak D, Le Toriellec E, Stern MH, et al. (2009). Molecular allelokaryotyping of T-cell prolymphocytic leukemia cells with high density single nucleotide polymorphism arrays identifies novel common genomic lesions and acquired uniparental disomy. Haematologica. 94:518–27. PMID:19278963
2902. Nowakowski GS, LaPlant B, Habermann TM, et al. (2011). Lenalidomide can be safely combined with R-CHOP (R2CHOP) in the initial chemotherapy for aggressive B-cell lymphomas: phase I study. Leukemia. 25:1877–81. PMID:21720383
2903. Nowakowski GS, LaPlant B, Macon WR, et al. (2015). Lenalidomide combined with R-CHOP overcomes negative prognostic impact of non-germinal center B-cell phenotype in newly diagnosed diffuse large B-Cell lymphoma: a phase II study. J Clin Oncol. 33:251–7. PMID:25135992
2905. Nowell PC, Hungerford DA (1960). Chromosome studies on normal and leukemic human leukocytes. J Natl Cancer Inst. 25:85–109. PMID:14427847
2906. Noy A, Lee JY, Cesarman E, et al. (2015). AMC 048: modified CODOX-M/IVAC-rituximab is safe and effective for HIV-associated Burkitt lymphoma. Blood. 126:160–6. PMID:25957391
2907. Nucifora G, Laricchia-Robbio L, Senyuk V (2006). EVI1 and hematopoietic disorders: history and perspectives. Gene. 368:1–11. PMID:16314052
2908. Nygren L, Baumgartner Wennerholm S, Klimkowska M, et al. (2012). Prognostic role of SOX11 in a population-based cohort of mantle cell lymphoma. Blood. 119:4215–23. PMID:22431568
2909. Nyman H, Jerkeman M, Karjalainen-Lindsberg ML, et al. (2009). Prognostic impact of activated B-cell focused classification in diffuse large B-cell lymphoma patients treated with R-CHOP. Mod Pathol. 22:1094–101. PMID:19448593
2910. O'Briain DS, Kennedy MJ, Daly PA, et al. (1989). Multiple lymphomatous polyposis of the gastrointestinal tract. A clinicopathologically distinctive form of non-Hodgkin's lymphoma of B-cell centrocytic type. Am J Surg Pathol. 13:691–9. PMID:2665536
2911. O'Brien S, Radich JP, Abboud CN, et al. (2014). Chronic myelogenous leukemia, version 1.2015. J Natl Compr Canc Netw. 12:1590–610. PMID:25361806
2912. O'Conor GT (1963). SIGNIFICANT ASPECTS OF CHILDHOOD LYMPHOMA IN AFRICA. Cancer Res. 23:1514–8. PMID:14072690
2913. O'Farrelly C, Feighery C, O'Briain DS, et al. (1986). Humoral response to wheat protein in patients with coeliac disease and enteropathy associated T cell lymphoma. Br Med J (Clin Res Ed). 293:908–10. PMID:3094712
2914. O'Mahony S, Howdle PD, Losowsky MS (1996). Review article: management of patients with non-responsive coeliac disease. Aliment Pharmacol Ther. 10:671–80. PMID:8899074
2915. O'Malley DP (2007). Benign extramedullary myeloid proliferations. Mod Pathol. 20:405–15. PMID:17334344
2916. O'Malley DP, Agrawal R, Grimm KE, et al. (2015). Evidence of BRAF V600E in indeterminate cell tumor and interdigitating dendritic cell sarcoma. Ann Diagn Pathol. 19:113–6. PMID:25787243
2917. O'Malley DP, Auerbach A, Weiss LM (2015). Practical Applications in Immunohistochemistry: Evaluation of Diffuse Large B-Cell Lymphoma and Related Large B-Cell Lymphomas. Arch Pathol Lab Med. 139:1094–107. PMID:25554969
2918. O'Malley DP, Kim YS, Perkins SL, et al. (2005). Morphologic and immunohistochemical evaluation of splenic hematopoietic proliferations in neoplastic and benign disorders. Mod Pathol. 18:1550–61. PMID:16118626
2919. O'Neil J, Shank J, Cusson N, et al. (2004). TAL1/SCL induces leukemia by inhibiting the transcriptional activity of E47/HEB. Cancer Cell. 5:587–96. PMID:15193261
2920. O'Shea JJ, Jaffe ES, Lane HC, et al. (1987). Peripheral T cell lymphoma presenting as hypereosinophilia with vasculitis. Clinical, pathologic, and immunologic features. Am J Med. 82:539–45. PMID:3493692
2921. Oakes CC, Seifert M, Assenov Y, et al. (2016). DNA methylation dynamics during B cell maturation underlie a continuum of disease phenotypes in chronic lymphocytic leukemia. Nat Genet. 48:253–64. PMID:26780610
2922. Obermann EC, Csato M, Dirnhofer S, et al. (2009). Aberrations of the MYC gene in unselected cases of diffuse large B-cell lymphoma are rare and unpredictable by morphological or immunohistochemical assessment. J Clin Pathol. 62:754–6. PMID:19638549
2923. Obermann EC, Diss TC, Hamoudi RA, et al. (2004). Loss of heterozygosity at chromosome 9p21 is a frequent finding in enteropathy-type T-cell lymphoma. J Pathol. 202:252–62. PMID:14743509
2924. Ocio EM, del Carpio D, Caballero Á, et al. (2011). Differential diagnosis of IgM MGUS and WM according to B-lymphoid infiltration by morphology and flow cytometry. Clin Lymphoma Myeloma Leuk. 11:93–5. PMID:21454201
2925. Ocio EM, Schop RF, Gonzalez B, et al. (2007). 6q deletion in Waldenström macroglobulinemia is associated with features of adverse prognosis. Br J Haematol. 136:80–6. PMID:17222197
2926. Ocqueteau M, Orfao A, Almeida J, et al. (1998). Immunophenotypic characterization of plasma cells from monoclonal gammopathy of undetermined significance patients. Implications for the differential diagnosis between MGUS and multiple myeloma. Am J Pathol. 152:1655–65. PMID:9626070
2927. Odame I, Li P, Lau L, et al. (2006). Pulmonary Langerhans cell histiocytosis: a variable disease in childhood. Pediatr Blood Cancer. 47:889–93. PMID:16276522
2928. Odejide O, Weigert O, Lane AA, et al. (2014). A targeted mutational landscape of angioimmunoblastic T-cell lymphoma. Blood. 123:1293–6. PMID:24345752
2929. Odenike O, Anastasi J, Le Beau MM (2011). Myelodysplastic syndromes. Clin Lab Med. 31:763–84. PMID:22118747
2930. Offit K, Lo Coco F, Louie DC, et al. (1994). Rearrangement of the bcl-6 gene as a prognostic marker in diffuse large-cell lymphoma. N

Engl J Med. 331:74–80. PMID:8208268
2931. Offit K, Parsa NZ, Gaidano G, et al. (1993). 6q deletions define distinct clinico-pathologic subsets of non-Hodgkin's lymphoma. Blood. 82:2157–62. PMID:8104536
2932. Offner F, Samoilova O, Osmanov E, et al. (2015). Frontline rituximab, cyclophosphamide, doxorubicin, and prednisone with bortezomib (VR-CAP) or vincristine (R-CHOP) for non-GCB DLBCL. Blood. 126:1893–901. PMID:26232170
2933. Ogata K, Della Porta MG, Malcovati L, et al. (2009). Diagnostic utility of flow cytometry in low-grade myelodysplastic syndromes: a prospective validation study. Haematologica. 94:1066–74. PMID:19546439
2934. Ogata K, Kakumoto K, Matsuda A, et al. (2012). Differences in blast immunophenotypes among disease types in myelodysplastic syndromes: a multicenter validation study. Leuk Res. 36:1229–36. PMID:22682984
2935. Ogata K, Kishikawa Y, Satoh C, et al. (2006). Diagnostic application of flow cytometric characteristics of CD34+ cells in low-grade myelodysplastic syndromes. Blood. 108:1037–44. PMID:16574954
2936. Ogata K, Nakamura K, Yokose N, et al. (2002). Clinical significance of phenotypic features of blasts in patients with myelodysplastic syndrome. Blood. 100:3887–96. PMID:12393641
2937. Ogwang MD, Bhatia K, Biggar RJ, et al. (2008). Incidence and geographic distribution of endemic Burkitt lymphoma in northern Uganda revisited. Int J Cancer. 123:2658–63. PMID:18767045
2938. Oh J, Yoon H, Shin DK, et al. (2012). A case of successful management of HHV-8, EBV germinotropic lymphoproliferative disorder (GLD). Int J Hematol. 95:107–11. PMID:22167655
2939. Ohanian M, Kantarjian HM, Quintas-Cardama A, et al. (2014). Tyrosine kinase inhibitors as initial therapy for patients with chronic myeloid leukemia in accelerated phase. Clin Lymphoma Myeloma Leuk. 14:155–162.e1. PMID:24332214
2940. Ohba R, Furuyama K, Yoshida K, et al. (2013). Clinical and genetic characteristics of congenital sideroblastic anemia: comparison with myelodysplastic syndrome with ring sideroblast (MDS-RS). Ann Hematol. 92:1–9. PMID:22983749
2941. Ohgami RS, Arber DA, Zehnder JL, et al. (2013). Indolent T-lymphoblastic proliferation (iT-LBP): a review of clinical and pathologic features and distinction from malignant T-lymphoblastic lymphoma. Adv Anat Pathol. 20:137–40. PMID:23574769
2942. Ohgami RS, Chisholm KM, Ma L, et al. (2014). E-cadherin is a specific marker for erythroid differentiation and has utility, in combination with CD117 and CD34, for enumerating myeloblasts in hematopoietic neoplasms. Am J Clin Pathol. 141:656–64. PMID:24713736
2943. Ohgami RS, Ma L, Merker JD, et al. (2015). Next-generation sequencing of acute myeloid leukemia identifies the significance of TP53, U2AF1, ASXL1, and TET2 mutations. Mod Pathol. 28:706–14. PMID:25412851
2944. Ohgami RS, Zhao S, Ohgami JK, et al. (2012). TdT+ T-lymphoblastic populations are increased in Castleman disease, in Castleman disease in association with follicular dendritic cell tumors, and in angioimmunoblastic T-cell lymphoma. Am J Surg Pathol. 36:1619–28. PMID:23060347
2945. Ohkura Y, Shindoh J, Haruta S, et al. (2015). Primary Adrenal Lymphoma Possibly Associated With Epstein-Barr Virus Reactivation Due to Immunosuppression Under Methotrexate Therapy. Medicine (Baltimore). 94:e1270. PMID:26252293
2946. Ohnishi H, Kandabashi K, Maeda Y, et al. (2006). Chronic eosinophilic leukaemia with FIP1L1-PDGFRA fusion and T6741 mutation that evolved from Langerhans cell histiocytosis with eosinophilia after chemotherapy. Br J Haematol. 134:547–9. PMID:16856885
2947. Ohno T, Stribley JA, Wu G, et al. (1997). Clonality in nodular lymphocyte-predominant Hodgkin's disease. N Engl J Med. 337:459–65. PMID:9250848
2948. Ohno Y, Amakawa R, Fukuhara S, et al. (1989). Acute transformation of chronic large granular lymphocyte leukemia associated with additional chromosome abnormality. Cancer. 64:63–7. PMID:2731121
2949. Ohsawa M, Tomita Y, Kanno H, et al. (1995). Role of Epstein-Barr virus in pleural lymphomagenesis. Mod Pathol. 8:848–53. PMID:8552574
2950. Ohshima K (2007). Pathological features of diseases associated with human T-cell leukemia virus type I. Cancer Sci. 98:772–8. PMID:17388788
2951. Ohshima K, Kimura H, Yoshino T, et al. (2008). Proposed categorization of pathological states of EBV-associated T/natural killer-cell lymphoproliferative disorder (LPD) in children and young adults: overlap with chronic active EBV infection and infantile fulminant EBV T-LPD. Pathol Int. 58:209–17. PMID:18324913
2952. Ohshima K, Mukai Y, Shiraki H, et al. (1997). Clonal integration and expression of human T-cell lymphotropic virus type I in carriers detected by polymerase chain reaction and inverse PCR. Am J Hematol. 54:306–12. PMID:9092686
2953. Ohshima K, Suzumiya J, Kato A, et al. (1997). Clonal HTLV-I-infected CD4+ T-lymphocytes and non-clonal non-HTLV-I-infected giant cells in incipient ATLL with Hodgkin-like histologic features. Int J Cancer. 72:592–8. PMID:9259396
2954. Ohshima K, Suzumiya J, Sato K, et al. (1999). Survival of patients with HTLV-I-associated lymph node lesions. J Pathol. 189:539–45. PMID:10629555
2955. Ohshima K, Suzumiya J, Shimazaki K, et al. (1997). Nasal T/NK cell lymphomas commonly express perforin and Fas ligand: important mediators of tissue damage. Histopathology. 31:444–50. PMID:9416485
2956. Ok CY, Li L, Xu-Monette ZY, et al. (2014). Prevalence and clinical implications of epstein-barr virus infection in de novo diffuse large B-cell lymphoma in Western countries. Clin Cancer Res. 20:2338–49. PMID:24583797
2957. Ok CY, Papathomas TG, Medeiros LJ, et al. (2013). EBV-positive diffuse large B-cell lymphoma of the elderly. Blood. 122:328–40. PMID:23649469
2958. Ok CY, Patel KP, Garcia-Manero G, et al. (2015). Mutational profiling of therapy-related myelodysplastic syndromes and acute myeloid leukemia by next generation sequencing, a comparison with de novo diseases. Leuk Res. 39:348–54. PMID:25573287
2959. Ok CY, Xu-Monette ZY, Tzankov A, et al. (2014). Prevalence and clinical implications of cyclin D1 expression in diffuse large B-cell lymphoma (DLBCL) treated with immunochemotherapy: a report from the International DLBCL Rituximab-CHOP Consortium Program. Cancer. 120:1818–29. PMID:24648050
2960. Okamoto A, Yanada M, Inaguma Y, et al. (2017). The prognostic significance of EBV DNA load and EBER status in diagnostic specimens from diffuse large B-cell lymphoma patients. Hematol Oncol. 35:87–93. PMID:26177728
2961. Okamoto A, Yanada M, Miura H, et al. (2015). Prognostic significance of Epstein-Barr virus DNA detection in pretreatment serum in diffuse large B-cell lymphoma. Cancer Sci. 106:1576–81. PMID:26353084
2962. Okamura D, Matsuda A, Ishikawa M, et al. (2014). Hematologic improvements in a myelodysplastic syndromes with myelofibrosis (MDS-F) patient treated with azacitidine. Leuk Res Rep. 3:24–7. PMID:24809010
2963. Okano M, Matsumoto S, Osato T, et al. (1991). Severe chronic active Epstein-Barr virus infection syndrome. Clin Microbiol Rev. 4:129–35. PMID:1848476
2964. Oki Y, Kantarjian HM, Zhou X, et al. (2006). Adult acute megakaryocytic leukemia: an analysis of 37 patients treated at M.D. Anderson Cancer Center. Blood. 107:880–4. PMID:16123215
2965. Oki Y, Younes A (2012). Brentuximab vedotin in systemic T-cell lymphoma. Expert Opin Biol Ther. 12:623–32. PMID:22428917
2966. Okosun J, Bödör C, Wang J, et al. (2014). Integrated genomic analysis identifies recurrent mutations and evolution patterns driving the initiation and progression of follicular lymphoma. Nat Genet. 46:176–81. PMID:24362818
2967. Okosun J, Wolfson RL, Wang J, et al. (2016). Recurrent mTORC1-activating RRAGC mutations in follicular lymphoma. Nat Genet. 48:183–8. PMID:26691987
2968. Oksenhendler E, Boulanger E, Galicier L, et al. (2002). High incidence of Kaposi sarcoma-associated herpesvirus-related non-Hodgkin lymphoma in patients with HIV infection and multicentric Castleman disease. Blood. 99:2331–6. PMID:11895764
2969. Oksenhendler E, Boutboul D, Beldjord K, et al. (2013). Human herpesvirus 8+ polyclonal IgMλ B-cell lymphocytosis mimicking plasmablastic leukemia/lymphoma in HIV-infected patients. Eur J Haematol. 91:497–503. PMID:23992152
2970. Okuda T, Sakamoto S, Deguchi T, et al. (1991). Hemophagocytic syndrome associated with aggressive natural killer cell leukemia. Am J Hematol. 38:321–3. PMID:1746541
2971. Olney HJ, Le Beau MM (2007). Evaluation of recurring cytogenetic abnormalities in the treatment of myelodysplastic syndromes. Leuk Res. 31:427–34. PMID:17161457
2972. Olsen E, Vonderheid E, Pimpinelli N, et al. (2007). Revisions to the staging and classification of mycosis fungoides and Sezary syndrome: a proposal of the International Society for Cutaneous Lymphomas (ISCL) and the cutaneous lymphoma task force of the European Organization of Research and Treatment of Cancer (EORTC). Blood. 110:1713–22. PMID:17540844
2973. Olteanu H, Harrington AM, Hari P, et al. (2011). CD200 expression in plasma cell myeloma. Br J Haematol. 153:408–11. PMID:21275968
2974. Olteanu H, Wang HY, Chen W, et al. (2008). Immunophenotypic studies of monoclonal gammopathy of undetermined significance. BMC Clin Pathol. 8:13. PMID:19040735
2975. Onaindia A, Montes-Moreno S, Rodríguez-Pinilla SM, et al. (2015). Primary cutaneous anaplastic large cell lymphomas with 6p25.3 rearrangement exhibit particular histological features. Histopathology. 66:846–55. PMID:25131361
2976. Onciu M, Behm FG, Downing JR, et al. (2003). ALK-positive plasmablastic B-cell lymphoma with expression of the NPM-ALK fusion transcript: report of 2 cases. Blood. 102:2642–4. PMID:12816858
2977. Ondrejka SL, Jegalian AG, Kim AS, et al. (2014). PDGFRB-rearranged T-lymphoblastic leukemia/lymphoma occurring with myeloid neoplasms: the missing link supporting a stem cell origin. Haematologica. 99:e148–51. PMID:24951465
2978. Onida F, Kantarjian HM, Smith TL, et al. (2002). Prognostic factors and scoring systems in chronic myelomonocytic leukemia: a retrospective analysis of 213 patients. Blood. 99:840–9. PMID:11806985
2979. Onnis A, De Falco G, Antonicelli G, et al. (2010). Alteration of microRNAs regulated by c-Myc in Burkitt lymphoma. PLoS One. 5:5. PMID:20930934
2980. Opelz G, Döhler B (2004). Lymphomas after solid organ transplantation: a collaborative transplant study report. Am J Transplant. 4:222–30. PMID:14974943
2981. Orazi A (2007). Histopathology in the diagnosis and classification of acute myeloid leukemia, myelodysplastic syndromes, and myelodysplastic/myeloproliferative diseases. Pathobiology. 74:97–114. PMID:17587881
2982. Orazi A, Albitar M, Heerema NA, et al. (1997). Hypoplastic myelodysplastic syndromes can be distinguished from acquired aplastic anemia by CD34 and PCNA immunostaining of bone marrow biopsy specimens. Am J Clin Pathol. 107:268–74. PMID:9052376
2983. Orazi A, Cattoretti G, Heerema NA, et al. (1993). Frequent p53 overexpression in therapy related myelodysplastic syndromes and acute myeloid leukemias: an immunohistochemical study of bone marrow biopsies. Mod Pathol. 6:521–5. PMID:8248107
2984. Orazi A, Cattoretti G, Soligo D, et al. (1993). Therapy-related myelodysplastic syndromes: FAB classification, bone marrow histology, and immunohistology in the prognostic assessment. Leukemia. 7:838–47. PMID:7684797
2985. Orazi A, Chiu R, O'Malley DP, et al. (2006). Chronic myelomonocytic leukemia: The role of bone marrow biopsy immunohistology. Mod Pathol. 19:1536–45. PMID:17041567
2986. Orazi A, Czader MB (2009). Myelodysplastic syndromes. Am J Clin Pathol. 132:290–305. PMID:19605823
2987. Orazi A, Germing U (2008). The myelodysplastic/myeloproliferative neoplasms: myeloproliferative diseases with dysplastic features. Leukemia. 22:1308–19. PMID:18480833
2988. Orazi A, Kahsai M, John K, et al. (1996). p53 overexpression in myeloid leukemic disorders is associated with increased apoptosis of hematopoietic marrow cells and ineffective hematopoiesis. Mod Pathol. 9:48–52. PMID:8821956
2989. Orazi A, Neiman RS, Cualing H, et al. (1994). CD34 immunostaining of bone marrow biopsy specimens is a reliable way to classify the phases of chronic myeloid leukemia. Am J Clin Pathol. 101:426–8. PMID:7512785
2990. Orazi A, Neiman RS, Ulbright TM, et al. (1993). Hematopoietic precursor cells within the yolk sac tumor component are the source of secondary hematopoietic malignancies in patients with mediastinal germ cell tumors. Cancer. 71:3873–81. PMID:8389653
2991. Orazi A, O'Malley DP, Jiang J, et al. (2005). Acute panmyelosis with myelofibrosis: an entity distinct from acute megakaryoblastic leukemia. Mod Pathol. 18:603–14. PMID:15578075
2992. Orchard J, Garand R, Davis Z, et al. (2003). A subset of t(11;14) lymphoma with mantle cell features displays mutated IgVH genes and includes patients with good prognosis, nonnodal disease. Blood. 101:4975–81. PMID:12609845
2993. Ortonne N, Dupuis J, Plonquet A, et al. (2007). Characterization of CXCL13+ neoplastic t cells in cutaneous lesions of angioimmunoblastic T-cell lymphoma (AITL). Am J Surg Pathol. 31:1068–76. PMID:17592274
2994. Osborne BM, Butler JJ, Gresik MV

(1992). Progressive transformation of germinal centers: comparison of 23 pediatric patients to the adult population. Mod Pathol. 5:135–40. PMID:1574490
2995. Oschlies I, Burkhardt B, Salaverria I, et al. (2011). Clinical, pathological and genetic features of primary mediastinal large B-cell lymphomas and mediastinal gray zone lymphomas in children. Haematologica. 96:262–8. PMID:20971819
2996. Oschlies I, Lisfeld J, Lamant L, et al. (2013). ALK-positive anaplastic large cell lymphoma limited to the skin: clinical, histopathological and molecular analysis of 6 pediatric cases. A report from the ALCL99 study. Haematologica. 98:50–6. PMID:22773605
2997. Oschlies I, Salaverria I, Mahn F, et al. (2010). Pediatric follicular lymphoma–a clinico-pathological study of a population-based series of patients treated within the Non-Hodgkin's Lymphoma–Berlin-Frankfurt-Munster (NHL-BFM) multicenter trials. Haematologica. 95:253–9. PMID:19679882
2998. Oschlies I, Simonitsch-Klupp I, Maldyk J, et al. (2015). Subcutaneous panniculitis-like T-cell lymphoma in children: a detailed clinicopathological description of 11 multifocal cases with a high frequency of haemophagocytic syndrome. Br J Dermatol. 172:793–7. PMID:25456748
2999. Oshimi K (1996). Lymphoproliferative disorders of natural killer cells. Int J Hematol. 63:279–90. PMID:8762811
3000. Oshimi K (2007). Progress in understanding and managing natural killer-cell malignancies. Br J Haematol. 139:532–44. PMID:17916099
3001. Oshimi K, Yamada O, Kaneko T, et al. (1993). Laboratory findings and clinical courses of 33 patients with granular lymphocyte-proliferative disorders. Leukemia. 7:782–8. PMID:8388971
3002. Ostergaard P, Simpson MA, Connell FC, et al. (2011). Mutations in GATA2 cause primary lymphedema associated with a predisposition to acute myeloid leukemia (Emberger syndrome). Nat Genet. 43:929–31. PMID:21892158
3002A. Ostronoff F, Othus M, Gerbing RB, et al. (2014). NUP98/NSD1 and FLT3/ITD coexpression is more prevalent in younger AML patients and leads to induction failure: a COG and SWOG report. Blood. 124:2400–7. PMID:25145343
3003. Osuji N, Beiske K, Randen U, et al. (2007). Characteristic appearances of the bone marrow in T-cell large granular lymphocyte leukaemia. Histopathology. 50:547–54. PMID:17394489
3004. Osuji N, Matutes E, Catovsky D, et al. (2005). Histopathology of the spleen in T-cell large granular lymphocyte leukemia and T-cell prolymphocytic leukemia: a comparative review. Am J Surg Pathol. 29:935–41. PMID:15958859
3005. Osuji N, Matutes E, Tjonnfjord G, et al. (2006). T-cell large granular lymphocyte leukemia: A report on the treatment of 29 patients and a review of the literature. Cancer. 107:570–8. PMID:16795070
3006. Otsuki T, Kumar S, Ensoli B, et al. (1996). Detection of HHV-8/KSHV DNA sequences in AIDS-associated extranodal lymphoid malignancies. Leukemia. 10:1358–62. PMID:8709643
3007. Ott G, Kalla J, Ott MM, et al. (1997). Blastoid variants of mantle cell lymphoma: frequent bcl-1 rearrangements at the major translocation cluster region and tetraploid chromosome clones. Blood. 89:1421–9. PMID:9028966
3008. Ott G, Katzenberger T, Lohr A, et al. (2002). Cytomorphologic, immunohistochemical, and cytogenetic profiles of follicular lymphoma: 2 types of follicular lymphoma grade 3. Blood. 99:3806–12. PMID:11986240
3009. Ott G, Ziepert M, Klapper W, et al. (2010). Immunoblastic morphology but not the immunohistochemical GCB/nonGCB classifier predicts outcome in diffuse large B-cell lymphoma in the RICOVER-60 trial of the DSHNHL. Blood. 116:4916–25. PMID:20736456
3010. Ottensmeier CH, Thompsett AR, Zhu D, et al. (1998). Analysis of VH genes in follicular and diffuse lymphoma shows ongoing somatic mutation and multiple isotype transcripts in early disease with changes during disease progression. Blood. 91:4292–9. PMID:9596678
3011. Oudejans JJ, Jiwa M, van den Brule AJ, et al. (1995). Detection of heterogeneous Epstein-Barr virus gene expression patterns within individual post-transplantation lymphoproliferative disorders. Am J Pathol. 147:923–33. PMID:7573368
3012. Ouillette P, Collins R, Shakhan S, et al. (2011). Acquired genomic copy number aberrations and survival in chronic lymphocytic leukemia. Blood. 118:3051–61. PMID:21795749
3013. Owaidah TM, Al Beihany A, Iqbal MA, et al. (2006). Cytogenetics, molecular and ultrastructural characteristics of biphenotypic acute leukemia identified by the EGIL scoring system. Leukemia. 20:620–6. PMID:16437134
3014. Owen C (2010). Insights into familial platelet disorder with propensity to myeloid malignancy (FPD/AML). Leuk Res. 34:141–2. PMID:19695705
3015. Owen C, Barnett M, Fitzgibbon J (2008). Familial myelodysplasia and acute myeloid leukaemia–a review. Br J Haematol. 140:123–32. PMID:18173751
3016. Owen RG, Barrans SL, Richards SJ, et al. (2001). Waldenström macroglobulinemia. Development of diagnostic criteria and identification of prognostic factors. Am J Clin Pathol. 116:420–8. PMID:11554171
3017. Owen RG, Treon SP, Al-Katib A, et al. (2003). Clinicopathological definition of Waldenstrom's macroglobulinemia: consensus panel recommendations from the Second International Workshop on Waldenstrom's Macroglobulinemia. Semin Oncol. 30:110–5. PMID:12720118
3018. Oyama T, Ichimura K, Suzuki R, et al. (2003). Senile EBV+ B-cell lymphoproliferative disorders: a clinicopathologic study of 22 patients. Am J Surg Pathol. 27:16–26. PMID:12502924
3019. Oyama T, Yamamoto K, Asano N, et al. (2007). Age-related EBV-associated B-cell lymphoproliferative disorders constitute a distinct clinicopathologic group: a study of 96 patients. Clin Cancer Res. 13:5124–32. PMID:17785567
3020. Oyarzo MP, Lin P, Glassman A, et al. (2004). Acute myeloid leukemia with t(6;9)(p23;q34) is associated with dysplasia and a high frequency of flt3 gene mutations. Am J Clin Pathol. 122:348–58. PMID:15362364
3021. Ozsan N, Bedke BJ, Law ME, et al. (2011). Clinicopathologic and genetic characterization of follicular lymphomas presenting in the ovary reveals 2 distinct subgroups. Am J Surg Pathol. 35:1691–9. PMID:21997689
3022. Pabst T, Eyholzer M, Fos J, et al. (2009). Heterogeneity within AML with CEBPA mutations; only CEBPA double mutations, but not single CEBPA mutations are associated with favourable prognosis. Br J Cancer. 100:1343–6. PMID:19277035
3023. Pabst T, Eyholzer M, Haefliger S, et al. (2008). Somatic CEBPA mutations are a frequent second event in families with germline CEBPA mutations and familial acute myeloid leukemia. J Clin Oncol. 26:5088–93. PMID:18768433
3024. Pacheco SE, Gottschalk SM, Gresik MV, et al. (2005). Chronic active Epstein-Barr virus infection of natural killer cells presenting as severe skin reaction to mosquito bites. J Allergy Clin Immunol. 116:470–2. PMID:16083813
3025. Padron E, Garcia-Manero G, Patnaik MM, et al. (2015). An international data set for CMML validates prognostic scoring systems and demonstrates a need for novel prognostication strategies. Blood Cancer J. 5:e333. PMID:26230957
3026. Pagano L, Valentini CG, Pulsoni A, et al. (2013). Blastic plasmacytoid dendritic cell neoplasm with leukemic presentation: an Italian multicenter study. Haematologica. 98:239–46. PMID:23065521
3027. Paietta E, Ferrando AA, Neuberg D, et al. (2004). Activating FLT3 mutations in CD117/KIT(+) T-cell acute lymphoblastic leukemias. Blood. 104:558–60. PMID:15044257
3028. Paietta E, Goloubeva O, Neuberg D, et al. (2004). A surrogate marker profile for PML/RAR alpha expressing acute promyelocytic leukemia and the association of immunophenotypic markers with morphologic and molecular subtypes. Cytometry B Clin Cytom. 59:1–9. PMID:15108165
3029. Paietta E, Racevskis J, Bennett JM, et al. (1998). Biologic heterogeneity in Philadelphia chromosome-positive acute leukemia with myeloid morphology: the Eastern Cooperative Oncology Group experience. Leukemia. 12:1881–5. PMID:9844918
3030. Paietta E, Racevskis J, Neuberg D, et al. (1997). Expression of CD25 (interleukin-2 receptor alpha chain) in adult acute lymphoblastic leukemia predicts for the presence of BCR/ABL fusion transcripts: results of a preliminary laboratory analysis of ECOG/MRC Intergroup Study E2993. Leukemia. 11:1887–90. PMID:9369422
3031. Paiva B, Chandia M, Vidriales MB, et al. (2014). Multiparameter flow cytometry for staging of solitary bone plasmacytoma: new criteria for risk of progression to myeloma. Blood. 124:1300–3. PMID:24876564
3032. Paiva B, Corchete LA, Vidriales MB, et al. (2015). The cellular origin and malignant transformation of Waldenström macroglobulinemia. Blood. 125:2370–80. PMID:25655603
3033. Paiva B, Gutiérrez NC, Chen X, et al. (2012). Clinical significance of CD81 expression by clonal plasma cells in high-risk smoldering and symptomatic multiple myeloma patients. Leukemia. 26:1862–9. PMID:22333880
3034. Paiva B, Montes MC, García-Sanz R, et al. (2014). Multiparameter flow cytometry for the identification of the Waldenström's clone in IgM-MGUS and Waldenström's Macroglobulinemia: new criteria for differential diagnosis and risk stratification. Leukemia. 28:166–73. PMID:23604227
3035. Paiva B, van Dongen JJ, Orfao A (2015). New criteria for response assessment: role of minimal residual disease in multiple myeloma. Blood. 125:3059–68. PMID:25838346
3036. Paiva B, Vidriales MB, Cerveró J, et al. (2008). Multiparameter flow cytometric remission is the most relevant prognostic factor for multiple myeloma patients who undergo autologous stem cell transplantation. Blood. 112:4017–23. PMID:18669875
3037. Pal S, Sullivan DG, Kim S, et al. (2006). Productive replication of hepatitis C virus in perihepatic lymph nodes in vivo: implications of HCV lymphotropism. Gastroenterology. 130:1107–16. PMID:16618405
3038. Palmi C, Vendramini E, Silvestri D, et al. (2012). Poor prognosis for P2RY8-CRLF2 fusion but not for CRLF2 over-expression in children with intermediate risk B-cell precursor acute lymphoblastic leukemia. Leukemia. 26:2245–53. PMID:22484421
3039. Palomero J, Vegliante MC, Rodríguez ML, et al. (2014). SOX11 promotes tumor angiogenesis through transcriptional regulation of PDGFA in mantle cell lymphoma. Blood. 124:2235–47. PMID:25092176
3040. Palomero T, Couronné L, Khiabanian H, et al. (2014). Recurrent mutations in epigenetic regulators, RHOA and FYN kinase in peripheral T cell lymphomas. Nat Genet. 46:166–70. PMID:24413734
3041. Palumbo A, Avet-Loiseau H, Oliva S, et al. (2015). Revised International Staging System for Multiple Myeloma: A Report From International Myeloma Working Group. J Clin Oncol. 33:2863–9. PMID:26240224
3042. Pan ST, Cheng CY, Lee NS, et al. (2014). Follicular Dendritic Cell Sarcoma of the Inflammatory Pseudotumor-like Variant Presenting as a Colonic Polyp. Korean J Pathol. 48:140–5. PMID:24868227
3043. Pan Z, Shen Y, Ge B, et al. (2007). Studies of a germinal centre B-cell expressed gene, GCET2, suggest its role as a membrane associated adapter protein. Br J Haematol. 137:578–90. PMID:17489982
3044. Pan ZG, Zhang QY, Lu ZB, et al. (2012). Extracavitary KSHV-associated large B-Cell lymphoma: a distinct entity or a subtype of primary effusion lymphoma? Study of 9 cases and review of an additional 43 cases. Am J Surg Pathol. 36:1129–40. PMID:22790853
3045. Panani AD (2006). Cytogenetic findings in untreated patients with essential thrombocythemia. In Vivo. 20:381–4. PMID:16724675
3046. Pandolfi F, Loughran TP Jr, Starkebaum G, et al. (1990). Clinical course and prognosis of the lymphoproliferative disease of granular lymphocytes. A multicenter study. Cancer. 65:341–8. PMID:2403836
3047. Pane F, Frigeri F, Camera A, et al. (1996). Complete phenotypic and genotypic lineage switch in a Philadelphia chromosome-positive acute lymphoblastic leukemia. Leukemia. 10:741–5. PMID:8618457
3048. Pane F, Frigeri F, Sindona M, et al. (1996). Neutrophilic-chronic myeloid leukemia: a distinct disease with a specific molecular marker (BCR/ABL with C3/A2 junction). Blood. 88:2410–4. PMID:8839830
3049. Papaemmanuil E, Cazzola M, Boultwood J, et al. (2011). Somatic SF3B1 mutation in myelodysplasia with ring sideroblasts. N Engl J Med. 365:1384–95. PMID:21995386
3050. Papaemmanuil E, Gerstung M, Malcovati L, et al. (2013). Clinical and biological implications of driver mutations in myelodysplastic syndromes. Blood. 122:3616–27, quiz 3699. PMID:24030381
3051. Papaemmanuil E, Hosking FJ, Vijayakrishnan J, et al. (2009). Loci on 7p12.2, 10q21.2 and 14q11.2 are associated with risk of childhood acute lymphoblastic leukemia. Nat Genet. 41:1006–10. PMID:19684604
3052. Papoudou-Bai A, Hatzimichael E, Kyriazopoulou L, et al. (2015). Rare variants in the spectrum of human herpesvirus 8/Epstein-Barr virus-copositive lymphoproliferations. Hum Pathol. 46:1566–71. PMID:26299509
3053. Paquette RL, Landaw EM, Pierre RV, et al. (1993). N-ras mutations are associated with poor prognosis and increased risk of leukemia in myelodysplastic syndrome. Blood. 82:590–9. PMID:8329714
3054. Pardanani A, Akin C, Valent P (2006). Pathogenesis, clinical features, and treatment advances in mastocytosis. Best Pract Res Clin Haematol. 19:595–615. PMID:16781490
3055. Pardanani A, Brockman SR, Paternoster SF, et al. (2004). FIP1L1-PDGFRA fusion: prevalence and clinicopathologic correlates in 89 consecutive patients with moderate to severe eosinophilia. Blood. 104:3038–45.

PMID:15284118

3056. Pardanani A, Lasho TL, Finke C, et al. (2007). Prevalence and clinicopathologic correlates of JAK2 exon 12 mutations in JAK2V617F-negative polycythemia vera. Leukemia. 21:1960–3. PMID:17597810

3057. Pardanani A, Lasho TL, Laborde RR, et al. (2013). CSF3R T618I is a highly prevalent and specific mutation in chronic neutrophilic leukemia. Leukemia. 27:1870–3. PMID:23604229

3058. Parikh SA, Kay NE, Shanafelt TD (2014). How we treat Richter syndrome. Blood. 123:1647–57. PMID:24421328

3059. Parikh SA, Leis JF, Chaffee KG, et al. (2015). Hypogammaglobulinemia in newly diagnosed chronic lymphocytic leukemia: Natural history, clinical correlates, and outcomes. Cancer. 121:2883–91. PMID:25931291

3060. Parikh SA, Rabe KC, Kay NE, et al. (2014). Chronic lymphocytic leukemia in young (≤ 55 years) patients: a comprehensive analysis of prognostic factors and outcomes. Haematologica. 99:140–7. PMID:23911703

3061. Park MJ, Park SH, Park PW, et al. (2015). Prognostic impact of concordant and discordant bone marrow involvement and cell-of-origin in Korean patients with diffuse large B-cell lymphoma treated with R-CHOP. J Clin Pathol. 68:733–8. PMID:25998512

3062. Park S, Ko YH (2014). Epstein-Barr virus-associated T/natural killer-cell lymphoproliferative disorders. J Dermatol. 41:29–39. PMID:24438142

3063. Park S, Lee J, Ko YH, et al. (2007). The impact of Epstein-Barr virus status on clinical outcome in diffuse large B-cell lymphoma. Blood. 110:972–8. PMID:17400912

3063A. Park SH, Lee HJ, Kim IS, et al. (2015). Incidences and prognostic impact of c-KIT, WT1, CEBPA, and CBL mutations, and mutations associated with epigenetic modification in core binding factor acute myeloid leukemia: a multicenter study in a Korean population. Ann Lab Med. 35:288–97. PMID:25932436

3064. Parker RI (2000). Hematologic aspects of systemic mastocytosis. Hematol Oncol Clin North Am. 14:557–68. PMID:10909040

3065. Parker TM, Klaassen RJ, Johnston DL (2008). Spontaneous remission of myelodysplastic syndrome with monosomy 7 in a young boy. Cancer Genet Cytogenet. 182:122–5. PMID:18406874

3066. Parkin JL, Arthur DC, Abramson CS, et al. (1982). Acute leukemia associated with the t(4;11) chromosome rearrangement: ultrastructural and immunologic characteristics. Blood. 60:1321–31. PMID:6958337

3067. Parmentier S, Schetelig J, Lorenz K, et al. (2012). Assessment of dysplastic hematopoiesis: lessons from healthy bone marrow donors. Haematologica. 97:723–30. PMID:22180437

3068. Parreira L, Tavares de Castro J, Hibbin JA, et al. (1986). Chromosome and cell culture studies in eosinophilic leukaemia. Br J Haematol. 62:659–69. PMID:3964559

3069. Parrilla Castellar ER, Jaffe ES, Said JW, et al. (2014). ALK-negative anaplastic large cell lymphoma is a genetically heterogeneous disease with widely disparate clinical outcomes. Blood. 124:1473–80. PMID:24894770

3070. Parry M, Rose-Zerilli MJ, Ljungström V, et al. (2015). Genetics and Prognostication in Splenic Marginal Zone Lymphoma: Revelations from Deep Sequencing. Clin Cancer Res. 21:4174–83. PMID:25779943

3071. Parry-Jones N, Matutes E, Morilla R, et al. (2007). Cytogenetic abnormalities additional to t(11;14) correlate with clinical features in leukaemic presentation of mantle cell lymphoma, and may influence prognosis: a study of 60 cases by FISH. Br J Haematol. 137:117–24. PMID:17391491

3072. Parsonnet J, Isaacson PG (2004). Bacterial infection and MALT lymphoma. N Engl J Med. 350:213–5. PMID:14724298

3073. Parvaneh N, Filipovich AH, Borkhardt A (2013). Primary immunodeficiencies predisposed to Epstein-Barr virus-driven haematological diseases. Br J Haematol. 162:573–86. PMID:23758097

3074. Parwaresch MR, Horny HP, Lennert K (1985). Tissue mast cells in health and disease. Pathol Res Pract. 179:439–61. PMID:2582403

3075. Pascal V, Schleinitz N, Brunet C, et al. (2004). Comparative analysis of NK cell subset distribution in normal and lymphoproliferative disease of granular lymphocyte conditions. Eur J Immunol. 34:2930–40. PMID:15368309

3076. Paschka P, Du J, Schlenk RF, et al. (2013). Secondary genetic lesions in acute myeloid leukemia with inv(16) or t(16;16): a study of the German-Austrian AML Study Group (AMLSG). Blood. 121:170–7. PMID:23115274

3077. Paschka P, Döhner K (2013). Core-binding factor acute myeloid leukemia: can we improve on HiDAC consolidation? Hematology Am Soc Hematol Educ Program. 2013:209–19. PMID:24319183

3078. Paschka P, Marcucci G, Ruppert AS, et al. (2006). Adverse prognostic significance of KIT mutations in adult acute myeloid leukemia with inv(16) and t(8;21): a Cancer and Leukemia Group B Study. J Clin Oncol. 24:3904–11. PMID:16921041

3078A. Paschka P, Marcucci G, Ruppert AS, et al. (2008). Wilms' tumor 1 gene mutations independently predict poor outcome in adults with cytogenetically normal acute myeloid leukemia: a cancer and leukemia group B study. J Clin Oncol. 26:4595–602. PMID:18559874

3078B. Paschka P, Schlenk RF, Gaidzik VI, et al. (2010). IDH1 and IDH2 mutations are frequent genetic alterations in acute myeloid leukemia and confer adverse prognosis in cytogenetically normal acute myeloid leukemia with NPM1 mutation without FLT3 internal tandem duplication. J Clin Oncol. 28:3636–43. PMID:20567020

3079. Paschka P, Schlenk RF, Gaidzik VI, et al. (2015). ASXL1 mutations in younger adult patients with acute myeloid leukemia: a study by the German-Austrian Acute Myeloid Leukemia Study Group. Haematologica. 100:324–30. PMID:25596267

3080. Pasqualetti P, Festuccia V, Collacciani A, et al. (1997). The natural history of monoclonal gammopathy of undetermined significance. A 5- to 20-year follow-up of 263 cases. Acta Haematol. 97:174–9. PMID:9066713

3081. Pasqualucci L, Dalla-Favera R (2014). SnapShot: diffuse large B cell lymphoma. Cancer Cell. 25:132–132.e1. PMID:24434215

3082. Pasqualucci L, Khiabanian H, Fangazio M, et al. (2014). Genetics of follicular lymphoma transformation. Cell Rep. 6:130–40. PMID:24388756

3083. Pasqualucci L, Liso A, Martelli MP, et al. (2006). Mutated nucleophosmin detects clonal multilineage involvement in acute myeloid leukemia: Impact on WHO classification. Blood. 108:4146–55. PMID:16926285

3084. Pasqualucci L, Migliazza A, Fracchiolla N, et al. (1998). BCL-6 mutations in normal germinal center B cells: evidence of somatic hypermutation acting outside Ig loci. Proc Natl Acad Sci U S A. 95:11816–21. PMID:9751748

3085. Pasqualucci L, Trifonov V, Fabbri G, et al. (2011). Analysis of the coding genome of diffuse large B-cell lymphoma. Nat Genet. 43:830–7. PMID:21804550

3086. Passamonti F, Cervantes F, Vannucchi AM, et al. (2010). A dynamic prognostic model to predict survival in primary myelofibrosis: a study by the IWG-MRT (International Working Group for Myeloproliferative Neoplasms Research and Treatment). Blood. 115:1703–8. PMID:20008785

3087. Passamonti F, Malabarba L, Orlandi E, et al. (2003). Polycythemia vera in young patients: a study on the long-term risk of thrombosis, myelofibrosis and leukemia. Haematologica. 88:13–8. PMID:12551821

3088. Passamonti F, Rumi E, Arcaini L, et al. (2008). Prognostic factors for thrombosis, myelofibrosis, and leukemia in essential thrombocythemia: a study of 605 patients. Haematologica. 93:1645–51. PMID:18790799

3089. Passamonti F, Rumi E, Arcaini L, et al. (2005). Leukemic transformation of polycythemia vera: a single center study of 23 patients. Cancer. 104:1032–6. PMID:16047334

3090. Passamonti F, Rumi E, Pungolino E, et al. (2004). Life expectancy and prognostic factors for survival in patients with polycythemia vera and essential thrombocythemia. Am J Med. 117:755–61. PMID:15541325

3091. Passamonti F, Vanelli L, Malabarba L, et al. (2003). Clinical utility of the absolute number of circulating CD34-positive cells in patients with chronic myeloproliferative disorders. Haematologica. 88:1123–9. PMID:14555308

3092. Passmore SJ, Chessells JM, Kempski H, et al. (2003). Paediatric myelodysplastic syndromes and juvenile myelomonocytic leukaemia in the UK: a population-based study of incidence and survival. Br J Haematol. 121:758–67. PMID:12780790

3093. Passmore SJ, Hann IM, Stiller CA, et al. (1995). Pediatric myelodysplasia: a study of 68 children and a new prognostic scoring system. Blood. 85:1742–50. PMID:7703482

3094. Pastore A, Jurinovic V, Kridel R, et al. (2015). Integration of gene mutations in risk prognostication for patients receiving first-line immunochemotherapy for follicular lymphoma: a retrospective analysis of a prospective clinical trial and validation in a population-based registry. Lancet Oncol. 16:1111–22. PMID:26256760

3095. Patel JP, Gönen M, Figueroa ME, et al. (2012). Prognostic relevance of integrated genetic profiling in acute myeloid leukemia. N Engl J Med. 366:1079–89. PMID:22417203

3096. Patel KP, Khokhar FA, Muzzafar T, et al. (2013). TdT expression in acute myeloid leukemia with minimal differentiation is associated with distinctive clinicopathological features and better overall survival following stem cell transplantation. Mod Pathol. 26:195–203. PMID:22936064

3097. Pati S, Foulke JS Jr, Barabitskaya O, et al. (2003). Human herpesvirus 8-encoded vGPCR activates nuclear factor of activated T cells and collaborates with human immunodeficiency virus type 1 Tat. J Virol. 77:5759–73. PMID:12719569

3098. Patnaik MM, Hanson CA, Hodnefield JM, et al. (2012). Differential prognostic effect of IDH1 versus IDH2 mutations in myelodysplastic syndromes: a Mayo Clinic study of 277 patients. Leukemia. 26:101–5. PMID:22033490

3099. Patnaik MM, Hanson CA, Sulai NH, et al. (2012). Prognostic irrelevance of ring sideroblast percentage in World Health Organization-defined myelodysplastic syndromes without excess blasts. Blood. 119:5674–7. PMID:22538853

3100. Patnaik MM, Itzykson R, Lasho TL, et al. (2014). ASXL1 and SETBP1 mutations and their prognostic contribution in chronic myelomonocytic leukemia: a two-center study of 466 patients. Leukemia. 28:2206–12. PMID:24695057

3101. Patnaik MM, Lasho TL, Finke CM, et al. (2010). WHO-defined 'myelodysplastic syndrome with isolated del(5q)' in 88 consecutive patients: survival data, leukemic transformation rates and prevalence of JAK2, MPL and IDH mutations. Leukemia. 24:1283–9. PMID:20485371

3102. Patnaik MM, Lasho TL, Finke CM, et al. (2016). Predictors of survival in refractory anemia with ring sideroblasts and thrombocytosis (RARS-T) and the role of next-generation sequencing. Am J Hematol. 91:492–8. PMID:26874914

3103. Patnaik MM, Lasho TL, Hodnefield JM, et al. (2012). SF3B1 mutations are prevalent in myelodysplastic syndromes with ring sideroblasts but do not hold independent prognostic value. Blood. 119:569–72. PMID:22096241

3104. Patnaik MM, Tefferi A (2015). Refractory anemia with ring sideroblasts and RARS with thrombocytosis. Am J Hematol. 90:549–59. PMID:25899435

3105. Patnaik MM, Wassie EA, Padron E, et al. (2015). Chronic myelomonocytic leukemia in younger patients: molecular and cytogenetic predictors of survival and treatment outcome. Blood Cancer J. 5:e270. PMID:25555161

3106. Patrick K, Wade R, Goulden N, et al. (2014). Outcome for children and young people with Early T-cell precursor acute lymphoblastic leukaemia treated on a contemporary protocol, UKALL 2003. Br J Haematol. 166:421–4. PMID:24708207

3107. Patsalides AD, Atac G, Hedge U, et al. (2005). Lymphomatoid granulomatosis: abnormalities of the brain at MR imaging. Radiology. 237:265–73. PMID:16100084

3108. Patterer V, Schnittger S, Kern W, et al. (2013). Hematologic malignancies with PCM1-JAK2 gene fusion share characteristics with myeloid and lymphoid neoplasms with eosinophilia and abnormalities of PDGFRA, PDGFRB, and FGFR1. Ann Hematol. 92:759–69. PMID:23400675

3109. Paul C, Le Tourneau A, Cayuela JM, et al. (1997). Epstein-Barr virus-associated lymphoproliferative disease during methotrexate therapy for psoriasis. Arch Dermatol. 133:867–71. PMID:9236525

3110. Paulli M, Berti E (2004). Cutaneous T-cell lymphomas (including rare subtypes). Current concepts. II. Haematologica. 89:1372–88. PMID:15531460

3111. Paulli M, Berti E, Rosso R, et al. (1995). CD30/Ki-1-positive lymphoproliferative disorders of the skin–clinicopathologic correlation and statistical analysis of 86 cases: a multicentric study from the European Organization for Research and Treatment of Cancer Cutaneous Lymphoma Project Group. J Clin Oncol. 13:1343–54. PMID:7751878

3112. Paulli M, Sträter J, Gianelli U, et al. (1999). Mediastinal B-cell lymphoma: a study of its histomorphologic spectrum based on 109 cases. Hum Pathol. 30:178–87. PMID:10029446

3113. Paulson K, Serebrin A, Lambert P, et al. (2014). Acute promyelocytic leukaemia is characterized by stable incidence and improved survival that is restricted to patients managed in leukaemia referral centres: a pan-Canadian epidemiological study. Br J Haematol. 166:660–6. PMID:24780059

3114. Paulus W, Jellinger K, Hallas C, et al. (1993). Human herpesvirus-6 and Epstein-Barr virus genome in primary cerebral lymphomas. Neurology. 43:1591–3. PMID:8394522

3115. Pawson R, Matutes E, Brito-Babapulle V, et al. (1997). Sezary cell leukaemia: a distinct T cell disorder or a variant form of T prolymphocytic leukaemia? Leukemia. 11:1009–13. PMID:9204983

3116. Pearson MG, Vardiman JW, Le Beau MM, et al. (1985). Increased numbers of marrow basophils may be associated with a t(6;9) in ANLL. Am J Hematol. 18:393–403.

PMID:3976650
3117. Pedersen MØ, Gang AO, Poulsen TS, et al. (2012). Double-hit BCL2/MYC translocations in a consecutive cohort of patients with large B-cell lymphoma - a single centre's experience. Eur J Haematol. 89:63–71. PMID:22510149
3118. Pedersen MØ, Gang AO, Poulsen TS, et al. (2014). MYC translocation partner gene determines survival of patients with large B-cell lymphoma with MYC- or double-hit MYC/BCL2 translocations. Eur J Haematol. 92:42–8. PMID:24118498
3119. Pedersen-Bjergaard J, Philip P (1991). Two different classes of therapy-related and de-novo acute myeloid leukemia? Cancer Genet Cytogenet. 55:119–24. PMID:1655239
3120. Peh SC, Kim LH, Poppema S (2002). Frequent presence of subtype A virus in Epstein-Barr virus-associated malignancies. Pathology. 34:446–50. PMID:12408344
3121. Pekarsky Y, Hallas C, Isobe M, et al. (1999). Abnormalities at 14q32.1 in T cell malignancies involve two oncogenes. Proc Natl Acad Sci U S A. 96:2949–51. PMID:10077617
3122. Peker D, Parekh V, Paluri R, et al. (2014). Clinicopathological and molecular features of myeloid sarcoma as initial presentation of therapy-related myeloid neoplasms: a single institution experience. Int J Hematol. 100:457–63. PMID:25209604
3123. Pellat-Deceunynck C, Barillé S, Jego G, et al. (1998). The absence of CD56 (NCAM) on malignant plasma cells is a hallmark of plasma cell leukemia and of a special subset of multiple myeloma. Leukemia. 12:1977–82. PMID:9844928
3124. Pellat-Deceunynck C, Bataille R (2004). Normal and malignant human plasma cells: proliferation, differentiation, and expansions in relation to CD45 expression. Blood Cells Mol Dis. 32:293–301. PMID:15003821
3125. Pellegrino B, Terrier-Lacombe MJ, Oberlin O, et al. (2003). Lymphocyte-predominant Hodgkin's lymphoma in children: therapeutic abstention after initial lymph node resection–a Study of the French Society of Pediatric Oncology. J Clin Oncol. 21:2948–52. PMID:12885814
3126. Peloponese JM Jr, Kinjo T, Jeang KT (2007). Human T-cell leukemia virus type 1 Tax and cellular transformation. Int J Hematol. 86:101–6. PMID:17875521
3127. Pels H, Montesinos-Rongen M, Schaller C, et al. (2005). VH gene analysis of primary CNS lymphomas. J Neurol Sci. 228:143–7. PMID:15694195
3128. Pels H, Schlegel U (2006). Primary central nervous system lymphoma. Curr Treat Options Neurol. 8:346–57. PMID:16942677
3129. Peng J, Zuo Z, Fu B, et al. (2016). Chronic myelomonocytic leukemia with nucleophosmin (NPM1) mutation. Eur J Haematol. 96:65–71 PMID:25809997
3130. Penn I (1991). The changing pattern of posttransplant malignancies. Transplant Proc. 23:1101–3. PMID:1899153
3131. Pérez B, Mechinaud F, Galambrun C, et al. (2010). Germline mutations of the CBL gene define a new genetic syndrome with predisposition to juvenile myelomonocytic leukaemia. J Med Genet. 47:686–91. PMID:20543203
3132. Perez Botero J, Oliveira JL, Chen D, et al. (2015). ASXL1 mutated chronic myelomonocytic leukemia in a patient with familial thrombocytopenia secondary to germline mutation in ANKRD26. Blood Cancer J. 5:e315. PMID:26001113
3133. Perez-Andreu V, Roberts KG, Harvey RC, et al. (2013). Inherited GATA3 variants are associated with Ph-like childhood acute lymphoblastic leukemia and risk of relapse. Nat Genet. 45:1494–8. PMID:24141364
3134. Perez-Garcia A, Ambesi-Impiombato A, Hadler M, et al. (2013). Genetic loss of SH2B3 in acute lymphoblastic leukemia. Blood. 122:2425–32. PMID:23908464
3135. Perez-Ordonez B, Erlandson RA, Rosai J (1996). Follicular dendritic cell tumor: report of 13 additional cases of a distinctive entity. Am J Surg Pathol. 20:944–55. PMID:8712294
3136. Perez-Ordoñez B, Rosai J (1998). Follicular dendritic cell tumor: review of the entity. Semin Diagn Pathol. 15:144–54. PMID:9606805
3137. Pérez-Persona E, Mateo G, García-Sanz R, et al. (2010). Risk of progression in smouldering myeloma and monoclonal gammopathies of unknown significance: comparative analysis of the evolution of monoclonal component and multiparameter flow cytometry of bone marrow plasma cells. Br J Haematol. 148:110–4. PMID:19821821
3138. Pérez-Persona E, Vidriales MB, Mateo G, et al. (2007). New criteria to identify risk of progression in monoclonal gammopathy of uncertain significance and smoldering multiple myeloma based on multiparameter flow cytometry analysis of bone marrow plasma cells. Blood. 110:2586–92. PMID:17576818
3139. Perkovic S, Basic-Kinda S, Gasparovic V, et al. (2012). Epstein-Barr virus-negative aggressive natural killer-cell leukaemia with high P-glycoprotein activity and phosphorylated extracellular signal-regulated protein kinases 1 and 2. Hematol Rep. 4:e16. PMID:23087805
3139A. Perrone S, D'Elia GM, Annechini G, et al. (2016). Splenic marginal zone lymphoma: Prognostic factors, role of watch and wait policy, and other therapeutic approaches in the rituximab era. Leuk Res. 44:53–60. PMID:27030961
3140. Perrone T, Frizzera G, Rosai J (1986). Mediastinal diffuse large-cell lymphoma with sclerosis. A clinicopathologic study of 60 cases. Am J Surg Pathol. 10:176–91. PMID:3953939
3141. Perry AM, Alvarado-Bernal Y, Laurini JA, et al. (2014). MYC and BCL2 protein expression predicts survival in patients with diffuse large B-cell lymphoma treated with rituximab. Br J Haematol. 165:382–91. PMID:24506200
3142. Perry AM, Aoun P, Coulter DW, et al. (2013). Early onset, EBV(-) PTLD in pediatric liver-small bowel transplantation recipients: a spectrum of plasma cell neoplasms with favorable prognosis. Blood. 121:1377–83. PMID:23255556
3143. Perry AM, Crockett D, Dave BJ, et al. (2013). B-cell lymphoma, unclassifiable, with features intermediate between diffuse large B-cell lymphoma and burkitt lymphoma: study of 39 cases. Br J Haematol. 162:40–9. PMID:23600716
3144. Perry AM, Nelson M, Sanger WG, et al. (2013). Cytogenetic abnormalities in follicular dendritic cell sarcoma: report of two cases and literature review. In Vivo. 27:211–4. PMID:23422480
3145. Perry AM, Warnke RA, Hu Q, et al. (2013). Indolent T-cell lymphoproliferative disease of the gastrointestinal tract. Blood. 122:3599–606. PMID:24009234
3146. Peters AM, Kohfink B, Martin H, et al. (1999). Defective apoptosis due to a point mutation in the death domain of CD95 associated with autoimmune lymphoproliferative syndrome, T-cell lymphoma, and Hodgkin's disease. Exp Hematol. 27:868–74. PMID:10340403
3147. Peterson LC, Brown BA, Crosson JT, et al. (1986). Application of the immunoperoxidase technic to bone marrow trephine biopsies in the classification of patients with monoclonal gammopathies. Am J Clin Pathol. 85:688–93. PMID:3085474
3148. Peterson LC, Parkin JL, Arthur DC, et al. (1991). Acute basophilic leukemia. A clinical, morphologic, and cytogenetic study of eight cases. Am J Clin Pathol. 96:160–70. PMID:1862771
3149. Peterson LF, Zhang DE (2004). The 8;21 translocation in leukemogenesis. Oncogene. 23:4255–62. PMID:15156181
3150. Petitjean B, Jardin F, Joly B, et al. (2002). Pyothorax-associated lymphoma: a peculiar clinicopathologic entity derived from B cells at late stage of differentiation and with occasional aberrant dual B- and T-cell phenotype. Am J Surg Pathol. 26:724–32. PMID:12023576
3151. Petrella T, Bagot M, Willemze R, et al. (2005). Blastic NK-cell lymphomas (agranular CD4+CD56+ hematodermic neoplasms): a review. Am J Clin Pathol. 123:662–75. PMID:15981806
3152. Petrella T, Comeau MR, Maynadié M, et al. (2002). 'Agranular CD4+ CD56+ hematodermic neoplasm' (blastic NK-cell lymphoma) originates from a population of CD56+ precursor cells related to plasmacytoid monocytes. Am J Surg Pathol. 26:852–62. PMID:12131152
3153. Petrella T, Dalac S, Maynadié M, et al. (1999). CD4+ CD56+ cutaneous neoplasms: a distinct hematological entity? Groupe Français d'Etude des Lymphomes Cutanés (GFELC). Am J Surg Pathol. 23:137–46. PMID:9989839
3154. Petrella T, Delfau-Larue MH, Caillot D, et al. (1996). Nasopharyngeal lymphomas: further evidence for a natural killer cell origin. Hum Pathol. 27:827–33. PMID:8760018
3155. Petrella T, Facchetti F (2010). Tumoral aspects of plasmacytoid dendritic cells: what do we know in 2009? Autoimmunity. 43:210–4. PMID:20166873
3156. Petrella T, Maubec E, Cornillet-Lefebvre P, et al. (2007). Indolent CD8-positive lymphoid proliferation of the ear: a distinct primary cutaneous T-cell lymphoma? Am J Surg Pathol. 31:1887–92. PMID:18043044
3157. Petrella T, Meijer CJ, Dalac S, et al. (2004). TCL1 and CLA expression in agranular CD4/CD56 hematodermic neoplasms (blastic NK-cell lymphomas) and leukemia cutis. Am J Clin Pathol. 122:307–13. PMID:15323148
3158. Petrich AM, Gandhi M, Jovanovic B, et al. (2014). Impact of induction regimen and stem cell transplantation on outcomes in double-hit lymphoma: a multicenter retrospective analysis. Blood. 124:2354–61. PMID:25161267
3159. Petruzziello F, Zeppa P, Catalano L, et al. (2010). Amyloid in bone marrow smears of patients affected by multiple myeloma. Ann Hematol. 89:469–74. PMID:19894050
3160. Pettirossi V, Santi A, Imperi E, et al. (2015). BRAF inhibitors reverse the unique molecular signature and phenotype of hairy cell leukemia and exert potent antileukemic activity. Blood. 125:1207–16. PMID:25480661
3161. Pfreundschuh M, Ho AD, Cavallin-Stahl E, et al. (2008). Prognostic significance of maximum tumour (bulk) diameter in young patients with good-prognosis diffuse large-B-cell lymphoma treated with CHOP-like chemotherapy with or without rituximab: an exploratory analysis of the MabThera International Trial Group (MInT) study. Lancet Oncol. 9:435–44. PMID:18400558
3162. Pham-Ledard A, Beylot-Barry M, Barbe C, et al. (2014). High frequency and clinical prognostic value of MYD88 L265P mutation in primary cutaneous diffuse large B-cell lymphoma, leg-type. JAMA Dermatol. 150:1173–9. PMID:25055137
3163. Pham-Ledard A, Cappellen D, Martinez F, et al. (2012). MYD88 somatic mutation is a genetic feature of primary cutaneous diffuse large B-cell lymphoma, leg type. J Invest Dermatol. 132:2118–20. PMID:22495176
3164. Pham-Ledard A, Cowppli-Bony A, Doussau A, et al. (2015). Diagnostic and prognostic value of BCL2 rearrangement in 53 patients with follicular lymphoma presenting as primary skin lesions. Am J Clin Pathol. 143:362–73. PMID:25696794
3165. Pham-Ledard A, Prochazkova-Carlotti M, Andrique L, et al. (2014). Multiple genetic alterations in primary cutaneous large B-cell lymphoma, leg type support a common lymphomagenesis with activated B-cell-like diffuse large B-cell lymphoma. Mod Pathol. 27:402–11. PMID:24030746
3166. Pham-Ledard A, Prochazkova-Carlotti M, Laharanne E, et al. (2010). IRF4 gene rearrangements define a subgroup of CD30-positive cutaneous T-cell lymphoma: a study of 54 cases. J Invest Dermatol. 130:816–25. PMID:19812605
3167. Piazza R, Valletta S, Winkelmann N, et al. (2013). Recurrent SETBP1 mutations in atypical chronic myeloid leukemia. Nat Genet. 45:18–24. PMID:23222956
3168. Picarsic J, Jaffe R, Mazariegos G, et al. (2011). Post-transplant Burkitt lymphoma is a more aggressive and distinct form of post-transplant lymphoproliferative disorder. Cancer. 117:4540–50. PMID:21446044
3169. Piccaluga PP, Agostinelli C, Califano A, et al. (2007). Gene expression analysis of peripheral T cell lymphoma, unspecified, reveals distinct profiles and new potential therapeutic targets. J Clin Invest. 117:823–34. PMID:17304354
3170. Piccaluga PP, Agostinelli C, Righi S, et al. (2007). Expression of CD52 in peripheral T-cell lymphoma. Haematologica. 92:566–7. PMID:17488672
3171. Piccaluga PP, De Falco G, Kustagi M, et al. (2011). Gene expression analysis uncovers similarity and differences among Burkitt lymphoma subtypes. Blood. 117:3596–608. PMID:21245480
3172. Piccaluga PP, Fuligni F, De Leo A, et al. (2013). Molecular profiling improves classification and prognostication of nodal peripheral T-cell lymphomas: results of a phase III diagnostic accuracy study. J Clin Oncol. 31:3019–25. PMID:23857971
3173. Piccaluga PP, Navari M, De Falco G, et al. (2016). Virus-encoded microRNA contributes to the molecular profile of EBV-positive Burkitt lymphomas. Oncotarget. 7:224–40 PMID:26325594
3174. Piccaluga PP, Rossi M, Agostinelli C, et al. (2014). Platelet-derived growth factor alpha mediates the proliferation of peripheral T-cell lymphoma cells via an autocrine regulatory pathway. Leukemia. 28:1687–97. PMID:24480986
3175. Pienkowska-Grela B, Rymkiewicz G, Grygalewicz B, et al. (2011). Partial trisomy 11, dup(11)(q23q13), as a defect characterizing lymphomas with Burkitt pathomorphology without MYC gene rearrangement. Med Oncol. 28:1589–95. PMID:20661666
3176. Pileri SA (2015). Follicular helper T-cell-related lymphomas. Blood. 126:1733–4. PMID:26450950
3177. Pileri SA, Ascani S, Cox MC, et al. (2007). Myeloid sarcoma: clinico-pathologic, phenotypic and cytogenetic analysis of 92 adult patients. Leukemia. 21:340–50. PMID:17170724
3178. Pileri SA, Ascani S, Leoncini L, et al. (2002). Hodgkin's lymphoma: the pathologist's viewpoint. J Clin Pathol. 55:162–76. PMID:11896065
3179. Pileri SA, Gaidano G, Zinzani PL, et al. (2003). Primary mediastinal B-cell lymphoma: high frequency of BCL-6 mutations and consistent expression of the transcription factors OCT-2, BOB.1, and PU.1 in the absence of immunoglobulins. Am J Pathol. 162:243–53.

PMID:12507907
3180. Pileri SA, Grogan TM, Harris NL, et al. (2002). Tumours of histiocytes and accessory dendritic cells: an immunohistochemical approach to classification from the International Lymphoma Study Group based on 61 cases. Histopathology. 41:1–29. PMID:12121233
3181. Pileri SA, Pulford K, Mori S, et al. (1997). Frequent expression of the NPM-ALK chimeric fusion protein in anaplastic large-cell lymphoma, lympho-histiocytic type. Am J Pathol. 150:1207–11. PMID:9094977
3182. Pilichowska ME, Fleming MD, Pinkus JL, et al. (2007). CD4+/CD56+ hematodermic neoplasm ("blastic natural killer cell lymphoma"): neoplastic cells express the immature dendritic cell marker BDCA-2 and produce interferon. Am J Clin Pathol. 128:445–53. PMID:17709319
3183. Pillai RK, Sathanoori M, Van Oss SB, et al. (2013). Double-hit B-cell lymphomas with BCL6 and MYC translocations are aggressive, frequently extranodal lymphomas distinct from BCL2 double-hit B-cell lymphomas. Am J Surg Pathol. 37:323–32. PMID:23348205
3184. Pillai RK, Surti U, Swerdlow SH (2013). Follicular lymphoma-like B cells of uncertain significance (in situ follicular lymphoma) may infrequently progress, but precedes follicular lymphoma, is associated with other overt lymphomas and mimics follicular lymphoma in flow cytometric studies. Haematologica. 98:1571–80. PMID:23831923
3185. Pillai V, Pozdnyakova O, Charest K, et al. (2013). CD200 flow cytometric assessment and semiquantitative immunohistochemical staining distinguishes hairy cell leukemia from hairy cell leukemia-variant and other B-cell lymphoproliferative disorders. Am J Clin Pathol. 140:536–43. PMID:24045551
3186. Pillay K, Solomon R, Daubenton JD, et al. (2004). Interdigitating dendritic cell sarcoma: a report of four paediatric cases and review of the literature. Histopathology. 44:283–91. PMID:14987233
3187. Pilozzi E, Müller-Hermelink HK, Falini B, et al. (1999). Gene rearrangements in T-cell lymphoblastic lymphoma. J Pathol. 188:267–70. PMID:10419594
3188. Pilozzi E, Pulford K, Jones M, et al. (1998). Co-expression of CD79a (JCB117) and CD3 by lymphoblastic lymphoma. J Pathol. 186:140–3. PMID:9924428
3189. Pincus LB, LeBoit PE, McCalmont TH, et al. (2009). Subcutaneous panniculitis-like T-cell lymphoma with overlapping clinicopathologic features of lupus erythematosus: coexistence of 2 entities? Am J Dermatopathol. 31:520–6. PMID:19590424
3190. Pingali SR, Mathiason MA, Lovrich SD, et al. (2009). Emergence of chronic myelogenous leukemia from a background of myeloproliferative disorder: JAK2V617F as a potential risk factor for BCR-ABL translocation. Clin Lymphoma Myeloma. 9:E25–9. PMID:19858050
3191. Pinkel D (1998). Differentiating juvenile myelomonocytic leukemia from infectious disease. Blood. 91:365–7. PMID:9414312
3192. Pinkus GS, Said JW (1985). Hodgkin's disease, lymphocyte predominance type, nodular–a distinct entity? Unique staining profile for L&H variants of Reed-Sternberg cells defined by monoclonal antibodies to leukocyte common antigen, granulocyte-specific antigen, and B-cell-specific antigen. Am J Pathol. 118:1–6. PMID:3155594
3193. Pinkus GS, Said JW (1988). Hodgkin's disease, lymphocyte predominance type, nodular–further evidence for a B cell derivation. L & H variants of Reed-Sternberg cells express L26, a pan B cell marker. Am J Pathol. 133:211–7. PMID:3263805
3194. Pinyol M, Bea S, Plà L, et al. (2007). Inactivation of RB1 in mantle-cell lymphoma detected by nonsense-mediated mRNA decay pathway inhibition and microarray analysis. Blood. 109:5422–9. PMID:17332242
3195. Pinyol M, Cobo F, Bea S, et al. (1998). p16(INK4a) gene inactivation by deletions, mutations, and hypermethylation is associated with transformed and aggressive variants of non-Hodgkin's lymphomas. Blood. 91:2977–84. PMID:9531609
3196. Pinyol M, Hernandez L, Cazorla M, et al. (1997). Deletions and loss of expression of p16INK4a and p21Waf1 genes are associated with aggressive variants of mantle cell lymphomas. Blood. 89:272–80. PMID:8978301
3197. Piris MA, Mollejo M, Campo E, et al. (1998). A marginal zone pattern may be found in different varieties of non-Hodgkin's lymphoma: the morphology and immunohistology of splenic involvement by B-cell lymphomas simulating splenic marginal zone lymphoma. Histopathology. 33:230–9. PMID:9777389
3198. Pitman SD, Huang Q, Zuppan CW, et al. (2006). Hodgkin lymphoma-like posttransplant lymphoproliferative disorder (HL-like PTLD) simulates monomorphic B-cell PTLD both clinically and pathologically. Am J Surg Pathol. 30:470–6. PMID:16625093
3199. Pittaluga S, Ayoubi TA, Wlodarska I, et al. (1996). BCL-6 expression in reactive lymphoid tissue and in B-cell non-Hodgkin's lymphomas. J Pathol. 179:145–50. PMID:8758205
3200. Pittaluga S, Verhoef G, Criel A, et al. (1996). Prognostic significance of bone marrow trephine and peripheral blood smears in 55 patients with mantle cell lymphoma. Leuk Lymphoma. 21:115–25. PMID:8907278
3201. Pittaluga S, Wlodarska I, Pulford K, et al. (1997). The monoclonal antibody ALK1 identifies a distinct morphological subtype of anaplastic large cell lymphoma associated with 2p23/ALK rearrangements. Am J Pathol. 151:343–51. PMID:9250148
3202. Piva R, Agnelli L, Pellegrino E, et al. (2010). Gene expression profiling uncovers molecular classifiers for the recognition of anaplastic large-cell lymphoma within peripheral T-cell neoplasms. J Clin Oncol. 28:1583–90. PMID:20159827
3203. Piva R, Deaglio S, Famà R, et al. (2015). The Krüppel-like factor 2 transcription factor gene is recurrently mutated in splenic marginal zone lymphoma. Leukemia. 29:503–7. PMID:25283840
3204. Pizzi M, Silver RT, Barel A, et al. (2015). Recombinant interferon-α in myelofibrosis reduces bone marrow fibrosis, improves its morphology and is associated with clinical response. Mod Pathol. 28:1315–23. PMID:26271725
3205. Plant AS, Venick RS, Farmer DG, et al. (2013). Plasmacytoma-like post-transplant lymphoproliferative disorder seen in pediatric combined liver and intestinal transplant recipients. Pediatr Blood Cancer. 60:E137–9. PMID:23813867
3206. Plaza JA, Sangueza M (2015). Hydroa vacciniforme-like lymphoma with primarily periorbital swelling: 7 cases of an atypical clinical manifestation of this rare cutaneous T-cell lymphoma. Am J Dermatopathol. 37:20–5. PMID:25162933
3207. Poirel HA, Bernheim A, Schneider A, et al. (2005). Characteristic pattern of chromosomal imbalances in posttransplantation lymphoproliferative disorders: correlation with histopathological subcategories and EBV status. Transplantation. 80:176–84. PMID:16041261
3207A. Pollard JA, Alonzo TA, Gerbing RB, et al. (2010). Prevalence and prognostic significance of KIT mutations in pediatric patients with core binding factor AML enrolled on serial pediatric cooperative trials for de novo AML. Blood. 115:2372–9. PMID:20056794
3208. Polprasert C, Schulze I, Sekeres MA, et al. (2015). Inherited and Somatic Defects in DDX41 in Myeloid Neoplasms. Cancer Cell. 27:658–70. PMID:25920683
3209. Polycythemia vera: the natural history of 1213 patients followed for 20 years; Gruppo Italiano Studio Policitemia (1995). Ann Intern Med. 123:656–64. PMID:7574220
3210. Pongpruttipan T, Sukpanichnant S, Assanasen T, et al. (2012). Extranodal NK/T-cell lymphoma, nasal type, includes cases of natural killer cell and αβ, γδ, and αβ/γδ T-cell origin: a comprehensive clinicopathologic and phenotypic study. Am J Surg Pathol. 36:481–99. PMID:22314189
3211. Ponti R, Quaglino P, Novelli M, et al. (2005). T-cell receptor gamma gene rearrangement by multiplex polymerase chain reaction/heteroduplex analysis in patients with cutaneous T-cell lymphoma (mycosis fungoides/Sézary syndrome) and benign inflammatory disease: correlation with clinical, histological and immunophenotypical findings. Br J Dermatol. 153:565–73. PMID:16120144
3212. Ponzoni M, Arrigoni G, Gould VE, et al. (2000). Lack of CD 29 (beta1 integrin) and CD 54 (ICAM-1) adhesion molecules in intravascular lymphomatosis. Hum Pathol. 31:220–6. PMID:10685637
3213. Ponzoni M, Berger F, Chassagne-Clement C, et al. (2007). Reactive perivascular T-cell infiltrate predicts survival in primary central nervous system B-cell lymphomas. Br J Haematol. 138:316–23. PMID:17555470
3214. Ponzoni M, Ferreri AJ (2006). Intravascular lymphoma: a neoplasm of 'homeless' lymphocytes? Hematol Oncol. 24:105–12. PMID:16721900
3215. Ponzoni M, Ferreri AJ, Campo E, et al. (2007). Definition, diagnosis, and management of intravascular large B-cell lymphoma: proposals and perspectives from an international consensus meeting. J Clin Oncol. 25:3168–73. PMID:17577023
3216. Ponzoni M, Kanellis G, Pouliou E, et al. (2012). Bone marrow histopathology in the diagnostic evaluation of splenic marginal-zone and splenic diffuse red pulp small B-cell lymphoma: a reliable substitute for spleen histopathology? Am J Surg Pathol. 36:1609–18. PMID:23073320
3217. Popovici C, Zhang B, Grégoire MJ, et al. (1999). The t(6;8)(q27;p11) translocation in a stem cell myeloproliferative disorder fuses a novel gene, FOP, to fibroblast growth factor receptor 1. Blood. 93:1381–9. PMID:9949182
3218. Poppema S (1980). The diversity of the immunohistological staining pattern of Sternberg-Reed cells. J Histochem Cytochem. 28:788–91. PMID:6777426
3219. Poppema S (1989). The nature of the lymphocytes surrounding Reed-Sternberg cells in nodular lymphocyte predominance and in other types of Hodgkin's disease. Am J Pathol. 135:351–7. PMID:2675617
3220. Porrata LF, Ristow KM, Habermann TM, et al. (2014). Peripheral blood absolute lymphocyte/monocyte ratio during rituximab, cyclophosphamide, doxorubicin, vincristine and prednisone treatment cycles predicts clinical outcomes in diffuse large B-cell lymphoma. Leuk Lymphoma. 55:2728–38. PMID:24547705
3221. Porwit A (2015). Is there a role for flow cytometry in the evaluation of patients with myelodysplastic syndromes? Curr Hematol Malig Rep. 10:309–17. PMID:26122389
3222. Porwit A, Béné MC (2015). Acute leukemias of ambiguous origin. Am J Clin Pathol. 144:361–76. PMID:26276768
3223. Porwit A, van de Loosdrecht AA, Bettelheim P, et al. (2014). Revisiting guidelines for integration of flow cytometry results in the WHO classification of myelodysplastic syndromes-proposal from the International/European LeukemiaNet Working Group for Flow Cytometry in MDS. Leukemia. 28:1793–8. PMID:24919805
3224. Porwit-MacDonald A, Janossy G, Ivory K, et al. (1996). Leukemia-associated changes identified by quantitative flow cytometry. IV. CD34 overexpression in acute myelogenous leukemia M2 with t(8;21). Blood. 87:1162–9. PMID:8562943
3225. Poulain S, Boyle EM, Roumier C, et al. (2014). MYD88 L265P mutation contributes to the diagnosis of Bing Neel syndrome. Br J Haematol. 167:506–13. PMID:25160558
3226. Powell BC, Jiang L, Muzny DM, et al. (2013). Identification of TP53 as an acute lymphocytic leukemia susceptibility gene through exome sequencing. Pediatr Blood Cancer. 60:E1–3. PMID:23255406
3227. Pozdnyakova O, Morgan EA, Li B, et al. (2012). Patterns of expression of CD56 and CD117 on neoplastic plasma cells and association with genetically distinct subtypes of plasma cell myeloma. Leuk Lymphoma. 53:1905–10. PMID:22423624
3228. Pozdnyakova O, Rodig S, Bhandarkar S, et al. (2015). The importance of central pathology review in international trials: a comparison of local versus central bone marrow reticulin grading. Leukemia. 29:241–4. PMID:25183285
3229. Pozzato G, Mazzaro C, Crovatto M, et al. (1994). Low-grade malignant lymphoma, hepatitis C virus infection, and mixed cryoglobulinemia. Blood. 84:3047–53. PMID:7949176
3230. Pozzi C, D'Amico M, Fogazzi GB, et al. (2003). Light chain deposition disease with renal involvement: clinical characteristics and prognostic factors. Am J Kidney Dis. 42:1154–63. PMID:14655186
3231. Prakash S, Fountaine T, Raffeld M, et al. (2006). IgD positive L&H cells identify a unique subset of nodular lymphocyte predominant Hodgkin lymphoma. Am J Surg Pathol. 30:585–92. PMID:16699312
3232. Prakash S, Hoffman R, Barouk S, et al. (2012). Splenic extramedullary hematopoietic proliferation in Philadelphia chromosome-negative myeloproliferative neoplasms: heterogeneous morphology and cytological composition. Mod Pathol. 25:815–27. PMID:22388763
3232A. Pratcorona M, Abbas S, Sanders MA, et al. (2012). Acquired mutations in ASXL1 in acute myeloid leukemia: prevalence and prognostic value. Haematologica. 97:388–92. PMID:22058207
3233. Pratcorona M, Brunet S, Nomdedéu J, et al. (2013). Favorable outcome of patients with acute myeloid leukemia harboring a low-allelic burden FLT3-ITD mutation and concomitant NPM1 mutation: relevance to post-remission therapy. Blood. 121:2734–8. PMID:23377436
3234. Preud'homme JL, Aucouturier P, Touchard G, et al. (1994). Monoclonal immunoglobulin deposition disease (Randall type). Relationship with structural abnormalities of immunoglobulin chains. Kidney Int. 46:965–72. PMID:7861722
3235. Preudhomme C, Renneville A, Bourdon V, et al. (2009). High frequency of RUNX1 biallelic alteration in acute myeloid leukemia secondary to familial platelet disorder. Blood. 113:5583–7. PMID:19357396
3236. Preudhomme C, Warot-Loze D, Roumier C, et al. (2000). High incidence of biallelic point mutations in the Runt domain of the AML1/PEBP2 alpha B gene in Mo acute myeloid leukemia and in myeloid malignancies with acquired trisomy 21. Blood. 96:2862–9.

PMID:11023523
3237. Preusser M, Woehrer A, Koperek O, et al. (2010). Primary central nervous system lymphoma: a clinicopathological study of 75 cases. Pathology. 42:547–52. PMID:20854073
3238. Prevot S, Hamilton-Dutoit S, Audouin J, et al. (1992). Analysis of African Burkitt's and high-grade B cell non-Burkitt's lymphoma for Epstein-Barr virus genomes using in situ hybridization. Br J Haematol. 80:27–32. PMID:1311194
3239. Price SK (1990). Immunoproliferative small intestinal disease: a study of 13 cases with alpha heavy-chain disease. Histopathology. 17:7–17. PMID:2227833
3240. Primignani M, Barosi G, Bergamaschi G, et al. (2006). Role of the JAK2 mutation in the diagnosis of chronic myeloproliferative disorders in splanchnic vein thrombosis. Hepatology. 44:1528–34. PMID:17133457
3241. Pro B, Advani R, Brice P, et al. (2012). Brentuximab vedotin (SGN-35) in patients with relapsed or refractory systemic anaplastic large-cell lymphoma: results of a phase II study. J Clin Oncol. 30:2190–6. PMID:22614995
3242. Pruneri G, Fabris S, Baldini L, et al. (2000). Immunohistochemical analysis of cyclin D1 shows deregulated expression in multiple myeloma with the t(11;14). Am J Pathol. 156:1505–13. PMID:10793062
3243. Przybylski GK, Wu H, Macon WR, et al. (2000). Hepatosplenic and subcutaneous panniculitis-like gamma/delta T cell lymphomas are derived from different Vdelta subsets of gamma/delta T lymphocytes. J Mol Diagn. 2:11–9. PMID:11272897
3244. Puente XS, Beà S, Valdés-Mas R, et al. (2015). Non-coding recurrent mutations in chronic lymphocytic leukaemia. Nature. 526:519–24. PMID:26200345
3245. Puente XS, Pinyol M, Quesada V, et al. (2011). Whole-genome sequencing identifies recurrent mutations in chronic lymphocytic leukaemia. Nature. 475:101–5. PMID:21642962
3246. Pui CH, Schrappe M, Ribeiro RC, et al. (2004). Childhood and adolescent lymphoid and myeloid leukemia. Hematology Am Soc Hematol Educ Program. 118–45. PMID:15561680
3246A. Puiggros A, Delgado J, Rodriguez-Vicente A, et al. (2013). Biallelic losses of 13q do not confer a poorer outcome in chronic lymphocytic leukaemia: analysis of 627 patients with isolated 13q deletion. Br J Haematol. 163:47–54. PMID:23869550
3247. Puiggros A, Venturas M, Salido M, et al. (2014). Interstitial 13q14 deletions detected in the karyotype and translocations with concomitant deletion at 13q14 in chronic lymphocytic leukemia: different genetic mechanisms but equivalent poorer clinical outcome. Genes Chromosomes Cancer. 53:788–97. PMID:24915757
3248. Pulford K, Banham AH, Lyne L, et al. (2006). The BCL11AXL transcription factor: its distribution in normal and malignant tissues and use as a marker for plasmacytoid dendritic cells. Leukemia. 20:1439–41. PMID:16710303
3249. Pulford K, Lamant L, Espinos E, et al. (2004). The emerging normal and disease-related roles of anaplastic lymphoma kinase. Cell Mol Life Sci. 61:2939–53. PMID:15583856
3250. Pulford K, Lamant L, Morris SW, et al. (1997). Detection of anaplastic lymphoma kinase (ALK) and nucleolar protein nucleophosmin (NPM)-ALK proteins in normal and neoplastic cells with the monoclonal antibody ALK1. Blood. 89:1394–404. PMID:9028963
3251. Purtilo DT, Strobach RS, Okano M, et al. (1992). Epstein-Barr virus-associated lymphoproliferative disorders. Lab Invest. 67:5–23. PMID:1320711
3252. Qian Z, Fernald AA, Godley LA, et al. (2002). Expression profiling of CD34+ hematopoietic stem/ progenitor cells reveals distinct subtypes of therapy-related acute myeloid leukemia. Proc Natl Acad Sci U S A. 99:14925–30. PMID:12417757
3253. Qian Z, Joslin JM, Tennant TR, et al. (2010). Cytogenetic and genetic pathways in therapy-related acute myeloid leukemia. Chem Biol Interact. 184:50–7. PMID:19958752
3254. Qin Y, Greiner A, Trunk MJ, et al. (1995). Somatic hypermutation in low-grade mucosa-associated lymphoid tissue-type B-cell lymphoma. Blood. 86:3528–34. PMID:7579460
3255. Qiu Y, Yang Y, Yang H (2014). The unique surface molecules on intestinal intraepithelial lymphocytes: from tethering to recognizing. Dig Dis Sci. 59:520–9. PMID:24248415
3256. Quaglino P, Pimpinelli N, Berti E, et al. (2012). Time course, clinical pathways, and long-term hazards risk trends of disease progression in patients with classic mycosis fungoides: a multicenter, retrospective follow-up study from the Italian Group of Cutaneous Lymphomas. Cancer. 118:5830–9. PMID:22674564
3257. Qubaja M, Marmey B, Le Tourneau A, et al. (2009). The detection of CD14 and CD16 in paraffin-embedded bone marrow biopsies is useful for the diagnosis of chronic myelomonocytic leukemia. Virchows Arch. 454:411–9. PMID:19242719
3258. Queiroga EM, Gualco G, Weiss LM, et al. (2008). Burkitt lymphoma in Brazil is characterized by geographically distinct clinicopathologic features. Am J Clin Pathol. 130:946–56. PMID:19019773
3259. Queirós AC, Villamor N, Clot G, et al. (2015). A B-cell epigenetic signature defines three biologic subgroups of chronic lymphocytic leukemia with clinical impact. Leukemia. 29:598–605. PMID:25151957
3260. Quelen C, Lippert E, Struski S, et al. (2011). Identification of a transforming MYB-GATA1 fusion gene in acute basophilic leukemia: a new entity in male infants. Blood. 117:5719–22. PMID:21474671
3261. Quentin S, Cuccuini W, Ceccaldi R, et al. (2011). Myelodysplasia and leukemia of Fanconi anemia are associated with a specific pattern of genomic abnormalities that includes cryptic RUNX1/AML1 lesions. Blood. 117:e161–70. PMID:21325596
3262. Quinlan SC, Pfeiffer RM, Morton LM, et al. (2011). Risk factors for early-onset and late-onset post-transplant lymphoproliferative disorder in kidney recipients in the United States. Am J Hematol. 86:206–9. PMID:21264909
3263. Quinn ER, Chan CH, Hadlock KG, et al. (2001). The B-cell receptor of a hepatitis C virus (HCV)-associated non-Hodgkin lymphoma binds the viral E2 envelope protein, implicating HCV in lymphomagenesis. Blood. 98:3745–9. PMID:11739181
3264. Quintanilla-Martinez L, Davies-Hill T, Fend F, et al. (2003). Sequestration of p27Kip1 protein by cyclin D1 in typical and blastic variants of mantle cell lymphoma (MCL): implications for pathogenesis. Blood. 101:3181–7. PMID:12515730
3265. Quintanilla-Martinez L, Fend F, Moguel LR, et al. (1999). Peripheral T-cell lymphoma with Reed-Sternberg-like cells of B-cell phenotype and genotype associated with Epstein-Barr virus infection. Am J Surg Pathol. 23:1233–40. PMID:10524524
3266. Quintanilla-Martinez L, Franklin JL, Guerrero I, et al. (1999). Histological and immunophenotypic profile of nasal NK/T cell lymphomas from Peru: high prevalence of p53 overexpression. Hum Pathol. 30:849–55. PMID:10414505
3267. Quintanilla-Martinez L, Jansen PM, Kinney MC, et al. (2013). Non-mycosis fungoides cutaneous T-cell lymphomas: report of the 2011 Society for Hematopathology/European Association for Haematopathology workshop. Am J Clin Pathol. 139:491–514. PMID:23525618
3268. Quintanilla-Martinez L, Kremer M, Keller G, et al. (2001). p53 Mutations in nasal natural killer/T-cell lymphoma from Mexico: association with large cell morphology and advanced disease. Am J Pathol. 159:2095–105. PMID:11733360
3269. Quintanilla-Martinez L, Kumar S, Fend F, et al. (2000). Fulminant EBV(+) T-cell lymphoproliferative disorder following acute/chronic EBV infection: a distinct clinicopathologic syndrome. Blood. 96:443–51. PMID:10887104
3270. Quintanilla-Martinez L, Pittaluga S, Miething C, et al. (2006). NPM-ALK-dependent expression of the transcription factor CCAAT/enhancer binding protein beta in ALK-positive anaplastic large cell lymphoma. Blood. 108:2029–36. PMID:16709933
3271. Quintanilla-Martinez L, Ridaura C, Nagl F, et al. (2013). Hydroa vacciniforme-like lymphoma: a chronic EBV+ lymphoproliferative disorder with risk to develop a systemic lymphoma. Blood. 122:3101–10. PMID:23982171
3272. Quintanilla-Martinez L, Sander B, Chan JK, et al. (2016). Indolent lymphomas in the pediatric population: follicular lymphoma, IRF4/MUM1+ lymphoma, nodal marginal zone lymphoma and chronic lymphocytic leukemia. Virchows Arch. 468:141–57 PMID:26416032
3273. Quintás-Cardama A, Gibbons DL, Cortes J, et al. (2008). Association of 3q21q26 syndrome and late-appearing Philadelphia chromosome in acute myeloid leukemia. Leukemia. 22:877–8. PMID:17928880
3274. Rabbani GR, Phyliky RL, Tefferi A (1999). A long-term study of patients with chronic natural killer cell lymphocytosis. Br J Haematol. 106:960–6. PMID:10519998
3275. Radaszkiewicz T, Dragosics B, Bauer P (1992). Gastrointestinal malignant lymphomas of the mucosa-associated lymphoid tissue: factors relevant to prognosis. Gastroenterology. 102:1628–38. PMID:1568573
3276. Raderer M, Streubel B, Woehrer S, et al. (2005). High relapse rate in patients with MALT lymphoma warrants lifelong follow-up. Clin Cancer Res. 11:3349–52. PMID:15867234
3277. Radich JP, Dai H, Mao M, et al. (2006). Gene expression changes associated with progression and response in chronic myeloid leukemia. Proc Natl Acad Sci U S A. 103:2794–9. PMID:16477019
3278. Raess PW, Mintzer D, Husson M, et al. (2013). BRAF V600E is also seen in unclassifiable splenic B-cell lymphoma/leukemia, a potential mimic of hairy cell leukemia. Blood. 122:3084–5. PMID:24159168
3279. Raffeld M, Wright JJ, Lipford E, et al. (1987). Clonal evolution of t(14;18) follicular lymphomas demonstrated by immunoglobulin genes and the 18q21 major breakpoint region. Cancer Res. 47:2537–42. PMID:3032407
3280. Rahal R, Frick M, Romero R, et al. (2014). Pharmacological and genomic profiling identifies NF-κB-targeted treatment strategies for mantle cell lymphoma. Nat Med. 20:87–92. PMID:24362935
3280A. Raghavan M, Steinrücken M, Harris K, et al. (2015). Population genetics. Genomic evidence for the Pleistocene and recent population history of Native Americans. Science. 349:aab3884. PMID:26198033
3281. Rahemtullah A, Reichard KK, Preffer FI, et al. (2006). A double-positive CD4+CD8+ T-cell population is commonly found in nodular lymphocyte predominant Hodgkin lymphoma. Am J Clin Pathol. 126:805–14. PMID:17050078
3282. Rahmé R, Thomas X, Recher C, et al. (2014). Early death in acute promyelocytic leukemia (APL) in French centers: a multicenter study in 399 patients. Leukemia. 28:2422–4. PMID:25142818
3283. Rai KR, Sawitsky A, Cronkite EP, et al. (1975). Clinical staging of chronic lymphocytic leukemia. Blood. 46:219–34. PMID:1139039
3284. Raimondi SC, Pui CH, Hancock ML, et al. (1996). Heterogeneity of hyperdiploid (51-67) childhood acute lymphoblastic leukemia. Leukemia. 10:213–24. PMID:8637229
3285. Rainey JJ, Omenah D, Sumba PO, et al. (2007). Spatial clustering of endemic Burkitt's lymphoma in high-risk regions of Kenya. Int J Cancer. 120:121–7. PMID:17019706
3286. Raja KR, Kovarova L, Hajek R (2010). Review of phenotypic markers used in flow cytometric analysis of MGUS and MM, and applicability of flow cytometry in other plasma cell disorders. Br J Haematol. 149:334–51. PMID:20201947
3287. Rajab A, Porwit A (2015). Screening bone marrow samples for abnormal lymphoid populations and myelodysplasia-related features with one 10-color 14-antibody screening tube. Cytometry B Clin Cytom. 88:253–60. PMID:25664445
3288. Rajala HL, Eldfors S, Kuusanmäki H, et al. (2013). Discovery of somatic STAT5b mutations in large granular lymphocytic leukemia. Blood. 121:4541–50. PMID:23596048
3289. Rajappa SJ, Uppin SG, Digumarti R (2007). Testicular relapse of primary central nervous system lymphoma. Leuk Lymphoma. 48:1023–5. PMID:17487747
3290. Rajkumar SV, Dimopoulos MA, Palumbo A, et al. (2014). International Myeloma Working Group updated criteria for the diagnosis of multiple myeloma. Lancet Oncol. 15:e538–48. PMID:25439696
3291. Rajkumar SV, Greipp PR (1999). Prognostic factors in multiple myeloma. Hematol Oncol Clin North Am. 13:1295–314, xi. [xi.] PMID:10626152
3292. Rajkumar SV, Kyle RA, Therneau TM, et al. (2005). Serum free light chain ratio is an independent risk factor for progression in monoclonal gammopathy of undetermined significance. Blood. 106:812–7. PMID:15855274
3293. Rajkumar SV, Landgren O, Mateos MV (2015). Smoldering multiple myeloma. Blood. 125:3069–75. PMID:25838344
3294. Ralfkiaer E, Delsol G, O'Connor NT, et al. (1990). Malignant lymphomas of true histiocytic origin. A clinical, histological, immunophenotypic and genotypic study. J Pathol. 160:9–17. PMID:2156039
3295. Rambaud JC, Halphen M, Galian A, et al. (1990). Immunoproliferative small intestinal disease (IPSID): relationships with alpha-chain disease and "Mediterranean" lymphomas. Springer Semin Immunopathol. 12:239–50. PMID:2205943
3296. Ramos E, Hernández F, Andres A, et al. (2013). Post-transplant lymphoproliferative disorders and other malignancies after pediatric intestinal transplantation: incidence, clinical features and outcome. Pediatr Transplant. 17:472–8. PMID:23730927
3297. Ramos F, Fernández-Ferrero S, Suárez D, et al. (1999). Myelodysplastic syndrome: a search for minimal diagnostic criteria. Leuk Res. 23:283–90. PMID:10071083
3298. Ramot B, Shahin N, Bubis JJ (1965). MALABSORPTION SYNDROME IN LYMPHOMA OF SMALL INTESTINE. A STUDY OF 13 CASES. Isr J Med Sci. 1:221–6. PMID:14279068
3299. Ramsay AD, Smith WJ, Isaacson PG (1988). T-cell-rich B-cell lymphoma. Am J Surg Pathol. 12:433–43. PMID:3287959
3300. Randall RE, Williamson WC Jr, Mullinax F, et al. (1976). Manifestations of systemic

light chain deposition. Am J Med. 60:293–9. PMID:814812
3301. Randen U, Trøen G, Tierens A, et al. (2014). Primary cold agglutinin-associated lymphoproliferative disease: a B-cell lymphoma of the bone marrow distinct from lymphoplasmacytic lymphoma. Haematologica. 99:497–504. PMID:24143001
3302. Randi ML, Geranio G, Bertozzi I, et al. (2015). Are all cases of paediatric essential thrombocythaemia really myeloproliferative neoplasms? Analysis of a large cohort. Br J Haematol. 169:584–9. PMID:25716342
3303. Randolph GJ, Angeli V, Swartz MA (2005). Dendritic-cell trafficking to lymph nodes through lymphatic vessels. Nat Rev Immunol. 5:617–28. PMID:16056255
3304. Ranganathan S, Webber S, Ahuja S, et al. (2004). Hodgkin-like posttransplant lymphoproliferative disorder in children: does it differ from posttransplant Hodgkin lymphoma? Pediatr Dev Pathol. 7:348–60. PMID:14564542
3305. Ranheim EA, Jones C, Zehnder JL, et al. (2000). Spontaneously relapsing clonal, mucosal cytotoxic T-cell lymphoproliferative disorder: case report and review of the literature. Am J Surg Pathol. 24:296–301. PMID:10680899
3306. Ranjan A, Penninga E, Jelsig AM, et al. (2013). Inheritance of the chronic myeloproliferative neoplasms. A systematic review. Clin Genet. 83:99–107. PMID:23094849
3307. Ranuncolo SM, Pittaluga S, Evbuomwan MO, et al. (2012). Hodgkin lymphoma requires stabilized NIK and constitutive RelB expression for survival. Blood. 120:3756–63. PMID:22968463
3308. Raoux D, Duband S, Forest F, et al. (2010). Primary central nervous system lymphoma: immunohistochemical profile and prognostic significance. Neuropathology. 30:232–40. PMID:19925562
3309. Raphael M, Gentilhomme O, Tulliez M, et al. (1991). Histopathologic features of high-grade non-Hodgkin's lymphomas in acquired immunodeficiency syndrome. Arch Pathol Lab Med. 115:15–20. PMID:1987908
3310. Raphael MM, Audouin J, Lamine M, et al. (1994). Immunophenotypic and genotypic analysis of acquired immunodeficiency syndrome-related non-Hodgkin's lymphomas. Correlation with histologic features in 36 cases. Am J Clin Pathol. 101:773–82. PMID:8209868
3310A. Rappaport H (1966). Tumors of the haematopoietic system. In: Atlas of tumor pathology. Washington (DC): AFIP.
3311. Rappaport H, Berard CW, Butler JJ, et al. (1971). Report of the Committee on Histopathological Criteria Contributing to Staging of Hodgkin's Disease. Cancer Res. 31:1864–5. PMID:5121696
3312. Rasmussen T, Kuehl M, Lodahl M, et al. (2005). Possible roles for activating RAS mutations in the MGUS to MM transition and in the intramedullary to extramedullary transition in some plasma cell tumors. Blood. 105:317–23. PMID:15339850
3313. Ratei R, Hummel M, Anagnostopoulos I, et al. (2010). Common clonal origin of an acute B-lymphoblastic leukemia and a Langerhans' cell sarcoma: evidence for hematopoietic plasticity. Haematologica. 95:1461–6. PMID:20421277
3314. Ratner N, Miller SJ (2015). A RASopathy gene commonly mutated in cancer: the neurofibromatosis type 1 tumour suppressor. Nat Rev Cancer. 15:290–301. PMID:25877329
3315. Ratterman M, Kruczek K, Sulo S, et al. (2014). Extramedullary chronic lymphocytic leukemia: systematic analysis of cases reported between 1975 and 2012. Leuk Res. 38:299–303. PMID:24064196
3316. Rauen KA (2013). The RASopathies. Annu Rev Genomics Hum Genet. 14:355–69. PMID:23875798
3317. Rauen KA, Schoyer L, McCormick F, et al. (2010). Proceedings from the 2009 genetic syndromes of the Ras/MAPK pathway: From bedside to bench and back. Am J Med Genet A. 152A:4–24. PMID:20014119
3318. Rauh MJ, Rahman F, Good D, et al. (2012). Blastic plasmacytoid dendritic cell neoplasm with leukemic presentation, lacking cutaneous involvement: Case series and literature review. Leuk Res. 36:81–6. PMID:21890199
3319. Rawstron AC, Bennett FL, O'Connor SJ, et al. (2008). Monoclonal B-cell lymphocytosis and chronic lymphocytic leukemia. N Engl J Med. 359:575–83. PMID:18687638
3320. Rawstron AC, Green MJ, Kuzmicki A, et al. (2002). Monoclonal B lymphocytes with the characteristics of "indolent" chronic lymphocytic leukemia are present in 3.5% of adults with normal blood counts. Blood. 100:635–9. PMID:12091358
3321. Rawstron AC, Shanafelt T, Lanasa MC, et al. (2010). Different biology and clinical outcome according to the absolute numbers of clonal B-cells in monoclonal B-cell lymphocytosis (MBL). Cytometry B Clin Cytom. 78 Suppl 1:S19–23. PMID:20839333
3322. Ray D, Kwon SY, Tagoh H, et al. (2013). Lineage-inappropriate PAX5 expression in t(8;21) acute myeloid leukemia requires signaling-mediated abrogation of polycomb repression. Blood. 122:759–69. PMID:23616623
3323. Raya JM, Martín-Santos T, Luño E, et al. (2015). Acute myeloid leukemia with inv(3)(q21q26.2) or t(3;3)(q21;q26.2): clinical and biological features and comparison with other acute myeloid leukemias with cytogenetic aberrations involving long arm of chromosome 3. Hematology. [Epub ahead of print]. PMID:25680074
3324. Rea D, Etienne G, Nicolini F, et al. (2012). First-line imatinib mesylate in patients with newly diagnosed accelerated phase-chronic myeloid leukemia. Leukemia. 26:2254–9. PMID:22460758
3325. Read JA, Koff JL, Nastoupil LJ, et al. (2014). Evaluating cell-of-origin subtype methods for predicting diffuse large B-cell lymphoma survival: a meta-analysis of gene expression profiling and immunohistochemistry algorithms. Clin Lymphoma Myeloma Leuk. 14:460–467.e2. PMID:25052052
3326. Reardon DA, Hanson CA, Roth MS, et al. (1994). Lineage switch in Philadelphia chromosome-positive acute lymphoblastic leukemia. Cancer. 73:1526–32. PMID:8111722
3327. Redaelli A, Laskin BL, Stephens JM, et al. (2005). A systematic literature review of the clinical and epidemiological burden of acute lymphoblastic leukaemia (ALL). Eur J Cancer Care (Engl). 14:53–62. PMID:15698386
3328. Ree HJ, Kadin ME, Kikuchi M, et al. (1998). Angioimmunoblastic lymphoma (AILD-type T-cell lymphoma) with hyperplastic germinal centers. Am J Surg Pathol. 22:643–55. PMID:9630171
3329. Reed JC (2008). Bcl-2-family proteins and hematologic malignancies: history and future prospects. Blood. 111:3322–30. PMID:18362212
3330. Reed M, McKenna RW, Bridges R, et al. (1981). Morphologic manifestations of monoclonal gammopathies. Am J Clin Pathol. 76:8–23. PMID:6789672
3331. Regev A, Stark P, Blickstein D, et al. (1997). Thrombotic complications in essential thrombocythemia with relatively low platelet counts. Am J Hematol. 56:168–72. PMID:9371529
3332. Reichard KK, Burks EJ, Foucar MK, et al. (2005). CD4(+) CD56(+) lineage-negative malignancies are rare tumors of plasmacytoid dendritic cells. Am J Surg Pathol. 29:1274–83. PMID:16160468
3333. Reichard KK, McKenna RW, Kroft SH (2007). ALK-positive diffuse large B-cell lymphoma: report of four cases and review of the literature. Mod Pathol. 20:310–9. PMID:17277765
3334. Reichel J, Chadburn A, Rubinstein PG, et al. (2015). Flow sorting and exome sequencing reveal the oncogenome of primary Hodgkin and Reed-Sternberg cells. Blood. 125:1061–72. PMID:25488972
3335. Reid AG, De Melo VA, Elderfield K, et al. (2009). Phenotype of blasts in chronic myeloid leukemia in blastic phase-Analysis of bone marrow trephine biopsies and correlation with cytogenetics. Leuk Res. 33:418–25. PMID:18760473
3336. Reilly JT (2002). Cytogenetic and molecular genetic aspects of idiopathic myelofibrosis. Acta Haematol. 108:113–9. PMID:12373082
3337. Reiter A, Walz C, Watmore A, et al. (2005). The t(8;9)(p22;p24) is a recurrent abnormality in chronic and acute leukemia that fuses PCM1 to JAK2. Cancer Res. 65:2662–7. PMID:15805263
3338. Reiter E, Greinix H, Rabitsch W, et al. (2000). Low curative potential of bone marrow transplantation for highly aggressive acute myelogenous leukemia with inversioin inv (3)(q21q26) or homologous translocation t(3;3) (q21;q26). Ann Hematol. 79:374–7. PMID:10965785
3339. Remacha AF, Nomdedéu JF, Puget G, et al. (2006). Occurrence of the JAK2 V617F mutation in the WHO provisional entity: myelodysplastic/myeloproliferative disease, unclassifiable-refractory anemia with ringed sideroblasts associated with marked thrombocytosis. Haematologica. 91:719–20. PMID:16670082
3340. Remstein ED, Dogan A, Einerson RR, et al. (2006). The incidence and anatomic site specificity of chromosomal translocations in primary extranodal marginal zone B-cell lymphoma of mucosa-associated lymphoid tissue (MALT lymphoma) in North America. Am J Surg Pathol. 30:1546–53. PMID:17122510
3341. Remstein ED, James CD, Kurtin PJ (2000). Incidence and subtype specificity of API2-MALT1 fusion translocations in extranodal, nodal, and splenic marginal zone lymphomas. Am J Pathol. 156:1183–8. PMID:10751343
3342. Ren M, Cowell JK (2011). Constitutive Notch pathway activation in murine ZMYM2-FGFR1-induced T-cell lymphomas associated with atypical myeloproliferative disease. Blood. 117:6837–47. PMID:21527531
3343. Renné C, Martín-Subero JI, Hansmann ML, et al. (2005). Molecular cytogenetic analyses of immunoglobulin loci in nodular lymphocyte predominant Hodgkin's lymphoma reveal a recurrent IGH-BCL6 juxtaposition. J Mol Diagn. 7:352–6. PMID:16049307
3343A. Renneville A, Boissel N, Nibourel O, et al. (2012). Prognostic significance of DNA methyltransferase 3A mutations in cytogenetically normal acute myeloid leukemia: a study by the Acute Leukemia French Association. Leukemia. 26:1247–54. PMID:22289988
3343B. Renneville A, Boissel N, Zurawski V, et al. (2009). Wilms tumor 1 gene mutations are associated with a higher risk of recurrence in young adults with acute myeloid leukemia: a study from the Acute Leukemia French Association. Cancer. 115:3719–27. PMID:19536888
3344. Renneville A, Quesnel B, Charpentier A, et al. (2006). High occurrence of JAK2 V617 mutation in refractory anemia with ringed sideroblasts associated with marked thrombocytosis. Leukemia. 20:2067–70. PMID:16990759
3345. Reshef R, Luskin MR, Kamoun M, et al. (2011). Association of HLA polymorphisms with post-transplant lymphoproliferative disorder in solid-organ transplant recipients. Am J Transplant. 11:817–25. PMID:21401872
3346. Reshef R, Vardhanabhuti S, Luskin MR, et al. (2011). Reduction of immunosuppression as initial therapy for posttransplantation lymphoproliferative disorder. Am J Transplant. 11:336–47. PMID:21219573
3347. Ribera-Cortada I, Martinez D, Amador V, et al. (2015). Plasma cell and terminal B-cell differentiation in mantle cell lymphoma mainly occur in the SOX11-negative subtype. Mod Pathol. 28:1435–47. PMID:26360498
3348. Riccardi A, Gobbi PG, Ucci G, et al. (1991). Changing clinical presentation of multiple myeloma. Eur J Cancer. 27:1401–5. PMID:1835856
3349. Ricci C, Fermo E, Corti S, et al. (2010). RAS mutations contribute to evolution of chronic myelomonocytic leukemia to the proliferative variant. Clin Cancer Res. 16:2246–56. PMID:20371679
3350. Rice L, Popat U (2005). Every case of essential thrombocythemia should be tested for the Philadelphia chromosome. Am J Hematol. 78:71–3. PMID:15609281
3351. Richard P, Vassallo J, Valmary S, et al. (2006). "In situ-like" mantle cell lymphoma: a report of two cases. J Clin Pathol. 59:995–6. PMID:16935977
3352. Richendollar BG, Hsi ED, Cook JR (2009). Extramedullary plasmacytoma-like posttransplantation lymphoproliferative disorders: clinical and pathologic features. Am J Clin Pathol. 132:581–8. PMID:19762536
3353. Richter J, Quintanilla-Martinez L, Bienemann K, et al. (2013). An unusual presentation of a common infection. Infection. 41:565–9. PMID:22926562
3354. Richter J, Schlesner M, Hoffmann S, et al. (2012). Recurrent mutation of the ID3 gene in Burkitt lymphoma identified by integrated genome, exome and transcriptome sequencing. Nat Genet. 44:1316–20. PMID:23143595
3355. Riemersma SA, Jordanova ES, Schop RF, et al. (2000). Extensive genetic alterations of the HLA region, including homozygous deletions of HLA class II genes in B-cell lymphomas arising in immune-privileged sites. Blood. 96:3569–77. PMID:11071656
3356. Riemersma SA, Oudejans JJ, Vonk MJ, et al. (2005). High numbers of tumour-infiltrating activated cytotoxic T lymphocytes, and frequent loss of HLA class I and II expression, are features of aggressive B cell lymphomas of the brain and testis. J Pathol. 206:328–36. PMID:15887291et al. (2004). SEER Cancer Statistics Review, 1975-2001. Bethesda: National Cancer Institute.
3358. Ries LAG, Kosary CL, Hankey BF, et al. (1999). SEER cancer statistics review, 1973-1996. Vol. NIH Publ. 99-2789. Bethesda: National Cancer Institute.
3359. Rigacci L, Vitolo U, Nassi L, et al. (2007). Positron emission tomography in the staging of patients with Hodgkin's lymphoma. A prospective multicentric study by the Intergruppo Italiano Linfomi. Ann Hematol. 86:897–903. PMID:17701410
3360. Rimsza LM, Roberts RA, Campo E, et al. (2006). Loss of major histocompatibility class II expression in non-immune-privileged site diffuse large B-cell lymphoma is highly coordinated and not due to chromosomal deletions. Blood. 107:1101–7. PMID:16239429
3361. Rimsza LM, Roberts RA, Miller TP, et al. (2004). Loss of MHC class II gene and protein expression in diffuse large B-cell lymphoma is

related to decreased tumor immunosurveillance and poor patient survival regardless of other prognostic factors: a follow-up study from the Leukemia and Lymphoma Molecular Profiling Project. Blood. 103:4251–8. PMID:14976040
3361A. Rinaldi A, Capello D, Scandurra M, et al. (2010). Single nucleotide polymorphism-arrays provide new insights in the pathogenesis of post-transplant diffuse large B-cell lymphoma. Br J Haematol. 149:569-77. PMID: 20230398.
3362. Rinaldi A, Mian M, Chigrinova E, et al. (2011). Genome-wide DNA profiling of marginal zone lymphomas identifies subtype-specific lesions with an impact on the clinical outcome. Blood. 117:1595–604. PMID:21115979
3362A. Ripp JA, Loiue DC, Chan W, et al. (2002). T-cell rich B-cell lymphoma: clinical distinctiveness and response to treatment in 45 patients. Leuk Lymphoma. 43:1573–80. PMID:12400599
3363. Ritz O, Guiter C, Castellano F, et al. (2009). Recurrent mutations of the STAT6 DNA binding domain in primary mediastinal B-cell lymphoma. Blood. 114:1236–42. PMID:19423726
3364. Ritz O, Rommel K, Dorsch K, et al. (2013). STAT6-mediated BCL6 repression in primary mediastinal B-cell lymphoma (PMBL). Oncotarget. 4:1093–102. PMID:23852366
3365. Rizvi MA, Evens AM, Tallman MS, et al. (2006). T-cell non-Hodgkin lymphoma. Blood. 107:1255–64. PMID:16210342
3366. Rizzo KA, Streubel B, Pittaluga S, et al. (2010). Marginal zone lymphomas in children and the young adult population; characterization of genetic aberrations by FISH and RT-PCR. Mod Pathol. 23:866–73. PMID:20305621
3367. Robak T (2006). Current treatment options in hairy cell leukemia and hairy cell leukemia variant. Cancer Treat Rev. 32:365–76. PMID:16781083
3368. Robbiani DF, Deroubaix S, Feldhahn N, et al. (2015). Plasmodium Infection Promotes Genomic Instability and AID-Dependent B Cell Lymphoma. Cell. 162:727–37. PMID:26276629
3368A. Roberti A, Dobay MP, Bisig B, et al. (2016). Type II enteropathy-associated T-cell lymphoma features a unique genomic profile with highly recurrent SETD2 alterations. Nat Commun. 7:12602. PMID:27600764
3369. Roberts I, Izraeli S (2014). Haematopoietic development and leukaemia in Down syndrome. Br J Haematol. 167:587–99. PMID:25155832
3370. Roberts KG, Li Y, Payne-Turner D, et al. (2014). Targetable kinase-activating lesions in Ph-like acute lymphoblastic leukemia. N Engl J Med. 371:1005–15. PMID:25207766
3371. Roberts KG, Pei D, Campana D, et al. (2014). Outcomes of children with BCR-ABL1–like acute lymphoblastic leukemia treated with risk-directed therapy based on the levels of minimal residual disease. J Clin Oncol. 32:3012–20. PMID:25049327
3372. Roberts MJ, Chadburn A, Ma S, et al. (2013). Nuclear protein dysregulation in lymphoplasmacytic lymphoma/waldenstrom macroglobulinemia. Am J Clin Pathol. 139:210–9. PMID:23355206
3373. Robertson PB, Neiman RS, Worapongpaiboon S, et al. (1997). 013 (CD99) positivity in hematologic proliferations correlates with TdT positivity. Mod Pathol. 10:277–82. PMID:9110287
3374. Robetorye RS, Bohling SD, Medeiros LJ, et al. (2000). Follicular lymphoma with monocytoid B-cell proliferation: molecular assessment of the clonal relationship between the follicular and monocytoid B-cell components. Lab Invest. 80:1593–9. PMID:11045576
3375. Robillard N, Avet-Loiseau H, Garand R, et al. (2003). CD20 is associated with a small mature plasma cell morphology and t(11;14) in multiple myeloma. Blood. 102:1070–1. PMID:12702507
3376. Robledo C, García JL, Benito R, et al. (2011). Molecular characterization of the region 7q22.1 in splenic marginal zone lymphomas. PLoS One. 6:e24939. PMID:21957467
3377. Robson A, Assaf C, Bagot M, et al. (2015). Aggressive epidermotropic cutaneous CD8(+) lymphoma: a cutaneous lymphoma with distinct clinical and pathological features. Report of an EORTC Cutaneous Lymphoma Task Force Workshop. Histopathology. 67:425–41. PMID:24438036
3378. Robyn J, Lemery S, McCoy JP, et al. (2006). Multilineage involvement of the fusion gene in patients with FIP1L1/PDGFRA-positive hypereosinophilic syndrome. Br J Haematol. 132:286–92. PMID:16409293
3379. Roccaro AM, Sacco A, Jimenez C, et al. (2014). C1013G/CXCR4 acts as a driver mutation of tumor progression and modulator of drug resistance in lymphoplasmacytic lymphoma. Blood. 123:4120–31. PMID:24711662
3380. Rocquain J, Carbuccia N, Trouplin V, et al. (2010). Combined mutations of ASXL1, CBL, FLT3, IDH1, IDH2, JAK2, KRAS, NPM1, NRAS, RUNX1, TET2 and WT1 genes in myelodysplastic syndromes and acute myeloid leukemias. BMC Cancer. 10:401. PMID:20678218
3381. Roden AC, Hu X, Kip S, et al. (2014). BRAF V600E expression in Langerhans cell histiocytosis: clinical and immunohistochemical study on 25 pulmonary and 54 extrapulmonary cases. Am J Surg Pathol. 38:548–51. PMID:24625419
3382. Roden AC, Macon WR, Keeney GL, et al. (2008). Seroma-associated primary anaplastic large-cell lymphoma adjacent to breast implants: an indolent T-cell lymphoproliferative disorder. Mod Pathol. 21:455–63. PMID:18223553
3383. Rodig SJ, Abramson JS, Pinkus GS, et al. (2006). Heterogeneous CD52 expression among hematologic neoplasms: implications for the use of alemtuzumab (CAMPATH-1H). Clin Cancer Res. 12:7174–9. PMID:17145843
3384. Rodig SJ, Savage KJ, LaCasce AS, et al. (2007). Expression of TRAF1 and nuclear c-Rel distinguishes primary mediastinal large cell lymphoma from other types of diffuse large B-cell lymphoma. Am J Surg Pathol. 31:106–12. PMID:17197926
3385. Rodig SJ, Vergilio JA, Shahsafaei A, et al. (2008). Characteristic expression patterns of TCL1, CD38, and CD44 identify aggressive lymphomas harboring a MYC translocation. Am J Surg Pathol. 32:113–22. PMID:18162778
3386. Rodríguez-Jurado R, Vidaurri-de la Cruz H, Durán-Mckinster C, et al. (2003). Indeterminate cell histiocytosis. Clinical and pathologic study in a pediatric patient. Arch Pathol Lab Med. 127:748–51. PMID:12741905
3387. Rodriguez-Justo M, Attygalle AD, Munson P, et al. (2009). Angioimmunoblastic T-cell lymphoma with hyperplastic germinal centres: a neoplasia with origin in the outer zone of the germinal centre? Clinicopathological and immunohistochemical study of 10 cases with follicular T-cell markers. Mod Pathol. 22:753–61. PMID:19329936
3388. Rodríguez-Pinilla SM, Barrionuevo C, García J, et al. (2011). Epstein-Barr virus-positive systemic NK/T-cell lymphomas in children: report of six cases. Histopathology. 59:1183–93. PMID:22175898
3389. Rodríguez-Pinilla SM, Barrionuevo C, Garcia J, et al. (2010). EBV-associated cutaneous NK/T-cell lymphoma: review of a series of 14 cases from peru in children and young adults. Am J Surg Pathol. 34:1773–82. PMID:21107082
3390. Rodríguez-Pinilla SM, Ortiz-Romero PL, Monsalvez V, et al. (2013). TCR-γ expression in primary cutaneous T-cell lymphomas. Am J Surg Pathol. 37:375–84. PMID:23348211
3391. Rodríguez Pinilla SM, Roncador G, Rodríguez-Peralto JL, et al. (2009). Primary cutaneous CD4+ small/medium-sized pleomorphic T-cell lymphoma expresses follicular T-cell markers. Am J Surg Pathol. 33:81–90. PMID:18987541
3391A. Roemer MG, Advani RH, Ligon AH, et al. (2016). PD-L1 and PD-L2 genetic alterations define classical Hodgkin lymphoma and predict outcome. J Clin Oncol. 34:2690–7. PMID:27069084
3392. Rogers HJ, Vardiman JW, Anastasi J, et al. (2014). Complex or monosomal karyotype and not blast percentage is associated with poor survival in acute myeloid leukemia and myelodysplastic syndrome patients with inv(3)(q21q26.2)/t(3;3)(q21;q26.2): a Bone Marrow Pathology Group study. Haematologica. 99:821–9. PMID:24463215
3393. Rogers SL, Zhao Y, Jiang X, et al. (2010). Expression of the leukemic prognostic marker CD7 is linked to epigenetic modifications in chronic myeloid leukemia. Mol Cancer. 9:41. PMID:20175919
3394. Rohatiner A, d'Amore F, Coiffier B, et al. (1994). Report on a workshop convened to discuss the pathological and staging classifications of gastrointestinal tract lymphoma. Ann Oncol. 5:397–400. PMID:8075046
3395. Rohr J, Guo S, Huo J, et al. (2015). Recurrent activating mutations of CD28 in peripheral T-cell lymphomas. Leukemia. 30:1062–70. PMID:26719098
3396. Roithmann S, Toledano M, Tourani JM, et al. (1991). HIV-associated non-Hodgkin's lymphomas: clinical characteristics and outcome. The experience of the French Registry of HIV-associated tumors. Ann Oncol. 2:289–95. PMID:1868025
3397. Rollison DE, Howlader N, Smith MT, et al. (2008). Epidemiology of myelodysplastic syndromes and chronic myeloproliferative disorders in the United States, 2001-2004, using data from the NAACCR and SEER programs. Blood. 112:45–52. PMID:18443215
3398. Roncador G, Garcia JF, Garcia JF, et al. (2005). FOXP3, a selective marker for a subset of adult T-cell leukaemia/lymphoma. Leukemia. 19:2247–53. PMID:16193085
3399. Roncador G, García Verdes-Montenegro JF, Tedoldi S, et al. (2007). Expression of two markers of germinal center T cells (SAP and PD-1) in angioimmunoblastic T-cell lymphoma. Haematologica. 92:1059–66. PMID:17640856
3400. Roos-Weil D, Dietrich S, Boumendil A, et al. (2013). Stem cell transplantation can provide durable disease control in blastic plasmacytoid dendritic cell neoplasm: a retrospective study from the European Group for Blood and Marrow Transplantation. Blood. 121:440–6. PMID:23203822
3401. Rosado FG, Morice WG, He R, et al. (2015). Immunophenotypic features by multiparameter flow cytometry can help distinguish low grade B-cell lymphomas with plasmacytic differentiation from plasma cell proliferative disorders with an unrelated clonal B-cell process. Br J Haematol. 169:368–76. PMID:25644063
3402. Rosado FG, Oliveira JL, Sohani AR, et al. (2015). Bone marrow findings of the newly described TEMPI syndrome: when erythrocytosis and plasma cell dyscrasia coexist. Mod Pathol. 28:367–72. PMID:25216227
3403. Rosales CM, Lin P, Mansoor A, et al. (2001). Lymphoplasmacytic lymphoma/Waldenström macroglobulinemia associated with Hodgkin disease. A report of two cases. Am J Clin Pathol. 116:34–40. PMID:11447749
3404. Rosati S, Mick R, Xu F, et al. (1996). Refractory cytopenia with multilineage dysplasia: further characterization of an 'unclassifiable' myelodysplastic syndrome. Leukemia. 10:20–6. PMID:8558932
3405. Roschewski M, Staudt LM, Wilson WH (2014). Diffuse large B-cell lymphoma-treatment approaches in the molecular era. Nat Rev Clin Oncol. 11:12–23. PMID:24217204
3406. Roschewski M, Wilson WH (2012). Lymphomatoid granulomatosis. Cancer J. 18:469–74. PMID:23006954
3407. Rosenberg AS, Morgan MB (2001). Cutaneous indeterminate cell histiocytosis: a new spindle cell variant resembling dendritic cell sarcoma. J Cutan Pathol. 28:531–7. PMID:11737523
3408. Rosenberg CL, Wong E, Petty EM, et al. (1991). PRAD1, a candidate BCL1 oncogene: mapping and expression in centrocytic lymphoma. Proc Natl Acad Sci U S A. 88:9638–42. PMID:1682919
3409. Rosenwald A, Alizadeh AA, Widhopf G, et al. (2001). Relation of gene expression phenotype to immunoglobulin mutation genotype in B cell chronic lymphocytic leukemia. J Exp Med. 194:1639–47. PMID:11733578
3410. Rosenwald A, Ott G, Pulford K, et al. (1999). t(1;2)(q21;p23) and t(2;3)(p23;q21): two novel variant translocations of the t(2;5)(p23;q35) in anaplastic large cell lymphoma. Blood. 94:362–4. PMID:10381534
3411. Rosenwald A, Wright G, Chan WC, et al. (2002). The use of molecular profiling to predict survival after chemotherapy for diffuse large-B-cell lymphoma. N Engl J Med. 346:1937–47. PMID:12075054
3412. Rosenwald A, Wright G, Leroy K, et al. (2003). Molecular diagnosis of primary mediastinal B cell lymphoma identifies a clinically favorable subgroup of diffuse large B cell lymphoma related to Hodgkin lymphoma. J Exp Med. 198:851–62. PMID:12975453
3413. Rosenwald A, Wright G, Wiestner A, et al. (2003). The proliferation gene expression signature is a quantitative integrator of oncogenic events that predicts survival in mantle cell lymphoma. Cancer Cell. 3:185–97. PMID:12620412
3414. Rosh JR, Gross T, Mamula P, et al. (2007). Hepatosplenic T-cell lymphoma in adolescents and young adults with Crohn's disease: a cautionary tale? Inflamm Bowel Dis. 13:1024–30. PMID:17480018
3415. Roshal M, Chien S, Othus M, et al. (2013). The proportion of CD34(+)CD38(low or neg) myeloblasts, but not side population frequency, predicts initial response to induction therapy in patients with newly diagnosed acute myeloid leukemia. Leukemia. 27:728–31. PMID:22926686
3416. Roshan B, Leffler DA, Jamma S, et al. (2011). The incidence and clinical spectrum of refractory celiac disease in a north american referral center. Am J Gastroenterol. 106:923–8. PMID:21468013
3416A. Rosier RN, Rosenberg AE (2000). Case records of the Massachusetts General Hospital. Weekly clinicopathological exercises. Case 9-2000. A 41-year-old man with multiple bony lesions and adjacent soft-tissue masses. N Engl J Med. 342:875–83. PMID:10727593
3417. Rosolen A, Perkins SL, Pinkerton CR, et al. (2015). Revised International Pediatric Non-Hodgkin Lymphoma Staging System. J Clin Oncol. 33:2112–8. PMID:25940716
3418. Rossbach HC (2006). Familial infantile myelofibrosis as an autosomal recessive disorder: preponderance among children from Saudi Arabia. Pediatr Hematol Oncol. 23:453–4. PMID:16728367
3419. Rossi D, Trifonov V, Fangazio M, et al.

(2012). The coding genome of splenic marginal zone lymphoma: activation of NOTCH2 and other pathways regulating marginal zone development. J Exp Med. 209:1537–51. PMID:22891273
3420. Rostagno A, Frizzera G, Ylagan L, et al. (2002). Tumoral non-amyloidotic monoclonal immunoglobulin light chain deposits ('aggregoma'): presenting feature of B-cell dyscrasia in three cases with immunohistochemical and biochemical analyses. Br J Haematol. 119:62–9. PMID:12358904
3421. Roth CG, Contis L, Gupta S, et al. (2011). De novo acute myeloid leukemia with Philadelphia chromosome (BCR-ABL) and inversion 16 (CBFB-MYH11): report of two cases and review of the literature. Leuk Lymphoma. 52:531–5. PMID:21281226
3422. Roth DE, Jones A, Smith L, et al. (2005). Severe chronic active Epstein-Barr virus infection mimicking steroid-dependent inflammatory bowel disease. Pediatr Infect Dis J. 24:261–4. PMID:15750464
3423. Roth MJ, Medeiros LJ, Elenitoba-Johnson K, et al. (1995). Extramedullary myeloid cell tumors. An immunohistochemical study of 29 cases using routinely fixed and processed paraffin-embedded tissue sections. Arch Pathol Lab Med. 119:790–8. PMID:7668936
3424. Roulland S, Faroudi M, Mamessier E, et al. (2011). Early steps of follicular lymphoma pathogenesis. Adv Immunol. 111:1–46. PMID:21970951
3425. Roulland S, Kelly RS, Morgado E, et al. (2014). t(14;18) Translocation: A predictive blood biomarker for follicular lymphoma. J Clin Oncol. 32:1347–55. PMID:24687831
3426. Roulland S, Navarro JM, Grenot P, et al. (2006). Follicular lymphoma-like B cells in healthy individuals: a novel intermediate step in early lymphomagenesis. J Exp Med. 203:2425–31. PMID:17043145
3427. Roullet MR, Cornfield DB (2006). Large natural killer cell lymphoma arising from an indolent natural killer cell large granular lymphocyte proliferation. Arch Pathol Lab Med. 130:1712–4. PMID:17076536
3428. Roullet MR, Martinez D, Ma L, et al. (2010). Coexisting follicular and mantle cell lymphoma with each having an in situ component: A novel, curious, and complex consultation case of coincidental, composite, colonizing lymphoma. Am J Clin Pathol. 133:584–91. PMID:20231612
3429. Roumiantsev S, Krause DS, Neumann CA, et al. (2004). Distinct stem cell myeloproliferative/T lymphoma syndromes induced by ZNF198-FGFR1 and BCR-FGFR1 fusion genes from 8p11 translocations. Cancer Cell. 5:287–98. PMID:15050920
3430. Roumier C, Eclache V, Imbert M, et al. (2003). M0 AML, clinical and biologic features of the disease, including AML1 gene mutations: a report of 59 cases by the Groupe Français d'Hématologie Cellulaire (GFHC) and the Groupe Français de Cytogénétique Hématologique (GFCH). Blood. 101:1277–83. PMID:12393381
3431. Rousselet MC, François S, Croué A, et al. (1994). A lymph node interdigitating reticulum cell sarcoma. Arch Pathol Lab Med. 118:183–8. PMID:8311662
3432. Rowe D, Cotterill SJ, Ross FM, et al. (2000). Cytogenetically cryptic AML1-ETO and CBF beta-MYH11 gene rearrangements: incidence in 412 cases of acute myeloid leukaemia. Br J Haematol. 111:1051–6. PMID:11167739
3433. Rowley JD (1973). Letter: A new consistent chromosomal abnormality in chronic myelogenous leukaemia identified by quinacrine fluorescence and Giemsa staining. Nature. 243:290–3. PMID:4126434
3434. Rowley JD (1988). Chromosome studies in the non-Hodgkin's lymphomas: the role of the 14;18 translocation. J Clin Oncol. 6:919–25. PMID:3284977
3435. Rowley JD, Olney HJ (2002). International workshop on the relationship of prior therapy to balanced chromosome aberrations in therapy-related myelodysplastic syndromes and acute leukemia: overview report. Genes Chromosomes Cancer. 33:331–45. PMID:11921269
3436. Rowlings PA, Curtis RE, Passweg JR, et al. (1999). Increased incidence of Hodgkin's disease after allogeneic bone marrow transplantation. J Clin Oncol. 17:3122–7. PMID:10506608
3437. Roy A, Roberts I, Norton A, et al. (2009). Acute megakaryoblastic leukaemia (AMKL) and transient myeloproliferative disorder (TMD) in Down syndrome: a multi-step model of myeloid leukaemogenesis. Br J Haematol. 147:3–12. PMID:19594743
3438. Roy A, Roberts I, Vyas P (2012). Biology and management of transient abnormal myelopoiesis (TAM) in children with Down syndrome. Semin Fetal Neonatal Med. 17:196–201. PMID:22421527
3439. Royo C, Navarro A, Clot G, et al. (2012). Non-nodal type of mantle cell lymphoma is a specific biological and clinical subgroup of the disease. Leukemia. 26:1895–8. PMID:22425896
3440. Royo C, Salaverria I, Hartmann EM, et al. (2011). The complex landscape of genetic alterations in mantle cell lymphoma. Semin Cancer Biol. 21:322–34. PMID:21945515
3441. Rozen L, Huybrechts S, Dedeken L, et al. (2014). Transient leukemia in a newborn without Down syndrome: case report and review of the literature. Eur J Pediatr. 173:1643–7. PMID:24253371
3442. Rozman M, Navarro JT, Arenillas L, et al. (2014). Multilineage dysplasia is associated with a poorer prognosis in patients with de novo acute myeloid leukemia with intermediate-risk cytogenetics and wild-type NPM1. Ann Hematol. 93:1695–703. PMID:24824767
3443. Rubenstein JL, Fridlyand J, Shen A, et al. (2006). Gene expression and angiotropism in primary CNS lymphoma. Blood. 107:3716–23. PMID:16418334
3444. Rubio-Moscardo F, Climent J, Siebert R, et al. (2005). Mantle-cell lymphoma genotypes identified with CGH to BAC microarrays define a leukemic subgroup of disease and predict patient outcome. Blood. 105:4445–54. PMID:15718413
3445. Rubio-Tapia A, Kelly DG, Lahr BD, et al. (2009). Clinical staging and survival in refractory celiac disease: a single center experience. Gastroenterology. 136:99–107, quiz 352–3. PMID:18996383
3446. Rubio-Tapia A, Murray JA (2010). Classification and management of refractory coeliac disease. Gut. 59:547–57. PMID:20332526
3447. Rubnitz JE, Onciu M, Pounds S, et al. (2009). Acute mixed lineage leukemia in children: the experience of St Jude Children's Research Hospital. Blood. 113:5083–9. PMID:19131545
3448. Rubnitz JE, Raimondi SC, Tong X, et al. (2002). Favorable impact of the t(9;11) in childhood acute myeloid leukemia. J Clin Oncol. 20:2302–9. PMID:11981001
3449. Ruchlemer R, Parry-Jones N, Brito-Babapulle V, et al. (2004). B-prolymphocytic leukaemia with t(11;14) revisited: a splenomegalic form of mantle cell lymphoma evolving with leukaemia. Br J Haematol. 125:330–6. PMID:15086413
3450. Rudzki Z, Giles L, Cross NC, et al. (2012). Myeloid neoplasm with rearrangement of PDGFRA, but with no significant eosinophilia: should we broaden the World Health Organization definition of the entity? Br J Haematol. 156:558. PMID:22224867
3451. Ruf S, Wagner HJ (2013). Determining EBV load: current best practice and future requirements. Expert Rev Clin Immunol. 9:139–51. PMID:23390945
3452. Ruggeri M, Tosetto A, Frezzato M, et al. (2003). The rate of progression to polycythemia vera or essential thrombocythemia in patients with erythrocytosis or thrombocytosis. Ann Intern Med. 139:470–5. PMID:13679323
3453. Rui L, Emre NC, Kruhlak MJ, et al. (2010). Cooperative epigenetic modulation by cancer amplicon genes. Cancer Cell. 18:590–605. PMID:21156283
3454. Ruiz A, Reischl U, Swerdlow SH, et al. (2007). Extranodal marginal zone B-cell lymphomas of the ocular adnexa: multiparameter analysis of 34 cases including interphase molecular cytogenetics and PCR for Chlamydia psittaci. Am J Surg Pathol. 31:792–802. PMID:17460465
3455. Ruiz-Ballesteros E, Mollejo M, Rodriguez A, et al. (2005). Splenic marginal zone lymphoma: proposal of new diagnostic and prognostic markers identified after tissue and cDNA microarray analysis. Blood. 106:1831–8. PMID:15914563
3456. Ruiz-Maldonado R, Parrilla FM, Orozco-Covarrubias ML, et al. (1995). Edematous, scarring vasculitic panniculitis: a new multisystemic disease with malignant potential. J Am Acad Dermatol. 32:37–44. PMID:7822515
3457. Rumi E (2008). Familial chronic myeloproliferative disorders: the state of the art. Hematol Oncol. 26:131–8. PMID:18484677
3458. Rumi E, Pietra D, Ferretti V, et al. (2014). JAK2 or CALR mutation status defines subtypes of essential thrombocythemia with substantially different clinical course and outcomes. Blood. 123:1544–51. PMID:24366362
3459. Ruskoné-Fourmestraux A, Delmer A, Lavergne A, et al. (1997). Multiple lymphomatous polyposis of the gastrointestinal tract: prospective clinicopathologic study of 31 cases. Groupe D'étude des Lymphomes Digestifs. Gastroenterology. 112:7–16. PMID:8978336
3460. Ruskova A, Thula R, Chan G (2004). Aggressive Natural Killer-Cell Leukemia: report of five cases and review of the literature. Leuk Lymphoma. 45:2427–38. PMID:15621755
3461. Ryan RJ, Akin C, Castells M, et al. (2013). Mast cell sarcoma: a rare and potentially under-recognized diagnostic entity with specific therapeutic implications. Mod Pathol. 26:533–43. PMID:23196796
3462. Ryder J, Wang X, Bao L, et al. (2007). Aggressive natural killer cell leukemia: report of a Chinese series and review of the literature. Int J Hematol. 85:18–25. PMID:17261497
3462A. Rücker FG, Schlenk RF, Bullinger L, et al. (2012). TP53 alterations in acute myeloid leukemia with complex karyotype correlate with specific copy number alterations, monosomal karyotype, and dismal outcome. Blood. 119:2114–21. PMID:22186996
3463. Rüdiger T, Ichinohasama R, Ott MM, et al. (2000). Peripheral T-cell lymphoma with distinct perifollicular growth pattern: a distinct subtype of T-cell lymphoma? Am J Surg Pathol. 24:117–22. PMID:10632495
3464. Rüdiger T, Weisenburger DD, Anderson JR, et al. (2002). Peripheral T-cell lymphoma (excluding anaplastic large-cell lymphoma): results from the Non-Hodgkin's Lymphoma Classification Project. Ann Oncol. 13:140–9. PMID:11863096
3465. Saarinen S, Kaasinen E, Karjalainen-Lindsberg ML, et al. (2013). Primary mediastinal large B-cell lymphoma segregating in a family: exome sequencing identifies MLL as a candidate predisposition gene. Blood. 121:3428–30. PMID:23457195
3466. Saarinen S, Pukkala E, Vahteristo P, et al. (2013). High familial risk in nodular lymphocyte-predominant Hodgkin lymphoma. J Clin Oncol. 31:938–43. PMID:23284040
3467. Sabattini E, Pizzi M, Tabanelli V, et al. (2013). CD30 expression in peripheral T-cell lymphomas. Haematologica. 98:e81–2. PMID:23716537
3468. Sabbah S, Jagne YJ, Zuo J, et al. (2012). T-cell immunity to Kaposi sarcoma-associated herpesvirus: recognition of primary effusion lymphoma by LANA-specific CD4+ T cells. Blood. 119:2083–92. PMID:22234686
3469. Sacchi S, Vinci G, Gugliotta L, et al. (2000). Diagnosis of essential thrombocythemia at platelet counts between 400 and 600x10(9)/L. Gruppo Italiano Malattie Mieloproliferative Croniche(GIMMC). Haematologica. 85:492–5. PMID:10800165
3470. Saffer H, Wahed A, Rassidakis GZ, et al. (2002). Clusterin expression in malignant lymphomas: a survey of 266 cases. Mod Pathol. 15:1221–6. PMID:12429802
3471. Safley AM, Sebastian S, Collins TS, et al. (2004). Molecular and cytogenetic characterization of a novel translocation t(4;22) involving the breakpoint cluster region and platelet-derived growth factor receptor-alpha genes in a patient with atypical chronic myeloid leukemia. Genes Chromosomes Cancer. 40:44–50. PMID:15034867
3472. Saft L, Karimi M, Ghaderi M, et al. (2014). p53 protein expression independently predicts outcome in patients with lower-risk myelodysplastic syndromes with del(5q). Haematologica. 99:1041–9. PMID:24682512
3473. Saggini A, Gulia A, Argenyi Z, et al. (2010). A variant of lymphomatoid papulosis simulating primary cutaneous aggressive epidermotropic CD8+ cytotoxic T-cell lymphoma. Description of 9 cases. Am J Surg Pathol. 34:1168–75. PMID:20661014
3474. Sahara N, Takeshita A, Shigeno K, et al. (2002). Clinicopathological and prognostic characteristics of CD56-negative multiple myeloma. Br J Haematol. 117:882–5. PMID:12060125
3475. Sai P, Kalavar M, Raval M, et al. (2004). A case of chronic neutrophilic leukemia with novel chromosomal abnormalities. Clin Adv Hematol Oncol. 2:543–5, discussion 545. PMID:16163234
3475A. Said J (2004). Multicentric Castleman disease: consensus at last? Blood. 129:1569-70. PMID:28336727
3476. Said JW (2007). Immunodeficiency-related Hodgkin lymphoma and its mimics. Adv Anat Pathol. 14:189–94. PMID:17452815
3477. Said JW, Shintaku IP, Asou H, et al. (1999). Herpesvirus 8 inclusions in primary effusion lymphoma: report of a unique case with T-cell phenotype. Arch Pathol Lab Med. 123:257–60. PMID:10086517
3478. Said JW, Tasaka T, Takeuchi S, et al. (1996). Primary effusion lymphoma in women: report of two cases of Kaposi's sarcoma herpes virus-associated effusion-based lymphoma in human immunodeficiency virus-negative women. Blood. 88:3124–8. PMID:8874212
3479. Said W, Chien K, Takeuchi S, et al. (1996). Kaposi's sarcoma-associated herpesvirus (KSHV or HHV8) in primary effusion lymphoma: ultrastructural demonstration of herpesvirus in lymphoma cells. Blood. 87:4937–43. PMID:8652805
3480. Saikia T, Advani S, Dasgupta A, et al. (1988). Characterisation of blast cells during blastic phase of chronic myeloid leukaemia by immunophenotyping–experience in 60 patients. Leuk Res. 12:499–506. PMID:3165486
3481. Sainati L, Matutes E, Mulligan S, et al.

(1990). A variant form of hairy cell leukemia resistant to alpha-interferon: clinical and phenotypic characteristics of 17 patients. Blood. 76:157–62. PMID:2364167
3482. Sainty D, Liso V, Cantù-Rajnoldi A, et al. (2000). A new morphologic classification system for acute promyelocytic leukemia distinguishes cases with underlying PLZF/RARA gene rearrangements. Blood. 96:1287–96. PMID:10942370
3483. Saito M, Gao J, Basso K, et al. (2007). A signaling pathway mediating downregulation of BCL6 in germinal center B cells is blocked by BCL6 gene alterations in B cell lymphoma. Cancer Cell. 12:280–92. PMID:17785208
3484. Sakaguchi H, Okuno Y, Muramatsu H, et al. (2013). Exome sequencing identifies secondary mutations of SETBP1 and JAK3 in juvenile myelomonocytic leukemia. Nat Genet. 45:937–41. PMID:23832011
3485. Sakata-Yanagimoto M, Enami T, Yoshida K, et al. (2014). Somatic RHOA mutation in angioimmunoblastic T cell lymphoma. Nat Genet. 46:171–5. PMID:24413737
3486. Salama ME, Lossos IS, Warnke RA, et al. (2009). Immunoarchitectural patterns in nodal marginal zone B-cell lymphoma: a study of 51 cases. Am J Clin Pathol. 132:39–49. PMID:19864232
3487. Salar A, Juanpere N, Bellosillo B, et al. (2006). Gastrointestinal involvement in mantle cell lymphoma: a prospective clinic, endoscopic, and pathologic study. Am J Surg Pathol. 30:1274–80. PMID:17001159
3488. Salaverria I, Beà S, Lopez-Guillermo A, et al. (2008). Genomic profiling reveals different genetic aberrations in systemic ALK-positive and ALK-negative anaplastic large cell lymphomas. Br J Haematol. 140:516–26. PMID:18275429
3489. Salaverria I, Martin-Guerrero I, Burkhardt B, et al. (2013). High resolution copy number analysis of IRF4 translocation-positive diffuse large B-cell and follicular lymphomas. Genes Chromosomes Cancer. 52:150–5. PMID:23073988
3490. Salaverria I, Martin-Guerrero I, Wagener R, et al. (2014). A recurrent 11q aberration pattern characterizes a subset of MYC-negative high-grade B-cell lymphomas resembling Burkitt lymphoma. Blood. 123:1187–98. PMID:24398325
3491. Salaverria I, Philipp C, Oschlies I, et al. (2011). Translocations activating IRF4 identify a subtype of germinal center-derived B-cell lymphoma affecting predominantly children and young adults. Blood. 118:139–47. PMID:21487109
3492. Salaverria I, Royo C, Carvajal-Cuenca A, et al. (2013). CCND2 rearrangements are the most frequent genetic events in cyclin D1(-) mantle cell lymphoma. Blood. 121:1394–402. PMID:23255553
3493. Salaverria I, Siebert R (2011). Follicular lymphoma grade 3B. Best Pract Res Clin Haematol. 24:111–9. PMID:21658612
3494. Salaverria I, Zettl A, Beà S, et al. (2007). Specific secondary genetic alterations in mantle cell lymphoma provide prognostic information independent of the gene expression-based proliferation signature. J Clin Oncol. 25:1216–22. PMID:17296973
3495. Salhany KE, Macon WR, Choi JK, et al. (1998). Subcutaneous panniculitis-like T-cell lymphoma: clinicopathologic, immunophenotypic, and genotypic analysis of alpha/beta and gamma/delta subtypes. Am J Surg Pathol. 22:881–93. PMID:9669350
3496. Saliba J, Saint-Martin C, Di Stefano A, et al. (2015). Germline duplication of ATG2B and GSKIP predisposes to familial myeloid malignancies. Nat Genet. 47:1131–40. PMID:26280900
3497. Salido M, Baró C, Oscier D, et al. (2010). Cytogenetic aberrations and their prognostic value in a series of 330 splenic marginal zone B-cell lymphomas: a multicenter study of the Splenic B-Cell Lymphoma Group. Blood. 116:1479–88. PMID:20479288
3498. Salloum E, Cooper DL, Howe G, et al. (1996). Spontaneous regression of lymphoproliferative disorders in patients treated with methotrexate for rheumatoid arthritis and other rheumatic diseases. J Clin Oncol. 14:1943–9. PMID:8656264
3499. Salomon-Nguyen F, Valensi F, Troussard X, et al. (1996). The value of the monoclonal antibody, DBA44, in the diagnosis of B-lymphoid disorders. Leuk Res. 20:909–13. PMID:9009248
3500. Samols MA, Su A, Ra S, et al. (2014). Intralymphatic cutaneous anaplastic large cell lymphoma/lymphomatoid papulosis: expanding the spectrum of CD30-positive lymphoproliferative disorders. Am J Surg Pathol. 38:1203–11. PMID:24805854
3501. Samoszuk M, Nansen L (1990). Detection of interleukin-5 messenger RNA in Reed-Sternberg cells of Hodgkin's disease with eosinophilia. Blood. 75:13–6. PMID:2403816
3502. Sanchorawala V, Sun F, Quillen K, et al. (2015). Long-term outcome of patients with AL amyloidosis treated with high-dose melphalan and stem cell transplantation: 20-year experience. Blood. 126:2345–7. PMID:26443620
3502A. Sandahl JD, Coenen EA, Forestier E, et al. (2014). t(6;9)(p22;q34)/DEK-NUP214-rearranged pediatric myeloid leukemia: an international study of 62 patients. Haematologica. 99865–72. PMID:24441146
3503. Sandahl JD, Kjeldsen E, Abrahamsson J, et al. (2015). The applicability of the WHO classification in paediatric AML. A NOPHO-AML study. Br J Haematol. 169:859–67. PMID:25819835
3504. Sandberg Y, Almeida J, Gonzalez M, et al. (2006). TCRgammadelta+ large granular lymphocyte leukemias reflect the spectrum of normal antigen-selected TCRgammadelta+ T-cells. Leukemia. 20:505–13. PMID:16437145
3505. Sander B, Quintanilla-Martinez L, Ott G, et al. (2015). Mantle cell lymphoma-a spectrum from indolent to aggressive disease. Virchows Arch. 468:245–57 PMID:26298543
3506. Sander CA, Jaffe ES, Gebhardt FC, et al. (1992). Mediastinal lymphoblastic lymphoma with an immature B-cell immunophenotype. Am J Surg Pathol. 16:300–5. PMID:1317999
3507. Sander CA, Medeiros LJ, Weiss LM, et al. (1992). Lymphoproliferative lesions in patients with common variable immunodeficiency syndrome. Am J Surg Pathol. 16:1170–82. PMID:1334378
3508. Sander CA, Yano T, Clark HM, et al. (1993). p53 mutation is associated with progression in follicular lymphomas. Blood. 82:1994–2004. PMID:8400252
3509. Sander S, Calado DP, Srinivasan L, et al. (2012). Synergy between PI3K signaling and MYC in Burkitt lymphomagenesis. Cancer Cell. 22:167–79. PMID:22897848
3510. Sanderson CJ (1992). Interleukin-5, eosinophils, and disease. Blood. 79:3101–9. PMID:1596561
3511. Sangle N, Cook J, Perkins S, et al. (2014). Myelofibrotic transformations of polycythemia vera and essential thrombocythemia are morphologically, biologically, and prognostically indistinguishable from primary myelofibrosis. Appl Immunohistochem Mol Morphol. 22:663–8. PMID:24897074
3512. Sangueza M, Plaza JA (2013). Hydroa vacciniforme-like cutaneous T-cell lymphoma: clinicopathologic and immunohistochemical study of 12 cases. J Am Acad Dermatol. 69:112–9. PMID:23541598
3513. Sangüeza OP, Salmon JK, White CR Jr, et al. (1995). Juvenile xanthogranuloma: a clinical, histopathologic and immunohistochemical study. J Cutan Pathol. 22:327–35. PMID:7499572
3513A. Sano H, Shimada A, Tabuchi K, et al. (2013). WT1 mutation in pediatric patients with acute myeloid leukemia: a report from the Japanese Childhood AML Cooperative Study Group. Int J Hematol. 98:437–45. PMID:23979985
3514. Sansonno D, De Vita S, Cornacchiulo V, et al. (1996). Detection and distribution of hepatitis C virus-related proteins in lymph nodes of patients with type II mixed cryoglobulinemia and neoplastic or non-neoplastic lymphoproliferation. Blood. 88:4638–45. PMID:8977256
3515. Sant M, Allemani C, Tereanu C, et al. (2010). Incidence of hematologic malignancies in Europe by morphologic subtype: results of the HAEMACARE project. Blood. 116:3724–34. PMID:20664057
3516. Santos FP, O'Brien S (2012). Small lymphocytic lymphoma and chronic lymphocytic leukemia: are they the same disease? Cancer J. 18:396–403. PMID:23006943
3517. Santucci M, Pimpinelli N, Arganini L (1991). Primary cutaneous B-cell lymphoma: a unique type of low-grade lymphoma. Clinicopathologic and immunologic study of 83 cases. Cancer. 67:2311–26. PMID:2013039
3518. Santucci M, Pimpinelli N, Massi D, et al. (2003). Cytotoxic/natural killer cell cutaneous lymphomas. Report of EORTC Cutaneous Lymphoma Task Force Workshop. Cancer. 97:610–27. PMID:12548603
3519. Sanz MA, Grimwade D, Tallman MS, et al. (2009). Management of acute promyelocytic leukemia: recommendations from an expert panel on behalf of the European LeukemiaNet. Blood. 113:1875–91. PMID:18812465
3520. Sapienza MR, Fuligni F, Agostinelli C, et al. (2014). Molecular profiling of blastic plasmacytoid dendritic cell neoplasm reveals a unique pattern and suggests selective sensitivity to NF-kB pathway inhibition. Leukemia. 28:1606–16. PMID:24504027
3521. Sargent RL, Cook JR, Aguilera NI, et al. (2008). Fluorescence immunophenotypic and interphase cytogenetic characterization of nodal lymphoplasmacytic lymphoma. Am J Surg Pathol. 32:1643–53. PMID:18670352
3522. Sarkozy C, Terré C, Jardin F, et al. (2014). Complex karyotype in mantle cell lymphoma is a strong prognostic factor for the time to treatment and overall survival, independent of the MCL international prognostic index. Genes Chromosomes Cancer. 53:106–16. PMID:24249260
3523. Sarkozy C, Traverse-Glehen A, Coiffier B (2015). Double-hit and double-protein-expression lymphomas: aggressive and refractory lymphomas. Lancet Oncol. 16:e555–67. PMID:26545844
3524. Sarris A, Jhanwar S, Cabanillas F (1999). Cytogenetics of Hodgkin's disease. In: Mauch P, Armitage JO, Diehl V, editors. Hodgkin's disease. Philadelphia: Lippincott Williams & Wilkins; p. 195.
3525. Sasajima Y, Yamabe H, Kobashi Y, et al. (1993). High expression of the Epstein-Barr virus latent protein EB nuclear antigen-2 on pyothorax-associated lymphomas. Am J Pathol. 143:1280–5. PMID:8238246
3526. Sashida G, Takaku TI, Shoji N, et al. (2003). Clinico-hematologic features of myelodysplastic syndrome presenting as isolated thrombocytopenia: an entity with a relatively favorable prognosis. Leuk Lymphoma. 44:653–8. PMID:12769343
3527. Sato A, Nakamura N, Kojima M, et al. (2014). Clinical outcome of Epstein-Barr virus-positive diffuse large B-cell lymphoma of the elderly in the rituximab era. Cancer Sci. 105:1170–5. PMID:24974976
3528. Sato H, Oka T, Shinnou Y, et al. (2010). Multi-step aberrant CpG island hyper-methylation is associated with the progression of adult T-cell leukemia/lymphoma. Am J Pathol. 176:402–15. PMID:20019193
3529. Sato T, Toki T, Kanezaki R, et al. (2008). Functional analysis of JAK3 mutations in transient myeloproliferative disorder and acute megakaryoblastic leukaemia accompanying Down syndrome. Br J Haematol. 141:681–8. PMID:18397343
3530. Sato Y, Ichimura K, Tanaka T, et al. (2008). Duodenal follicular lymphomas share common characteristics with mucosa-associated lymphoid tissue lymphomas. J Clin Pathol. 61:377–81. PMID:17601964
3531. Satou A, Asano N, Nakazawa A, et al. (2015). Epstein-Barr virus (EBV)-positive sporadic burkitt lymphoma: an age-related lymphoproliferative disorder? Am J Surg Pathol. 39:227–35. PMID:25321330
3532. Satou Y, Yasunaga J, Yoshida M, et al. (2006). HTLV-I basic leucine zipper factor gene mRNA supports proliferation of adult T cell leukemia cells. Proc Natl Acad Sci U S A. 103:720–5. PMID:16407133
3532A. Sausville EA, Worsham GF, Matthews MJ, et al. (1985). Histologic assessment of lymph nodes in mycosis fungoides/Sézary syndrome (cutaneous T-cell lymphoma): clinical correlations and prognostic import of a new classification system. Hum Pathol. 16:1098–109. PMID:3876976
3533. Sausville JE, Salloum RG, Sorbara L, et al. (2003). Minimal residual disease detection in hairy cell leukemia. Comparison of flow cytometric immunophenotyping with clonal analysis using consensus primer polymerase chain reaction for the heavy chain gene. Am J Clin Pathol. 119:213–7. PMID:12579991
3534. Savage DG, Szydlo RM, Goldman JM (1997). Clinical features at diagnosis in 430 patients with chronic myeloid leukaemia seen at a referral centre over a 16-year period. Br J Haematol. 96:111–6. PMID:9012696
3535. Savage KJ, Al-Rajhi N, Voss N, et al. (2006). Favorable outcome of primary mediastinal large B-cell lymphoma in a single institution: the British Columbia experience. Ann Oncol. 17:123–30. PMID:16236753
3536. Savage KJ, Harris NL, Vose JM, et al. (2008). ALK- anaplastic large-cell lymphoma is clinically and immunophenotypically different from both ALK+ ALCL and peripheral T-cell lymphoma, not otherwise specified: report from the International Peripheral T-Cell Lymphoma Project. Blood. 111:5496–504. PMID:18385450
3537. Savage KJ, Johnson NA, Ben-Neriah S, et al. (2009). MYC gene rearrangements are associated with a poor prognosis in diffuse large B-cell lymphoma patients treated with R-CHOP chemotherapy. Blood. 114:3533–7. PMID:19704118
3538. Savage KJ, Monti S, Kutok JL, et al. (2003). The molecular signature of mediastinal large B-cell lymphoma differs from that of other diffuse large B-cell lymphomas and shares features with classical Hodgkin lymphoma. Blood. 102:3871–9. PMID:12933571
3539. Savage KJ, Slack GW, Mottok A, et al. (2016). Impact of dual expression of MYC and BCL2 by immunohistochemistry on the risk of CNS relapse in DLBCL. Blood. 127:2182–8. PMID:26834242
3540. Savilo E, Campo E, Mollejo M, et al. (1998). Absence of cyclin D1 protein expression in splenic marginal zone lymphoma. Mod

Pathol. 11:601–6. PMID:9688179
3541. Sawyer JR, Waldron JA, Jagannath S, et al. (1995). Cytogenetic findings in 200 patients with multiple myeloma. Cancer Genet Cytogenet. 82:41–9. PMID:7627933
3542. Sayed RH, Wechalekar AD, Gilbertson JA, et al. (2015). Natural history and outcome of light chain deposition disease. Blood. 126:2805–10. PMID:26392598
3543. Saygin C, Uzunaslan D, Ozguroglu M, et al. (2013). Dendritic cell sarcoma: a pooled analysis including 462 cases with presentation of our case series. Crit Rev Oncol Hematol. 88:253–71. PMID:23755890
3544. Scandura JM, Boccuni P, Cammenga J, et al. (2002). Transcription factor fusions in acute leukemia: variations on a theme. Oncogene. 21:3422–44. PMID:12032780
3545. Scandurra M, Mian M, Greiner TC, et al. (2010). Genomic lesions associated with a different clinical outcome in diffuse large B-Cell lymphoma treated with R-CHOP-21. Br J Haematol. 151:221–31. PMID:20813005
3546. Scarisbrick JJ, Woolford AJ, Calonje E, et al. (2002). Frequent abnormalities of the p15 and p16 genes in mycosis fungoides and sezary syndrome. J Invest Dermatol. 118:493–9. PMID:11874489
3547. Scarisbrick JJ, Woolford AJ, Russell-Jones R, et al. (2000). Loss of heterozygosity on 10q and microsatellite instability in advanced stages of primary cutaneous T-cell lymphoma and possible association with homozygous deletion of PTEN. Blood. 95:2937–42. PMID:10779442
3548. Scarpa A, Moore PS, Rigaud G, et al. (1999). Molecular features of primary mediastinal B-cell lymphoma: involvement of p16INK4A, p53 and c-myc. Br J Haematol. 107:106–13. PMID:10520030
3549. Schade AE, Wlodarski MW, Maciejewski JP (2006). Pathophysiology defined by altered signal transduction pathways: the role of JAK-STAT and PI3K signaling in leukemic large granular lymphocytes. Cell Cycle. 5:2571–4. PMID:17172839
3549A. Schafernak KT, Variakojis D, Goolsby CL, et al. (2014). Clonality assessment of cutaneous B-cell lymphoid proliferations: a comparison of flow cytometry immunophenotyping, molecular studies, and immunohistochemistry/in situ hybridization and review of the literature. Am J Dermatopathol. 36:781–95. PMID:24335516
3550. Schaffner C, Idler I, Stilgenbauer S, et al. (2000). Mantle cell lymphoma is characterized by inactivation of the ATM gene. Proc Natl Acad Sci U S A. 97:2773–8. PMID:10706620
3551. Schanz J, Tüchler H, Solé F, et al. (2012). New comprehensive cytogenetic scoring system for primary myelodysplastic syndromes (MDS) and oligoblastic acute myeloid leukemia after MDS derived from an international database merge. J Clin Oncol. 30:820–9. PMID:22331955
3552. Schatz JH, Horwitz SM, Teruya-Feldstein J, et al. (2015). Targeted mutational profiling of peripheral T-cell lymphoma not otherwise specified highlights new mechanisms in a heterogeneous pathogenesis. Leukemia. 29:237–41. PMID:25257991
3552A. Scheffer E, Meijer CJ, van Vloten WA (1980). Dermatopathic lymphadenopathy and lymph node involvement in mycosis fungoides. Cancer. 45:137–48. PMID:7350998
3553. Scheffer E, Meijer CJ, van Vloten WA, et al. (1986). A histologic study of lymph nodes from patients with the Sézary syndrome. Cancer. 57:2375–80. PMID:2938724
3554. Schemenau J, Baldus S, Anlauf M, et al. (2015). Cellularity, characteristics of hematopoietic parameters and prognosis in myelodysplastic syndromes. Eur J Haematol. 95:181–9. PMID:25600827
3555. Schifferli A, Hitzler J, Bartholdi D, et al. (2015). Transient myeloproliferative disorder in neonates without Down syndrome: case report and review. Eur J Haematol. 94:456–62. PMID:24853125
3556. Schlegel U (2009). Primary CNS lymphoma. Ther Adv Neurol Disord. 2:93–104. PMID:21180644
3557. Schlegelberger B, Weber-Matthiesen K, Himmler A, et al. (1994). Cytogenetic findings and results of combined immunophenotyping and karyotyping in Hodgkin's disease. Leukemia. 8:72–80. PMID:8289502
3558. Schlegelberger B, Zhang Y, Weber-Matthiesen K, et al. (1994). Detection of aberrant clones in nearly all cases of angioimmunoblastic lymphadenopathy with dysproteinemia-type T-cell lymphoma by combined interphase and metaphase cytogenetics. Blood. 84:2640–8. PMID:7919378
3559. Schlenk RF, Benner A, Krauter J, et al. (2004). Individual patient data-based meta-analysis of patients aged 16 to 60 years with core binding factor acute myeloid leukemia: a survey of the German Acute Myeloid Leukemia Intergroup. J Clin Oncol. 22:3741–50. PMID:15289486
3560. Schlenk RF, Döhner K, Krauter J, et al. (2008). Mutations and treatment outcome in cytogenetically normal acute myeloid leukemia. N Engl J Med. 358:1909–18. PMID:18450602
3561. Schlenk RF, Kayser S, Bullinger L, et al. (2014). Differential impact of allelic ratio and insertion site in FLT3-ITD-positive AML with respect to allogeneic transplantation. Blood. 124:3441–9. PMID:25270908
3562. Schlenk RF, Taskesen E, van Norden Y, et al. (2013). The value of allogeneic and autologous hematopoietic stem cell transplantation in prognostically favorable acute myeloid leukemia with double mutant CEBPA. Blood. 122:1576–82. PMID:23863898
3563. Schlette E, Bueso-Ramos C, Giles F, et al. (2001). Mature B-cell leukemias with more than 55% prolymphocytes. A heterogeneous group that includes an unusual variant of mantle cell lymphoma. Am J Clin Pathol. 115:571–81. PMID:11293906
3564. Schmatz AI, Streubel B, Kretschmer-Chott E, et al. (2011). Primary follicular lymphoma of the duodenum is a distinct mucosal/submucosal variant of follicular lymphoma: a retrospective study of 63 cases. J Clin Oncol. 29:1445–51. PMID:21383289
3565. Schmid C, Pan L, Diss T, et al. (1991). Expression of B-cell antigens by Hodgkin's and Reed-Sternberg cells. Am J Pathol. 139:701–7. PMID:1656757
3566. Schmid C, Sargent C, Isaacson PG (1991). L and H cells of nodular lymphocyte predominant Hodgkin's disease show immunoglobulin light-chain restriction. Am J Pathol. 139:1281–9. PMID:1721489
3567. Schmidt J, Federmann B, Schindler N, et al. (2015). MYD88 L265P and CXCR4 mutations in lymphoplasmacytic lymphoma identify cases with high disease activity. Br J Haematol. 169:795–803. PMID:25819228
3567A. Schmidt J, Gong S, Marafioti T, et al. (2016). Genome-wide analysis of pediatric-type follicular lymphoma reveals low genetic complexity and recurrent alterations of TNFRSF14 gene. Blood. 128:1101–11. PMID:27257180
3567B. Schmidt J, Ramis-Zaldivar JE, Nadeu F, et al. (2017). Mutations of MAP2K1 are frequent in pediatric-type follicular lymphoma and result in ERK pathway activation. Blood. 22. pii: blood-2017-03-776278. doi: 10.1182/blood-2017-03-776278. PMID:28533310
3568. Schmidt J, Salaverria I, Haake A, et al. (2014). Increasing genomic and epigenomic complexity in the clonal evolution from in situ to manifest t(14;18)-positive follicular lymphoma. Leukemia. 28:1103–12. PMID:24153014
3569. Schmitt-Graeff A, Thiele J, Zuk I, et al. (2002). Essential thrombocythemia with ringed sideroblasts: a heterogeneous spectrum of diseases, but not a distinct entity. Haematologica. 87:392–9. PMID:11940483
3570. Schmitt-Graeff AH, Teo SS, Olschewski M, et al. (2008). JAK2V617F mutation status identifies subtypes of refractory anemia with ringed sideroblasts associated with marked thrombocytosis. Haematologica. 93:34–40. PMID:18166783
3571. Schmitz F, Tjon JM, Lai Y, et al. (2013). Identification of a potential physiological precursor of aberrant cells in refractory coeliac disease type II. Gut. 62:509–19. PMID:22760007
3572. Schmitz LL, McClure JS, Litz CE, et al. (1994). Morphologic and quantitative changes in blood and marrow cells following growth factor therapy. Am J Clin Pathol. 101:67–75. PMID:7506481
3572A. Schmitz R, Hansmann ML, Bohle V, et al. (2009). TNFAIP3 (A20) is a tumor suppressor gene in Hodgkin lymphoma and primary mediastinal B cell lymphoma. J Exp Med. 206:981–9. PMID:19380639
3573. Schmitz R, Young RM, Ceribelli M, et al. (2012). Burkitt lymphoma pathogenesis and therapeutic targets from structural and functional genomics. Nature. 490:116–20. PMID:22885699
3574. Schneider RK, Ademà V, Heckl D, et al. (2014). Role of casein kinase 1A1 in the biology and targeted therapy of del(5q) MDS. Cancer Cell. 26:509–20. PMID:25242043
3574A. Schneider RK, Schenone M, Ferreira MV et al. (2016). Rps14 haploinsufficiency causes a block in erythroid differentiation mediated by S100A8 and S100A9. Nat Med. 22:288–97. PMID: 26878232
3575. Schnittger S, Bacher U, Haferlach C, et al. (2008). Detection of an MPLW515 mutation in a case with features of both essential thrombocythemia and refractory anemia with ringed sideroblasts and thrombocytosis. Leukemia. 22:453–5. PMID:17713548
3576. Schnittger S, Dicker F, Kern W, et al. (2011). RUNX1 mutations are frequent in de novo AML with noncomplex karyotype and confer an unfavorable prognosis. Blood. 117:2348–57. PMID:21148331
3576A. Schnittger S, Eder C, Jeromin S, et al. (2013). ASXL1 exon 12 mutations are frequent in AML with intermediate risk karyotype and are independently associated with an adverse outcome. Leukemia. 27:82–91. PMID:23018865
3576B. Schnittger S, Kohl TM, Haferlach T, et al. (2006). KIT-D816 mutations in AML1-ETO-positive AML are associated with impaired event-free and overall survival. Blood. 107:1791–9. PMID:16254134
3577. Schnittger S, Schoch C, Kern W, et al. (2005). Nucleophosmin gene mutations are predictors of favorable prognosis in acute myelogenous leukemia with a normal karyotype. Blood. 106:3733–9. PMID:16076867
3578. Scholtysik R, Kreuz M, Hummel M, et al. (2015). Characterization of genomic imbalances in diffuse large B-cell lymphoma by detailed SNP-chip analysis. Int J Cancer. 136:1033–42. PMID:25042405
3579. Scholtysik R, Kreuz M, Klapper W, et al. (2010). Detection of genomic aberrations in molecularly defined Burkitt's lymphoma by array-based, high resolution, single nucleotide polymorphism analysis. Haematologica. 95:2047–55. PMID:20823134
3580. Schommers P, Hentrich M, Hoffmann C, et al. (2015). Survival of AIDS-related diffuse large B-cell lymphoma, Burkitt lymphoma, and plasmablastic lymphoma in the German HIV Lymphoma Cohort. Br J Haematol. 168:806–10. PMID:25403997
3581. Schooley RT, Flaum MA, Gralnick HR, et al. (1981). A clinicopathologic correlation of the idiopathic hypereosinophilic syndrome. II. Clinical manifestations. Blood. 58:1021–6. PMID:7197566
3582. Schop RF, Van Wier SA, Xu R, et al. (2006). 6q deletion discriminates Waldenström macroglobulinemia from IgM monoclonal gammopathy of undetermined significance. Cancer Genet Cytogenet. 169:150–3. PMID:16938573
3583. Schraders M, de Jong D, Kluin P, et al. (2005). Lack of Bcl-2 expression in follicular lymphoma may be caused by mutations in the BCL2 gene or by absence of the t(14;18) translocation. J Pathol. 205:329–35. PMID:15682435
3584. Schrappe M, Valsecchi MG, Bartram CR, et al. (2011). Late MRD response determines relapse risk overall and in subsets of childhood T-cell ALL: results of the AIEOP-BFM-ALL 2000 study. Blood. 118:2077–84. PMID:21719599
3585. Schroyens W, O'Connell C, Sykes DB (2012). Complete and partial responses of the TEMPI syndrome to bortezomib. N Engl J Med. 367:778–80. PMID:22913703
3585A. Schuback HL, Alonzo TA, Gerbing RB, et al. (2014). CBFA2T3-GLIS2 fusion is prevalent in younger patients with acute myeloid leukemia and associated with high-risk of relapse and poor outcome: a Children's Oncology Group report [meeting abstract]. Blood. 124:13.
3586. Schubbert S, Zenker M, Rowe SL, et al. (2006). Germline KRAS mutations cause Noonan syndrome. Nat Genet. 38:331–6. PMID:16474405
3587. Schuler E, Schroeder M, Neukirchen J, et al. (2014). Refined medullary blast and white blood cell count based classification of chronic myelomonocytic leukemias. Leuk Res. 38:1413–9. PMID:25444076
3588. Schultz KR, Carroll A, Heerema NA, et al. (2014). Long-term follow-up of imatinib in pediatric Philadelphia chromosome-positive acute lymphoblastic leukemia: Children's Oncology Group study AALL0031. Leukemia. 28:1467–71. PMID:24441288
3589. Schultz KR, Pullen DJ, Sather HN, et al. (2007). Risk- and response-based classification of childhood B-precursor acute lymphoblastic leukemia: a combined analysis of prognostic markers from the Pediatric Oncology Group (POG) and Children's Cancer Group (CCG). Blood. 109:926–35. PMID:17003380
3590. Schwarting R, Gerdes J, Dürkop H, et al. (1989). BER-H2: a new anti-Ki-1 (CD30) monoclonal antibody directed at a formol-resistant epitope. Blood. 74:1678–89. PMID:2477085
3591. Schwartz LB, Sakai K, Bradford TR, et al. (1995). The alpha form of human tryptase is the predominant type present in blood at baseline in normal subjects and is elevated in those with systemic mastocytosis. J Clin Invest. 96:2702–10. PMID:8675637
3592. Schwarzmann F, von Baehr R, Jäger M, et al. (1999). A case of severe chronic active infection with Epstein-Barr virus: immunologic deficiencies associated with a lytic virus strain. Clin Infect Dis. 29:626–31. PMID:10530459
3593. Schweitzer J, Zimmermann M, Rasche M, et al. (2015). Improved outcome of pediatric patients with acute megakaryoblastic leukemia in the AML-BFM 04 trial. Ann Hematol. 94:1327–36. PMID:25913479
3594. Schwering I, Bräuninger A, Klein U, et al. (2003). Loss of the B-lineage-specific gene expression program in Hodgkin and Reed-Sternberg cells of Hodgkin lymphoma. Blood. 101:1505–12. PMID:12393731

3594A. Schwind S, Maharry K, Radmacher MD, et al. (2010). Prognostic significance of expression of a single microRNA, miR-181a, in cytogenetically normal acute myeloid leukemia: a Cancer and Leukemia Group B study. J Clin Oncol. 28:5257–64. PMID:21079133
3594B. Schwind S, Marcucci G, Kohlschmidt J, et al. (2011). Low expression of MN1 associates with better treatment response in older patients with de novo cytogenetically normal acute myeloid leukemia. Blood. 118:4188–98. PMID:21828125
3594C. Schwind S, Marcucci G, Maharry K, et al. (2010). BAALC and ERG expression levels are associated with outcome and distinct gene and microRNA expression profiles in older patients with de novo cytogenetically normal acute myeloid leukemia: a Cancer and Leukemia Group B study. Blood. 116:5660–9. PMID:20841507
3595. Schwindt H, Vater I, Kreuz M, et al. (2009). Chromosomal imbalances and partial uniparental disomies in primary central nervous system lymphoma. Leukemia. 23:1875–84. PMID:19494841
3596. Schwyzer R, Sherman GG, Cohn RJ, et al. (1998). Granulocytic sarcoma in children with acute myeloblastic leukemia and t(8;21). Med Pediatr Oncol. 31:144–9. PMID:9722895
3597. Sciallis AP, Law ME, Inwards DJ, et al. (2012). Mucosal CD30-positive T-cell lymphoproliferations of the head and neck show a clinicopathologic spectrum similar to cutaneous CD30-positive T-cell lymphoproliferative disorders. Mod Pathol. 25:983–92. PMID:22388754
3598. Score J, Curtis C, Waghorn K, et al. (2006). Identification of a novel imatinib responsive KIF5B-PDGFRA fusion gene following screening for PDGFRA overexpression in patients with hypereosinophilia. Leukemia. 20:827–32. PMID:16498388
3599. Scott AA, Head DR, Kopecky KJ, et al. (1994). HLA-DR-, CD33+, CD56+, CD16- myeloid/natural killer cell acute leukemia: a previously unrecognized form of acute leukemia potentially misdiagnosed as French-American-British acute myeloid leukemia-M3. Blood. 84:244–55. PMID:7517211
3600. Scott DW, Gascoyne RD (2014). The tumour microenvironment in B cell lymphomas. Nat Rev Cancer. 14:517–34. PMID:25008267
3601. Scott DW, Mottok A, Ennishi D, et al. (2015). Prognostic Significance of Diffuse Large B-Cell Lymphoma Cell of Origin Determined by Digital Gene Expression in Formalin-Fixed Paraffin-Embedded Tissue Biopsies. J Clin Oncol. 33:2848–56. PMID:26240231
3602. Scott DW, Mungall KL, Ben-Neriah S, et al. (2012). TBL1XR1/TP63: a novel recurrent gene fusion in B-cell non-Hodgkin lymphoma. Blood. 119:4949–52. PMID:22496164
3603. Scott DW, Wright GW, Williams PM, et al. (2014). Determining cell-of-origin subtypes of diffuse large B-cell lymphoma using gene expression in formalin-fixed paraffin-embedded tissue. Blood. 123:1214–7. PMID:24398326
3604. Scott LM, Tong W, Levine RL, et al. (2007). JAK2 exon 12 mutations in polycythemia vera and idiopathic erythrocytosis. N Engl J Med. 356:459–68. PMID:17267906
3605. Scquizzato E, Teramo A, Miorin M, et al. (2007). Genotypic evaluation of killer immunoglobulin-like receptors in NK-type lymphoproliferative disease of granular lymphocytes. Leukemia. 21:1060–9. PMID:17361229
3606. Seaman V, Jumaan A, Yanni E, et al. (2009). Use of molecular testing to identify a cluster of patients with polycythemia vera in eastern Pennsylvania. Cancer Epidemiol Biomarkers Prev. 18:534–40. PMID:19190168
3607. Sebastián E, Alcoceba M, Martín-García D, et al. (2016). High-resolution copy number analysis of paired normal-tumor samples from diffuse large B cell lymphoma. Ann Hematol. 95:253–62. PMID:26573278
3608. Secker-Walker LM, Mehta A, Bain B (1995). Abnormalities of 3q21 and 3q26 in myeloid malignancy: a United Kingdom Cancer Cytogenetic Group study. Br J Haematol. 91:490–501. PMID:8547101
3609. Seegmiller AC, Xu Y, McKenna RW, et al. (2007). Immunophenotypic differentiation between neoplastic plasma cells in mature B-cell lymphoma vs plasma cell myeloma. Am J Clin Pathol. 127:176–81. PMID:17210522
3610. Sehn LH, Berry B, Chhanabhai M, et al. (2007). The revised International Prognostic Index (R-IPI) is a better predictor of outcome than the standard IPI for patients with diffuse large B-cell lymphoma treated with R-CHOP. Blood. 109:1857–61. PMID:17105812
3611. Sehn LH, Gascoyne RD (2015). Diffuse large B-cell lymphoma: optimizing outcome in the context of clinical and biologic heterogeneity. Blood. 125:22–32. PMID:25499448
3612. Sehn LH, Scott DW, Chhanabhai M, et al. (2011). Impact of concordant and discordant bone marrow involvement on outcome in diffuse large B-cell lymphoma treated with R-CHOP. J Clin Oncol. 29:1452–7. PMID:21383296
3613. Seif AE (2011). Pediatric leukemia predisposition syndromes: clues to understanding leukemogenesis. Cancer Genet. 204:227–44. PMID:21665176
3614. Seitz V, Hummel M, Marafioti T, et al. (2000). Detection of clonal T-cell receptor gamma-chain gene rearrangements in Reed-Sternberg cells of classic Hodgkin disease. Blood. 95:3020–4. PMID:10807764
3615. Seki R, Ohshima K, Fujisaki T, et al. (2009). Prognostic impact of immunohistochemical biomarkers in diffuse large B-cell lymphoma in the rituximab era. Cancer Sci. 100:1842–7. PMID:19656156
3616. Seliem RM, Griffith RC, Harris NL, et al. (2007). HHV-8+, EBV+ multicentric plasmablastic microlymphoma in an HIV+ Man: the spectrum of HHV-8+ lymphoproliferative disorders expands. Am J Surg Pathol. 31:1439–45. PMID:17721201
3617. Seligmann M (1975). Immunochemical, clical, and pathological features of alpha-chain disease. Arch Intern Med. 135:78–82. PMID:1089398
3618. Selimoglu-Buet D, Wagner-Ballon O, Saada V, et al. (2015). Characteristic repartition of monocyte subsets as a diagnostic signature of chronic myelomonocytic leukemia. Blood. 125:3618–26. PMID:25852055
3619. Selves J, Meggetto F, Brousset P, et al. (1996). Inflammatory pseudotumor of the liver. Evidence for follicular dendritic reticulum cell proliferation associated with clonal Epstein-Barr virus. Am J Surg Pathol. 20:747–53. PMID:8651355
3620. Semenzato G, Zambello R, Starkebaum G, et al. (1997). The lymphoproliferative disease of granular lymphocytes: updated criteria for diagnosis. Blood. 89:256–60. PMID:8978299
3621. Sena Teixeira Mendes L, D Attygalle A, C Wotherspoon A (2014). Helicobacter pylori infection in gastric extranodal marginal zone lymphoma of mucosa-associated lymphoid tissue (MALT) lymphoma: a re-evaluation. Gut. 63:1526–7. PMID:24951256
3622. Senent L, Arenillas L, Luño E, et al. (2013). Reproducibility of the World Health Organization 2008 criteria for myelodysplastic syndromes. Haematologica. 98:568–75. PMID:23065505
3623. Senff NJ, Hoefnagel JJ, Jansen PM, et al. (2007). Reclassification of 300 primary cutaneous B-Cell lymphomas according to the new WHO-EORTC classification for cutaneous lymphomas: comparison with previous classifications and identification of prognostic markers. J Clin Oncol. 25:1581–7. PMID:17353548
3624. Senff NJ, Noordijk EM, Kim YH, et al. (2008). European Organization for Research and Treatment of Cancer and International Society for Cutaneous Lymphoma consensus recommendations for the management of cutaneous B-cell lymphomas. Blood. 112:1600–9. PMID:18567836
3625. Senff NJ, Zoutman WH, Vermeer MH, et al. (2009). Fine-mapping chromosomal loss at 9p21: correlation with prognosis in primary cutaneous diffuse large B-cell lymphoma, leg type. J Invest Dermatol. 129:1149–55. PMID:19020554
3626. Serpell LC, Sunde M, Blake CC (1997). The molecular basis of amyloidosis. Cell Mol Life Sci. 53:871–87. PMID:9447239
3627. Seto M, Yamamoto K, Iida S, et al. (1992). Gene rearrangement and overexpression of PRAD1 in lymphoid malignancy with t(11;14)(q13;q32) translocation. Oncogene. 7:1401–6. PMID:1535701
3628. Setoodeh R, Schwartz S, Papenhausen P, et al. (2013). Double-hit mantle cell lymphoma with MYC gene rearrangement or amplification: a report of four cases and review of the literature. Int J Clin Exp Pathol. 6:155–67. PMID:23330001
3629. Shah N, Leaker MT, Teshima I, et al. (2008). Late-appearing Philadelphia chromosome in childhood acute myeloid leukemia. Pediatr Blood Cancer. 50:1052–3. PMID:18213712
3630. Shah S, Schrader KA, Waanders E, et al. (2013). A recurrent germline PAX5 mutation confers susceptibility to pre-B cell acute lymphoblastic leukemia. Nat Genet. 45:1226–31. PMID:24013638
3631. Shanafelt TD, Ghia P, Lanasa MC, et al. (2010). Monoclonal B-cell lymphocytosis (MBL): biology, natural history and clinical management. Leukemia. 24:512–20. PMID:20090778
3632. Shao H, Calvo KR, Grönborg M, et al. (2013). Distinguishing hairy cell leukemia variant from hairy cell leukemia: development and validation of diagnostic criteria. Leuk Res. 37:401–9. PMID:23347903
3633. Shao H, Xi L, Raffeld M, et al. (2011). Clonally related histiocytic/dendritic cell sarcoma and chronic lymphocytic leukemia/small lymphocytic lymphoma: a study of seven cases. Mod Pathol. 24:1421–32. PMID:21666687
3634. Shao H, Xi L, Raffeld M, et al. (2010). Nodal and extranodal plasmacytomas expressing immunoglobulin a: an indolent lymphoproliferative disorder with a low risk of clinical progression. Am J Surg Pathol. 34:1425–35. PMID:20871216
3635. Shapiro RS (2011). Malignancies in the setting of primary immunodeficiency: Implications for hematologists/oncologists. Am J Hematol. 86:48–55. PMID:21120868
3636. Shapiro RS, McClain K, Frizzera G, et al. (1988). Epstein-Barr virus associated B cell lymphoproliferative disorders following bone marrow transplantation. Blood. 71:1234–43. PMID:2833957
3637. Sharaiha RZ, Lebwohl B, Reimers L, et al. (2012). Increasing incidence of enteropathy-associated T-cell lymphoma in the United States, 1973-2008. Cancer. 118:3786–92. PMID:22169928
3638. Sharpe RW, Bethel KJ (2006). Hairy cell leukemia: diagnostic pathology. Hematol Oncol Clin North Am. 20:1023–49. PMID:16990105
3639. Shaughnessy JD Jr, Zhan F, Burington BE, et al. (2007). A validated gene expression model of high-risk multiple myeloma is defined by deregulated expression of genes mapping to chromosome 1. Blood. 109:2276–84. PMID:17105813
3640. Shen Q, Ouyang J, Tang G, et al. (2015). Flow cytometry immunophenotypic findings in chronic myelomonocytic leukemia and its utility in monitoring treatment response. Eur J Haematol. 95:168–76. PMID:25354960
3641. Shen ZX, Shi ZZ, Fang J, et al. (2004). All-trans retinoic acid/As2O3 combination yields a high quality remission and survival in newly diagnosed acute promyelocytic leukemia. Proc Natl Acad Sci U S A. 101:5328–35. PMID:15044693
3642. Shepherd PC, Ganesan TS, Galton DA (1987). Haematological classification of the chronic myeloid leukaemias. Baillieres Clin Haematol. 1:887–906. PMID:3332855
3643. Sherman MJ, Hanson CA, Hoyer JD (2011). An assessment of the usefulness of immunohistochemical stains in the diagnosis of hairy cell leukemia. Am J Clin Pathol. 136:390–9. PMID:21846914
3644. Shi G, Weh HJ, Dührsen U, et al. (1997). Chromosomal abnormality inv(3)(q21q26) associated with multilineage hematopoietic progenitor cells in hematopoietic malignancies. Cancer Genet Cytogenet. 96:58–63. PMID:9209472
3645. Shi M, Roemer MG, Chapuy B, et al. (2014). Expression of programmed cell death 1 ligand 2 (PD-L2) is a distinguishing feature of primary mediastinal (thymic) large B-cell lymphoma and associated with PDCD1LG2 copy gain. Am J Surg Pathol. 38:1715–23. PMID:25025450
3646. Shi R, Munker R (2015). Survival of patients with mixed phenotype acute leukemias: A large population-based study. Leuk Res. 39:606–16. PMID:25858895
3647. Shi Y, Rand AJ, Crow JH, et al. (2015). Blast phase in chronic myelogenous leukemia is skewed toward unusual blast types in patients treated with tyrosine kinase inhibitors: a comparative study of 67 cases. Am J Clin Pathol. 143:105–19. PMID:25511149
3648. Shia J, Teruya-Feldstein J, Pan D, et al. (2002). Primary follicular lymphoma of the gastrointestinal tract: a clinical and pathologic study of 26 cases. Am J Surg Pathol. 26:216–24. PMID:11812943
3649. Shiels MS, Koritzinsky EH, Clarke CA, et al. (2014). Prevalence of HIV Infection among U.S. Hodgkin lymphoma cases. Cancer Epidemiol Biomarkers Prev. 23:274–81. PMID:24326629
3650. Shigesada K, van de Sluis B, Liu PP (2004). Mechanism of leukemogenesis by the inv(16) chimeric gene CBFB/PEBP2B-MHY11. Oncogene. 23:4297–307. PMID:15156186
3651. Shih AH, Abdel-Wahab O, Patel JP, et al. (2012). The role of mutations in epigenetic regulators in myeloid malignancies. Nat Rev Cancer. 12:599–612. PMID:22898539
3652. Shih AH, Chung SS, Dolezal EK, et al. (2013). Mutational analysis of therapy-related myelodysplastic syndromes and acute myelogenous leukemia. Haematologica. 98:908–12. PMID:23349305
3653. Shih LY, Liang DC, Fu JF, et al. (2006). Characterization of fusion partner genes in 114 patients with de novo acute myeloid leukemia and MLL rearrangement. Leukemia. 20:218–23. PMID:16341046
3653A. Shih LY, Liang DC, Huang CF, et al. (2008). Cooperating mutations of receptor tyrosine kinases and Ras genes in childhood core-binding factor acute myeloid leukemia and a comparative analysis on paired diagnosis and relapse samples. Leukemia. 22:303–7. PMID:17960171
3654. Shimabukuro-Vornhagen A, Haverkamp H, Engert A, et al. (2005). Lymphocyte-rich

classical Hodgkin's lymphoma: clinical presentation and treatment outcome in 100 patients treated within German Hodgkin's Study Group trials. J Clin Oncol. 23:5739–45. PMID:16009944
3655. Shimada K, Kinoshita T, Naoe T, et al. (2009). Presentation and management of intravascular large B-cell lymphoma. Lancet Oncol. 10:895–902. PMID:19717091
3656. Shimada K, Matsue K, Yamamoto K, et al. (2008). Retrospective analysis of intravascular large B-cell lymphoma treated with rituximab-containing chemotherapy as reported by the IVL study group in Japan. J Clin Oncol. 26:3189–95. PMID:18506023
3657. Shimada K, Murase T, Matsue K, et al. (2010). Central nervous system involvement in intravascular large B-cell lymphoma: a retrospective analysis of 109 patients. Cancer Sci. 101:1480–6. PMID:20412122
3657A. Shimada A, Taki T, Tabuchi K, et al. (2006). KIT mutations, and not FLT3 internal tandem duplication, are strongly associated with a poor prognosis in pediatric acute myeloid leukemia with t(8;21): a study of the Japanese Childhood AML Cooperative Study Group. Blood. 107:1806–9. PMID:16291592
3658. Shimamura A, Alter BP (2010). Pathophysiology and management of inherited bone marrow failure syndromes. Blood Rev. 24:101–22. PMID:20417588
3659. Shimizu H, Yokohama A, Hatsumi N, et al. (2014). Philadelphia chromosome-positive mixed phenotype acute leukemia in the imatinib era. Eur J Haematol. 93:297–301. PMID:24750307
3660. Shimoyama M (1991). Diagnostic criteria and classification of clinical subtypes of adult T-cell leukaemia-lymphoma. A report from the Lymphoma Study Group (1984-87). Br J Haematol. 79:428–37. PMID:1751370
3661. Shimoyama Y, Yamamoto K, Asano N, et al. (2008). Age-related Epstein-Barr virus-associated B-cell lymphoproliferative disorders: special references to lymphomas surrounding this newly recognized clinicopathologic disease. Cancer Sci. 99:1085–91. PMID:18429953
3662. Shiota M, Nakamura S, Ichinohasama R, et al. (1995). Anaplastic large cell lymphomas expressing the novel chimeric protein p80NPM/ALK: a distinct clinicopathologic entity. Blood. 86:1954–60. PMID:7655022
3663. Shiozawa E, Yamochi-Onizuka T, Takimoto M, et al. (2007). The GCB subtype of diffuse large B-cell lymphoma is less frequent in Asian countries. Leuk Res. 31:1579–83. PMID:17448534
3664. Shiseki M, Kitagawa Y, Wang YH, et al. (2007). Lack of nucleophosmin mutation in patients with myelodysplastic syndrome and acute myeloid leukemia with chromosome 5 abnormalities. Leuk Lymphoma. 48:2141–4. PMID:17990177
3665. Shlush LI, Zandi S, Mitchell A, et al. (2014). Identification of pre-leukaemic haematopoietic stem cells in acute leukaemia. Nature. 506:328–33. PMID:24522528
3666. Shoffner JM, Lott MT, Wallace DC (1991). MERRF: a model disease for understanding the principles of mitochondrial genetics. Rev Neurol (Paris). 147:431–5. PMID:1962048
3667. Shustik J, Han G, Farinha P, et al. (2010). Correlations between BCL6 rearrangement and outcome in patients with diffuse large B-cell lymphoma treated with CHOP or R-CHOP. Haematologica. 95:96–101. PMID:19797725
3668. Shustik J, Quinn M, Connors JM, et al. (2011). Follicular non-Hodgkin lymphoma grades 3A and 3B have a similar outcome and appear incurable with anthracycline-based therapy. Ann Oncol. 22:1164–9. PMID:21062969
3669. Sibaud V, Beylot-Barry M, Thiébaut R, et al. (2003). Bone marrow histopathologic and molecular staging in epidermotropic T-cell lymphomas. Am J Clin Pathol. 119:414–23. PMID:12645344
3670. Sibon D, Fournier M, Brière J, et al. (2012). Long-term outcome of adults with systemic anaplastic large-cell lymphoma treated within the Groupe d'Etude des Lymphomes de l'Adulte trials. J Clin Oncol. 30:3939–46. PMID:23045585
3670A. Siddiqi IN, Friedman J, Barry-Holson KQ, et al. (2016). Characterization of a variant of t(14;18) negative nodal diffuse follicular lymphoma with CD23 expression, 1p36/TNFRSF14 abnormalities, and STAT6 mutations. Mod Pathol. 29:570-81. PMID:26965583
3671. Siddiqui N, Ayub B, Badar F, et al. (2006). Hodgkin's lymphoma in Pakistan: a clinico epidemiological study of 658 cases at a cancer center in Lahore. Asian Pac J Cancer Prev. 7:651–5. PMID:17250446
3672. Sidoroff A, Zelger B, Steiner H, et al. (1996). Indeterminate cell histiocytosis–a clinicopathological entity with features of both X- and non-X histiocytosis. Br J Dermatol. 134:525–32. PMID:8731682
3673. Siegel RL, Miller KD, Jemal A (2015). Cancer statistics, 2015. CA Cancer J Clin. 65:5–29. PMID:25559415
3674. Siegert W, Nerl C, Agthe A, et al. (1995). Angioimmunoblastic lymphadenopathy (AILD)-type T-cell lymphoma: prognostic impact of clinical observations and laboratory findings at presentation. Ann Oncol. 6:659–64. PMID:8664186
3675. Sieniawski M, Angamuthu N, Boyd K, et al. (2010). Evaluation of enteropathy-associated T-cell lymphoma comparing standard therapies with a novel regimen including autologous stem cell transplantation. Blood. 115:3664–70. PMID:20197551
3676. Silano M, Volta U, Vincenzi AD, et al. (2008). Effect of a gluten-free diet on the risk of enteropathy-associated T-cell lymphoma in celiac disease. Dig Dis Sci. 53:972–6. PMID:17934841
3677. Silver RT, Chow W, Orazi A, et al. (2013). Evaluation of WHO criteria for diagnosis of polycythemia vera: a prospective analysis. Blood. 122:1881–6. PMID:23900239
3678. Silver SR, Bertke SJ, Hines CJ, et al. (2015). Cancer incidence and metolachlor use in the Agricultural Health Study: An update. Int J Cancer. 137:2630–43. PMID:26033014
3679. Silverman LB, Sallan SE (2003). Newly diagnosed childhood acute lymphoblastic leukemia: update on prognostic factors and treatment. Curr Opin Hematol. 10:290–6. PMID:12799535
3680. Simon HU, Plötz SG, Dummer R, et al. (1999). Abnormal clones of T cells producing interleukin-5 in idiopathic eosinophilia. N Engl J Med. 341:1112–20. PMID:10511609
3681. Simon TA, Thompson A, Gandhi KK, et al. (2015). Incidence of malignancy in adult patients with rheumatoid arthritis: a meta-analysis. Arthritis Res Ther. 17:212. PMID:26271620
3682. Simonitsch-Klupp I, Hauser I, Ott G, et al. (2004). Diffuse large B-cell lymphomas with plasmablastic/plasmacytoid features are associated with TP53 deletions and poor clinical outcome. Leukemia. 18:146–55. PMID:14603341
3683. Simpson HM, Khan RZ, Song C, et al. (2015). Concurrent Mutations in ATM and Genes Associated with Common γ Chain Signaling in Peripheral T Cell Lymphoma. PLoS One. 10:e0141906. PMID:26536348
3684. Singh A, Schabath R, Ratei R, et al. (2014). Peripheral blood sCD3□ CD4□ T cells: a useful diagnostic tool in angioimmunoblastic T cell lymphoma. Hematol Oncol. 32:16–21. PMID:23798351
3685. Singh J, Dudley AW Jr, Kulig KA (1990). Increased incidence of monoclonal gammopathy of undetermined significance in blacks and its age-related differences with whites on the basis of a study of 397 men and one woman in a hospital setting. J Lab Clin Med. 116:785–9. PMID:2246554
3686. Singh ZN, Huo D, Anastasi J, et al. (2007). Therapy-related myelodysplastic syndrome: morphologic subclassification may not be clinically relevant. Am J Clin Pathol. 127:197–205. PMID:17210514
3687. Singleton TP, Yin B, Teferra A, et al. (2015). Spectrum of Clonal Large Granular Lymphocytes (LGLs) of αβ T Cells: T-Cell Clones of Undetermined Significance, T-Cell LGL Leukemias, and T-Cell Immunoclones. Am J Clin Pathol. 144:137–44. PMID:26071471
3688. Siu LL, Chan V, Chan JK, et al. (2000). Consistent patterns of allelic loss in natural killer cell lymphoma. Am J Pathol. 157:1803–9. PMID:11106552
3689. Siu LL, Wong KF, Chan JK, et al. (1999). Comparative genomic hybridization analysis of natural killer cell lymphoma/leukemia. Recognition of consistent patterns of genetic alterations. Am J Pathol. 155:1419–25. PMID:10550295
3690. Skibola CF, Berndt SI, Vijai J, et al. (2014). Genome-wide association study identifies five susceptibility loci for follicular lymphoma outside the HLA region. Am J Hum Genet. 95:462–71. PMID:25279986
3691. Skibola CF, Bracci PM, Nieters A, et al. (2010). Tumor necrosis factor (TNF) and lymphotoxin-alpha (LTA) polymorphisms and risk of non-Hodgkin lymphoma in the InterLymph Consortium. Am J Epidemiol. 171:267–76. PMID:20047977
3692. Skinnider BF, Connors JM, Sutcliffe SB, et al. (1999). Anaplastic large cell lymphoma: a clinicopathologic analysis. Hematol Oncol. 17:137–48. PMID:10725869
3693. Skinnider BF, Elia AJ, Gascoyne RD, et al. (2002). Signal transducer and activator of transcription 6 is frequently activated in Hodgkin and Reed-Sternberg cells of Hodgkin lymphoma. Blood. 99:618–26. PMID:11781246
3694. Skokowa J, Steinemann D, Katsman-Kuipers JE, et al. (2014). Cooperativity of RUNX1 and CSF3R mutations in severe congenital neutropenia: a unique pathway in myeloid leukemogenesis. Blood. 123:2229–37. PMID:24523240
3695. Slack GW, Ferry JA, Hasserjian RP, et al. (2009). Lymphocyte depleted Hodgkin lymphoma: an evaluation with immunophenotyping and genetic analysis. Leuk Lymphoma. 50:937–43. PMID:19455461
3696. Slack GW, Steidl C, Sehn LH, et al. (2014). CD30 expression in de novo diffuse large B-cell lymphoma: a population-based study from British Columbia. Br J Haematol. 167:608–17. PMID:25135752
3697. Slager SL, Caporaso NE, de Sanjose S, et al. (2013). Genetic susceptibility to chronic lymphocytic leukemia. Semin Hematol. 50:296–302. PMID:24246697
3698. Sloand EM, Wu CO, Greenberg P, et al. (2008). Factors affecting response and survival in patients with myelodysplasia treated with immunosuppressive therapy. J Clin Oncol. 26:2505–11. PMID:18413642
3699. Slovak ML, Bedell V, Popplewell L, et al. (2002). 21q22 balanced chromosome aberrations in therapy-related hematopoietic disorders: report from an international workshop. Genes Chromosomes Cancer. 33:379–94. PMID:11921272
3700. Slovak ML, Gundacker H, Bloomfield CD, et al. (2006). A retrospective study of 69 patients with t(6;9)(p23;q34) AML emphasizes the need for a prospective, multicenter initiative for rare 'poor prognosis' myeloid malignancies. Leukemia. 20:1295–7. PMID:16628187
3701. Slovak ML, Kopecky KJ, Cassileth PA, et al. (2000). Karyotypic analysis predicts outcome of preremission and postremission therapy in adult acute myeloid leukemia: a Southwest Oncology Group/Eastern Cooperative Oncology Group Study. Blood. 96:4075–83. PMID:11110676
3702. Smalberg JH, Arends LR, Valla DC, et al. (2012). Myeloproliferative neoplasms in Budd-Chiari syndrome and portal vein thrombosis: a meta-analysis. Blood. 120:4921–8. PMID:23043069
3703. Smalberg JH, Darwish Murad S, Braakman E, et al. (2006). Myeloproliferative disease in the pathogenesis and survival of Budd-Chiari syndrome. Haematologica. 91:1712–3. PMID:17145613
3704. Smedby KE, Foo JN, Skibola CF, et al. (2011). GWAS of follicular lymphoma reveals allelic heterogeneity at 6p21.32 and suggests shared genetic susceptibility with diffuse large B-cell lymphoma. PLoS Genet. 7:e1001378. PMID:21533074
3705. Smith DB, Harris M, Gowland E, et al. (1986). Non-secretory multiple myeloma: a report of 13 cases with a review of the literature. Hematol Oncol. 4:307–13. PMID:3549511
3706. Smith JR, Braziel RM, Paoletti S, et al. (2003). Expression of B-cell-attracting chemokine 1 (CXCL13) by malignant lymphocytes and vascular endothelium in primary central nervous system lymphoma. Blood. 101:815–21. PMID:12393412
3707. Smith MC, Cohen DN, Greig B, et al. (2014). The ambiguous boundary between EBV-related hemophagocytic lymphohistiocytosis and systemic EBV-driven T cell lymphoproliferative disorder. Int J Clin Exp Pathol. 7:5738–49. PMID:25337215
3708. Smith ML, Cavenagh JD, Lister TA, et al. (2004). Mutation of CEBPA in familial acute myeloid leukemia. N Engl J Med. 351:2403–7. PMID:15575056
3709. Smith SM, Le Beau MM, Huo D, et al. (2003). Clinical-cytogenetic associations in 306 patients with therapy-related myelodysplasia and myeloid leukemia: the University of Chicago series. Blood. 102:43–52. PMID:12623843
3710. Smith WJ, Price SK, Isaacson PG (1987). Immunoglobulin gene rearrangement in immunoproliferative small intestinal disease (IPSID). J Clin Pathol. 40:1291–7. PMID:3121678
3711. Sneller MC, Wang J, Dale JK, et al. (1997). Clincal, immunologic, and genetic features of an autoimmune lymphoproliferative syndrome associated with abnormal lymphocyte apoptosis. Blood. 89:1341–8. PMID:9028957
3712. Snuderl M, Kolman OK, Chen YB, et al. (2010). B-cell lymphomas with concurrent IGH-BCL2 and MYC rearrangements are aggressive neoplasms with clinical and pathologic features distinct from Burkitt lymphoma and diffuse large B-cell lymphoma. Am J Surg Pathol. 34:327–40. PMID:20118770
3713. Sobin LH, Gospodarowicz MK, Wittekind Ch, editors. (2009). International Union against Cancer (UICC): TNM classification of malignant tumors. 7th ed. Oxford: Wiley-Blackwell.
3714. Sojitra P, Gandhi P, Fitting P, et al. (2013). Chronic myelomonocytic leukemia monocytes uniformly display a population of monocytes with CD11c underexpression. Am J Clin Pathol. 140:686–92. PMID:24124148
3715. Sojka DK, Huang YH, Fowell DJ (2008). Mechanisms of regulatory T-cell suppression - a diverse arsenal for a moving target. Immunology. 124:13–22. PMID:18346152
3716. Sokal JE, Cox EB, Baccarani M, et al.

(1984). Prognostic discrimination in "good-risk" chronic granulocytic leukemia. Blood. 63:789–99. PMID:6584184
3717. Sokol L, Caceres G, Rocha K, et al. (2010). JAK2(V617F) mutation in myelodysplastic syndrome (MDS) with del(5q) arises in genetically discordant clones. Leuk Res. 34:821–3. PMID:19819015
3718. Sokolowska-Wojdylo M, Wenzel J, Gaffal E, et al. (2005). Absence of CD26 expression on skin-homing CLA+ CD4+ T lymphocytes in peripheral blood is a highly sensitive marker for early diagnosis and therapeutic monitoring of patients with Sézary syndrome. Clin Exp Dermatol. 30:702–6. PMID:16197392
3719. Solal-Celigny P, Desaint B, Herrera A, et al. (1984). Chronic myelomonocytic leukemia according to FAB classification: analysis of 35 cases. Blood. 63:634–8. PMID:6582939
3720. Solal-Céligny P, Roy P, Colombat P, et al. (2004). Follicular lymphoma international prognostic index. Blood. 104:1258–65. PMID:15126323
3721. Soldini D, Valera A, Solé C, et al. (2014). Assessment of SOX11 expression in routine lymphoma tissue sections: characterization of new monoclonal antibodies for diagnosis of mantle cell lymphoma. Am J Surg Pathol. 38:86–93. PMID:24145648
3722. Soler J, Bordes R, Ortüno F, et al. (1994). Aggressive natural killer cell leukaemia/lymphoma in two patients with lethal midline granuloma. Br J Haematol. 86:659–62. PMID:8043452
3724. Soligo D, Delia D, Oriani A, et al. (1991). Identification of CD34+ cells in normal and pathological bone marrow biopsies by QBEND10 monoclonal antibody. Leukemia. 5:1026–30. PMID:1723130
3725. Song JY, Jaffe ES (2013). HHV-8-positive but EBV-negative primary effusion lymphoma. Blood. 122:3712. PMID:24427809
3726. Song JY, Pittaluga S, Dunleavy K, et al. (2015). Lymphomatoid granulomatosis–a single institute experience: pathologic findings and clinical correlations. Am J Surg Pathol. 39:141–56. PMID:25321327
3727. Song MK, Chung JS, Joo YD, et al. (2011). Clinical importance of Bcl-6-positive non-deep-site involvement in non-HIV-related primary central nervous system diffuse large B-cell lymphoma. J Neurooncol. 104:825–31. PMID:21380743
3728. Song SY, Kim WS, Ko YH, et al. (2002). Aggressive natural killer cell leukemia: clinical features and treatment outcome. Haematologica. 87:1343–5. PMID:12495907
3729. Song WJ, Sullivan MG, Legare RD, et al. (1999). Haploinsufficiency of CBFA2 causes familial thrombocytopenia with propensity to develop acute myelogenous leukaemia. Nat Genet. 23:166–75. PMID:10508512
3730. Sonke GS, Ludwig I, van Oosten H, et al. (2008). Poor outcomes of chronic active Epstein-Barr virus infection and hemophagocytic lymphohistiocytosis in non-Japanese adult patients. Clin Infect Dis. 47:105–8. PMID:18491961
3731. Sonnex TS, Hawk JL (1988). Hydroa vacciniforme: a review of ten cases. Br J Dermatol. 118:101–8. PMID:3342168
3732. Sorà F, Autore F, Chiusolo P, et al. (2014). Extreme thrombocytosis in chronic myeloid leukemia in the era of tyrosine kinase inhibitors. Leuk Lymphoma. 55:2958–60. PMID:24684229
3733. Sordillo PP, Epremian B, Koziner B, et al. (1982). Lymphomatoid granulomatosis: an analysis of clinical and immunologic characteristics. Cancer. 49:2070–6. PMID:6978760
3734. Sotlar K, Cerny-Reiterer S, Petat-Dutter K, et al. (2011). Aberrant expression of CD30 in neoplastic mast cells in high-grade mastocytosis. Mod Pathol. 24:585–95. PMID:21186345
3735. Sotlar K, Fridrich C, Mall A, et al. (2002). Detection of c-kit point mutation Asp-816 -> Val in microdissected pooled single mast cells and leukemic cells in a patient with systemic mastocytosis and concomitant chronic myelomonocytic leukemia. Leuk Res. 26:979–84. PMID:12363464
3736. Sotlar K, Horny HP, Simonitsch I, et al. (2004). CD25 indicates the neoplastic phenotype of mast cells: a novel immunohistochemical marker for the diagnosis of systemic mastocytosis (SM) in routinely processed bone marrow biopsy specimens. Am J Surg Pathol. 28:1319–25. PMID:15371947
3737. Soubrier M, Dubost JJ, Serre AF, et al. (1997). Growth factors in POEMS syndrome: evidence for a marked increase in circulating vascular endothelial growth factor. Arthritis Rheum. 40:786–7. PMID:9125266
3738. Soubrier MJ, Dubost JJ, Sauvezie BJ; French Study Group on POEMS Syndrome (1994). POEMS syndrome: a study of 25 cases and a review of the literature. Am J Med. 97:543–53. PMID:7985714
3739. Soumelis V, Liu YJ (2006). From plasmacytoid to dendritic cell: morphological and functional switches during plasmacytoid pre-dendritic cell differentiation. Eur J Immunol. 36:2286–92. PMID:16892183
3740. Soupir CP, Vergilio JA, Dal Cin P, et al. (2007). Philadelphia chromosome-positive acute myeloid leukemia: a rare aggressive leukemia with clinicopathologic features distinct from chronic myeloid leukemia in myeloid blast crisis. Am J Clin Pathol. 127:642–50. PMID:17369142
3741. Soussain C, Patte C, Ostronoff M, et al. (1995). Small noncleaved cell lymphoma and leukemia in adults. A retrospective study of 65 adults treated with the LMB pediatric protocols. Blood. 85:664–74. PMID:7833470
3742. Soutar R, Lucraft H, Jackson G, et al. (2004). Guidelines on the diagnosis and management of solitary plasmacytoma of bone and solitary extramedullary plasmacytoma. Br J Haematol. 124:717–26. PMID:15009059
3743. Soverini S, de Benedittis C, Mancini M, et al. (2015). Mutations in the BCR-ABL1 Kinase Domain and Elsewhere in Chronic Myeloid Leukemia. Clin Lymphoma Myeloma Leuk. 15 Suppl:S120–8. PMID:26297264
3743A. Soverini S, Branford S, Nicolini FE, et al. (2014). Implications of BCR-ABL1 kinase domain-mediated resistance in chronic myeloid leukemia. Leuk Res. 38:10–20. PMID:24131888
3744. Specht K, Haralambieva E, Bink K, et al. (2004). Different mechanisms of cyclin D1 overexpression in multiple myeloma revealed by fluorescence in situ hybridization and quantitative analysis of mRNA levels. Blood. 104:1120–6. PMID:15090460
3745. Specht L, Hasenclever D (1999). Prognostic factors of Hodgkin's disease. In: Mauch P, Armitage JO, Diehl V, editors. Hodgkin's disease. Philadelphia: Lippincott Williams & Wilkins; p. 295.
3746. Speck NA, Gilliland DG (2002). Core-binding factors in haematopoiesis and leukaemia. Nat Rev Cancer. 2:502–13. PMID:12094236
3747. Speedy HE, Di Bernardo MC, Sava GP, et al. (2014). A genome-wide association study identifies multiple susceptibility loci for chronic lymphocytic leukemia. Nat Genet. 46:56–60. PMID:24292274
3748. Spencer J, Cerf-Bensussan N, Jarry A, et al. (1988). Enteropathy-associated T cell lymphoma (malignant histiocytosis of the intestine) is recognized by a monoclonal antibody (HML-1) that defines a membrane molecule on human mucosal lymphocytes. Am J Pathol. 132:1–5. PMID:3260750
3749. Spencer J, Finn T, Pulford KA, et al. (1985). The human gut contains a novel population of B lymphocytes which resemble marginal zone cells. Clin Exp Immunol. 62:607–12. PMID:3910320
3750. Sperr WR, Escribano L, Jordan JH, et al. (2001). Morphologic properties of neoplastic mast cells: delineation of stages of maturation and implication for cytological grading of mastocytosis. Leuk Res. 25:529–36. PMID:11377677
3751. Sperr WR, Horny HP, Valent P (2002). Spectrum of associated clonal hematologic non-mast cell lineage disorders occurring in patients with systemic mastocytosis. Int Arch Allergy Immunol. 127:140–2. PMID:11919425
3752. Spiegel A, Paillard C, Ducassou S, et al. (2014). Paediatric anaplastic large cell lymphoma with leukaemic presentation in children: a report of nine French cases. Br J Haematol. 165:545–51. PMID:24666317
3753. Spiers AS, Bain BJ, Turner JE (1977). The peripheral blood in chronic granulocytic leukaemia. Study of 50 untreated Philadelphia-positive cases. Scand J Haematol. 18:25–38. PMID:265093
3754. Spina M, Vaccher E, Nasti G, et al. (2000). Human immunodeficiency virus-associated Hodgkin's disease. Semin Oncol. 27:480–8. PMID:10950375
3755. Spinner MA, Sanchez LA, Hsu AP, et al. (2014). GATA2 deficiency: a protean disorder of hematopoiesis, lymphatics, and immunity. Blood. 123:809–21. PMID:24227816
3756. Spiro IJ, Yandell DW, Li C, et al. (1993). Brief report: lymphoma of donor origin occurring in the porta hepatis of a transplanted liver. N Engl J Med. 329:27–9. PMID:8505941
3757. Spits H, Lanier LL, Phillips JH (1995). Development of human T and natural killer cells. Blood. 85:2654–70. PMID:7742523
3758. Spivak JL (2002). Polycythemia vera: myths, mechanisms, and management. Blood. 100:4272–90. PMID:12393615
3759. Spry CJ, Davies J, Tai PC, et al. (1983). Clinical features of fifteen patients with the hypereosinophilic syndrome. Q J Med. 52:1–22. PMID:6878618
3760. Srinivas SK, Sample JT, Sixbey JW (1998). Spontaneous loss of viral episomes accompanying Epstein-Barr virus reactivation in a Burkitt's lymphoma cell line. J Infect Dis. 177:1705–9. PMID:9607853
3761. Staal-Viliare A, Latger-Cannard V, Didion J, et al. (2007). CD203c /CD117-, an useful phenotype profile for acute basophilic leukaemia diagnosis in cases of undifferentiated blasts. Leuk Lymphoma. 48:439–41. PMID:17325915
3762. Staal-Viliare A, Latger-Cannard V, Rault JP, et al. (2006). [A case of de novo acute basophilic leukaemia: diagnostic criteria and review of the literature]. Ann Biol Clin (Paris). 64:361–5. PMID:16829481
3763. Stachurski D, Miron PM, Al-Homsi S, et al. (2007). Anaplastic lymphoma kinase-positive diffuse large B-cell lymphoma with a complex karyotype and cryptic 3' ALK gene insertion to chromosome 4 q22-24. Hum Pathol. 38:940–5. PMID:17509395
3763A. Staffas A, Kanduri M, Hovland R, et al. (2011). Presence of FLT3-ITD and high BAALC expression are independent prognostic markers in childhood acute myeloid leukemia. Blood. 118:5905–13. PMID:21967978
3764. Standen GR, Jasani B, Wagstaff M, et al. (1990). Chronic neutrophilic leukemia and multiple myeloma. An association with lambda light chain expression. Cancer. 66:162–6. PMID:2112978
3765. Standen GR, Steers FJ, Jones L (1993). Clonality of chronic neutrophilic leukaemia associated with myeloma: analysis using the X-linked probe M27 beta. J Clin Pathol. 46:297–8. PMID:8098719
3766. Stanley M, McKenna RW, Ellinger G, et al. (1985). Classification of 358 cases of acute myeloid leukemia by FAB criteria: analysis of clinical and morphologic features. In: Bloomfield CD, editor. Chronic and acute leukemias in adults. Boston: Martin Nijhoff Publishers; pp. 147–74.
3767. Starczynowski DT, Kuchenbauer F, Argiropoulos B, et al. (2010). Identification of miR-145 and miR-146a as mediators of the 5q- syndrome phenotype. Nat Med. 16:49–58. PMID:19898489
3768. Stark B, Resnitzky P, Jeison M, et al. (1995). A distinct subtype of M4/M5 acute myeloblastic leukemia (AML) associated with t(8:16)(p11:p13), in a patient with the variant t(8:19)(p11:q13)–case report and review of the literature. Leuk Res. 19:367–79. PMID:7596149
3768A. Starr AG, Caimi PF, Fu P, et al. (2017). Splenic marginal zone lymphoma: excellent outcomes in 64 patients treated in the rituximab era. Hematology. [Epub ahead of print]. PMID: 28105889
3769. Starzl TE, Nalesnik MA, Porter KA, et al. (1984). Reversibility of lymphomas and lymphoproliferative lesions developing under cyclosporin-steroid therapy. Lancet. 1:583–7. PMID:6142304
3770. Stasik CJ, Nitta H, Zhang W, et al. (2010). Increased MYC gene copy number correlates with increased mRNA levels in diffuse large B-cell lymphoma. Haematologica. 95:597–603. PMID:20378577
3771. Steelman LS, Pohnert SC, Shelton JG, et al. (2004). JAK/STAT, Raf/MEK/ERK, PI3K/Akt and BCR-ABL in cell cycle progression and leukemogenesis. Leukemia. 18:189–218. PMID:14737178
3772. Steensma DP, Bejar R, Jaiswal S, et al. (2015). Clonal hematopoiesis of indeterminate potential and its distinction from myelodysplastic syndromes. Blood. 126:9–16. PMID:25931582
3773. Steensma DP, Caudill JS, Pardanani A, et al. (2006). MPL W515 and JAK2 V617 mutation analysis in patients with refractory anemia with ringed sideroblasts and an elevated platelet count. Haematologica. 91:ECR57. PMID:17194663
3774. Steensma DP, Dewald GW, Hodnefield JM, et al. (2003). Clonal cytogenetic abnormalities in bone marrow specimens without clear morphologic evidence of dysplasia: a form fruste of myelodysplasia? Leuk Res. 27:235–42. PMID:12537976
3775. Steensma DP, Dewald GW, Lasho TL, et al. (2005). The JAK2 V617F activating tyrosine kinase mutation is an infrequent event in both "atypical" myeloproliferative disorders and myelodysplastic syndromes. Blood. 106:1207–9. PMID:15860661
3776. Steer EJ, Cross NC (2002). Myeloproliferative disorders with translocations of chromosome 5q31-35: role of the platelet-derived growth factor receptor Beta. Acta Haematol. 107:113–22. PMID:11919393
3777. Steidl C, Gascoyne RD (2011). The molecular pathogenesis of primary mediastinal large B-cell lymphoma. Blood. 118:2659–69. PMID:21700770
3778. Steidl C, Lee T, Shah SP, et al. (2010). Tumor-associated macrophages and survival in classic Hodgkin's lymphoma. N Engl J Med. 362:875–85. PMID:20220182
3779. Steidl C, Shah SP, Woolcock BW, et al. (2011). MHC class II transactivator CIITA is a recurrent gene fusion partner in lymphoid cancers. Nature. 471:377–81. PMID:21368758

3780. Steidl C, Telenius A, Shah SP, et al. (2010). Genome-wide copy number analysis of Hodgkin Reed-Sternberg cells identifies recurrent imbalances with correlations to treatment outcome. Blood. 116:418–27. PMID:20339089
3781. Stein H, Diehl V, Marafioti T, et al. (1999). The nature of Reed-Sternberg cells, lymphocytic and histiocytic cells and their molecular biology in Hodgkin's disease. In: Mauch P, Armitage JO, Diehl V, editors. Hodgkin's disease. Philadelphia: Lippincott Williams & Wilkins; p. 121.
3782. Stein H, Foss HD, Dürkop H, et al. (2000). CD30(+) anaplastic large cell lymphoma: a review of its histopathologic, genetic, and clinical features. Blood. 96:3681–95. PMID:11090048
3783. Stein H, Gerdes J, Kirchner H, et al. (1981). Hodgkin and sternberg-reed cell antigen(s) detected by an antiserum to a cell line (L428) derived from Hodgkin's disease. Int J Cancer. 28:425–9. PMID:6946981
3784. Stein H, Hansmann ML, Lennert K, et al. (1986). Reed-Sternberg and Hodgkin cells in lymphocyte-predominant Hodgkin's disease of nodular subtype contain J chain. Am J Clin Pathol. 86:292–7. PMID:3529924
3785. Stein H, Marafioti T, Foss HD, et al. (2001). Down-regulation of BOB.1/OBF.1 and Oct2 in classical Hodgkin disease but not in lymphocyte predominant Hodgkin disease correlates with immunoglobulin transcription. Blood. 97:496–501. PMID:11154228
3786. Stein H, Marafioti T, Foss HD, et al. (2001). Down-regulation of BOB.1/OBF.1 and Oct2 in classical Hodgkin disease but not in lymphocyte predominant Hodgkin disease correlates with immunoglobulin transcription. Blood. 97:496–501. PMID:11154228
3787. Stein H, Mason DY, Gerdes J, et al. (1985). The expression of the Hodgkin's disease associated antigen Ki-1 in reactive and neoplastic lymphoid tissue: evidence that Reed-Sternberg cells and histiocytic malignancies are derived from activated lymphoid cells. Blood. 66:848–58. PMID:3876124
3788. Stein H, Uchánska-Ziegler B, Gerdes J, et al. (1982). Hodgkin and Sternberg-Reed cells contain antigens specific to late cells of granulopoiesis. Int J Cancer. 29:283–90. PMID:6175588
3789. Steinhoff M, Hummel M, Anagnostopoulos I, et al. (2002). Single-cell analysis of CD30+ cells in lymphomatoid papulosis demonstrates a common clonal T-cell origin. Blood. 100:578–84. PMID:12091351
3790. Steinman RM, Hemmi H (2006). Dendritic cells: translating innate to adaptive immunity. Curr Top Microbiol Immunol. 311:17–58. PMID:17048704
3791. Steinway SN, LeBlanc F, Loughran TP Jr (2014). The pathogenesis and treatment of large granular lymphocyte leukemia. Blood Rev. 28:87–94. PMID:24679833
3792. Renneville A, Roumier C, Biggio V, et al. (2008). Cooperating gene mutations in acute myeloid leukemia: a review of the literature. Leukemia 22:915-31. PMID:18288131
3793. Stellmacher F, Sotlar K, Balleisen L, et al. (2004). Bone marrow mastocytosis associated with IgM kappa plasma cell myeloma. Leuk Lymphoma. 45:801–5. PMID:15160959
3794. Stengel A, Kern W, Zenger M, et al. (2016). Genetic characterization of T-PLL reveals two major biologic subgroups and JAK3 mutations as prognostic marker. Genes Chromosomes Cancer. 55:82–94 PMID:26493028
3795. Stenzinger A, Endris V, Pfarr N, et al. (2014). Targeted ultra-deep sequencing reveals recurrent and mutually exclusive mutations of cancer genes in blastic plasmacytoid dendritic cell neoplasm. Oncotarget. 5:6404–13. PMID:25115387
3796. Stephens K, Weaver M, Leppig KA, et al. (2006). Interstitial uniparental isodisomy at clustered breakpoint intervals is a frequent mechanism of NF1 inactivation in myeloid malignancies. Blood. 108:1684–9. PMID:16690971
3797. Stern MH, Soulier J, Rosenzwajg M, et al. (1993). MTCP-1: a novel gene on the human chromosome Xq28 translocated to the T cell receptor alpha/delta locus in mature T cell proliferations. Oncogene. 8:2475–83. PMID:8361760
3798. Stewart AK, Bergsagel PL, Greipp PR, et al. (2007). A practical guide to defining high-risk myeloma for clinical trials, patient counseling and choice of therapy. Leukemia. 21:529–34. PMID:17230230
3799. Stewart K, Carstairs KC, Dubé ID, et al. (1990). Neutrophilic myelofibrosis presenting as Philadelphia chromosome negative BCR non-rearranged chronic myeloid leukemia. Am J Hematol. 34:59–63. PMID:2327406
3800. Stieglitz E, Loh ML (2013). Genetic predispositions to childhood leukemia. Ther Adv Hematol. 4:270–90. PMID:23926459
3801. Stieglitz E, Taylor-Weiner AN, Chang TY, et al. (2015). The genomic landscape of juvenile myelomonocytic leukemia. Nat Genet. 47:1326–33. PMID:26457647
3802. Stieglitz E, Ward AF, Gerbing RB, et al. (2015). Phase II/III trial of a pre-transplant farnesyl transferase inhibitor in juvenile myelomonocytic leukemia: a report from the Children's Oncology Group. Pediatr Blood Cancer. 62:629–36. PMID:25704135
3803. Stilgenbauer S, Schaffner C, Litterst A, et al. (1997). Biallelic mutations in the ATM gene in T-prolymphocytic leukemia. Nat Med. 3:1155–9. PMID:9334731
3804. Stiller CA, Chessells JM, Fitchett M (1994). Neurofibromatosis and childhood leukaemia/lymphoma: a population-based UKCCSG study. Br J Cancer. 70:969–72. PMID:7947106
3805. Storniolo AM, Moloney WC, Rosenthal DS, et al. (1990). Chronic myelomonocytic leukemia. Leukemia. 4:766–70. PMID:2232890
3806. Stover EH, Chen J, Lee BH, et al. (2005). The small molecule tyrosine kinase inhibitor AMN107 inhibits TEL-PDGFRbeta and FIP1L1-PDGFRalpha in vitro and in vivo. Blood. 106:3206–13. PMID:16030188
3807. Strahm B, Locatelli F, Bader P, et al. (2007). Reduced intensity conditioning in unrelated donor transplantation for refractory cytopenia in childhood. Bone Marrow Transplant. 40:329–33. PMID:17589538
3808. Strahm B, Nöllke P, Zecca M, et al. (2011). Hematopoietic stem cell transplantation for advanced myelodysplastic syndrome in children: results of the EWOG-MDS 98 study. Leukemia. 25:455–62. PMID:21212791
3809. Straus SE (1988). The chronic mononucleosis syndrome. J Infect Dis. 157:405–12. PMID:2830340
3810. Straus SE, Jaffe ES, Puck JM, et al. (2001). The development of lymphomas in families with autoimmune lymphoproliferative syndrome with germline Fas mutations and defective lymphocyte apoptosis. Blood. 98:194–200. PMID:11418480
3811. Strauss A, Furlan I, Steinmann S, et al. (2015). Unmistakable morphology? Infantile malignant osteopetrosis resembling juvenile myelomonocytic leukemia in infants. J Pediatr. 167:486–8. PMID:25982139
3812. Streubel B, Huber D, Wöhrer S, et al. (2004). Frequency of chromosomal aberrations involving MALT1 in mucosa-associated lymphoid tissue lymphoma in patients with Sjögren's syndrome. Clin Cancer Res. 10:476–80. PMID:14760068
3813. Streubel B, Simonitsch-Klupp I, Müllauer L, et al. (2004). Variable frequencies of MALT lymphoma-associated genetic aberrations in MALT lymphomas of different sites. Leukemia. 18:1722–6. PMID:15356642
3814. Streubel B, Vinatzer U, Willheim M, et al. (2006). Novel t(5;9)(q33;q22) fuses ITK to SYK in unspecified peripheral T-cell lymphoma. Leukemia. 20:313–8. PMID:16341044
3815. Strom SS, Gu Y, Gruschkus SK, et al. (2005). Risk factors of myelodysplastic syndromes: a case-control study. Leukemia. 19:1912–8. PMID:16167059
3816. Strom SS, Vélez-Bravo V, Estey EH (2008). Epidemiology of myelodysplastic syndromes. Semin Hematol. 45:8–13. PMID:18179964
3817. Strullu M, Caye A, Lachenaud J, et al. (2014). Juvenile myelomonocytic leukaemia and Noonan syndrome. J Med Genet. 51:689–97. PMID:25097206
3818. Strupp C, Gattermann N, Giagounidis A, et al. (2003). Refractory anemia with excess of blasts in transformation: analysis of reclassification according to the WHO proposals. Leuk Res. 27:397–404. PMID:12620291
3819. Strupp C, Germing U, Trommer I, et al. (2000). Pericardial effusion in chronic myelomonocytic leukemia (CMML): a case report and review of the literature. Leuk Res. 24:1059–62. PMID:11077120
3820. Stuhlmann-Laeisz C, Borchert A, Quintanilla-Martinez L, et al. (2016). In Europe expression of EBNA2 is associated with poor survival in EBV-positive diffuse large B-cell lymphoma of the elderly. Leuk Lymphoma. 57:39–44. PMID:25899404
3821. Stuhlmann-Laeisz C, Szczepanowski M, Borchert A, et al. (2015). Epstein-Barr virus-negative diffuse large B-cell lymphoma hosts intra- and peritumoral B-cells with activated Epstein-Barr virus. Virchows Arch. 466:85–92. PMID:25339301
3822. Su IJ, Chen RL, Lin DT, et al. (1994). Epstein-Barr virus (EBV) infects T lymphocytes in childhood EBV-associated hemophagocytic syndrome in Taiwan. Am J Pathol. 144:1219–25. PMID:8203462
3823. Suarez F, Mahlaoui N, Canioni D, et al. (2015). Incidence, presentation, and prognosis of malignancies in ataxia-telangiectasia: a report from the French national registry of primary immune deficiencies. J Clin Oncol. 33:202–8. PMID:25488969
3824. Subramaniam K, D'Rozario J, Pavli P (2013). Lymphoma and other lymphoproliferative disorders in inflammatory bowel disease: a review. J Gastroenterol Hepatol. 28:24–30. PMID:23094824
3825. Subramaniam K, Yeung D, Grimpen F, et al. (2014). Hepatosplenic T-cell lymphoma, immunosuppressive agents and biologicals: what are the risks? Intern Med J. 44:287–90. PMID:24621284
3826. Such E, Cervera J, Costa D, et al. (2011). Cytogenetic risk stratification in chronic myelomonocytic leukemia. Haematologica. 96:375–83. PMID:21109693
3827. Such E, Germing U, Malcovati L, et al. (2013). Development and validation of a prognostic scoring system for patients with chronic myelomonocytic leukemia. Blood. 121:3005–15. PMID:23372164
3828. Suchak R, O'Connor S, McNamara C, et al. (2010). Indolent CD8-positive lymphoid proliferation on the face: part of the spectrum of primary cutaneous small-/medium-sized pleomorphic T-cell lymphoma or a distinct entity? J Cutan Pathol. 37:977–81. PMID:19891656
3829. Sugaya N, Kimura H, Hara S, et al. (2004). Quantitative analysis of Epstein-Barr virus (EBV)-specific CD8+ T cells in patients with chronic active EBV infection. J Infect Dis. 190:985–8. PMID:15295706
3830. Sulak LE, Clare CN, Morale BA, et al. (1990). Biphenotypic acute leukemia in adults. Am J Clin Pathol. 94:54–8. PMID:1694392
3831. Sultan C, Sigaux F, Imbert M, et al. (1981). Acute myelodysplasia with myelofibrosis: a report of eight cases. Br J Haematol. 49:11–6. PMID:7272222
3832. Sun J, Lu Z, Yang D, et al. (2011). Primary intestinal T-cell and NK-cell lymphomas: a clinicopathological and molecular study from China focused on type II enteropathy-associated T-cell lymphoma and primary intestinal NK-cell lymphoma. Mod Pathol. 24:983–92. PMID:21423155
3833. Sun X, Chang KC, Abruzzo LV, et al. (2003). Epidermal growth factor receptor expression in follicular dendritic cells: a shared feature of follicular dendritic cell sarcoma and Castleman's disease. Hum Pathol. 34:835–40. PMID:14562277
3834. Sundrud MS, Trivigno C (2013). Identity crisis of Th17 cells: many forms, many functions, many questions. Semin Immunol. 25:263–72. PMID:24239567
3835. Sutcliffe MJ, Shuster JJ, Sather HN, et al. (2005). High concordance from independent studies by the Children's Cancer Group (CCG) and Pediatric Oncology Group (POG) associating favorable prognosis with combined trisomies 4, 10, and 17 in children with NCI Standard-Risk B-precursor Acute Lymphoblastic Leukemia: a Children's Oncology Group (COG) initiative. Leukemia. 19:734–40. PMID:15789069
3836. Suttorp M, Eckardt L, Tauer JT, et al. (2012). Management of chronic myeloid leukemia in childhood. Curr Hematol Malig Rep. 7:116–24. PMID:22395816
3837. Suvajdzic N, Marisavljevic D, Kraguljac N, et al. (2004). Acute panmyelosis with myelofibrosis: clinical, immunophenotypic and cytogenetic study of twelve cases. Leuk Lymphoma. 45:1873–9. PMID:15223649
3838. Suzuki K, Ohshima K, Karube K, et al. (2004). Clinicopathological states of Epstein-Barr virus-associated T/NK-cell lymphoproliferative disorders (severe chronic active EBV infection) of children and young adults. Int J Oncol. 24:1165–74. PMID:15067338
3839. Suzuki R, Nakamura S, Suzumiya J, et al. (2005). Blastic natural killer cell lymphoma/leukemia (CD56-positive blastic tumor): prognostication and categorization according to anatomic sites of involvement. Cancer. 104:1022–31. PMID:15999368
3840. Suzuki R, Suzumiya J, Nakamura S, et al. (2004). Aggressive natural killer-cell leukemia revisited: large granular lymphocyte leukemia of cytotoxic NK cells. Leukemia. 18:763–70. PMID:14961041
3841. Suzuki R, Yamamoto K, Seto M, et al. (1997). CD7+ and CD56+ myeloid/natural killer cell precursor acute leukemia: a distinct hematolymphoid disease entity. Blood. 90:2417–28. PMID:9310493
3842. Suzumiya J, Ohshima K, Takeshita M, et al. (1999). Nasal lymphomas in Japan: a high prevalence of Epstein-Barr virus type A and deletion within the latent membrane protein gene. Leuk Lymphoma. 35:567–78. PMID:10609794
3843. Swan N, Skinner M, O'Hara CJ (2003). Bone marrow core biopsy specimens in AL (primary) amyloidosis. A morphologic and immunohistochemical study of 100 cases. Am J Clin Pathol. 120:610–6. PMID:14560572
3844. Sweet DL, Golomb HM, Rowley JD, et al. (1979). Acute myelogenous leukemia and thrombocythemia associated with an abnormality of chromosome no. 3. Cancer Genet

Cytogenet. 1:33–7.
3845. Swerdlow SH (2007). T-cell and NK-cell posttransplantation lymphoproliferative disorders. Am J Clin Pathol. 127:887–95. PMID:17509986
3846. Swerdlow SH (2014). Diagnosis of 'double hit' diffuse large B-cell lymphoma and B-cell lymphoma, unclassifiable, with features intermediate between DLBCL and Burkitt lymphoma: when and how, FISH versus IHC. Hematology Am Soc Hematol Educ Program. 2014:90–9. PMID:25696840
3847. Swerdlow SH (2014). Diagnosis of 'double hit' diffuse large B-cell lymphoma and B-cell lymphoma, unclassifiable, with features intermediate between DLBCL and Burkitt lymphoma: when and how, FISH versus IHC. Hematology Am Soc Hematol Educ Program. 2014:90–9. PMID:25696840
3848. Swerdlow SH, Campo E, Harris NL, et al., editors. (2008). WHO classification of tumours of haematopoietic and lymphoid tissues. 4th ed. Lyon: IARC.
3848A. Swerdlow SH, Campo E, Pileri SA, et al. (2016). The 2016 revision of the World Health Organization classification of lymphoid neoplasms. Blood. 127:2375–90. PMID:26980727
3849. Swerdlow SH, Habeshaw JA, Murray LJ, et al. (1983). Centrocytic lymphoma: a distinct clinicopathologic and immunologic entity. A multiparameter study of 18 cases at diagnosis and relapse. Am J Pathol. 113:181–97. PMID:6416075
3850. Swerdlow SH, Jaffe ES, Brousset P, et al. (2014). Cytotoxic T-cell and NK-cell lymphomas: current questions and controversies. Am J Surg Pathol. 38:e60–71. PMID:25025449
3851. Swerdlow SH, Kuzu I, Dogan A, et al. (2016). The many faces of small B cell lymphomas with plasmacytic differentiation and the contribution of MYD88 testing. Virchows Arch. 468:259–75 PMID:26454445
3852. Swerdlow SH, Quintanilla-Martinez L, Willemze R, et al. (2013). Cutaneous B-cell lymphoproliferative disorders: report of the 2011 Society for Hematopathology/European Association for Haematopathology workshop. Am J Clin Pathol. 139:515–35. PMID:23525619
3853. Swerdlow SH, Utz GL, Williams ME (1993). Bcl-2 protein in centrocytic lymphoma; a paraffin section study. Leukemia. 7:1456–8. PMID:8371594
3854. Swerdlow SH, Williams ME (2002). From centrocytic to mantle cell lymphoma: a clinicopathologic and molecular review of 3 decades. Hum Pathol. 33:7–20. PMID:11823969
3855. Swerdlow SH, Yang WI, Zukerberg LR, et al. (1995). Expression of cyclin D1 protein in centrocytic/mantle cell lymphomas with and without rearrangement of the BCL1/cyclin D1 gene. Hum Pathol. 26:999–1004. PMID:7545645
3855A. Swerdlow SH, Zukerberg LR, Yang WI, et al. (1996). The morphologic spectrum of non-Hodgkin's lymphomas with BCL1/cyclin D1 gene rearrangements. Am J Surg Pathol. 20:627–40. PMID:8619427
3856. Swick BL, Baum CL, Venkat AP, et al. (2011). Indolent CD8+ lymphoid proliferation of the ear: report of two cases and review of the literature. J Cutan Pathol. 38:209–15. PMID:21083681
3857. Swinson CM, Slavin G, Coles EC, et al. (1983). Coeliac disease and malignancy. Lancet. 1:111–5. PMID:6129425
3858. Sykes DB, Schroyens W, O'Connell C (2011). The TEMPI syndrome–a novel multisystem disease. N Engl J Med. 365:475–7. PMID:21812700
3859. Szablewski V, Ingen-Housz-Oro S, Baia M, et al. (2016). Primary Cutaneous Follicle Center Lymphomas Expressing BCL2 Protein Frequently Harbor BCL2 Gene Break and May Present 1p36 Deletion: A Study of 20 Cases. Am J Surg Pathol. 40:127–36. PMID:26658664
3860. Szczepański T, Pongers-Willemse MJ, Langerak AW, et al. (1999). Ig heavy chain gene rearrangements in T-cell acute lymphoblastic leukemia exhibit predominant DH6-19 and DH7-27 gene usage, can result in complete V-D-J rearrangements, and are rare in T-cell receptor alpha beta lineage. Blood. 93:4079–85. PMID:10361104
3861. Szpurka H, Jankowska AM, Makishima H, et al. (2010). Spectrum of mutations in RARS-T patients includes TET2 and ASXL1 mutations. Leuk Res. 34:969–73. PMID:20334914
3862. Szpurka H, Tiu R, Murugesan G, et al. (2006). Refractory anemia with ringed sideroblasts associated with marked thrombocytosis (RARS-T), another myeloproliferative condition characterized by JAK2 V617F mutation. Blood. 108:2173–81. PMID:16741247
3863. Tabanelli V, Valli R, Righi S, et al. (2014). A unique case of an indolent myometrial T-cell lymphoproliferative disorder with phenotypic features resembling uterine CD8+ resident memory T cells. Pathobiology. 81:176–82. PMID:25138577
3864. Tack GJ, van Wanrooij RL, Langerak AW, et al. (2012). Origin and immunophenotype of aberrant IEL in RCDII patients. Mol Immunol. 50:262–70. PMID:22364936
3865. Taddesse-Heath L, Meloni-Ehrig A, Scheerle J, et al. (2010). Plasmablastic lymphoma with MYC translocation: evidence for a common pathway in the generation of plasmablastic features. Mod Pathol. 23:991–9. PMID:20348882
3866. Taddesse-Heath L, Pittaluga S, Sorbara L, et al. (2003). Marginal zone B-cell lymphoma in children and young adults. Am J Surg Pathol. 27:522–31. PMID:12657939
3867. Taegtmeyer AB, Halil O, Bell AD, et al. (2005). Neutrophil dysplasia (acquired pseudo-pelger anomaly) caused by ganciclovir. Transplantation. 80:127–30. PMID:16003243
3868. Tai YC, Kim LH, Peh SC (2004). High frequency of EBV association and 30-bp deletion in the LMP-1 gene in CD56 lymphomas of the upper aerodigestive tract. Pathol Int. 54:158–66. PMID:14989738
3869. Tajima K, Hinuma Y (1992). Epidemiology of HTLV-I/II in Japan and the world. In: Takatsuki K, Hinuma Y, Yoshida M, editors. Advances in adult T-cell leukemia and HTLV-I research (Gann Monograph on Cancer Research). Tokyo: Japan Scientific Societies Press; pp. 129–49.
3870. Tajima S, Takanashi Y, Koda K, et al. (2015). Methotrexate-associated lymphoproliferative disorder presenting as extranodal NK/T-cell lymphoma arising in the lungs. Pathol Int. 65:661–5. PMID:26459854
3871. Takahashi E, Kajimoto K, Fukatsu T, et al. (2005). Intravascular large T-cell lymphoma: a case report of CD30-positive and ALK-negative anaplastic type with cytotoxic molecule expression. Virchows Arch. 447:1000–6. PMID:16189700
3872. Takahashi K, Pemmaraju N, Strati P, et al. (2013). Clinical characteristics and outcomes of therapy-related chronic myelomonocytic leukemia. Blood. 122:2807–11, quiz 2920. PMID:23896412
3873. Takakuwa T, Ham MF, Luo WJ, et al. (2006). Loss of expression of Epstein-Barr virus nuclear antigen-2 correlates with a poor prognosis in cases of pyothorax-associated lymphoma. Int J Cancer. 118:2782–9. PMID:16385574
3874. Takakuwa T, Luo WJ, Ham MF, et al. (2003). Establishment and characterization of unique cell lines derived from pyothorax-associated lymphoma which develops in long-standing pyothorax and is strongly associated with Epstein-Barr virus infection. Cancer Sci. 94:858–63. PMID:14556658
3875. Takakuwa T, Tresnasari K, Rahadiani N, et al. (2008). Cell origin of pyothorax-associated lymphoma: a lymphoma strongly associated with Epstein-Barr virus infection. Leukemia. 22:620–7. PMID:18079737
3876. Takata K, Okada H, Ohmiya N, et al. (2011). Primary gastrointestinal follicular lymphoma involving the duodenal second portion is a distinct entity: a multicenter, retrospective analysis in Japan. Cancer Sci. 102:1532–6. PMID:21561531
3877. Takata K, Sato Y, Nakamura N, et al. (2009). Duodenal and nodal follicular lymphomas are distinct: the former lacks activation-induced cytidine deaminase and follicular dendritic cells despite ongoing somatic hypermutations. Mod Pathol. 22:940–9. PMID:19396151
3878. Takata K, Sato Y, Nakamura N, et al. (2013). Duodenal follicular lymphoma lacks AID but expresses BACH2 and has memory B-cell characteristics. Mod Pathol. 26:22–31. PMID:22899287
3879. Takata K, Tanino M, Ennishi D, et al. (2014). Duodenal follicular lymphoma: comprehensive gene expression analysis with insights into pathogenesis. Cancer Sci. 105:608–15. PMID:24602001
3880. Takatsuki K, Yamaguchi K, Watanabe T, et al. (1992). Adult T-cell leukemia and HTLV-1 related disease. Gann Mono Can Res. 32:1–15.
3881. Takenokuchi M, Kawano S, Nakamachi Y, et al. (2012). FLT3/ITD associated with an immature immunophenotype in PML-RARα leukemia. Hematol Rep. 4:e22. PMID:23355940
3882. Takeshita M, Akamatsu M, Ohshima K, et al. (1995). CD30 (Ki-1) expression in adult T-cell leukaemia/lymphoma is associated with distinctive immunohistological and clinical characteristics. Histopathology. 26:539–46. PMID:7665144
3882A. Takeuchi K, Yokoyama M, Ishizawa S, et al. (2010). Lymphomatoid gastropathy: a distinct clinicopathologic entity of self-limited pseudomalignant NK-cell proliferation. Blood. 116:5631–7. PMID:20829373
3883. Talaulikar D, Dahlstrom JE, Shadbolt B, et al. (2007). Occult bone marrow involvement in patients with diffuse large B-cell lymphoma: results of a pilot study. Pathology. 39:580–5. PMID:18027262
3884. Talaulikar D, Shadbolt B, Dahlstrom JE, et al. (2009). Routine use of ancillary investigations in staging diffuse large B-cell lymphoma improves the International Prognostic Index (IPI). J Hematol Oncol. 2:49. PMID:19930611
3885. Tallman MS, Andersen JW, Schiffer CA, et al. (1997). All-trans-retinoic acid in acute promyelocytic leukemia. N Engl J Med. 337:1021–8. PMID:9321529
3886. Tallman MS, Kim HT, Paietta E, et al. (2004). Acute monocytic leukemia (French-American-British classification M5) does not have a worse prognosis than other subtypes of acute myeloid leukemia: a report from the Eastern Cooperative Oncology Group. J Clin Oncol. 22:1276–86. PMID:14970186
3887. Tan BT, Warnke RA, Arber DA (2006). The frequency of B- and T-cell gene rearrangements and epstein-barr virus in T-cell lymphomas: a comparison between angioimmunoblastic T-cell lymphoma and peripheral T-cell lymphoma, unspecified with and without associated B-cell proliferations. J Mol Diagn. 8:466–75, quiz 527. PMID:16931587
3888. Tan DE, Foo JN, Bei JX, et al. (2013). Genome-wide association study of B cell non-Hodgkin lymphoma identifies 3q27 as a susceptibility locus in the Chinese population. Nat Genet. 45:804–7. PMID:23749188
3889. Tan SY, Chuang SS, Tang T, et al. (2013). Type II EATL (epitheliotropic intestinal T-cell lymphoma): a neoplasm of intra-epithelial T-cells with predominant CD8αα phenotype. Leukemia. 27:1688–96. PMID:23399895
3890. Tan SY, Ooi AS, Ang MK, et al. (2011). Nuclear expression of MATK is a novel marker of type II enteropathy-associated T-cell lymphoma. Leukemia. 25:555–7. PMID:21233830
3891. Tanaka M, Suda T, Haze K, et al. (1996). Fas ligand in human serum. Nat Med. 2:317–22. PMID:8612231
3892. Tanaka Y, Kurata M, Togami K, et al. (2006). Chronic eosinophilic leukemia with the FIP1L1-PDGFRalpha fusion gene in a patient with a history of combination chemotherapy. Int J Hematol. 83:152–5. PMID:16513534
3893. Tandon B, Peterson L, Gao J, et al. (2011). Nuclear overexpression of lymphoid-enhancer-binding factor 1 identifies chronic lymphocytic leukemia/small lymphocytic lymphoma in small B-cell lymphomas. Mod Pathol. 24:1433–43. PMID:21685909
3894. Tandon B, Swerdlow SH, Hasserjian RP, et al. (2015). Chronic lymphocytic leukemia/small lymphocytic lymphoma: another neoplasm related to the B-cell follicle? Leuk Lymphoma. 56:3378–86. PMID:25860247
3895. Tang G, Jorgensen LJ, Zhou Y, et al. (2012). Multi-color CD34+ progenitor-focused flow cytometric assay in evaluation of myelodysplastic syndromes in patients with post cancer therapy cytopenia. Leuk Res. 36:974–81. PMID:22626984
3895A. Tang G, Wang SA, Menon M, et al. (2011). High-level CD34 expression on megakaryocytes independently predicts an adverse outcome in patients with myelodysplastic syndromes. Leuk Res. 35:766-70. PMID:21367453
3896. Tang G, Zhang L, Fu B, et al. (2014). Cytogenetic risk stratification of 417 patients with chronic myelomonocytic leukemia from a single institution. Am J Hematol. 89:813–8. PMID:24782398
3897. Tang JL, Hou HA, Chen CY, et al. (2009). AML1/RUNX1 mutations in 470 adult patients with de novo acute myeloid leukemia: prognostic implication and interaction with other gene alterations. Blood. 114:5352–61. PMID:19808697
3898. Tangye SG, Phillips JH, Lanier LL, et al. (2000). Functional requirement for SAP in 2B4-mediated activation of human natural killer cells as revealed by the X-linked lymphoproliferative syndrome. J Immunol. 165:2932–6. PMID:10975798
3899. Tanière P, Thivolet-Béjui F, Vitrey D, et al. (1998). Lymphomatoid granulomatosis–a report on four cases: evidence for B phenotype of the tumoral cells. Eur Respir J. 12:102–6. PMID:9701422
3900. Taniguchi K, Takata K, Chuang SS, et al. (2016). Frequent MYD88 L265P and CD79B Mutations in Primary Breast Diffuse Large B-Cell Lymphoma. Am J Surg Pathol. 40:324–34. PMID:26752547
3901. Tao J, Valderrama E (1999). Epstein-Barr virus-associated polymorphic B-cell lymphoproliferative disorders in the lungs of children with AIDS: a report of two cases. Am J Surg Pathol. 23:560–6. PMID:10328088
3902. Tapia G, Lopez R, Muñoz-Mármol AM, et al. (2011). Immunohistochemical detection of MYC protein correlates with MYC gene status in aggressive B cell lymphomas. Histopathology. 59:672–8. PMID:22014048
3903. Tari A, Asaoku H, Takata K, et al. (2016). The role of "watch and wait" in intestinal follicular lymphoma in rituximab era. Scand J Gastroenterol. 51:321–8. PMID:26382560

3904. Taris M, de Mascarel A, Riols M, et al. (2014). [KHSV/EBV associated germinotropic lymphoproliferative disorder: a rare entity, case report and review of the literature]. Ann Pathol. 34:373–7. PMID:25439990

3905. Tarlock K, Alonzo TA, Moraleda PP, et al. (2014). Acute myeloid leukaemia (AML) with t(6;9)(p23;q34) is associated with poor outcome in childhood AML regardless of FLT3-ITD status: a report from the Children's Oncology Group. Br J Haematol. 166:254–9. PMID:24661089

3905A. Tarlock K, Meshinchi S (2015). Pediatric acute myeloid leukemia: biology and therapeutic implications of genomic variants. Pediatr Clin North Am. 62:75–93. PMID:25435113

3906. Tartaglia M, Niemeyer CM, Fragale A, et al. (2003). Somatic mutations in PTPN11 in juvenile myelomonocytic leukemia, myelodysplastic syndromes and acute myeloid leukemia. Nat Genet. 34:148–50. PMID:12717436

3907. Tashiro H, Shirasaki R, Noguchi M, et al. (2006). Molecular analysis of chronic eosinophilic leukemia with t(4;10) showing good response to imatinib mesylate. Int J Hematol. 83:433–8. PMID:16787876

3908. Taskesen E, Bullinger L, Corbacioglu A, et al. (2011). Prognostic impact, concurrent genetic mutations, and gene expression features of AML with CEBPA mutations in a cohort of 1182 cytogenetically normal AML patients: further evidence for CEBPA double mutant AML as a distinctive disease entity. Blood. 117:2469–75. PMID:21177436

3909. Tawana K, Wang J, Renneville A, et al. (2015). Disease evolution and outcomes in familial AML with germline CEBPA mutations. Blood. 126:1214–23. PMID:26162409

3910. Taylor AM, Metcalfe JA, Thick J, et al. (1996). Leukemia and lymphoma in ataxia telangiectasia. Blood. 87:423–38. PMID:8555463

3911. Taylor CR, Siddiqi IN, Brody GS (2013). Anaplastic large cell lymphoma occurring in association with breast implants: review of pathologic and immunohistochemical features in 103 cases. Appl Immunohistochem Mol Morphol. 21:13–20. PMID:23235342

3912. Tebit DM, Arts EJ (2011). Tracking a century of global expansion and evolution of HIV to drive understanding and to combat disease. Lancet Infect Dis. 11:45–56. PMID:21126914

3913. Tedeschi A, Baratè C, Minola E, et al. (2007). Cryoglobulinemia. Blood Rev. 21:183–200. PMID:17289231

3914. Tefferi A (2000). Myelofibrosis with myeloid metaplasia. N Engl J Med. 342:1255–65. PMID:10781623

3915. Tefferi A (2010). Novel mutations and their functional and clinical relevance in myeloproliferative neoplasms: JAK2, MPL, TET2, ASXL1, CBL, IDH and IKZF1. Leukemia. 24:1128–38. PMID:20428194

3916. Tefferi A (2014). Primary myelofibrosis: 2014 update on diagnosis, risk-stratification, and management. Am J Hematol. 89:915–25. PMID:25124313

3917. Tefferi A, Barbui T (2015). Polycythemia vera and essential thrombocythemia: 2015 update on diagnosis, risk-stratification and management. Am J Hematol. 90:162–73. PMID:25611051

3918. Tefferi A, Elliott M, Pardanani A (2015). Chronic neutrophilic leukemia: novel mutations and their impact on clinical practice. Curr Opin Hematol. 22:171–6. PMID:25575036

3919. Tefferi A, Elliott MA, Pardanani A (2006). Atypical myeloproliferative disorders: diagnosis and management. Mayo Clin Proc. 81:553–63. PMID:16610578

3920. Tefferi A, Guglielmelli P, Larson DR, et al. (2014). Long-term survival and blast transformation in molecularly annotated essential thrombocythemia, polycythemia vera, and myelofibrosis. Blood. 124:2507–13, quiz 2615. PMID:25037629

3921. Tefferi A, Guglielmelli P, Lasho TL, et al. (2014). CALR and ASXL1 mutations-based molecular prognostication in primary myelofibrosis: an international study of 570 patients. Leukemia. 28:1494–500. PMID:24496303

3922. Tefferi A, Hoagland HC, Therneau TM, et al. (1989). Chronic myelomonocytic leukemia: natural history and prognostic determinants. Mayo Clin Proc. 64:1246–54. PMID:2593715

3923. Tefferi A, Huang J, Schwager S, et al. (2007). Validation and comparison of contemporary prognostic models in primary myelofibrosis: analysis based on 334 patients from a single institution. Cancer. 109:2083–8. PMID:17407134

3924. Tefferi A, Lasho TL, Finke CM, et al. (2014). CALR vs JAK2 vs MPL-mutated or triple-negative myelofibrosis: clinical, cytogenetic and molecular comparisons. Leukemia. 28:1472–7. PMID:24402162

3925. Tefferi A, Li CY, Witzig TE, et al. (1994). Chronic natural killer cell lymphocytosis: a descriptive clinical study. Blood. 84:2721–5. PMID:7919384

3926. Tefferi A, Mesa RA, Schroeder G, et al. (2001). Cytogenetic findings and their clinical relevance in myelofibrosis with myeloid metaplasia. Br J Haematol. 113:763–71. PMID:11380468

3927. Tefferi A, Murphy S (2001). Current opinion in essential thrombocythemia: pathogenesis, diagnosis, and management. Blood Rev. 15:121–31. PMID:11735160

3928. Tefferi A, Pardanani A (2004). Clinical, genetic, and therapeutic insights into systemic mast cell disease. Curr Opin Hematol. 11:58–64. PMID:14676628

3929. Tefferi A, Rumi E, Finazzi G, et al. (2013). Survival and prognosis among 1545 patients with contemporary polycythemia vera: an international study. Leukemia. 27:1874–81. PMID:23739289

3930. Tefferi A, Skoda R, Vardiman JW (2009). Myeloproliferative neoplasms: contemporary diagnosis using histology and genetics. Nat Rev Clin Oncol. 6:627–37. PMID:19806146

3931. Tefferi A, Thiele J, Orazi A, et al. (2007). Proposals and rationale for revision of the World Health Organization diagnostic criteria for polycythemia vera, essential thrombocythemia, and primary myelofibrosis: recommendations from an ad hoc international expert panel. Blood. 110:1092–7. PMID:17488875

3932. Tefferi A, Thiele J, Vannucchi AM, et al. (2014). An overview on CALR and CSF3R mutations and a proposal for revision of WHO diagnostic criteria for myeloproliferative neoplasms. Leukemia. 28:1407–13. PMID:24441292

3933. Tefferi A, Vainchenker W (2011). Myeloproliferative neoplasms: molecular pathophysiology, essential clinical understanding, and treatment strategies. J Clin Oncol. 29:573–82. PMID:21220604

3934. Tefferi A, Wassie EA, Guglielmelli P, et al. (2014). Type 1 versus Type 2 calreticulin mutations in essential thrombocythemia: a collaborative study of 1027 patients. Am J Hematol. 89:E121–4. PMID:24753125

3935. Tefferi A, Wassie EA, Lasho TL, et al. (2014). Calreticulin mutations and long-term survival in essential thrombocythemia. Leukemia. 28:2300–3. PMID:24791854

3936. Tehranchi R, Invernizzi R, Grandien A, et al. (2005). Aberrant mitochondrial iron distribution and maturation arrest characterize early erythroid precursors in low-risk myelodysplastic syndromes. Blood. 106:247–53. PMID:15755901

3937. Tembhare PR, Yuan CM, Venzon D, et al. (2014). Flow cytometric differentiation of abnormal and normal plasma cells in the bone marrow in patients with multiple myeloma and its precursor diseases. Leuk Res. 38:371–6. PMID:24462038

3938. ten Berge RL, de Bruin PC, Oudejans JJ, et al. (2003). ALK-negative anaplastic large-cell lymphoma demonstrates similar poor prognosis to peripheral T-cell lymphoma, unspecified. Histopathology. 43:462–9. PMID:14636272

3939. ten Berge RL, Oudejans JJ, Ossenkoppele GJ, et al. (2003). ALK-negative systemic anaplastic large cell lymphoma: differential diagnostic and prognostic aspects–a review. J Pathol. 200:4–15. PMID:12692835

3940. ten Berge RL, Oudejans JJ, Ossenkoppele GJ, et al. (2000). ALK expression in extranodal anaplastic large cell lymphoma favours systemic disease with (primary) nodal involvement and a good prognosis and occurs before dissemination. J Clin Pathol. 53:445–50. PMID:10911802

3941. Terré C, Nguyen-Khac F, Barin C, et al. (2006). Trisomy 4, a new chromosomal abnormality in Waldenström's macroglobulinemia: a study of 39 cases. Leukemia. 20:1634–6. PMID:16838026

3942. Teruya-Feldstein J, Chiao E, Filippa DA, et al. (2004). CD20-negative large-cell lymphoma with plasmablastic features: a clinically heterogenous spectrum in both HIV-positive and -negative patients. Ann Oncol. 15:1673–9. PMID:15520070

3943. Teruya-Feldstein J, Jaffe ES, Burd PR, et al. (1997). The role of Mig, the monokine induced by interferon-gamma, and IP-10, the interferon-gamma-inducible protein-10, in tissue necrosis and vascular damage associated with Epstein-Barr virus-positive lymphoproliferative disease. Blood. 90:4099–105. PMID:9354680

3944. Teruya-Feldstein J, Jaffe ES, Burd PR, et al. (1999). Differential chemokine expression in tissues involved by Hodgkin's disease: direct correlation of eotaxin expression and tissue eosinophilia. Blood. 93:2463–70. PMID:10194423

3945. Teruya-Feldstein J, Temeck BK, Sloas MM, et al. (1995). Pulmonary malignant lymphoma of mucosa-associated lymphoid tissue (MALT) arising in a pediatric HIV-positive patient. Am J Surg Pathol. 19:357–63. PMID:7872434

3946. Teruya-Feldstein J, Zauber P, Setsuda JE, et al. (1998). Expression of human herpesvirus-8 oncogene and cytokine homologues in an HIV-seronegative patient with multicentric Castleman's disease and primary effusion lymphoma. Lab Invest. 78:1637–42. PMID:9881964

3947. Testoni M, Kwee I, Greiner TC, et al. (2011). Gains of MYC locus and outcome in patients with diffuse large B-cell lymphoma treated with R-CHOP. Br J Haematol. 155:274–7. PMID:21488860

3948. Testoni N, Borsaru G, Martinelli G, et al. (1999). 3q21 and 3q26 cytogenetic abnormalities in acute myeloblastic leukemia: biological and clinical features. Haematologica. 84:690–4. PMID:10457403

3949. The World Health Organization classification of malignant lymphomas in Japan: incidence of recently recognized entities; Lymphoma Study Group of Japanese Pathologists (2000). Pathol Int. 50:696–702. PMID:11012982

3950. Thelander EF, Walsh SH, Thorsélius M, et al. (2005). Mantle cell lymphomas with clonal immunoglobulin V(H)3-21 gene rearrangements exhibit fewer genomic imbalances than mantle cell lymphomas utilizing other immunoglobulin V(H) genes. Mod Pathol. 18:331–9. PMID:15257315

3951. Theoharides TC, Valent P, Akin C (2015). Mast Cells, Mastocytosis, and Related Disorders. N Engl J Med. 373:163–72. PMID:26154789

3952. Thieblemont C, Bastion Y, Berger F, et al. (1997). Mucosa-associated lymphoid tissue gastrointestinal and nongastrointestinal lymphoma behavior: analysis of 108 patients. J Clin Oncol. 15:1624–30. PMID:9193362

3953. Thieblemont C, Berger F, Dumontet C, et al. (2000). Mucosa-associated lymphoid tissue lymphoma is a disseminated disease in one third of 158 patients analyzed. Blood. 95:802–6. PMID:10648389

3954. Thieblemont C, Bertoni F, Copie-Bergman C, et al. (2014). Chronic inflammation and extra-nodal marginal-zone lymphomas of MALT-type. Semin Cancer Biol. 24:33–42. PMID:24333758

3955. Thieblemont C, Felman P, Berger F, et al. (2002). Treatment of splenic marginal zone B-cell lymphoma: an analysis of 81 patients. Clin Lymphoma. 3:41–7. PMID:12141954

3956. Thieblemont C, Felman P, Callet-Bauchu E, et al. (2003). Splenic marginal-zone lymphoma: a distinct clinical and pathological entity. Lancet Oncol. 4:95–103. PMID:12573351

3957. Thieblemont C, Nasser V, Felman P, et al. (2004). Small lymphocytic lymphoma, marginal zone B-cell lymphoma, and mantle cell lymphoma exhibit distinct gene-expression profiles allowing molecular diagnosis. Blood. 103:2727–37. PMID:14630827

3958. Thiede C, Koch S, Creutzig E, et al. (2006). Prevalence and prognostic impact of NPM1 mutations in 1485 adult patients with acute myeloid leukemia (AML). Blood. 107:4011–20. PMID:16455956

3959. Thiele J, Bennewitz FG, Bertsch HP, et al. (1993). Splenic haematopoiesis in primary (idiopathic) osteomyelofibrosis: immunohistochemical and morphometric evaluation of proliferative activity of erytro- and endoreduplicative capacity of megakaryopoiesis (PCNA- and Ki-67 staining). Virchows Arch B Cell Pathol Incl Mol Pathol. 64:281–6. PMID:7904516

3960. Thiele J, Kvasnicka HM (2002). CD34+ stem cells in chronic myeloproliferative disorders. Histol Histopathol. 17:507–21. PMID:11962756

3961. Thiele J, Kvasnicka HM (2003). Chronic myeloproliferative disorders with thrombocythemia: a comparative study of two classification systems (PVSG, WHO) on 839 patients. Ann Hematol. 82:148–52. PMID:12634946

3962. Thiele J, Kvasnicka HM (2003). Diagnostic differentiation of essential thrombocythaemia from thrombocythaemias associated with chronic idiopathic myelofibrosis by discriminate analysis of bone marrow features–a clinicopathological study on 272 patients. Histol Histopathol. 18:93–102. PMID:12507288

3963. Thiele J, Kvasnicka HM (2004). Prefibrotic chronic idiopathic myelofibrosis–a diagnostic enigma? Acta Haematol. 111:155–9. PMID:15034237

3964. Thiele J, Kvasnicka HM (2005). Diagnostic impact of bone marrow histopathology in polycythemia vera (PV). Histol Histopathol. 20:317–28. PMID:15578448

3965. Thiele J, Kvasnicka HM (2005). Hematopathologic findings in chronic idiopathic myelofibrosis. Semin Oncol. 32:380–94. PMID:16202684

3966. Thiele J, Kvasnicka HM (2006). Clinicopathological criteria for differential diagnosis of thrombocythemias in various myeloproliferative disorders. Semin Thromb Hemost. 32:219–30. PMID:16673276

3967. Thiele J, Kvasnicka HM (2006). Grade

of bone marrow fibrosis is associated with relevant hematological findings-a clinicopathological study on 865 patients with chronic idiopathic myelofibrosis. Ann Hematol. 85:226–32. PMID:16421727
3968. Thiele J, Kvasnicka HM (2007). Myelofibrosis–what's in a name? Consensus on definition and EUMNET grading. Pathobiology. 74:89–96. PMID:17587880
3969. Thiele J, Kvasnicka HM (2009). The 2008 WHO diagnostic criteria for polycythemia vera, essential thrombocythemia, and primary myelofibrosis. Curr Hematol Malig Rep. 4:33–40. PMID:20425436
3970. Thiele J, Kvasnicka HM, Czieslick C (2002). CD34+ progenitor cells in idiopathic (primary) myelofibrosis: a comparative quantification between spleen and bone marrow tissue. Ann Hematol. 81:86–9. PMID:11907788
3971. Thiele J, Kvasnicka HM, Diehl V (2005). Bone marrow CD34+ progenitor cells in Philadelphia chromosome-negative chronic myeloproliferative disorders–a clinicopathological study on 575 patients. Leuk Lymphoma. 46:709–15. PMID:16019508
3972. Thiele J, Kvasnicka HM, Diehl V (2005). Initial (latent) polycythemia vera with thrombocytosis mimicking essential thrombocythemia. Acta Haematol. 113:213–9. PMID:15983426
3973. Thiele J, Kvasnicka HM, Diehl V (2005). Standardization of bone marrow features–does it work in hematopathology for histological discrimination of different disease patterns? Histol Histopathol. 20:633–44. PMID:15736066
3974. Thiele J, Kvasnicka HM, Dietrich H, et al. (2005). Dynamics of bone marrow changes in patients with chronic idiopathic myelofibrosis following allogeneic stem cell transplantation. Histol Histopathol. 20:879–89. PMID:15944939
3975. Thiele J, Kvasnicka HM, Facchetti F, et al. (2005). European consensus on grading bone marrow fibrosis and assessment of cellularity. Haematologica. 90:1128–32. PMID:16079113
3976. Thiele J, Kvasnicka HM, Fischer R (1999). Bone marrow histopathology in chronic myelogenous leukemia (CML)–evaluation of distinctive features with clinical impact. Histol Histopathol. 14:1241–56. PMID:10506940
3977. Thiele J, Kvasnicka HM, Müllauer L, et al. (2011). Essential thrombocythemia versus early primary myelofibrosis: a multicenter study to validate the WHO classification. Blood. 117:5710–8. PMID:21447832
3978. Thiele J, Kvasnicka HM, Orazi A (2005). Bone marrow histopathology in myeloproliferative disorders–current diagnostic approach. Semin Hematol. 42:184–95. PMID:16210032
3979. Thiele J, Kvasnicka HM, Schmitt-Graeff A, et al. (2003). Bone marrow histopathology following cytoreductive therapy in chronic idiopathic myelofibrosis. Histopathology. 43:470–9. PMID:14636273
3980. Thiele J, Kvasnicka HM, Schmitt-Graeff A, et al. (2003). Dynamics of fibrosis in chronic idiopathic (primary) myelofibrosis during therapy: a follow-up study on 309 patients. Leuk Lymphoma. 44:949–53. PMID:12854892
3981. Thiele J, Kvasnicka HM, Schmitt-Graeff A, et al. (2002). Follow-up examinations including sequential bone marrow biopsies in essential thrombocythemia (ET): a retrospective clinicopathological study of 120 patients. Am J Hematol. 70:283–91. PMID:12210809
3982. Thiele J, Kvasnicka HM, Schmitt-Graeff A, et al. (2000). Bone marrow features and clinical findings in chronic myeloid leukemia–a comparative, multicenter, immunohistological and morphometric study on 614 patients. Leuk Lymphoma. 36:295–308. PMID:10674901
3983. Thiele J, Kvasnicka HM, Vardiman J (2006). Bone marrow histopathology in the diagnosis of chronic myeloproliferative disorders: a forgotten pearl. Best Pract Res Clin Haematol. 19:413–37. PMID:16781481
3984. Thiele J, Kvasnicka HM, Zankovich R, et al. (2000). Relevance of bone marrow features in the differential diagnosis between essential thrombocythemia and early stage idiopathic myelofibrosis. Haematologica. 85:1126–34. PMID:11064463
3985. Thiele J, Kvasnicka HM, Zankovich R, et al. (2001). The value of bone marrow histology in differentiating between early stage Polycythemia vera and secondary (reactive) Polycythemias. Haematologica. 86:368–74. PMID:11325641
3986. Thiele J, Kvasnicka HM, Zerhusen G, et al. (2004). Acute panmyelosis with myelofibrosis: a clinicopathological study on 46 patients including histochemistry of bone marrow biopsies and follow-up. Ann Hematol. 83:513–21. PMID:15173958
3987. Thiele J, Quitmann H, Wagner S, et al. (1991). Dysmegakaryopoiesis in myelodysplastic syndromes (MDS): an immunomorphometric study of bone marrow trephine biopsy specimens. J Clin Pathol. 44:300–5. PMID:2030148
3987A. Thol F, Damm F, Lüdeking A, et al. (2011). Incidence and prognostic influence of DNMT3A mutations in acute myeloid leukemia. J Clin Oncol. 29:2889–96. PMID:21670448
3987B. Thol F, Damm F, Wagner K, et al. (2010). Prognostic impact of IDH2 mutations in cytogenetically normal acute myeloid leukemia. Blood. 116:614–6. PMID:20421455
3988. Thol F, Kade S, Schlarmann C, et al. (2012). Frequency and prognostic impact of mutations in SRSF2, U2AF1, and ZRSR2 in patients with myelodysplastic syndromes. Blood. 119:3578–84. PMID:22389253
3989. Thomas E, Brewster DH, Black RJ, et al. (2000). Risk of malignancy among patients with rheumatic conditions. Int J Cancer. 88:497–502. PMID:11054684
3990. Thompsett AR, Ellison DW, Stevenson FK, et al. (1999). V(H) gene sequences from primary central nervous system lymphomas indicate derivation from highly mutated germinal center B cells with ongoing mutational activity. Blood. 94:1738–46. PMID:10477699
3991. Thompson MA, Stumph J, Henrickson SE, et al. (2005). Differential gene expression in anaplastic lymphoma kinase-positive and anaplastic lymphoma kinase-negative anaplastic large cell lymphomas. Hum Pathol. 36:494–504. PMID:15948116
3992. Thorns C, Bastian B, Pinkel D, et al. (2007). Chromosomal aberrations in angioimmunoblastic T-cell lymphoma and peripheral T-cell lymphoma unspecified: A matrix-based CGH approach. Genes Chromosomes Cancer. 46:37–44. PMID:17044049
3993. Thornton PD, Bellas C, Santon A, et al. (2005). Richter's transformation of chronic lymphocytic leukemia. The possible role of fludarabine and the Epstein-Barr virus in its pathogenesis. Leuk Res. 29:389–95. PMID:15725472
3994. Tiacci E, Liso A, Piris M, et al. (2006). Evolving concepts in the pathogenesis of hairy-cell leukaemia. Nat Rev Cancer. 6:437–48. PMID:16723990
3995. Tiacci E, Park JH, De Carolis L, et al. (2015). Targeting Mutant BRAF in Relapsed or Refractory Hairy-Cell Leukemia. N Engl J Med. 373:1733–47. PMID:26352686
3996. Tiacci E, Pileri S, Orleth A, et al. (2004). PAX5 expression in acute leukemias: higher B-lineage specificity than CD79a and selective association with t(8;21)-acute myelogenous leukemia. Cancer Res. 64:7399–404. PMID:15492262
3997. Tiacci E, Schiavoni G, Forconi F, et al. (2012). Simple genetic diagnosis of hairy cell leukemia by sensitive detection of the BRAF-V600E mutation. Blood. 119:192–5. PMID:22028477
3998. Tiacci E, Trifonov V, Schiavoni G, et al. (2011). BRAF mutations in hairy-cell leukemia. N Engl J Med. 364:2305–15. PMID:21663470
3998A. Tian X, Xu Y, Yin J, et al. (2014). TET2 gene mutation is unfavorable prognostic factor in cytogenetically normal acute myeloid leukemia patients with NPM1+ and FLT3-ITD - mutations. Int J Hematol. 100:96–104. PMID:24859829
3999. Tiede C, Maecker-Kolhoff B, Klein C, et al. (2013). Risk factors and prognosis in T-cell posttransplantation lymphoproliferative diseases: reevaluation of 163 cases. Transplantation. 95:479–88. PMID:23296147
4000. Tiedemann RE, Gonzalez-Paz N, Kyle RA, et al. (2008). Genetic aberrations and survival in plasma cell leukemia. Leukemia. 22:1044–52. PMID:18216867
4000A. Tiemann M, Riener MO, Claviez A, et al. (2005). Proliferation rate and outcome in children with T-cell rich B-cell lymphoma: a clinicopathologic study from the NHL-BFM-study group. Leuk Lymphoma. 46:1295–300. PMID:16109606
4001. Tiemann M, Schrader C, Klapper W, et al. (2005). Histopathology, cell proliferation indices and clinical outcome in 304 patients with mantle cell lymphoma (MCL): a clinicopathological study from the European MCL Network. Br J Haematol. 131:29–38. PMID:16173960
4002. Tien HF, Su IJ, Tang JL, et al. (1997). Clonal chromosomal abnormalities as direct evidence for clonality in nasal T/natural killer cell lymphomas. Br J Haematol. 97:621–5. PMID:9207410
4003. Tierney RJ, Shannon-Lowe CD, Fitzsimmons L, et al. (2015). Unexpected patterns of Epstein-Barr virus transcription revealed by a high throughput PCR array for absolute quantification of viral mRNA. Virology. 474:117–30. PMID:25463610
4004. Tiesinga JJ, Wu CD, Inghirami G (2000). CD5+ follicle center lymphoma. Immunophenotyping detects a unique subset of "floral" follicular lymphoma. Am J Clin Pathol. 114:912–21. PMID:11338480
4005. Tilly H, Rossi A, Stamatoullas A, et al. (1994). Prognostic value of chromosomal abnormalities in follicular lymphoma. Blood. 84:1043–9. PMID:8049424
4006. Timár B, Fülöp Z, Csernus B, et al. (2004). Relationship between the mutational status of VH genes and pathogenesis of diffuse large B-cell lymphoma in Richter's syndrome. Leukemia. 18:326–30. PMID:14671632
4007. Tinguely M, Vonlanthen R, Müller E, et al. (1998). Hodgkin's disease-like lymphoproliferative disorders in patients with different underlying immunodeficiency states. Mod Pathol. 11:307–12. PMID:9578079
4008. Tirelli U, Vaccher E, Zagonel V, et al. (1995). CD30 (Ki-1)-positive anaplastic large-cell lymphomas in 13 patients with and 27 patients without human immunodeficiency virus infection: the first comparative clinicopathologic study from a single institution that also includes 80 patients with other human immunodeficiency virus-related systemic lymphomas. J Clin Oncol. 13:373–80. PMID:7844598
4009. Titgemeyer C, Grois N, Minkov M, et al. (2001). Pattern and course of single-system disease in Langerhans cell histiocytosis data from the DAL-HX 83- and 90-study. Med Pediatr Oncol. 37:108–14. PMID:11496348
4010. Titmarsh GJ, Duncombe AS, McMullin MF, et al. (2014). How common are myeloproliferative neoplasms? A systematic review and meta-analysis. Am J Hematol. 89:581–7. PMID:24971434
4011. Tiu RV, Sekeres MA (2014). Making sense of the myelodysplastic/myeloproliferative neoplasms overlap syndromes. Curr Opin Hematol. 21:131–40. PMID:24378705
4012. Toki T, Kanezaki R, Kobayashi E, et al. (2013). Naturally occurring oncogenic GATA1 mutants with internal deletions in transient abnormal myelopoiesis in Down syndrome. Blood. 121:3181–4. PMID:23440243
4013. Tokita K, Maki K, Tadokoro J, et al. (2007). Chronic idiopathic myelofibrosis expressing a novel type of TEL-PDGFRB chimaera responded to imatinib mesylate therapy. Leukemia. 21:190–2. PMID:17122866
4014. Tokuhira M, Watanabe R, Nemoto T, et al. (2012). Clinicopathological analyses in patients with other iatrogenic immunodeficiency-associated lymphoproliferative diseases and rheumatoid arthritis. Leuk Lymphoma. 53:616–23. PMID:21933041
4015. Tokura Y, Ishihara S, Tagawa S, et al. (2001). Hypersensitivity to mosquito bites as the primary clinical manifestation of a juvenile type of Epstein-Barr virus-associated natural killer cell leukemia/lymphoma. J Am Acad Dermatol. 45:569–78. PMID:11568749
4016. Tokura Y, Tamura Y, Takigawa M, et al. (1990). Severe hypersensitivity to mosquito bites associated with natural killer cell lymphocytosis. Arch Dermatol. 126:362–8. PMID:1689990
4017. Tolani B, Gopalakrishnan R, Punj V, et al. (2014). Targeting Myc in KSHV-associated primary effusion lymphoma with BET bromodomain inhibitors. Oncogene. 33:2928–37. PMID:23792448
4018. Tolksdorf G, Stein H, Lennert K (1980). Morphological and immunological definition of a malignant lymphoma derived from germinal-centre cells with cleaved nuclei (centrocytes). Br J Cancer. 41:168–82. PMID:7370158
4019. Tomita N (2011). BCL2 and MYC dual-hit lymphoma/leukemia. J Clin Exp Hematop. 51:7–12. PMID:21628855
4020. Tomita N, Tokunaka M, Nakamura N, et al. (2009). Clinicopathological features of lymphoma/leukemia patients carrying both BCL2 and MYC translocations. Haematologica. 94:935–43. PMID:19535347
4021. Tomita S, Kikuti YY, Carreras J, et al. (2015). Genomic and immunohistochemical profiles of enteropathy-associated T-cell lymphoma in Japan. Mod Pathol. 28:1286–96. PMID:26226842
4022. Tomita S, Mori KL, Sakajiri S, et al. (2003). B-cell marker negative (CD7+, CD19-) Epstein-Barr virus-related pyothorax-associated lymphoma with rearrangement in the JH gene. Leuk Lymphoma. 44:727–30. PMID:12769353
4023. Tomita Y, Ohsawa M, Qiu K, et al. (1997). Epstein-Barr virus in lymphoproliferative diseases in the sino-nasal region: close association with CD56+ immunophenotype and polymorphic-reticulosis morphology. Int J Cancer. 70:9–13. PMID:8985084
4024. Topka S, Vijai J, Walsh MF, et al. (2015). Germline ETV6 Mutations Confer Susceptibility to Acute Lymphoblastic Leukemia and Thrombocytopenia. PLoS Genet. 11:e1005262. PMID:26102509
4025. Tordjman R, Macintyre E, Emile JF, et al. (1996). Aggressive acute CD3+, CD56- T cell large granular lymphocyte leukemia with two stages of maturation arrest. Leukemia. 10:1514–9. PMID:8751472
4026. Torlakovic E, Nielsen S, Vyberg M (2005). Antibody selection in immunohistochemical detection of cyclin D1 in mantle cell lymphoma. Am J Clin Pathol. 124:782–9. PMID:16203276
4027. Torlakovic E, Tierens A, Dang HD, et al. (2001). The transcription factor PU.1, necessary for B-cell development is expressed in

lymphocyte predominance, but not classical Hodgkin's disease. Am J Pathol. 159:1807–14. PMID:11696441

4028. Torlakovic E, Torlakovic G, Nguyen PL, et al. (2002). The value of anti-pax-5 immunostaining in routinely fixed and paraffin-embedded sections: a novel pan pre-B and B-cell marker. Am J Surg Pathol. 26:1343–50. PMID:12360049

4029. Torlakovic EE, Aamot HV, Heim S (2006). A marginal zone phenotype in follicular lymphoma with t(14;18) is associated with secondary cytogenetic aberrations typical of marginal zone lymphoma. J Pathol. 209:258–64. PMID:16583359

4030. Toro JR, Beaty M, Sorbara L, et al. (2000). gamma delta T-cell lymphoma of the skin: a clinical, microscopic, and molecular study. Arch Dermatol. 136:1024–32. PMID:10926739

4031. Toro JR, Liewehr DJ, Pabby N, et al. (2003). Gamma-delta T-cell phenotype is associated with significantly decreased survival in cutaneous T-cell lymphoma. Blood. 101:3407–12. PMID:12522013

4032. Tort F, Camacho E, Bosch F, et al. (2004). Familial lymphoid neoplasms in patients with mantle cell lymphoma. Haematologica. 89:314–9. PMID:15020270

4033. Tort F, Pinyol M, Pulford K, et al. (2001). Molecular characterization of a new ALK translocation involving moesin (MSN-ALK) in anaplastic large cell lymphoma. Lab Invest. 81:419–26. PMID:11310834

4034. Touati M, Delage-Corre M, Monteil J, et al. (2015). CD68-positive tumor-associated macrophages predict unfavorable treatment outcomes in classical Hodgkin lymphoma in correlation with interim fluorodeoxyglucose-positron emission tomography assessment. Leuk Lymphoma. 56:332–41. PMID:24766492

4035. Touhy EL (1920). A case of splenomegaly with polymorphonuclear neutrophil hyperleukocytosis. Am J Med Sci. 160:18–25.

4036. Toujani S, Dessen P, Ithzar N, et al. (2009). High resolution genome-wide analysis of chromosomal alterations in Burkitt's lymphoma. PLoS One. 4:e7089. PMID:19759907

4037. Touriol C, Greenland C, Lamant L, et al. (2000). Further demonstration of the diversity of chromosomal changes involving 2p23 in ALK-positive lymphoma: 2 cases expressing ALK kinase fused to CLTCL (clathrin chain polypeptide-like). Blood. 95:3204–7. PMID:10807789

4038. Toya T, Yoshimi A, Morioka T, et al. (2014). Development of hairy cell leukemia in familial platelet disorder with predisposition to acute myeloid leukemia. Platelets. 25:300–2. PMID:23971860

4039. Tracey L, Villuendas R, Dotor AM, et al. (2003). Mycosis fungoides shows concurrent deregulation of multiple genes involved in the TNF signaling pathway: an expression profile study. Blood. 102:1042–50. PMID:12689942

4040. Tracy RP, Kyle RA, Leitch JM (1984). Alpha heavy-chain disease presenting as goiter. Am J Clin Pathol. 82:336–9. PMID:6431799

4041. Traina F, Visconte V, Elson P, et al. (2014). Impact of molecular mutations on treatment response to DNMT inhibitors in myelodysplasia and related neoplasms. Leukemia. 28:78–87. PMID:24045501

4042. Trappe R, Zimmermann H, Fink S, et al. (2011). Plasmacytoma-like post-transplant lymphoproliferative disorder, a rare subtype of monomorphic B-cell post-transplant lymphoproliferation, is associated with a favorable outcome in localized as well as in advanced disease: a prospective analysis of 8 cases. Haematologica. 96:1067–71. PMID:21719885

4043. Traverse-Glehen A, Baseggio L, Bauchu EC, et al. (2008). Splenic red pulp lymphoma with numerous basophilic villous lymphocytes: a distinct clinicopathologic and molecular entity? Blood. 111:2253–60. PMID:18042795

4044. Traverse-Glehen A, Baseggio L, Salles G, et al. (2012). Splenic diffuse red pulp small-B cell lymphoma: toward the emergence of a new lymphoma entity. Discov Med. 13:253–65. PMID:22541613

4045. Traverse-Glehen A, Davi F, Ben Simon E, et al. (2005). Analysis of VH genes in marginal zone lymphoma reveals marked heterogeneity between splenic and nodal tumors and suggests the existence of clonal selection. Haematologica. 90:470–8. PMID:15820942

4046. Traverse-Glehen A, Felman P, Callet-Bauchu E, et al. (2006). A clinicopathological study of nodal marginal zone B-cell lymphoma. A report on 21 cases. Histopathology. 48:162–73. PMID:16405665

4047. Traverse-Glehen A, Pittaluga S, Gaulard P, et al. (2005). Mediastinal gray zone lymphoma: the missing link between classic Hodgkin's lymphoma and mediastinal large B-cell lymphoma. Am J Surg Pathol. 29:1411–21. PMID:16224207

4047A. Traverse-Glehen A1, Verney A, Gazzo S, et al. (2017). Splenic diffuse red pulp lymphoma has a distinct pattern of somatic mutations amongst B-cell malignancies. Leuk Lymphoma. 58:666-75. PMID:27347751

4048. Travert M, Huang Y, de Leval L, et al. (2012). Molecular features of hepatosplenic T-cell lymphoma unravels potential novel therapeutic targets. Blood. 119:5795–806. PMID:22510872

4049. Traweek ST, Arber DA, Rappaport H, et al. (1993). Extramedullary myeloid cell tumors. An immunohistochemical and morphologic study of 28 cases. Am J Surg Pathol. 17:1011–9. PMID:8372941

4050. Trempat P, Villalva C, Laurent G, et al. (2003). Chronic myeloproliferative disorders with rearrangement of the platelet-derived growth factor alpha receptor: a new clinical target for STI571/Glivec. Oncogene. 22:5702–6. PMID:12944919

4051. Treon SP (2015). How I treat Waldenström macroglobulinemia. Blood. 126:721–32. PMID:26002963

4052. Treon SP, Cao Y, Xu L, et al. (2014). Somatic mutations in MYD88 and CXCR4 are determinants of clinical presentation and overall survival in Waldenstrom macroglobulinemia. Blood. 123:2791–6. PMID:24553177

4053. Treon SP, Hunter ZR, Aggarwal A, et al. (2006). Characterization of familial Waldenstrom's macroglobulinemia. Ann Oncol. 17:488–94. PMID:16357024

4054. Treon SP, Tripsas C, Hanzis C, et al. (2012). Familial disease predisposition impacts treatment outcome in patients with Waldenström macroglobulinemia. Clin Lymphoma Myeloma Leuk. 12:433–7. PMID:23084402

4055. Treon SP, Tripsas CK, Meid K, et al. (2015). Ibrutinib in previously treated Waldenström's macroglobulinemia. N Engl J Med. 372:1430–40. PMID:25853747

4056. Treon SP, Xu L, Hunter Z (2015). MYD88 Mutations and Response to Ibrutinib in Waldenström's Macroglobulinemia. N Engl J Med. 373:584–6. PMID:26244327

4057. Treon SP, Xu L, Yang G, et al. (2012). MYD88 L265P somatic mutation in Waldenström's macroglobulinemia. N Engl J Med. 367:826–33. PMID:22931316

4058. Trimoreau F, Donnard M, Turlure P, et al. (2003). The CD4+ CD56+ CD116- CD123+ CD45RA+ CD45RO- profile is specific of DC2 malignancies. Haematologica. 88:ELT10. PMID:12651292

4059. Trinei M, Lanfrancone L, Campo E, et al. (2000). A new variant anaplastic lymphoma kinase (ALK)-fusion protein (ATIC-ALK) in a case of ALK-positive anaplastic large cell lymphoma. Cancer Res. 60:793–8. PMID:10706082

4060. Trinh DL, Scott DW, Morin RD, et al. (2013). Analysis of FOXO1 mutations in diffuse large B-cell lymphoma. Blood. 121:3666–74. PMID:23460611

4061. Trofe J, Buell JF, Beebe TM, et al. (2005). Analysis of factors that influence survival with post-transplant lymphoproliferative disorder in renal transplant recipients: the Israel Penn International Transplant Tumor Registry experience. Am J Transplant. 5:775–80. PMID:15760401

4062. Trotter MJ, Whittaker SJ, Orchard GE, et al. (1997). Cutaneous histopathology of Sézary syndrome: a study of 41 cases with a proven circulating T-cell clone. J Cutan Pathol. 24:286–91. PMID:9194581

4063. Truong F, Smith BR, Stachurski D, et al. (2009). The utility of flow cytometric immunophenotyping in cytopenic patients with a non-diagnostic bone marrow: a prospective study. Leuk Res. 33:1039–46. PMID:19232722

4064. Trøen G, Nygaard V, Jenssen TK, et al. (2004). Constitutive expression of the AP-1 transcription factors c-jun, junD, junB, and c-fos and the marginal zone B-cell transcription factor Notch2 in splenic marginal zone lymphoma. J Mol Diagn. 6:297–307. PMID:15507668

4065. Tsagarakis NJ, Kentrou NA, Papadimitriou KA, et al. (2010). Acute lymphoplasmacytoid dendritic cell (DC2) leukemia: results from the Hellenic Dendritic Cell Leukemia Study Group. Leuk Res. 34:438–46. PMID:19793612

4066. Tsai DE, Hardy CL, Tomaszewski JE, et al. (2001). Reduction in immunosuppression as initial therapy for posttransplant lymphoproliferative disorder: analysis of prognostic variables and long-term follow-up of 42 adult patients. Transplantation. 71:1076–88. PMID:11374406

4067. Tsang P, Cesarman E, Chadburn A, et al. (1996). Molecular characterization of primary mediastinal B-cell lymphoma. Am J Pathol. 148:2017–25. PMID:8669486

4068. Tsang RW, Gospodarowicz MK, Pintilie M, et al. (2001). Solitary plasmacytoma treated with radiotherapy: impact of tumor size on outcome. Int J Radiat Oncol Biol Phys. 50:113–20. PMID:11316553

4069. Tsang WY, Chan JK, Ng CS, et al. (1996). Utility of a paraffin section-reactive CD56 antibody (123C3) for characterization and diagnosis of lymphomas. Am J Surg Pathol. 20:202–10. PMID:8554110

4070. Tse E, Gill H, Loong F, et al. (2012). Type II enteropathy-associated T-cell lymphoma: a multicenter analysis from the Asia Lymphoma Study Group. Am J Hematol. 87:663–8. PMID:22641357

4070A. Tsirigotis P, Economopoulos T, Rontogianni D, et al. (2001). T-cell-rich B-cell lymphoma. Analysis of clinical features, response to treatment, survival and comparison with diffuse large B-cell lymphoma. Oncology. 61:257–64. PMID:11721171

4071. Tsuge I, Morishima T, Kimura H, et al. (2001). Impaired cytotoxic T lymphocyte response to Epstein-Barr virus-infected NK cells in patients with severe chronic active EBV infection. J Med Virol. 64:141–8. PMID:11360246

4072. Tsuge I, Morishima T, Morita M, et al. (1999). Characterization of Epstein-Barr virus (EBV)-infected natural killer (NK) cell proliferation in patients with severe mosquito allergy; establishment of an IL-2-dependent NK-like cell line. Clin Exp Immunol. 115:385–92. PMID:10193407

4073. Tsukamoto H, Yoshinari M, Okamura K, et al. (1992). Meningioma developed 25 years after radiation therapy for Cushing's disease. Intern Med. 31:629–32. PMID:1504425

4074. Tsukamoto Y, Katsunobu Y, Omura Y, et al. (2006). Subcutaneous panniculitis-like T-cell lymphoma: successful initial treatment with prednisolone and cyclosporin A. Intern Med. 45:21–4. PMID:16467600

4075. Tsukasaki K, Tsushima H, Yamamura M, et al. (1997). Integration patterns of HTLV-I provirus in relation to the clinical course of ATL: frequent clonal change at crisis from indolent disease. Blood. 89:948–56. PMID:9028326

4076. Turakhia S, Lanigan C, Hamadeh F, et al. (2015). Immunohistochemistry for BRAF V600E in the Differential Diagnosis of Hairy Cell Leukemia vs Other Splenic B-Cell Lymphomas. Am J Clin Pathol. 144:87–93. PMID:26071465

4077. Turakhia SK, Hill BT, Dufresne SD, et al. (2014). Aggressive B-cell lymphomas with translocations involving BCL6 and MYC have distinct clinical-pathologic characteristics. Am J Clin Pathol. 142:339–46. PMID:25125624

4078. Turesson I, Kovalchik SA, Pfeiffer RM, et al. (2014). Monoclonal gammopathy of undetermined significance and risk of lymphoid and myeloid malignancies: 728 cases followed up to 30 years in Sweden. Blood. 123:338–45. PMID:24222331

4079. Tursz T, Flandrin G, Brouet JC, et al. (1974). [Coexistence of a myeloma and a granulocytic leukemia in the absence of any treatment. Study of 4 cases]. Nouv Rev Fr Hematol. 14:693–704. PMID:4377020

4080. Tutt AN, Brada M, Sampson SA (1997). Enteropathy associated T cell lymphoma presenting as an isolated CNS lymphoma three years after diagnosis of coeliac disease: T cell receptor polymerase chain reaction studies failed to show the original enteropathy to be a clonal disorder. Gut. 40:801–3. PMID:9245937

4081. Twa DD, Chan FC, Ben-Neriah S, et al. (2014). Genomic rearrangements involving programmed death ligands are recurrent in primary mediastinal large B-cell lymphoma. Blood. 123:2062–5. PMID:24497532

4082. Twa DD, Mottok A, Chan FC, et al. (2015). Recurrent genomic rearrangements in primary testicular lymphoma. J Pathol. 236:136–41. PMID:25712539

4083. Tzankov A, Bourgau C, Kaiser A, et al. (2005). Rare expression of T-cell markers in classical Hodgkin's lymphoma. Mod Pathol. 18:1542–9. PMID:16056244

4084. Tzankov A, Matter MS, Dirnhofer S (2010). Refined prognostic role of CD68-positive tumor macrophages in the context of the cellular micromilieu of classical Hodgkin lymphoma. Pathobiology. 77:301–8. PMID:21266828

4085. Tzankov A, Xu-Monette ZY, Gerhard M, et al. (2014). Rearrangements of MYC gene facilitate risk stratification in diffuse large B-cell lymphoma patients treated with rituximab-CHOP. Mod Pathol. 27:958–71. PMID:24336156

4086. Tzankov A, Zimpfer A, Pehrs AC, et al. (2003). Expression of B-cell markers in classical hodgkin lymphoma: a tissue microarray analysis of 330 cases. Mod Pathol. 16:1141–7. PMID:14614054

4087. Uccini S, Al-Jadiry MF, Scarpino S, et al. (2015). Epstein-Barr virus-positive diffuse large B-cell lymphoma in children: a disease reminiscent of Epstein-Barr virus-positive diffuse large B-cell lymphoma of the elderly. Hum Pathol. 46:716–24. PMID:25704629

4088. Uckun FM, Sather HN, Gaynon PS, et al. (1997). Clinical features and treatment outcome of children with myeloid antigen positive acute lymphoblastic leukemia: a report from the Children's Cancer Group. Blood. 90:28–35. PMID:9207434

4089. Uldrick TS, Little RF (2015). How I treat

classical Hodgkin lymphoma in patients infected with human immunodeficiency virus. Blood. 125:1226–35, quiz 1355. PMID:25499453
4090. Uldrick TS, Polizzotto MN, Yarchoan R (2012). Recent advances in Kaposi sarcoma herpesvirus-associated multicentric Castleman disease. Curr Opin Oncol. 24:495–505. PMID:22729151
4091. Ungewickell A, Bhaduri A, Rios E, et al. (2015). Genomic analysis of mycosis fungoides and Sézary syndrome identifies recurrent alterations in TNFR2. Nat Genet. 47:1056–60. PMID:26258847
4092. Urayama KY, Jarrett RF, Hjalgrim H, et al. (2012). Genome-wide association study of classical Hodgkin lymphoma and Epstein-Barr virus status-defined subgroups. J Natl Cancer Inst. 104:240–53. PMID:22286212
4093. Urosevic M, Conrad C, Kamarashev J, et al. (2005). CD4+CD56+ hematodermic neoplasms bear a plasmacytoid dendritic cell phenotype. Hum Pathol. 36:1020–4. PMID:16153467
4094. Vaandrager JW, Schuuring E, Raap T, et al. (2000). Interphase FISH detection of BCL2 rearrangement in follicular lymphoma using breakpoint-flanking probes. Genes Chromosomes Cancer. 27:85–94. PMID:10564590
4095. Vaandrager JW, Schuuring E, Zwikstra E, et al. (1996). Direct visualization of dispersed 11q13 chromosomal translocations in mantle cell lymphoma by multicolor DNA fiber fluorescence in situ hybridization. Blood. 88:1177–82. PMID:8695834
4096. Vaghefi P, Martin A, Prévot S, et al. (2006). Genomic imbalances in AIDS-related lymphomas: relation with tumoral Epstein-Barr virus status. AIDS. 20:2285–91. PMID:17117014
4097. Vaidyanathan G, Ngamphaiboon N, Hernandez-Ilizaliturri FJ (2011). Clinical spectrum and prognosis of follicular lymphoma with blastoid transformation: case series and a review of the literature. Ann Hematol. 90:955–62. PMID:21286717
4098. Vaishampayan UN, Mohamed AN, Dugan MC, et al. (2001). Blastic mantle cell lymphoma associated with Burkitt-type translocation and hypodiploidy. Br J Haematol. 115:66–8. PMID:11722412
4099. Vajdic CM, Mao L, van Leeuwen MT, et al. (2010). Are antibody deficiency disorders associated with a narrower range of cancers than other forms of immunodeficiency? Blood. 116:1228–34. PMID:20466855
4100. Vakiani E, Basso K, Klein U, et al. (2008). Genetic and phenotypic analysis of B-cell post-transplant lymphoproliferative disorders provides insights into disease biology. Hematol Oncol. 26:199–211. PMID:18457340
4101. Vakiani E, Nandula SV, Subramaniyam S, et al. (2007). Cytogenetic analysis of B-cell posttransplant lymphoproliferations validates the World Health Organization classification and suggests inclusion of florid follicular hyperplasia as a precursor lesion. Hum Pathol. 38:315–25. PMID:17134734
4102. Valbuena JR, Medeiros LJ, Rassidakis GZ, et al. (2006). Expression of B cell-specific activator protein/PAX5 in acute myeloid leukemia with t(8;21)(q22;q22). Am J Clin Pathol. 126:235–40. PMID:16891199
4103. Valent P (2013). Mast cell activation syndromes: definition and classification. Allergy. 68:417–24. PMID:23409940
4104. Valent P, Akin C, Arock M, et al. (2012). Definitions, criteria and global classification of mast cell disorders with special reference to mast cell activation syndromes: a consensus proposal. Int Arch Allergy Immunol. 157:215–25. PMID:22041891
4105. Valent P, Akin C, Escribano L, et al. (2007). Standards and standardization in mastocytosis: consensus statements on diagnostics, treatment recommendations and response criteria. Eur J Clin Invest. 37:435–53. PMID:17537151
4106. Valent P, Bain BJ, Bennett JM, et al. (2012). Idiopathic cytopenia of undetermined significance (ICUS) and idiopathic dysplasia of uncertain significance (IDUS), and their distinction from low risk MDS. Leuk Res. 36:1–5. PMID:21920601
4107. Valent P, Horny HP, Escribano L, et al. (2001). Diagnostic criteria and classification of mastocytosis: a consensus proposal. Leuk Res. 25:603–25. PMID:11377686
4108. Valent P, Sotlar K, Sperr WR, et al. (2014). Refined diagnostic criteria and classification of mast cell leukemia (MCL) and myelomastocytic leukemia (MML): a consensus proposal. Ann Oncol. 25:1691–700. PMID:24675021
4109. Valentino C, Kendrick S, Johnson N, et al. (2013). Colorimetric in situ hybridization identifies MYC gene signal clusters correlating with increased copy number, mRNA, and protein in diffuse large B-cell lymphoma. Am J Clin Pathol. 139:242–54. PMID:23355209
4110. Valera A, Balagué O, Colomo L, et al. (2010). IG/MYC rearrangements are the main cytogenetic alteration in plasmablastic lymphomas. Am J Surg Pathol. 34:1686–94. PMID:20962620
4111. Valera A, Colomo L, Martínez A, et al. (2013). ALK-positive large B-cell lymphomas express a terminal B-cell differentiation program and activated STAT3 but lack MYC rearrangements. Mod Pathol. 26:1329–37. PMID:23599149
4112. Valera A, Colomo L, Martínez A, et al. (2013). ALK-positive large B-cell lymphomas express a terminal B-cell differentiation program and activated STAT3 but lack MYC rearrangements. Mod Pathol. 26:1329–37. PMID:23599149
4113. Valera A, López-Guillermo A, Cardesa-Salzmann T, et al. (2013). MYC protein expression and genetic alterations have prognostic impact in patients with diffuse large B-cell lymphoma treated with immunochemotherapy. Haematologica. 98:1554–62. PMID:23716551
4114. Valli R, Froio E, Alvarez de Celis MI, et al. (2014). Diffuse large B-cell lymphoma occurring in an ovarian cystic teratoma: expanding the spectrum of large B-cell lymphoma associated with chronic inflammation. Hum Pathol. 45:2507–11. PMID:25439346
4115. Valli R, Piana S, Capodanno I, et al. (2011). Diffuse large B-cell lymphoma associated with chronic inflammation arising in a renal pseudocyst. Int J Surg Pathol. 19:117–9. PMID:21131315
4116. van de Donk NW, Palumbo A, Johnsen HE, et al. (2014). The clinical relevance and management of monoclonal gammopathy of undetermined significance and related disorders: recommendations from the European Myeloma Network. Haematologica. 99:984–96. PMID:24658815
4117. van de Loosdrecht AA, Alhan C, Béné MC, et al. (2009). Standardization of flow cytometry in myelodysplastic syndromes: report from the first European LeukemiaNet working conference on flow cytometry in myelodysplastic syndromes. Haematologica. 94:1124–34. PMID:19546437
4118. van de Loosdrecht AA, Ireland R, Kern W, et al. (2013). Rationale for the clinical application of flow cytometry in patients with myelodysplastic syndromes: position paper of an International Consortium and the European LeukemiaNet Working Group. Leuk Lymphoma. 54:472–5. PMID:22916713
4119. van de Loosdrecht AA, Westers TM (2013). Cutting edge: flow cytometry in myelodysplastic syndromes. J Natl Compr Canc Netw. 11:892–902. PMID:23847222
4120. van den Berg A, Visser L, Poppema S (1999). High expression of the CC chemokine TARC in Reed-Sternberg cells. A possible explanation for the characteristic T-cell infiltratein Hodgkin's lymphoma. Am J Pathol. 154:1685–91. PMID:10362793
4121. van den Bosch C (2012). A Role for RNA Viruses in the Pathogenesis of Burkitt's Lymphoma: The Need for Reappraisal. Adv Hematol. 2012:494758. PMID:22550493
4122. van den Bosch CA (2004). Is endemic Burkitt's lymphoma an alliance between three infections and a tumour promoter? Lancet Oncol. 5:738–46. PMID:15581545
4123. van den Brand M, van Krieken JH (2013). Recognizing nodal marginal zone lymphoma: recent advances and pitfalls. A systematic review. Haematologica. 98:1003–13. PMID:23813646
4124. van den Oord JJ, de Wolf-Peeters C, Desmet VJ (1989). Marginal zone lymphocytes in the lymph node. Hum Pathol. 20:1225–7. PMID:2591956
4125. van der Veer A, Waanders E, Pieters R, et al. (2013). Independent prognostic value of BCR-ABL1-like signature and IKZF1 deletion, but not high CRLF2 expression, in children with B-cell precursor ALL. Blood. 122:2622–9. PMID:23974192
4126. van der Velden VH, Brüggemann M, Hoogeveen PG, et al. (2004). TCRB gene rearrangements in childhood and adult precursor-B-ALL: frequency, applicability as MRD-PCR target, and stability between diagnosis and relapse. Leukemia. 18:1971–80. PMID:15470492
4127. van der Velden VH, Hoogeveen PG, de Ridder D, et al. (2014). B-cell prolymphocytic leukemia: a specific subgroup of mantle cell lymphoma. Blood. 124:412–9. PMID:24891323
4128. van der Velden WJ, Nissen L, van Rijn M, et al. (2015). Identification of IG-clonality status as a pre-treatment predictor for mortality in patients with immunodeficiency-associated Epstein-Barr virus-related lymphoproliferative disorders. Haematologica. 100:e152–4. PMID:25527569
4129. van Dongen JJ, Seriu T, Panzer-Grümayer ER, et al. (1998). Prognostic value of minimal residual disease in acute lymphoblastic leukaemia in childhood. Lancet. 352:1731–8. PMID:9848348
4130. van Doorn R, Dijkman R, Vermeer MH, et al. (2004). Aberrant expression of the tyrosine kinase receptor EphA4 and the transcription factor twist in Sézary syndrome identified by gene expression analysis. Cancer Res. 64:5578–86. PMID:15313894
4131. van Doorn R, Scheffer E, Willemze R (2002). Follicular mycosis fungoides, a distinct disease entity with or without associated follicular mucinosis: a clinicopathologic and follow-up study of 51 patients. Arch Dermatol. 138:191–8. PMID:11843638
4132. van Doorn R, Van Haselen CW, van Voorst Vader PC, et al. (2000). Mycosis fungoides: disease evolution and prognosis of 309 Dutch patients. Arch Dermatol. 136:504–10. PMID:10768649
4132A. Van Dyke DL, Shanafelt TD, Call TG, et al. (2010). A comprehensive evaluation of the prognostic significance of 13q deletions in patients with B-chronic lymphocytic leukaemia. Br J Haematol. 148:544-50. PMID:19895615
4133. van Gorp J, Weiping L, Jacobse K, et al. (1994). Epstein-Barr virus in nasal T-cell lymphomas (polymorphic reticulosis/midline malignant reticulosis) in western China. J Pathol. 173:81–7. PMID:7522272
4134. van Kester MS, Borg MK, Zoutman WH, et al. (2012). A meta-analysis of gene expression data identifies a molecular signature characteristic for tumor-stage mycosis fungoides. J Invest Dermatol. 132:2050–9. PMID:22513784
4135. van Kester MS, Tensen CP, Vermeer MH, et al. (2010). Cutaneous anaplastic large cell lymphoma and peripheral T-cell lymphoma NOS show distinct chromosomal alterations and differential expression of chemokine receptors and apoptosis regulators. J Invest Dermatol. 130:563–75. PMID:19710685
4136. van Krieken JH (2004). Lymphoproliferative disease associated with immune deficiency in children. Am J Clin Pathol. 122 Suppl:S122–7. PMID:15690648
4137. van Maldegem F, van Dijk R, Wormhoudt TA, et al. (2008). The majority of cutaneous marginal zone B-cell lymphomas expresses class-switched immunoglobulins and develops in a T-helper type 2 inflammatory environment. Blood. 112:3355–61. PMID:18687986
4138. Van Neer FJ, Toonstra J, Van Voorst Vader PC, et al. (2001). Lymphomatoid papulosis in children: a study of 10 children registered by the Dutch Cutaneous Lymphoma Working Group. Br J Dermatol. 144:351–4. PMID:11251571
4139. van Nierop K, de Groot C (2002). Human follicular dendritic cells: function, origin and development. Semin Immunol. 14:251–7. PMID:12163300
4140. van Rhee F, Hochhaus A, Lin F, et al. (1996). p190 BCR-ABL mRNA is expressed at low levels in p210-positive chronic myeloid and acute lymphoblastic leukemias. Blood. 87:5213–7. PMID:8652835
4141. van Spronsen DJ, Vrints LW, Hofstra G, et al. (1997). Disappearance of prognostic significance of histopathological grading of nodular sclerosing Hodgkin's disease for unselected patients, 1972-92. Br J Haematol. 96:322–7. PMID:9029020
4142. Van Vlierberghe P, Ambesi-Impiombato A, Perez-Garcia A, et al. (2011). ETV6 mutations in early immature human T cell leukemias. J Exp Med. 208:2571–9. PMID:22162831
4143. Van Vlierberghe P, Pieters R, Beverloo HB, et al. (2008). Molecular-genetic insights in paediatric T-cell acute lymphoblastic leukaemia. Br J Haematol. 143:153–68. PMID:18691165
4144. Van Weyenberg SJ, Meijerink MR, Jacobs MA, et al. (2011). MR enteroclysis in refractory celiac disease: proposal and validation of a severity scoring system. Radiology. 259:151–61. PMID:21330559
4145. VanBuskirk AM, Malik V, Xia D, et al. (2001). A gene polymorphism associated with posttransplant lymphoproliferative disorder. Transplant Proc. 33:1834. PMID:11267533
4146. Vandenberghe E, De Wolf-Peeters C, van den Oord J, et al. (1991). Translocation (11;14): a cytogenetic anomaly associated with B-cell lymphomas of non-follicle centre cell lineage. J Pathol. 163:13–8. PMID:2002419
4147. Vandenberghe P, Wlodarska I, Michaux L, et al. (2004). Clinical and molecular features of FIP1L1-PDFGRA (+) chronic eosinophilic leukemias. Leukemia. 18:734–42. PMID:14973504
4148. Vang R, Medeiros LJ, Ha CS, et al. (2000). Non-Hodgkin's lymphomas involving the uterus: a clinicopathologic analysis of 26 cases. Mod Pathol. 13:19–28. PMID:10658906
4149. Vannucchi AM, Lasho TL, Guglielmelli P, et al. (2013). Mutations and prognosis in primary myelofibrosis. Leukemia. 27:1861–9. PMID:23619563
4150. Vaqué JP, Gómez-López G, Monsálvez V, et al. (2014). PLCG1 mutations in cutaneous T-cell lymphomas. Blood. 123:2034–43. PMID:24497536

4151. Vardiman JW (2003). The new World Health Organization classification of myeloid neoplasms: Q&A with James W. Vardiman, MD. Clin Adv Hematol Oncol. 1:18, 21. PMID:16227955

4152. Vardiman JW (2004). Myelodysplastic/ myeloproliferative diseases. Cancer Treat Res. 121:13–43. PMID:15217205

4153. Vardiman JW, Coelho A, Golomb HM, et al. (1983). Morphologic and cytochemical observations on the overt leukemic phase of therapy-related leukemia. Am J Clin Pathol. 79:525–30. PMID:6188364

4154. Vardiman JW, Golomb HM, Rowley JD, et al. (1978). Acute nonlymphocytic leukemia in malignant lymphoma: a morphologic study. Cancer. 42:229–42. PMID:276415

4155. Varettoni M, Arcaini L, Zibellini S, et al. (2013). Prevalence and clinical significance of the MYD88 (L265P) somatic mutation in Waldenstrom's macroglobulinemia and related lymphoid neoplasms. Blood. 121:2522–8. PMID:23355535

4156. Varettoni M, Zibellini S, Arcaini L, et al. (2013). MYD88 (L265P) mutation is an independent risk factor for progression in patients with IgM monoclonal gammopathy of undetermined significance. Blood. 122:2284–5. PMID:24072850

4157. Varghese AM, Rawstron AC, Ashcroft AJ, et al. (2009). Assessment of bone marrow response in Waldenström's macroglobulinemia. Clin Lymphoma Myeloma. 9:53–5. PMID:19362973

4158. Varon R, Vissinga C, Platzer M, et al. (1998). Nibrin, a novel DNA double-strand break repair protein, is mutated in Nijmegen breakage syndrome. Cell. 93:467–76. PMID:9590180

4159. Vase MØ, Maksten EF, Bendix K, et al. (2015). Occurrence and prognostic relevance of CD30 expression in post-transplant lymphoproliferative disorders. Leuk Lymphoma. 56:1677–85. PMID:25248878

4160. Vasef MA, Zaatari GS, Chan WC, et al. (1995). Dendritic cell tumors associated with low-grade B-cell malignancies. Report of three cases. Am J Clin Pathol. 104:696–701. PMID:8526215

4161. Vasmatzis G, Johnson SH, Knudson RA, et al. (2012). Genome-wide analysis reveals recurrent structural abnormalities of TP63 and other p53-related genes in peripheral T-cell lymphomas. Blood. 120:2280–9. PMID:22855598

4162. Vassallo J, Lamant L, Brugieres L, et al. (2006). ALK-positive anaplastic large cell lymphoma mimicking nodular sclerosis Hodgkin's lymphoma: report of 10 cases. Am J Surg Pathol. 30:223–9. PMID:16434897

4163. Vater I, Montesinos-Rongen M, Schlesner M, et al. (2015). The mutational pattern of primary lymphoma of the central nervous system determined by whole-exome sequencing. Leukemia. 29:677–85. PMID:25189415

4164. Vega F, Chang CC, Medeiros LJ, et al. (2005). Plasmablastic lymphomas and plasmablastic plasma cell myelomas have nearly identical immunophenotypic profiles. Mod Pathol. 18:806–15. PMID:15578069

4165. Vega F, Coombes KR, Thomazy VA, et al. (2006). Tissue-specific function of lymph node fibroblastic reticulum cells. Pathobiology. 73:71–81. PMID:16943687

4166. Vega F, Medeiros LJ, Bueso-Ramos C, et al. (2001). Hepatosplenic gamma/delta T-cell lymphoma in bone marrow. A sinusoidal neoplasm with blastic cytologic features. Am J Clin Pathol. 116:410–9. PMID:11554170

4167. Vega F, Medeiros LJ, Bueso-Ramos CE, et al. (2015). Hematolymphoid neoplasms associated with rearrangements of PDGFRA,

PDGFRB, and FGFR1. Am J Clin Pathol. 144:377–92. PMID:26276769

4168. Vega F, Medeiros LJ, Gaulard P (2007). Hepatosplenic and other gammadelta T-cell lymphomas. Am J Clin Pathol. 127:869–80. PMID:17509984

4169. Vegliante MC, Palomero J, Pérez-Galán P, et al. (2013). SOX11 regulates PAX5 expression and blocks terminal B-cell differentiation in aggressive mantle cell lymphoma. Blood. 121:2175–85. PMID:23321250

4170. Vela-Chávez T, Adam P, Kremer M, et al. (2011). Cyclin D1 positive diffuse large B-cell lymphoma is a post-germinal center-type lymphoma without alterations in the CCND1 gene locus. Leuk Lymphoma. 52:458–66. PMID:21281227

4171. Velusamy T, Kiel MJ, Sahasrabuddhe AA, et al. (2014). A novel recurrent NPM1-TYK2 gene fusion in cutaneous CD30-positive lymphoproliferative disorders. Blood. 124:3768–71. PMID:25349176

4172. Venditti A, Del Poeta G, Buccisano F, et al. (1998). Prognostic relevance of the expression of Tdt and CD7 in 335 cases of acute myeloid leukemia. Leukemia. 12:1056–63. PMID:9665190

4173. Vener C, Fracchiolla NS, Gianelli U, et al. (2008). Prognostic implications of the European consensus for grading of bone marrow fibrosis in chronic idiopathic myelofibrosis. Blood. 111:1862–5. PMID:18029552

4174. Vener C, Soligo D, Berti E, et al. (2007). Indeterminate cell histiocytosis in association with later occurrence of acute myeloblastic leukaemia. Br J Dermatol. 156:1357–61. PMID:17459045

4175. Venkataraman G, Raffeld M, Pittaluga S, et al. (2011). CD15-expressing nodular lymphocyte-predominant Hodgkin lymphoma. Histopathology. 58:803–5. PMID:21457163

4176. Venkataraman G, Song JY, Tzankov A, et al. (2013). Aberrant T-cell antigen expression in classical Hodgkin lymphoma is associated with decreased event-free survival and overall survival. Blood. 121:1795–804. PMID:23305738

4177. Verbeek WH, Van De Water JM, Al-Toma A, et al. (2008). Incidence of enteropathy-associated T-cell lymphoma: a nation-wide study of a population-based registry in The Netherlands. Scand J Gastroenterol. 43:1322–8. PMID:18618372

4178. Verbeek WH, von Blomberg BM, Coupe VM, et al. (2009). Aberrant T-lymphocytes in refractory coeliac disease are not strictly confined to a small intestinal intraepithelial localization. Cytometry B Clin Cytom. 76:367–74. PMID:19444812

4179. Verburgh E, Achten R, Louw VJ, et al. (2007). A new disease categorization of low-grade myelodysplastic syndromes based on the expression of cytopenia and dysplasia in one versus more than one lineage improves on the WHO classification. Leukemia. 21:668–77. PMID:17301818

4180. Verburgh E, Achten R, Maes B, et al. (2003). Additional prognostic value of bone marrow histology in patients subclassified according to the International Prognostic Scoring System for myelodysplastic syndromes. J Clin Oncol. 21:273–82. PMID:12525519

4181. Vereide DT, Seto E, Chiu YF, et al. (2014). Epstein-Barr virus maintains lymphomas via its miRNAs. Oncogene. 33:1258–64. PMID:23503461

4182. Vergara-Lluri ME, Piatek CI, Pullarkat V, et al. (2014). Autoimmune myelofibrosis: an update on morphologic features in 29 cases and review of the literature. Hum Pathol. 45:2183–91. PMID:25282037

4183. Vergier B, Belaud-Rotureau MA, Benassy MN, et al. (2004). Neoplastic cells do not carry

bcl2-JH rearrangements detected in a subset of primary cutaneous follicle center B-cell lymphomas. Am J Surg Pathol. 28:748–55. PMID:15166666

4184. Vergier B, de Muret A, Beylot-Barry M, et al. (2000). Transformation of mycosis fungoides: clinicopathological and prognostic features of 45 cases. Blood. 95:2212–8. PMID:10733487

4185. Verhaak RG, Goudswaard CS, van Putten W, et al. (2005). Mutations in nucleophosmin (NPM1) in acute myeloid leukemia (AML): association with other gene abnormalities and previously established gene expression signatures and their favorable prognostic significance. Blood. 106:3747–54. PMID:16109776

4186. Verkarre V, Asnafi V, Lecomte T, et al. (2003). Refractory coeliac sprue is a diffuse gastrointestinal disease. Gut. 52:205–11. PMID:12524401

4187. Verkarre V, Romana SP, Cellier C, et al. (2003). Recurrent partial trisomy 1q22-q44 in clonal intraepithelial lymphocytes in refractory celiac sprue. Gastroenterology. 125:40–6. PMID:12851869

4188. Vermeer MH, Geelen FA, Kummer JA, et al. (1999). Expression of cytotoxic proteins by neoplastic T cells in mycosis fungoides increases with progression from plaque stage to tumor stage disease. Am J Pathol. 154:1203–10. PMID:10233858

4189. Vermeer MH, Geelen FA, van Haselen CW, et al. (1996). Primary cutaneous large B-cell lymphomas of the legs. A distinct type of cutaneous B-cell lymphoma with an intermediate prognosis. Arch Dermatol. 132:1304–8. PMID:8915307

4190. Vermeer MH, van Doorn R, Dijkman R, et al. (2008). Novel and highly recurrent chromosomal alterations in Sézary syndrome. Cancer Res. 68:2689–98. PMID:18413736

4191. Vermi W, Facchetti F, Rosati S, et al. (2004). Nodal and extranodal tumor-forming accumulation of plasmacytoid monocytes/ interferon-producing cells associated with myeloid disorders. Am J Surg Pathol. 28:585–95. PMID:15105645

4192. Vermi W, Lonardi S, Bosisio D, et al. (2008). Identification of CXCL13 as a new marker for follicular dendritic cell sarcoma. J Pathol. 216:356–64. PMID:18792075

4192A. Veyssier-Belot C, Cacoub P, Caparros-Lefebvre D, et al. (1996). Erdheim-Chester disease. Clinical and radiologic characteristics of 59 cases. Medicine (Baltimore). 75:157–69. PMID:8965684

4193. Vicente C, Cools J (2015). The genomic landscape of adult T cell leukemia/lymphoma. Nat Genet. 47:1226–7. PMID:26506901

4194. Vie H, Chevalier S, Garand R, et al. (1989). Clonal expansion of lymphocytes bearing the gamma delta T-cell receptor in a patient with large granular lymphocyte disorder. Blood. 74:285–90. PMID:2546620

4195. Vijay A, Gertz MA (2007). Waldenström macroglobulinemia. Blood. 109:5096–103. PMID:17303694

4196. Villano JL, Koshy M, Shaikh H, et al. (2011). Age, gender, and racial differences in incidence and survival in primary CNS lymphoma. Br J Cancer. 105:1414–8. PMID:21915121

4197. Vinh DC, Patel SY, Uzel G, et al. (2010). Autosomal dominant and sporadic monocytopenia with susceptibility to mycobacteria, fungi, papillomaviruses, and myelodysplasia. Blood. 115:1519–29. PMID:20040766

4197A. Virappane P, Gale R, Hills R, et al. (2008). Mutation of the Wilms' tumor 1 gene is a poor prognostic factor associated with chemotherapy resistance in normal karyotype

acute myeloid leukemia: the United Kingdom Medical Research Council Adult Leukaemia Working Party. J Clin Oncol. 26:5429–35. PMID:18591546

4198. Virgilio L, Lazzeri C, Bichi R, et al. (1998). Deregulated expression of TCL1 causes T cell leukemia in mice. Proc Natl Acad Sci U S A. 95:3885–9. PMID:9520462

4199. Visco C, Li Y, Xu-Monette ZY, et al. (2012). Comprehensive gene expression profiling and immunohistochemical studies support application of immunophenotypic algorithm for molecular subtype classification in diffuse large B-cell lymphoma: a report from the International DLBCL Rituximab-CHOP Consortium Program Study. Leukemia. 26:2103–13. PMID:22437443

4200. Visco C, Tzankov A, Xu-Monette ZY, et al. (2013). Patients with diffuse large B-cell lymphoma of germinal center origin with BCL2 translocations have poor outcome, irrespective of MYC status: a report from an International DLBCL rituximab-CHOP Consortium Program Study. Haematologica. 98:255–63. PMID:22929980

4201. Visconte V, Rogers HJ, Singh J, et al. (2012). SF3B1 haploinsufficiency leads to formation of ring sideroblasts in myelodysplastic syndromes. Blood. 120:3173–86. PMID:22826563

4202. Visconte V, Tabarroki A, Hasrouni E, et al. (2016). Molecular and phenotypic heterogeneity of refractory anemia with ring sideroblasts associated with marked thrombocytosis. Leuk Lymphoma. 57:212–5. PMID:25926061

4203. Visconte V, Tabarroki A, Zhang L, et al. (2014). Splicing factor 3b subunit 1 (Sf3b1) haploinsufficient mice display features of low risk Myelodysplastic syndromes with ring sideroblasts. J Hematol Oncol. 7:89. PMID:25481243

4204. Viswanatha DS, Foucar K, Berry BR, et al. (2000). Blastic mantle cell leukemia: an unusual presentation of blastic mantle cell lymphoma. Mod Pathol. 13:825–33. PMID:10912944

4205. Vitolo U, Ferreri AJ, Zucca E (2008). Primary testicular lymphoma. Crit Rev Oncol Hematol. 65:183–9. PMID:17962036

4206. Vitte F, Fabiani B, Bénet C, et al. (2012). Specific skin lesions in chronic myelomonocytic leukemia: a spectrum of myelomonocytic and dendritic cell proliferations: a study of 42 cases. Am J Surg Pathol. 36:1302–16. PMID:22895265

4207. Vizmanos JL, Hernández R, Vidal MJ, et al. (2004). Clinical variability of patients with the t(6;8)(q27;p12) and FGFR1OP-FGFR1 fusion: two further cases. Hematol J. 5:534–7. PMID:15570299

4208. Vogt N, Klapper W (2013). Variability in morphology and cell proliferation in sequential biopsies of mantle cell lymphoma at diagnosis and relapse: clinical correlation and insights into disease progression. Histopathology. 62:334–42. PMID:23240716

4208A. von Bergh AR, van Drunen E, van Wering ER, et al. (2006). High incidence of t(7;12) (q36;p13) in infant AML but not in infant ALL, with a dismal outcome and ectopic expression of HLXB9. Genes Chromosomes Cancer. 45:731–9. PMID:16646086

4209. von Neuhoff C, Reinhardt D, Sander A, et al. (2010). Prognostic impact of specific chromosomal aberrations in a large group of pediatric patients with acute myeloid leukemia treated uniformly according to trial AML-BFM 98. J Clin Oncol. 28:2682–9. PMID:20439630

4210. von Wasielewski S, Franklin J, Fischer R, et al. (2003). Nodular sclerosing Hodgkin disease: new grading predicts prognosis in intermediate and advanced stages. Blood. 101:4063–9. PMID:12543871

4211. Vonderheid EC (2006). On the diagnosis of erythrodermic cutaneous T-cell

lymphoma. J Cutan Pathol. 33 Suppl 1:27–42. PMID:16412210
4212. Vonderheid EC, Pavlov I, Delgado JC, et al. (2014). Prognostic factors and risk stratification in early mycosis fungoides. Leuk Lymphoma. 55:44–50. PMID:23547839
4213. Vonderheid EC, Pena J, Nowell P (2006). Sézary cell counts in erythrodermic cutaneous T-cell lymphoma: implications for prognosis and staging. Leuk Lymphoma. 47:1841–56. PMID:17064997
4214. Voorhees PM, Carder KA, Smith SV, et al. (2004). Follicular lymphoma with a burkitt translocation–predictor of an aggressive clinical course: a case report and review of the literature. Arch Pathol Lab Med. 128:210–3. PMID:14736281
4215. Vorechovský I, Luo L, Dyer MJ, et al. (1997). Clustering of missense mutations in the ataxia-telangiectasia gene in a sporadic T-cell leukaemia. Nat Genet. 17:96–9. PMID:9288106
4216. Vos JA, Abbondanzo SL, Barekman CL, et al. (2005). Histiocytic sarcoma: a study of five cases including the histiocyte marker CD163. Mod Pathol. 18:693–704. PMID:15696128
4217. Vose J, Armitage J, Weisenburger D; International T-Cell Lymphoma Project (2008). International peripheral T-cell and natural killer/T-cell lymphoma study: pathology findings and clinical outcomes. J Clin Oncol. 26:4124–30. PMID:18626005
4218. Vose JM (2015). Mantle cell lymphoma: 2015 update on diagnosis, risk-stratification, and clinical management. Am J Hematol. 90:739–45. PMID:26103436
4219. Voso MT, Fenu S, Latagliata R, et al. (2013). Revised International Prognostic Scoring System (IPSS) predicts survival and leukemic evolution of myelodysplastic syndromes significantly better than IPSS and WHO Prognostic Scoring System: validation by the Gruppo Romano Mielodisplasie Italian Regional Database. J Clin Oncol. 31:2671–7. PMID:23796988
4220. Voss MH, Lunning MA, Maragulia JC, et al. (2013). Intensive induction chemotherapy followed by early high-dose therapy and hematopoietic stem cell transplantation results in improved outcome for patients with hepatosplenic T-cell lymphoma: a single institution experience. Clin Lymphoma Myeloma Leuk. 13:8–14. PMID:23107915
4221. Vrana JA, Gamez JD, Madden BJ, et al. (2009). Classification of amyloidosis by laser microdissection and mass spectrometry-based proteomic analysis in clinical biopsy specimens. Blood. 114:4957–9. PMID:19797517
4222. Vyas P, Crispino JD (2007). Molecular insights into Down syndrome-associated leukemia. Curr Opin Pediatr. 19:9–14. PMID:17224656
4223. Wada DA, Law ME, Hsi ED, et al. (2011). Specificity of IRF4 translocations for primary cutaneous anaplastic large cell lymphoma: a multicenter study of 204 skin biopsies. Mod Pathol. 24:596–605. PMID:21169992
4224. Wada T, Toga A, Sakakibara Y, et al. (2012). Clonal expansion of Epstein-Barr virus (EBV)-infected γδ T cells in patients with chronic active EBV disease and hydroa vacciniforme-like eruptions. Int J Hematol. 96:443–9. PMID:22886572
4225. Wagener R, Aukema SM, Schlesner M, et al. (2015). The PCBP1 gene encoding poly(rC) binding protein I is recurrently mutated in Burkitt lymphoma. Genes Chromosomes Cancer. 54:555–64. PMID:26173642
4226. Wagner SD, Martinelli V, Luzzatto L (1994). Similar patterns of V kappa gene usage but different degrees of somatic mutation in hairy cell leukemia, prolymphocytic leukemia, Waldenstrom's macroglobulinemia, and myeloma. Blood. 83:3647–53. PMID:8204889
4227. Wagner-Johnston ND, Link BK, Byrtek M, et al. (2015). Outcomes of transformed follicular lymphoma in the modern era: a report from the National LymphoCare Study (NLCS). Blood. 126:851–7. PMID:26105149
4228. Wahlin BE, Yri OE, Kimby E, et al. (2012). Clinical significance of the WHO grades of follicular lymphoma in a population-based cohort of 505 patients with long follow-up times. Br J Haematol. 156:225–33. PMID:22126847
4229. Wahner-Roedler DL, Kyle RA (1992). Mu-heavy chain disease: presentation as a benign monoclonal gammopathy. Am J Hematol. 40:56–60. PMID:1566748
4230. Wahner-Roedler DL, Kyle RA (2005). Heavy chain diseases. Best Pract Res Clin Haematol. 18:729–46. PMID:16026747
4231. Wahner-Roedler DL, Witzig TE, Loehrer LL, et al. (2003). Gamma-heavy chain disease: review of 23 cases. Medicine (Baltimore). 82:236–50. PMID:12861101
4232. Walter MJ, Shen D, Ding L, et al. (2012). Clonal architecture of secondary acute myeloid leukemia. N Engl J Med. 366:1090–8. PMID:22417201
4233. Walter RB, Othus M, Burnett AK, et al. (2013). Significance of FAB subclassification of "acute myeloid leukemia, NOS" in the 2008 WHO classification: analysis of 5848 newly diagnosed patients. Blood. 121:2424–31. PMID:23325837
4234. Walts AE, Shintaku IP, Said JW (1990). Diagnosis of malignant lymphoma in effusions from patients with AIDS by gene rearrangement. Am J Clin Pathol. 94:170–5. PMID:2371971
4235. Walz C, Curtis C, Schnittger S, et al. (2006). Transient response to imatinib in a chronic eosinophilic leukemia associated with ins(9;4)(q33;q12q25) and a CDK5RAP2-PDGFRA fusion gene. Genes Chromosomes Cancer. 45:950–6. PMID:16845659
4236. Walz C, Metzgeroth G, Haferlach C, et al. (2007). Characterization of three new imatinib-responsive fusion genes in chronic myeloproliferative disorders generated by disruption of the platelet-derived growth factor receptor beta gene. Haematologica. 92:163–9. PMID:17296564
4237. Wandt H, Schäkel U, Kroschinsky F, et al. (2008). MLD according to the WHO classification in AML has no correlation with age and no independent prognostic relevance as analyzed in 1766 patients. Blood. 111:1855–61. PMID:18056840
4238. Wang C, McKeithan TW, Gong Q, et al. (2015). IDH2R172 mutations define a unique subgroup of patients with angioimmunoblastic T-cell lymphoma. Blood. 126:1741–52. PMID:26268241
4239. Wang C, Sashida G, Saraya A, et al. (2014). Depletion of Sf3b1 impairs proliferative capacity of hematopoietic stem cells but is not sufficient to induce myelodysplasia. Blood. 123:3336–43. PMID:24735968
4240. Wang J, Bu DF, Li T, et al. (2005). Autoantibody production from a thymoma and a follicular dendritic cell sarcoma associated with paraneoplastic pemphigus. Br J Dermatol. 153:558–64. PMID:16120143
4241. Wang L, Chen S, Ma H, et al. (2015). Intravascular NK/T-cell lymphoma: a report of five cases with cutaneous manifestation from China. J Cutan Pathol. 42:610–7. PMID:25931234
4242. Wang L, Lawrence MS, Wan Y, et al. (2011). SF3B1 and other novel cancer genes in chronic lymphocytic leukemia. N Engl J Med. 365:2497–506. PMID:22150006
4243. Wang L, Peters JM, Fuda F, et al. (2015). Acute megakaryoblastic leukemia associated with trisomy 21 demonstrates a distinct immunophenotype. Cytometry B Clin Cytom. 88:244–52. PMID:25361478
4244. Wang RC, Chang ST, Hsieh YC, et al. (2014). Spectrum of Epstein-Barr virus-associated T-cell lymphoproliferative disorder in adolescents and young adults in Taiwan. Int J Clin Exp Pathol. 7:2430–7. PMID:24966953
4245. Wang SA, Galili N, Cerny J, et al. (2006). Chronic myelomonocytic leukemia evolving from preexisting myelodysplasia shares many features with de novo disease. Am J Clin Pathol. 126:789–97. PMID:17050076
4246. Wang SA, Hasserjian RP (2012). Erythroid proliferations in myeloid neoplasms. Hum Pathol. 43:153–64. PMID:22154053
4247. Wang SA, Hasserjian RP (2015). Acute Erythroleukemias, Acute Megakaryoblastic Leukemias, and Reactive Mimics: A Guide to a Number of Perplexing Entities. Am J Clin Pathol. 144:44–60. PMID:26071461
4248. Wang SA, Hasserjian RP, Fox PS, et al. (2014). Atypical chronic myeloid leukemia is clinically distinct from unclassifiable myelodysplastic/myeloproliferative neoplasms. Blood. 123:2645–51. PMID:24627528
4249. Wang SA, Hasserjian RP, Loew JM, et al. (2006). Refractory anemia with ringed sideroblasts associated with marked thrombocytosis harbors JAK2 mutation and shows overlapping myeloproliferative and myelodysplastic features. Leukemia. 20:1641–4. PMID:16871284
4249A. Wang SA, Olson N, Zukerberg L, et al. (2006). Splenic marginal zone lymphoma with micronodular T-cell rich B-cell lymphoma. Am J Surg Pathol. 30:128–32. PMID:16330953
4249B. Wang SA, Tam W, Tsai AG, et al. (2016). Targeted next-generation sequencing identifies a subset of idiopathic hypereosinophilic syndrome with features similar to chronic eosinophilic leukemia, not otherwise specified. Mod Pathol. 29:854–64. PMID:27174585
4250. Wang SA, Wang L, Hochberg EP, et al. (2005). Low histologic grade follicular lymphoma with high proliferation index: morphologic and clinical features. Am J Surg Pathol. 29:1490–6. PMID:16224216
4251. Wang SS, Cozen W, Cerhan JR, et al. (2007). Immune mechanisms in non-Hodgkin lymphoma: joint effects of the TNF G308A and IL10 T3575A polymorphisms with non-Hodgkin lymphoma risk factors. Cancer Res. 67:5042–54. PMID:17510437
4252. Wang SS, Vajdic CM, Linet MS, et al. (2015). Associations of non-Hodgkin Lymphoma (NHL) risk with autoimmune conditions according to putative NHL loci. Am J Epidemiol. 181:406–21. PMID:25713336
4253. Wang T, Feldman AL, Wada DA, et al. (2014). GATA-3 expression identifies a high-risk subset of PTCL, NOS with distinct molecular and clinical features. Blood. 123:3007–15. PMID:24497534
4254. Wang W, Hu S, Lu X, et al. (2015). Triple-hit B-cell Lymphoma With MYC, BCL2, and BCL6 Translocations/Rearrangements: Clinicopathologic Features of 11 Cases. Am J Surg Pathol. 39:1132–9. PMID:25828391
4255. Wang X, Prakash S, Lu M, et al. (2012). Spleens of myelofibrosis patients contain malignant hematopoietic stem cells. J Clin Invest. 122:3888–99. PMID:23023702
4256. Wang Y, Gu M, Mi Y, et al. (2011). Clinical characteristics and outcomes of mixed phenotype acute leukemia with Philadelphia chromosome positive and/or bcr-abl positive in adult. Int J Hematol. 94:552–5. PMID:22015493
4257. Wang ZY, Liu QF, Wang H, et al. (2012). Clinical implications of plasma Epstein-Barr virus DNA in early-stage extranodal nasal-type NK/T-cell lymphoma patients receiving primary radiotherapy. Blood. 120:2003–10. PMID:22826562
4258. Warnke RA, Jones D, Hsi ED (2007). Morphologic and immunophenotypic variants of nodal T-cell lymphomas and T-cell lymphoma mimics. Am J Clin Pathol. 127:511–27. PMID:17369127
4259. Warren HS, Christiansen FT, Witt CS (2003). Functional inhibitory human leucocyte antigen class I receptors on natural killer (NK) cells in patients with chronic NK lymphocytosis. Br J Haematol. 121:793–804. PMID:12780796
4260. Warsame R, Gertz MA, Lacy MQ, et al. (2012). Trends and outcomes of modern staging of solitary plasmacytoma of bone. Am J Hematol. 87:647–51. PMID:22549792
4261. Warzynski MJ, White C, Golightly MG, et al. (1989). Natural killer lymphocyte blast crisis of chronic myelogenous leukemia. Am J Hematol. 32:279–86. PMID:2816923
4262. Wasco MJ, Fullen D, Su L, et al. (2008). The expression of MUM1 in cutaneous T-cell lymphoproliferative disorders. Hum Pathol. 39:557–63. PMID:18234282
4263. Washington LT, Doherty D, Glassman A, et al. (2002). Myeloid disorders with deletion of 5q as the sole karyotypic abnormality: the clinical and pathologic spectrum. Leuk Lymphoma. 43:761–5. PMID:12153162
4264. Wassie EA, Itzykson R, Lasho TL, et al. (2014). Molecular and prognostic correlates of cytogenetic abnormalities in chronic myelomonocytic leukemia: a Mayo Clinic-French Consortium Study. Am J Hematol. 89:1111–5. PMID:25195656
4265. Watanabe N, Noh JY, Narimatsu H, et al. (2011). Clinicopathological features of 171 cases of primary thyroid lymphoma: a long-term study involving 24553 patients with Hashimoto's disease. Br J Haematol. 153:236–43. PMID:21371004
4266. Watanabe O, Maruyama I, Arimura K, et al. (1998). Overproduction of vascular endothelial growth factor/vascular permeability factor is causative in Crow-Fukase (POEMS) syndrome. Muscle Nerve. 21:1390–7. PMID:9771661
4267. Waterfall JJ, Arons E, Walker RL, et al. (2014). High prevalence of MAP2K1 mutations in variant and IGHV4-34-expressing hairy-cell leukemias. Nat Genet. 46:8–10. PMID:24241536
4268. Watkins AJ, Hamoudi RA, Zeng N, et al. (2012). An integrated genomic and expression analysis of 7q deletion in splenic marginal zone lymphoma. PLoS One. 7:e44997. PMID:23028731
4269. Webb D, Roberts I, Vyas P (2007). Haematology of Down syndrome. Arch Dis Child Fetal Neonatal Ed. 92:F503–7. PMID:17804520
4270. Webber SA (1999). Post-transplant lymphoproliferative disorders: a preventable complication of solid organ transplantation? Pediatr Transplant. 3:95–9. PMID:10389129
4271. Webber SA, Naftel DC, Fricker FJ, et al. (2006). Lymphoproliferative disorders after paediatric heart transplantation: a multi-institutional study. Lancet. 367:233–9. PMID:16427492
4272. Wechalekar AD, Lachmann HJ, Goodman HJ, et al. (2008). AL amyloidosis associated with IgM paraproteinemia: clinical profile and treatment outcome. Blood. 112:4009–16. PMID:18708629
4273. Weiler-Sagie M, Bushelev O, Epelbaum R, et al. (2010). (18)F-FDG avidity in lymphoma readdressed: a study of 766 patients. J Nucl Med. 51:25–30. PMID:20009002
4274. Weinberg OK, Rodig SJ, Pozdnyakova O, et al. (2015). Surface Light Chain Expression in Primary Mediastinal Large B-Cell Lymphomas by Multiparameter Flow Cytometry. Am J Clin Pathol. 144:635–41. PMID:26386085
4275. Weinberg OK, Seetharam M, Ren L, et al. (2014). Mixed phenotype acute leukemia: A study of 61 cases using World

Health Organization and European Group for the Immunological Classification of Leukaemias criteria. Am J Clin Pathol. 142:803–8. PMID:25389334

4276. Weinberg OK, Seetharam M, Ren L, et al. (2009). Clinical characterization of acute myeloid leukemia with myelodysplasia-related changes as defined by the 2008 WHO classification system. Blood. 113:1906–8. PMID:19131546

4277. Weinreb M, Day PJ, Niggli F, et al. (1996). The consistent association between Epstein-Barr virus and Hodgkin's disease in children in Kenya. Blood. 87:3828–36. PMID:8611709

4278. Weinreb M, Day PJ, Niggli F, et al. (1996). The role of Epstein-Barr virus in Hodgkin's disease from different geographical areas. Arch Dis Child. 74:27–31. PMID:8660041

4279. Weir EG, Ali Ansari-Lari M, Batista DA, et al. (2007). Acute bilineal leukemia: a rare disease with poor outcome. Leukemia. 21:2264–70. PMID:17611554

4280. Weir EG, Cowan K, LeBeau P, et al. (1999). A limited antibody panel can distinguish B-precursor acute lymphoblastic leukemia from normal B precursors with four color flow cytometry: implications for residual disease detection. Leukemia. 13:558–67. PMID:10214862

4281. Weisberg E, Manley PW, Cowan-Jacob SW, et al. (2007). Second generation inhibitors of BCR-ABL for the treatment of imatinib-resistant chronic myeloid leukaemia. Nat Rev Cancer. 7:345–56. PMID:17457302

4282. Weisenburger DD, Anderson J, Armitage J, et al. (1998). Grading of follicular lymphoma: diagnostic accuracy, reproducibility, and clinical relevance. Mod Pathol. 11:142a.

4283. Weisenburger DD, Savage KJ, Harris NL, et al. (2011). Peripheral T-cell lymphoma, not otherwise specified: a report of 340 cases from the International Peripheral T-cell Lymphoma Project. Blood. 117:3402–8. PMID:21270441

4284. Weiss BM, Abadie J, Verma P, et al. (2009). A monoclonal gammopathy precedes multiple myeloma in most patients. Blood. 113:5418–22. PMID:19234139

4285. Weiss LM (2000). Epstein-Barr virus and Hodgkin's disease. Curr Oncol Rep. 2:199–204. PMID:11122844

4286. Weiss LM, Berry GJ, Dorfman RF, et al. (1990). Spindle cell neoplasms of lymph nodes of probable reticulum cell lineage. True reticulum cell sarcoma? Am J Surg Pathol. 14:405–14. PMID:2158241

4287. Weiss LM, Bindl JM, Picozzi VJ, et al. (1986). Lymphoblastic lymphoma: an immunophenotype study of 26 cases with comparison to T cell acute lymphoblastic leukemia. Blood. 67:474–8. PMID:3080041

4288. Weiss LM, Jaffe ES, Liu XF, et al. (1992). Detection and localization of Epstein-Barr viral genomes in angioimmunoblastic lymphadenopathy and angioimmunoblastic lymphadenopathy-like lymphoma. Blood. 79:1789–95. PMID:1373088

4289. Weiss LM, Movahed LA, Warnke RA, et al. (1989). Detection of Epstein-Barr viral genomes in Reed-Sternberg cells of Hodgkin's disease. N Engl J Med. 320:502–6. PMID:2536894

4290. Weissmann DJ, Ferry JA, Harris NL, et al. (1995). Posttransplantation lymphoproliferative disorders in solid organ recipients are predominantly aggressive tumors of host origin. Am J Clin Pathol. 103:748–55. PMID:7785662

4290A. Weissmann S, Alpermann T, Grossmann V, et al. (2012). Landscape of TET2 mutations in acute myeloid leukemia. Leukemia. 26:934–42. PMID:22116554

4291. Weller PF, Bubley GJ (1994). The idiopathic hypereosinophilic syndrome. Blood. 83:2759–79. PMID:8180373

4292. Wellmann A, Thieblemont C, Pittaluga S, et al. (2000). Detection of differentially expressed genes in lymphomas using cDNA arrays: identification of clusterin as a new diagnostic marker for anaplastic large-cell lymphomas. Blood. 96:398–404. PMID:10887098

4293. Wendum D, Sebban C, Gaulard P, et al. (1997). Follicular large-cell lymphoma treated with intensive chemotherapy: an analysis of 89 cases included in the LNH87 trial and comparison with the outcome of diffuse large B-cell lymphoma. Groupe d'Etude des Lymphomes de l'Adulte. J Clin Oncol. 15:1654–63. PMID:9193366

4294. Weng AP, Ferrando AA, Lee W, et al. (2004). Activating mutations of NOTCH1 in human T cell acute lymphoblastic leukemia. Science. 306:269–71. PMID:15472075

4295. Weng AP, Millholland JM, Yashiro-Ohtani Y, et al. (2006). c-Myc is an important direct target of Notch1 in T-cell acute lymphoblastic leukemia/lymphoma. Genes Dev. 20:2096–109. PMID:16847353

4296. Weniger MA, Gesk S, Ehrlich S, et al. (2007). Gains of REL in primary mediastinal B-cell lymphoma coincide with nuclear accumulation of REL protein. Genes Chromosomes Cancer. 46:406–15. PMID:17243160

4297. Weniger MA, Melzner I, Menz CK, et al. (2006). Mutations of the tumor suppressor gene SOCS-1 in classical Hodgkin lymphoma are frequent and associated with nuclear phospho-STAT5 accumulation. Oncogene. 25:2679–84. PMID:16532038

4298. Went P, Agostinelli C, Gallamini A, et al. (2006). Marker expression in peripheral T-cell lymphoma: a proposed clinical-pathologic prognostic score. J Clin Oncol. 24:2472–9. PMID:16636342

4299. Went P, Ascani S, Strøm E, et al. (2004). Nodal marginal-zone lymphoma associated with monoclonal light-chain and heavy-chain deposition disease. Lancet Oncol. 5:381–3. PMID:15172359

4300. Wessendorf S, Barth TF, Viardot A, et al. (2007). Further delineation of chromosomal consensus regions in primary mediastinal B-cell lymphomas: an analysis of 37 tumor samples using high-resolution genomic profiling (array-CGH). Leukemia. 21:2463–9. PMID:17728785

4301. West AH, Godley LA, Churpek JE (2014). Familial myelodysplastic syndrome/acute leukemia syndromes: a review and utility for translational investigations. Ann N Y Acad Sci. 1310:111–8. PMID:24467820

4302. West DS, Dogan A, Quint PS, et al. (2013). Clonally related follicular lymphomas and Langerhans cell neoplasms: expanding the spectrum of transdifferentiation. Am J Surg Pathol. 37:978–86. PMID:23759932

4303. West RR, Hsu AP, Holland SM, et al. (2014). Acquired ASXL1 mutations are common in patients with inherited GATA2 mutations and correlate with myeloid transformation. Haematologica. 99:276–81. PMID:24077845

4304. Westers TM, Alhan C, Chamuleau ME, et al. (2010). Aberrant immunophenotype of blasts in myelodysplastic syndromes is a clinically relevant biomarker in predicting response to growth factor treatment. Blood. 115:1779–84. PMID:20038788

4305. Westers TM, Ireland R, Kern W, et al. (2012). Standardization of flow cytometry in myelodysplastic syndromes: a report from an international consortium and the European LeukemiaNet Working Group. Leukemia. 26:1730–41. PMID:22307178

4306. Weston BW, Hayden MA, Roberts KG, et al. (2013). Tyrosine kinase inhibitor therapy induces remission in a patient with refractory EBF1-PDGFRB-positive acute

lymphoblastic leukemia. J Clin Oncol. 31:e413–6. PMID:23835704

4307. Westwood NB, Gruszka-Westwood AM, Pearson CE, et al. (2000). The incidences of trisomy 8, trisomy 9 and D20S108 deletion in polycythaemia vera: an analysis of blood granulocytes using interphase fluorescence in situ hybridization. Br J Haematol. 110:839–46. PMID:11054066

4307A. Whitman SP, Archer KJ, Feng L, et al. (2001). Absence of the wild-type allele predicts poor prognosis in adult de novo acute myeloid leukemia with normal cytogenetics and the internal tandem duplication of FLT3: a cancer and leukemia group B study. Cancer Res. 61:7233–9. PMID:11585760

4307B. Whitman SP, Caligiuri MA, Maharry K, et al. (2012). The MLL partial tandem duplication in adults aged 60 years and older with de novo cytogenetically normal acute myeloid leukemia. Leukemia. 26:1713–7. PMID:22382894

4307C. Whitman SP, Maharry K, Radmacher MD, et al. (2010). FLT3 internal tandem duplication associates with adverse outcome and gene- and microRNA-expression signatures in patients 60 years of age or older with primary cytogenetically normal acute myeloid leukemia: a Cancer and Leukemia Group B study. Blood. 116:3622–6. PMID:20656931

4307D. Whitman SP, Ruppert AS, Marcucci G, et al. (2007). Long-term disease-free survivors with cytogenetically normal acute myeloid leukemia and MLL partial tandem duplication: a Cancer and Leukemia Group B study. Blood. 109:5164–7. PMID:17341662

4308. Whittaker SJ, Smith NP (1992). Diagnostic value of T-cell receptor beta gene rearrangement analysis on peripheral blood lymphocytes of patients with erythroderma. J Invest Dermatol. 99:361–2. PMID:1324964

4309. Whittaker SJ, Smith NP, Jones RR, et al. (1991). Analysis of beta, gamma, and delta T-cell receptor genes in mycosis fungoides and Sezary syndrome. Cancer. 68:1572–82. PMID:1654197

4310. Wickert RS, Weisenburger DD, Tierens A, et al. (1995). Clonal relationship between lymphocytic predominance Hodgkin's disease and concurrent or subsequent large-cell lymphoma of B lineage. Blood. 86:2312–20. PMID:7662978

4311. Wiemels JL, Cazzaniga G, Daniotti M, et al. (1999). Prenatal origin of acute lymphoblastic leukaemia in children. Lancet. 354:1499–503. PMID:10551495

4312. Wiesner T, Obenauf AC, Cota C, et al. (2010). Alterations of the cell-cycle inhibitors p27(KIP1) and p16(INK4a) are frequent in blastic plasmacytoid dendritic cell neoplasms. J Invest Dermatol. 130:1152–7. PMID:19924135

4313. Wijlhuizen TJ, Vrints LW, Jairam R, et al. (1989). Grades of nodular sclerosis (NSI-NSII) in Hodgkin's disease. Are they of independent prognostic value? Cancer. 63:1150–3. PMID:2917317

4314. Wilcox RA, Ristow K, Habermann TM, et al. (2011). The absolute monocyte and lymphocyte prognostic score predicts survival and identifies high-risk patients in diffuse large-B-cell lymphoma. Leukemia. 25:1502–9. PMID:21606957

4315. Wilder RB, Ha CS, Cox JD, et al. (2002). Persistence of myeloma protein for more than one year after radiotherapy is an adverse prognostic factor in solitary plasmacytoma of bone. Cancer. 94:1532–7. PMID:11920511

4316. Wilkins BS, Radia D, Woodley C, et al. (2013). Resolution of bone marrow fibrosis in a patient receiving JAK1/JAK2 inhibitor treatment with ruxolitinib. Haematologica. 98:1872–6. PMID:24056820

4317. Wilks S (1856). Cases of lardaceous

disease and some allied affections, with remarks. Guys Hosp Rep. 17:103.

4318. Wilks S (1856). Enlargement of the lymphatic glands and spleen (or, Hodgkin's disease) with remarks. Guys Hosp Rep. 11:56.

4319. Willemse MJ, Seriu T, Hettinger K, et al. (2002). Detection of minimal residual disease identifies differences in treatment response between T-ALL and precursor B-ALL. Blood. 99:4386–93. PMID:12036866

4320. Willemze R, Jaffe ES, Burg G, et al. (2005). WHO-EORTC classification for cutaneous lymphomas. Blood. 105:3768–85. PMID:15692063

4321. Willemze R, Jansen PM, Cerroni L, et al. (2008). Subcutaneous panniculitis-like T-cell lymphoma: definition, classification, and prognostic factors: an EORTC Cutaneous Lymphoma Group Study of 83 cases. Blood. 111:838–45. PMID:17934071

4322. Willemze R, Kerl H, Sterry W, et al. (1997). EORTC classification for primary cutaneous lymphomas: a proposal from the Cutaneous Lymphoma Study Group of the European Organization for Research and Treatment of Cancer. Blood. 90:354–71. PMID:9207472

4323. Williams ME, Swerdlow SH, Rosenberg CL, et al. (1993). Chromosome 11 translocation breakpoints at the PRAD1/cyclin D1 gene locus in centrocytic lymphoma. Leukemia. 7:241–5. PMID:8426477

4324. Williams ME, Westermann CD, Swerdlow SH (1990). Genotypic characterization of centrocytic lymphoma: frequent rearrangement of the chromosome 11 bcl-1 locus. Blood. 76:1387–91. PMID:2207314

4325. Williams ME, Whitefield M, Swerdlow SH (1997). Analysis of the cyclin-dependent kinase inhibitors p18 and p19 in mantle-cell lymphoma and chronic lymphocytic leukemia. Ann Oncol. 8 Suppl 2:71–3. PMID:9209645

4326. Williams ME, Woytowitz D, Finkelstein SD, et al. (1995). MTS1/MTS2 (p15/p16) deletions and p53 mutations in mantle cell (centrocytic) lymphoma. Blood. 86:747a.

4327. Williamson PJ, Kruger AR, Reynolds PJ, et al. (1994). Establishing the incidence of myelodysplastic syndrome. Br J Haematol. 87:743–5. PMID:7986716

4328. Willis MS, McKenna RW, Peterson LC, et al. (2005). Low blast count myeloid disorders with Auer rods: a clinicopathologic analysis of 9 cases. Am J Clin Pathol. 124:191–8. PMID:16040288

4329. Willman CL (1998). Molecular genetic features of myelodysplastic syndromes (MDS). Leukemia. 12 Suppl 1:S2–6. PMID:9777886

4330. Willman CL, Busque L, Griffith BB, et al. (1994). Langerhans'-cell histiocytosis (histiocytosis X)–a clonal proliferative disease. N Engl J Med. 331:154–60. PMID:8008029

4331. Wilson MS, Weiss LM, Gatter KC, et al. (1990). Malignant histiocytosis. A reassessment of cases previously reported in 1975 based on paraffin section immunophenotyping studies. Cancer. 66:530–6. PMID:2194647

4332. Wilson WH, Kingma DW, Raffeld M, et al. (1996). Association of lymphomatoid granulomatosis with Epstein-Barr viral infection of B lymphocytes and response to interferon-alpha 2b. Blood. 87:4531–7. PMID:8639820

4333. Wilson WH, Pittaluga S, Nicolae A, et al. (2014). A prospective study of mediastinal gray-zone lymphoma. Blood. 124:1563–9. PMID:25024303

4334. Wilson WH, Young RM, Schmitz R, et al. (2015). Targeting B cell receptor signaling with ibrutinib in diffuse large B cell lymphoma. Nat Med. 21:922–6. PMID:26193343

4335. Wiltshaw E (1976). The natural history of extramedullary plasmacytoma and its relation to solitary myeloma of bone and

myelomatosis. Medicine (Baltimore). 55:217–38. PMID:1272069
4336. Wimazal F, Fonatsch C, Thalhammer R, et al. (2007). Idiopathic cytopenia of undetermined significance (ICUS) versus low risk MDS: the diagnostic interface. Leuk Res. 31:1461–8. PMID:17507091
4337. Winter JN, Weller EA, Horning SJ, et al. (2006). Prognostic significance of Bcl-6 protein expression in DLBCL treated with CHOP or R-CHOP: a prospective correlative study. Blood. 107:4207–13. PMID:16449523
4338. Winton EF, Chan WC, Check I, et al. (1986). Spontaneous regression of a monoclonal proliferation of large granular lymphocytes associated with reversal of anemia and neutropenia. Blood. 67:1427–32. PMID:3754473
4339. Wlodarska I, De Wolf-Peeters C, Falini B, et al. (1998). The cryptic inv(2)(p23q35) defines a new molecular genetic subtype of ALK-positive anaplastic large-cell lymphoma. Blood. 92:2688–95. PMID:9763551
4340. Wlodarska I, Martin-Garcia N, Achten R, et al. (2002). Fluorescence in situ hybridization study of chromosome 7 aberrations in hepatosplenic T-cell lymphoma: isochromosome 7q as a common abnormality accumulating in forms with features of cytologic progression. Genes Chromosomes Cancer. 33:243–51. PMID:11807981
4341. Wlodarska I, Stul M, De Wolf-Peeters C, et al. (2004). Heterogeneity of BCL6 rearrangements in nodular lymphocyte predominant Hodgkin's lymphoma. Haematologica. 89:965–72. PMID:15339680
4342. Wlodarski MW, Hirabayashi S, Pastor V, et al. (2016). Prevalence, clinical characteristics, and prognosis of GATA2-related myelodysplastic syndromes in children and adolescents. Blood. 127:1387–97 PMID:26702063
4343. Wlodarski MW, O'Keefe C, Howe EC, et al. (2005). Pathologic clonal cytotoxic T-cell responses: nonrandom nature of the T-cell-receptor restriction in large granular lymphocyte leukemia. Blood. 106:2769–80. PMID:15914562
4344. Wobser M, Kerstan A, Kneitz H, et al. (2013). Primary cutaneous marginal zone lymphoma with sequential development of nodal marginal zone lymphoma in a patient with selective immunoglobulin A deficiency. J Cutan Pathol. 40:1035–41. PMID:24274426
4345. Wobser M, Roth S, Reinartz T, et al. (2015). CD68 expression is a discriminative feature of indolent cutaneous CD8-positive lymphoid proliferation and distinguishes this lymphoma subtype from other CD8-positive cutaneous lymphomas. Br J Dermatol. 172:1573–80. PMID:25524664
4346. Woessmann W, Lisfeld J, Burkhardt B; NHL-BFM Study Group (2013). Therapy in primary mediastinal B-cell lymphoma. N Engl J Med. 369:282. PMID:23863060
4347. Wolach O, Stone RM (2015). How I treat mixed-phenotype acute leukemia. Blood. 125:2477–85. PMID:25605373
4348. Wolanskyj AP, Schwager SM, McClure RF, et al. (2006). Essential thrombocythemia beyond the first decade: life expectancy, long-term complication rates, and prognostic factors. Mayo Clin Proc. 81:159–66. PMID:16471068
4349. Wolf BC, Kumar A, Vera JC, et al. (1986). Bone marrow morphology and immunology in systemic amyloidosis. Am J Clin Pathol. 86:84–8. PMID:3524195
4350. Wolf D, Sopper S, Pircher A, et al. (2015). Treg(s) in cancer: friends or foe? J Cell Physiol. 230:2598–605. PMID:25913194
4351. Wolf T, Brodt HR, Fichtlscherer S, et al. (2005). Changing incidence and prognostic factors of survival in AIDS-related non-Hodgkin's lymphoma in the era of highly active antiretroviral therapy (HAART). Leuk Lymphoma. 46:207–15. PMID:15621803
4352. Wolfe F, Michaud K (2007). The effect of methotrexate and anti-tumor necrosis factor therapy on the risk of lymphoma in rheumatoid arthritis in 19,562 patients during 89,710 person-years of observation. Arthritis Rheum. 56:1433–9. PMID:17469100
4353. Wolff K, Komar M, Petzelbauer P (2001). Clinical and histopathological aspects of cutaneous mastocytosis. Leuk Res. 25:519–28. PMID:11377676
4354. Woll PS, Kjällquist U, Chowdhury O, et al. (2014). Myelodysplastic syndromes are propagated by rare and distinct human cancer stem cells in vivo. Cancer Cell. 25:794–808. PMID:24835589
4355. Wong AK, Kerkoutian S, Said J, et al. (2012). Risk of lymphoma in patients receiving antitumor necrosis factor therapy: a meta-analysis of published randomized controlled studies. Clin Rheumatol. 31:631–6. PMID:22147207
4356. Wong KF, Chan JK, Cheung MM, et al. (2001). Bone marrow involvement by nasal NK cell lymphoma at diagnosis is uncommon. Am J Clin Pathol. 115:266–70. PMID:11211616
4357. Wong KF, Chan JK, Ng CS, et al. (1992). CD56 (NKH1)-positive hematolymphoid malignancies: an aggressive neoplasm featuring frequent cutaneous/mucosal involvement, cytoplasmic azurophilic granules, and angiocentricity. Hum Pathol. 23:798–804. PMID:1377163
4358. Wong KF, So CC, Chan JK (2002). Nucleolated variant of mantle cell lymphoma with leukemic manifestations mimicking prolymphocytic leukemia. Am J Clin Pathol. 117:246–51. PMID:11865846
4359. Wong KF, Zhang YM, Chan JK (1999). Cytogenetic abnormalities in natural killer cell lymphoma/leukaemia–is there a consistent pattern? Leuk Lymphoma. 34:241–50. PMID:10439361
4360. Wong TN, Ramsingh G, Young AL, et al. (2015). Role of TP53 mutations in the origin and evolution of therapy-related acute myeloid leukaemia. Nature. 518:552–5. PMID:25487151
4361. Woo DK, Jones CR, Vanoli-Storz MN, et al. (2009). Prognostic factors in primary cutaneous anaplastic large cell lymphoma: characterization of clinical subset with worse outcome. Arch Dermatol. 145:667–74. PMID:19528422
4362. Wood BL, Winter SS, Dunsmore KP, et al. (2014). T-lymphoblastic leukemia (T-ALL) shows excellent outcome, lack of significance of the early thymic precursor (ETP) immunophenotype, and validation of the prognostic value of end-induction minimal residual disease (MRD) in Children's Oncology Group (COG) Study AALL0434. Blood. 124(21):1.
4363. Wood GS, Hu CH, Beckstead JH, et al. (1985). The indeterminate cell proliferative disorder: report of a case manifesting as an unusual cutaneous histiocytosis. J Dermatol Surg Oncol. 11:1111–9. PMID:3902927
4364. Woodlock TJ, Seshi B, Sham RL, et al. (1994). Use of cell surface antigen phenotype in guiding therapeutic decisions in chronic myelomonocytic leukemia. Leuk Res. 18:173–81. PMID:7511190
4365. Worsley A, Oscier DG, Stevens J, et al. (1988). Prognostic features of chronic myelomonocytic leukaemia: a modified Bournemouth score gives the best prediction of survival. Br J Haematol. 68:17–21. PMID:3422815
4366. Wotherspoon AC, Doglioni C, Diss TC, et al. (1993). Regression of primary low-grade B-cell gastric lymphoma of mucosa-associated lymphoid tissue type after eradication of Helicobacter pylori. Lancet. 342:575–7. PMID:8102719
4367. Wotherspoon AC, Ortiz-Hidalgo C, Falzon MR, et al. (1991). Helicobacter pylori-associated gastritis and primary B-cell gastric lymphoma. Lancet. 338:1175–6. PMID:1682595
4368. Wouters BJ, Löwenberg B, Erpelinck-Verschueren CA, et al. (2009). Double CEBPA mutations, but not single CEBPA mutations, define a subgroup of acute myeloid leukemia with a distinctive gene expression profile that is uniquely associated with a favorable outcome. Blood. 113:3088–91. PMID:19171880
4369. Wright DH (1971). Burkitt's lymphoma: a review of the pathology, immunology, and possible etiologic factors. Pathol Annu. 6:337–63. PMID:4342309
4370. Wright DH (1997). Enteropathy associated T cell lymphoma. Cancer Surv. 30:249–61. PMID:9547996
4371. Wright DH, Jones DB, Clark H, et al. (1991). Is adult-onset coeliac disease due to a low-grade lymphoma of intraepithelial T lymphocytes? Lancet. 337:1373–4. PMID:1674763
4372. Wright G, Tan B, Rosenwald A, et al. (2003). A gene expression-based method to diagnose clinically distinct subgroups of diffuse large B cell lymphoma. Proc Natl Acad Sci U S A. 100:9991–6. PMID:12900505
4373. Wu B, Li F, Zou S (2014). MLL-AF9 rearrangement in myeloid sarcomas involving the breast. Ann Hematol. 93:709–10. PMID:23900528
4374. Wu CD, Wickert RS, Williamson JE, et al. (1999). Using fluorescence-based human androgen receptor gene assay to analyze the clonality of microdissected dendritic cell tumors. Am J Clin Pathol. 111:105–10. PMID:9894460
4375. Wu H, Wasik MA, Przybylski G, et al. (2000). Hepatosplenic gamma-delta T-cell lymphoma as a late-onset posttransplant lymphoproliferative disorder in renal transplant recipients. Am J Clin Pathol. 113:487–96. PMID:10761449
4376. Wu SS, Brady K, Anderson JJ, et al. (1991). The predictive value of bone marrow morphologic characteristics and immunostaining in primary (AL) amyloidosis. Am J Clin Pathol. 96:95–9. PMID:1712547
4377. Wu TT, Swerdlow SH, Locker J, et al. (1996). Recurrent Epstein-Barr virus-associated lesions in organ transplant recipients. Hum Pathol. 27:157–64. PMID:8617457
4378. Wu W, Youm W, Rezk SA, et al. (2013). Human herpesvirus 8-unrelated primary effusion lymphoma-like lymphoma: report of a rare case and review of 54 cases in the literature. Am J Clin Pathol. 140:258–73. PMID:23897264
4379. Wu Y, Slovak ML, Snyder DS, et al. (2006). Coexistence of inversion 16 and the Philadelphia chromosome in acute and chronic myeloid leukemias : report of six cases and review of literature. Am J Clin Pathol. 125:260–6. PMID:16393682
4380. Wuchter C, Harbott J, Schoch C, et al. (2000). Detection of acute leukemia cells with mixed lineage leukemia (MLL) gene rearrangements by flow cytometry using monoclonal antibody 7.1. Leukemia. 14:1232–8. PMID:10914547
4381. Wöhrer S, Streubel B, Bartsch R, et al. (2004). Monoclonal immunoglobulin production is a frequent event in patients with mucosa-associated lymphoid tissue lymphoma. Clin Cancer Res. 10:7179–81. PMID:15534090
4382. Xi L, Arons E, Navarro W, et al. (2012). Both variant and IGHV4-34-expressing hairy cell leukemia lack the BRAF V600E mutation. Blood. 119:3330–2. PMID:22210875
4383. Xia ZG, Xu ZZ, Zhao WL, et al. (2010). The prognostic value of immunohistochemical subtyping in Chinese patients with de novo diffuse large B-cell lymphoma undergoing CHOP or R-CHOP treatment. Ann Hematol. 89:171–7. PMID:19669764
4384. Xiao R, Cerny J, Devitt K, et al. (2014). MYC protein expression is detected in plasma cell myeloma but not in monoclonal gammopathy of undetermined significance (MGUS). Am J Surg Pathol. 38:776–83. PMID:24705315
4385. Xie J, Zhou X, Zhang X, et al. (2015). Primary intravascular natural killer/T cell lymphoma of the central nervous system. Leuk Lymphoma. 56:1154–6. PMID:25248881
4386. Xie M, Lu C, Wang J, et al. (2014). Age-related mutations associated with clonal hematopoietic expansion and malignancies. Nat Med. 20:1472–8. PMID:25326804
4387. Xing KH, Connors JM, Lai A, et al. (2014). Advanced-stage nodular lymphocyte predominant Hodgkin lymphoma compared with classical Hodgkin lymphoma: a matched pair outcome analysis. Blood. 123:3567–73. PMID:24713929
4388. Xing KH, Kahlon A, Skinnider BF, et al. (2015). Outcomes in splenic marginal zone lymphoma: analysis of 107 patients treated in British Columbia. Br J Haematol. 169:520–7. PMID:25854936
4389. Xing X, Feldman AL (2015). Anaplastic large cell lymphomas: ALK positive, ALK negative, and primary cutaneous. Adv Anat Pathol. 22:29–49. PMID:25461779
4390. Xochelli A, Kalpadakis C, Gardiner A, et al. (2014). Clonal B-cell lymphocytosis exhibiting immunophenotypic features consistent with a marginal-zone origin: is this a distinct entity? Blood. 123:1199–206. PMID:24300853
4391. Xochelli A, Sutton LA, Agathangelidis A, et al. (2015). Molecular evidence for antigen drive in the natural history of mantle cell lymphoma. Am J Pathol. 185:1740–8. PMID:25843681
4392. Xu L, Gu ZH, Li Y, et al. (2014). Genomic landscape of CD34+ hematopoietic cells in myelodysplastic syndrome and gene mutation profiles as prognostic markers. Proc Natl Acad Sci U S A. 111:8589–94. PMID:24850867
4393. Xu L, Hunter ZR, Yang G, et al. (2013). MYD88 L265P in Waldenström macroglobulinemia, immunoglobulin M monoclonal gammopathy, and other B-cell lymphoproliferative disorders using conventional and quantitative allele-specific polymerase chain reaction. Blood. 121:2051–8. PMID:23321251
4394. Xu X, Zhang L, Wang Y, et al. (2013). Double-hit and triple-hit lymphomas arising from follicular lymphoma following acquisition of MYC: report of two cases and literature review. Int J Clin Exp Pathol. 6:788–94. PMID:23573328
4395. Xu Y, Dolan MM, Nguyen PL (2003). Diagnostic significance of detecting dysgranulopoiesis in chronic myeloid leukemia. Am J Clin Pathol. 120:778–84. PMID:14608906
4396. Xu Y, McKenna RW, Karandikar NJ, et al. (2005). Flow cytometric analysis of monocytes as a tool for distinguishing chronic myelomonocytic leukemia from reactive monocytosis. Am J Clin Pathol. 124:799–806. PMID:16203279
4397. Xu Z, Lian S (2010). Epstein-Barr virus-associated hydroa vacciniforme-like cutaneous lymphoma in seven Chinese children. Pediatr Dermatol. 27:463–9. PMID:20497358
4398. Xu-Monette ZY, Dabaja BS, Wang X, et al. (2015). Clinical features, tumor biology, and prognosis associated with MYC rearrangement and Myc overexpression in diffuse large B-cell lymphoma patients treated with rituximab-CHOP. Mod Pathol. 28:1555–73. PMID:26541272
4399. Xu-Monette ZY, Tu M, Jabbar KJ, et al. (2015). Clinical and biological significance of de novo CD5+ diffuse large B-cell lymphoma in Western countries. Oncotarget. 6:5615–33. PMID:25760242
4400. Xu-Monette ZY, Wu L, Visco C, et al.

(2012). Mutational profile and prognostic significance of TP53 in diffuse large B-cell lymphoma patients treated with R-CHOP: report from an International DLBCL Rituximab-CHOP Consortium Program Study. Blood. 120:3986–96. PMID:22955915
4401. Yagyu S, Morimoto A, Kakazu N, et al. (2008). Late appearance of a Philadelphia chromosome in a patient with therapy-related acute myeloid leukemia and high expression of EVI1. Cancer Genet Cytogenet. 180:115–20. PMID:18206536
4402. Yam LT, Yam CF, Li CY (1980). Eosinophilia in systemic mastocytosis. Am J Clin Pathol. 73:48–54. PMID:7352423
4403. Yamada K, Oshiro Y, Okamura S, et al. (2015). Clinicopathological characteristics and rituximab addition to cytotoxic therapies in patients with rheumatoid arthritis and methotrexate-associated large B lymphoproliferative disorders. Histopathology. 67:70–80. PMID:25429725
4404. Yamada O, Kitahara K, Imamura K, et al. (1998). Clinical and cytogenetic remission induced by interferon-alpha in a patient with chronic eosinophilic leukemia associated with a unique t(3;9;5) translocation. Am J Hematol. 58:137–41. PMID:9625582
4405. Yamaguchi K (1994). Human T-lymphotropic virus type I in Japan. Lancet. 343:213–6. PMID:7904671
4406. Yamaguchi M, Seto M, Okamoto M, et al. (2002). De novo CD5+ diffuse large B-cell lymphoma: a clinicopathologic study of 109 patients. Blood. 99:815–21. PMID:11806981
4407. Yamaguchi M, Takata K, Yoshino T, et al. (2014). Prognostic biomarkers in patients with localized natural killer/T-cell lymphoma treated with concurrent chemoradiotherapy. Cancer Sci. 105:1435–41. PMID:25181936
4408. Yamakawa N, Fujimoto M, Kawabata D, et al. (2014). A clinical, pathological, and genetic characterization of methotrexate-associated lymphoproliferative disorders. J Rheumatol. 41:293–9. PMID:24334644
4409. Yamamoto JF, Goodman MT (2008). Patterns of leukemia incidence in the United States by subtype and demographic characteristics, 1997-2002. Cancer Causes Control. 19:379–90. PMID:18064533
4410. Yamamura M, Yamada Y, Momita S, et al. (1998). Circulating interleukin-6 levels are elevated in adult T-cell leukaemia/lymphoma patients and correlate with adverse clinical features and survival. Br J Haematol. 100:129–34. PMID:9450801
4411. Yamashita Y, Nakamura S, Kagami Y, et al. (2000). Lennert's lymphoma: a variant of cytotoxic T-cell lymphoma? Am J Surg Pathol. 24:1627–33. PMID:11117783
4412. Yamato H, Ohshima K, Suzumiya J, et al. (2001). Evidence for local immunosuppression and demonstration of c-myc amplification in pyothorax-associated lymphoma. Histopathology. 39:163–71. PMID:11493333
4413. Yamazaki H, Suzuki M, Otsuki A, et al. (2014). A remote GATA2 hematopoietic enhancer drives leukemogenesis in inv(3)(q21;q26) by activating EVI1 expression. Cancer Cell. 25:415–27. PMID:24703906
4414. Yan L, Ping N, Zhu M, et al. (2012). Clinical, immunophenotypic, cytogenetic, and molecular genetic features in 117 adult patients with mixed-phenotype acute leukemia defined by WHO-2008 classification. Haematologica. 97:1708–12. PMID:22581002
4415. Yan LX, Liu YH, Luo DL, et al. (2014). MYC expression in concert with BCL2 and BCL6 expression predicts outcome in Chinese patients with diffuse large B-cell lymphoma, not otherwise specified. PLoS One. 9:e104068. PMID:25090026
4416. Yanada M, Suzuki M, Kawashima K, et al. (2005). Long-term outcomes for unselected patients with acute myeloid leukemia categorized according to the World Health Organization classification: a single-center experience. Eur J Haematol. 74:418–23. PMID:15813916
4417. Yanagisawa K, Ohminami H, Sato M, et al. (1998). Neoplastic involvement of granulocytic lineage, not granulocytic-monocytic, monocytic, or erythrocytic lineage, in a patient with chronic neutrophilic leukemia. Am J Hematol. 57:221–4. PMID:9495373
4418. Yang W, Zhang P, Hama A, et al. (2012). Diagnosis of acquired bone marrow failure syndrome during childhood using the 2008 World Health Organization classification system. Int J Hematol. 96:34–8. PMID:22562435
4419. Yang Y, Shaffer AL 3rd, Emre NC, et al. (2012). Exploiting synthetic lethality for the therapy of ABC diffuse large B cell lymphoma. Cancer Cell. 21:723–37. PMID:22698399
4420. Yano T, Jaffe ES, Longo DL, et al. (1992). MYC rearrangements in histologically progressed follicular lymphomas. Blood. 80:758–67. PMID:1638027
4421. Ye H, Liu H, Attygalle A, et al. (2003). Variable frequencies of t(11;18)(q21;q21) in MALT lymphomas of different sites: significant association with CagA strains of H pylori in gastric MALT lymphoma. Blood. 102:1012–8. PMID:12676782
4422. Ye Q, Xu-Monette ZY, Tzankov A, et al. (2016). Prognostic impact of concurrent MYC and BCL6 rearrangements and expression in de novo diffuse large B-cell lymphoma. Oncotarget. 7:2401–16. PMID:26573234
4423. Yeoh EJ, Ross ME, Shurtleff SA, et al. (2002). Classification, subtype discovery, and prediction of outcome in pediatric acute lymphoblastic leukemia by gene expression profiling. Cancer Cell. 1:133–43. PMID:12086872
4424. Yilmaz AF, Saydam G, Sahin F, et al. (2013). Granulocytic sarcoma: a systematic review. Am J Blood Res. 3:265–70. PMID:24396704
4425. Yin CC, Medeiros LJ, Cromwell CC, et al. (2007). Sequence analysis proves clonal identity in five patients with typical and blastoid mantle cell lymphoma. Mod Pathol. 20:1–7. PMID:17057651
4426. Yong AS, Melo JV (2009). The impact of gene profiling in chronic myeloid leukaemia. Best Pract Res Clin Haematol. 22:181–90. PMID:19698927
4427. Yong AS, Szydlo RM, Goldman JM, et al. (2006). Molecular profiling of CD34+ cells identifies low expression of CD7, along with high expression of proteinase 3 or elastase, as predictors of longer survival in patients with CML. Blood. 107:205–12. PMID:16144796
4428. Yoo HY, Kim P, Kim WS, et al. (2016). Frequent CTLA4-CD28 gene fusion in diverse types of T cell lymphoma. Haematologica. haematol.2015.139253. PMID:26819049
4429. Yoo HY, Sung MK, Lee SH, et al. (2014). A recurrent inactivating mutation in RHOA GTPase in angioimmunoblastic T cell lymphoma. Nat Genet. 46:371–5. PMID:24584070
4430. Yoon DH, Choi DR, Ahn HJ, et al. (2010). Ki-67 expression as a prognostic factor in diffuse large B-cell lymphoma patients treated with rituximab plus CHOP. Eur J Haematol. 85:149–57. PMID:20477862
4431. Yoon H, Park S, Ju H, et al. (2015). Integrated copy number and gene expression profiling analysis of Epstein-Barr virus-positive diffuse large B-cell lymphoma. Genes Chromosomes Cancer. 54:383–96. PMID:25832818
4432. Yoon SO, Jeon YK, Paik JH, et al. (2008). MYC translocation and an increased copy number predict poor prognosis in adult diffuse large B-cell lymphoma (DLBCL), especially in germinal centre-like B cell (GCB) type. Histopathology. 53:205–17. PMID:18752503
4433. Yoshida K, Sanada M, Shiraishi Y, et al. (2011). Frequent pathway mutations of splicing machinery in myelodysplasia. Nature. 478:64–9. PMID:21909114
4434. Yoshida K, Toki T, Okuno Y, et al. (2013). The landscape of somatic mutations in Down syndrome-related myeloid disorders. Nat Genet. 45:1293–9. PMID:24056718
4435. Yoshimatsu H (1974). [Development in the diagnosis of lung tumor. (5) Mediastinoscopy]. Nihon Kyobu Shikkan Gakkai Zasshi. 12:659–64. PMID:4477877
4436. Yoshimi A, Kamachi Y, Imai K, et al. (2013). Wiskott-Aldrich syndrome presenting with a clinical picture mimicking juvenile myelomonocytic leukaemia. Pediatr Blood Cancer. 60:836–41. PMID:23023736
4437. Yoshimi A, Niemeyer C, Baumann I, et al. (2013). High incidence of Fanconi anaemia in patients with a morphological picture consistent with refractory cytopenia of childhood. Br J Haematol. 160:109–11. PMID:23043447
4438. Yoshimi A, van den Heuvel-Eibrink MM, Baumann I, et al. (2014). Comparison of horse and rabbit antithymocyte globulin in immunosuppressive therapy for refractory cytopenia of childhood. Haematologica. 99:656–63. PMID:24162791
4439. Yoshino T, Miyake K, Ichimura K, et al. (2000). Increased incidence of follicular lymphoma in the duodenum. Am J Surg Pathol. 24:688–93. PMID:10800987
4440. Yoshizato T, Dumitriu B, Hosokawa K, et al. (2015). Somatic Mutations and Clonal Hematopoiesis in Aplastic Anemia. N Engl J Med. 373:35–47. PMID:26132940
4441. You W, Weisbrot IM (1979). Chronic neutrophilic leukemia. Report of two cases and review of the literature. Am J Clin Pathol. 72:233–42. PMID:289288
4442. Younes A, Bartlett NL, Leonard JP, et al. (2010). Brentuximab vedotin (SGN-35) for relapsed CD30-positive lymphomas. N Engl J Med. 363:1812–21. PMID:21047225
4443. Younes A, Gopal AK, Smith SE, et al. (2012). Results of a pivotal phase II study of brentuximab vedotin for patients with relapsed or refractory Hodgkin's lymphoma. J Clin Oncol. 30:2183–9. PMID:22454421
4444. Young KH, Chan WC, Fu K, et al. (2006). Mantle cell lymphoma with plasma cell differentiation. Am J Surg Pathol. 30:954–61. PMID:16861965
4445. Young KH, Leroy K, Møller MB, et al. (2008). Structural profiles of TP53 gene mutations predict clinical outcome in diffuse large B-cell lymphoma: an international collaborative study. Blood. 112:3088–98. PMID:18559976
4446. Young KH, Xie Q, Zhou G, et al. (2008). Transformation of follicular lymphoma to precursor B-cell lymphoblastic lymphoma with c-myc gene rearrangement as a critical event. Am J Clin Pathol. 129:157–66. PMID:18089500
4447. Young NS (2006). Pathophysiologic mechanisms in acquired aplastic anemia. Hematology Am Soc Hematol Educ Program. 72–7. PMID:17124043
4448. Young NS, Calado RT, Scheinberg P (2006). Current concepts in the pathophysiology and treatment of aplastic anemia. Blood. 108:2509–19. PMID:16778145
4449. Yousem SA, Colby TV, Chen YY, et al. (2001). Pulmonary Langerhans' cell histiocytosis: molecular analysis of clonality. Am J Surg Pathol. 25:630–6. PMID:11342775
4450. Yu H, Gibson JA, Pinkus GS, et al. (2007). Podoplanin (D2-40) is a novel marker for follicular dendritic cell tumors. Am J Clin Pathol. 128:776–82. PMID:17951199
4450A. Yu L, Tu M, Cortes J,et al. (2017). Clinical and pathological characteristics of HIV- and HHV-8-negative Castleman disease. Blood. 129:1658-68. PMID:28100459
4451. Yu RC, Chu C, Buluwela L, et al. (1994). Clonal proliferation of Langerhans cells in Langerhans cell histiocytosis. Lancet. 343:767–8. PMID:7510816
4452. Yuan J, Wright G, Rosenwald A, et al. (2015). Identification of Primary Mediastinal Large B-cell Lymphoma at Nonmediastinal Sites by Gene Expression Profiling. Am J Surg Pathol. 39:1322–30. PMID:26135560
4453. Yue G, Hao S, Fadare O, et al. (2008). Hypocellularity in myelodysplastic syndrome is an independent factor which predicts a favorable outcome. Leuk Res. 32:553–8. PMID:17888511
4454. Zajdel M, Rymkiewicz G, Chechlinska M, et al. (2015). miR expression in MYC-negative DLBCL/BL with partial trisomy 11 is similar to classical Burkitt lymphoma and different from diffuse large B-cell lymphoma. Tumour Biol. 36:5377–88. PMID:25677902
4455. Zamagni E, Cavo M (2012). The role of imaging techniques in the management of multiple myeloma. Br J Haematol. 159:499–513. PMID:22881361
4456. Zambello R, Falco M, Della Chiesa M, et al. (2003). Expression and function of KIR and natural cytotoxicity receptors in NK-type lymphoproliferative diseases of granular lymphocytes. Blood. 102:1797–805. PMID:12750175
4457. Zambello R, Loughran TP Jr, Trentin L, et al. (1995). Serologic and molecular evidence for a possible pathogenetic role of viral infection in CD3-negative natural killer-type lymphoproliferative disease of granular lymphocytes. Leukemia. 9:1207–11. PMID:7630196
4458. Zambello R, Loughran TP Jr, Trentin L, et al. (1997). Spontaneous resolution of p58/EB6 antigen restricted NK-type lymphoproliferative disease of granular lymphocytes: role of Epstein Barr virus infection. Br J Haematol. 99:215–21. PMID:9359527
4459. Zambello R, Trentin L, Ciccone E, et al. (1993). Phenotypic diversity of natural killer (NK) populations in patients with NK-type lymphoproliferative disease of granular lymphocytes. Blood. 81:2381–5. PMID:8481518
4460. Zamò A, Malpeli G, Scarpa A, et al. (2005). Expression of TP73L is a helpful diagnostic marker of primary mediastinal large B-cell lymphomas. Mod Pathol. 18:1448–53. PMID:15920542
4461. Zanelli M, Ragazzi M, Valli R, et al. (2016). Transformation of IGHV4-34+ hairy cell leukaemia-variant with U2AF1 mutation into a clonally-related high grade B-cell lymphoma responding to immunochemotherapy. Br J Haematol. 173:491–5 PMID:26303517
4462. Zangwill SD, Hsu DT, Kichuk MR, et al. (1998). Incidence and outcome of primary Epstein-Barr virus infection and lymphoproliferative disease in pediatric heart transplant recipients. J Heart Lung Transplant. 17:1161–6. PMID:9883755
4463. Zarate-Osorno A, Medeiros LJ, Longo DL, et al. (1992). Non-Hodgkin's lymphomas arising in patients successfully treated for Hodgkin's disease. A clinical, histologic, and immunophenotypic study of 14 cases. Am J Surg Pathol. 16:885–95. PMID:1415907
4464. Zelent A, Guidez F, Melnick A, et al. (2001). Translocations of the RARalpha gene in acute promyelocytic leukemia. Oncogene. 20:7186–203. PMID:11704847
4465. Zelger B, Cerio R, Orchard G, et al. (1994). Juvenile and adult xanthogranuloma. A histological and immunohistochemical comparison. Am J Surg Pathol. 18:126–35. PMID:8291651
4466. Zeller B, Gustafsson G, Forestier E, et al.

(2005). Acute leukaemia in children with Down syndrome: a population-based Nordic study. Br J Haematol. 128:797–804. PMID:15755283

4467. Zeng W, Fu K, Quintanilla-Fend L, et al. (2012). Cyclin D1-negative blastoid mantle cell lymphoma identified by SOX11 expression. Am J Surg Pathol. 36:214–9. PMID:22251940

4468. Zeng W, Nava VE, Cohen P, et al. (2012). Indolent CD8-positive T-cell lymphoid proliferation of the ear: a report of two cases. J Cutan Pathol. 39:696–700. PMID:22612273

4469. Zenz T, Mertens D, Küppers R, et al. (2010). From pathogenesis to treatment of chronic lymphocytic leukaemia. Nat Rev Cancer. 10:37–50. PMID:19956173

4470. Zettl A, Lee SS, Rüdiger T, et al. (2002). Epstein-Barr virus-associated B-cell lymphoproliferative disorders in angioimmunoblastic T-cell lymphoma and peripheral T-cell lymphoma, unspecified. Am J Clin Pathol. 117:368–79. PMID:11888076

4471. Zettl A, Ott G, Makulik A, et al. (2002). Chromosomal gains at 9q characterize enteropathy-type T-cell lymphoma. Am J Pathol. 161:1635–45. PMID:12414511

4472. Zettl A, Rüdiger T, Konrad MA, et al. (2004). Genomic profiling of peripheral T-cell lymphoma, unspecified, and anaplastic large T-cell lymphoma delineates novel recurrent chromosomal alterations. Am J Pathol. 164:1837–48. PMID:15111330

4473. Zettl A, Rüdiger T, Marx A, et al. (2005). Composite marginal zone B-cell lymphoma and classical Hodgkin's lymphoma: a clinicopathological study of 12 cases. Histopathology. 46:217–28. PMID:15693895

4474. Zhan F, Huang Y, Colla S, et al. (2006). The molecular classification of multiple myeloma. Blood. 108:2020–8. PMID:16728703

4475. Zhang J, Ding L, Holmfeldt L, et al. (2012). The genetic basis of early T-cell precursor acute lymphoblastic leukaemia. Nature. 481:157–63. PMID:22237106

4476. Zhang J, Grubor V, Love CL, et al. (2013). Genetic heterogeneity of diffuse large B-cell lymphoma. Proc Natl Acad Sci U S A. 110:1398–403. PMID:23292937

4477. Zhang J, Jima D, Moffitt AB, et al. (2014). The genomic landscape of mantle cell lymphoma is related to the epigenetically determined chromatin state of normal B cells. Blood.

123:2988–96. PMID:24682267

4478. Zhang L, Padron E, Lancet J (2015). The molecular basis and clinical significance of genetic mutations identified in myelodysplastic syndromes. Leuk Res. 39:6–17. PMID:25465125

4479. Zhang L, Wang SA (2014). A focused review of hematopoietic neoplasms occurring in the therapy-related setting. Int J Clin Exp Pathol. 7:3512–23. PMID:25120730

4480. Zhang MY, Churpek JE, Keel SB, et al. (2015). Germline ETV6 mutations in familial thrombocytopenia and hematologic malignancy. Nat Genet. 47:180–5. PMID:25581430

4481. Zhang MY, Keel SB, Walsh T, et al. (2015). Genomic analysis of bone marrow failure and myelodysplastic syndromes reveals phenotypic and diagnostic complexity. Haematologica. 100:42–8. PMID:25239263

4482. Zhang Q, Jing W, Ouyang J, et al. (2014). Six cases of aggressive natural killer-cell leukemia in a Chinese population. Int J Clin Exp Pathol. 7:3423–31. PMID:25031771

4483. Zhang S, Kipps TJ (2014). The pathogenesis of chronic lymphocytic leukemia. Annu Rev Pathol. 9:103–18. PMID:23987584

4484. Zhang Y, Nagata H, Ikeuchi T, et al. (2003). Common cytological and cytogenetic features of Epstein-Barr virus (EBV)-positive natural killer (NK) cells and cell lines derived from patients with nasal T/NK-cell lymphomas, chronic active EBV infection and hydroa vacciniforme-like eruptions. Br J Haematol. 121:805–14. PMID:12780797

4485. Zhang Y, Sanjose SD, Bracci PM, et al. (2008). Personal use of hair dye and the risk of certain subtypes of non-Hodgkin lymphoma. Am J Epidemiol. 167:1321–31. PMID:18408225

4486. Zhao J, Niu X, Wang Z, et al. (2015). Histiocytic sarcoma combined with acute monocytic leukemia: a case report. Diagn Pathol. 10:110. PMID:26187047

4487. Zhao T, Matsuoka M (2012). HBZ and its roles in HTLV-1 oncogenesis. Front Microbiol. 3:247. PMID:22787458

4488. Zhong X, Wang N, Hu D, et al. (2014). Sequence analysis of cytb gene in Echinococcus granulosus from Western China. Korean J Parasitol. 52:205–9. PMID:24850967

4489. Zhou XG, Sandvej K, Li PJ, et al. (2001). Epstein-Barr virus (EBV) in Chinese pediatric

Hodgkin disease: Hodgkin disease in young children is an EBV-related lymphoma. Cancer. 92:1621–31. PMID:11745241

4490. Zhou Y, Jorgensen JL, Wang SA, et al. (2012). Usefulness of CD11a and CD18 in flow cytometric immunophenotypic analysis for diagnosis of acute promyelocytic leukemia. Am J Clin Pathol. 138:744–50. PMID:23086776

4491. Zhou Z, Sehn LH, Rademaker AW, et al. (2014). An enhanced International Prognostic Index (NCCN-IPI) for patients with diffuse large B-cell lymphoma treated with the rituximab era. Blood. 123:837–42. PMID:24264230

4492. Zhu YM, Zhao WL, Fu JF, et al. (2006). NOTCH1 mutations in T-cell acute lymphoblastic leukemia: prognostic significance and implication in multifactorial leukemogenesis. Clin Cancer Res. 12:3043–9. PMID:16707600

4493. Zibellini S, Capello D, Forconi F, et al. (2010). Stereotyped patterns of B-cell receptor in splenic marginal zone lymphoma. Haematologica. 95:1792–6. PMID:20511668

4494. Ziino O, Rondelli R, Micalizzi C, et al. (2006). Acute lymphoblastic leukemia in children with associated genetic conditions other than Down's syndrome. The AIEOP experience. Haematologica. 91:139–40. PMID:16434385

4495. Zimmermann H, Reinke P, Neuhaus R, et al. (2012). Burkitt post-transplantation lymphoma in adult solid organ transplant recipients: sequential immunochemotherapy with rituximab (R) followed by cyclophosphamide, doxorubicin, vincristine, and prednisone (CHOP) or R-CHOP is safe and effective in an analysis of 8 patients. Cancer. 118:4715–24. PMID:22392525

4496. Zingone A, Kuehl WM (2011). Pathogenesis of monoclonal gammopathy of undetermined significance and progression to multiple myeloma. Semin Hematol. 48:4–12. PMID:21232653

4497. Zintzaras E, Voulgarelis M, Moutsopoulos HM (2005). The risk of lymphoma development in autoimmune diseases: a meta-analysis. Arch Intern Med. 165:2337–44. PMID:16287762

4498. Zinzani PL, Martelli M, Poletti V, et al. (2008). Practice guidelines for the management of extranodal non-Hodgkin's lymphomas of adult non-immunodeficient patients. Part I: primary lung and mediastinal lymphomas. A project of the Italian Society of Hematology,

the Italian Society of Experimental Hematology and the Italian Group for Bone Marrow Transplantation. Haematologica. 93:1364–71. PMID:18603558

4499. Zinzani PL, Quaglino P, Pimpinelli N, et al. (2006). Prognostic factors in primary cutaneous B-cell lymphoma: the Italian Study Group for Cutaneous Lymphomas. J Clin Oncol. 24:1376–82. PMID:16492713

4500. Zipursky A, Brown EJ, Christensen H, et al. (1999). Transient myeloproliferative disorder (transient leukemia) and hematologic manifestations of Down syndrome. Clin Lab Med. 19:157–67, vii. [vii.] PMID:10403079

4501. Zittoun R, Réa D, Ngoc LH, et al. (1994). Chronic neutrophilic leukemia. A study of four cases. Ann Hematol. 68:55–60. PMID:8148416

4502. Zoi K, Cross NC (2015). Molecular pathogenesis of atypical CML, CMML and MDS/MPN-unclassifiable. Int J Hematol. 101:229–42. PMID:25212680

4503. Zuckerman E, Zuckerman T, Levine AM, et al. (1997). Hepatitis C virus infection in patients with B-cell non-Hodgkin lymphoma. Ann Intern Med. 127:423–8. PMID:9312998

4504. Zukerberg LR, Collins AB, Ferry JA, et al. (1991). Coexpression of CD15 and CD20 by Reed-Sternberg cells in Hodgkin's disease. Am J Pathol. 139:475–83. PMID:1716042

4505. Zukerberg LR, Medeiros LJ, Ferry JA, et al. (1993). Diffuse low-grade B-cell lymphomas. Four clinically distinct subtypes defined by a combination of morphologic and immunophenotypic features. Am J Clin Pathol. 100:373–85. PMID:8213632

4506. Zuo Z, Medeiros LJ, Chen Z, et al. (2012). Acute myeloid leukemia (AML) with erythroid predominance exhibits clinical and molecular characteristics that differ from other types of AML. PLoS One. 7:e41485. PMID:22844482

4507. Zutter MM, Martin PJ, Sale GE, et al. (1988). Epstein-Barr virus lymphoproliferation after bone marrow transplantation. Blood. 72:520–9. PMID:2840986

4508. Zvulunov A, Barak Y, Metzker A (1995). Juvenile xanthogranuloma, neurofibromatosis, and juvenile chronic myelogenous leukemia. World statistical analysis. Arch Dermatol. 131:904–8. PMID:7632061

Subject index

Isochromosome 7q 382

J

JAK2 SV617F 22, 23, 38, 39, 41, 43, 45, 49, 53, 89, 93, 94, 96, 115
JAK2 SV617F mutation 22, 45, 89, 93, 94, 96
JAK3 91, 171, 347, 371, 378, 445
JAK/STAT signalling pathway 35, 195, 295, 306, 316, 347, 348, 371, 378, 382, 391, 399, 417, 429
JMML 77, 89-92
Juvenile chronic myelomonocytic leukaemia 89
Juvenile myelomonocytic leukaemia (JMML) 77, 89-92, 123
JXG 480

K

Kahler disease 243
KANK1-PDGFRB 77
KANSL1 171
Kaposi sarcoma 323, 325, 326, 328
Kaposi sarcoma-associated herpesvirus 323, 325
KAT6A-CREBBP 131
Ki-1 lymphoma 413
KIR genes 352
KIT SD816V mutation 63, 66-69
KLF2 225
KMT2A-AFDN 131
KMT2A-AFF1 204
KMT2A-MLLT1 fusion 204
KMT2A-MLLT3 131, 136, 168
KMT2A-MLLT10 131
KMT2A-MLLT11 131
KMT2A-rearranged 136, 183, 203, 204
KMT2D 234, 271, 272, 279, 288, 295, 371

L

Langerhans cell granulomatosis 470
Langerhans cell histiocytosis (LCH) **470**
Langerhans cell (LC) sarcoma **473**
Large B-cell lymphoma with IRF4 rearrangement **280**
LBCL 280, 314, 319, 321, 322
LDCHL 424, 425, 429, 441, 442
Lennert lymphoma 403, 404
Lethal midline granuloma 368, 369
Letterer-Siwe disease 470
Leukaemic non-nodal mantle cell lymphoma **290**
Leukaemic reticuloendotheliosis 226
LIG4 syndrome 119
Light and heavy chain deposition disease (LHCDD) **255**
Lipid (cholesterol) granulomatosis 481
Lipogranulomatosis 481
Lipoid granulomatosis 481
LMO2 191, 211, 264, 269, 293, 302

LPL 195, 232-236
LRCHL 424, 425, 438-440
LRRFIP1-FGFR1 78
LYG See Lymphomatoid granulomatosis
Lymphocyte-depleted CHL 424, 425, 435, 440
Lymphocyte-depleted classic Hodgkin lymphoma (LDCHL) **441**
Lymphocyte predominant Hodgkin lymphoma (NLPHL) 424
Lymphocyte-rich classic Hodgkin lymphoma (LRCHL) 424, 425, 432, 435, **438**, 439
Lymphoepithelioid lymphoma 403, 404, 409
Lymphogranulomatosis 408
Lymphomas associated with HIV infection **449**
Lymphomatoid granulomatosis (LYG) 291, **312**, 313, 446
Lymphomatoid papulosis (LyP) **392**, 393-395
Lymphomatosis cerebri 300
Lymphoplasmacytic lymphoma (LPL) **232**, 233, 234, 236, 463
Lymphoproliferative diseases associated with primary immune disorders (PID) **444**
LyP See Lymphomatoid papulosis

M

M2, NOS 158
M4 86, 159
M5 86, 160
Maculopapular cutaneous mastocytosis 62, 65
MAFB 247, 248
Malignant angioendotheliomatosis 317
Malignant histiocytosis 467
Malignant histiocytosis of the intestine 372
Malignant lymphoma, centrocytic 285
Malignant lymphoma, lymphocytic, intermediate differentiation, diffuse 285
Malignant lymphoma, lymphoplasmacytoid 232
Malignant lymphoma, small non-cleaved, Burkitt type 330
Malignant lymphomatous polyposis 285
Malignant mast cell tumour 69
Malignant mastocytoma 69
Malignant midline reticulosis 368
Malignant myelosclerosis 165
Malignant reticulosis 368
Malignant reticulosis, NOS 368
MALT1 194, 225, 234, 240, 262, 272, 302, 303, 451
MALT lymphoma **259**
Mantle cell lymphoma **285**-289
Mantle zone lymphoma 285
MAP2K1 mutations 228, 231, 279, 472
MAP3K14 430
Marginal zone lymphoma (MZL) 251, 263
Mast cell activation syndrome 63

Mast cell leukaemia 10, 62, 68, 69
Mast cell sarcoma (MCS) 62, **69**, 530, 536
Mastocytosis 22, **62**
Mature T follicular helper (TFH) cells 408
MBL 220, 221
MCAS See Mast cell activation syndrome
MCCHL 424, 425, 429, 440
MCD 325-329
MCS See Mast cell sarcoma
MDS/AML 122-128
MDS-EB 100, 101, 104, 113, 114
MDS-MLD 101, 107, 108, 111-113
MDS/MPN-RS-T 93, 95
MDS/MPN-U 95, 96
MDS-RS 93, 94, 101, 106-113
MDS-SLD 101, 106-109
MDS-U 101, 116
MECOM 36, 136-138, 149
Mediastinal diffuse large cell lymphoma with sclerosis 314
Mediastinal grey-zone lymphoma (MGZL) 342
Mediterranean lymphoma 240
Medullary plasmacytoma 243
MEF2B 271, 295
Megakaryocytic leukaemia 162
Megakaryocytic lineage 50, 169-171
Megakaryocytic myelosclerosis 44
Methotrexate 302, 307, 350, 447, 452, 463, 464
MGUS See IgM monoclonal gammopathy of undetermined significance
MGZL See Mediastinal grey-zone lymphoma
Mixed cellularity classic Hodgkin lymphoma (MCCHL) **424**, 425, 429, 435, 437, 439-441
Mixed myeloproliferative/myelodysplastic syndrome, unclassifiable 95
Mixed-phenotype acute leukaemia 20, 77, 78, 140, 157, 168, 180, 181, 183-187, 211, 212
Mixed-phenotype acute leukaemia (MPAL) with t(v;11q23.3) 183
Mixed-phenotype acute leukaemia, NOS, rare types **186**
Mixed-phenotype acute leukaemias with gene rearrangements 179
Mixed-phenotype acute leukaemia, B/myeloid, NOS **184**
Mixed-phenotype acute leukaemia, T/myeloid, NOS **185**
Mixed-phenotype acute leukaemia with MLL rearrangement 183
Mixed-phenotype acute leukaemia with t(9;22)(q34.1;q11.2); BCR-ABL1 **182**
Mixed-phenotype acute leukaemia with t(v;11q23.3); KMT2A-rearranged **183**
MLH1 177
MLL rearranged 183
MLLT1 137, 204, 211

List of abbreviations

AIDS	acquired immunodeficiency syndrome
ATP	adenosine triphosphate
CHOP	cyclophosphamide, hydroxydaunorubicin, oncovin (vincristine), prednisone
CI	confidence interval
CNS	central nervous system
CT	computed tomography
DNA	deoxyribonucleic acid
EBV	Epstein–Barr virus
EORTC	European Organisation for Research and Treatment of Cancer
FISH	fluorescence in situ hybridization
FLAIR	fluid-attenuated inversion recovery
GDP	guanosine diphosphate
GTP	guanosine-5'-triphosphate
HAART	highly active antiretroviral therapy
H&E	haematoxylin and eosin
HHV	human herpesvirus
HIV	human immunodeficiency virus
HLA	human leukocyte antigen
HTLV-1	human T-lymphotropic virus type 1
ICD-O	International Classification of Diseases for Oncology
Ig	immunoglobulin
IG gene	immunoglobulin gene
KSHV	Kaposi sarcoma–associated herpesvirus – an alternative name for human herpesvirus 8 (HHV8)
LMP1	latent membrane protein 1 (of Epstein–Barr virus)
LOH	loss of heterozygosity
MALT	mucosa-associated lymphoid tissue
MAPK	mitogen-activated protein kinase
MHC	major histocompatibility complex
MRI	magnetic resonance imaging
mRNA	messenger ribonucleic acid
N:C ratio	nuclear-to-cytoplasmic ratio
NK cell	natural killer cell
NOS	not otherwise specified
PAS	periodic acid–Schiff
PCR	polymerase chain reaction
PET	positron emission tomography
RB	retinoblastoma
RBC	red blood cell
R-CHOP	the CHOP chemotherapy regimen plus rituximab
RNA	ribonucleic acid
RT-PCR	reverse transcriptase polymerase chain reaction
SEER	Surveillance, Epidemiology, and End Results
SNP	single nucleotide polymorphism
TdT	terminal deoxynucleotidyl transferase
TNM	tumour, node, metastasis
TR gene	T-cell receptor gene
WBC	white blood cell

A note on gene and protein nomenclature: Throughout this volume, we have used the Human Genome Organisation (HUGO) Gene Nomenclature Committee (HGNC) Guidelines (http://www.genenames.org/) for citing genes and proteins. For immunoglobulin (IG) and T-cell receptor (TR) alleles, we have used the nomenclature assigned by the ImMunoGeneTics (IMGT) Nomenclature Committee (http://www.imgt.org/), as recommended by HGNC.